Mosby's
Pharmacy Technician

PRINCIPLES AND PRACTICE

Mosby's
Pharmacy Technician

PRINCIPLES AND PRACTICE

THIRD EDITION

Teresa Hopper, BS, CPhT

Instructor of Pharmacy Technology
Boston Reed College
Napa, California

ELSEVIER
SAUNDERS

3251 Riverport Lane
St. Louis, Missouri 63043

MOSBY'S PHARMACY TECHNICIAN: PRINCIPLES
AND PRACTICE

ISBN: 978-1-4377-0670-3

Copyright © 2012, 2007, 2004 by Saunders, an imprint of Elsevier Inc.

Notices

Previous editions copyrighted 2007, 2004

Publisher: Andrew Allen
Senior Acquisitions Editor: Jennifer Janson
Developmental Editor: Kelly Brinkman
Publishing Services Manager: Julie Eddy
Senior Project Manager: Rich Barber
Senior Designer: Amy Buxton

Printed in China

Last digit is the print number: 9 8 7 6 5 4 3 2 1

Preface

YOU ARE ABOUT TO EMBARK on an exciting journey into one of today's fastest-growing fields in health care. Whether you will end up working in a hospital pharmacy, a community pharmacy, mail order pharmacy, internet pharmacy, or another location, the knowledge you will gain from this textbook and its supplements will prepare you well for your new career. The author and publisher have made every effort to equip you with all of the background knowledge and tools you will need to succeed on the job. To this end, *Mosby's Pharmacy Technician: Principles & Practice* was designed as a fundamental yet comprehensive resource that represents the very latest information available for preparing pharmacy technician students for today's challenging job environment.

Who Will Benefit From This Book?

Pharmacy technicians are increasingly called upon to perform duties traditionally fulfilled by pharmacists. This is because of new federal regulations that now require pharmacists to spend more time with patients providing patient education. As the number of pharmacy technicians in the United States and Canada continues to grow, the need to outline a scope of practice for the pharmacy technician profession has become more urgent. *Mosby's Pharmacy Technician: Principles and Practice* provides students a solid coverage of information needed to be successful, while also giving the instructor the tools needed to present the information effectively and easily.

Why is This Book Important to the Profession?

Although there is no standardization for the qualifications or set job descriptions for pharmacy technicians at this time, this textbook covers all the theory and skills set forth by several national certifying bodies, including the Pharmacy Technician Certification Board (PTCB), the Institute for the Certification of Pharmacy Technicians (ICPT), the American Society of Health System Pharmacists (ASHP), and the American Pharmaceutical Association (APA), the last two of which created the criteria for the Pharmacy Technician Certification Board's certification exam. In Canada the Canadian Council for Accreditation of Pharmacy Programs (CCAPP) accredits pharmacy technician programs. The criteria that are required of technician programs are designed to help pharmacy technicians work more effectively with pharmacists, provide greater patient care and services, and create a minimum standard of knowledge across all 50 states and providences throughout Canada, to help employers determine a knowledge base for employment. Although there are some differences in pharmacy law and drug terms between the U.S. and Canada much of the information that is related to the pharmacy technician's requirements remain the same.

Organization

Mosby's Pharmacy Technician: Principles and Practice is a reliable and understandable resource written specifically for the pharmacy technician student and for those technicians already on the job, including those who are preparing for the PCTB, ExCPT (issued by the ICPT) in the U.S., or the pharmacy examination board of Canada (PEBC). The writing style, content, and organization guide the student to a better understanding of anatomy and physiology, diseases, and, most importantly, drugs and agents used to treat these diseases. Pharmacologic information is presented in a thorough, yet basic and concise, manner. The text is divided into four sections—**General Pharmacy, Body Systems, Classifications of Drugs, Basic Sciences for the Pharmacy Technician.**

Section One, General Pharmacy, provides an overview of pharmacy practice as it relates to pharmacy technicians. Highlights of Section One include history, law and ethics, drug calculations and dosage forms, abbreviations, routes of administration, filling prescriptions, over-the-counter medications, and the differences in the roles of pharmacists and pharmacy technicians. *Mosby's Pharmacy Technician* is the only book on the market that devotes an entire chapter each to alternative and complementary medicine and medication safety and error prevention.

Section Two, Body Systems, provides a brief overview of each body system and the medications used to treat common conditions that afflict these systems. Unique to this section are detailed discussions of anatomy and physiology, as well as photographs of a number of drugs used to treat various conditions of each body system. In addition each chapter lists the most common drugs within each classification and how to pronounce them as well as a medical terminology list related to the body systems being discussed.

Section Three, Classifications of Drugs, discusses five major drug classifications, anti-infectives, anti-inflammatories, antihistamines, vaccines, and oncology agents. A description of these drug classifications helps the pharmacy technician student understand how similar agents work. Section Three also includes a chapter on vitamins and minerals, their importance and possible drug interactions.

Section Four, Basic Sciences for the Pharmacy Technician, includes two chapters—on microbiology and chemistry—that are indeed unique to this textbook. They give the pharmacy student a basic overview of both fields that will greatly help technicians understand the method of action.

Distinctive Features of this Edition

DRUG NAMES AND PRONUNCIATIONS

A list of the drugs (generic and trade names) discussed within a chapter, along with the pronunciation, appear at the beginning of each body system chapter. This helps familiarize students with the spelling and pronunciation of drugs that they need to be familiar with on the job. It is essential that students be proficient in this area.

COMMON DRUGS USED FOR PSYCHOTHERAPEUTIC CONDITIONS

Trade Name	Generic Name	Pronunciation	Trade Name	Generic Name	Pronunciation
Agents for Psychosis and Bipolar Disorder			Seroquel	quetiapine	(kwe-**tye**-a-peen)
Atypical Antipsychotics			Zyprexa	olanzapine	(oh-lan-**zah**-peen)
Abilify	aripiprazole	(**ar**-i-**pip**-ra-zole)			
Clozaril, FazaClo	clozapine	(**kloe**-za-peen)	**Phenothiazine Antipsychotics**		
Fanapt	iloperidone	(**eye**-low-**per**-i-done)	Mellaril	thioridazine	(thy-oh-**rid**-ah-zeen)
Geodon	ziprasidone	(zi-**praz**-ih-dohn)	Prolixin	fluphenazine	(flew-**fen**-ah-zeen)
Invega	paliperidone	(**pal**-ee-**per**-i-done)	Serentil	mesoridazine	(meh-zoe-**rih**-da-zeen)
Risperdal	risperidone	(ris-**per**-ih-done)	Stelazine	trifluoperazine	(try-flew-**per**-ah-zeen)

TECH NOTES

Helpful pharmacy technician notes appear interspersed throughout the chapters, providing interesting historical facts, drug cautions, hints, and safety information. These notes enhance students' knowledge of practical information that they will need to know in a pharmacy setting.

TECH ALERTS

Tech Alerts can be found in the margins throughout the text. These boxes indicate important information the tech needs to remember when in the pharmacy. A lot of times, Tech Alerts will be medication safety reminders or proper drug names.

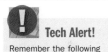

Tech Alert!

Remember the following sound-alike/look-alike drugs:

dopamine versus dobutamine
levodopa versus methyldopa
clonazepam, lorazepam, and clorazepate
esmolol versus Osmitrol
Trandate versus Tridrate

MINI DRUG MONOGRAPHS

Drug monograph information with pill photos is provided in every body systems and drug classification chapter. These monographs include drug class, generic and trade names, strength of medication, route of administration, dosage, and photos of drugs, providing students with quick, easy to understand information about specific drugs.

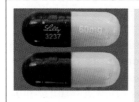

GENERIC NAME: duloxetine
TRADE NAME: Cymbalta
INDICATION: antidepressant, fibromyalgia
ROUTE OF ADMINISTRATION: oral
COMMON ADULT DOSAGE: 40 or 60 mg once daily
SIDE EFFECTS: nausea, vomiting, dizziness, insomnia, dry mouth, headache, diarrhea, loss of appetite
AUXILIARY LABEL:
■ May cause dizziness and drowsiness.

PHARMACIST'S PERSPECTIVE

Written by a practicing pharmacist on specific topics related to content, these boxes provide students with more information on content from the point of view of the pharmacist, making the content more interesting by relating the content information to on-the-job situations.

TECHNICIAN'S CORNER

Technician's Corner boxes appear at the end of each chapter, providing critical thinking questions to help students prepare for on-the-job experiences.

New to This Edition

NEW CHAPTER! CHAPTER 14: MEDICATION SAFETY AND ERROR PREVENTION

This textbook is the only pharmacy technician text that looks into the growing concern of medication errors by taking a compressive look into the history of medication errors and how handling them has changed over the years. Topics covered in this chapter are agencies involved in drug enforcement, new technologies used to deter common drug errors, real life cases of drug errors and the lives they have affected. Tools are also given to the students to further enlighten their perspective on drug errors with several scenarios given within the chapter.

MEDICAL TERMINOLOGY

Basic medical terminology is covered in this textbook which gives the student a basic foundation onto which they can expand their knowledge base in Chapter 5. In addition, each body system chapter lists the most common terms used in medical terminology and conditions. This will greatly enhance the student's comprehension of the materials covered in each chapter and ultimately in the workplace.

PSYCHOPHARMACOLOGY TERMINOLOGY

Word Combinations

Claustr/o	Barrier
Agor/a	Marketplace
Acr/o	Top
Pyr/o	Fire
Trichotill/o	Related to hair
Anxi/o	Anxiety
Somn	Sleep

APPENDIX A: REVIEW FOR THE PTCB, EXPCT, OR PEBC EXAMINATION

This appendix presents a 150-question practice certification exam with multiple choice questions, assisting students as they prepare for taking the PTCB or ExCPT exam in the United States or, The Canadian Pharmacy Examining Board of Canada (PEBC). Certification is now a requirement in several U.S. States and is required throughout Canada.

UPDATED PILL IMAGES

Updated pill images have been added to the third edition, assisting the pharmacy technician in identifying pills on sight and avoiding pharmacy errors.

ADDITIONAL MATH EXERCISES

Additional math exercises have been added to the textbook, as well as to the Evolve site. These additional math exercises will help students strengthen their math skills in the appropriate areas.

OVERALL CONTENT UPDATE

Mosby's Pharmacy Technician provides the student with the most up-to-date pharmacy information available. New drugs added, including indications and pill photos, provide pharmacy technicians with the most current information.

Learning Aids

FOUR-COLOR DESIGN

The colorful design, figures, and pill images help to present a difficult subject in an inviting and unintimidating manner.

EXTENSIVE VISUAL AIDS

Mosby's Pharmacy Technician contains over 500 line drawings and photos in full color, helping students see concepts and procedures in visual form, while greatly enhancing learning of this new information that can be difficult to learn.

CHAPTER OBJECTIVES

Chapter objectives appear at the beginning of each chapter, clearly outlining key concepts covered.

KEY TERMS

Key terms with definitions appear at the beginning of each chapter, identifying new terminology for the student and making it easier to learn.

DO YOU REMEMBER THESE KEY POINTS?

This review of key points appears at the end of each chapter, providing students the opportunity to quickly revisit the main concepts of the chapter before attempting to answer the review questions.

Ancillaries

Considering the broad range of students, instructors, programs, and institutions for which this textbook was designed, we have developed an extensive package of supplements designed to complement *Mosby's Pharmacy Technician: Principles and Practice,* third edition. Each of these comprehensive supplements has been thoughtfully developed with the shared goals of students and instructors in mind: producing students who are well prepared for a career in pharmacy, as well as for earning their certification. All these supplements and their inventive features can be found on the Evolve website (http://evolve.elsevier.com/Hopper/), and include:

FOR THE INSTRUCTOR

TEACH Instructor Resource
TEACH for Mosby's Pharmacy Technician is designed to help the pharmacy technician instructor prepare for class by reducing preparation time, providing new and innovative ideas to promote student learning, and helping to make full use of the rich array of resources available. This completely revised manual includes:

- Lecture Outlines to correspond with the PowerPoint presentations
- Detailed lesson plans
- Chapter-specific PowerPoint presentations
- Instructor's Resource with additional tools to use in the classroom (discussed below)

Instructor's Resource. This product, included with *TEACH for Mosby's Pharmacy Technician,* includes:

- Additional Classroom Activities
- Sample Class Syllabus
- Sample Program Outline
- All textbook review question answers
- Answers to the workbook/lab manual exercises

TEACH Online Pharmacy Technician Program Guide. The TEACH Online Pharmacy Technician Program Guide assists instructors seeking to start or expand a pharmacy technician program. The Program Guide is accessible via this textbook's Evolve web site at http://evolve.elsevier.com/Hopper/.

Additional Instructor Ancillaries
- Examview Test Bank
- Image Collection
- Supplemental Canadian Material

FOR THE STUDENT

Ancillaries Available on the Evolve Companion Web Site
- Interactive crossword puzzles, drag and drop, and flashcard activities for each chapter
- Additional math review
- Appendices on abbreviations, HIPPA, and proper hand care for pharmacy
- Answer key to odd numbered review questions in the text
- Anatomy Animations
- English/Spanish Audio Glossary
- Mosby's Essential Drug List
- WebLinks

Student Workbook/Lab Manual
The student workbook/lab manual has been completely revised and is a combination traditional workbook, and enhanced with lab exercises for the student to perform in class. This valuable product includes:

- Exercises to **Reinforce** key concepts taught in the Hopper, 3rd edition text
- **Reflect** critically on topics to assist students as they develop critical thinking and decision-making skills.
- Complete lab activities that will **relate** to practice.

Acknowledgments

To ENSURE THE ACCURACY of the material presented throughout this textbook, an extensive review and development process was used. This included evaluation by a variety of knowledgeable pharmacy technicians and pharmacists. We are deeply grateful to the numerous people who have shared their comments and suggestions. Reviewing a book or supplement takes an incredible amount of energy, time and attention, and we are glad so many colleagues were able to take time out of their busy schedules to help ensure the validity and appropriateness of content in this new edition. The reviewers provided us with additional viewpoints and opinions that combine to make this text an incredible learning tool.

We wish to thank the following Editorial and Technical Review Team:

REVIEWERS

Julette Barta, CPhT, BSIT, MA Ed
Pharmacy Technician Instructor/Curriculum
  Specialist
Colton-Redlands-Yucaipa Regional Occupational
  Program
Redlands, California

James Mizner Jr., MBA, RPh
Pharmacy Technician Program Director
ACT College
Arlington, Virginia

MaryAnne Hochadels, PharmD, BCPS
Clinical Pharmacist
Bayfront Medical Center
Saint Petersburg, Florida

Terri. L. Levien, PharmD
Clinical Associate Professor
Washington State University–Spokane
Spokane, Washington

John J. Smith, EdD
AVP, Curriculum and Instructor
Corinthian Colleges, Inc.
Santa Ana, California

CONTRIBUTORS

Deby Harris
Sacramento, California

This book is dedicated to
all student technicians who have chosen a career in the healthcare field.
As the population grows more experienced technicians are desperately needed.
You are an important component in future pharmacy.

My thanks to my family who always keep my spirits lifted;
Tracy, Jeni, Tiffy, and Christo.
To my grandchildren—Nathan, Reiley, Carter, Wyatt,
Christopher, and Hayden.

A special thanks to
Larry Cacace, PharmD; Tina Goldberg, PharmD;
Mary Lehman, RN; Sue Wong, PharmD; and Tracy Lee Crum, BSN.

Contents

SECTION TWO Body Systems

SECTION THREE Classification of Drugs

SECTION

one

General Pharmacy

History of Medicine and Pharmacy

Objectives

UPON COMPLETING THIS CHAPTER, YOU SHOULD BE ABLE TO DO THE FOLLOWING:

■ Discuss ancient beliefs of illness and medicine from 440 BC through AD 1600.

■ List common ancient treatments that prevailed in Western civilization.

■ Describe nineteenth-century medicine, and identify influences that major wars had on medicine.

■ Describe the wide use of opium and the problems surrounding opium use.

■ Differentiate between opiates and opioids.

■ Describe how the first pharmacies began in the United States.

■ Identify the role that early pharmacists played in society.

■ Describe the first technicians in pharmacy.

■ List major ways pharmacy has changed over the past 100 years.

■ List important current trends in pharmacy in relation to pharmacy technicians.

■ Identify the resistance to technicians that parallels the historical resistance to pharmacists.

Aristotle	Greek scientist, philosopher
Asclepius	Early physician and hero in Greece who was eventually considered the God of healing and medicine
Bacon, Roger	English scientist responsible for scientific methods
Domagk, Gerhard	Discovered sulfonamide, first synthetic antibiotic
Fleming, Alexander	Discovered penicillin, first antibiotic
Galen, Claudius	Greek physician
Hippocrates	Greek physician and philosopher, considered to be the father of medicine
Mendel, Gregor	Scientist and monk known as the father of genetics
Paracelsus	Swiss physician, philosopher, and scientist
Pasteur, Louis	French scientist, discovered several vaccines and invented pasteurization

TERMS AND DEFINITIONS

Apothecary *Latin term for pharmacist; also, a place where drugs are sold*

Bloodletting *The practice of draining blood; believed to release illness*

Caduceus *Often confused as the symbol of the medical field; it is a staff with two entwined snakes and two wings at the top*

Dogma *Code of beliefs based on ideology, religion, or authoritative tradition rather than factual evidence*

Hippocratic Oath *An oath taken by physicians concerning the ethics and practice of medicine*

Inpatient pharmacy *A pharmacy in a hospital or institutional setting*

Laudanum *A mixture of opium and alcohol used to treat dozens of illnesses through the 1800s*

Leeches *A type of segmented worm with suckers that attach to the skin of a host and engorge themselves on the host's blood*

Maggots *Fly larvae that feed on dead tissue; used in medicine to clean wounds not responding to routine antibiotics*

Medicine *The science and art dealing with the maintenance of health and the prevention, alleviation, or cure of disease*

Opioid *Any agent that binds to opioid receptors*

Opium *An analgesic that is made from the poppy plant*

Outpatient pharmacy *Pharmacies that serve patients in their communities; pharmacies that are not in inpatient facilities*

Pharmacist *Person who dispenses drugs and counsels patients on medication use and any interactions it may have with food or other drugs*

Pharmacy *Drug or remedy (Greek word pharmakon); place where drugs are sold*

Pharmacy clerk *Person who assists the pharmacist at the front counter of the pharmacy; the person who accepts payment for medications*

Pharmacy technician *Person who assists a pharmacist by filling prescriptions and performing other nondiscretionary tasks*

Pharmacy Technician Certification Board (PTCB) *Issues a national exam for pharmacy technicians*

Placebo effect *A person suffering symptoms from illness experiences relief through faith in a treatment that provides no tangible medicinal or treatment value*

Shaman *A person who holds a high place of honor in a tribe as a healer and spiritual mediator*

Staff of Asclepius *The symbol of the medical profession; it is a wingless staff with one snake wrapped around it*

Trephining *A practice of making an opening in the head to allow disease to leave the body*

History of Medicine

ANCIENT BELIEFS AND TREATMENTS

Medicine has been practiced for thousands of years. Archaeological discoveries have unearthed civilizations that have documented the use of minerals, animals, and plant parts to heal the sick. Certain remedies, such as herbals, have been used consistently throughout history. For example, herbs have been used for centuries for minor ailments such as intestinal problems, arthritis, and gout.

Many ancient treatments for illness were based on the dreams or visions of the believers. A **dogma,** such as gods being able to both cause and cure illnesses, is based on a set of beliefs (e.g., religious or ideological doctrines) proposed by authoritarians. These beliefs are based on writings from respected spiritual authorities rather than scientific evidence. One belief surrounding healing the sick was the idea that severe illness was caused by evil spirits. To rid oneself of an evil spirit, a cut was made into the skull to give the spirit a portal through which to leave. This type of treatment was called **trephining** and often was performed by a tribal **shaman** (a spiritual person in a tribe who cares for the spiritual, medicinal, and physical health of the tribe). Tribal shamans were believed to have the gift of being able to communicate with spirits. Other shamans believed that they were connected with a special spirit who helped them render the evil spirits harmless through the use of prayer, herbs, or potions. Shamans were prevalent throughout societies in ancient times. Some still exist in various societies throughout the world. In North America, various Eskimo and Native American tribes held shamans in high esteem. However, many of the popular beliefs of the past have mostly disappeared.

THE MEDICAL STAFF

The **staff of Asclepius** is the formal symbol of medicine, and is associated with **Asclepius**, a great physician and hero of his time in ancient Greece. From his lifetime and beyond through the fourth century AD, Asclepius was worshipped as a Greek God associated with healing. The staff of Asclepius is a wingless walking stick with a single serpent wrapped around it. Because snakes shed their skin, the single snake was believed to signify renewal of youth. The staff of **caduceus** is often mistakenly used as a symbol of medicine. The caduceus was the staff of Hermes, a Greek god; the staff represented magic and had two serpents wrapped around it, usually with two wings at the top (Figure 1-1). For example, in 1902 the U.S. Army erroneously adopted the caduceus as an emblem of the Medical Corps, leading to its mistaken use as a symbol of medicine. While many organizations still use the caduceus to represent medicine, the true staff of Asclepius is adopted as a symbol by authoritative health organizations such as the World Health Organization and the American Medical Association.

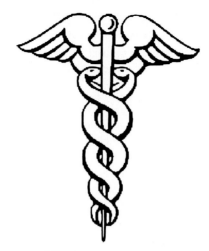

FIGURE 1-1 Medical staff.

MEDICINE IN ITS INFANCY

The infancy of medicine was not a smooth road. Throughout the ages, many plagues killed thousands of people. The existence of microbes, unseen by the eye, was not known to be responsible for many of the diseases that caused death and despair. Despite advancements made through early history, most remedies for physical ailments tended to be extreme. Other ancient remedies have been used for hundreds of years. Prevalent thoughts included one that sickness was an entity within the body that needed a means to leave the body. Another widely held belief was that spirits were responsible for illness. The most common form of treatment, prayer, still has remained in many cultures as the only way to cure illness.

Hippocrates (460-357 BC) was born on the small island of Cos near Greece, and he was a third-generation physician. He taught at Cos School of Medicine, which was one of the first medical schools established. He believed in the prevailing concept of that era: life consisted of a balance of four elements that were linked to qualities of good health. These four elements were wet, dry, hot, and cold. In addition, he believed that illness resulted from an imbalance of the four humors of the body system: blood, phlegm, yellow bile, and black bile. These four humors were linked to the four basic elements: blood is air, phlegm is water, yellow bile is fire, and black bile is earth. Methods used to treat imbalance of the humors included bloodletting and natural laxatives.

Hippocrates was responsible for much advancement in the world of medicine. Some of his observations included the effects of food, climate, and other influences on illness. He was one of the first physicians to record his patients' medical illnesses. This new way of viewing the causes of illnesses eventually led to the belief that sickness originated from something other than the supernatural. Hippocrates believed that the spirit of the patient should be as important as the condition being treated, and he promoted being kind to the sick. He also believed in letting nature do the healing and promoted resting and eating light foods. He taught that doctors needed to rebalance the four humors. Most of his teachings have been documented in a collection of books called the *Corpus Hippocraticum*. Although many of the writings are now believed to be from different authors, they still reflect the teachings of Hippocrates.

Today's medical schools still use the **Hippocratic Oath** as part of their graduation ceremony. See Box 1-1 to read the revised version of the Hippocratic Oath used today. The Hippocratic Oath outlines the physician's responsibility to

BOX 1-1 THE HIPPOCRATIC OATH

"I swear to fulfill, to the best of my ability and judgment, this covenant:

I will respect the hard-won scientific gains of those physicians in whose steps I walk, and gladly share such knowledge as is mine with those who are to follow.

I will apply, for the benefit of the sick, all measures [that] are required, avoiding those twin traps of overtreatment and therapeutic nihilism.

I will remember that there is art to medicine as well as science, and that warmth, sympathy, and understanding may outweigh the surgeon's knife or the chemist's drug.

I will not be ashamed to say "I know not," nor will I fail to call in my colleagues when the skills of another are needed for a patient's recovery.

I will respect the privacy of my patients, for their problems are not disclosed to me that the world may know. Most especially must I tread with care in matters of life and death. If it is given me to save a life, all thanks. But it may also be within my power to take a life; this awesome responsibility must be faced with great humbleness and awareness of my own frailty. Above all, I must not play at God.

I will remember that I do not treat a fever, chart a cancerous growth, but a sick human being, whose illness may affect the person's family and economic stability. My responsibility includes these related problems, if I am to care adequately for the sick.

I will prevent disease whenever I can, for prevention is preferable to cure.

I will remember that I remain a member of society, with special obligations to all my fellow human beings, those sound of mind and body as well as the infirm.

If I do not violate this oath, may I enjoy life and art, respected while I live and remembered with affection thereafter. May I always act so as to preserve the finest traditions of my calling and may I long experience the joy of healing those who seek my help."

Written in 1964 by Louis Lasagna, Academic Dean of the School of Medicine at Tufts University, and used in many medical schools today.

Tech Note!

The origin of the term *black humor* stems from the belief that too much of the black bile humor resulted in a person showing signs of melancholy.

the patient. Hippocrates practiced what he preached with respect to exercise, rest, diet, and overall moderation in one's lifestyle. Various records have documented his death at 377 BC, whereas others record his death at 357 BC. Considering that the average human life span was no more than 40 years at that time, living between 83 and 103 years was astonishing. Because of the advancements he promoted in the world of medicine, it is not surprising that Hippocrates is known as the Father of Medicine. Before the existence of Hippocrates and other innovative scientists, people believed that they were at the mercy of the gods or supernatural forces.

Later in history, the Greek philosopher and scientist **Aristotle** (384-322 BC) was responsible for many advancements in the areas of biology and medicine. His main area of interest was biology and the study and classification of various organisms. He classified human beings as animals. Because the Grecian belief system in those times did not allow dissection of the dead, he described much of human anatomy from observations he made from dissections of other animals. This included in-depth descriptions of the brain, heart, lungs, and blood vessels.

Claudius Galen (AD 129-210) began to study medicine at the age of 16. He attended medical schools in Greece and the famous Alexandria School of Medicine in Egypt. He later resided in Rome and was the personal physician of the Roman imperial family. Although he was born nearly 600 years after Hippocrates, he followed many of the same beliefs, such as eating a balanced diet, exercising, and practicing good hygiene. He contributed greatly to the study of medicine, writing more than 100 books on topics such as physiology, anatomy, pathology, diagnosis, and pharmacology. Many of his books were used in medical schools for 1500 years. He proved that blood flowed through arteries rather than air.

Philosopher and alchemist **Roger Bacon** (AD 1214-1294) further refined and explained the importance of experimental methods, moving even further away from the dogmatic beliefs of the era.

Paracelsus (AD 1493-1541), a Swiss physician and alchemist, believed that it was important to treat illness with one medication at a time. At the end of the Middle Ages, it was a common practice to give multiple remedies or large quantities of agents that had not been tested previously. Through the use of experimentation and documentation of the effectiveness and dosage of each individual agent, Paracelsus was able to produce many medications. He introduced one of the most popular tonics of that time—laudanum, which was used to deaden pain. Table 1-1 lists major figures and their influences throughout medical history.

Ancient Herbal Remedies

Over the millennia, some prevalent treatments consisted of multiple mixtures of plants, roots, and other concoctions. Digestion of the type of plant that resembled the organ affected by disease also was believed to cure illnesses. For example, those with liver problems ingested a plant called liverwort (named because the leaves were shaped like a liver). Other popular treatments included using garlic for inflammation of the bronchial tubes, wine and pepper for various

TABLE 1-1 Advancements in Medicine

Name	Year	Advancement
William Harvey	1628	Writes first book on blood circulation through the heart
James Lind	1747	Discovers that citrus fruits prevent scurvy
Rene Laennec	1816	Invents stethoscope
James Blundell	1818	Performs first blood transfusion
Crawford W. Long	1842	Uses ether as a general anesthetic
Joseph Lister	1867	Publishes *Antiseptic Principle of the Practice of Surgery*
Louis Pasteur	1870s	Establishes germ theory of disease
Wilhelm Roentgen	1895	Discovers x-ray
Ronald Ross	1897	Demonstrates that malaria is transmitted by mosquitoes
Felix Hoffman	1899	Develops aspirin
Karl Landsteiner	1901	First describes ABO, B, AB, and O blood groups
Sir Frederick Gowland Hopkins	1906	Suggests existence of vitamins and concludes they are essential to health
Dr. Paul Dudley White	1913	One of the first cardiologists; pioneers use of electrocardiograph
Edward Mellanby	1921	Discovers lack of vitamin D causes rickets
	1922	First uses insulin to treat diabetes
Sir Alexander Fleming	1928	Discovers penicillin*
Gerhard Domagk	1932	Discovers sulfonamides
Dr. John H. Gibbon, Jr.	1935	Successfully uses heart-lung machine (on cat) to continue circulating blood while patient was in surgery
Selman A. Waksman	1943	Discovers streptomycin
Paul Zoll	1952	Develops first cardiac pacemaker
James Watson, Francis Crick	1953	Describes double-helical structure of DNA
Dr. Joseph E. Murray	1954	Performs first kidney transplant
Dr. Luc Montagnier and Dr. Anthony Galo	1983	HIV, the virus that causes AIDS, is discovered
James Thomson	2007	Scientists discover how to use human skin cells to create embryonic stem cells; study was performed in laboratory at University of Wisconsin

*Although discovered in 1928, it was not isolated and used as an antibiotic until 1938.
http://www.infoplease.com/ipa/A0932661.html.

stomach ailments, onions for worms, and tiger fat for joint pain. It was difficult to detect which, if any, of the ingredients administered actually worked because many concoctions contained a multitude of ingredients. As strange as many of these archaic remedies seem, there were many people who were "cured" because of their strong belief in the treatment given or their belief in the person treating them. This outcome is called the **placebo effect** and is still evident today; there is still no conclusive explanation of why or how it works.

Throughout history, popular religious beliefs revolved around the idea that evil spirits were the cause of illness in a person who had sinned. This belief may have persisted partially because no one had the slightest idea about germs or genetics. Many times, through trial and error (error sometimes causing death), certain treatments were found to be fairly effective.

Any time new theories are proposed, they can be met with some skepticism and disbelief. Eventually, medicine and science discovered methods to answer this need for corroboration, leading to modern approaches and effective treatments for disease. A new hypothesis should be treated as a possible answer that has not been disproved. As new scientists emerge and new methods are devised to test hypotheses, the results can lead to medical advancements. This was especially evident throughout the golden age of microbiology (see Chapter 30).

EIGHTEENTH- AND NINETEENTH-CENTURY MEDICINE

From the time of Galen, it was widely believed that the four humors could be rebalanced through the use of cathartics to clean out the bowels, diuretics to lessen the imbalance of body fluids, emetics to empty the stomach, and bloodletting to lessen body fluids, heart rate, and temperature. Physicians brought this theory to America, where such techniques were widely used, especially **bloodletting.**

Bloodletting had its origins in Egypt more than 3000 years ago and spread into all areas of Europe later through the Middle Ages. Just as trephination of the skull was believed to relieve evil spirits, bloodletting was thought to be an effective way of lessening excess body fluids that were believed to cause illness. Artifacts such as sharp bones, sharks' teeth, thorns, and sharpened sticks were believed to be the earliest instruments used in bloodletting. During the nineteenth century some even used bloodletting as preventative medicine to ensure good health. A well-known victim of bloodletting in America during the eighteenth century was George Washington, who suffered from an infection and died of complications from bloodletting. At that time it was wrongly believed that the body contained 12 quarts of blood; however, it only contains 6 quarts, and President Washington was bled 4 quarts over a 24-hour period.

One bloodletting treatment involved using **leeches.** These blood-sucking worms were gathered, stored, and used to remove blood from patients. The leech has the ability to latch onto the skin with sharp teethlike appendages and engorge itself to nearly twice its size on a person's blood. They also emit a natural anticoagulant called hirudin that allows the blood to flow freely. Leeches were used in specific places such as the vagina to treat menorrhea. Once the leeches were finished eating, they would normally detach themselves; if not, they were encouraged to detach with the use of salt. Bleeding would continue until it was necessary to manually stop the flow of blood with bandages.

Another form of bloodletting, venesection (phlebotomy or drawing blood) was widely used in the 1700s and 1800s for those who did not want leeches applied. The physician would heat the air inside a small cup and place it on the skin, which would draw up the skin tissue along with its blood flow (called wet cupping). At this point, a lancet would be used to cut into the skin, the cup would be removed, and 1 to 4 ounces of blood would be collected. Many patients succumbed to this type of treatment until the early 1900s when this type of treat-

BOX 1-2 EXAMPLE OF PRESCRIPTION COMPOUND FROM THE 1900s

Infusion of Dandelion, &c. Interpretation of order

Infusi Taraxaci, f℥iv.	4 fluid ounces of infusion of dandelion
Extracti Taraxaci, f℥ij.	2 fluid drachms of extract of dandelion
Sodæ Carbonatis, ℥ß.	½ drachm of sodium carbonate
Potasse Tartratis, ℥iij.	3 drachms of potassium tartrate
Tincturæ Rhei, f℥iij.	3 fluid drachms of tincture of rhubarb
Hyoscyami, gtt. xx.	20 drops[19] of henbane tincture

Signa.—One third part to be taken three times a day. In dropsical and visceral affections.

ment was declared quackery. For an update on these types of treatments, see "Old Remedies Making a Comeback?" on page 12.

Fortunately, medicine did advance through the nineteenth century in many ways. Medical schools arose throughout Europe, specifically in France and Germany. Many of the doctors trained in these schools came to America and brought with them this European influence in medicine. Medicinal recipes were written in Latin until the 1900s. An example of a common prescription to be compounded is listed in Box 1-2. Because Latin was used in medicine and **apothecary** products, this order could be interpreted by most practitioners. Although there have been many changes in the accepted abbreviations and weights in medicine, the fluid ounce can still be seen on pharmacy bottles. Table 1-1 lists several important medical advancements that have changed medical treatments and life span.

Throughout the nineteenth century, the church became active in scientific research as well. A monk named **Gregor Mendel** experimented on plants and noticed the changes in plants from generation to generation with respect to their color, size, and appearance. He used pea plants to determine how traits were transferred from one to another and in doing so determined the basics of genetics. In 1822 he determined how stronger plants could be propagated through heredity. It was not until the 1900s that other scientists were able to continue his work and enlightened the science world with the theory of genetics. As a result of his work, Mendel became known as the Father of Genetics.

North American Medicine

In early North America, as new immigrants brought their families from Europe and other parts of the world, disease followed. At that time, doctors were responsible not only for diagnosing conditions but also for preparing the necessary remedies to cure patients. Disease was widespread in the colonies; many persons did not survive the voyage across the sea from Europe, succumbing to diseases such as scurvy and severe intestinal infection. Patients were at a disadvantage throughout the colonies because there were few doctors and even fewer hospitals. The first pharmacists, known as druggists at the time, were doctors until pharmacy became a specialty. The term "druggist" was widely used from the 1700s until the mid-1800s to describe the practitioners of pharmacy, eventually leading to the title pharmacist.

Remedies used in early American history included cinchona bark (quinine) for the treatment of malaria; more unconventional and dangerous treatments were also employed, such as using mercury to treat syphilis. Many persons died of mercury poisoning because of its toxicity. Many people also died of typhoid fever, malaria, diphtheria, and dysentery. The need for doctors and treatments increased dramatically. The average life expectancy was approximately 40 years,

Tech Note!

and many families lost several children to childhood diseases such as smallpox, for which there were no vaccines available. Most treatments were concoctions handed down through family tradition. If a person were to use a doctor, he or she most likely would be treated at home or in a doctor's office, with treatments ranging from minor procedures to surgery. See typical remedies in Box 1-3.

Opium and Alcohol. One of the most popular tonics made for medicinal use in early America contained opium and alcohol. Its effectiveness was surpassed only by its addictiveness. This tonic was given as a sedative and to dull the sensation of pain. Paracelsus (as mentioned earlier in this chapter) introduced the opium-alcohol mixture called **laudanum** in the sixteenth century, and laudanum was used as a medicinal remedy. Laudanum was used widely throughout Europe in the Victorian era. During the Civil War laudanum not only was used to treat painful wounds from the battlefield but also found its way into households throughout the United States for less severe problems. See Box 1-4 for more information on Civil War medical treatments. Laudanum was used mostly by white middle to upper class women for a host of problems including nervousness, diabetes, diarrhea, gastric problems, menstrual pain, and even morning sickness. Laudanum was also used to calm screaming babies. Individuals became addicted at an alarming rate. Many mortalities and miscarriages were attributed to this agent. Even though it was well-known by the eighteenth century that opium and alcohol were addictive, alternative remedies were hard to find. An example of a laudanum recipe from 1669 is given in Box 1-5 as a remedy for

BOX 1-3   TYPICAL REMEDIES OF THE 1800s IN AMERICA

To stop earaches	Blow tobacco smoke into the ear.
To treat a cold	Combine a mixture of sugar, mineral oil, sulfur, ginger, lemon, and whisky in 8 oz of water; drink this and go to bed.
For baldness	Rub the head with an onion in the morning and at night before bed until the skin becomes red, and then rub it with honey.
For worms	Take a tablespoon of molasses and mix it with tin rust and ingest.
For stomach aches	Mix strychnine and other alkaline additives into an oral solution.
For cough and cold	Mix terpin of hydrate with codeine or heroin into an oral solution.
For eye infections	Add mercury to other ingredients such as eye drops.

BOX 1-4   THE CIVIL WAR

From 1861 through 1865 the Civil War claimed more lives than any other war in American history. More than 1 million soldiers died on the battlefield. Soldiers who did not die of their wounds succumbed to tuberculosis, typhoid fever, dysentery, and a host of other diseases, including measles, mumps, and chickenpox. Diseases spread rapidly as a result of the overcrowded and close quarters of men who had never been exposed to these diseases. Field hospitals were unsanitary and overcrowded. Many men died of infections caused by amputations and gunshot wounds. Medication was not available most of the time and anesthesia was limited to chloroform, from which many men died as a result of an overdose of the drug. Those who were hurt on the battlefield received care from undertrained medical staff with less than adequate equipment in nonsterile conditions. Most of the doctors (in the states) had minimal training; usually they completed an apprenticeship in lieu of formal training.

BOX 1-5 LAUDANUM RECIPE FROM THE 1700s

16 ounces of sherry wine
2 ounces of opium
1 ounce of saffron
1 ounce powder of cinnamon
1 ounce powder of cloves

Tech Note!

Alcohol use has been dated back to 3500 BC in Egypt. Opium has long been a part of human history; opium plants have been found as part of neolithic burial sites. Cultivated opium made its appearance in Egypt about 1300 BC; from Egypt, opium was then traded to Greece and eventually other parts of Europe.

dysentery. Another alcohol-based liquid was absinthe. This herb (*Artemisia absinthium*) was mixed with alcohol and other additives. Absinthe was served with water and sugar and was purported to rid oneself of tapeworms, among other ailments.

Origin of Opium (Opiates). **Opium** has a long history in the medicinal relief of pain and in recreational use. Opium is a byproduct gathered from the plant *Papaver somniferum,* commonly known as the opium poppy. The sap is taken from the head of the poppy. The raw opium then is precipitated from the sap. The result from this process is a potent drug that causes an analgesic effect. Although opiates was a term used for drugs derived from opium, the more common term used is opioid, which refers to both synthetic and semisynthetic medications. Both opiates and opioids react on the same opioid receptor sites, which are located in the central nervous system and gastrointestinal tract (see Chapter 16). The effects associated with the opioid receptors include analgesia, respiratory depression, pupil constriction, reduced gastrointestinal motility, euphoria, dysphoria, sedation, and physical dependence. Opioids and opiates share many of the same side effects, including nausea and vomiting. When used properly, the opioid drugs are effective and help many patients who otherwise would suffer extreme pain. Not until 1909, under the Opium Exclusion Act, did the prohibition of opium importation (except for medicinal purposes) begin in the United States (see Chapter 2).

TWENTIETH CENTURY MEDICINE

In the 1900s many new medicines were discovered; some of the earlier, groundbreaking discoveries were for those medicines that were useful in treating infections. The Scottish physician and bacteriologist **Alexander Fleming** accidentally contaminated a plate of bacteria with penicillium mold while working in his lab in 1928; the mold inhibited the growth of the bacteria and he named the mold "penicillin." Many years of failed and successful experimentation by many scientists followed before penicillin would be recognized as a useful medicine. It was not until after 1938 that penicillin would undergo mass production and be used worldwide as a helpful antibiotic. Penicillin was the first antibiotic discovered and is still in use today. The first synthetic drug, a sulfonamide, was discovered by **Gerhard Domagk** in 1938 and was derived from a chemical dye found to inhibit bacterial growth. This sulfonamide was used extensively during World War II to treat infections that were a result of battle wounds. Today, sulfonamides are primarily used to treat urinary tract infections. Many antibiotics were discovered in the years following penicillin and sulfa (see Chapter 30, Microbiology).

ADVANCEMENTS IN DRUG THERAPY AND VACCINATIONS

Many of the most famous chemists, biologists, and doctors who contributed to science were from European countries, such as Germany, England, France, and

TABLE 1-2 Examples of Important Vaccine Advancements in Medicine*

Scientist	Year of Discovery	Disease Identified	Vaccine
Edward Jenner (England)	1796 (acknowledged in 1800)	Smallpox	Smallpox vaccine
Robert Koch (Germany)	1876	Anthrax, tuberculosis	BioThrax[†] vaccine[†]
Louis Pasteur (France)	1877-1887	Staphylococcus, streptococcus, pneumococcus	Rabies, chickenpox, cholera, anthrax vaccines
Emil von Behring (Germany)	1890	Discovers antitoxins	Tetanus/diphtheria/ typhoid fever vaccine (DPT)
	1896	Typhoid fever	
	1926	Whooping cough	Pertussis vaccine
	1945	Influenza	Various vaccines used currently: Fluarix, Fluvirin, Fluzone, FluLaval intranasal, FluMist
Jonas Salk (America)	1955	Polio	First polio vaccine
Albert Sabin (America)	1962	Polio[§]	First oral polio vaccine
	1964	Measles	Vaccine combo (MMR)
	1967	Mumps	Vaccine combo (MMR)
	1970	Rubella	Vaccine combo (MMR)
	1974	Chickenpox[¶]	Varicella (Varivax) vaccine
	1977	Pneumonia	Pneumovax vaccine
	1978	Meningitis	Menactra, Menomune vaccines
	1981	Hepatitis B	HepB (Engerix-B, Recombivax HB)
	1992	Hepatitis A	HepA (Havrix, Vaqta) HepA/HepB combo (Twinrix)
	1998	Lyme disease	Vaccine removed from U.S. market in 2002 because of low demand
	2009	Swine flu	H1N1 vaccine

*For more information on vaccines, refer to Chapter 28.
[†]For military use only.
[‡]Not used in the United States.
[§]Oral polio vaccine no longer used for routine vaccination in United States because of its eradication in this country.
[¶]Given to persons born after 1956.

Poland. **Louis Pasteur** (France), most well known for the pasteurization process, was also responsible for inventing vaccinations such as the anthrax vaccine. Table 1-2 provides a list of the diseases that were discovered along with vaccines administered to prevent them.

Old Remedies Making a Comeback?
Many archaic treatments fell out of favor during the middle to late nineteenth century, yet certain ones prevail. For instance, patients are bled daily in all types of medical settings. For example, if a doctor orders a blood lab to be done on a patient, up to 30 mL of blood will be taken from the patient's vein. This, of course, is used to diagnose an illness rather than as a curative purpose, yet these techniques originated in the distant past and today no one would question such a technique. The disorder hemochromatosis is a hereditary condition in which the body absorbs too much iron, which is stored in organs and can cause serious damage. The current treatment used to treat this disorder is to remove blood (phlebotomy) on a regular basis. The FDA approved the use of both leeches and maggots in the medical setting in 1976. This may seem strange and not much of an advancement in medicine. The origins of this type of treatment stem from

research in the repair of tissue that has been severely damaged, such as that found in patients who have undergone reconstructive surgery, skin grafts, or infections. However, surgical reattachment of veins can cause coagulation before blood flow is reestablished to the affected part, killing the affected tissues. Leeches are used to siphon excess blood from the area and prevent coagulation from taking place too soon. They are applied one at a time over 20 minutes for up to 2 days as necessary. Leeches are cared for and stored in the refrigerator in the pharmacy. They may not be the first choice of a physician, but they have been used successfully in many cases as a means of avoiding amputation.

Because dead skin is the main dietary intake of **maggots,** they have the ability to remove dead skin. Antibiotics are normally used as the first course of treatment; however, when they are ineffective, physicians have used maggots to do the manual work of restoring the wound to a recoverable stage. Maggots only eat the dead tissue but they also have the ability to kill the bacteria that are the cause of the infection. Treatments from both leeches and maggots are very inexpensive compared to other treatments.

Other remedies are being studied, such as the honey produced by bees (Manuka). The medicinal attributes of this type of honey include the ability to heal wounds. Manuka keeps the wound moist, is bacteria free, and has a high sugar content along with minerals, vitamins, and amino acids that are thought to promote healing. In 2007 the FDA and Health Canada approved its use for wounds and burns. It is believed there are more uses for Manuka and studies are continuing. As medicine advances it is wise not to forget the past, because many historical treatments and remedies may be the answer to future cures. Pharmacy plays a part in both the historical and futuristic advancements in medicine and treatments because the roots of medicinal knowledge run deep. (See Chapter 9, Complementary and Alternative Medicine, for more nontraditional medicine treatments.)

History of Pharmacy

EARLY PHARMACISTS

The expanding population and the subsequent increasing need for trained medical personnel influenced the need for specialists such as veterinarians, eye doctors, and **pharmacists**. In addition, the shipping of medicines to America from England was becoming difficult as the colonies separated from England. After the Civil War, apothecaries (pharmacies) began to emerge in towns across America. Manufacturing plants were built, and persons were trained to prepare medications accurately. As the physician's role changed from distributing drugs to diagnosing disease and performing surgery, the role of the pharmacist emerged. The first pharmacy school opened in 1821 at the College of Pharmacy and Sciences in Philadelphia. The school is now called the University of the Sciences in Philadelphia. Through the 1800s, the pharmacist compounded nearly every drug ordered by physicians. Various sizes of ornate apothecary jars were used to store herbs and ingredients (Figure 1-2). The instructions for preparing remedies were contained in medical recipe books. Ingredients such as chalk for heartburn; rose petals for headaches; and oils, herbs, and spices filled containers in the apothecary. Although many of the ingredients in early compounded remedies are no longer used, there are several still in use today, such as aspirin, digoxin, and others.

Another type of interesting container associated with the pharmacy was the show globe. Show globes have been the beacons for pharmacy dating back as far as the early 1600s. It is believed that they were placed in the apothecary stores of the town to let visitors know the status of the health of the town. Red meant there was illness or that the town was in quarantine because of disease, whereas

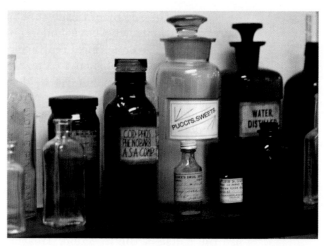

FIGURE 1-2 Medications were compounded by hand using a variety of compounds.

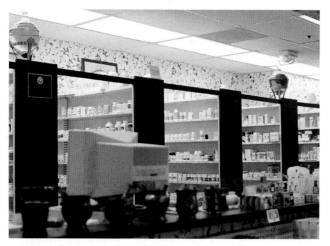

FIGURE 1-3 Large show globes (seen on top of shelf). An assortment of different mortars and pestles (seen on countertop).

green meant the town was healthy and thus that it was safe to come into the town. It is also said that signs were posted on the doors of the contagious persons rather than relying on globes. Decorative globes (Figure 1-3) showed patrons the pharmacist's competencies in chemical mixtures. More ornate globes were layered in various colors, resulting in a striped appearance. This was done by using various liquids of differing densities, causing a layered effect. These types of jars are now displayed in many pharmacies, along with other artifacts from the past.

EARLY PHARMACY IN AMERICA

The first **pharmacy** managed by a registered pharmacist opened in New Orleans in 1823. Starting in the mid-1800s and early 1900s the soda fountain became an extension of the town drugstore. The first soda fountain pharmacy began in the mid-1800s and gained popularity in the early 1900s. Prohibition in 1919 also helped with the proliferation of soda fountains. With the invention by a pharmacist, Jacob Baur (1921), of a soda fountain that also dispensed carbon dioxide, soda fountain units could easily prepare all types of carbonated drinks.

BOX 1-6 FAMOUS PHARMACISTS

Charles Alderton: Invented Dr Pepper
Caleb Bradham: Invented Pepsi-Cola
Charles Elmer Hires: Invented Hires Root Beer
John Pemberton: Invented Coca-Cola
William Proctor, Jr.: Father of American Pharmacy; founded American Pharmaceutical
 Association in 1852
James Vernor: Invented Vernors Ginger Ale
Harvey A.K. Whitney: Founder and first president of the American Society of Hospital
 Pharmacists in 1942

Pharmacists would make and market their own recipes to be used for various treatments. It was common to find drugs mixed with flavorings along with effervescent soda water to treat ailments or provide a boost of energy. Both caffeine and cocaine were also often used in sodas. Some of the many conditions mineral water was supposed to cure were obesity, upset stomach, depression, and nervous disorders. Pharmacists sold phosphate sodas and ice cream favorites, worked the lunch counter, and filled the prescriptions for the day. The first 7-Up drink was made with lithium and was sold from soda fountains for conditions such as gout, uremia, and rheumatism. In 1886 Coca Cola was invented by Doctor John Pemberton, who was a pharmacist in Georgia. The soft drink was marketed as a tonic and contained extracts of cocaine and caffeine until 1905, when cocaine was removed from the recipe because of changing public opinion regarding its use. It was not until later, after the Harrison Narcotic Drug Act of 1914 (see Chapter 2), that pharmacists were prohibited from making cocaine-containing preparations and began to sell plain soda drinks.

A list of pharmacists/inventors can be seen in Box 1-6. By the late 1800s, the soda shop/pharmacy was so popular that persons came to drink the sweet concoctions whether they were ailing or not. This type of pharmacy setting undoubtedly added to the image of the friendly neighborhood pharmacist as a person who could be trusted. The stereotypic local neighborhood pharmacist who wore a white jacket, packaged medications, and sometimes worked the soda machine has all but disappeared, except in a few shops where a person may still purchase an old-fashioned malt or shake while waiting for a prescription to be filled.

Early Pharmacy Technicians

The first **pharmacy technicians** were those enlisted in the military because of the high demand for medications to treat injuries and illness. These individuals were trained on the job not only to fill prescriptions but also to perform many of the functions of a pharmacist. To this day, military technicians have a broader scope of training than civilian technicians. Technicians also were employed by pharmacists who owned drugstores. Family members helped behind the counters, filled stock, and waited on customers. These early **pharmacy clerks** then moved on to become what we now call pharmacy technicians.

An urgent need for standardized training arose in the 1960s as pharmacist organizations such as the American Society of Health-System Pharmacists (ASHP), the Michigan Pharmacists Association (MPA), and the American Pharmacists Association (APhA) realized that technicians would be able to better serve the patient with additional training. Technicians play such an important role in the health care of patients, it is important that they understand all aspects of their required tasks within pharmacy. At the first conference on pharmacy technicians held by ASHP in 1988, although many of the topics involved pharmacy technician training, other important aspects of the pharmacy setting, such as the lack of technician involvement in the workplace, were also discussed. In 1995 the **Pharmacy Technician Certification Board (PTCB)** was formed, responsible for creating a national exam for technicians (see Chapter 3).

Although the transition from clerk to technician is fairly recent in history, forecasts indicate that the pharmacy technician will play a critical role in the future pharmacy setting. New job positions are constantly being created for those technicians who have the necessary skills and knowledge to fulfill them. Clinical technicians now assist the pharmacist with a variety of tasks such as anticoagulation monitoring. They may also manage the automation and pharmacy coordination systems within certain pharmacies. Table 1-3 contains an outline of the important chronological events that have molded the position of pharmacy technician into what it is today.

As of June 30, 2009, the PTCB has certified more than 345,929 technicians nationwide. This demonstrates the seriousness of this profession and the need for standardized competencies in the workplace. Up until the PTCB exam most technicians had a high school diploma, although it was not mandatory; also,

TABLE 1-3 Advancements in the Field of Pharmacy Technology

Date	Description of Change in Pharmacy
1940s	The origins of a training program for technicians began in the military (U.S. Army).
1968	National support and development of curriculum in junior colleges and other institutions by the Bureau of Health Manpower (U.S. Department of Health) began.
1969	ASHP began to establish national guidelines for pharmacy technicians to improve standards.
1973	NACDS began support of technicians and on-the-job training programs.
1975	ASHP created a set of guidelines for the hospital pharmacy technician.
1977	ASHP created competencies for technicians in organized health care settings and qualifications for entry-level technicians in hospitals.
1979	Massachusetts College of Pharmacy started a pharmacy technician training program.
1979	American Association of Pharmacy Technicians formed.
1981	The Michigan Pharmacists Association (MPA) started the first examination program for certifying pharmacy technicians. ASHP created a bulletin for technical assistance on training guidelines for pharmacy technician training programs.
1982	ASHP created accreditation standards for training programs.
1987	The Illinois Council of Hospital Pharmacists (ICHP) began an examination program to certify technicians.
1988	ASHP Research and Education Foundation had a conference on the use of technicians in pharmacy. This addressed on-the-job training, quality care, voluntary certification of technicians, and roles and responsibilities of a pharmacy technician in the hospital setting.
1991	The Pharmacy Technician Education Council (PTEC) was formed.
1994	A project called The Scope of Pharmacy Practice Project was completed. This addressed the task analysis of pharmacy technicians.
1995	The Pharmacy Technician Certification Board (PTCB) was created by ASHP, APhA, ICHP, and Michigan Pharmacists Association (MPA).
1996	ASHP and APhA published the first *White Paper on Pharmacy Technicians*. This addressed the need for national standards in training pharmacy technicians.
1997	ASHP, APhA, AACP, AAPT, and PTEC collaborated on a model curriculum for training courses for pharmacy technicians.
1999	NPTA was founded in Houston, Texas.
2000	PTCB updated the task analysis of pharmacy technicians.
2001	The second edition of the *Model Curriculum for Pharmacy Technician Training* was published.
2002	The second *White Paper on Pharmacy Technicians: Needed Changes Can No Longer Wait* was published (see Chapter 3).

background checks were not done in every state. After the PTCB was established, not only educational standards were instituted but also salaries were increased for many certified technicians. Attitudes have changed over time as well. Although technicians were once viewed as incompetent in many areas of pharmacy but still threatening the replacement of pharmacists with cheap labor, views now have changed as even with the increase in technicians in the workplace pharmacists are still in high demand. Technicians are now a part of the health care team and most pharmacists are confident they can delegate tasks to technicians knowing that the job will be done correctly. It is no coincidence that as higher standards and educational requirements are required for the pharmacy technician, the pharmacists' trust in technicians also increases.

CHANGING PHARMACY

Times have changed and so have the requirements of today's pharmacist. As a requirement for licensure, most states now require new pharmacists to obtain a doctor of pharmacy degree (PharmD), which requires 6 years of education in an accredited school of pharmacy. Those pharmacists who received a bachelor of science in pharmacy before this change have been allowed to work in pharmacy without attaining a doctor of pharmacy. Pharmacist licensure also requires examination through the National Association of Boards of Pharmacy (NABP) as well as examination according to the state's pharmacy laws; candidates for licensure must demonstrate competency through the passing of these examinations. Today's pharmacist also needs in-depth and broad communication skills to effectively communicate with doctors and with customers. Today's typical pharmacy technician is required to do an array of tasks, all of which require competencies in many areas. Thus in some states, today's technicians are required to complete additional education in addition to on-the-job training. Currently, there are no nationally standardized requirements for pharmacy technicians. Technicians help the pharmacist by preparing prescriptions and compounding (Figure 1-4). In a hospital setting, also known as an inpatient pharmacy, tasks include supplying floor stock to the hospital floors, preparing parenteral medications, transcribing doctors' orders, and filling patients' medication cassettes. Other specialized technicians may be responsible for the ordering of all drugs and supplies. As always, the need for strong communication skills is required by the technician in all pharmacy settings (see Chapter 3).

Pharmacists can obtain specialty certifications and may participate in providing specialty services. In some cases, participation may be governed by state

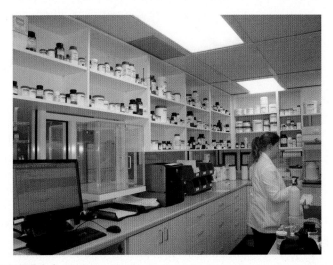

FIGURE 1-4 Pharmacy technician working in the pharmacy setting.

law, professional licensing boards, and certifying bodies. For example, some pharmacists participate in anticoagulation or pharmacokinetics services, where they interpret patients' laboratory results to determine the drug concentration and its relation to the therapeutic response of the patient. These pharmacists then are allowed to write the necessary change in medication strength based on the laboratory results. Other specialty duties include, but are not limited to, oncology, pediatrics, geriatrics, and compounding services.

Trust in Pharmacists/Trust in Technicians

Over the decades, pharmacists have become known as persons who can be trusted to provide truthful information, and someone with whom a person can be comfortable confiding. Although some traditions continue, times have changed concerning the role of the pharmacist. The most prevalent change can be seen in the inpatient setting of the hospital. As the competency of a pharmacist has become more "clinical," pharmacists are becoming more involved alongside doctors in the appropriate prescribing of medications and their dosages. These clinical pharmacists are found in the community pharmacy as well as hospital settings. Another important change in pharmacy concerns the laws governing patient consultation. The Omnibus Budget Reconciliation Act of 1990 (OBRA '90, Chapter 2) addressed several issues concerning patient education and monitoring of medications. Although initially consultation was mandated to be offered to only Medicaid patients, most states have developed statutes that require pharmacists to provide written and/or oral consultation to all patients who are prescribed new or changed medications. Consultation is meant to inform and educate the patient about the medication he or she is taking. Because of these changes in the way pharmacies function, virtually every pharmacy employs pharmacy technicians. There are thousands of technicians used to help lighten the load of filling prescriptions and performing other nondiscretionary tasks. Therefore it is important that the patient can trust a technician to provide the best care by filling the correct medication and referring the patient to the pharmacist for appropriate counseling. Most pharmacists agree it is important that pharmacy technicians have and maintain a standard of knowledge concerning pharmacy practice. The use of national certification is so far one of the best markers to ensure a minimum level of competency in pharmacy.

Pharmacists have earned the trust of their patients over many decades and it will take technicians time to earn the same trust. This takes a true commitment to the profession of pharmacy on the part of the pharmacy technician. Through education, training, and good communication skills, technicians will gain the trust of the patients whom they serve.

Technicians of the Twenty-First Century and Beyond

In the new millennium with the roles of pharmacists, technicians, and clerks becoming more clearly defined, new concerns arise. We must be aware that just as the advancement of medicine through the ages met with much resistance, so has the profession of pharmacy. The changing roles of pharmacists, technicians, and even clerks have had their share of blockades, mostly from within the medical community. Some doctors are not eager to have pharmacists writing orders, even if the medications are simple. Likewise, technicians have been perceived as posing a threat to pharmacy. Some pharmacists believe that technicians may take jobs away from pharmacists or increase the liability to the pharmacist if someone who is not properly trained makes a mistake. Therefore there is disparity across the United States regarding the duties of a pharmacy technician. In some states, pharmacies limit technicians' duties to a clerk level. In other states, technicians are required to be certified as pharmacy technicians before they are employed. All technicians must be aware of the legislative laws within their state. To find out more information on the laws in your state pertaining to pharmacy technicians, visit the website www.nabp.net. Each year more pharmacies are requiring a certain level of education from their technicians. This in turn allows expansion of job duties and higher pay for the technician.

Clerks' duties also are expanding and changing. In some pharmacies, clerks regularly enter new prescription orders into the computer. This task previously was done exclusively by a pharmacist or technician. The pharmacist is moving into a more highly clinical role, not only counseling patients but also working with medical staff. To a degree, the technician has become what the traditional pharmacist once was—one who transcribes orders, pulls medications, and fills prescriptions. Finally, the clerk has replaced the early technicians. Some colleges are offering specialized training programs for pharmacy clerks. Education in understanding trade/generic drug names and instruction in billing procedures are some of the curricula provided specifically for future pharmacy clerks.

DO YOU REMEMBER THESE KEY POINTS?

- Terms and definitions used within this chapter
- Common ancient beliefs, including the dogmas of those eras
- Common treatments used for conditions in earlier times
- Early American medicine practices and challenges during the Civil War
- Major persons who influenced the changes of dogmas in medicine
- The use of leeches and maggots throughout history
- The beginnings of pharmacists and pharmacy technicians
- How the roles have changed for pharmacists, pharmacy technicians, and pharmacy clerks
- Competencies required of today's technicians
- The use of opium in the nineteenth century
- Advancements in medicine over the centuries
- The effects of a placebo on curing illnesses

REVIEW QUESTIONS

Multiple choice questions

1. During the Civil War many soldiers died due to:
   A. Unsanitary conditions
   B. Postsurgical infections
   C. Gunshot wounds
   D. All of the above

2. Which of the following choices best describes sources of materials for remedies in ancient times?
   A. Chemicals, minerals, vitamins
   B. Minerals, animals, prayer
   C. Minerals, animals, plants
   D. Plants, seeds, minerals

3. Which of the following statements are not true?
   A. Sulfonamides are synthetic antibiotics.
   B. Sulfonamides are used for urinary tract infections.
   C. Gerhard Domagk discovered sulfonamide.
   D. Sulfonamide was one of many new antibiotic classes discovered in the 1800s.

4. Taking new prescriptions and entering them into the computer are tasks a _____ can do.
   A. Pharmacist
   B. Pharmacy technician
   C. Pharmacy clerk
   D. All of the above

5. Leeches are used for the following conditions except:
   A. To remove dead tissue
   B. Tissue infection
   C. Reconstructive surgery
   D. Skin grafts

6. The PTCB was founded by the following entities:
   A. ASHP, MPA, CPhA, PTEC
   B. MPA, ICHP, APhA, ASHP
   C. Federal agencies
   D. State and federal agencies

7. Opium and alcohol were once used to:
   A. Desensitize a person from pain
   B. Help ease depression
   C. Treat anxiety
   D. All of the above

8. Apothecary means:
   A. Pharmacist
   B. Store
   C. Drug
   D. Both A and B

9. _____ is known as the Father of Medicine.
   A. Hippocrates
   B. Paracelsus
   C. Mendel
   D. Aristotle

10. Trephining was the technique of:
   A. Bloodletting to rid the body of toxins
   B. Praying to rid the body of sickness
   C. Making an incision into the skull to release poison and/or evil spirits
   D. Manufacturing opium and alcohol

11. The placebo effect often worked through the use of:
   A. Faith
   B. Medicine
   C. Animal guts
   D. None of the above

12. Which of the following treatments are no longer used in mainstream medicine?
   A. Leeches
   B. Opiates
   C. Maggots
   D. Venesection

13. Pharmacy technicians perform the following functions except:
   A. Filling prescriptions
   B. Compounding medications
   C. Counseling patients
   D. Occupying clinical positions

14. The PTCB is an organization that:
   A. Regulates all pharmacy technicians
   B. Gives a national exam for pharmacy technicians
   C. Was founded by several pharmacist associations
   D. Both B and C

15. Which scientist was responsible for studies in anatomy, physiology, and pharmacology among other topics?

A. Galen

B. Aristotle

C. Bacon

D. Paracelsus

True/False

If a statement is false, then change it to make it true.

_____ **1.** In ancient times, plants were the only available remedies for illness.

_____ **2.** Bloodletting was a short-lived treatment because of many deaths.

_____ **3.** Sometimes families of the "early" pharmacists assisted behind the counter.

_____ **4.** Shamans were medicine men who communicated with the spirits.

_____ **5.** The roles of pharmacy technicians have changed little since their beginning.

_____ **6.** Plants given to ill patients in early times resembled the organ being treated.

_____ **7.** Pharmacists have little contact with patients in today's pharmacy.

_____ **8.** Only pharmacists can fill prescriptions.

_____ **9.** Over the years, the pharmacy technician's job description has remained the same.

_____ **10.** The concept of the four basic elements of life (air, water, fire, and earth) was created by Hippocrates in the late fifth century BC.

_____ **11.** The first pharmacy technician training took place in the military in the 1940s.

_____ **12.** In 1982 ASHP created the first accreditation standards for technician training programs.

_____ **13.** Clinical pharmacists are those who work only in hospitals.

_____ **14.** The first medical schools for physicians arose in Europe in the nineteenth century.

_____ **15.** Clinical pharmacy technician is a term used for different job descriptions other than the traditional duties of a technician.

TECHNICIAN'S CORNER

Write a brief summary about the new types of advancements that are occurring in medicine today. Do any of the dogmas that plagued ancient civilizations affect current beliefs?

BIBLIOGRAPHY

Anderson MJ, Stephenson KF: *Scientists of the ancient world*, Springfield, NJ, 1999, Enslow.

Ballington DA: *Pharmacy practice for technicians*, ed 3, St Paul, Minn, 2006, EMC/Paradigm.

Moulton C, editor: *Ancient Greece and Rome*, vol 3, New York, 1998, Simon & Schuster.

Narcto D: *The complete history of ancient Greece*, San Diego, 2001, Greenhaven.

Suplee C: *Milestones of science*, Washington, DC, 2000, National Geographic.

WEBSITES REFERENCED

"Asclepius." Encyclopedia Mythica. 2009. Encyclopedia Mythica Online. 23 Aug. 2009 (Referenced August 20, 2009) www.pantheon.org/articles/a/asclepius.html

Asclepius. Mythology, Cult, The Staff of Asclepius and The Hippocratic Oath. (Referenced July 23, 2009) www-structmed.cimr.cam.ac.uk/Asclepius.html

Sultz S: Epidemics in Colonial Philadelphia from 1699–1799 and The Risk of Dying. Archiving Early America. (Referenced July 29, 2009) www.earlyamerica.com/review/2007_winter_spring/epidemics.html

Vivian J, Fink J: OBRA90 at Sweet Sixteen: A Retrospective Review. US Pharm. 2008: 33(3):59-65. 3/20/08. (Referenced August 21, 2009) www.uspharmacist.com/content/t/pain_management,miscellaneous/c/10126/

Hemochromatos.Mayo Clinic staff. 9/12/08 Mayo Foundation for Medical Education and Research. (Referenced May 18, 2009) www.mayoclinic.com/health/hemochromatosis/DS00455/

PTCB website. Active PTCB CPhTs and State Regulations as of June 30, 2009(Referenced August 23, 2009) www.ptcb.org

The National Alliance of Advocates for Buprenorphine Treatment. Opiates/Opioids. 5/10/2008. (Referenced July 3, 2009) www.naabt.org/education/opiates_opioids.cfm

Rainey L: Who discovered HIV: Gallo, Montagnier or both? July 6, 2006. Last updated May 22, 2009. (Referenced August 15, 2009) www.dallasvoice.com/artman/publish/article_2666.php

University of Wisconsin-Madison. "Scientists Guide Human Skin Cells To Embryonic State." ScienceDaily 21 November 2007. (Referenced 23 August 2009) www.sciencedaily.com-/releases/2007/11/071120092709.htm

Centers for Disease Control and Prevention. List of Vaccines used in United States. Last reviewed May 8, 2009. (Referenced 6/23/09)

Melancholy and black humor. Mirrors of Melancholy: Models, History and Reception (Referenced 8/2/09) http://web.uvic.ca/~histmed/mirrors.pdf

FOR MORE INFORMATION ON TOPICS COVERED

http://nobelprize.org/nobel_prizes/medicine/laureates/
www.nida.nih.gov
www.pasteur.fr/ip/easysite/go/03b-00002j-000/en
www.drugstoremuseum.com

Pharmacy Federal Laws and Regulations

Objectives

UPON COMPLETING THIS CHAPTER, YOU SHOULD BE ABLE TO DO THE FOLLOWING:

- List the history of federal drug laws in chronological order.
- Explain which law prevails among state, federal, and local laws.
- List the current laws pertaining to ordering controlled stock and required record keeping.
- Define the functions of the Food and Drug Administration (FDA) and Drug Enforcement Administration (DEA).
- Perform the function of verifying a DEA number.
- Explain the verification process for Internet pharmacies.
- Describe the FDA reporting process for adverse reactions.
- Describe the reasoning behind the creation of the DEA term "drug diversion."
- List who can prescribe medications/devices.
- Explain the OSHA guidelines as they pertain to pharmacy.
- Explain the necessary forms and regulations used for controlled substances.
- Explain the difference between technicians' tasks and pharmacists' responsibilities.
- Identify the major laws within which technicians need to work when performing nondiscretionary functions in a pharmacy.
- Describe the implications of the Health Insurance Portability and Accountability Act of 1996 (HIPAA).
- Describe the regulations and guidelines under the provisions of USP 797.

TERMS AND DEFINITIONS

Act *A statutory plan passed by Congress or any legislature that is a "bill" until it is enacted and becomes law*

Adulteration *The mishandling of medication that can lead to contamination/impurity, falsification of contents, or loss of drug quality or potency. Adulteration may cause injury or illness to the consumer*

Amendment *A change in the original act or law*

Barbiturate *A drug derived from barbituric acid; a barbiturate acts as a central nervous system depressant. Barbiturates are often employed in the treatment of seizures and as sedative and hypnotic agents*

Board of pharmacy *State board that regulates the practice of pharmacy within the state*

Boxed warning *Drug warning that is placed in the prescribing information or package insert of the product and indicates a significant risk of potentially dangerous side effects. It is the strongest warning the FDA can give. It is common in the pharmacy profession to call these warnings "Black Box Warnings" because of their appearance in a drug label; the warning is often enclosed in a black outlined box to draw attention to the content.*

Controlled substance *Any drug or other substance that is scheduled I through V and regulated by the Drug Enforcement Administration*

Drug diversion *The intentional misuse of a drug intended for medical purposes; the Drug Enforcement Administration usually defines diversion as the recreational use of a prescription or scheduled drug. Diversion can also refer to the channeling of the prescription drug supply away from legal distribution and to the illegal street market.*

Drug Enforcement Administration (DEA) *Federal agency within the U.S. Department of Justice that enforces U.S. laws and regulations related to controlled substances*

Drug Facts and Comparisons *Reference book found in pharmacies that contains detailed information on medications*

Drug utilization evaluation (DUE) *A process employed to ensure prescribed drugs are utilized appropriately. The main desired outcome of any DUE program is an increase in medication-related efficacy and safety*

Food and Drug Administration (FDA) *The agency within the U.S. Department of Health and Human Services responsible for assuring the safety, efficacy, and security of human and veterinary drugs, biological products, medical devices, the national food supply, cosmetics, and radioactive products*

Health Insurance Portability and Accountability Act of 1996 (HIPAA) *Federal act for protecting patients' rights, establishing national standards for electronic health care communication, and ensuring the security and privacy of health data*

Legend drug *Drug that requires a prescription for dispensing*

Material Safety Data Sheet (MSDS) *A document providing chemical product information. A MSDS includes the product name, composition (chemicals in the product), hazards, toxicology, and other information regarding the proper steps to take with spills, accidental exposure, handling, and storage of the product. The filing of a MSDS within the pharmacy or workplace is usually a requirement to meet Occupational Safety and Health Administration (OSHA) standards.*

Medicaid *Federal- and state-operated insurance program that covers health care costs and prescription drugs for low-income children, adults, and elderly and those with disabilities*

Medicare *Federal- and state-managed insurance program that covers health care costs and prescription drugs for individuals older than 65, persons younger than 65 with long-term disabilities, or those persons with end-stage renal disease*

Misbranding *Labeling of a product that is false or misleading; label information must include directions for use; safe and/or unsafe dosages; manufacturer, packer, or distributor; quantity, and weight.*

Monograph *Comprehensive information on a medication's actions within that class of drugs. Also lists generic and trade names, ingredients, dosages, side effects, adverse effects, how the patient should take the medication, and foods or other drugs (e.g., OTC medications, herbals) to avoid while taking the medication.*

Narcotic *A nonspecific term used to describe a drug (such as opium) that in moderate doses dulls the senses, relieves pain, and induces profound sleep but in excessive doses causes stupor, coma, or convulsions, and may lead to addiction. From the standpoint of U.S. law, opium, opiates (derivatives of opium), and opioids, as well as cocaine and coca leaves, are "narcotics."*

National Drug Code (NDC) *A 10-digit number that indicates specifics of a prescription drug or an insulin product. The NDC specifies the drug manufacturer, the drug product (drug strength, dosage form, and formulation), and the package size.*

Negligence *A legal concept that describes an action taken without the forethought that should have been taken by a reasonable person of similar competency*

Occupational Safety and Health Administration (OSHA) *U.S. government–managed agency that oversees safety in the workplace; created MSDS requirements*

Omnibus Budget Reconciliation Act of 1990 (OBRA '90) *Congressional act that changed reimbursement limits and mandated drug utilization evaluation, pharmacy patient consultation, and educational outreach programs*

Over-the-counter (OTC) medication *Medication that can be purchased without a prescription; nonlegend medications*

Physicians' Desk Reference (PDR) *One of the many reference books of medications, this reference compiles and publishes select manufacturer-provided package inserts and prescribing information useful for health professionals.*

Pregnancy Category *A system in use by the FDA to describe five levels of assessment of the fetal effects caused by a drug, a required section of current prescription drug labeling. First introduced in 1979, the system is currently under reevaluation for usefulness and inclusion in the prescription label.*

Protected Health Information (PHI) *A term used to describe a patient's personal health data. Under HIPAA this information is protected from being shared or distributed without permission*

The Joint Commission (TJC) *An independent nonprofit organization that accredits hospitals and other health care organizations in the United States. Accreditation is required to accept Medicare and Medicaid payment.*

Tort *To cause harm or injury to a person intentionally or because of negligence*

United States Pharmacopeia (USP) *An independent nonprofit organization that establishes documentation on product quality standards, drug quality and information, and health care information on medications, over-the-counter products, dietary supplements, and food ingredients to ensure the appropriate purity, quality, and strength are met*

United States Pharmacopeia-National Formulary (USP-NF) *A publication of the USP that contains standards for medications, dosage forms, drug substances, excipients, medical devices, and dietary supplements*

Introduction

The practice of pharmacy is governed by a series of laws, regulations, and rules enforced by federal, state, and local government. The practice of pharmacy is also subject to policies and procedures made by institutions and/or pharmacy management at each pharmacy site. The number of rules and regulations is staggering, and most of us cannot easily decipher the legal tangle of words; however, we are required to follow these rules and regulations. Therefore this chapter presents the most basic laws and regulations that pertain to pharmacy, pharmacists, and especially the technician. A good understanding of these laws is necessary to pass the Pharmacy Technician Certification Board examination, and more important, it is necessary to know your responsibilities when working in pharmacy. An overview of the history of the **Food and Drug Administration (FDA)** is given and its present-day functions will be described. The laws are listed in chronological order along with a short description of how and why each one was established. Common record-keeping practices are covered. The legal liabilities of pharmacists and technicians are explained. Morals and ethics are discussed at the end of this section because they play a vital role in the decisions that technicians will make in pharmacy.

FDA History

The Food and Drug Administration (FDA) was established in 1862 along with the U.S. Department of Agriculture. The FDA is the oldest consumer protection agency in the U.S. federal government. The FDA's Division of Chemistry consists of a staff composed of several disciplines, including chemists, physicians, veterinarians, pharmacists, microbiologists, and lawyers. Until 1901 the Division of Chemistry evaluated applications for new drugs for use in humans or animals, food and color additives, medical devices, and infant formulas. The chief chemist within the Division of Chemistry, Harvey Wiley, changed the direction of the division, establishing scientific authority by researching the effects of chemical preservatives used in the production of foods and drugs, exposing potential hazards in products, focusing on consumer safety, and eventually paving the way for government regulation. Inspectors within the department visited thousands of food and other manufacturing facilities each year. In 1901 the Division of Chemistry was renamed the Bureau of Chemistry. Wiley's efforts led to the first major passage of legislation, the **Federal Food and Drugs Act of 1906.** This new agency was to make many more changes in its authority and scope as it grew. In 1927 the agency's name was changed to the Food, Drug, and Insecticide Administration, and in 1930 the name was shortened to the Food and Drug Administration (FDA). The FDA remained under the authority of the U.S. Department of Agriculture until 1940, when the agency became part of the Federal Security Agency. As the FDA continued to regulate new applications for drugs, devices, and other products, the agency was transferred to the Department of Health, Education, and Welfare (HEW) in 1953 and eventually was placed under the authority of the U.S. Public Health Service within HEW in 1968. Ultimately the FDA's final destination occurred in 1980 when it was moved from HEW to a newly created U.S. Department of Health and Human Services, where it still remains today.

EARLY ACTIVITY OF THE FDA

Since the FDA's founding, they have investigated the **adulteration** and **misbranding** of agriculture goods used for food and drugs. Hundreds of bills were introduced to Congress to regulate standards to protect the health of consumers, yet the FDA's ability to regulate and enforce standards remained limited, leaving the primary control of domestically produced foods and drugs to each individual state. The laws varied widely between states. Meanwhile, horrible incidents continued to occur, such as the death of 13 children and 9 babies in 1902 after being injected with a tainted batch of tetanus diphtheria antitoxins. In June of 1906 President Theodore Roosevelt signed the Federal Food and Drugs Act of 1906, also known as the Wiley Act. This important act gave the FDA the power to administer and prohibit the interstate transport of unlawful food and drugs. Drugs had to meet the standards of strength, quality, and purity in the **United States Pharmacopeia (USP)** and the *National Formulary* guidelines; any variations from the guidelines needed to be plainly listed on the product label. The label could not mislead the consumer and all ingredients had to be listed on the label. The law also prohibited the addition of any ingredients to a food that would substitute for the food, conceal damage, pose a health hazard, or constitute a filthy or decomposed substance.

Wiley's authority was challenged and undercut many times by the Supreme Court as attempts were made to form standards in regards to food and drug manufacturers. The FDA suffered a severe setback when the Supreme Court in 1912 determined that the law enforcing the regulation of drugs did not apply to false therapeutic claims. The controversy lay in the attempt to prove that the drug companies "intended" to defraud the consumer. This Supreme Court ruling undermined the Wiley Act and many manufacturers won court cases, allowing their products to be sold to consumers. In 1912 Wiley resigned from the FDA, and at this point the bureau focused more closely on drug regulation, as this was a great concern.

With a new presidential administration taking over in 1933 under Franklin D. Roosevelt, the FDA was able to change its authority to include both quality and identity standards for food and drugs, prohibition of false therapeutic claims for drugs, and coverage of cosmetics and medical devices. The FDA had the right to inspect factories and control the advertising of products. The FDA countered advertisements of drug claims by exposing the horrible but true results of certain drugs. For example, an eyelash dye that blinded some women as a result of dangerous additives had been widely advertised to consumers. A medication tonic made with radium as an additive was found to cause a slow and painful death to the user. All products were protected under the previous laws. For the next 5 years a bill that would replace the 1906 revised law was stalled in Congress. It took tremendous effort to pass new standards enforceable by the FDA. In 1937 a Tennessee drug company advertised a new sulfanilamide elixir specifically aimed toward children. The toxic solvent was untested (per then current laws) and more than 100 people, mostly children, died. It was later determined that the solvent was similar to antifreeze, which is deadly to humans. Unfortunately this type of deadly scenario was repeated several times before the necessary changes in the laws of that time were made. As a result of public pressure, Congress finally passed the 1938 Food, Drug, and Cosmetic Act. The act required manufacturers to prove to the FDA that a drug was safe for use before marketing, and the manufacturers had to provide directions on the drug's label for its safe use. The act also mandated standards for foods, set tolerances for certain poisonous substances, and authorized factory inspections. The FDA was given authority to enforce the standards. Just a few months after its passing, the FDA identified that sulfa and other drugs required a prescription from physicians before they could be purchased. Clarification of what constituted a prescription drug versus an over-the-counter drug was determined in 1951 with the enactment of the Durham-Humphrey Amendment. Other laws passed in the 1950s banned carcinogenic additives to foods.

Another potential tragedy was averted in the United States in the 1960s when the drug thalidomide, a sedative used in Europe, was found to cause severe birth defects, including grossly deformed limbs, when administered during pregnancy. The drug was never approved for use in the United States. The Kefauver-Harris Drug Amendments of 1962 were revolutionary in their scope to ensure the safety and effectiveness of medications in the U.S. market. Another growing concern was the use and abuse of amphetamines, **barbiturates**, and other potentially addictive agents. The FDA was given more control over these agents with the enactment of the Drug Abuse Control Amendments of 1965. This control was eventually delegated to the Drug Enforcement Administration (DEA) in 1968. In 1973 some of the responsibilities of the FDA were given to the Consumer Product Safety Commission. These included oversight of hazardous toys, flammable fabrics, and potential poisons in consumer products. Other provisions in the 1960s allowed for greater FDA oversight to ensure the safety and effectiveness of veterinary drugs and additives to animal feed.

Before 1938 the Post Office Department and Federal Trade Commission were in charge of ensuring the safety of cosmetics and medical devices; after 1938 regulating cosmetics and medical devices became the responsibility of the FDA. The advertising of various quack products was widespread throughout the country; claims such as increasing life span, curing conditions, and protecting one's health were unfounded in many cases. However, in 1976 another disaster occurred when an intrauterine device, which claimed to prevent pregnancy, caused serious injury to thousands of women. Only then did the **1976 Medical Device Amendments** allow the FDA to regulate and approve these types of devices, as well as recall ineffective or dangerous devices.

With continued consumer and political pressure the FDA has influenced new laws such as the **Orphan Drug Act,** which was passed in 1983 and targeted all rare diseases. The Orphan Drug Act influenced expanded research and availability of new treatments for AIDS, cancer, and genetic diseases. An overview of several acts and **amendments** is discussed under the section titled Description of Laws. In recent years the FDA has continued its mission to ensure public safety, including the necessary oversight of dietary supplements that present safety problems, have false or misleading claims, or are otherwise adulterated or misbranded.

Description of Laws

What is an **act**? An act is a statutory plan passed by Congress or any legislature that is called a "bill" until it is enacted, at which point it becomes a law. An amendment is a change in the original act or law. The following examples are brief because the various acts and amendments encompass broader descriptions. Further reading is suggested to gain a deeper insight into the laws that pertain to pharmacy and patient rights. Also see Box 2-1 for a list of well-known federal laws in chronological order that are discussed in this chapter.

1906 FEDERAL FOOD AND DRUGS ACT

The 1906 Federal Food and Drugs Act was one of the first laws enacted to stop the sale of inaccurately labeled drugs. All manufacturers were required to have truthful information on the label before selling their drugs. Although this act was well intentioned, there were many drugs that still made their way onto the market because of continued false claims regarding their effectiveness. Additional changes were made to this act that ultimately required manufacturers to prove the effectiveness of the drugs through methods such as scientific studies.

1914 HARRISON NARCOTICS ACT

By 1912 international meetings were being held to curb the increase in trafficking of controlled substances. The International Opium Convention of 1912 was

BOX 2-1 WELL-KNOWN FEDERAL LAWS

1906	Federal Food and Drugs Act
1912	International Opium Convention
1914	Harrison Narcotics Act
1938	Food, Drug, and Cosmetic Act
1951	Durham-Humphrey Amendment
1962	Kefauver-Harris Amendments (thalidomide disaster)
1970	Comprehensive Drug Abuse Prevention and Control Act
1970	Poison Prevention Packaging Act
1972	Drug Listing Act
1983	Orphan Drug Act
1987	Prescription Drug Marketing Act
1990	Anabolic Steroids Control Act
1990	Omnibus Budget Reconciliation Act of 1990 (OBRA '90)
1994	Dietary Supplement Health and Education Act (DSHEA)
1996	Health Insurance Portability and Accountability Act of 1996 (HIPAA)
2000	Drug Addiction Treatment Act (DATA 2000)
2003	Medicare Modernization Act (MMA)
2005	Combat Methamphetamine Epidemic Act (CMEA)
2006	Dietary Supplement and Nonprescription Drug Consumer Protection Act

one of these meetings. Limitations on opium transport and recreational use were attempted. The Harrison Narcotics Act of 1914 was enacted in the United States in parallel with international treaties to curb recreational use of opium. Individuals could no longer purchase opium without a prescription, and it became harder to obtain opium for nonmedical purposes. The Harrison Narcotics Act required practitioner registration, documentation regarding prescriptions and dispensing, and implementation of restrictions regarding the importation, sale, and distribution of opium, coca leaves, and any derivative products. See Chapter 1, History of Medicine and Pharmacy.

1938 FOOD, DRUG, AND COSMETIC ACT

The 1938 Food, Drug, and Cosmetic Act was enacted because the earlier Federal Food and Drugs Act of 1906 was not worded strictly enough and did not include cosmetics. Two important concepts introduced in this new act were adulteration and misbranding. For example, false or exaggerated claims commonly were placed on new drug labels and often misled the consumer. This was considered misbranding. All controlled substances were required to be labeled "Warning: May be habit forming." This act also provided the legal status for the Food and Drug Administration (FDA). Adulteration deals with the preparation and/or storage of a medication. Mishandling of the food or drug may cause injury or even death to a consumer. This act described the exact labeling for products and defined misbranding and adulteration as being illegal. The new law also required drug companies to include package inserts and directions to the consumer regarding safe use (see more information under the section titled Food and Drug Administration/Drug Enforcement Administration).

1951 DURHAM-HUMPHREY AMENDMENT

The 1951 Durham-Humphrey Amendment added more instructions for drug companies and required the labeling "Caution: Federal law prohibits dispensing without a prescription." Under this amendment, certain drugs require a physician's order and supervision. This amendment also made the initial distinction between legend drugs (by prescription only) and **over-the-counter (OTC)** medications that do not require a physician's order (also known as nonlegend or nonprescription drugs).

1962 KEFAUVER-HARRIS AMENDMENTS

The Kefauver-Harris Amendments enacted in 1962 were groundbreaking in their attempts to ensure the safety and effectiveness of all new drugs on the U.S. market. The amendments gave the FDA specific authority to approve a manufacturer's marketing application before a drug could be available for commercial use. Firms now had to prove safety and provide substantial evidence of effectiveness for the drug's intended use. The required evidence had to consist of adequate and well-controlled studies. The amendments helped establish rules of clinical drug investigation and the informed consent of study subjects. The amendments also required that drug-related adverse events be reported to the FDA. The regulation of prescription drug advertising was transferred from the Federal Trade Commission to the FDA, and the burden was put on the drug manufacturing companies to ensure quality as "good manufacturing practice" (GMP) standards were established. One example of the effectiveness of the FDA is illustrated by its role in preventing the sale of thalidomide in the United States. In Europe, persons were taking this new medication to help them sleep. In Europe in the early 1960s, women who had taken thalidomide while pregnant gave birth to children with severe defects including the absence of limbs. The FDA postponed approving thalidomide until just before the birth defects across Europe were reported. Very few cases were reported in America; those reported were due to women obtaining thalidomide from outside the United States. Consumers became aware that drug companies were not doing enough to test the drugs they were marketing. More laws ensued after the thalidomide tragedy to better safeguard the public and greatly increase the time and money spent on testing a drug for its safety and effectiveness.

1970 COMPREHENSIVE DRUG ABUSE PREVENTION AND CONTROL ACT

The Drug Enforcement Administration (DEA) was formed to enforce the laws concerning controlled substances and their distribution. A stair-step schedule of controlled substances was introduced, based on the drug's intended medical use, the propensity of a drug to be abused, and safety and dependency concerns. The five-level stair-step schedule of controlled substances requires stricter rules as the drug rating intensifies. Schedule I is the most restrictive and is defined as those drugs with no medically accepted use in the United States. Therefore the prescription of a schedule V drug is less restricted and requires less documentation than that required for a schedule II drug (see Controlled Substances section of this chapter).

1970 THE POISON PREVENTION PACKAGING ACT (PPPA)

The Poison Prevention Packaging Act of 1970 required manufacturers and pharmacies to place all medications in containers with childproof caps or packaging. This includes both over-the-counter and legend drugs. The standard specifies that medication should not be able to be opened by at least 80% of children under the age of 5 and that at least 90% of adults should be able to open the medication. Exceptions to this act include physician requests for non-childproof caps for their patients, certain legend medications, hospitalized patients, or at the specific request of the patient.

BOX 2-2 PPPA GUIDELINES (EXEMPT DRUGS)*

All medications must be dispensed with a childproof cap, with the exception of the following:

Anhydrous cholestyramine powder
Betamethasone tablets 12.6 mg or less contained in dispenser packages
Colestipol no more than 5 g
Conjugated estrogens containing no more than 32 mg
Contraceptives in daily dispensing sets
Erythromycin ethylsuccinate tablet packages not containing more than 16 g
Hormone replacement therapy products that contain one or more progestin or estrogen
    substances
Mebendazole containing no more than 600 mg in dispenser packages
Medroxyprogesterone tablets
Methylprednisolone tablets containing no more than 84 mg
Norethindrone numonic packages containing no more than 50 mg
No more than 8 g of erythromycin granules in suspension
Pancrelipase powder, capsule or tablet forms
Prednisone package containing no more than 105 mg
Sacrosidase preparations in glycerin and water
Sodium fluoride containing no more than 264 mg per package
Sublingual forms of isosorbide dinitrate 10 mg or less
Sublingual forms of nitroglycerin

or

All medications dispensed in a hospital or nursing home do not require childproof
    packaging

or

Customer requests medication not be dispensed with childproof cap; may be a "blanket"
    request for all prescription medications

or

Physician requests medication not be dispensed with a childproof cap; may be a
    "blanket" request for all prescription medications

*National Poison Control Center: 1-800-222-1222.

Before the implementation of this act there were hundreds of unintentional deaths of children under the age of 5 years as a result of ingestion of either drugs or household chemicals. The first attempt to prevent these tragic outcomes included the Hazardous Substances Labeling Act of 1960. A pharmacist by the name of Homer George of Mississippi was the driving force behind the first National Poison Prevention Week (occurring yearly in March). Individual states followed by implementing poison control centers. It was not until 1970 that the PPPA was enacted and is now under the authority of the Consumer Product Safety Commission (CPSC). It was estimated that more than 1.4 million childhood deaths were prevented annually because of childproof caps (www.cpsc.gov/cpscpub/pubs/384.pdf). See Box 2-2 for PPPA Guidelines Exempt Drugs.

1983 ORPHAN DRUG ACT

The 1983 Orphan Drug Act encouraged drug companies to develop drugs for rare diseases by providing research assistance, grants, and cost incentives to manufacturers. Before this act, companies had no incentive to develop medications and spend millions of dollars and many years of trials to treat a disease that affected a small portion of the population. Therefore several regulatory restrictions were waived for diseases that affected fewer than 200,000 persons in the United States. The act also covered diseases that affected more than 200,000 persons if it could be proved that the cost of developing and testing a drug could not be recovered by the eventual sales. The act also encouraged manufacturers to develop drugs for rare diseases by providing marketing exclusivity for orphan drugs for a period of 7 years after FDA approval.

1987 PRESCRIPTION DRUG MARKETING ACT

The 1987 Prescription Drug Marketing Act (PDMA) addressed issues related to the distribution and wholesale pedigree of human prescription drugs. The intent of the act was to solidify the legal supply channel of prescription drugs from manufacturers to authorized distributors and wholesalers. The act helps to avoid counterfeit drugs and ingredients in the supply chain and also helps limit diversion of pharmaceutical samples and prescription drugs.

1990 OMNIBUS BUDGET RECONCILIATION ACT (OBRA '90)

The origins of the **Omnibus Budget Reconciliation Act** began in 1987 when the U.S. Congress addressed the problems regarding health care quality for the elderly. With increasing numbers of elderly entering nursing homes, great concern arose over the substandard care being provided, high nursing-to-patient ratios, and unhealthy conditions present. Requirements were set for those facilities participating in Medicare/Medicaid programs and addressed enforcement mechanisms. A minimum standard of care was required and a change began to take place, transitioning nursing homes from uncomfortable institutions to a comfortable homelike environment providing higher quality care. However, the provisions under OBRA '87 did not address individual privacy rights. OBRA '90 affected the responsibilities of practicing pharmacists and health care personnel in general (see Chapter 13). The act outlines specifics for pharmacies to participate in the Medicaid Drug Rebate Program. Medicaid is a state- and federally-managed program that provides medical coverage for low-income persons (see Chapter 13). OBRA '90 has profoundly affected pharmacy responsibilities. This act states that a pharmacist must offer to counsel (at the time of purchase) all patients who receive new prescriptions. OBRA '90 also required **drug utilization evaluation (DUE)**. The intent of DUE under OBRA '90 was to ensure that all medications being prescribed to patients would be reviewed for appropriateness. Three important provisions of OBRA '90 include:

1. Evaluation of drug therapy: completed before filling a prescription (prospectively). Pharmacists must review drugs for appropriateness, possible drug interactions, contraindications, and correctness of drug dosage and duration of therapy to ensure patient safety.
2. Review of drug therapy: This is a long-term review of provision 1 through the use of software programs and includes educational interventions intended to ensure the quality of prescribing by physicians.
3. DUE board review: The board reviews, evaluates, and develops strategies to improve patient care and reduce costs for those covered under the Medicaid program.

In addition the DUE must include systems such as computer programs that alert the pharmacist to possible drug interactions, precautions, and other pertinent information that the patient should know. Pharmacies must document and maintain records to track consultations and outcomes. Although OBRA '90 is specific to **Medicaid** coverage, pharmacies usually now counsel all patients on medications that have been prescribed. If these provisions are not met, the pharmacy cannot receive federal reimbursement for medication and may face civil liability proceedings. The Board of Pharmacy within each state oversees OBRA '90 compliance. They can also impose fines on both pharmacies and pharmacists for noncompliance. A patient may refuse counseling.

1996 HEALTH INSURANCE PORTABILITY AND ACCOUNTABILITY ACT (HIPAA)

HIPAA is also referred to as **protected health information** or PHI. The privacy rules are meant to protect certain health information. Standards of PHI address the use and disclosure of an individual's health information. Entities that are covered by PHI are obligated to comply with all requirements within the rules of HIPAA, which became effective in 2003. A HIPAA-covered entity is either a health care provider, a health plan, or a health care clearinghouse. This includes entities that process nonstandard health information they receive from another entity into a standard format (e.g., standard electronic format or data content, or vice versa).

Patient Confidentiality

Confidentiality is another aspect of ethical work. The definition of confidentiality is to keep privileged information about a customer from being disclosed without his or her consent. This includes information that may cause the patient embarrassment or harm. Under federal law, patients have the right to privacy concerning their medications, treatment, or any aspect of their health care. These laws affect all areas of medicine, including pharmacy, concerning issues of obtaining, transferring, and accessing patient information. Changes have been made throughout all medical facilities and medical information centers that limit access to patient information in charts and computer databases. A patient's approval is required for any information concerning the patient to be released to any third party, including insurance companies, physicians, and pharmacies. Because pharmacy technicians and other health care professionals have access to information about a patient's condition, medications, and other personal information, they are responsible for keeping the patient's information confidential.

What Information Is Protected?

The Privacy Rule protects all *"individually identifiable health information"* held or transmitted by a covered entity or its business associate, in any form or media, whether electronic, paper, or oral.

What Does This Mean for the Pharmacy?

Patient information must be communicated on a need-to-know basis with the provisions that the entity is covered under the HIPAA health information rules and regulations. This means the physician can call and request information about his or her patient. The patient's health insurance company can request information on their participant. The pharmacist can share information with the patient about his or her own coverage or medications.

How Is Information Protected via the Computer?

There are several safeguards in place that help protect electronically transmitted patient information. For the sender of electronic protected health information, it is required that encryption converts the information into a nonreadable format. Decryption is the reverse process. The encryption technology must be approved by the National Institute of Standards and Technologies to ensure its effectiveness in protecting patients' rights.

What Are the Rights of the Patient?

Under HIPAA, as a patient you have the following rights:

- Ask to see and get a copy of your health records.
- Have corrections added to your health information.
- Receive a notice that tells you how your health information may be used and shared.
- Decide if you want to give your permission before your health information can be used or shared for certain purposes, such as for marketing.
- Obtain a report on when and why your health information was shared for certain purposes.
- If you believe your rights are being denied or your health information is not being protected, you can do the following:
    - File a complaint with your provider or health insurer.
    - File a complaint with the U.S. Government.
    - Either authorize or not authorize any sharing of your personal or medical information.
    - Change or rescind this permission any time you desire.

The HIPAA Privacy Rule specifically permits certain persons identified by the patient, such as a spouse, family members, or friends, to receive information that is directly relevant to the patient's care or the patient's payment for health care. If the patient is present or is otherwise available before the disclosure and has the capacity to make health care decisions, the covered entity may discuss this information with the family and these other persons if the patient agrees or, when given the opportunity, does not object.

For example, when a person comes to a pharmacy and requests to pick up a prescription on behalf of an individual he or she identifies by name, a pharmacist, based on professional judgment and experience with common practice, may allow the person to do so.

Examples of What You (the Technician) Cannot Do

As a pharmacy technician, you may not do the following:

- Offer any personal or medical information pertaining to the patient to any entity not covered under HIPAA rules and regulations.
- Share any information with any family member or friend, co-worker, manager, or any entity not covered under the HIPAA rules and regulations.

See Box 2-3 for examples.

BOX 2-3 EXAMPLES OF BREACHING CONFIDENTIALITY

Describe why the examples below are in violation of HIPAA regulations

Example 1: Ms. K has cancer. Two pharmacy technicians discuss her condition and the medications that she is taking. A co-worker of Ms. K overhears this information and tells her employer.

Example 2: A computer screen is left on that shows a patient's health information and can be seen by other patients.

Example 3: A regular customer of the pharmacy asks the technician for another patient's phone number; the customer knows that patient.

Example 4: A technician looks up personal patient information because the technician is curious about the patient.

Example 5: A technician gives drug information over the phone to a family member of the patient.

Examples of What Is Not Covered under HIPAA Patient Rights

If you work for a health plan or covered health care provider:

- The Privacy Rule does not apply to your employment records.
- The Rule *does* protect your medical or health plan records if you are a patient of the provider or a member of the health plan.

Public Health Activities

Covered entities may disclose protected health information to the following:

1. Public health authorities authorized by law to collect or receive such information for preventing or controlling disease, injury, or disability and to public health or other government authorities authorized to receive reports of child abuse and neglect
2. Entities subject to FDA regulation regarding FDA-regulated products or activities for purposes such as adverse event reporting, tracking of products, product recalls, and postmarketing surveillance
3. Individuals who may have contracted or been exposed to a communicable disease when notification is authorized by law
4. Employers, regarding employees, for information concerning a work-related illness or injury or workplace-related medical surveillance to comply with the Occupational Safety and Health Administration (OHSA) or similar state law.

Law Enforcement Purposes

Covered entities may disclose protected health information to law enforcement officials for law enforcement purposes under the following six circumstances, and subject to specified conditions:

1. As required by law, such as court orders
2. To identify or locate a suspect, fugitive, material witness, or missing person
3. In response to a law enforcement official's request for information about a victim or suspected victim of a crime
4. To alert law enforcement of a person's death, if the covered entity suspects that criminal activity caused the death
5. When a covered entity believes that protected health information is evidence of a crime that occurred on its premises
6. By a covered health care provider in a medical emergency not occurring on its premises, when necessary to inform law enforcement about the nature of a crime, the location of the crime or crime victims, and the perpetrator of the crime

Examples

1. Can I have a friend pick up my medications and medical supplies for me?
   - Yes; under HIPAA pharmacists are allowed to give prescription medications and supplies to a family member, friend, or any person you send to pick up the medications or supplies.
2. If my daughter calls the pharmacy to ask about whether my medications are ready, can they tell her?
   - Yes; but no other information can be given out.
3. If I cannot speak the language and a stranger offers to interpret the exchange between myself and the pharmacist, is this okay?
   - Yes; as long as you do not object.

4. Is a pharmacist permitted to have the customer acknowledge receipt of the notice by signing or initialing the log book when picking up prescriptions?

• Yes; provided that the individual is clearly informed on the log book of what he or she is acknowledging and the acknowledgment is not also used as a waiver or permission for something else that also appears on the log book (such as a waiver to consult with the pharmacist). The HIPAA Privacy Rule provides covered health care providers with discretion to design an acknowledgment process that works best for their businesses (see www.hhs.gov/ocr/privacy/psa/understanding/index.html).

2000 DRUG ADDICTION TREATMENT ACT (DATA 2000)

The Drug Addiction Treatment Act of 2000 permits physicians to prescribe controlled substances (preapproved by the DEA) in schedules C-III, C-IV, or C-V to persons suffering from opioid addiction, for the purpose of maintenance or detoxification treatments. This act is different from the regulations that oversee methadone maintenance treatments for opioid addiction. Certain controlled substances have been found to effectively attenuate the craving for opioids and also prevent withdrawal symptoms. Patients must be in a treatment program that provides additional support services. Physicians must complete a training course and be registered/certified with the DEA in order to prescribe these agents. If the physician is in private practice they may only treat up to 30 patients at one time. After 1 year they may apply to treat up to 100 patients.

2003 MEDICARE MODERNIZATION ACT (MMA)

Medicare is a government-managed insurance program that provides assistance to people older than age 65. In addition, those who are younger than age 65 with disabilities and persons with end-stage renal failure are covered under this program. Medicare has a long history, starting in 1965. In 2003 a major change took place with the addition of the Medicare Modernization Act for millions of Americans. This new revision provided a drug discount card to beneficiaries with low incomes who require pharmacy company assistance for obtaining medications. The new program is under the Medicare Advantage program that began in 2006. This allows Medicare participants to offset high drug costs, which should also reduce preventable hospitalizations resulting from lack of medication treatment. For complete information on Medicare's history and provisions, see Chapter 13.

2005 COMBAT METHAMPHETAMINE EPIDEMIC ACT

Until 2004 the drug pseudoephedrine was sold OTC as a decongestant and was not limited in quantity for purchase by the consumer. Several different manufacturers produce this drug, and it was stocked outside the pharmacy on the shelves of every store that carried cold remedies. The OTC status of pseudoephedrine has changed since the U.S. government has become aware of its diversion and use as an ingredient in the preparation of methamphetamines (see Figure 2-1).

Congress passed a bill named the Combat Methamphetamine Epidemic Act (CMEA) of 2005 in response to this problem. This bill addresses all areas of the manufacturing, law enforcement, and sale of this drug. Although pseudoephedrine is still labeled as a "non-controlled substance," the manufacture, distribution, and sale of this drug must follow several strict guidelines. According to

U.S. Department of Justice
Drug Enforcement Administration
Office of Diversion Control

Problem
Pseudoephedrine and ephedrine, both List 1 chemicals, are highly coveted by drug traffickers who use them to manufacture methamphetamine, a Schedule II controlled substance, for the illicit market. The diversion of over-the-counter, pseudoephedrine-containing products is one of the major contributing factors to the methamphetamine problem in the United States. Inappropriate retail level purchases by individuals attempting to procure pseudoephedrine for the illicit manufacture of methamphetamine have been documented as a source of much of the pseudoephedrine found in clandestine methamphetamine laboratories. These purchases, which are accomplished by methods such as "*smurfing*" and *shelf sweeping*, violate Federal law and may expose the seller to criminal and civil penalties.

Common Pseudoephedrine Products
Common cold products including, but not limited to Sudafed®, Tylenol®Cold, Advil®Cold, Drixoral®, Benadryl® Allergy & Cold Tablets, Robitussin®Cold Sinus & Congestion, as well as many generic brands.

Retail Thresholds
The Methamphetamine Anti-Proliferation Act (MAPA) limits the thresholds of pseudoephedrine drug products to 9-gram single transactions with the package size not to exceed 3 grams.

Nine (9) Gram Single Transactions--Three (3) Grams per Package
- 120 mg pseudoephedrine HCl = 92 tablets
- 120 mg pseudoephedrine HCl = 31 tablets
- 60 mg pseudoephedrine HCl = 184 tablets
- 60 mg pseudoephedrine HCl = 62 tablets
- 30 mg pseudoephedrine HCl = 367 tablets
- 30 mg pseudoephedrine HCl = 123 tablets

Common Methods of Diversion
- *Smurfing* involves the retail purchase of sub-threshold amounts by organized groups of individuals that either send in multiple purchasers into the same location or visit a large number of different locations.
- *Shelf sweeping* occurs when individuals or groups remove all the shelf stock and exit the store, similar to a "smash and grab" shoplifting technique.
- *Shoplifting* occurs when individuals remove stock from the shelves and exit the store without paying.

All of the above methods can be prevented by limiting access to products or by utilizing mirrors or other surveillance equipment such as cameras.

Suspicious Purchase Items
Camping fuel, lithium batteries, large quantities of matches, iodine, coffee filters, rock salt, battery acid, swimming pool acid (when purchased in unusual quantities or under unusual circumstances).

Theft or Loss of List I Chemicals
The DEA reminds List I chemical handlers of the regulatory requirement: "A regulated chemical handler must immediately report thefts or losses to the nearest DEA office and should notify state/local law enforcement and regulatory agencies. A written report must be submitted to the DEA within 15 days of discovery of the theft or loss." (CFR 21 §1310.05)

Improper Sales
"Any person who possesses or distributes a listed chemical knowing or having reasonable cause to believe that the listed chemical will be used to manufacture a controlled substance, except as authorized by this title, shall be fined in accordance with Title 18, or imprisoned not more than 20 years, or both." (Title 21 U.S.C. 841 (c)(2))

FIGURE 2-1 DEA poster on the misuse of pseudoephedrine. (Courtesy of Drug Enforcement Administration.)

BOX 2-4 COMBAT METHAMPHETAMINE EPIDEMIC ACT 2005

Pseudoephedrine storage: Behind counter or locked in a cabinet.
The maximum amount sold may not exceed 3.6 g in a calendar day or 7.5 g per 30 days.
Purchaser's identification must be provided.
Documentation may be done electronically or via log book. If a log book is used it must be a bound book.
Records of all information must be kept for at least 2 years.
Documentation required:
  Drug name
  Drug strength
  Drug amount
  Date/time of sale
  Customer's name
  Customer's address
  Customer's signature

these guidelines, only a licensed pharmacist or technician may dispense, sell, or distribute this drug (see Box 2-4). Each state has responded by enforcing controls over the sale of pseudoephedrine. Many of the pharmacy regulations range from requiring photo identification and having the consumer sign a log book for the amount purchased to requiring a prescription. Even so, the court systems are battling over the final judgment of this drug because it is a popular and effective

TABLE 2-1 Additional Pharmacy-Related Acts

Date	Act	Abbreviation	Brief Description
1967	Fair Packaging and Labeling Act	FPLA	Label must show net contents; name and place of business of manufacturer, packer, or distributor; and net quantity of contents in terms of weight, measure, or numeric count. Measurement must be in metric and U.S. units.
1972	Drug Listing Act	DLA	Provides the FDA an accurate list of all drugs manufactured, prepared, propagated, compounded, or processed by a drug establishment regulated under the FDA. This act amends the Food, Drug, and Cosmetic Act and prevents unfair or deceptive packaging and labeling.
1990	Anabolic Steroids Control Act	ASCA	Because of anabolic steroid misuse by athletes, this act helped enforce regulations on abuse.
1990	The Humanitarian Device Exemption—Safe Medical Devices Act	SMDA	This act encourages discovery and use of devices intended to benefit patients in treatment and diagnosis of diseases or conditions that affect fewer than 4000 individuals in the U.S.
1990	Nutrition Labeling and Education Act	NLEA	This act covers food items and their labeling; vitamins, minerals, or other nutrients are on the label and in some cases are highlighted.
1994	Dietary Supplement Health and Education Act	DSHEA	This act better defines the term *dietary supplements* to include herbs such as ginseng, garlic, fish oil, psyllium, enzymes, glandulars, and mixtures of these. Consumers must be informed of health-related benefits. Manufacturers of these supplements are held under same regulations. Labels cannot mislead consumer. Labels must include nutritional values.
1997	Food and Drug Administration Modernization Act	FDAMA	New drugs are being reviewed and released into the public faster. Millions of persons have a wider and more timely access to information on new medications.

decongestant. Drug companies will certainly be adversely affected if more constraints are placed on the purchase of pseudoephedrine. Drug enforcement also is taking place worldwide across many countries such as Canada, Germany, Australia, and the United Kingdom. The Netherlands pulled pseudoephedrine from the market in 1989 because of concerns of cardiac safety. Within the United States, many states—such as Alabama, Arizona, Georgia, Illinois, Tennessee, Washington, and Wyoming—restrict sales of pseudoephedrine products to pharmacies and require customers to show photo ID and sign a log book during purchase. States such as California, Maryland, Maine, and New Mexico have enacted degrees of controlled access to OTC pseudoephedrine products. The state of Oregon now requires a prescription for pseudoephedrine. For a quick overview of other pharmacy-related acts, see Table 2-1.

Food and Drug Administration/Drug Enforcement Administration

Two government agencies that are important with respect to pharmacy are the FDA and DEA. The FDA was created under the U.S. Department of Health and Human Services; refer to earlier in this chapter for the history of the FDA. The main functions of the FDA are to enforce the guidelines for manufacturers to ensure the safety and effectiveness of medications. Under the Food, Drug, and

Cosmetic Act are standards that prohibit misbranding and adulteration or misleading labeling of any products before they are provided to consumers. Any food, drug, or product that contains any avoidable, added, poisonous, or harmful substance is unsafe and is considered adulteration. To prevent misbranding, manufacturers must meet the following package standards under the Food, Drug, and Cosmetic Act:

1. Mandatory drug labeling (see Monographs section)
2. Standards of identity
3. Imitation foods
4. Nutritional information for special dietary foods
5. Manufacturers may not advertise false or misleading statements about their product

Examples of misleading information of product labeling would be the following:

1. Incorrect, inadequate, or incomplete identification
2. Unsubstantiated claims of therapeutic value
3. Inaccuracies concerning condition, state, treatment size, shape, or style
4. Substitution of parts or material
5. Ambiguity, half-truths, and trade puffery
6. Failure to reveal material facts, consequences that may result from use, or existence of difference of opinion

The other enforcement department is the DEA. This entity was created later under the Department of Justice. The function of the DEA is to prevent illegal distribution and misuse of controlled substances. The DEA also issues licenses to practitioners, pharmacies, and manufacturers of controlled substances. Each agency plays a different part in law enforcement, but the agencies work together when the DEA must evaluate new drugs and the level at which they should be controlled.

1972 DRUG LISTING ACT; NATIONAL DRUG CODE (NDC)

In 1972 the Drug Listing Act (**National Drug Code**) was implemented under the authority of the FDA. Every drug has a unique 10-digit number divided into 3 segments. The numbers identify the labeler, product, and trade package size (Figure 2-2). The first set of numbers (labeler code) is assigned by the FDA. The second set (product code) identifies the specifics of the product. The third set of numbers (package code) identifies the specifics of the package size and types.

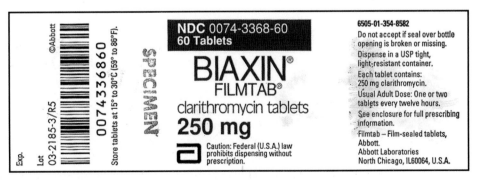

FIGURE 2-2 Example of NDC label. (From Ogden SJ: *Calculation of drug dosages*, ed 8, St Louis, 2007, Mosby.)

BOX 2-5 NDC NUMBER SPECIFICS

NDC 50580-449-05

50580: First five positions indicate the **labeler code;** this identifies any firm that manufactures or distributes (under its own name) the drug (includes **repackers** or **relabelers**).

449: Second set of numbers indicates the **product code;** this identifies a specific strength, dosage form, and formulation for a particular drug. Examples include active ingredients and size, shape, color, or imprinted code on drug, as well as any other distinguishing markings on the drug.

05: Third set of numbers indicates the **package code** and identifies package types and sizes. For example, drug is in a bottle, vial, or box; drug's quantity or amount, such as in milliliters, ounces, or pints for liquids.

If the NDC number contains **two asterisks** at the end, this identifies the product as a bulk, raw, nonformulated controlled substance.

Although the NDC directory is limited to both prescription and insulin drugs, there are certain products that may not be listed. Reasons include the following:

- The product is not a prescription or insulin.
- The manufacturer has notified the FDA that the drug is no longer being produced.
- The manufacturer has not complied with all obligations necessary; therefore it is not included until all information is provided to the FDA.

Both product and package codes are set by the drug company. See the example in Box 2-5 for a specific overview of each code.

FDA REPORTING PROCESS AND ADVERSE REACTIONS

The FDA has a toll-free number (1-800-FDA-1088) for reporting any defect found in OTC medications or any drug problem noted by a person. A technician or pharmacist also has this number available to report any problems with a drug, whether it is OTC or legend (prescription). A product that looks different from its normal package should be reported. Adverse reactions also should be reported to the FDA's MedWatch program. Any medication reaction that may cause disability, hospitalization, or death should be reported along with any less disabling type of reaction, such as fainting, or other types of reactions that may not have been listed in the drug monograph. MedWatch is the program under the FDA that allows consumers and health care professionals to report discrepancies or adverse reactions with medications. The MedWatch form for such reports may be found in many drug reference publications and drug compendia databases, or online (www.fda.gov/medwatch/how.htm). The reporting persons identity is kept confidential (Figure 2-3).

RECALLED DRUGS

The FDA does not typically order recalls but instead may request (in writing) a recall from the manufacturer. Only if the manufacturer refuses and there is clear evidence that there is a risk to human health may the FDA enforce such a request. The manufacturer voluntarily recalls items that have been found to be defective or somehow tainted. This is done by several means, such as television news or newspapers, and can be downloaded from the FDA website. In addition, the manufacturer must notify via e-mail, phone, or fax all entities that may have dispensed the product. They must include how to handle each type of recall (Box 2-6). Once the product is recalled it is destroyed and an investigation of why the product was defective is conducted.

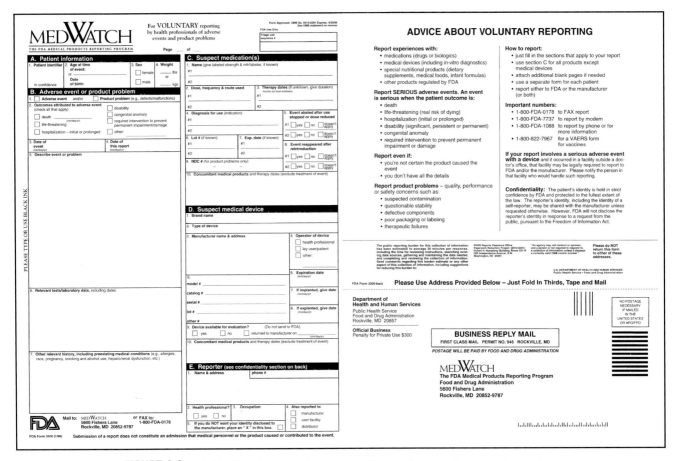

FIGURE 2-3 FDA MedWatch form. (Courtesy of Drug Enforcement Administration.)

All stock must be pulled from the shelves following the guidelines of the manufacturing company. In addition, the manufacturer will supply a return form with instructions for reimbursement. The three classes of recalls are as follows:

- **Class 1:** the highest level of recall dealing with products that could cause serious or even fatal harm. This includes life-saving drugs. This level also includes foods that contain toxins or labels that do not list ingredients that may cause allergies.
- **Class 2:** the next level dealing with products found to cause a temporary health problem or cause a slight threat of serious harm. This level includes drugs that are dispensed at less than the strength labeled on the container; it does not include drugs used in life-threatening events.
- **Class 3:** the lowest level used for products that may have a minor defect or other condition that would not harm the patient, but the drugs cannot be resold. This level includes a drug container defect (such as a faulty cap), a product with a strange color or taste, or the lack of English labeling on retail food items.

Controlled Substances

Controlled substances, such as barbiturates, opioids, benzodiazepines, and central nervous system stimulants, are substances that are addictive and have

BOX 2-6 SAMPLE RECALL NOTIFICATION

The FDA posts press releases and other notices of recalls and market withdrawals from the firms involved as a service to consumers, the media, and other interested parties. The FDA does not endorse either the product or the company.

Recall—Firm Press Release

Qualitest Pharmaceuticals, Inc., issues a voluntary nationwide recall of Accusure insulin syringes (1/2 cc, 31 G, short needle) Lot #6JCB1 and Accusure insulin syringes (1 cc, 31 G, short needle) Lot #7CPT1.

Contact: Qualitest Pharmaceuticals, Larry Kass: 1 (800) 444-4011.

FOR IMMEDIATE RELEASE—August 21, 2009—Huntsville, AL: Qualitest Pharmaceuticals, Inc., today has issued a voluntary nationwide recall of Accusure insulin syringes (1/2 cc, 31 G, short needle) with lot number 6JCB1 (expiration 10/2011), NDC 0603-7001-21. This lot was distributed between January 2007 and June 2007 to wholesalers and retail pharmacies nationwide (including Puerto Rico). Also today, Qualitest has issued a voluntary nationwide recall of Accusure insulin syringes (1 cc, 31 G, short needle) with lot number 7CPT1 (expiration 03/2012), NDC 0603-7002-21. This lot was distributed between May 2007 and June 2008 to wholesalers and retail pharmacies nationwide (including Puerto Rico). The syringes in these lots have been found to have needles that can detach from the syringe.

When the needle becomes detached from the syringe during use, it can become stuck in the insulin vial, push back into the syringe, or remain in the skin after an injection.

Consumers who have any Accusure insulin syringes (1/2 cc, 31 G, short needle) with lot number 6JCB1 or Accusure insulin syringes (1 cc, 31 G, short needle) with lot number 7CPT1 should stop using them and contact Qualitest at 1-800-444-4011 for product replacement instructions. You can find the lot number on the white paper backing of each individual syringe.

Qualitest is notifying all customers who received the product and arranging for return of any affected product.

This recall is being made with the knowledge of the Food and Drug Administration.

Consumers with questions may contact Qualitest at 1-800-444-4011 for more information.

Adverse reactions or quality problems experienced with the use of this product may be reported to FDA's MedWatch Adverse Event Reporting program either online, by regular mail, or by fax.

Online: www.accessdata.fda.gov/scripts/medwatch/medwatch-online.htm

Regular mail: use postage-paid FDA Form 3500; available at www.fed.gov/MedWatch/getforms.htm

Mail to: MedWatch, 5600 Fishers Lane, Rockville, MD 20852-9787

Fax: 1-800-FDA-0178

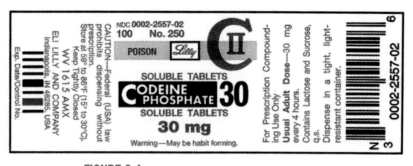

FIGURE 2-4 Codeine label showing C-II imprint.

a potential to be abused. Opioids, such as codeine and morphine, are substances created from opium and are addictive. When consumed over time, a person can build up a tolerance to their effects and require increased doses. Each type of controlled substance is assigned a rating that depends on its addiction and abuse potential. Figure 2-4 gives an example of a labeled **narcotic**.

TABLE 2-2 Typical Controlled Substances

| Drug Level | Type of Medication | | Potential for Abuse |
	Generic Name	Trade Name	
C-I		LSD Cocaine Mescaline Heroin	Drugs that have no accepted medical use in U.S. and have very high abuse potential
C-II	Meperidine Oxycodone/APAP* Oxycodone/ASA Hydromorphone Methylphenidate Fentanyl Codeine Morphine Amphetamines Methadone Opium	Demerol Percocet Percodan Dilaudid Ritalin Duragesic	High potential for abuse; used for medicinal purposes; abuse may lead to severe psychological or physical dependence
C-III	Hydrocodone/APAP Acetaminophen/ codeine #2, #3, #4 Hydrocodone/ibuprofen	Vicodin Tylenol/codeine Vicoprofen	Potential for abuse under this schedule is less than that of controlled substances under C-II; abuse may lead to moderate or low physical dependence or high psychological dependence; most schedule III drugs are combination narcotics
C-IV	Diazepam Lorazepam Pentazocine Chlordiazepoxide Flurazepam Chloral hydrate Phenobarbital	Valium Ativan Talwin Librium Dalmane	Potential for abuse is low compared to C-III drugs; abuse may lead to limited physical or psychological dependence
C-V	Diphenoxylate/atropine Guaifenesin/codeine Promethazine/codeine	Lomotil Robitussin AC Phenergan/codeine	Low potential for abuse in relation to C-IV drugs; abuse may lead to limited physical or psychological dependence

*APAP, Acetyl-*p*-aminophenol (acetaminophen); *ASA*, acetylsalicylic acid (aspirin).

RATINGS OF SCHEDULED (CONTROLLED) SUBSTANCES

The letter C (meaning controlled substance) is used in addition to Roman numerals to indicate the addictiveness and abuse potential of controlled substances. In 1970 the U.S. Congress established five levels of control based on the potential for abuse. The strongest level in terms of abuse potential are C-I drugs; these drugs have been determined to have a high potential for abuse and to have no acceptable medical purpose, and also are deemed unsafe for use under medical supervision. These include such drugs as D-lysergic acid diethylamide (LSD) and heroin. Pharmacies do not stock drugs in the C-I class because they do not have any medicinal use in the United States. Therefore physicians cannot prescribe C-I drugs for their patients. All medicinal controlled substances are placed in the following four categories: C-II, C-III, C-IV, and C-V. Table 2-2 shows the schedule, types of medications, and abuse potential for each level of controlled substances.

Individual states establish certain rules concerning controlled substances, such as storage and record keeping. Schedule C-V medications (referred to as exempt controlled substances) may be kept OTC in some states because of the low potential of abuse, whereas many states require C-II through C-III drugs to be kept (before filling) in locked storage areas because of their high potential of abuse. However, for exempt controlled substances there are specific rules governing the quantity kept on hand and records that need to be retained by the pharmacy when these substances are purchased by consumers.

The U.S. Attorney General has the authority to decide under which schedule a drug should be placed. The decision is made after careful consideration is given to scientific findings and after receiving input from various authorities on the possible dependency potential of each agent. Some drugs may be labeled under two different schedules because the dose may alter the dependency of the drug. Sometimes, controlled substances can be reevaluated; for example, dronabinol (Marinol) previously was rated as a C-II drug but is now a C-III drug. In contrast, certain narcotics are used primarily for procedures in hospitals; for example, topical cocaine is used locally to stop bleeding and provide anesthesia before suturing.

TAMPER-PROOF PRESCRIPTIONS

Many states have changed to a new type of controlled substance prescriptions. These new prescriptions have up to eight different tamper-proof security marks on them. These features were designed to stop forgery and/or fraud to a prescriber's intended order. There are several deterrents that eliminate photocopying the prescription order. The prescriptions can be ordered with any or all of the features. The DEA must approve the printer company that prints the new prescriptions but there is no specific format because each state may adopt its own features, colors, or size. Check with your individual state Board of Pharmacy for more information. The individual features are listed in Box 2-7. See Figure 2-5 for a sample prescription form.

BOX 2-7 TAMPER-PROOF FEATURES

- Tamper-resistant background ink shows attempts to alter script by patient.
- Thermochromatic ink box shows "SECURE" when rubbed or heated.
- Each prescription sheet has an individual numeric identifier so lost or stolen prescription pads can be invalidated.
- Each sheet is sequentially numbered for internal and state-mandated record keeping.
- Security feature warning bands are on the front of each script to detail security features.
- Penetrating magnetic ink is used to print your information on the script, preventing chemical "lifting" of information during forgery.
- Secure prescriptions have "coin reactive" ink. Message appears when the back of the pad is rubbed with a coin
- Photocopied features:
  - Hidden security "VOID" appears when photocopied on most high-end photocopiers.
  - Reverse printed RX (lighter colored) notations in upper corners of pad drop out when photocopied to appear white.
  - All secure prescriptions have a high security watermark on reverse side that cannot be copied and can only be seen when held to a light source at an angle.
  - MicroPrint security borders are present, which are tiny printings of a security message along the edges of a pad that combine to form a solid line when digitally scanned or copied.

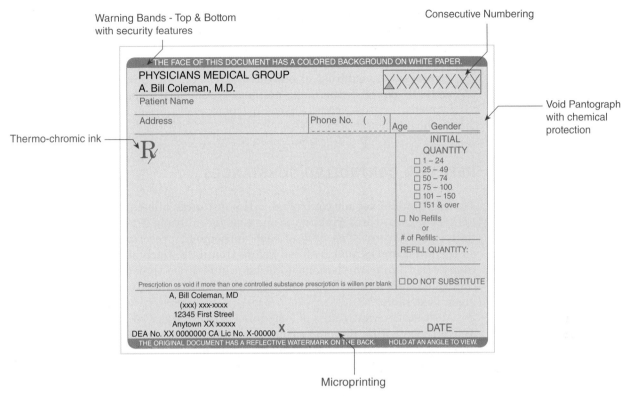

FIGURE 2-5 Sample of tamper-proof prescription.

REGISTRATION REQUIRED FOR MAINTAINING NARCOTICS

The DEA has three main registration forms used in the regulation of controlled substances. Only Form 224 is needed by the pharmacy to dispense controlled substances. The following is a list of form numbers issued by the DEA along with additional requirements:

1. To manufacture or distribute controlled substances: Form 225.
2. To manage a controlled substances' treatment program or compound controlled substances: Form 363.
3. To dispense controlled substances: Form 224 (must be renewed every 3 years using Form 224a).
4. To order or transfer schedule II substances: Form 222. This must be done by the receiving registrant to the registrant transferring the drugs. A final count of the drugs must be completed on the day of transfer. No copy needs to be sent to the DEA but a copy should be kept on file for 2 years for DEA inspection.
5. Authorization to destroy damaged, outdated, or unwanted controlled substances: Form 41. Retail pharmacies can only request this form from the DEA once a year. (Hospitals may request a "blanket destruction" permission form, which allows them to destroy a controlled substance multiple times throughout the year.) For retail pharmacies a letter must be sent to the DEA for approval along with the completed Form 41 at least 2 weeks before destruction. The request letter must contain the names of at least two people who will witness the destruction as well as the proposed date and method of destruction. The disposal of the scheduled drug(s) must be witnessed by either a licensed physician, pharmacist, registered nurse (RN), or law enforcement officer. Signed copies of DEA Form 41 must then be forwarded to the DEA.

6. Retail pharmacies who want to engage in wholesale distribution of bulk quantities of drugs containing pseudoephedrine, phenylpropanolamine, or ephedrine must register with the DEA: Form 510.
7. For loss or theft of a controlled substance: Form 106. Information required includes name/address of pharmacy, DEA registration number, date of loss or theft, police department notified, type of loss or theft, drug name, and symbols or cost codes used by pharmacy in marking containers (if applicable).

REFILLING CONTROLLED SUBSTANCES

The DEA guidelines for controlled C-II substances allow physicians to write up to three separate prescriptions at one time for multiple drugs, to be filled sequentially over 90 days. The date of each subsequent prescription must be written on the order and cannot be filled before that date. Each state's **board of pharmacy** (BOP) may implement additional guidelines that control the amount of controlled substances that can be refilled; representative state examples are given (see Table 2-3).

Most states limit refills of schedule C-III through C-V drugs to a maximum of five times within 6 months from the original order, whichever comes first. In addition, the amount ordered on the refills may not exceed the original order. The length of time for keeping records may also vary per state, but a record must be kept of controlled substance refills indicating the pharmacist's initials and the date it was dispensed. (A list of each state's BOP can be found at www.nabp.net.)

ORDERING CONTROLLED SUBSTANCES

A pharmacy has two ways to obtain schedule II controlled substances from a distributor. A DEA Form 222 (Figure 2-6) must be filled out by the receiving pharmacist. This form must be completed only with a pen, a typewriter, or an indelible pencil. The top copy and the middle (DEA) copy with the carbon paper are sent to the supplier or manufacturer by the pharmacy receiving the drugs. Filing electronically is also possible. This electronic order can be submitted online. Digital signatures are issued by the DEA and include a unique number that the purchaser assigns to track the order. The number is in a nine-character format—the last two digits of the year, X, and the six characters as selected by the purchaser. An electronic order can include controlled substances that are

TABLE 2-3 **Examples of State Regulations for C-II Refills and C-III to C-V Refills**

State	C-II Refills	C-III to C-V Refills
Colorado	No refills	Same as C-II
Florida	No refills	May not be filled or refilled more than 6 months after date written or be refilled more than 5 times
Montana	No refills	May be filled up to 1 year from date written
Utah	No refills	May not be filled or refilled more than 6 months after date written or be refilled more than 5 times
Arkansas	No refills	May not be filled or refilled more than 6 months after date written or be refilled more than 5 times

See Reverse of PURCHASER'S Copy for Instructions	No order form may be issued for Schedule I and II substances unless a completed application form has been received, (21 CFR 1305.04).	OMB APPROVAL No. 1117-0010

TO: *(Name of Supplier)* — STREET ADDRESS

CITY and STATE — DATE — **TO BE FILLED IN BY SUPPLIER** / SUPPLIERS DEA REGISTRATION No.

LINE No.	No. of Packages	Size of Package	Name of Item	National Drug Code	Packages Shipped	Date Shipped
1						
2						
3						
4						
5						
6						
7						
8						
9						
10						

TO BE FILLED IN BY PURCHASER

◄ **LAST LINE COMPLETED** *(MUST BE 10 OR LESS)* — SIGNATURE OF PURCHASER OR ATTORNEY OR AGENT

Date Issued	DEA Registration No.	Name and Address of Registrant
20010101	DEAREGNO	VOID VOID VOID

Schedules XXXXXXXXXXXX — VOID VOID VOID

Registered as a	No. of this Order Form
XXXXXXXXXXXX	000000005

VOID VOID VOID
VOID VOID VOID
VOID VOID VOID

DEA Form -222 (Oct. 2004)

U.S. OFFICIAL ORDER FORMS - SCHEDULES I & II
DRUG ENFORCEMENT ADMINISTRATION
SUPPLIER'S Copy 1

107051797

FIGURE 2-6 Drug Enforcement Administration Form 222.

Tech Note!

Under the authority of the Controlled Substances Act of 1970, the Controlled Substances Ordering Systems (CSOS) now allow electronic filing of DEA Form 222. This allows more stock to be ordered than possible by using the paper form. Less controlled stock will usually need to be kept in the pharmacy since ordering is quicker and stock can be ordered more often.

not in schedules I and II and non–controlled substances. The purchaser must create a record of the quantity received and the date received. This record must be linked electronically to the original order and archived.

The pharmacy retains the bottom copy. When the medication is shipped to the pharmacy, the middle (DEA) copy is forwarded to the DEA to prove that the medication has been properly received. When the pharmacy receives the controlled substances, the pharmacist compares the pharmacy's copy of Form 222 with the invoice and signs and dates both. The invoice and the form are stapled together and retained for 7 years. If any error is made, the form becomes invalid but must be retained for reference; therefore the pharmacy cannot erase mistakes or throw away the form. When returning any C-II drugs, the pharmacy must have the manufacturer or wholesaler fill out the same form (Form 222) to request the controlled substance, and the pharmacy then is the provider who retains the top copy and sends the middle copy to the DEA. Other controlled substances (C-III, C-IV, and C-V) are ordered on normal invoice forms, but invoices must be filed and retained for possible DEA or state Board of Pharmacy inspection. These should be kept separate from other nonscheduled drugs for easy retrieval. Once the scheduled drugs are received, the invoice forms for schedules III to V must be kept for no less than 2 years.

RECORD KEEPING

A pharmacy has three methods of filing controlled substances and legend drugs, as shown in Table 2-4. Although federal law allows any one of these three methods to be used, a state's Board of Pharmacy may require a specific method. In addition to the filing of controlled medications, every time a controlled substance is issued to a patient or nursing station, it must be logged out of the pharmacy stock (Figure 2-7, *A, B*) as required under state law. Levels are first counted; the amount of each drug must be correct. Then the technician or pharmacist will subtract the amount taken. Again, the remaining stock is double-checked for accuracy. This same standard holds true for returning items or adding new stock to the inventory.

TABLE 2-4 Three Methods of Filing Controlled Substances and Legend Drugs

System	Drawer I	Drawer II	Drawer III
1	C-II separate	C-III, C-IV, C-V	All other prescriptions
2	C-II separate	C-III, C-IV, C-V,* and all legend drugs	
3	C-II, C-III, C-IV, C-V*		All other prescriptions

*If any C-III, C-IV, or C-V controlled drugs are kept with non–controlled drugs (system 2) or mixed with C-II drugs (system 3), they must be stamped with a red "C" for easy identification. All records must be kept on site for no less than 2 years. Many states, however, have longer requirements for keeping records; remember that the strictest law is the one that must be followed. When taking inventory, one must have exact counts of C-II substances at all times. The final count can be inventoried only by a *licensed pharmacist.*

Oxycodone/apap 5/325mg Tablets

Date	Prescription/Invoice#	Quantity	Patient/Supplier	Balance	Initials	Current Inventory Count	Discrepancy
4/8/xx	Rx#12345	25	10	15	jj	15	0
4/9/xx	Invoice# 9876	100	Glaxo	115	Kb	115	0

A

			Codeine 30mg	Diazepam 5mg	Hydrocodone/ APAP 5/325mg	Lorazepam 5mg	Oxazepam 15mg	Oxycodone ER 10mg	Meperidine 25mg/mL	Meperidine 75mg/mL	Diazepam 5mg/mL	Hydromorphone 5mg/5mL	Morphine 1mg/mL	Morphine 10mg/mL	
Previous Days Count			20	15	35	2	12	9	21	25	5	19	4	16	
Date	Patient	Dispensed	Oral						Inj						SIGNATURE
9/21 /xx	Jane Smith	10mg Meperidine							20						Paul James RN
9/21 /xx	Add to stock-	John Whey CPhT		25		27	24				25		29		Sean Ray RN

B

FIGURE 2-7 A, Pharmacy log sheet. **B,** Nursing floor log sheet.

NARCOTIC INVENTORY

Narcotics are at high risk for **drug diversion** and must be inventoried differently than normal nonscheduled drugs. Pharmacy maintains a perpetual inventory of these medications. This means that once the inventory is started it does not end; instead, it continues until the drug is no longer stocked. The basic principle is to identify an initial count of all controlled substances and to monitor the count as drugs are dispensed by subtracting the amount taken out of stock and adding to the count all drugs received by the pharmacy and placed into stock. This can be done either in pen in a ledger or through the use of software. The type of ledger or software differs between community and institutional pharmacies although basic information is required. Although the technician may be responsible for keeping track of all transactions, a pharmacist must validate all counts. In addition, overall periodic counts are done weekly or monthly by pharmacists. The DEA requires an inventory to be taken every 2 years; the DEA does not require a copy of the inventory taken. Any discrepancies that are identified must be investigated and explained.

REVERSE DISTRIBUTOR

The term reverse distributor indicates all controlled substances that are unwanted, unusable, or outdated that are returned to the distributor. These must be dealt with in accordance with DEA regulations. All transactions must be under the control of a person authorized by the DEA to handle controlled substances; this process is meant to deter the loss or misuse of drugs, also known as drug diversion. If a controlled substance becomes outdated or damaged, the pharmacy must return the substance to the manufacturer or return the substance to a company that collects controlled substances and then either returns them to the manufacturer or arranges for their disposal. These authorized companies may call themselves reverse distributors or returns processors. In the case of a nurse or pharmacy personnel using a partial dose of a controlled substance, it is required that two parties witness and sign off the destruction or waste of the drug. All liquid and solid medications must have proper documentation that is kept for 2 years. To destroy medication, DEA Form 41 must be filed. This is determined by an agent of the DEA who will instruct the applicant how to proceed. The completed form must include the following:

* Date
* Name of substance
* Dosage form
* Number of units
* Reason for destruction
* Manner of destruction
* Applicant's signature

Records must be kept on all drugs destroyed as determined by state law.

FILLING, REFILLING, AND TRANSFERRING PRESCRIPTIONS FOR CONTROLLED DRUGS

Original Filling of C-II through C-V

Schedule II through V drug prescriptions can be accepted by the pharmacy in written, oral, or fax form following certain DEA provisions and/or circumstances. Although the following regulations are outlined according to the DEA, each state normally has additional restrictions that must be followed. For information on

Tech Note!

Because opioids in general are used widely to treat patients for pain, technicians, pharmacists, and nurses come into contact with them daily. This has led to many cases of addiction by health care workers. All narcotics such as opioids and other controlled medications must be accounted for and not left out in the open where they could be misused. All controlled substances must be signed in and out of stock in pen to serve as a permanent mark.

your specific state's guidelines, visit your state's board of pharmacy website, which can be found at www.nabp.net.

Schedule C-II drugs require a prescription signed by the prescriber. An order may be called or faxed ahead of time to the pharmacy, but the original prescription must be presented for comparison at the time it is actually dispensed.

Emergency Filling of C-II

An oral order in place of a written prescription is permitted only in emergency situations. The guidelines are as follows:

1. The physician determines that the patient needs the C-II drug and considers it to be an emergency with no alternative treatment possible.
2. The physician cannot give a written prescription to the pharmacist. This may be because the physician is away from the office.
3. The pharmacist must obtain all information from the physician, including the drug name, strength, dosage form, and route of administration. The physician's name, address, phone number, and DEA number are required. All information must be recorded in written form.
4. The amount of the drug can only be enough to sustain the patient through the emergency period. The pharmacist should indicate on the prescription that it is being filled because of an emergency.
5. The pharmacist must make every effort to verify the physician's authority unless he or she knows the physician personally.
6. The prescriber has 7 days to produce the written and signed prescription to the pharmacist. Each state may impose lesser time limits. In addition, the prescription must have written on its face "Authorization for Emergency Dispensing." If this is not done, the pharmacist must notify the DEA. The written prescription must be attached to the oral record of the prescription.
7. There is no time limit when a C-II drug must be filled after being signed by the prescriber; however, the pharmacist must determine if the patient still needs the medication (for example, as in a drug filled several weeks after the order was written).
8. No quantity limits are placed on the quantity of C-II drugs.
9. There may be additional provisions per state BOP regulations.

Schedule C-III, C-IV, and C-V drugs may be reduced to written form if called into the pharmacy. All required prescription information must be attained by the pharmacist including the prescriber's DEA number.

Refilling of C-II through C-V

When it comes to refilling prescriptions per DEA regulations, controlled substances are placed into the following three categories: C-II; C-III and C-IV; C-V.

1. Schedule C-II drugs may not be refilled.
2. Schedule C-III and C-IV may only be refilled up to five times within 6 months after the date the prescription was written, whichever occurs first. Patients are allowed to request refills via e-mail or by phone.
3. Schedule C-V drugs can be refilled as often as prescribed on the prescription.

When C-III, C-IV, and C-V drugs are refilled, the following required information must be provided on the back of the prescription: pharmacist's initials, refill date, and the amount of drug that is refilled. In addition, a pharmacy may use a data-processing system to store and retrieve C-III, C-IV, and C-V prescription refill information. To meet DEA regulations, the following criteria must be met:

1. Pharmacies must use one of two methods: manual or computerized log for refills.
2. A daily hard copy is printed and pharmacists verify all refills they have authorized.
3. A log book is kept in which all controlled refills are verified by the pharmacist.
4. A computer system is used to print a refill-by-refill audit for any specific strength, dosage, or form, retrievable by either generic or trade name.
5. In case the computer system is not functioning, the pharmacy must have an alternative procedure for authorizing documentation. These data are entered into the computer system as soon as possible.

Partial Filling of C-II through C-V

Schedule III, IV, and V drugs may be partially filled if the pharmacist does not have enough in stock. The pharmacist must note on the prescription the amount filled, and the remaining amount must be dispensed within 6 months.

Schedule II drugs may be partially filled if the pharmacist does not have the full quantity in stock. The pharmacist must note on the prescription the amount filled, and the remaining amount may be dispensed within 72 hours of the first fill. If the amount cannot be filled within 72 hours, the pharmacist must notify the prescribing physician because no further quantity may be supplied after this time.

Transferring Controlled Drug Prescriptions C-II through C-V

Schedule III, IV, and V prescriptions may be transferred to another pharmacy one time only. The receiving pharmacy must have all of the information required on an original prescription, including the prescriber's DEA number, and the information must be transcribed into written form. Schedule II prescriptions are not transferrable because they can only be filled once.

Dispensing Without a Prescription

Schedule V drugs that are sold over-the-counter in some states are required to be dispensed by the pharmacist. The pharmacist must determine if the medication is necessary as well as follow the following guidelines:

1. The purchaser must be at least 18 years of age.
2. The purchaser must show identification, including proof of age.
3. No more than 240 mL or 48 solid doses of opium can be sold.
4. No more than 120 mL or 24 solid doses of any other controlled substance can be sold.
5. No more than a 48-hour supply may be sold without a prescription to any one purchaser.
6. A schedule V log book is kept with the purchaser's name and address, name and quantity of medication sold, date dispensed, and pharmacist's initials.
7. The log book must be kept for 2 years.
8. If there are no federal or state laws that require a prescription to dispense schedule V drugs, then it is permitted.

Lending or Transferring Schedule C-II through C-V Drugs to Another Pharmacy

A pharmacy may lend scheduled drugs to another pharmacy as long as the following guidelines are met:

1. The pharmacy to be lent medication is registered with the DEA to dispense controlled substances.

2. The pharmacy must record that it lent the medication and the receiving pharmacy records that it obtained the medication.
3. If a scheduled II drug is lent, it must be documented on a DEA Form 222 by the pharmacy lending the C-II drug. The form must indicate the name, dosage form, and quantity of the drug and the name, address, and DEA registration number of the pharmacy that is receiving the drug.
4. No more than 5% of the total number of dosage units of controlled substances can be dispensed by a pharmacy within a calendar year unless the pharmacy is registered as a distributor.

Mailing Controlled Substances C-II through C-V

A pharmacy is allowed to mail any controlled substance as long as it is mailed in a container that is not marked with the content's information. The inner container must be labeled to indicate the name and address of the dispensing pharmacy.

Monographs

Under the FDA labeling regulations, the following information must be available in **monographs**, also known as package inserts or official prescribing information, because of the lack of space on most drug containers. Physicians often refer to this information as published in the *Physicians' Desk Reference,* and it also is contained in free online resources such as the National Library of Medicine's DailyMed (http://dailymed.nlm.nih.gov/dailymed/about.cfm), which provides files from the FDA database. The concepts of the package labeling are also found in the monographs published in many print and online nationally recognized drug compendia (see Chapter 6). All official label information is required to give the date of the most recent revision. As new information is found or reported, new monographs are written or revised. Thus it is important to have an updated copy of the required information within the pharmacy's referencing materials. If you do not have one available, you always can read the package insert from the medication container to find the most recent information. The type of information contained in a package insert follows:

- FDA monograph information
- FDA prescription drug labeling contains a summary of the essential scientific information for the safe and effective use of the drug and should meet the following specific requirements:
  - Be informative and accurate.
  - Use language that is not promotional in tone, false, or misleading.
  - Not make claims or suggested uses for drugs when there is insufficient evidence of safety and unsubstantiated evidence of effectiveness.
  - Contain information based whenever possible on data derived from human experience.
- The information on prescription drug labeling is also referred to as:
  - Prescribing information
  - Package insert
  - Professional labeling

The Highlights section of the official prescribing information is approximately one-half page in length and provides a quick reference summary of the most important information about the prescription drug. The drug manufacturer is required to include a list of all changes made within the past year to ensure the most updated information is available for the prescriber. The Highlights of the label cover the following topics in a quick reference format and are cross-referenced to the corresponding full prescribing information section for additional details:

- Boxed Warning
- Major Recent Changes
- Indications and Usage
- Dosage and Administration
- Dosage Forms and Strengths
- Contraindications
- Warnings and Precautions
- Adverse Reactions
- Drug Interactions
- Use in Specific Populations
- Patient Counseling Information Statement

Full prescribing information now includes the following:

- Table of contents section (new change). This easy-to-use reference helps practitioners quickly locate specific information rather than having to scan the whole document
- Generic and trade names and date of initial U.S. approval
- Boxed warning section: each drug may or may not have one
- Uses bullets limited to 20 lines for ease of reading
- Complete prescribing information can be accessed using a cross-referencing number or the hyperlink given (see Boxed Warning section)

1. INDICATIONS AND USAGE

The following information may be found in this section:

- The conditions the drug is approved to treat
- Listed in bulleted form for ease of reading
- Pharmacological class of the drug (to remind prescriber about the drug's mechanism of action)
- Also all limitations are included, such as patients who should not use the drug

2. DOSAGE AND ADMINISTRATION

Presented in this section are the recommended dosage regimen, dosage range, the manner in which the medication should be administered, and pharmacological information.

3. DOSAGE FORMS AND STRENGTHS

This section lists all the dosage forms and their strengths. Product identification information, such as color and scoring, is also listed under the "How Supplied" section.

4. CONTRAINDICATIONS

This bulleted section lists clear situations in which the drug should absolutely not be used. It describes specific conditions in which the risk of taking the medication clearly outweighs any possible therapeutic benefit, as well as known hazards of the drug. The order in which contraindications are listed is based on the likelihood of occurrence and the size of the population studied.

5. WARNINGS AND PRECAUTIONS

This section is an abbreviated summary of the most clinically adverse reactions as well as actions to take when such reactions occur. Additionally, information is given on the monitoring parameters of these side effects.

6. ADVERSE REACTIONS

This section lists the most commonly occurring adverse reactions and the incidence of these effects. Separate listings are required for adverse reactions reported from clinical trials or from postmarketing experience. Additional details are given on the nature, severity, and frequency of adverse reactions, as well as the relationship to dose and demographics. This section also provides advice on how to report adverse reactions to manufacturers by using MedWatch to telephonically or electronically (or both) record reactions.

7. DRUG INTERACTIONS

Both food and drug interactions are listed as well as instructions on how to prevent or lessen the interaction. Also included in this section are conditions in which the drug interaction necessitates a dosage adjustment (also found in the "Clinical Pharmacology" section).

8. USE IN SPECIFIC POPULATIONS

This section is a bulleted summary on use of the medication in various patient populations, including the following: pregnant patients (see Pregnancy Categories section), patients in labor and delivery units, pediatric patients, geriatric patients, patients with renal impairment, and patients with hepatic impairment. Also included are cross-references to sections that can be reviewed to determine necessary prescribing adjustments.

9. DRUG ABUSE AND DEPENDENCE

If patients have shown any tendency to become addicted to the medication or if the medication has been found to be abused by patients, the information is listed in this section.

10. OVERDOSAGE

Information on toxicity and use of antidotes is provided in this section.

11. DESCRIPTION

This section lists specifics about chemical agents and ingredients, such as the drug's chemical formula.

12. CLINICAL PHARMACOLOGY

This section describes how other drugs can interact with the medication, and alerts the prescriber to adverse reactions. Also included is a "Microbiology" data subsection for the drug, if applicable. Drug interaction data may be found in section 7 (Drug Interactions) as well.

13. NONCLINICAL TOXICOLOGY

This section contains information on studies conducted during the development of the drug, including in vitro (i.e., in test tubes) studies, drug formulation, and in vivo (e.g., in live animals) efficacy studies.

14. CLINICAL STUDIES

This section summarizes the most important studies that establish the effectiveness and safety of the drug in humans. Not all studies are included.

15. REFERENCES

A list of reference materials that may be accessed for further information specific to the drug is presented in this section.

16. HOW SUPPLIED/STORAGE AND HANDLING

Information about how the medication is supplied often is given in chart format because it lists the varying strengths, amount of drug per container, dosage form, and whether the medication should be given any special considerations, such as protection from light or storage in a refrigerator.

17. PATIENT COUNSELING INFORMATION

This section contains suggested pertinent information about the drug that professionals should convey to their patients. The FDA-approved patient labeling is written for a lay audience. Even drugs given in the hospital by a health care professional may have patient counseling information.

Hyperlinks can be used to access specific information. In 2005 the FDA required structured product labeling in a standardized electronic file format and the use of embedded computer tags to help health professionals improve patient care.

The FDA and the National Library of Medicine created the DailyMed labeling resource; it can easily be downloaded and is available to professionals and patients electronically free of charge (see http://dailymed.nlm.nih.gov). Figure 2-8 is a sample of important information found within a drug monograph.

BOXED WARNING

A **boxed warning** is encased in a bold border within the manufacturer's insert; health care professionals often refer to the boxed warning as a "Black Box Warning," even though this is not the official labeling term for the warning. This type of warning is required on medications and other products that carry a high risk potential to the consumer. The label indicates the necessary proper use of a drug to avoid or decrease the possibility of serious or even life-threatening side effects. Warnings can be very specific or may include an entire class of drugs, such as antidepressants. Antidepressants have been found to cause an increase in suicidal behavior in adolescents, especially those with prior psychiatric disorders. See Box 2-8, part A, for an example of a boxed warning and Box 2-8, part B, for a sample list of agents with boxed warnings.

HIGHLIGHTS OF PRESCRIBING INFORMATION

These highlights do not include all the information needed to use Imdicon safely and effectively. See full prescribing information for Imdicon.

IMDICON

® (cholinasol) CAPSULES

Initial U.S. Approval: 2000

WARNING: LIFE-THREATENING HEMATOLOGICAL ADVERSE REACTIONS

See full prescribing information for complete boxed warning.

Monitor for hematological adverse reactions every 2 weeks for first 3 months of treatment (5.2). Discontinue Imdicon immediately if any of the following occur:

- Neutropenia/agranulocytosis (5.1)
- Thrombotic thrombocytopenic purpura (5.1)
- Aplastic anemia (5.1)

—————————————————RECENT MAJOR CHANGES—————————————————

Indications and Usage, Coronary Stenting (1.2) 2/200X
Dosage and Administration, Coronary Stenting (2.2) 2/200X

—————————————————INDICATIONS AND USAGE—————————————————

Imdicon is an adenosine diphosphate (ADP) antagonist platelet aggregation inhibitor indicated for:

- Reducing the risk of thrombotic stroke in patients who have experienced stroke precursors or who have had a completed thrombotic stroke (1.1)
- Reducing the incidence of subacute coronary stent thrombosis, when used with aspirin (1.2)
Important limitations:
- For stroke, Imdicon should be reserved for patients who are intolerant of or allergic to aspirin or who have failed aspirin therapy (1.1)

—————————————————DOSAGE AND ADMINISTRATION—————————————————

- Stroke: 50 mg once daily with food. (2.1)
- Coronary Stenting: 50 mg once daily with food, with antiplatelet doses of aspirin, for up to 30 days following stent implantation (2.2)
Discontinue in renally impaired patients if hemorrhagic or hematopoietic problems are encountered (2.3, 8.6, 12.3)

—————————————————DOSAGE FORMS AND STRENGTHS—————————————————

Capsules: 50 mg (3)

—————————————————CONTRAINDICATIONS—————————————————

- Hematopoietic disorders or a history of TTP or aplastic anemia (4)
- Hemostatic disorder or active bleeding (4)
- Severe hepatic impairment (4, 8.7)

—————————————————WARNINGS AND PRECAUTIONS—————————————————

- Neutropenia (2.4% incidence; may occur suddenly; typically resolves within 1-2 weeks of discontinuation), thrombotic thrombocytopenic purpura (TTP), aplastic anemia, agranulocytosis, pancytopenia, leukemia, and thrombocytopenia can occur (5.1)
- Monitor for hematological adverse reactions every 2 weeks through the third month of treatment (5.2)

—————————————————ADVERSE REACTIONS—————————————————

Most common adverse reactions (incidence 2%) are diarrhea, nausea, dyspepsia, rash, gastrointestinal pain, neutropenia, and purpura (6.1).

To report SUSPECTED ADVERSE REACTIONS, contact (manufacturer) at (phone # and Web address) or FDA at 1-800-FDA-1088 or *www.fda.gov/medwatch*.

—————————————————DRUG INTERACTIONS—————————————————

- Anticoagulants: Discontinue prior to switching to Imdicon (5.3, 7.1)
- Phenytoin: Elevated phenytoin levels have been reported. Monitor levels. (7.2)

—————————————————USE IN SPECIFIC POPULATIONS—————————————————

- Hepatic impairment: Dose may need adjustment. Contraindicated in severe hepatic disease (4, 8.7, 12.3)
- Renal impairment: Dose may need adjustment (2.3, 8.6, 12.3)

See 17 for PATIENT COUNSELING INFORMATION and FDA-approved patient labeling

Revised: 5/200X

FIGURE 2-8 Highlights of a drug monograph.

FULL PRESCRIBING INFORMATION: CONTENTS*

WARNING–LIFE-THREATENING HEMATOLOGICAL ADVERSE REACTIONS

1 INDICATIONS AND USAGE
  1.1 Thrombotic Stroke
  1.2 Coronary Stenting
2 DOSAGE AND ADMINISTRATION
  2.1 Thrombotic Stroke
  2.2 Coronary Stenting
  2.3 Renally Impaired Patients
3 DOSAGE FORMS AND STRENGTHS
4 CONTRAINDICATIONS
5 WARNINGS AND PRECAUTIONS
  5.1 Hematological Adverse Reactions
  5.2 Monitoring for Hematological Adverse Reactions
  5.3 Anticoagulant Drugs
  5.4 Bleeding Precautions
  5.5 Monitoring: Liver Function Tests
6 ADVERSE REACTIONS
  6.1 Clinical Studies Experience
  6.2 Postmarketing Experience
7 DRUG INTERACTIONS
  7.1 Anticoagulant Drugs
  7.2 Phenytoin
  7.3 Antipyrine and Other Drugs Metabolized Hepatically
  7.4 Aspirin and Other Non-Steroidal Anti-Inflammatory Drugs
  7.5 Cimetidine
  7.6 Theophylline
  7.7 Propranolol
  7.8 Antacids
  7.9 Digoxin
  7.10 Phenobarbital
  7.11 Other Concomitant Drug Therapy
  7.12 Food Interaction
8 USE IN SPECIFIC POPULATIONS
  8.1 Pregnancy
  8.3 Nursing Mothers
  8.4 Pediatric Use
  8.5 Geriatric Use
  8.6 Renal Impairment
  8.7 Hepatic Impairment
10 OVERDOSAGE
11 DESCRIPTION
12 CLINICAL PHARMACOLOGY
  12.1 Mechanism of Action
  12.2 Pharmacodynamics
  12.3 Pharmacokinetics
13 NONCLINICAL TOXICOLOGY
  13.1 Carcinogenesis, Mutagenesis, Impairment of Fertility
14 CLINICAL STUDIES
  14.1 Thrombotic Stroke
  14.2 Coronary Stenting
16 HOW SUPPLIED/STORAGE AND HANDLING
17 PATIENT COUNSELING INFORMATION
  17.1 Importance of Monitoring
  17.2 Bleeding
  17.3 Hematological Adverse Reactions
  17.4 FDA-Approved Patient Labeling

*Sections or subsections omitted from the full prescribing information are not listed.
http://www.fda.gov/ohrms/dockets/ac/06/briefing/2006-4210b_13_01_physician%20labeling%20rule.pdf

FIGURE 2-8, cont'd.

BOX 2-8

(A) Special Warnings and Information

Explanation of what types of serious side effects may occur

Monitoring recommendations, such as blood labs and pregnancy tests before and while using the medication; signs and symptoms that may occur during treatment

Indication of other medications that cannot be taken at the same time

Instructions to the prescriber about what information needs to be given to the patient before dosing

What steps are to be taken if a possible adverse reaction may have occurred (MedWatch: 1-800-FDA-1088).

(B) Example of Drugs Requiring Boxed Warning

Amitriptyline

Antidepressants

Bupropion

Clozapine

Estrogens

Fenoprofen

Fluoroquinolones

Nonsteroidal antiinflammatory drugs (NSAIDs)

Pioglitazone, rosiglitazone

Stavudine

Tamoxifen

Zidovudine

MEDGUIDES

MedGuides are paper handouts that are available with many prescription medicines. Many medications with boxed warnings also come with MedGuides. The guides address issues that are specific to particular drugs and drug classes, and they contain FDA-approved information that can help patients avoid serious adverse events. A MedGuide is distributed by the pharmacy with each prescription and each prescription refill, because the information for the patient may change frequently.

The FDA requires that MedGuides be issued with certain prescribed drugs and biological products when the FDA determines the following:

- Certain information is necessary to prevent serious adverse effects.
- The patient should be informed about a known serious side effect with a product.
- Patient adherence to directions for use of a product is essential to the product's effectiveness.

PREGNANCY CATEGORIES

A pregnant woman's fetus is susceptible to the effects of drugs taken by the mother. The drug may be transmitted to the fetus during its developmental stages, causing birth defects. The FDA established five **pregnancy categories** that indicate the potential of a drug to cause fetal defects; the categories are based on the ratio of risks versus benefits. These categories are set for each drug based on extensive clinical trials by the manufacturer. Both the prescriber and the pharmacist must counsel the patient to make sure the patient understands the risks involved before taking the agent. The categories are listed in Box 2-9.

BOX 2-9 PREGNANCY CATEGORIES

Category A
Adequate and well-controlled studies have failed to demonstrate a risk to the fetus in the first trimester of pregnancy (and there is no evidence of risk in later trimesters).

Category B
Animal reproduction studies have failed to demonstrate a risk to the fetus and there are no adequate and well-controlled studies in pregnant women.

Category C
Animal reproduction studies have shown an adverse effect on the fetus and there are no adequate and well-controlled studies in humans, but potential benefits may warrant use of the drug in pregnant women despite potential risks.

Category D
There is positive evidence of human fetal risk based on adverse reaction data from investigational or marketing experience or studies in humans, but potential benefits may warrant use of the drug in pregnant women despite potential risks.

Category X
Studies in animals or humans have demonstrated fetal abnormalities and/or there is positive evidence of human fetal risk based on adverse reaction data from investigational or marketing experience, and the risks involved in use of the drug in pregnant women clearly outweigh potential benefits.

Prescription Regulation

WHO CAN PRESCRIBE?

The FDA and DEA have no authority in determining prescribers. Physicians and other medical prescribers are licensed by their individual state boards. The scope of practice is determined by the person's degree. For example, a podiatrist, a physician of feet, can prescribe medications and devices that are used in treating foot conditions; a podiatrist would not and should not be prescribing heart medication. The same is true for dentists, veterinarians, and optometrists because each is an expert in a specialty and not in others. The prescribers can vary from state to state (Box 2-10); therefore the specific laws governing them are not covered. However, more states are allowing professionals such as nurse practitioners and physician assistants to prescribe a limited number of medications and/or devices. These practitioners are regulated at the state level; some are required to be supervised by a physician, who assumes responsibility for their prescribing methods and scope of knowledge. In 12 states nurse practitioners are allowed to prescribe medications independently (including controlled substances). Each state also regulates whether it will accept out-of-state prescriptions written by practitioners who are not licensed within the state. Persons who are able to prescribe controlled drugs must be registered as a midlevel practitioner with DEA Form 224.

WHO CAN RECEIVE A PRESCRIPTION?

Clearly, a pharmacy technician takes in prescriptions, enters them, and fills them; the pharmacist is responsible for interpreting and reviewing the prescription before dispensing the medication. Most states prohibit pharmacy

BOX 2-10 PRESCRIBING AUTHORITY

Except for the following footnoted prescribers, each state varies on prescriber authorization as well as specific exceptions, requirements, and limitations for prescribing medications.

Advanced practice RN
Certified RN anesthetist
Chiropractors*
Clinical RN specialist
Dentist†
Doctor of homeopathy
Doctor of osteopathy
Doctor of podiatry†
DVM (veterinarian)†
Emergency medical technician-paramedic
Licensed certified social worker (LCSW)
Medical physicians†
Midwife, nurse-midwife
Neuropathic MD
Nurse practitioner
OB/Gyn RN
Optometrist
Pediatric RN practitioners
Physicians' assistants
Psychiatric RN practitioners
Psychologists

*Have no prescribing authority in any state.
†Have independent prescribing authority limited to their specific course of practice in every state.
†Have unlimited, independent prescribing authority in every state.
For a list of specifics, refer to National Board of Pharmacy. www.nabp.net

Tech Note!

In the state of Tennessee additional functions of a certified pharmacy technician include receiving new or transferred oral medical and prescription orders; however, this is uncommon at this time and most states do not allow technicians to take verbal orders.

technicians from taking phone orders for **legend drugs**. All states require a pharmacist to authorize a phoned-in prescription for a controlled substance per DEA regulations. Often prescriptions are called in, faxed or transmitted via computer from the physician's office by the physician or nurse. A pharmacist must translate any verbal orders into written form. Also, if a patient wants a prescription transferred to another pharmacy, this must occur between licensed pharmacists or pharmacy interns under the supervision of a pharmacist. A pharmacy intern also can receive prescriptions by phone.

PRESCRIPTION LABELS

The information on a prescription label differs from what is required on a prescription order. Two necessary components for the prescription label are the pharmacy information and patient information. Samples of labels are given in Figure 2-9, *A, B*. The components that differ between orders and labels are listed as follows:

Prescriber's prescription order
1. Name of prescriber
2. Address/phone number of prescriber
3. License number of prescriber (DEA number if applicable)
4. Date prescription was written
5. Prescriber's signature

Dr. Tracy Crum
DEA#AC1243170
LIC#44550

11287 E Villanova Drive
Aurora, CO 30358
Phone: 303-555-1212

Date: *12/12/07*

Patient's name: Billie Jones   Age: *83 yrs*
Address: 125 Grand Canyon Drive, Tucson, Arizona 85707

Rx:

K-Dur 20 mEq tab
1 daily   #90

Substitution permitted Ⓨ N
Refills 1 2 3 4 5 ⑥ 7 8 9   Signature____Tracy L Crum, MD

A

Thomas Pharmacy
519 Barney Lane
Clarksville, TN 03542
Phone: 931-555-1122

Patient: Christopher Gilbert
RX # G03011984

Dosage: Clonazepam 1mg tablets   Quantity #30

Take 1 tablet by mouth at bedtime

Refills 0
Filled: 12/12/10   Expiration date: 09/25/12
Dr. Ronald Belham

B

FIGURE 2-9 **A,** Sample of information necessary on a physician's prescription order. **B,** Sample of information on a medication label.

Medication label
 1. Name of pharmacy
 2. Address and phone number of pharmacy
 3. Name of prescriber
 4. Date prescription was filled
 5. Prescription number
 6. Any cautions described or provided on auxiliary labels

Special Labeling
Certain drugs require that additional manufacturer-provided information be given to a patient because of the possibility of adverse effects from the medication; interactions between food, drugs, and/or supplements; and teratogenicity (genetic harm) to an unborn fetus. These instructions are known as patient package inserts and are distributed by the prescriber or the pharmacy dispensing the medication and/or device (Box 2-11).

RECORDS AND LABELING REQUIREMENTS

Hospitals and community pharmacies differ in the length of time that patient records are to be kept. Record keeping is regulated by state law. Both hospitals

BOX 2-11 DRUGS REQUIRING ADDITIONAL INFORMATION

- Estrogens
- Injectable contraceptives
- Intrauterine devices
- Oral contraceptives
- Progestational drugs
- Retinoids

TABLE 2-5 Required Prescription Information*

Type of Facility	Patient's Full Name	Prescriber's Name	Name and Strength of Drug	Date of Issue	Prescription Number	Expiration Date	Lot and Control Number of Drug	Manufacturer	Name of Drug Dispensed
Hospital	X	X	X	X	—†	X	—†	—†	X
Community	X	X	X	X	X	X	X	X	X
Home health	X	X	X	X	X	X	X	X	X

*Each medication sent to the floor has manufacturer name, lot number, and expiration date on each unit dose medication. Hospital patients are not given prescription numbers; instead, orders are listed in the computer under their medical record number, and a hard copy, often called the medication administration record (MAR), is made daily of all medications for the patient's chart.
†These areas represent information not transcribed onto the patient's computer record.

and community pharmacies are required to keep complete and accurate records of patients. For the purpose of simplicity, Table 2-5 lists community patient information separately from institutional requirements.

REPACKAGING

Unit dose medication that is prepared in the pharmacy requires the following record-keeping rules. Technicians traditionally prepare most of the unit dose medications in a pharmacy setting; the pharmacist verifies the preparations (except in states that allow tech-check-tech). Any medication taken from bulk packages and placed into blister packs or unit-dosing devices (e.g., oral syringes) must have the following information on each individual label:

1. Drug name (trade/generic)
2. Strength
3. Dosage form
4. Manufacturer
5. Lot number
6. Expiration date

All information must be logged into a binder or a system in which such information can be retrieved easily. For more information on repackaging, refer to Chapter 11.

DRUG ENFORCEMENT ADMINISTRATION VERIFICATION

All prescribers must be registered with the DEA to write prescriptions for controlled substances. When approved, the prescribers are given a nine-character

BOX 2-12 DRUG ENFORCEMENT ADMINISTRATION VERIFICATION PROCESS OF PRESCRIBER'S DEA NUMBER

Dr. Tom Johnston writes an order for Tylenol #3. The physician's DEA number is AJ1234892.

To verify physician's DEA number:

Step 1: Make sure the first letter is either A, B, F, or M (for nurse practitioners).

Step 2: The second letter must be the first letter of the prescriber's last name (in this case, J for Johnston).

Step 3: Add the first, third, and fifth numbers in the DEA set (1 + 3 + 8 = 12).

Step 4: Add the second, fourth, and sixth numbers and then multiply by 2 (2 + 4 + 9 = 15; 15 × 2 = 30).

Step 5: Add the two sums together (12 + 30 = 42).

Step 6: The last digit from your total (i.e., 2) must match the last number in the DEA set. In this case all steps match; therefore the number is good.

TABLE 2-6 Prescription Drugs That Can Be Packaged in Non–Child-Resistant Bottles

Drug	Dosage Form	Restriction on Strength of Drug
Betamethasone	Tablet	X
Cholestyramine	Powder	X
Colestipol	Powder	X
Erythromycin (EES)	Tablet, granules	X
Isosorbide dinitrate (less than 10 mg)	Sublingual, chewable tablets	X
Mebendazole	Tablet	X
Methylprednisolone	Tablet	X
Nitroglycerin*	Sublingual	
Prednisone	Tablet	X
Sodium fluoride	Package	X

*Nitroglycerin is the only medication that does not have a strength limit on filling it without a childproof cap.

Tech Alert!

Hospital physicians are assigned an internal code number that is attached to their DEA registration number. This information must be kept by the institution for verification purposes; for example: AB1234567-045.

identification code. This code is different for each prescriber. There is a method of verifying DEA numbers. The first two characters are composed of letters. The first letter is an A, B, F, M, or X followed by the first letter of the prescriber's last name. Prescribers who are qualified to order medications to treat opioid addiction are assigned an X. The letter M is assigned to mid-level practitioners (MLPs) such as a nurse practitioner. For example, for Dr. D. Wong, MD, the DEA number could begin with AW or BW. The next seven digits are composed of numbers that are added together. Following the six steps laid out in Box 2-12, one can verify a DEA number.

NON–CHILD-RESISTANT CAPS

Most medications are required to be packaged in containers that are exceptionally hard for children to open. Hence, childproof caps were created. Unfortunately, the caps can be difficult for some adults to open as well. Therefore some exceptions to this regulation were made because of the necessity for patients to access their medications easily (Table 2-6). In addition to these exceptions, medications can be packaged in non–child-resistant containers if certain requirements have been met. Either the prescriber, such as a physician, will order the medication to be filled without a childproof cap, or the patient will request that the medication be filled without a childproof cap. Usually this information will be entered into the patient's medical record for future reference. Some pharmacies may require the patient to sign a release form that is kept in the patient record.

Special Prescribing Programs

PROGRAMS FOR OPIOID MAINTENANCE

Methadone Maintenance Treatment (MMT)

Methadone is a schedule II controlled substance and is used to treat persons addicted to opiates. Patients are to receive specialized treatment while taking this medication. No more than 1 day's supply may be filled by a pharmacy and the medication must be taken in a physician's office or drug treatment center. Other brand names for methadone include Dolophine and Methadose. Although methadone is more commonly used for treatment of opioid addiction, it can also be prescribed by physicians (with appropriate DEA registration) as an analgesic to treat chronic pain and to alleviate pain in cancer patients.

Suboxone and Subutex

These two agents are both sublingual tablets, schedule III controlled substances that require special consent forms to be completed by the patient. While most treatments are supervised either in a physician's office or in a clinical setting, a pharmacy may receive orders for small amounts to be delivered to a physician's office or to be picked up by a family member of the patient. Under federal law prescribers must meet certain criteria. When all conditions are met the DEA issues a special number with an X identifying them as qualified prescribers (see www.deadiversion.usdoj.gov/drugreg/reg_apps/new_reg_number110906.htm).

RISK MANAGEMENT PROGRAMS FOR PRESCRIPTION DRUGS

iPledge Program under the FDA

The FDA regulates isotretinoin (Accutane, Amnesteem, Claravis, Sotret) under a special program because of the severe adverse effects of the drug. It causes birth defects; therefore it is important that the user understands that she cannot become pregnant. In addition, possible side effects of suicidal thoughts and signs of depression are now being associated with this drug. This agent requires a boxed warning.

Tech Alert!

The special programs listed are not inclusive; there are others. These are examples of the three most common programs found in either hospital or retail settings.

Pharmacy Sites

BRICK AND MORTAR AND MAIL-ORDER PHARMACIES

The term brick and mortar refers to a building such as a retail pharmacy. A common practice is to mail medications through the post office or other authorized mailing system. This option will always be available for patients since the introduction of online pharmacies and mail-order pharmacies. Rules govern the way in which drugs are mailed. When drugs are sent to the patient's home, they must be unmarked on the outside (that is, the contents should not be listed). The mailing requirements between pharmacies and the manufacturer are different. In this case, all medications and even controlled substances are allowed to be mailed as long as the recipient (pharmacy) is registered with the DEA.

ONLINE PHARMACIES (E-PHARMACY)

In the 1990s E-pharmacies began to appear on the Internet, which led to the opportunity for drugs to be illegally ordered as well as for consumers to be defrauded, when E-pharmacies charged credit cards but did not mail the drugs ordered. The National Association of Boards of Pharmacies (NABP) began to accredit sites in 1999 to allow consumers to discern between legal and illegal sites. VIPPS (Verified Internet Pharmacy Practice Sites) is a label that indicates to the public that the website from which they are ordering drugs is both legitimate and licensed (obtain more information at www.nabp.net/verify). When linking onto a pharmacy Internet site the customer should click into the label for authentication. At this time the VIPPS is a voluntary accreditation. Although verification is done by the NABP, they do not regulate the sites; instead, the websites are regulated by the state in which the pharmacy is physically located along with federal guidelines. E-pharmacies have the same regulations as both retail and mail-order pharmacies with regard to dispensing to out-of-state pharmacy locations, and they are also required to adhere to HIPAA regulations. There are many advantages to ordering medications via the web, including ease of ordering, lower prices, and easy accessibility to online information, which lessens wait time when trying to ask a pharmacist for information. In retrospect, illegal pharmacies are a constant struggle for both state and federal agencies. If a suspicious E-pharmacy is found, it should be reported to the NABP. If the wrong medication or label is dispensed then it should be reported to the state's board of pharmacy.

Signs of a probable *illegal* pharmacy site include:

- Dispensing medications without having the customer mail in the prescription
- Faxing a prescription that cannot be confirmed as a valid prescription
- Dispensing medications upon completion of a questionnaire
- Not having a preexisting exam or patient-prescriber relationship
- Being unable to contact a pharmacist at the website for consultation

Occupational Safety and Health Administration

The purpose of the **Occupational Safety and Health Administration (OSHA)** is to make the workplace safe for employees (for an outline of common safety and health topics, see Box 2-13). A safe workplace includes having safe equipment and materials, being able to safely perform tasks, and ensuring that policies and procedures are safe within a company, including pharmacy. In 1986

BOX 2-13 COMMON SAFETY AND HEALTH TOPICS

- Hazard Communication Standards
- Hazardous Drugs During Preparation
- Hazardous Drugs During Storage
- Hazardous Drugs During Administration
- Hazardous Drugs During Care Giving
- Handling Practices
- Disposal of Hazardous Drugs
- Latex Allergy
- Ergonomics
- Workplace Violence

OSHA began requiring **material safety data sheet** (MSDS) information on all potentially dangerous chemicals used in the workplace.

MATERIAL SAFETY DATA SHEETS (MSDS)

Almost all chemicals can be dangerous if either ingested or spilled. In all workplaces, including pharmacy, all chemicals must have an MSDS on file in an MSDS binder, or available electronically through a database. The binders are normally bright yellow and black. The type of information contained on these sheets includes the storage requirements, handling procedures, and actions to take if the chemical is either spilled or sprayed into the eyes or comes into contact with the skin. It is important to know where the binder or database is kept and that every chemical has a sheet on file. For example, phenol is a very dangerous antiseptic agent often used in nerve blocks; it is stored in many institutional pharmacies. If spilled, it is important not to breathe in the fumes but to contain the spill as quickly as possible and call the appropriate department for clean-up. Normally environmental services in a hospital will respond and handle the clean-up. It is extremely easy to get MSDS information to protect the employees who will handle the agent. The phone number is always given by the manufacturer and they are required by law to distribute the information to the requesting party within 24 hours. This is normally accomplished by the manufacturer faxing the MSDS directly to the business. For more information, go to www.osha.gov. The MSDS information not only is important but also is required by law.

The Joint Commission

The **Joint Commission** was first created in 1910; its original mission was to improve the safety and quality of care via accreditation of health care organizations. To this day their mission remains the same. The Joint Commission sets standards of care for patients to ensure their treatment while in a hospital. In 1951 several medical associations created the Joint Commission on Accreditation of Healthcare Organizations (JCAHO) as an independent, nonprofit organization that voluntarily accredited hospitals. In 1959 Canada withdrew from JCAHO to form its own accrediting organization. It was not until 1964 that JCAHO began to charge for its surveys. The following year hospitals were required to be accredited in order to participate in the Medicare and Medicaid programs. Over the following years JCAHO expanded its range of compliances over hospitals and institutions. For many years this organization was known as JCAHO but in 2007 it changed its identity to The Joint Commission (TJC). The Joint Commission meets 3 times annually and has 29 board members, consisting of physicians, administrators, nurses, employers, a labor representative, health plan leaders, quality experts, ethicists, educators, and a consumer advocate. They accredit more than 16,000 health care organizations and programs throughout the United States. Organizations must be surveyed at least every 3 years. Once accredited the organization may display the seal of approval; ratings of all institutions can be found on the website for TJC (www.jointcommission.org). The benefits of accreditation and certification include the following:

- Provides the community with confidence in the quality and safety of care, treatment, and other institutional services
- Identifies and addresses risk management and reduction
- Provides professional advice and staff education to improve services
- Recognized by many health care insurers and other third parties (Medicare and Medicaid)
- Meets regulatory requirements in specific states

The Joint Commission surveys all aspects of hospital services including pharmacy. Areas of concern within pharmacy include how look-a-like, sound-a-like drugs are identified; communication, allergy notification, conflicting prescriptions, verbal orders, and other areas that may create an avenue for errors are addressed. When the pharmacy is visited by The Joint Commission all employees should be very aware of their policies and procedures within the pharmacy department if asked. If you do not know the answer to any question given by The Joint Commission, give an honest answer; do not try to make up an answer. They may collect pharmacy data in order to monitor its performance, identify adverse drug reactions, and determine how the pharmacy identifies and has attempted to improve problems in these areas. In 2004 TJC created the "do not use" list of abbreviations (see Chapter 5) as a requirement. This requirement has met with resistance because surveys reveal that as of 2006, 22% of accredited organizations were still noncompliant with their standards.

Legal Standards

STATE LAWS

Each state has its own set of laws that pharmacists, interns, pharmacy technicians, and clerks must follow when working in the pharmacy. You must know the regulations of your state. All pharmacy personnel should become familiar with the laws by obtaining the regulations' booklet from their state Board of Pharmacy. You will notice that many states have laws that differ from federal law. Remember that the strictest law is the one you follow. Therefore if the FDA states that you must keep records for no less than 2 years but your state regulations require 7 years for inpatient records, then you would follow the strictest regulation, in this case your state regulation. To learn more about your specific state regulations and laws, go to your state's Board of Pharmacy (BOP) website, which can be found at www.napb.net.

LIABILITIES

You also should be aware of federal and state liability laws pertaining to pharmacy technicians. A patient can make various charges against a pharmacy technician if the pharmacy technician caused damage because of **negligence** or intentional action in the workplace. A **tort** is defined as causing injury to a person intentionally or because of negligence. The word negligence may describe an action taken without the forethought that should have been taken by a reasonable person of similar competency; a mistake was made. For an intentional mistake, the penalty can range from criminal charges to the awarding of damages, which usually means that money is paid to the person or persons who were wrongly affected. A negligent mistake can affect a person's ability to continue to work as a technician and also may result in punitive damages (i.e., monetary payment).

Mistakes occur for many reasons. Some are because of excessive workload or possibly staffing shortages that can lead to a mishap and could be classified as a negligent tort. Criminal behavior, such as false insurance claims or diverting drugs, could be called an intentional tort and could result in imprisonment. One of the questions you should ask your employer is whether you are covered under the company's legal department. If a lawsuit were to be filed with you as the plaintiff, do you know who would represent you? Many companies have lawyers that represent the company, although you should not assume that they would represent you. If you are not covered by your employer, you may want to purchase malpractice insurance. Most technicians do not have such insurance, and it is a personal preference. At the very least, be aware of what your rights and responsibilities are, including legal considerations, before entering a workplace. Depending on the state in which the technician works, laws vary as they pertain to the liability of the technician. Therefore you must check your state laws as they pertain to you. If you are involved in or witness any incidents in the workplace, you should follow these guidelines:

1. Review your state's regulations.
2. Understand your employer's rules and practices.
3. Define your scope of employment.

If an "event" occurs in the pharmacy, you should be prepared in the following ways:

1. Know the name of your attorney.
2. Always be careful of what you say and to whom you say it if you are ever questioned by state or federal investigators pertaining to an incident.
3. Write down in-depth notes on the facts of the event (as soon as possible) and keep them for reference.

PHARMACY EMPLOYEE REQUIREMENTS: REQUEST FOR WAIVER

Under the restrictions of the DEA, a pharmacy registrant cannot employ a person to handle or have access to any controlled substances if the person has been convicted of a felony related to scheduled drugs or if the person's DEA application for registration has been revoked, surrendered, or denied. However, if a pharmacy wants to hire such a person, they must apply for a waiver through the DEA. Certain factors will be considered when deciding to grant such a waiver (see www.deadiversion.usdoj.gov:80/pubs/manuals/pharm2/pharm_content.htm), including the following:

1. A detailed description of the nature and extent of the applicant's past controlled substances' violations
2. Activities of the applicant since the violation
3. Current status of the applicant's state licensure
4. Extent of applicant's proposed access to controlled substances
5. Registrant's proposed physical and professional safeguards to prevent diversion by the applicant if employed
6. Status of employing registrant regarding handling of controlled substances
7. Other pertinent information uncovered by the DEA in its investigation of the applicant's or registrant's handling of controlled substances

Such a waiver should not be considered unless there are valid reasons to believe that diversion is unlikely to occur.

Both federal and state laws change frequently; therefore it is your responsibility to keep up with the current regulations in place. Pharmacy departments keep close track of these changes and will notify employees of changes, but it is you who carries out these laws on a daily basis. Be acquainted with the specifics of a new rule or regulation and obtain clarification if necessary, because not understanding a new rule or regulation and not seeking further guidance are unacceptable excuses. Because pharmacy technicians can be held accountable for their actions, this is a fundamental competency of all pharmacy technicians. In addition, the PTCB does require at least 1 continuing education (CE) unit to be taken in current law for recertification within a 2-year period.

Tech Alert!

More states are enacting laws to make technicians accountable for their actions in the pharmacy. Previously, pharmacists would have to take the responsibility for any mistakes, even if the mistake was caused by the technician. This is not true any longer; A technician can lose his or her license, certification, and job and may have to pay court fees. Of course, this is in addition to the possibility of having to spend time in jail, depending on the severity of the crime. Such cases are listed in pharmacy journals and on the FDA website.

DO YOU REMEMBER THESE KEY POINTS?

- Terms and definitions covered in this chapter
- Major federal laws affecting pharmacists and pharmacy
- The differences between functions of the DEA and FDA
- Filing systems required for stock and controlled substances' inventory
- Filing requirements for patients' information
- Who can write a prescription
- The legal limitations of pharmacy technicians
- Labeling requirements for repackaged medications
- How to decipher a DEA number
- Regulations and authentication of E-pharmacies
- The segments of an NDC number
- MSDS guidelines
- Drug recalls and how to handle them
- The functions and authority of your state's Board of Pharmacy
- OSHA guidelines
- Which medications require package inserts when dispensed

REVIEW QUESTIONS

Multiple choice questions

1. The amendment that required the labeling "Caution: Federal law prohibits dispensing without a prescription" was the:
   A. Durham-Humphrey Amendment
   B. Kefauver-Harris Amendments
   C. OBRA '90
   D. None of the above

2. What is the purpose of the Orphan Drug Act?
   A. Enacts stricter rules concerning sales and distribution of controlled substances.
   B. Allows drug companies to bypass lengthy testing to treat persons who have a rare disease.
   C. Stops the use of drug testing in animals.
   D. Ensures safety and effectiveness of manufacturing practices.

3. The law that requires pharmacists to counsel patients on new medications is:
   A. OBRA '90
   B. Comprehensive Drug Abuse Prevention and Control Act
   C. Prescription Drug Marketing Act
   D. Durham-Humphrey Amendment

4. The main purpose of the FDA is to:
   A. Make arrests
   B. Ensure the safety and effectiveness of medications are met by manufacturers
   C. Prevent the distribution and illegal use of controlled substances
   D. Make sure all laws pertaining to physicians and pharmacists are met

5. A pharmacy that will be dispensing controlled drugs must have which one of the following forms on file with the DEA?
   A. Form 222
   B. Form 224
   C. Form 363
   D. Form 225

6. All adverse reactions should be reported to the:
   A. FDA
   B. DEA
   C. CIA
   D. Pharmacy management

7. The five categories of controlled substances are rated on the basis of:
   A. Cost
   B. Strength
   C. Conditions that they treat
   D. Potential for abuse

8. Of the information contained in a monograph of a medication, which of the following sections would have information related to the mechanism of action of the drug?
   A. Description
   B. Clinical Pharmacology
   C. Adverse Reactions
   D. Indications and Usage

9. Which of the following health care providers is NOT one of the standard practitioners that all states accept?
   A. Doctor of podiatry
   B. Dentists
   C. Chiropractors
   D. Veterinarians

10. Which of the components listed is NOT required on a prescription label?
    A. Name, address, and phone number of the pharmacy
    B. Name, address, and phone number of the prescriber
    C. Date prescription was filled
    D. Any auxiliary stickers and/or warnings

11. MSDS contain information on:
    A. Storage of a chemical
    B. Actions to take in case of a spill
    C. The combustion and stability of a chemical
    D. All of the above

12. Drug diversion is:
    A. Intentionally misusing a drug intended for medical purposes
    B. Taking a drug at the wrong time or in the wrong amount
    C. Transporting drugs
    D. Using illicit drugs for illicit purposes

13. All of the following letters are used for the beginning of a DEA number EXCEPT:
    A. C
    B. F
    C. M
    D. Both A and B

14. Common methods of drug diversion include all of the following EXCEPT:
    A. Shoplifting
    B. Smurfing
    C. Shop-shifting
    D. Shelf-sweeping

15. The three sections of an NDC number include:
    A. The manufacturer, expiration date, and storage requirements
    B. The manufacturer or distributor; the remaining two sections are developed by the manufacturer and indicate package information
    C. The manufacturer or distributor; the remaining two sections are developed by the FDA and indicate the drug's effectiveness and dosage form and strength
    D. None of the above

True/False

If a statement is false, then change it to make it true.

_____ **1.** Only a physician with an FDA number may write a prescription for Suboxone or Subutex.

_____ **2.** DEA Form 222 is used to obtain controlled substances from the manufacturer or distributor.

_____ **3.** Drugs such as LSD and heroin are C-I medications prescribed by physicians on rare occasions.

_____ **4.** Monographs can be found with the drug and may be published in the *Physicians' Desk Reference*.

_____ **5.** The Contraindications section of the monograph explains the abuse and dependence dangers of the medication.

_____ **6.** Physicians should order only medications within their scope of practice.

_____ **7.** Pharmacy technicians can take oral prescriptions as long as there is a pharmacist on duty who gives permission for them to do so.

_____ **8.** Only pharmacists can fill out Form 222 required by the DEA; it should be completed in pencil.

_____ **9.** Isosorbide and nitroglycerin can be dispensed without childproof caps.

_____ **10.** A recall that is classified as Class 1 means that it is the lowest level of a recall and is used for products that contain only a minor defect.

_____ **11.** E-pharmacies and mail-order pharmacies are not covered under the same DEA regulations as traditional pharmacies.

_____ **12.** Pharmacy technicians are required to know FDA laws and regulations that pertain to the pharmacy.

_____ **13.** Pharmacists are solely responsible for all mistakes made by the technicians on duty under their supervision.

_____ **14.** Only estrogens and oral contraceptives require a patient package insert with every order filled.

_____ **15.** C-II and C-III drugs are equally addictive under the DEA's definition.

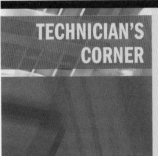

TECHNICIAN'S CORNER

Dr. Beth Golden writes an order for the following prescription:

DEA#BG1958366
Disp: hydrocodone/acetaminophen tablets #50
Sig: Take 1 tablet q8h prn severe pain
10 refills

Determine whether this DEA number is correct, and explain each step of the checking process.
List how many mistakes, if any, you find on all parts of this order.

BIBLIOGRAPHY

Ballington DA: *Pharmacy practice for technicians*, ed 2, St Paul, Minn, 2002, EMC/Paradigm.

Gray Morris D: *Calculate with confidence*, ed 5, St Louis, 2009, Elsevier.

National Association of Boards of Pharmacy: *Survey of pharmacy law*, Mount Prospect, Ill, 2005, The Association.

Nielsen JR, James JD: *Handbook of federal drug law*, ed 2, Philadelphia, 1992, Williams & Wilkins.

Potter PA, Perry AG: *Fundamentals of nursing*, ed 7, St Louis, 2008, Elsevier.

Shargel L, Mutnick A, Souney P, et al: *Comprehensive pharmacy review*, ed 5, Baltimore, 2003, Lippincott Williams & Wilkins.

REFERENCED WEBSITES

American Family Physician. April 1, 2005. Methadone use. (Referenced 3/13/09) www.aafp.org/afp/20050401/1353.html

Encyclopedia of Surgery. Barbiturates. (Referenced 4/8/09) www.surgeryencyclopedia.com/A-Ce/Barbiturates.html

FDA website. National Drug Code Directory. Last updated: 8/17/09) (Referenced 8/21/09). www.fda.gov/Drugs/InformationOnDrugs/ucm142438.htm

FDA website. New Requirements for Prescribing Information. (Referenced 8/23/09). www.fda.gov/Drugs/GuidanceComplianceRegulatoryInformation/LawsActsandRules/ucm084159.htm

FDA website. Recall Firm Press Release. (Referenced 8/20/09). www.fda.gov/Safety/Recalls/ucm179943.htm

Gieringer D: The Safety and Efficacy of New Drug Approval. Page 201. (Referenced 8/9/09). www.cato.org/pubs/journal/cj5n1/cj5n1-10.pdf

Life Science Services. Outsourcing-Pharm.com. Pseudoephedrine drugs still OTC. (Referenced 8/21/09) www.outsourcing-pharma.com/Contract-Manufacturing/Pseudoephedrine-drugs-still-OTC

OTC-Meds.com. Home: Controlled Substances Act: Federal Regulation of Pseudoephedrine. (Referenced 8/23/09) www.otcmeds.com/Controlled_Substances_Act::Federal_regulation_of_pseudoephedrine/encyclopedia.htm

Safety Emporium: Sample MSDS for Benzoic Acid. (Referenced 8/19/09). http://www.ilpi.com/msds/benzoic.html

USP information. (Referenced 7/13/09) www.usp.org/aboutUSP/

USP_NF website. (Referenced 6/2/09) www.usp.org/USPNF/

WHO Pain & Palliative Care Communications Program: Expanding nurses' role in pain management: International news on nurse prescribing. (Referenced 8/16/09). http://whocancerpain.wisc.edu/?q=node/180

3

Pharmacy Ethics, Competencies, Associations, and Settings for Technicians

Objectives

UPON COMPLETING THIS CHAPTER, YOU SHOULD BE ABLE TO DO THE FOLLOWING:

- Discuss historical data on technicians.

- Describe the competencies involved in the pharmacy setting.

- Explain the term *nondiscretionary duties*.

- Explore various settings for technicians.

- Describe various pharmacy setting requirements as they apply to technicians.

- Describe how pharmacy has expanded onto the Internet.

- List the new position openings for technicians that are available in the health care field.

- Explain how networking is important in the search for a pharmacy position.

- List the associations available to technicians.

- Determine which attributes each pharmacy association has that are important to the technician.

- Describe the various national certification examinations and their requirements.
- Determine the ways to approach job searching.
- Explain how the Internet can be used for research and information pertaining to pharmacy.
- List ways in which the PTCB national exam differs from the ICPT national exam.
- Differentiate between licensing, registration, and certification.
- State the pharmacy code of ethics.
- Explore the various websites that can be used to attain continuing education credits.

TERMS AND DEFINITIONS

American Association of Pharmacy Technicians (AAPT) *First pharmacy technician association; founded in 1979*

American Pharmacists Association (APhA) *Oldest pharmacy association; founded in 1852*

American Society of Health-System Pharmacists (ASHP) *Pharmacy association founded in 1942*

Board of Pharmacy (BOP) *State-managed agency that licenses pharmacists and may either register or license pharmacy technicians to work in pharmacy*

Certified pharmacy technician *A technician who has passed the national certification examination; the technician can use the abbreviation CPhT after his or her name*

Closed door pharmacy *A pharmacy where medications are called in from institutions such as long-term care facilities and are then delivered; closed door pharmacies are not open to the public*

Communication *The ability to express oneself in such a way that one is readily and clearly understood*

Competency *The capability or proficiency to perform a function*

Confidentiality *The practice of keeping privileged customer information from being disclosed without the customer's consent*

Continuing education (CE) *Education beyond the basic technical education, usually required for license or certification renewal*

Ethics *The values and morals that are used within a profession*

Hyperalimentation *Parenteral (intravenous) nutrition for patients who are unable to eat solids or liquids*

Inpatient pharmacy *A pharmacy in a hospital or institutional setting*

Institute for the Certification of Pharmacy Technicians (ICPT) *National board for the certification of pharmacy technicians*

Licensed pharmacy technician *A pharmacy technician who is licensed by the state board; licensing ensures that an individual has at least the minimum degree of competency required by the profession, unlike a registered pharmacy technician*

Morals *Ethics; honorable beliefs*

National Association of Boards of Pharmacy (NABP) *National organization for members of state boards of pharmacy*

National Pharmacy Technician Association (NPTA) *Pharmacy association primarily for technicians; founded in 1999*

Outpatient pharmacies *Pharmacies that serve patients in their communities; pharmacies that are not in inpatient facilities*

Parenteral medications *Most commonly used to describe medications administered by injection, such as intravenously or intramuscularly*

Pharmacy Technician Certification Board (PTCB) *National board for the certification of pharmacy technicians*

Professionalism *Conforming to the right principles of conduct (work ethics) as accepted by others in the profession*

Protocol *A standard that is to be met by all employees; governs specific duties*

Registered pharmacy technician *A pharmacy technician who is registered through the state board of pharmacy; registration process helps maintain list of those working in pharmacy and usually requires a background check through the legal system; registration process does not guarantee degree of registrant's knowledge or skills*

Introduction

Because of the rapidly changing health care system, job descriptions and educational requirements of pharmacy technicians are quickly changing. Among the changes are increased responsibilities, the need for higher education, more legal responsibility, and even continuing education. This trend can be seen across the United States as more states require a high school diploma or general equivalency diploma in order for a person to become a registered technician, and more states have accepted certification as their measure of the knowledge base of pharmacy technicians. Positive aspects of these changes include a wider range of jobs available, bonuses, salary increases, and better benefits for technicians.

Each of America's 50 states has not standardized the qualifications and job descriptions for the pharmacy technician. This is also true for pharmacists because each state has different laws to which pharmacists must adhere, although the laws do not vary as much as the requirements for technicians. Therefore each state board of pharmacy determines what standards will be required and how they must be met by technicians. This one area of discrepancy is an issue that will become more defined through the continuing efforts of the boards of pharmacy over the next decade.

This chapter begins with a brief overview of the history of pharmacy, and then explores each area in the health care field pertaining to pharmacy such as communication, ethics, and morals. Necessary job qualifications, expectations, and trends in pharmacy are also explored along with the importance of national pharmacy organizations and the benefits of pharmacy technician certification. This chapter also provides information about the preparation necessary before conducting a job search as well as the possible future roles of the pharmacy technician. This will help the student technician determine the best path to follow, understand the various positions that are available, and attain the ultimate goals and benefits of this profession.

Historical Data

Historically, technicians have answered to a variety of titles. These include pharmacy clerk, pharmacist assistant, or pharmacy aide. Technicians have held a variety of positions. Some of the job responsibilities have been billing, ordering, stocking medications, typing, answering the phone, greeting customers, trouble-shooting, cashiering, and running errands. Technicians have been a part of the pharmacy field since the beginning of pharmacy (see Chapter 1). However, more recently, pharmacy managers and their respective state boards of pharmacy have been attempting to classify and clearly define the role of the pharmacy technician as the needs of pharmacy change. Pharmacists' duties have been changing from filling prescriptions and compounding simple agents to counseling patients and interacting with other medical professionals such as physicians and nurses. This change can especially be seen in the hospital setting, where pharmacists are responsible for managing dosing of medications and participating on committees. The change in responsibility has been addressed many times over the course of pharmacy technician history (see Chapter 1) by the **American Society of Health-System Pharmacists (ASHP),** the **American Pharmacists Association** (APhA), and other pharmacy associations. This expanding career field will make many more changes in the future because the scope of pharmacy technicians is increasing. The need for skilled personnel has never been greater.

In 2002 the *American Journal of Health-System Pharmacists* addressed many of the challenges pharmacy faces by publishing the *White paper on pharmacy technicians 2002: needed changes can no longer wait.* A white paper argues a specific position or solution to a problem. The paper explores the diversity of pharmacy technician qualifications, knowledge, and responsibilities (see Box 3-1). The white paper was endorsed by a panel of pharmacy organizations and comprehensively discussed issues pertinent to the promotion and growth of a competent pharmacy technician workforce.

Competencies

Because of the varying types of settings in which technicians may work, technicians have many different duties as well. Box 3-2 references chapters that cover common responsibilities and **competencies** necessary to function in various settings. To fulfill the duties of a technician, one must become competent in those areas. The competencies are outlined in this chapter. Although certain areas of pharmacy require direct technician-patient contact, others do not. However, the technician converses with co-workers and other health care workers daily under various circumstances. Because of this, the technician must exercise competencies and communication skills daily.

CURRENT QUALIFICATIONS

Each state in the United States has its own **board of pharmacy (BOP)** that is overseen by the **National Association of Boards of Pharmacy (NABP).**

BOX 3-1 WHITE PAPER ON PHARMACY TECHNICIANS 2002

1. Education and training: Encompasses the history of training techniques and programs. Explores the need for adjusting the length of the training program based on the functions of the technician. Course curriculum adjustments and adequacy are discussed.
2. Accreditation of training programs and institutions: Describes the types of training programs and the need for institutional accreditation. Explains why it is important to oversee these programs because there are no nationally recognized ones.
3. Certification: Covers the history and growth of the national certification process; describes the importance of certification, both for the establishment of minimum levels of competency and for the recognition of pharmacy technicians as para-professionals.

BOX 3-2 CHAPTER REFERENCES CITING COMMON RESPONSIBILITIES AND COMPETENCIES OF A PHARMACY TECHNICIAN

Pharmacy Federal Laws and Regulations	Chapter 2
Conversions and Calculations Used by Pharmacy Technicians	Chapter 4
Dosage Forms, Routes of Administration, Drug Classifications, Drug Abbreviations & Medical Terminology	Chapter 5
Drug Information References	Chapter 6
Prescription Processing	Chapter 7
Hospital Pharmacy	Chapter 10
Repackaging and Compounding	Chapter 11
Aseptic Technique	Chapter 12
Pharmacy Stock and Billing	Chapter 13
Medication Safety and Error Prevention	Chapter 14

Each state's BOP serves many functions besides registering technicians and licensing pharmacists. The board also provides consumers with a way to file a complaint or report any problems or illegal actions they have experienced in a pharmacy. BOPs also review and update current rules and regulations pertaining to pharmacy practice. When new standards are implemented BOP inspectors may visit any pharmacy to determine its compliance with these new standards. If the pharmacy is found guilty of noncompliance, the BOP has the authority not only to impose fines but also to close the pharmacy until compliance is attained. The National Association of Boards of Pharmacy and also state BOPs are currently studying the expanded use of technicians in the pharmacy field. For example, in 2008 technicians in California who had achieved a specific level of competency were granted the additional job duty of monitoring other pharmacy technicians. In Tennessee, technicians can take verbal physicians' orders over the phone. More states are requiring technicians to be registered, certified, and/or licensed. This examination of the current uses of technicians no doubt will reveal the skill level necessary for various types of pharmacy tasks, and ultimately changes will be made throughout each state board of pharmacy. Boards of pharmacy also may change technician-to-pharmacist ratios in pharmacy settings. Knowledge of pharmacy law is essential before working in a pharmacy environment. The basics are listed in Box 3-3 (for more examples, see Chapter 2). Federal laws govern all 50 states. In addition, each state's BOP also has specific laws, regulations, and guidelines that pertain to pharmacy practice in that state. State laws may differ from federal laws. (For more information on the legal requirements of pharmacy technicians, see Chapter 2.)

NONDISCRETIONARY DUTIES

All technicians, regardless of their title, can and do perform many types of **nondiscretionary** duties in the pharmacy setting. This means they can perform repetitive tasks that do not require any advanced pharmacy knowledge. Examples include repackaging medications, ordering stock, and billing insurance plans. All of these tasks are clearly defined and should be easy to follow. This does not mean that anyone can do the job, because prior knowledge of pharmacy terms, drugs, and procedures is required. As job classifications within pharmacy expand, so will the level of pharmacology knowledge required for pharmacy technicians. Historically, the pharmacist was responsible for the final approval of any task completed in a pharmacy setting, although this is also changing; some states now allow "tech-check-tech" approval procedures. In addition, more states are requiring extensive background checks to ensure

BOX 3-3 EXAMPLES OF FEDERAL LAWS GOVERNING PHARMACY

Prescription Records

A record of all prescriptions dispensed should be maintained for 2 years after last refill. All systems used for maintaining records of any prescriptions must include:

Prescription number
Date of issuance
Patient's identification (name, address)
Name, strength, dosage form of medication
Quantity dispensed
Practitioner's identification (DEA registration, if applicable)
Pharmacist's identification

Patient Consultation (OBRA '90)

Pharmacists must screen entire drug profile of all Medicaid recipients before their prescriptions are filled. Each patient must be given counseling on the medication that has been prescribed, including topics such as how to take the drug, storage of the drug, and side effects of the medication. Most states have passed regulations that require counseling of all patients according to the same processes, although different requirements regarding the provision of written and/or oral consultation may exist among the states.

For more information on pharmacy law, refer to Chapter 2.

technicians do not have a criminal record (see Chapter 2). Nondiscretionary duties do limit technicians from interpreting scientific studies, counseling patients about their current or adjunct medications, and conferring with other medical personnel regarding proper treatments.

BASIC NONDISCRETIONARY SKILLS

Typing

The typing speed required by most pharmacy employers is a minimum of at least 35 words per minute. A technician who has speed and a good knowledge of medications is cherished within the pharmacy setting. The number of prescriptions processed per day in a pharmacy directly relates to the speed and accuracy of the typist. This makes a fast and accurate pharmacy technician typist a greatly appreciated pharmacy asset.

Computers

One of the requirements imposed on pharmacies by the federal government is the reduction of pharmacy errors (Chapter 14). This has influenced pharmacies to use computers for dispensing medications and keeping inventory. Dispensing medication systems accurately count and dispense medications and directly have led to a decrease in the rate of errors. Although these systems increase accurate dosing, human error still occurs. Nothing replaces the knowledge of a skilled pharmacy technician to decrease error rates.

Reports and Documentation

Many pharmacies expect technicians to prepare various reports. Knowledge of computers and programs such as Microsoft Word and Excel can make a technician a valuable asset to the pharmacy. Because all pharmacies have integrated computers into their ordering, filling, and documentation procedures, technicians must be computer savvy.

Ordering Supplies

The task of ordering stock is the responsibility of a specific person within the pharmacy, although everyone should know how to order stock when necessary.

Tech Note!

In very rare cases a pharmacy technician may be given power of attorney for a pharmacy and may register or return controlled substances for the pharmacy.

Tech Note!

The bottom line when working in any area of pharmacy is the following: "Always make sure the pharmacist has checked all drugs and/or devices before they leave the pharmacy." If this step is taken, the technician is working within the scope of practice and fewer mistakes will occur.

Learning how to order stock, return expired or damaged stock, and handle recalled items are among the duties in which pharmacy technicians should be competent. This skill is normally taught on-the-job as each pharmacy has its own way of handling stock inventory. An important aspect of an inventory technician is the storage requirements of the medications that arrive in pharmacy. For more information on this topic, refer to Chapter 13.

INPATIENT SETTING REQUIREMENTS

Inpatient pharmacy usually refers to those pharmacies located in hospitals or institutions in which patients stay overnight or longer, depending on the procedures they require. Most departments in a hospital have medications and supplies that are specific to their department. These are supplied by the inpatient pharmacy. Therefore inpatient pharmacies traditionally have a wider range of stock than outpatient pharmacies so that they can provide all the necessary supplies required of each department. For example, the labor and delivery unit stocks a large amount of the drug oxytocin (induces labor), whereas the intensive care unit and coronary care unit require a wide variety of cardiac medications in their stock areas. The cancer units may stock high amounts of morphine and other analgesics, whereas the pediatrics department stocks many drugs in liquid form for children. Stocking all of these areas is just one of the responsibilities of an inpatient pharmacy technician.

Other important tasks, for example, include preparing intravenous medications and hyperalimentation products (i.e., parenteral nutrition) and performing nonsterile compounding of ointments and creams. The pharmacy loads patient medication drawers and/or automated dispensing systems that allow nurses to access medications. Various persons in the health care institution are responsible for proper documentation of controlled substances and floor stock disposition; however, the inpatient pharmacy oversees the process. For more information on hospital job descriptions and competency requirements, see Chapter 10.

In addition to knowing the various drugs, strengths, and dosage forms, the technician must be able to immediately and appropriately react when emergency (stat) orders are received by the pharmacy. The dynamics of an inpatient pharmacy can fluctuate minute to minute depending on the flow of patients into and out of the hospital. "Stat" doses are to be delivered within 15 minutes or less to the area requesting them, such as the emergency department, operating room, intensive care unit, or cardiac care unit. This duty includes preparing any intravenous solutions (Figure 3-1).

Another aspect of the inpatient pharmacy is the preparation of unit dose medications (see Chapter 11), which are widely used in many hospital settings. Medications need to be repackaged because either (1) the drug companies do not have the medication available in unit dose or (2) the hospital has chosen to prepare its own unit dose medication for cost-saving reasons.

The following are common job descriptions of inpatient technicians, along with some new responsibilities that have been incorporated in the pharmacy setting. The jobs listed do not require any additional educational training other than the training provided by each pharmacy setting. Most inpatient pharmacy technicians who are interested in the following areas in pharmacy will receive additional on-the-job training to prepare them for these additional tasks:

- Inventory technician: Orders all stock, handles billing, talks to drug representatives, and may be responsible for ordering lowest-cost items.
- Robot filler: Many pharmacies are installing robots to fill patient medication drawers each day. Technicians must be trained to load these million-dollar mechanical robots and to keep them running smoothly.

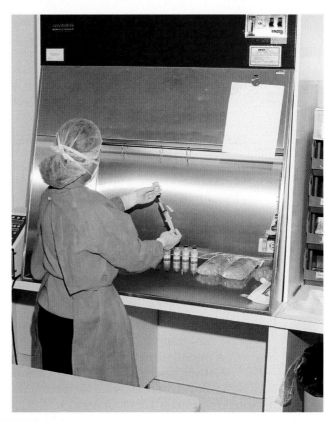

FIGURE 3-1 Room for preparing intravenous solutions for inpatients.

- IV technician: Interprets orders and prepares all **parenteral medications**, both large and small volumes, including controlled substance drips, **hyperalimentation** products, insulin drips, and any other special-order intravenous or intramuscular drugs.
- Chemotherapy technician: Receives orders and prepares all chemotherapeutic agents and their adjunct medications, such as antiemetics.
- Anticoagulant technician: Assists the anticoagulant pharmacist in contacting patients when patient follow-up is necessary or the patient's anticoagulation medication (e.g., warfarin) or dosage needs to be changed.
- Tech-check-tech: This specially trained technician checks the work of other technicians, including filling patient cassettes (plastic containers) and preparing floor stock.
- Clinical technician: Assists the clinical pharmacist with tracking patients' medications. The clinical technician may compile important data—such as patient demographics, medication records, or laboratory results—that are needed by the pharmacist to monitor and evaluate patient outcomes or the appropriateness of drug therapies, or to monitor formulary compliance.
- Supervisory technician: Schedules other technicians and may even hire prospective technicians by reviewing their skills and backgrounds.

In addition, many facilities have specific levels for technicians' responsibilities. The lowest level is tech I, followed by tech II and tech III. Each level requires a minimum amount of time spent working in the previous level. This type of structure allows for career advancement and salary increases based on responsibilities. In the community pharmacy, the structure of responsibilities is quite different.

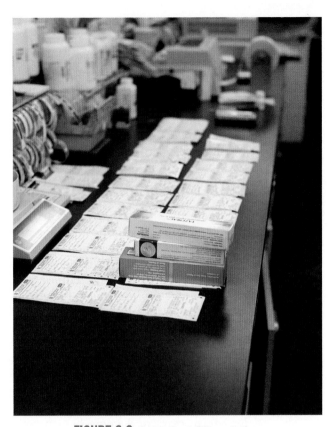

FIGURE 3-2 Outpatient filling station.

COMMUNITY (OUTPATIENT) SETTING REQUIREMENTS

Working in **outpatient pharmacy** is one of the most difficult tasks in pharmacy because of the close interaction with patients. This job tests communication skills and stress levels of the technicians who work with the public. The job has a high volume of interaction on the telephone, registering refill prescriptions and answering questions pertaining to various types of insurance coverage. Computer skills are often necessary to find specific patient information and assist the customer over the phone or in person. Many neighborhood pharmacies fill a high volume of prescriptions daily (Figure 3-2). For a midsize pharmacy to fill 300+ prescriptions in a day, answer phone calls, and address patients' problems is not uncommon. In addition to filling prescriptions, the outpatient technician must be able to order stock in a timely manner. Smaller community pharmacies may keep minimal stock because of limited space and the limited variety of drugs prescribed by physicians in the area. Billing various insurance companies is another skill the outpatient technician must master. This includes understanding the various rules, regulations, and special codes that may accompany each type of prescription claim.

The following list includes job descriptions of outpatient pharmacy technicians as well as those for some of the new positions being filled by technicians in community pharmacies. In addition, larger drug companies that are community-based have recognized the positive aspects of hiring technicians to fill certain positions:

- Insurance billing technician: This person must know the guidelines of Medicare, Blue Cross, Medicaid, and other insurance companies.
- Retail technician: This person must have excellent communication skills, phone skills, and prescription-filling abilities.

- Stock inventory technician: This person must know contacts for fast service, be able to obtain products and drugs as soon as possible, and perform proper billing functions for the pharmacy, including processing returns, recalled drugs, and controlled substances.
- Technician recruiter: Some outpatient pharmacies and/or temporary agencies employ these technicians to recruit other technicians into their company.
- Technician trainer: Various outpatient pharmacies employ technicians to train newly hired technicians on computer programs and to master other necessary skills relevant to their specific pharmacy.

CLOSED DOOR PHARMACY REQUIREMENTS

A **closed door pharmacy** is exactly what its name implies. These pharmacies are not open to the public and they are normally based away from institutional sites (Figure 3-3). Depending on the types of service the closed door pharmacy provides, couriers deliver the medications to home health clients, inpatient hospital pharmacies, specialty clinics, and assisted living or long-term care facilities. Home health pharmacy technicians have job descriptions that incorporate some of the duties of both inpatient and outpatient pharmacy technicians. On one hand, the technicians usually are processing prescription medications for patients weekly or monthly, which is similar to an outpatient setting. However, there are no patients, physicians, nurses, or other health care providers in the facility. Closed door pharmacies are different in that the oral prescriptions usually are packaged differently. Flat cardboard blister packs are prepared by technicians for use by nurses, who administer the drugs in the assisted living, long-term care, and home health settings (see Chapter 11). Other technician responsibilities include preparing parenteral medications. Usually a few days to

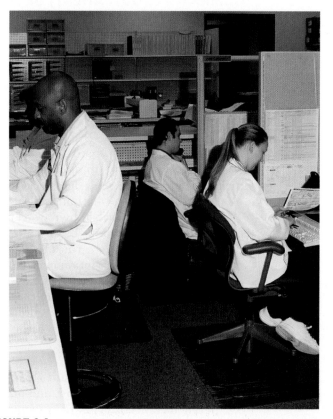

FIGURE 3-3 Home health and long-term pharmacy industry setting.

a 1-month supply is filled each time instead of only a 24-hour dose of medication. A licensed pharmacist checks all medications filled for a home care patient before they are delivered. Home health nurses may receive supplies from the pharmacy clinic, or the patient's family may pick up or have supplies delivered. Examples of patients who may receive care at home include kidney dialysis patients undergoing peritoneal dialysis and hospice patients.

Mail-Order Pharmacy and E-Pharmacy

The mail-order pharmacy and E-pharmacy are growing as the "baby boomers" reach maturity. The need to fill prescriptions expeditiously has increased as more medications have become available to treat commonly acquired illnesses specific to older persons. Large distribution centers process new prescriptions and refills. Technicians are used in these settings as well. This is a relatively new area of pharmacy that is growing steadily. This growth is occurring partially because many aging Americans are living longer and are taking multiple medications that can be costly. By using mail order, they normally receive drugs at lesser cost.

Ethics and Communication in the Workplace

PROFESSIONALISM

Pharmacy technicians are paraprofessionals, which means they work in conjunction with professionals and require specialized training. Because of the vast changes that have taken place during the last decade, pharmacy technicians are moving into an emerging field of pharmacy. As technicians assume more roles—such as clinical pharmacy technicians, inventory specialists, nuclear medication technicians, and other specialized roles—they must be knowledgeable in many areas of pharmacy. More technical colleges are offering associate's degrees for pharmacy technicians. The field of pharmacy technician is becoming a profession.

Although it is good that the job of a pharmacy technician is beginning to be considered a profession, there is a difference between a profession and professionalism. A profession is a job, occupation, or line of work that becomes a career; a profession is founded upon specialized training. **Professionalism** is conforming to the right principles of conduct (work ethics) as accepted by others in the profession. It takes time, hard work, and consistency to be respected as a professional. Because of the increasing depth of education and training that a pharmacy technician needs, today's technicians are the first generation of pharmacy technicians who have been considered professionals. If they do not meet certain responsibilities, they will remain pharmacy assistants and not professionals in the eyes of other health care professionals. Measuring professionalism includes projecting the correct behavior. This includes your attitude and interpersonal skills, in addition to meeting the requirements of your state's BOP. Pharmacy technicians work daily with patients, pharmacists, physicians, and nurses. How technicians conduct themselves in various situations reveals their competencies in the pharmacy and their personal maturity. Probably one of the most prevalent concerns of pharmacy managers and pharmacists is the need for pharmacy technicians who are competent in the area of **communication**.

MORALS VERSUS ETHICS IN THE WORKPLACE

Work **ethics** are a set of standards that should be followed by anyone working in the medical field. Work ethics are often outlined in pharmacy protocol. One important factor that the pharmacy technician must remember is that he or she has a clear responsibility to the patient on many levels. Patients are consumers, and as consumers they have the right to receive goods that have been handled properly and are in good condition. They also trust the pharmacy personnel with their personal information, expecting that their information will be treated as confidential. Many times within a pharmacy or any work setting, employees will express their opinions concerning various medical procedures such as abortion, surgery, or a type of treatment. These are controversial topics, and the opinions that each person has are a part of personal morals or beliefs. Although each person has his or her own set of morals, many morals tend to coincide with the beliefs of others (e.g., stealing is wrong).

In the workplace, however, technicians, pharmacists, and other health care workers are faced with patients who might have different morals. In these situations, ethics include the professional behavior of a technician regardless of a patient's morals. Ethics tend to overlap many morals and need to be separated in the workplace and in the public domain. When you assume the responsibility of serving the public in a setting such as the pharmacy, you accept work ethics that will guide your behavior. For instance, in a hospital setting there may be a need for medication that is used for the termination of pregnancy, emergency contraception, or other controversial treatments. The responsibility of the pharmacy staff is to provide services for all patients. If providing the service is in conflict with your morals and your beliefs prohibit you from participating in servicing patients, you must communicate this to your supervisor.

On a lighter side, just keeping small matters in perspective can help you make the right choice in many decisions. Keeping patients' information confidential and working within pharmacy laws and guidelines, including policies and procedures, will ensure that patients are receiving the best service possible. One should remember that pharmacists, technicians, and clerks are present to serve patients and customers in a professional manner at all times as outlined in the pharmacy technician's code of ethics (Box 3-4).

PROTOCOL

Protocols are a set of standardized rules and guidelines within which a facility functions. This can encompass behavior and tasks required, as well as how drugs will be dispensed and ordered. All medical personnel must abide by the protocols of their workplace. Some hospitals have specialty pharmacists called drug education coordinators. These individuals meet to discuss various new medications that have become available. The drug education coordinators are part of a hospital committee along with physicians, dietitians, and other medical staff. Each new drug is reviewed, and the committee determines whether the drug is better and more cost-effective than current medications being used. These types of pharmacists can be considered clinical pharmacists. Other information that the committee takes into consideration is any literature about the medication that drug companies produce or other published information concerning the best use of their medication. The best medication for the institution is then placed on the formulary or list of medications that can be prescribed. For example, if a physician writes a prescription order for ceftriaxone every 6 hours (normally given once or twice daily), the pharmacist on duty will contact the physician to determine whether the patient had the proper diagnosis for this dosing regimen. In another institution, the pharmacist may have the ability to change the physician's orders when necessary to another medication or dosage as long as the change is predetermined per protocol and adheres to the formulary. The usual hospital protocol will not always preside over treatment decisions. Special procedures can be used to bypass certain formulary medications if the patient's needs require them.

BOX 3-4 PHARMACY TECHNICIAN CODE OF ETHICS

Preamble

Pharmacy technicians are health care professionals who assist pharmacists in providing the best possible care for patients. The principles of this code, which apply to pharmacy technicians working in any and all settings, are based on the application and support of the moral obligations that guide the pharmacy profession in relationships with patients, health care professionals, and society.

Principles

- A pharmacy technician's first consideration is to ensure the health and safety of the patient, and to use knowledge and skills to the best of his/her ability in serving patients.
- A pharmacy technician supports and promotes honesty and integrity in the profession, which includes a duty to observe the law, maintain the highest moral and ethical conduct at all times, and uphold the ethical principles of the profession.
- A pharmacy technician assists and supports the pharmacist in the safe, efficacious, and cost-effective distribution of health services and health care resources.
- A pharmacy technician respects and values the abilities of pharmacists, colleagues, and other health care professionals.
- A pharmacy technician maintains competency in his/her practice and continually enhances his/her professional knowledge and expertise.
- A pharmacy technician respects and supports the patient's individuality, dignity, and confidentiality.
- A pharmacy technician respects the confidentiality of a patient's records and discloses pertinent information only with proper authorization.
- A pharmacy technician never assists in dispensing, promoting, or distribution of medication or medical devices that are not of good quality or do not meet the standards required by law.
- A pharmacy technician does not engage in any activity that will discredit the profession, and will expose, without fear or favor, illegal or unethical conduct in the profession.
- A pharmacy technician associates with and engages in the support of organizations that promote the profession of pharmacy through the utilization and enhancement of pharmacy technicians.

See www.nationaltechexam.org/pdf/code-of-ethics.pdf.

COMMUNICATION

Pharmacy technicians communicate daily with family, friends, strangers, acquaintances, and customers (Figure 3-4). Good communication skills are required for a pharmacy technician. For example, a competent pharmacy technician must possess effective communication skills not only to order medications but also to successfully relate with both pharmacy team members and customers. Communication is defined as the ability to express oneself in such a way that one is understood readily and clearly; however, one of the major complaints from customers and managers is the lack of good communication skills. Most schools do not teach students to be good communicators; however, virtually all jobs require good communication skills. One of the most important areas in which effective communication is needed is in the pharmacy and other health care settings, because these are settings in which life and death issues are often confronted. Good communication skills include diplomacy, compassion, sensitivity, responsibility, tact, and patience. Communication skills, or interpersonal skills, also can be referred to as the ability to relate to another person, verbally or nonverbally.

Health is a serious concern to most people. Seeing the physician is not enjoyable but is done out of necessity. Feeling sick or unable to perform can cause

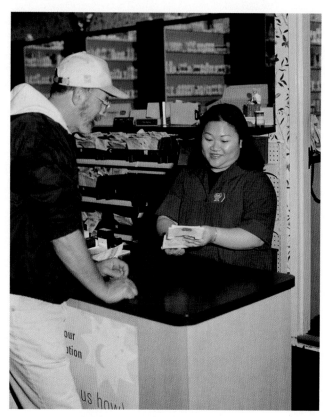

FIGURE 3-4 Technician helping customer.

sadness and depression. After visiting the physician, a person may have to start taking medication or add another medication to the many that the person already is taking. On arrival to the pharmacy, the first person with whom the customer may have to interact may be the pharmacy technician. This direct and personal interaction reveals the best and worst communication skills of the pharmacy technician. One must consider several areas when assessing interpersonal skills, such as the different ways in which we communicate.

It is often difficult to implement good communication skills. Working in a pharmacy is very different than other positions because of the large number of ill people who interact within the pharmacy setting. The lady who seems scatterbrained and not "with it" may have just been told her mother has only 1 year to live. The man who is mad and loud and abrasive may have a severe case of shingles and is in terrible pain and wants his medication as soon as possible. There are many people who do not feel comfortable in a hospital or medical setting; they become scared and these feelings can be projected in different ways. It is not your responsibility to counsel patients but to help them through the process of getting their medications quickly and safely.

Listening Skills

Listen, listen, and listen. Sometimes just listening to a person is all that is required. If a customer is angry about a medication, regardless of the problem, just listening can ease the person's frustration. Instead of talking over the person or telling the person that he or she is wrong, try to listen until the person is finished and empathize with the dilemma. Most persons know a problem with a medication is not the fault of the pharmacy technician, but they want to be heard. A professional does not allow himself or herself to be directed by another person's inappropriate behavior. Pharmacy technicians must remember the final outcome and behave professionally.

BOX 3-5 EXAMPLE OF NEGATIVE BODY LANGUAGE

Ms. Lehman walks up to the counter to have her prescription filled and asks whether it can be done within 5 minutes because her bus will be leaving. Pharmacy technician John rolls his eyes and shakes his head in disbelief, wondering why everyone thinks they should not have to wait. He turns and walks away without saying a word.

Alternate response: John shows concern for Ms. Lehman and tells her they will fill her prescription as soon as possible. John can ask the pharmacist to please fill the prescription as quickly as possible.

Body Language

Everyone communicates on a daily basis; however, rarely do we take a step back and evaluate how effectively we are communicating. One important aspect of communication is facial expressions. The old phrase "Actions speak louder than words" is very true. When working closely with customers in the pharmacy setting or with co-workers, it is important to maintain a caring but professional attitude at all times. In many instances the pharmacy technician may encounter stressful and even embarrassing situations with customers.

Many persons make an instant judgment of others within the first 30 seconds of meeting. This is also true with respect to the pharmacy setting. The primary goal of pharmacy personnel is to help others, which can be accomplished by being friendly and remaining calm. Facial expressions can show many different emotions, thoughts, and biases. As a paraprofessional it is imperative that the only body language that should be conveyed is that of a helpful and concerned pharmacy staff member. A professional should not bring his or her outside personal problems to work. Stress manifests in various ways, such as frowning, tensing the shoulders, biting one's lip, raising eyebrows, folding arms, placing hands on hips, or other idiosyncrasies. If and when stress begins to transform into this type of body language, it is time to take a step back and maybe a deep breath to help regain focus. In these instances it is necessary to think before you react with a typical "common reaction." Remember, the goal is to help customers to the extent that when customers leave the pharmacy, they believe they have received the best service possible. See an example in Box 3-5.

Verbal Communications

Verbal communication is an important tool in pharmacy. It is a skill that has to be learned and practiced. To be an effective communicator, you must remember that both your words and your voice are not always in agreement. Each is a separate entity and can be used to work for or against you. There are two parts to verbal communication skills: vocal and verbal; each will be discussed separately.

Vocal: How You Sound. Your voice is a powerful tool that affects the customer or person to whom you are talking. Words alone do not necessarily convey your meaning or feelings; the inflection (pitch), tone, speed, and volume add multitudes of information that is being picked up by the listener. As an example of the use of inflection, in the following statements stress the boldfaced word while you say each sentence to a partner, and notice your partner's response to each statement.

- **IF** you'll wait a moment, I'll get the information you need.
- If you'll **WAIT** a moment, I'll get the information you need.
- If you'll wait a moment, I'll get the information you need.

As you can see, or hear in this case, the way in which you emphasize a word within a sentence makes a big difference in how it is perceived.

How to Improve Your Vocal Communication Skills

- Try not to talk using the same tone all the time (monotone voice) because it loses the listener's interest and attention.
- Do not talk too rapidly to a customer; the customer may not be able to follow what you are saying.
- Talking very slow indicates you do not know the answer; if this is the case, contact the pharmacist.
- People prefer a lower pitched voice; high, squeaky tones can annoy the listener and they can result in the listener taking you less seriously.
- A loud or extremely soft voice can annoy and irritate people; speak in a medium tone of voice so you can be heard.
- Articulation is extremely important; either mumbling, mispronouncing words, or using slang is one of the fastest ways of sounding unprofessional. Speak in clear, crisp words and sentences.

Verbal: What You Say. Words are also a strong tool that can calm or escalate a situation between you and a customer or patient. Using intimidating words, belittling a person's opinion, or leaving the customer feeling embarrassed, angry, or sad are not goals of effective communication.

Be careful of the words you use while addressing a customer. If the customer is definitely wrong, do not tell the person that he or she is wrong. Instead, after carefully listening to the customer, point out the misconception to let the customer know that you understand how this point could be easily confused. Determine which of the following scenarios is best handled.

First Way of Handling a Problem

Customer: When I called earlier they said the prescriptions would be done by noon; now you tell me they aren't ready; why do you guys lie like that?
Technician: We don't lie; you probably called in late.
Customer: Oh no; I think I called in around 10 AM.
Technician: Well either way, you'll have to wait.
Customer: Let me talk to your manager.

Second Way of Handling the Same Problem

Customer: When I called earlier they said the prescriptions would be done by noon; now you tell me they aren't ready; why do you guys lie like that?
Technician: I'm sorry; I know the phone recorder said they would be done by noon but that's for prescriptions that were called in by a certain time. Did you call in your prescription before 9 AM?
Customer: Oh no; I think I called it in around 10 AM.
Technician: That's okay; let me go take a look to see if we can get your prescription ready for you as soon as possible.
Customer: Thanks.

How to Improve Your Verbal Skills

- Reading will increase your vocabulary.
- Take a course in communication.
- There are several types of communication aids that you can use to increase your vocabulary, such as CDs, DVDs, and Internet sites.
- Always try to put yourself in the customer's position when talking to him or her; many times the customer is sick or in pain and cannot control his or her emotions; however, you can. Even if the customer is wrong, arguing will

BOX 3-6 EXAMPLE OF UNACCEPTABLE PHONE ETIQUETTE

Patient: Hello, I'm calling because my medication looks different than before and I need to know if it's the same drug or not.
Pharmacy technician: Would you please hold?
Patient: No, I need to know now because ...
Pharmacy technician: [Places the patient on hold and forgets to get back to the patient.]
Alternate response: The technician waits to hear the patient's response to the question. When the patient says she cannot wait, the technician waits to hear why and then proceeds to help her.

not help the situation; instead, it will energize the discussion with negativity. However, if a customer is abusive, the technician should not engage in this type of communication and should notify the pharmacist in charge immediately. If the pharmacist cannot rectify the problem, security is normally called, and the patient would be escorted from the premises.

Phone Etiquette

Another area of communication that can stimulate an upset customer is phone communication. It is common to be placed on hold for long periods of time and to even be disconnected. If the call must be placed on hold, then check back with the caller in 1- to 2-minute intervals to reassure the caller that you have not forgotten him or her. If customers raise their voices, let them air their complaint; do not react negatively or try to place blame on them. Ask them what you can do to help them resolve the situation. The tone in one's voice either can easily resolve a problem or can escalate a problem into a long, drawn-out argument. Talk in an even tone and always be pleasant and professional. If you argue with the customer this will fuel the fire and the situation may get out of hand with no resolution (Box 3-6).

Written Communication

Many times handwriting is not considered a type of communication; however, in pharmacy it is extremely important to relate the correct information, or medication errors can result. Many of the drug errors that have been reported in the news and in medical journals are due to poor handwriting (Box 3-7). Taking notes is another opportunity for drug errors in the pharmacy. In hospitals, nurses often call into the pharmacy and the technician will answer the phone. It is necessary not only to record all the pertinent information but also to write it legibly so that a pharmacist or other technician can understand the note completely.

CONFIDENTIALITY

Confidentiality is another aspect of working ethically. The definition of confidentiality is to keep privileged information about a customer from being disclosed without his or her consent. This includes information that may cause the patient embarrassment or harm. Patients have a right to privacy concerning their medications, treatment, or any aspect of their health care. The Health Insurance Portability and Accountability Act (HIPAA) addresses patient confidentiality in the pharmacy (see Appendix E). HIPAA affects all areas of medicine, including pharmacy, because they all involve the practice of obtaining, transferring, and accessing patient information. Changes have been made throughout all medical facilities and medical information centers that limit access to patient

BOX 3-7 EXAMPLE OF POOR WRITTEN COMMUNICATION SKILLS

Nurse Black calls the pharmacist to ask if the two drugs she is about to administer are compatible. She is in a hurry. Joe North, CPhT, scribbles down the question but does not get the nurse's name or telephone extension. By the time the nurse calls back to contact the pharmacist, the dose is late and the patient has been in pain while waiting for a response.

Alternate response: The technician, Joe North, tells the nurse he will ask the pharmacist to return her call and then proceeds to ask for the nurse's name, station, and extension as well as the patient's name and medical record number.

Information That Should Be Obtained and Written Down in the Message:
- Nurse's or caller's name
- Floor location and extension in a hospital setting, or the physician's office in a community pharmacy, or the patient's preferred call-back number
- The purpose of the call written in a concise question
- The time of the call
- The initials of the technician who took the call
- How soon the information is needed

Only then can a pharmacist quickly and easily relay the correct information to the appropriate person. If your handwriting is illegible, it can cost time and possibly result in a preventable error. There is no excuse for poor handwriting. Poor handwriting is one of the reasons that physicians now are transitioning to electronic medication ordering. Thousands of preventable errors can be overcome through the use of computer ordering.

BOX 3-8 EXAMPLE OF BREACH OF CONFIDENTIALITY

Ms. K has cancer. Two pharmacy technicians discuss her condition and the medications that she is taking. A co-worker of Ms. K overhears this information and tells her employer.

information in charts and computer bases. A patient's approval is required for any information concerning the patient to be released to any third party, including insurance companies, physicians, and pharmacies. Because pharmacy technicians and other health care professionals have access to a patient's condition, medications, and other personal information, they are responsible for keeping the patient's information confidential (Box 3-8).

TERMINALLY ILL PATIENTS

Special consideration should be given to those patients who are terminally ill. This can prove difficult. Although each person copes with his or her own mortality differently, there are "normal" progressive steps that persons experience. The five stages that terminally ill patients experience are as follows:

Stages	Example
Denial	"This can't be happening ..."
Anger	"It isn't fair. I don't deserve this ..."
Bargaining	"Please make me better, and I promise ..."
Depression	"I will never be able to see you again ..."
Acceptance	"I can do this, everyone does ..."

Normally the first stage is denial. This is a defense mechanism in which the situation does not seem real. Perhaps the reality is too harsh for the person to accept. The next stage is anger. Sometimes one may have a feeling of unfairness. Bargaining usually follows anger. The person makes promises to himself or herself or to a higher power in the hope of a miracle. Depression may take over at this point with the realization that nothing is going to change concerning the prognosis. The final phase is acceptance, in which the person concedes his or her own mortality and prepares for eventual death.

Each of these stages can manifest at any time and last for different lengths of time. Therefore it is important that the technician be compassionate to the patient's situation. Most health care workers do not hesitate to help a dying patient; however, the problem is how to identify these patients. Unfortunately, unless the patient decides to share this information, the pharmacy staff does not necessarily know. Some medications indicate an advancing medical condition. These include pain medications, such as fentanyl patches or morphine; however, these drugs do not definitively identify a fatal condition. Therefore the pharmacy technician must be objective about each person who enters the pharmacy and realize that he or she does not know what each person is experiencing.

If the technician treats persons equally regardless of their disposition, then the pharmacy technician is behaving appropriately and professionally. The pharmacy technician can influence the development of a positive atmosphere within the pharmacy setting. Allowing customers to express frustration, being a good listener, and doing one's best to help others are important components of acting professionally.

Training Programs for the Pharmacy Technician Student

Since 1982, when pharmacy technician accreditation programs were first established, the American Society of Health-System Pharmacists (ASHP) has been the leader in providing course curriculum and standards and offering students the best foundation for becoming technicians. Before the formation of technician schools, ASHP's training guidelines and standards were used in hospitals for training pharmacy interns. ASHP accreditation is a voluntary process at this time. Program accreditation is given to those colleges and technical schools that apply and meet the minimum requirements set by ASHP. The following is an outline of topics that need to be addressed in order for a program to meet the minimum standard requirements necessary for ASHP accreditation (Box 3-9).

DIFFERENT LEVELS OF PHARMACY TECHNICIANS

There are four levels of pharmacy technicians: pharmacy technicians who have no specialized training or credentials, licensed, registered, and certified technicians. Each level has different qualifications and may differ from state to state. The following list provides descriptions of the various levels.

Technician: There are states that require their pharmacy technicians to attain minimum standards. Some states require a high school diploma; others do not. For example, the Kentucky Board of Pharmacy has an online registration that requires only a valid driver's license/state ID number or Social Security number; the pharmacy name and address; and the permit numbers of all pharmacies at which you will be employed.

Licensed: A license is the process in which an agency of the government grants permission to an individual to engage in a given occupation based on the findings that the applicant has attained the minimum degree of competency necessary to ensure that the public health, safety, and welfare will

BOX 3-9 ASHP COURSE CURRICULUM REQUIREMENTS

1. Orientation to Pharmacy Practice
2. Therapeutic Agents for the Nervous System
3. Therapeutic Agents for the Skeletal System
4. Therapeutic Agents for the Muscular System
5. Therapeutic Agents for the Cardiovascular System
6. Therapeutic Agents for the Respiratory System
7. Therapeutic Agents for the Gastrointestinal System
8. Therapeutic Agents for the Renal System
9. Therapeutic Agents for the Reproductive Systems
10. Therapeutic Agents for the Immune System
11. Therapeutic Agents for Eyes, Ears, Nose, and Throat
12. Therapeutic Agents for the Dermatologic System
13. Therapeutic Agents for the Hematologic System
14. Collecting, Organizing, and Evaluating Information
15. Purchase of Pharmaceuticals, Devices, and Supplies
16. Control of Inventory
17. Assessment of Medication Orders/Prescriptions
18. Preparation of Noncompounded Products
19. Preparation of Nonsterile Compounded Products
20. Preparation of Sterile Compounded Products
21. Preparation of Cytotoxic and Hazardous Medication Products
22. Medication Distribution
23. Identification of Patients for Counseling
24. Medication Safety
25. Collection of Payment (Billing)
26. Monitoring Medication Therapy
27. Maintenance of Equipment and Facilities
28. Investigational Medication Products
29. Personal Qualities of Technicians
30. Certification
31. Pharmacy Organizations
32. Management of Change
33. Acute Care Practice (Option Long-Term Care) Experience
34. Home Care Practice Experience
35. Ambulatory Clinic with Infusion Services Practice Experience
36. Community or Outpatient Pharmacy Practice Experience

In addition, programs must have a minimum of 600 contact hours and last no less than 15 weeks. The technician must complete an externship in a pharmacy setting for no less than the required amount predetermined by the state board of pharmacy.

See www.ashp.org/s_ashp/docs/files/RTP_TechModuleDesc.pdf.

be reasonably well protected. Very few states require **licensure of a technician**; those that do follow the recommendations of the National Association of Boards of Pharmacy (NABP). Each state determines if continuing education is required of technicians to renew their license.

Registered: A technician is registered through the state board of pharmacy. It is the process of making a list or being enrolled in an existing list; registration should be used to help safeguard the public via tracking of the technician workforce and preventing individuals with documented problems from serving as pharmacy technicians. Registration carries no indication or guarantee of the registrant's knowledge or skills. Each state determines if continuing education is required of technicians to renew their registration.

Certified: A **certified technician** is one who has been granted recognition by a nongovernmental agency or association; certification indicates that the person has met predetermined qualifications specified by that agency or association (PTCB or ICPT). CPhT is the only credential available to pharmacy technicians. Certification is an indication of the mastery of a specific core of knowledge. Certified technicians must renew their certification every 2 years and complete at least 20 hours of pharmacy-related continuing education, including 1 hour of pharmacy law, during that time. (See ashp.org for a description of uniform state laws and regulations regarding pharmacy technicians.)

NATIONAL CERTIFICATION FOR TECHNICIANS

During the infancy of any profession, there is a lack of regular guidelines and standards, or continuity. Currently there are five types of verification that may be required or pursued by technicians; these include registration, licensing, certification, associate of science (AS) degree in pharmacy technology, or certificate in pharmacy technology. As outlined above, registration is given by the state and requires that the applicant pass a standard background check as well as meet BOP standards. Licensing may also be required by the state, but is not currently required in all states. A certified pharmacy technician is given a certificate that acknowledges the technician has a basic understanding of all areas of pharmacy including federal law. Maintaining certification also requires continuing education to keep skills at a minimum level.

Pharmacy technicians work throughout the United States and in all types of pharmacy settings under different rules determined by the individual states, which makes this profession challenging. At some point in the near future a national minimum standard for the profession must be met and agreed on across the United States. Although there will always be some variations from state to state, the overall skill level of a pharmacy technician should be a well-known standard. Currently, there is a wide range of skill levels, experience, pay, and belief systems. One of the most basic aspects is the lack of a common title. Pharmacy technicians also are known as pharmacy clerks and pharmacy assistants.

There are two national groups that certify technicians and are recognized by various states: the Pharmacy Technician Certification Board and the Institute for the Certification of Pharmacy Technicians. The **Pharmacy Technician Certification Board (PTCB)** is an organization that was founded in 1995 by four organizations with the intent of implementing an examination that would certify that a technician has met a basic skill level (Box 3-10). These

BOX 3-10 GOALS OF PTCB AND EXAM REQUIREMENTS

Goals
- To work more effectively with pharmacists
- To provide better patient care and service
- To create a minimum standard of knowledge of pharmacy technicians
- To help employers determine the knowledge base of pharmacy technicians

Eligibility Requirements to Take the Exam Include the Following:
- A high school diploma or general equivalency diploma
- Never been convicted of a drug-related felony
- Exam questions encompass the following topics:
  - Assisting the pharmacist in serving patients, 64%
  - Maintaining medication and inventory control systems, 25%
  - Participating in the administration and management of pharmacy practice, 11%

organizations are the American Society of Health-System Pharmacists, the American Pharmacists Association, the Illinois Council of Health-System Pharmacists, and the Michigan Pharmacists Association.

The PTCB offers 4 different sample exams consisting of 50 multiple choice questions to be taken within 60 minutes. They cover both calculations and medication usage and administration. The cost is $29.00 per exam. The actual certification exam, administered by PTCB is given at a professional testing center and is computerized. Testing can take place once an appointment is made. Participants are given 2 hours to take the survey and exam. Computers have a calculator available or one may be brought to the test center, and scratch pads are provided by the testing center. Scoring is done by an independent group that grades the various areas of pharmacy knowledge. The results are immediately calculated at the end of the examination. The scope of pharmacy knowledge that is tested includes the following:

- Pharmacy math
- Pharmacy law (federal only)
- Pharmacy operations
- Drug names (trade/generic)
- Drug classifications

For more information, visit www.PTCB.org.

The Institute for the Certification of Pharmacy Technicians (ICPT) is accredited by boards of the NCPA (National Community Pharmacists Association), NCCA (National Commission for Certifying Agencies), and NACDS (National Association of Chain Drug Stores). For more information, visit www.icpt.org. The ICPT has a certification exam that is also given in all states. The exam administered by ICPT is called ExCPT and is given at preestablished times throughout the country at various proctored testing sites. These sites can be located via www.Lasergrade.com and clicking into "locate a test center." From there the closest testing site is found based on the zip code entered. Once a site is found you call the provided phone number and register to take the 2-hour exam. There are two 50-question sample exams at $25 each (one is just math while the other covers various areas of pharmacy) to practice online. ICPT also offers a study manual covering a wide variety of information pertaining to pharmacy requirements for technicians. The cost of the guide is $54.00, except in Virginia where the cost is $49.00 (as of January 2009).

Table 3-1 compares the PTCB and ExCPT examinations.

CONTINUING EDUCATION

Technicians who meet the requirements of national certification may use the initials *CPhT* on their identification tag, indicating that they are a certified pharmacy technician. To maintain their certification they must earn **continu-**

TABLE 3-1 Comparisons of National Certification Examinations

National Certification Organization	Cost	Questions	CE Requirements	Cost of Recertification	Cost of Retaking Exam	Online Practice Exam & Cost	Endorsement
PTCB	$129.00	90	20 CE per 2 years/ 1 unit in law	$40	Must wait 90 days	Yes/$29.00	NABP
ICPT	$95.00	110	20 CE per 2 years/ 1 unit in law	$40	Must wait 1 month	Yes/$25.00	NACDS* & NCPA

*National Association of Chain Drug Stores (NACDS) and National Community Pharmacists Association (NCPA), updated Jan 2009.

Tech Note!

While not always a condition of employment, many employers may encourage certification and formally recognize achievement. Some pharmacy technicians may receive a raise in pay or expanded career responsibilities after completion of the pharmacy technician certification examination, although some pharmacies do not formally recognize national certification as a career incentive.

Tech Alert!

Many states still do not require certification of their technicians but have different guidelines for their responsibilities in the pharmacy. Not all states' requirements are standardized. Certain states require **licensing** but not national certification while others require registration. States such as Texas require certification of all new technicians but do have exemptions for certain pharmacy technicians. Alabama does not require certification, but the state does require that all pharmacy technicians receive continuing education each year. California only requires **registration.** In this case a background check is done before a pharmacy technician applies for registration. However, most, if not all, states now require technicians to have a high school diploma. Each student must visit the website of his or her board of pharmacy to become familiar with the current state laws pertaining to pharmacy technicians.

TABLE 3-2 Examples of Continuing Education Website Portals for Technicians

CE Website/Portal	Internet CE	Live CE	Cost*
www.uspharmacist.com	X		None
www.rxschool.com	X	X	None
www.powerpak.com	X		None
www.freece.com/freece/index.asp	X	X	None
www.abbottpharmacy.com	X	X	None
www.cecity.com/	X		None

*Many programs are available at no charge; occasionally, fee-based programs may also be available, depending on the session provider.

ing education (CE) credits. All valid CE credits must be approved by ACPE (Accreditation Council for Pharmacy Education), which is indicated on each CE course. As of 2007 ACPE offers CE courses specifically for pharmacy technicians. While technicians can still take CE courses meant for pharmacists, the technician versions are easier to understand. The letter "P" indicates the CE course is designed for pharmacists whereas a "T" indicates the course is for technicians. In addition to the two levels of CE courses (i.e., "P" and "T"), current courses may also have "05" added to their name, which designates the CE course is a topic on patient safety. CE can be obtained through pharmacy organizations that offer free continuing education to members, journals that include continuing education units, or seminars. Continuing education is less expensive for association members, and many drug companies offer free continuing education units to pharmacists. Technicians can use the same continuing education units as pharmacists, although certain courses can be difficult to understand. Independent pharmacists and other small businesses offer low-cost continuing education credit on the Internet (refer to Table 3-2).

Box 3-11 lists both qualifications and common duties of certified technicians according to the PTCB organization.

According to the current statistics, there are more than 399,000 technicians nationwide. Many states are beginning to recognize the importance of certification to guarantee that the technicians hired are competent in all areas of pharmacy (see Chapter 14, Emily's Act). More information about this credential, and schools that offer it, can be obtained at www.nhanow.com. Employers increasingly are using these credentials as a requirement for hiring technicians.

In May of 2009, the National Association of Boards of Pharmacy (NABP) sent a letter to all state boards of pharmacy encouraging them to require certification of all technicians by the year 2015. This recommendation was made by their Task Force on Standardized Pharmacy Technician Education and Training, and the initiative was announced at the 2009 national meeting of the NABP. The Task Force's recommendation was to use the PTCB exam as the method of technician certification, given its acceptance by the members of NABP since the year 2000.

OPPORTUNITIES FOR TECHNICIANS

Pharmacies use computers daily; therefore software must be developed for pharmacy personnel. Some pharmacy-related fields do require more education in specific areas such as computers. With the proper educational training, such as an associate of science (AS) or bachelor of science (BS) degree in computer science, the pharmacy technician is well equipped to write software or supply support. Also, as many technicians are granted the responsibility of training

BOX 3-11 PTCB QUALIFICATIONS AND COMMON DUTIES OF CERTIFIED TECHNICIANS

Job Duties

This is a representation of the types of responsibilities technicians should have. It will depend on the pharmacy setting and scope of practice.

- Assist pharmacist in labeling and filling prescriptions
- Assist patients in dropping off and picking up prescriptions
- Enter prescriptions into the computer
- Verify that customer receives correct prescription(s)
- Compound oral solutions, ointments, and creams
- Schedule and maintain workflow
- Prepackage bulk medications
- Screen calls for pharmacists
- Order medication(s)
- Work with insurance carriers to obtain payments and refilling authority
- Prepare medication inventories
- Prepare chemotherapeutic agents
- Compound total parenteral nutrition solutions
- Compound large volumes of intravenous mixtures
- Assist in outpatient dispensing
- Assist in inpatient dispensing
- Prepare IV mixtures
- Assist in purchasing and billing

Knowledge, Skills, Training, and Education

State practice acts and employer policies determine training and education requirements. Below is a list of some characteristics that are commonly desired:

- Professional attitude
- Strong communication skills
- Ability to work in teams
- Previous customer service experience
- Ability to type 35 words per minute
- Understanding of medical terminology and calculations
- Attention to detail
- Outgoing
- Hard working
- Quick learner
- PTCB certification may be desired or mandatory

This information was obtained from the Pharmacy Technician Certification Board website (www.PTCB.org).

technicians, their expertise may help them write curriculums, articles, and even books for pharmacy technicians. Many vocational schools hire experienced pharmacy technicians to teach students the necessary requirements to be a competent pharmacy technician. Completion of such training programs offers different degrees, such as certificates, an associate's degree (associate of arts [AA] or AS), or a bachelor's degree (bachelor of arts [BA] or BS).

Pharmacy technicians can fill many other (not well-known) positions. The following is a list of various nontraditional jobs:

- Pharmacy business management operators—Pharmacy business management companies are beginning to realize the importance of knowing not only the trade and generic names of drugs but also the classifications of drugs. They are hiring technicians, rather than registered pharmacists, to help pharmacy customers over the phone, which is a cost savings for the company.

- Computer support technician (PYXIS, SUREMED)—Large companies that supply hospitals, community pharmacies, and other facilities with automated medication dispensing systems are employing technicians as support personnel.
- Software writer—Some pharmacy software writers are using technicians with additional computer background and/or training to prepare software services. Technicians use their terminology and drug knowledge in creating new software programs.
- Poison control call center operator—Some poison control centers are using technicians to triage calls coming into the 911 stations. If the call is in regard to something life-threatening, then technicians transfer the call to a pharmacist or poison specialist. If the call is something less critical, technicians are authorized to take the call.
- Nuclear pharmacy technician—The technician may assist the pharmacist with handling and preparing physicians' orders for radioactive medications used in diagnosis and treatment.
- Director/instructor—Pharmacy technicians can oversee technician training programs and/or instruct in schools around the country. Some require a bachelor of science degree or vocational education teaching credentials.
- Corporate pharmacy analysis—Working through an independent management service, a technician surveys the efficiency in all areas of the pharmacy and recommends changes to help the pharmacy operate more productively and efficiently. The analyst may travel and even work on The Joint Commission standards to prepare pharmacies for inspection.
- Pharmacy supervisors—Supervisors oversee as many as 20 to 30 technicians and pharmacist interns within the pharmacy. They are responsible for training them on all software and may organize work schedules.
- Clinical coordinator—The coordinator's responsibilities may include scheduling patients for educational classes, such as disease management training with the pharmacist, or they may refer individuals to the pharmacist, nurse practitioner, or physician managed clinic for individualized medication consultation.

In addition to the positions listed, technicians may continue their education and apply for pharmacy school. Many pharmacists were once technicians. New positions are being developed by different pharmacy settings specifically for technicians. Although these positions currently may be nontraditional, their numbers are growing. It would not be surprising if these positions became commonly held positions for future technicians.

Examples Include	Setting
Clinical pharmacy technician	Hospital
Anticoagulant pharmacy technician	Hospital; assists pharmacist
Program director—pharmacy technician	Vocational/technical school
Medical billing specialist—pharmacy technician	Health care services
Certified pharmacy technician—loader, driver	Long-term care facility
Implementation pharmacy technician	Pharmacy benefits service
Data entry pharmacy technician	Institutional pharmacy

INCENTIVE PROGRAMS

Pharmacies sometimes have an incentive program for employees who want to further their careers in pharmacy. Many pharmacists that began their careers as technicians have used this company benefit to their advantage. Many pharmacy employers provide incentives to their technicians for returning to school and becoming a pharmacist. They may reimburse tuition costs or give pay incentives for agreeing to be employed by the pharmacy a certain number of years upon graduation from pharmacy school. Whether a company does support and partially fund a school program is something one should consider when inquiring about a pharmacy position.

As the geriatric community increases in number over the next decades, so will the need for qualified medical personnel. Pharmacy technicians are very knowledgeable about the challenges and benefits that pharmacy has to offer. The future of technicians still is being determined, but judging from the advances currently being made by technicians, the only limitations to pharmacy technicians are self-imposed. Many pharmacy companies reimburse their technicians after they pass the PTCB examination. This is more likely to take place in states in which certification is not mandatory, but preferred. Attaining increased skill levels, including becoming certified pharmacy technicians, opens more doors for technicians in pharmacy.

The Professional Technician Associations

There are several pharmacy associations that pharmacy technicians can join. Although each association has requisite yearly dues, each has different benefits. A brief history of each of the national associations is given. Throughout history it has become clear that professions that form associations provide the participants an avenue to make changes and advance their careers. It is important that pharmacy technicians not only join pharmacy associations to keep abreast of new information but also become active participants. In the state of California in 2008, the state chapter of ASHP allowed a pharmacy technician to vote on policies along with pharmacists for the first time. Besides the benefits of association membership, such as free CE courses and access to journals, are the networking possibilities. Not enough can be said about networking to advance one's career, and life-long acquaintances can be made. Table 3-3 shows the information for each of the following organizations listed. Each organization has continuing education programs, association fees, and regular conferences or seminars.

AMERICAN PHARMACISTS ASSOCIATION (APhA)

This is the oldest and largest pharmacist association, founded in 1852. It participates in pharmacy issues from around the world and its membership includes pharmacists, technicians, pharmacy students, scientists, and other interested parties. The association holds annual meetings where CE courses can be taken. They participate in several important government policies such as Medicare Part D.

AMERICAN SOCIETY OF HEALTH-SYSTEM PHARMACISTS (ASHP)

In 1942 the American Society of Hospital Pharmacists with 154 members separated from the APhA. In 1945 this group established focus areas on minimum standards of pharmaceutical services in the hospital and education about new techniques and medications. The group expanded over time, and in 1950 it published its journal, *Mirror of Hospital Pharmacy*. After receiving feedback from more than 3000 hospitals, the journal began to publish recommendations to enhance the development of hospital pharmacy. In 1995 it expanded its outreach to areas other than hospital pharmacists. With the new name American Society of Health-System Pharmacists, the association now includes other pharmacy settings, such as home care and ambulatory care; however, most of its members are pharmacists based in hospital settings.

TABLE 3-3 Organizations/Associations for Pharmacy Technicians*

Name of Organization/ Association	Technicians	Pharmacists	Educators	Annual Fees	Special Category/ Technician Student Fees	Journal or Magazine Included	Website
ASHP (has state chapters)	Yes	Yes	n/a	$70/yr without subscription; $180.00 with journal[†]	No/state chapters vary	*AJHP Journal*[†]	www.ashp.org
APhA (has state chapters)	Yes	Yes	n/a	$62.00; $139.00 with journal[†]	No	*JAPhA Journal*[†]	www.pharmacist. com
AAPT	Yes	Yes	n/a	$47.50 (e-mail correspondence); $50.00 (mail correspondence)	$23.75 (e-mail); $25.00 (mail)	None	www.pharmacyte clinician.com
NPTA	Yes	No	n/a	$69.00/yr; $128.00/2 yr; $187.00/3 yr	No	*Today's Technician* magazine	www.pharmacy technician.org
NCPA	Yes	Yes	n/a	$75.00	No	None	www.ncpanet.org
PTEC[§]	Yes	Yes	Yes	$55.00; $80.00 without journal	No	*Journal of Pharmacy Technology*	www.rxptec.org

*Updated 8/23/09.
[†]Fees may vary based on state.
[‡]Included for fee.
n/a, Not applicable; *PTEC,* Pharmacy Technician Educators Council.

They also have a technician division. In addition, there are state chapters that can be joined.

AMERICAN ASSOCIATION OF PHARMACY TECHNICIANS (AAPT)

This was the first pharmacy technician association formed, established in 1979. It has always been managed by volunteer pharmacy technicians and serves to participate in the advancement of pharmacy technicians.

NATIONAL COMMUNITY PHARMACISTS ASSOCIATION (NCPA)

This organization was founded in 1898 under the National Association of Retail Druggists. Members include pharmacists, pharmacy owners, managers, pharmacy students, and pharmacy technicians.

NATIONAL PHARMACY TECHNICIAN ASSOCIATION (NPTA)

NPTA began in 1999 in Houston, Texas. In 2000 they released the *Today's Technician* magazine and also had their first convention. In 2004 they gained American Council for Pharmacy Education (ACPE) approval and began offering their own CE courses. In 2005 this association joined the membership of CEPT (Committee of European Pharmacy Technicians), a European technicians' association. The association also is part of an advocacy group that serves to advance education and acknowledgement for technicians.

BOX 3-12 INTERNET SITES FOR JOBS

The following is a list of websites that can be used to search for pharmacy technician jobs:

http://pharmacyjobs.rxcareercenter.com
www.allpharmacyjobs.com/infusion_pharmacy_jobs.htm
www.healthjobsusa.com/
www.indeed.com
www.maximstaffing.com/allied/career-opportunities/pharmacy-jobs.aspx
www.monster.com
www.pharmacy.org/job.html
www.pharmacychoice.com/careers/pharmtech.cfm
www.pharmacyjobsnationwide.com/
www.righthealth.com
http://certified.pharmacy.technician.jobs.com/

The Job Search

Many websites are available that provide tips for preparing resumes and cover letters and that explain the interview process. Remember that as a student, your work experience is not a strong point because this is a new vocation for you. Instead, you must focus on your educational background. It is important that the program you attend supplies you with an adequate knowledge base to prepare you for this important vocation in pharmacy. The importance of attitude, attendance, and punctuality in pharmacy cannot be stressed enough. Arrive early for interviews and a few minutes early every day to work. This shows your dedication to your profession. When searching for your first job or subsequent jobs, be sure to explore every avenue. Besides the obvious newspaper ads, check out websites and job fairs, and remember to ask friends in the pharmacy business if they know of any positions that are available. Attending pharmacy seminars can be another way to find a job opening. For a sample of websites available when job searching, see Box 3-12.

Why not start your career while in school? Many student technicians are employed as pharmacy clerks. The benefits are endless; being employed as a pharmacy clerk not only can strengthen and expand the student's knowledge base about drugs but also can provide insight into the business of pharmacy, and even a possible future job as a technician.

THE RESUME

One of the first encounters you will have with your future employer is through your resume. This is why it is so important to make your resume noticeable, easily distinguished when compared to other resumes. Some students have been employed in multiple jobs while other students may be recent high school graduates and have no employment experience. If a resume is prepared correctly and if the student has good grades and attendance, it should not make too much difference. On a resume, list jobs in which you have had customer service or those where you managed yourself or others, because these are highly valuable skills. Make sure you can obtain references from those jobs. Any job that encompasses skills used in pharmacy is good to cite, but only list a few because the resume should not be more than 1 page. For those who have no employment history, your strengths are going to be academic only. In both cases list your academic study areas first on the resume because this is the first information

BOX 3-13 RESUME HELP

The following is a list of websites that help with resumes and letters of interest:

http://msn.careerbuilder.com
www.1st-writer.com/free_resume_examples.htm
www.collegegrad.com/resume/freeresumetemplate.shtml
www.e-resume.us/ma/resume.asp?ref=g_uscvc_[res]_s2
www.resume-help.org
www.resumeimproved.com
www.jobstar.org/tools/resume

that will be seen. When pharmacy managers have many resumes to check, they look from the top down; if all they read is a list of former jobs, they may dismiss the resume. Get help in writing your resume and have others look at it to see if it looks professional (see Box 3-13). Never get fancy with the format and always have references ready on a separate page for your future employer. Larger pharmacy companies may even have a standardized format to automate the filing of your resume online. In such cases, it may be helpful for you to familiarize yourself with the information they desire before submitting your application.

PROFESSIONAL DRESS

Pharmacy is predominantly a conservative profession. Dressing professionally includes proper clothing, shoes, and hairstyle; off-colored hair, facial jewelry, visible tattoos, or any other feature that detracts attention from your personality should be avoided. Medical personnel should appear to be professional, knowledgeable, and competent; they should not frighten patients. There are few physicians with strange haircuts or nurses who have pierced noses and pop bubble gum at the patient's bedside. It is just as important that the pharmacy technician show the public that he or she is professional and does not view the vocation as just a job. You show this directly and immediately by appearance and demeanor. Although some pharmacies do not have strict dress and appearance guidelines, most professionals want to project themselves as conscientious employees and dress appropriately.

Tech Note!

Each year pharmacy technicians celebrate their profession. National Pharmacy Technician Day is observed on the Tuesday within National Pharmacy Week, which is always the third week of October.

The Possibilities

Although it is impossible to foresee the future of any profession, there are clear indications regarding the direction a profession is taking. Reviewing the history of pharmacy, one can see a trend. The education requirements of pharmacists have increased from a bachelor of science degree in pharmacy (requiring 5 years of college) to a physician of pharmacy degree (requiring 6 years) because of the necessary skill level needed in today's pharmacy practice. The pharmacist's role is more clinically oriented, ranging from consulting patients to providing information services to medical staff. The roles of pharmacy technicians are changing as well. The technician's role has evolved from a clerk, cashier, and shelf-stocker to such specialties as a clinical technician, chemotherapy technician, nuclear medicine pharmacy technician, and inventory specialist technician. In addition to the change in duties are the changing guidelines that all states are researching to provide a base level of training for pharmacy technicians in the future.

DO YOU REMEMBER THESE KEY POINTS?

- The major pharmacy associations and their resources for technicians
- Nontraditional jobs that pharmacy technicians can perform
- Where technicians can find the current state requirements necessary to work as a pharmacy technician
- The differences between the functions of inpatient (hospital), outpatient (community), and home health pharmacies
- New expanding areas of pharmacy, such as mail order and E-pharmacy, that are incorporating pharmacy technicians
- Various duties that pharmacy technicians can perform under the supervision of a pharmacist
- The various competencies required of a pharmacy technician
- The importance of good communication skills and the protection of patient privacy
- The type of information that the Pharmacy Technician Certification Board includes when testing prospective pharmacy technicians
- The importance of national certification and the benefits for technicians
- The types of associations available to pharmacy technicians and their benefits
- The importance of submitting a well-written resume and how to search for job positions
- Additional degrees for pharmacy technicians that can lead them into other areas of pharmacy
- The requirements of national certification after passing the examination

REVIEW QUESTIONS

Multiple choice questions

1. The pharmacy association organized for technicians and managed solely by technicians is the:
   A. National Pharmacy Technician Association
   B. American Association of Pharmacy Technicians
   C. American Society of Health-System Pharmacists
   D. American Pharmacists Association

2. Certified technicians must meet which of the following Pharmacy Technician Certification Board standards?
   A. Continuing education
   B. State registration requirements
   C. Membership in a pharmacy association
   D. All of the above

3. All of the following statements are true concerning national certification EXCEPT:
   A. The PTCB exam may be taken after an appointment is made with a testing center
   B. Results are given to the tester immediately after the exam is finished
   C. The certification is good for 2 years
   D. Pharmacy technicians must take 10 CE units within 2 years for recertification

4. All of the following statements are true concerning pharmacy technicians in general EXCEPT:
   A. Dressing professionally can increase the chance of being hired
   B. Punctuality is important when working in pharmacy
   C. The pharmacy technician is expected to take the Pharmacy Technician Certification Board examination before employment
   D. Communication is an essential skill for pharmacy technicians

5. The following reasons to become involved in pharmacy organizations are true EXCEPT:
   A. For networking possibilities
   B. For new information on the future of pharmacy technicians
   C. To increase knowledge about new pharmaceuticals through continuing education
   D. For the tax deduction

6. Boards of pharmacy serve what function?
   A. Licensing and registration of pharmacists and technicians
   B. Writing and enforcing the rules and regulations of pharmacy practice
   C. Being an avenue for consumer complaints
   D. All of the above

7. All pharmacies in their respective states are overseen by:
   A. Each state's National Association of Boards of Pharmacy
   B. Each state's board of pharmacy
   C. Pharmacy managers
   D. Consumer advocacy groups

8. Nondiscretionary duties of a technician include all of the following EXCEPT:
   A. Requiring all work to be checked by a pharmacist
   B. Duties that do not require interpretation of reference materials
   C. Duties that assist the pharmacist in preparing and dispensing medication
   D. Counseling patients on all nonprescription medications

9. All of the following duties may be required of an inpatient technician EXCEPT:
   A. Supplying stock to emergency clinics
   B. Repackaging medications into unit dose packages
   C. Helping deliver medications to patient's homes
   D. Preparing chemotherapy medications

10. An important aspect of outpatient pharmacy is the need to keep a lesser amount of frequently used drugs on the shelf but in stock at all times. This is because of:
    A. The lack of shelf space
    B. The need to keep employee hours limited
    C. Changes in medication usage by physicians
    D. Both A and C

11. Most hospital jobs can be found via:
    A. Using the Internet
    B. Networking
    C. Reading the newspaper
    D. Applying in person

12. The most important aspect of landing a job would depend upon:
    A. Professional dress
    B. Experience
    C. Personality
    D. All of the above

13. Once nationally certified as a technician it is necessary to attain _____ CE units in law every 2 years.
    A. 1
    B. 2
    C. 3
    D. None of the above

14. A person's voice can influence how the information is perceived based on:
    A. Voice inflection
    B. Voice speed
    C. Voice tone
    D. Both A and C

15. Characteristics that may be required of a pharmacy technician include:
   A. Detail-oriented
   B. Professional attitude
   C. Quick learner
   D. All of the above

True/False

If the statement is false, then change it to make it true.

_____ **1.** The National Association of Boards of Pharmacy determines regulations in each state pertaining to technicians.

_____ **2.** Technicians currently hold the same positions that they have held historically.

_____ **3.** Most pharmacies that hire technicians require the same basic skills.

_____ **4.** Most companies that use pharmacy technicians outside of the pharmacy require a college degree.

_____ **5.** Most prescription orders filled in a hospital pharmacy are for 24 hours, whereas a community pharmacy fills the full length of the prescription order.

_____ **6.** Inpatient technicians assist inpatient pharmacists to monitor patients who are taking certain medications.

_____ **7.** Stat doses are to be delivered within 3 minutes.

_____ **8.** A technician giving advice to a nurse on the proper dosage to use for a patient is nonjudgmental.

_____ **9.** Most states require technicians to be certified.

_____ **10.** Certification renewal for a pharmacy technician requires 30 hours of continuing education per year.

_____ **11.** Pharmacy technicians are represented equally in all pharmacy associations.

_____ **12.** Joining an association can lead to a future job because of networking capabilities.

_____ **13.** APhA is one of the founders of PTCB, which certifies pharmacy technicians.

_____ **14.** All national certification exams are given electronically.

_____ **15.** Both national exams have the same number of questions.

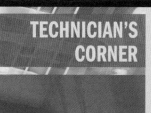

TECHNICIAN'S CORNER

Internet assignment: Log onto the Internet and visit the National Association of Boards of Pharmacy (www.nabp.org). List the board objectives, and find the listing for your state and another state of your choice. Visit the two BOP sites, and find the current requirements for technicians. Print your findings and submit them to your instructor. Write a 1-page summary on the differences between the two states as they pertain to the description of a pharmacy technician.

BIBLIOGRAPHY

Accreditation Council for Pharmacy Education www.acpe-accredit.org/ (Referenced 8/21/09)

American Society of Healthcare Pharmacists. Model Curriculum for Pharmacy Technician Training. (Referenced 8/21/09). www.ashp.org

Center for Drug Evaluation and Research. (Reference 8/19/09). www.fda.gov/cder

EruptinMind Self Improvement Tips website. Verbal communication skills. (Referenced 8/22/09). www.eruptingmind.com/verbal-communication-skills/

ExCPT. ICPT creates on-demand testing, the preferred method for certification exams. (Referenced 8/22/09). www.nationaltechexam.org/documents/On-demand-testing-090908.pdf

Franco M, et al. The National Association of Boards of Pharmacy (NABP). Moves to Next Phase of Technician Recognition and Regulation. May 27, 2009. www.ptcb.org/AM/Template.cfm?Section=Press_Releases1&TEMPLATE=/CM/ContentDisplay.cfm&CONTENTID=3444

Harteker LR: *The pharmacy technician companion*, Washington, DC, 1998, American Pharmacists Association.

Institute for the Certification of Pharmacy Technicians. Code of Ethics for Pharmacy Technicians. (Referenced 8/21/09). www.nationaltechexam.org/pdf/code-of-ethics.pdf

Koln LT, Corrigan JM, Donaldson MS: To err is human: building a safer health system. Retrieved March 2, 2003, from http://books.nap.edu/books/030906837/html/R1.html

Manual for pharmacy technicians, ed 3, Bethesda, Md, 2004, American Society of Health-System Pharmacists.

Nordenberg T: Make no mistake: medical errors can be deadly serious. FDA Consumer Sep-Oct 2000. Retrieved March 2, 2003, from www.fda.gov/fdac/features/2000/500_err.html

Phillips J: Generic name confusion. FDA Safety Page, Drug Topics 10-6-2003; 147:90

U.S. Food and Drug Administration. Website. Laws (Referenced 8/19/09) www.fda.gov

Western Career College curriculum, Sacramento, Calif, Western Career College.

White paper on pharmacy technicians 2002: "Needed changes can no longer wait. Am J Health-Syst Pharm; 2003; 60:37-51. Available at: www.acpe-accredit.org/pdf/whitePaper.pdf Accessed November 15, 2009.

Conversions and Calculations Used by Pharmacy Technicians

Objectives

UPON COMPLETING THIS CHAPTER, YOU SHOULD BE ABLE TO DO THE FOLLOWING:

- Describe the history of the International System of Units.

- Convert Arabic numbers into Roman numerals.

- Convert traditional time into military time.

- Employ mathematical calculations to determine dosage using:
  Multiplication/division
  Fractions
  Decimals
  Percentages
  Ratios

- Demonstrate the ability to convert between the various systems of measurement used in the practice of pharmacy:
  Apothecary system
  Avoirdupois system
  Metric system
  Common household measurements

- Calculate pediatric and geriatric dosages.

- Understand the process of dilution.

- Understand alligation.

- Calculate drip rates.

TERMS AND DEFINITIONS

Alligation *A mathematical method of solving problems that involves the mixing of solutions or mixtures of solids possessing different percentage weights*

Apothecary system *A system of measurement once used in the practice of pharmacy to measure both volume and weight; has been replaced by the metric system*

Avoirdupois system *A system of measurement previously used in pharmacy for the determination of weight in ounces and pounds; has been replaced by the metric system*

Diluent *An inert product, either liquid or solid, that is added to a preparation and reduces the strength of the original product*

Dilution *The process of adding a diluent or solvent to a compound, resulting in a product of increased volume or weight and lower concentration*

Household system *A system of measurement commonly used in the United States; measures volumes using household utensils*

International time *A 24-hour method of keeping time in which hours are not distinguished between AM and PM but are counted continuously through the entire day*

International System of Units (SI) *The prefixes for the modern metric system are taken from the French Système International d'Unités and were adopted to provide a single worldwide system of weights and measures. This system of measurement is based upon multiples of 10.*

Metric system *The approved system of measurement for pharmacy in the United States based on multiples of 10. The basic units of measurement are the gram (g) for weight, the liter (L) for volume, and the meter (m) for length.*

Solvent *An inert product, either liquid or solid, that is added to a preparation and reduces the strength of the original product*

Volume *The amount of liquid enclosed within a container*

Tech Note!

Although a pharmacist needs to check all transcriptions and calculations, it is important that the technician have a good understanding to avoid medication errors.

Introduction

The ability to manipulate conversions and make calculations is a requirement of pharmacy technicians. Unfortunately, in many cases when math is mentioned to new pharmacy technicians it can trigger instant stress by reminding students of previous bad experiences. However, the calculations performed in pharmacy are performed on a daily basis and applied to the drugs prepared in class and at work. The repetitiveness of these conversions and calculations reinforces one's knowledge. It is important to learn the basic conversions and feel comfortable with them.

This chapter describes the types of calculations used throughout history, explains Roman numerals and military time, and presents common math problems involving multiplication, division, fractions, decimals, percentages, and ratios. Other areas of focus in this chapter are the following:

- Ratio/proportion
- Metric system
- Household system
- Apothecary system

- Avoirdupois system
- Drip rates and drop factors
- Dilution
- Alligation
- Pediatric dosing using:
  - mg/kg/day and mg/kg/dose
  - mg/m^2/day and mg/m^2/dose

Calculations for infants, children, and senior citizens will also be discussed; these patient populations deserve special consideration because of the metabolic differences that exist before adolescence and after menopause. Medication dosing will be discussed for the following medications and therapies:

- Insulin
- Heparin
- Chemotherapy
- Parenteral and enteral nutrition

Make sure you understand each section before moving onto the next. Answers for all practice question and quizzes are located on Evolve.

History of Pharmacy

Pharmacy has a long history (see Chapter 1), and throughout its history various measurement systems were used. Many of these measurement systems are not converted precisely but are approximations. The pharmacy technician should have an understanding of these systems; however, in the United States, the *United States Pharmacopeia (USP)* recognizes the metric system as the official system of measurement for pharmacy. The metric system is based on multiples of 10 and is easy to remember; it will be discussed later in this chapter. As a technician, you may encounter prescriptions expressed in household, apothecary, or avoirdupois units.

A good way to become familiar with common pharmacy measurements is to start with what you know and then slowly build on that knowledge. For example, most persons are familiar with the **household** measurement of a teaspoon. In fact, most persons could gauge a teaspoonful by eye alone. Some doctors may prefer not to write instructions for 1 teaspoon when ordering a prescription; instead, you will see the measurement for 1 teaspoon in one of the other systems. The pharmacy technician must translate the doctor's orders into terms an average person can understand. You must make the instructions easy enough for a child to understand. Remember always to read what will be printed on the label to consider whether it will make sense to the patient. Do not assume that a person understands the meaning of 1 milliliter or 1 ounce. This will decrease the chance of any misreading of the instructions.

Roman Numerals

The number system commonly used in the United States is the Arabic system, consisting of the numbers 1, 2, 3, and so forth. This system is not always used by physicians when ordering medications. Instead, they may use Roman numerals to indicate the quantity of tablets or capsules, the number of fluid ounces, or the number of refills. Roman numerals may be either upper case or lower case. When using Roman numerals, begin with I to III; then write IV (1 less than 5) to equal 4. Repeat the process at 9 by writing IX (1 less than 10) to equal 9. In the same way, if you were to write 49, you would write IL (1 less than 50)

TABLE 4-1 Arabic and Roman Numerals

1	I	22	XXII
2	II	23	XXIII
3	III	24	XXIV
4	IV	25	XXV
5	V	26	XXVI
6	VI	27	XXVII
7	VII	28	XXVIII
8	VIII	29	XXIX
9	IX	30	XXX
10	X	40	XL
11	XI	50	L
12	XII	60	LX
13	XII	70	LXX
14	XIV	80	LXXX
15	XV	90	XC
16	XVI	100	C
17	XVII	500	D
18	XVIII	600	DC
19	XIX	700	DCC
20	XX	800	DCCC
21	XXI	900	CM
		1000	M

to equal 49. See Table 4-1 for a comparison of Roman numerals and Arabic numbers.

RULES FOR DETERMINING ROMAN NUMERALS

1. When a numeral is repeated, its value is repeated.
   Example: II = 2
2. A numeral may not be repeated more than 3 times.
   Example: XL = 40, not XXXX
3. V, L, and D are never repeated. LL is incorrect.
4. When a smaller numeral is placed before a larger numeral, it is subtracted from the larger numeral.
   Example: XC = 100 − 10 = 90
5. When a smaller numeral is placed after a larger numeral, it is added to the larger numeral.
   Example: CL = 100 + 50 = 150
6. V, L, and D are never subtracted. LC is incorrect.
7. Never subtract more than one numeral.
   Example: 8 = VIII, not IIX
8. When subtracting, only use a numeral before the next two higher-value numerals. For example, use I before V and X, X before L and C, and C before D and M.

EXAMPLE 4-1 WORKING WITH ROMAN NUMERALS

When working with Roman numerals, remember that if a larger number is placed in front of a smaller one, you must add both to determine the value.

$$X (10) + V (5) = XV (15)$$

However, if there is a smaller number placed before a larger number, then you must subtract.

$$X (10) - I (1) = IX (9)$$

EXERCISE 4-1 QUICK CHECK

Interpret the following:
1. XIV = _____
2. XC = _____
3. CIV = _____
4. XL = _____
5. VIII = _____
6. C = _____
7. IV = _____
8. LX = _____
9. IX = _____
10. XX = _____
11. XXIV = _____
12. LXXV = _____
13. XXXIX = _____
14. CXX = _____
15. VIIss— = _____

International Time (Military Time)

In a hospital or institutional setting, **international time**, also known as military time, is used exclusively. Orders are written 24 hours a day and a system is needed to ensure that all medical-related caretakers understand exactly when the order was written and when the medication or treatment is to take place. The system is based on 100. Starting with the first hour of the day, the clock begins at 0100 (1 AM) through 0000 (or midnight) (Figure 4-1). This system is easy for most persons to use through 1200 (noon), but then it can become confusing. As the clock hands begin to make their second trip around the face of the clock, the numbers continue. For example, 1300 is 1 PM, and 1400 is 2 PM. When the pharmacy receives orders, the receiver needs to check date and time against previous orders to ensure that the most recent order is in effect. By using this system, one never has any question as to when an order was written or which order supersedes another (Box 4-1).

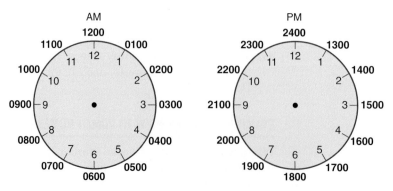

FIGURE 4-1 Military clock versus traditional clock.

BOX 4-1 TIME CONVERSIONS

Midnight (12:00 AM) = 0000 hr	12:00 PM = 1200 hr
1:00 AM = 0100 hr	1:00 PM = 1300 hr
2:00 AM = 0200 hr	2:00 PM = 1400 hr
3:00 AM = 0300 hr	3:00 PM = 1500 hr
4:00 AM = 0400 hr	4:00 PM = 1600 hr
5:00 AM = 0500 hr	5:00 PM = 1700 hr
6:00 AM = 0600 hr	6:00 PM = 1800 hr
7:00 AM = 0700 hr	7:00 PM = 1900 hr
8:00 AM = 0800 hr	8:00 PM = 2000 hr
9:00 AM = 0900 hr	9:00 PM = 2100 hr
10:00 AM = 1000 hr	10:00 PM = 2200 hr
11:00 AM = 1100 hr	11:00 PM = 2300 hr

EXERCISE 4-2 QUICK CHECK

Convert each time to either international or standard time:

1. 12:00 AM = _____
2. 4:30 PM = _____
3. 7:00 AM = _____
4. 1:30 AM = _____
5. 9:45 AM = _____
6. 11:11 AM = _____
7. 9:15 PM = _____
8. 2:30 PM = _____
9. 4:40 PM = _____
10. 2000 = _____
11. 1417 = _____
12. 2101 = _____
13. 2359 = _____
14. 0614 = _____
15. 1025 = _____

PRACTICE QUIZ #1 (ROMAN NUMERALS AND TIME)

Fill in the blanks:

1. From 0800 to 1500 hours is _____ hours.
2. A dose given at 0600, 1400, and 2200 hours is _____ hours apart.
3. A dose given at 0005, 1430, and 2045 would be given at _____, _____, and _____ on a 12-hour clock.
4. Write 4:20 PM, 7:15 PM, and 12:00 AM in international time: _____, _____, _____.
5. 0630 =
6. 1800 =
7. 2400 =
8. 0230 =
9. 0005 =
10. 4:20 PM =
11. 7 PM =
12. 5:40 PM =
13. 2:30 PM =
14. 9:20 PM =

15. VL =
16. CIX =
17. IX =
18. XXII =
19. VC =
20. 24 =
21. 59 =
22. 2011 =
23. 150 =
24. 55 =

Multiplication/Division

Multiplication is used constantly in performing pharmacy calculations (Table 4-2). Sometimes it is necessary to enlarge or reduce your recipe. Division is used to determine a part or portion of a recipe too. For the next math sets, use the multiplication and division tables for reference if necessary. However, you should memorize them before continuing.

EXERCISE 4-3 QUICK CHECK

Multiply the following numbers:
1. 12 × 9 =
2. 8 × 8 =
3. 6 × 9 =
4. 7 × 6 =
5. 4 × 9 =
6. 11 × 12 =
7. 12 × 7 =
8. 9 × 8 =
9. 5 × 6 =
10. 4 × 7 =

TABLE 4-2 Multiplication Chart

1	2	3	4	5	6	7	8	9	10	11	12
2	4	6	8	10	12	14	16	18	20	22	24
3	6	9	12	15	18	21	24	27	30	33	36
4	8	12	16	20	24	28	32	36	40	44	48
5	10	15	20	25	30	35	40	45	50	55	60
6	12	18	24	30	36	42	48	54	60	66	72
7	14	21	28	35	42	49	56	63	70	77	84
8	16	24	32	40	48	56	64	72	80	88	96
9	18	27	36	45	54	63	72	81	90	99	108
10	20	30	40	50	60	70	80	90	100	110	120
11	22	33	44	55	66	77	88	99	110	121	132
12	24	36	48	60	72	84	96	108	120	132	144

Fractions, Decimals, Percentages, Ratios, and Proportions

CONVERTING FRACTIONS TO DECIMALS

A fraction consists of a numerator and denominator: the numerator is the top number in a fraction and the denominator the bottom number. The numerator of a fraction shows the number of equivalent parts in the whole and the denominator shows how many are being considered. There are three types of fractions: proper, improper, and mixed. In a proper fraction, the numerator is smaller than the denominator while in an improper fraction the numerator is greater than or equal to the denominator. A mixed number consists of both a whole number and a proper fraction. Follow the steps outlined below for each type then complete the sets as indicated.

Proper	Improper	Mixed
$\frac{1}{2}$	$\frac{5}{2}$	$3\frac{1}{2}$

When fractions are converted they are represented in decimal form. An example of each type of fraction conversion is given.

To convert a proper fraction to a decimal:

$\frac{1}{2}$ [Divide the numerator (1) by the denominator (2)]

$$\frac{1}{2} = 0.5$$

To convert an improper fraction to a decimal:

$\frac{5}{2}$ [Divide the numerator (5) by the denominator (2)]

$$\frac{5}{2} = 2.5$$

To convert a mixed fraction to a decimal:

$3\frac{1}{2}$ [Convert into improper fraction ($3 \times 2 + 1 = 7$; or 7/2); then divide the numerator (7) by the denominator (2)]

$$\frac{7}{2} = 3.5$$

EXERCISE 4-4 **QUICK CHECK**

Convert the following fractions to decimals:

1. $\frac{1}{2}$ =
2. $5\frac{10}{9}$ =
3. $8\frac{11}{7}$ =
4. $\frac{3}{4}$ =
5. $\frac{9}{7}$ =
6. $4\frac{5}{8}$ =
7. $\frac{7}{8}$ =
8. $2\frac{1}{2}$ =
9. $2\frac{1}{3}$ =
10. $\frac{22}{48}$ =
11. $1\frac{1}{8}$ =
12. $\frac{3}{2}$ =
13. $\frac{2}{12}$ =
14. $\frac{5}{20}$ =
15. $\frac{9}{5}$ =

CONVERTING FRACTIONS TO PERCENTAGES

Fractions can be expressed as percentages because both fractions and percentages are expressions of a part of a whole. We will begin with an easy one, such as ½. Simple division is used. Take the numerator and divide it by the denominator, that is, 1 divided by 2. Because 100 is used to represent the whole, carry out the division to a minimum of three spaces to the right of the decimal point. For example, ⅓ converts into 0.33333333 ...; this would be reduced to 0.333 in order to get the closest rounded number when performing calculations. When rounding a number you must determine to what whole number or decimal place the number is to be rounded. You must look at the number to the right of the value being rounded. If that number is a 0, 1, 2, 3, or 4, the value remains the same in that column. If the value to the right of the column to be rounded is 5 or greater, you add 1 to the column being rounded and change all the values to the right of this new number to zero. In this chapter, we will be rounding numbers to the nearest hundredth.

$$\frac{1}{2} = 0.5$$

CONVERTING RATIOS TO PERCENTAGES

A ratio is an expression that compares two quantities or measurements. A ratio is sometimes defined as the quotient of two like numbers. These measurements may be expressed with the same type of units. A ratio expresses a relationship between two numbers. The following expression is written as a ratio: 1:2, which is read "one is to two." A ratio can be written as a fraction where the first number is the numerator and the second number is the denominator. In the previous example, the ratio 1:2 can be written as the fraction ½. Once the ratio is expressed as a fraction, it can then be converted to both a decimal and a percentage. All rules governing common fractions apply to a ratio. If two ratios have the same value, they are considered equivalent.

CONVERTING DECIMALS TO PERCENTAGES

The term percent and its corresponding sign (%) mean "in a hundred." Percentages represent a portion of a whole. The number 100 is used to represent the whole; therefore 100% equals the whole. This whole could be anything—a pie, a cup of water, or a 1-L intravenous solution. If 100% is a whole, what is one half of a whole, two tenths of a whole, or six thousandths of a whole?

To convert a fraction to a percent, divide the numerator by the denominator and multiply by 100, which results in the decimal point moving two spaces to the right; then add a percent sign (%). Each decimal place represents "10"; therefore if you have the number 10,000 and you move the decimal point one place to the left, you will decrease the number to 1,000 or 10 times less than the original number. Likewise, if you move the decimal point to the right by one place, you increase the number by 10 times, to 100,000.

$$0.5 \times 100\% = 50\%$$

Percentages are used in the pharmacy to identify the strength or concentration of a medication, to perform dilution problems, and to calculate the markup on prices, payment discounts, net profits, and gross profits. Both the Pharmacy Technician Certification Board (PTCB) exam and the Exam for the Certification of Pharmacy Technicians (ExCPT) contain math problems using percentages.

EXERCISE 4-5 **QUICK CHECK**

Calculate the dollar amount by using the following percentages:
1. $200.00 = _____ (25%) _____ (50%) _____ (75%)
2. $956.00 = _____ (15%) _____ (55%) _____ (85%)
3. $2050.00 = _____ (20%) _____ (40%) _____ (60%)
4. 10,449.00 = _____ (2.5%) _____ (5.5%) _____ (7.5%)
5. The following products are on sale for 15% off the regular price. Determine the total amount of savings to the customer:
   Tylenol 325 mg tablets #100 @ $5.50
   Benadryl 25 mg capsules #50 @ $4.25
6. 62% of a $2,100.00 bill will be given as a discount if paid before the 15th of the month. What is the savings to the pharmacy if paid early?
7. 75% of a $12,000.00 bill will be given as a discount from the manufacturer if paid within 5 days. What is the savings to the pharmacy if paid early?
8. These products are on sale for 20% off the regular price. Calculate the total amount of savings to the customer:
   Milk of Magnesia 4 oz ($3.25)
   Pepcid AC 10 mg tablets ($10.95)
   Motrin suspension 120 mL ($6.50)
   Vitamin C 250 mg tablets #100 ($2.95)

RATIOS/PROPORTIONS

A ratio is a relationship between two parts of a whole or between one part and the whole. A ratio can be written either as 1/2 or as 1:2. When technicians compound certain products, they may be required to solve problems using ratios, which can be considered parts or fractions. For example, a concentration of 1:1000 means there is 1 part to 1000 parts, or 1 gram (g) of drug dissolved in 1000 mL of solution. If you have 25 g of drug dissolved in 100 mL of solution, this can be written as the ratio 25:100, which can be reduced to 1:4.

A proportion is a relationship between two ratios. A proportion may be written as 1/2 = 2/4 or 1:2 : 2:4. The majority of all pharmaceutical calculations performed in either retail or institutional settings can be accomplished by using proportion. There are two ways to solve proportion problems. The first involves cross multiplying and dividing, while the second method is described as "means and extremes." Both methods will yield the same answer if set up correctly.

One of the first things to remember is to dismiss the unnecessary information. Second, find what strength you have in stock and what strength you need (what the doctor is ordering). Next, set up the equation and double-check the calculations. It is important to remember to place the correct units into the correct position. For example, if one side of the equation has milligrams divided by milliliters then the opposite side of the equation must be expressed as milligrams divided by milliliters. The following drug label examples are provided for interpretation and to aid in calculations.

EXAMPLE 4-2

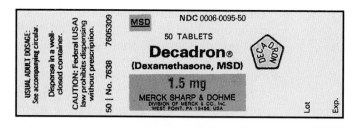

You receive an order for erythromycin suspension 125 mg to be taken 3 times a day for 10 days. How many milliliters (mL) do you need to fill this order?

You have 200 mg/5 mL.

You need 125 mg to be taken 3 times per day for 10 days.

You need to solve for milliliters needed.

Set up your equation:

$$\text{Have} = \text{Need}$$
$$200 \text{ mg}/5 \text{ mL} = 125 \text{ mg}/x$$
$$5 \times 125 = 625/200 = 3.125 \text{ mL per dose}$$
$$3 \times 3.125 = 9.375 \text{ mL per day}$$
$$10 \text{ (days)} \times 9.375 \text{ mL} = 93.75 \text{ mL}$$

EXAMPLE 4-3

Tech Note!

Remember: You must place the proper units (such as mL, L, mg, or g) next to the number amount. This cannot be stressed enough, because you may be working with various systems of measurement. Including the units on all numbers can help reduce mistakes.

You receive an order for Decadron 3 mg twice daily for 30 days. How many tablets do you need to fill this order?

You have 1.5-mg tablets.

You need 3 mg to be taken 2 times a day for 30 days.

You need to solve for the total amount of tablets needed for the month.

Set up your equation:

$$\text{Have} = \text{Need}$$
$$1.5 \text{ mg/tablet} = 3 \text{ mg}/x \text{ tablets}$$
$$1 \text{ tablet} \times 3 \text{ mg} = 3/1.5 \text{ mg} = 2 \text{ tablets are needed}$$
$$2 \text{ tablets/dose} \times 2 \text{ (doses per day)} = 4 \text{ tablets per day}$$
$$4 \times 30 = 120 \text{ tablets total}$$

Solve the following proportions:
1. 2/10 = 4/x
2. 4/40 = x/100
3. 55/82 = 35/x
4. 250/500 = 750/x
5. 1/25 = 40/x

OTHER EXAMPLES OF PROPORTION PROBLEMS

EXAMPLE 4-4

Prepare 240 mg of gentamicin IVPB (intravenous piggyback) using the pharmacy stock concentration of 40 mg/mL bid.

In this case, you need to determine how many milliliters of the stock solution are needed to fill the 240-mg order. Write your stock strength or given concentration on the left and the needed amount on the right. Make sure that milligrams are in the numerator and milliliters are in the denominator. Then cross multiply by the quantity on the side of the x and divide by the numerator of your concentration; this will give you the necessary milliliters to draw from the vial.

$$240 \text{ mg}/1 \text{ mL} = 40 \text{ mg}/x \text{ mL}$$
$$240 = 40x$$

Divide both sides by 40:

$$6 \text{ mL} = x$$

Answer: You will need to withdraw 12 mL of solution to equal 240 mg of drug for a dose given twice daily.

EXAMPLE 4-5

You receive an order for clindamycin 450 mg IVPB q12h. To set up your equation, you need to know what you have on hand or in stock. Clindamycin is available in different volumes, but all of the volumes have the same concentration (strength). The strength for clindamycin is 150 mg/mL. For each milliliter in the vial, there is 150 mg of drug (clindamycin). We now have all the components we need to begin.

You are solving for x because you do not know how much clindamycin to draw up into a syringe. To solve for x, you *cross multiply and divide.*

$$150 \text{ mg}/\text{mL} = 450 \text{ mg}/x$$
$$150x = 450$$
$$x = 3 \text{ mL}$$

EXAMPLE 4-6

You receive an order for erythromycin 200 mg/5 mL suspension. Give 100 mg q6h × 10 days.

1. How many milliliters of suspension will be given per dose?
2. How many milliliters of suspension will be given per day?

3. How many milliliters of suspension will be given over the course of the treatment?
4. How much suspension will be discarded, if any?

To solve, do the following:
You have on hand a 200-mL container of 200 mg/5 mL. You need 100 mg/*x* mL (*x* mL = the volume).

Answer to question 1

$$x = 2.5 \text{ mL per dose}$$

Answer to question 2
Multiply the dose by times per day.

$$2.5 \text{ mL per dose} \times 4 \text{ doses/day} = 10 \text{ mL/day}$$

Answer to question 3
This requires a straight multiplication to get the answer.

$$10 \text{ mL (per day)} \times 10 \text{ (amount of days)} = 100 \text{ mL over 10 days}$$

Answer to question 4
This requires subtraction of the total volume minus the used portion.

$$\text{Erythromycin suspension } 200 \text{ mL} - 100 \text{ mL} = 100 \text{ mL that will be discarded by the patient}$$

★ Tech Note!

Always pay attention to the dosage form. If you have a capsule, you cannot take one and a half capsules, but you can take a scored tablet, which is a tablet that is marked so that it can be split into equal parts. Also remember that not all tablets can be split, such as sustained-release tablets.

EXAMPLE 4-7

You need to fill cimetidine 600 mg tid (3 times a day) for 30 days.
    You have 400-mg tablets.
    How many 400-mg tablets will you need to fill this order?
    To solve, do the following:

$$600 \text{ mg} \times 3 \text{ doses} = 1800 \text{ mg per day}$$
$$4.5 \text{ tablets (per day)} \times 30\text{-day supply} = 135 \text{ tablets to fill this order}$$

Directions: The label would read as follows:
Take 1 & ½ tablets 3 times daily for 30 days.

EXAMPLE OF PROPORTIONS IN COMPOUNDING

Order: You need to prepare 1 pint (pt) of 40 g of medicated lotion. How many milliliters of the stock solution (5 g/mL) will it take to prepare the final product? Write your stock or given concentration on the left and your volume needed on the right. Make sure your milligrams and milliliters match across from one another. Do not forget to cross multiply and divide by the quantity on the side of the *x*, and you will have your necessary volume to draw from the container.

$$40 \text{ g} \div 5 \text{ g} = x$$
$$x = 8 \text{ mL of medicated solution}$$

Answer: You need a total volume of 8 mL of drug mixed into the lotion to equal 1 pt, and 1 pt (30 mL/oz × 16 oz/pt) = 480 mL. Therefore you subtract the amount of drug to be added from the total volume:

$$480 \text{ mL} - 8 \text{ mL} = 472 \text{ mL}$$

Answer: You will add 8 g of drug to 472 mL of lotion to get a 40-g medicated bottle of lotion.

Working with Word Problems

Many pharmacy technicians experience difficulty interpreting word problems that require calculations to be performed. Equations are not given to you and therefore you must set up the calculation from the information given to you. One way in which you can lessen the confusion of a word problem is by asking yourself what is known and what is being asked. Sometimes there is extra information that is not necessary and can be ignored; other times a problem must be calculated in a specific order, or there may be more than one step that needs to be performed. For example, let us decipher the following word problem:

> Jane, the inventory tech, was calculating the totals for the day after the pharmacy closed. She calculated $3,409.23 as the total income for the day, with $872.00 in cash; the rest of the income consisted of charges from either debit or credit cards. The pharmacy has an outstanding bill of $8,345.00 with a drug vendor. The vendor requires a minimum payment of 5% of the outstanding bill each month.

> If the pharmacy makes their payment from today's total income, what dollar amount will be paid and how much will Jane take to the bank? What will be the pharmacy's required payment next month?

The $872.00 in cash can be ignored because it has nothing to do with the amount due. The only questions that need to be answered are the following: What is 5% of the bill? How much is left over for the deposit? How much money will be due next month? Let us answer each one in the following order:

- First: Change 5% into a decimal by dividing by 100; $5 \div 100 = 0.05$.

  Determine the amount due by multiplying $0.05 \times \$8345.00 = \$417.25$ due to the vendor

- Second: Subtract the amount to be paid from today's total for the amount to be deposited.

  $$\$8345.00 - \$417.25 = \$7,927.75 \text{ will be deposited by Jane}$$

- Lastly: Next month 5% of the balance of the bill will be due.

  0.05% of $\$7,927.75 = \$396.39$ will be due next month

EXAMPLE 4-8

An invoice from the supplier claims the pharmacy will receive a 1.5% discount if the invoice is paid within 10 days, but the entire amount is due within 30 days. How is the discount determined? Let us solve this problem:

To begin, we will say the amount due is $500.00.

Convert the percentage 1.5% into a decimal; $1.5 \div 100 = 0.015$

Multiply the amount due: $\$500.00$ by $0.015 = \$7.50$

Subtract this discount from the $\$500.00 - \$7.50 = \$492.50$

(this is the amount due if paid within 10 days)

EXAMPLE 4-9

If the amount due is $744.00 within 30 days and the supplier will allow a 0.5% discount if paid within 7 days, how much will be due with the discount?

Convert the percentage into a decimal by dividing by 100; $0.5 \div 100 = 0.005$

Multiply the amount due; $744.00 by $0.005 = \$3.72$ (less)

Subtract $3.72 from $744.00 to determine the final amount due of $740.28

For example, you are responsible for figuring out how much your community pharmacy can save on invoices if they are paid quickly. The total amount of an invoice is $3500.00 and the pharmacy is to receive a 2.5% discount. Calculating the discount requires two steps. First, convert the percentage to a decimal. Second, multiply the invoice total and the decimal number to obtain the discount. First, convert 2.5% to a decimal:

$$2.5\% \div 100 = 0.025$$

Now multiply the decimal and the invoice total:

$$\$3500.00 \times 0.025 = \$87.50$$

The discount would be $87.50. It does not sound like a big discount, but remember that this is only one invoice. A pharmacy could save thousands of dollars a year just by paying the invoices quickly.

Another use of percentages is to calculate the markup necessary so the pharmacy can make a profit. Remember, the pharmacy has to make a profit so that it can pay you, pay for rent and utilities, and provide the owner with a profit. Let us do a few practice exercises on how to determine markup.

The pharmacy must increase the costs of all cold medicines by 56% to make a profit. The following is an example of three different products at different prices: Determine the markup of each product and then calculate the total cost of the product.

Daytime cold and cough liquid, $4.25: $4.25 \times 0.56 = \$2.38$ (markup)

Total cost of this medication would be $4.25 + \$2.38 = \$6.63$

Tylenol cold and cough liquid, $5.50: $5.50 \times 0.56 = \$3.08$ (markup)

Total cost of this medication would be $5.50 + \$3.08 = \$8.58$

Pseudoephedrine tablets, $2.95: $2.95 \times 0.56 = \$1.65$ (markup)

Total cost of this medication would be $2.95 + \$1.65 = \$4.60$

EXERCISE 4-7 **QUICK CHECK**

1. You receive an order for erythromycin 1.5-g dose stat to the hospital floor. You have 500-mg tablets in stock. How many 500-mg tablets will you need to fill this order? How many would you need for three doses?

2. Order 1: metoprolol tartrate 100-mg tablet twice a day for 30 days. You have 50-mg tablets. How many tablets will it take to fill this 30-day supply?

3. Order 2: ranitidine 75 mg of syrup at bedtime. You have 1 pt of a 15 mg/mL bottle available. How many milliliters will it take to fill a 30-day supply? Do you have enough?

Determine 1 Dose

4. Stock: 250 mg tabs; dose 125 mg; give _____ tabs

5. Stock: gr X tabs; dose 325 mg; give _____ tabs

6. Stock: 1 g tabs; dose 500 mg; give _____ tabs
7. Stock: 10 mg/mL; dose 25 mg; give _____ L
8. Stock: 10 mg/mL; dose 3000 mcg; give _____ mL
9. Stock: 100 units/10 mL; dose 25 units; give _____ mL
10. Stock: 25,000 units/2 mL; dose 20,000; give _____ mL
11. Stock: 40 mg/mL; dose 25 mg; give _____ mL
12. Stock: 3.375 g; dose 6.75 g; give _____ mL
13. Stock: gr $\frac{1}{400}$ SL tab; dose 0.2 mg; give _____ SL tabs
14. Stock: 125 mcg tab; dose 3 bid = _____ mg
15. Stock: gr VIII caps; dose 2 caps = _____ mg
16. Stock: 500 mg tab; dose 4 tabs = _____ g
17. Stock: 1.5 g/mL; dose 600 mg = _____ mL
18. Stock: 25 mg/mL; dose 0.5 g = _____ mL
19. Stock: 50,000 units/mL; dose 0.25 mL = _____ units
20. Stock: 75 mcg/cap; dose 3 caps = _____ mg

PRACTICE QUIZ #2 (DECIMALS, FRACTIONS, PERCENTAGES)

Convert the following percents to decimals.

1. 50% = _____
2. 12% = _____
3. 175% = _____
4. 2.5% = _____
5. 33% = _____

Convert the following fractions to percents.

6. 1/8 = _____ %
7. 5/2 = _____ %
8. 3/4 = _____ %
9. 4/10 = _____ %
10. 2/3 = _____ %

11. Your drug wholesaler will give you a discount of 2% if paid within 1 week; calculate the final bill if the amount due is $6,544.00
12. Your pharmacy is having a big sale on all first aid supplies; take 20% off the following purchase and total the bill.
Tylenol cold and cough, $8.95
Bayer aspirin, $1.95
Pepcid antacid, $18.00
Vicks Formula 44, $2.95
Imodium chewable tablets, $8.50
13. Your pharmacy received an order that contained 144 bottles; 25% of the bottles that were shipped to the pharmacy were damaged. How many damaged bottles are being returned?
14. All new prescriptions are being given a 15% discount to the customer. What is the dollar amount lost by the pharmacy if all the new prescriptions for the day added up to $2,339.00?
15. Your pharmacy is giving a 12.5% discount on all vitamins and the manufacturer is giving a 5% discount to the pharmacy for all vitamins sold. If you sell $865.00 in vitamins over the weekend, how much will the pharmacy lose after the 5% manufacturer's discount?

Metric System

The *United States Pharmacopeia (USP)* has established the **international system of units** (SI), or, metric system as the official system of measurement for pharmacy in the United States. The metric system can be used to measure

TABLE 4-3 Metric Prefixes

Prefix	Meaning
nano-	One-billionth of the basic unit
micro-	One-millionth of the basic unit
milli-	One-thousandth of the basic unit
centi-	One-hundredth of the basic unit
deci-	One-tenth of the basic unit
deka-	10 times the basic unit
hecto-	100 times the basic unit
kilo-	1000 times the basic unit

Tech Alert!

One of the most common errors made in pharmacy is the improper use of the decimal point. Doctors who write medication orders without using a leading zero (for example, .5 g) risk the order being mistaken for 5 g. A leading zero clarifies that the value is less than 1 and will help reduce pharmacy errors (for example, 0.5 g). Always seek clarification of an order when it seems that the dose is extremely high or low. When the pharmacy technician performs calculations, he or she must use leading zeros if the number is less than 1. Certain medications given in wrong strengths can harm or even kill the patient. See the examples below. For more information on drug errors, see Chapter 14.

Wrong way	.1 mg could be mistaken for 1 mg
Right way	0.1 mg very clear because of leading zero
Wrong way	25.0 mg could be mistaken for 250 mg
Right way	25 mg very clear because of lack of decimals or zeros

weight, volume, and distance. The basic unit of measurement for weight is the gram (g); the liter (L) is the basic unit of measurement for volume, and the meter (m) is the basic unit of measurement for length. A pharmacy technician needs to memorize the prefixes used in the metric system (refer to Table 4-3). In the metric system, each unit of measurement is a multiple of 10. In other words, to go from a larger unit of measurement to a smaller unit of measurement, you would multiply by a multiple of 10. On the other hand, if you were converting from a smaller unit of measurement to a larger unit of measurement, you would divide by a multiple of 10. A technician must know the difference between the various units used in the metric system. For example, if a prescription was filled with 1 g of drug when only 1 mg was ordered, the patient would overdose by 1000 times the ordered dose. A 1000-unit difference exists between each measurement. This means that 1000 micrograms (mcg) equals 1 mg.

METRIC MEASUREMENTS

1. The more commonly used measurements of weight in the metric system include the microgram (mcg), the milligram (mg), the gram (g), and the kilogram (kg).
2. When measuring volumes, a pharmacy technician will see both milliliters (mL) and liters (L). There are some physicians who may use cubic centimeter (cc) as a volume; 1 cubic centimeter (cc) is equal to 1 milliliter (mL).

1 mL = 1 cc

* cc is not commonly used anymore per the ISMP guidelines (see Chapter 14) as it can be confused with 00 when written by hand.
3. The use of millimeters is reserved for drug calculations that are based on body surface areas and would be calculated by a physician or pharmacist using a surface area calculation chart.

The metric system can be easily converted into household liquid measurements, which will be discussed next.

EXERCISE 4-8 QUICK CHECK

Solve the following problems using the appropriate conversions:
1. You receive a doctor's order for 0.88 mcg of drug A.
   What is the equivalent in milligrams?
2. You receive a doctor's order for 5 g of drug B.
   What is the equivalent in kilograms?
3. You receive an order for 250 mg of drug C.
   What is the equivalent in micrograms?

TABLE 4-4 Metric-Household Conversion Measurements

Metric (Volume)	Household Equivalent
5 mL	1 teaspoon (tsp)
15 mL	3 tsp or 1 tablespoon (Tbsp)
30 mL	6 tsp or 2 Tbsp or 1 fluid ounce (fl oz)
240 mL	48 tsp or 16 Tbsp or 8 fl oz or 1 cup
480 mL	96 tsp or 32 Tbsp or 16 fl oz or 2 cups or 1 pint (pt)
960 mL	192 tsp or 64 Tbsp or 32 fl oz or 4 cups or 2 pt or 1 quart (qt)
3840 mL	768 tsp or 256 Tbsp or 128 fl oz or 16 cups or 8 pt or 4 qt or 1 gallon

4. You receive a doctor's order for 250 mg of drug D. What is the equivalent in grams?
5. You receive a doctor's order to prepare 0.5 kg of drug E. What is the equivalent in grams?

Household Measurements

Other common measurements include tablespoons and cups. Conversions for household measurements are listed in Table 4-4.

EXAMPLE 4-10

How many milliliters are in 2 tablespoons?
We know there are 5 mL per teaspoon and 3 teaspoons in 1 tablespoon.

$$5 \text{ mL} \times 3 \text{ teaspoons} = 15 \text{ mL}$$
$$2 \text{ tablespoons} \times 15 \text{ mL} = 30 \text{ mL}$$

EXAMPLE 4-11

How many milliliters are in 5 ounces (oz)?
We know there are 30 mL per ounce.

$$30 \text{ mL} \times 5 \text{ oz} = 150 \text{ mL}$$

EXAMPLE 4-12

How many ounces in ½ cup and how many mLs is this?
We know there are 8 ounces to a cup.

$$\frac{1}{2} \times 8 \text{ oz} = 4 \text{ oz}$$

We know there are 30 mL per ounce.

$$4 \text{ oz} \times 30 \text{ mL} = 120 \text{ mL}$$

 Tech Note!

If you have measuring cups and spoons in your kitchen, pull them out and convert them into milliliters and ounces.

EXERCISE 4-9 QUICK CHECK

1. 3 teaspoons = _____ tablespoons = _____ mL
2. 1 ounce = _____ tablespoons = _____ mL
3. 1 cup = _____ ounces = _____ mL

4. 1 pint = _____ tablespoons = _____ mL
5. 1 quart = _____ pints = _____ mL
6. 1 gallon = _____ teaspoons = _____ mL
7. 40 ounces = _____ tablespoons = _____ mL
8. 32 ounces = _____ cups = _____ mL
9. 2 pints = _____ ounces = _____ mL
10. 3 quarts = _____ teaspoons = _____ mL
11. 1 quart = _____ teaspoons = _____ mL
12. 1 pint = _____ ounces = _____ teaspoons = _____ mL
13. 1 quart = _____ ounces = _____ teaspoons = _____ mL
14. 1 gallon = _____ quarts = _____ pints = _____ tablespoons = _____ mL
15. ½ gallon = _____ tablespoons = _____ teaspoons = _____ mL

Apothecary System

The **apothecary system** originated in Europe, where it was used extensively by physicians and apothecaries for medical recipes. The apothecary system of measurement is the traditional system of pharmacy; although it is now largely of historic significance, some components of this system may still be found on some prescriptions, although it is rare. The units used in this system include grain (gr), scruple* (℈), dram (ʒ), ounce, and pound for dry weight; and fluid ounce (℥), dram, and minim (♏) for volume. When using the apothecary system, place the unit of measurement before the amount; for example, 1 gr is written gr i. How do you write ½ gr? Historically the most common way was gr s̄s̄ (s̄s̄ means ½). However, now that s̄s̄ is indicated as a potentially dangerous abbreviation on the ISMP list, you should write out gr ½ daily.

The most common pharmacy units are converted into metric and household measurements (see Table 4-4). Be sure to learn these conversions before continuing. See Figure 4-2 for examples of conversions between household, metric, and apothecary systems in medication cups.

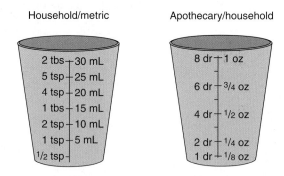

One-ounce medicine cups (30 mL)

FIGURE 4-2 Oral cups show equivalent volumes between household to metric and household to apothecary units. (From Gray Morris D: *Calculate with confidence*, ed 4, St Louis, 2008, Elsevier.)

*Scruples are not used anymore in pharmacy, although it is part of the apothecary system.

EXAMPLE 4-13

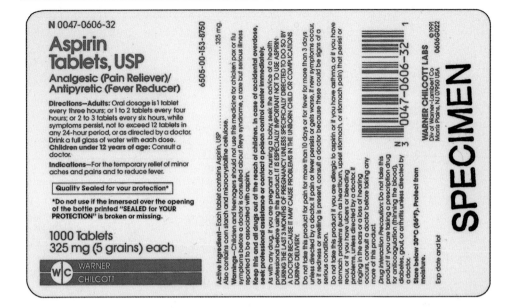

Using 65 mg/grain

How many grains are in 325 mg of aspirin?

$$65 \text{ mg}/1 \text{ grain} = 325 \text{ mg}/x$$

$$1 \times 325 \text{ mg} = 325 \text{ mg}/65 \text{ mg} = 5 \text{ grains or gr V}$$

EXAMPLE 4-14

Using 65 mg/grain

How many milligrams are in gr $\frac{1}{150}$ of nitroglycerin sublingual (SL) tablets?

$$\frac{1}{150} = 0.006666$$

$$0.005 \text{ gr} \times 65 \text{ mg} = 0.325 \text{ mg}$$

EXERCISE 4-10 QUICK CHECK

Solve the following conversions (use 65 mg/grain):

1. $\frac{1}{150}$ gr = _____ mg
2. $\frac{1}{9}$ gr = _____ mg
3. $\frac{1}{200}$ gr = _____ mg
4. $\frac{1}{2}$ gr = _____ mg
5. $\frac{5}{120}$ gr = _____ mg
6. 500 mg = _____ gr
7. 325 mg = _____ gr
8. 120 mg = _____ gr
9. 1500 mg = _____ gr
10. 130 mg = _____ gr

Tech Note!

The weight of a grain in the apothecary system may vary between 60 mg, 64.8 mg, and 65 mg. Why? When the grain was used in ancient times to determine weight, real grains of wheat were used, and the weight depended on that year's harvest. If the crop was good, then it took fewer grains because each piece weighed more. If the crops were bad that year, then it may have taken more grains to equal the same weight. Therefore be aware that some medication labels will state that there is 60 mg/gr, whereas others might have 64.8 mg/gr or even 65 mg/gr. However, when performing calculations, the use of 60 mg/gr or 65 mg/gr is preferred.

TABLE 4-5 Standard Weights and Volumes: Avoirdupois/Metric*

Avoirdupois	Metric Equivalent
Dry Weights	
1 lb	454 g
1 oz	30 g
1 gr	64.8 mg
Liquids	
1 fl oz	30 mL
1 pt	473 mL
1 gal	3785 mL

*Conversions: 60 minims (℞) = 1 fluidrachm or fluid dram (··); 8 fluidrachms (480 minims) = 1 fluid ounce (ʒ); 16 fl oz = 1 pint (pt); 2 pt (32 fl oz) = 1 quart (qt); 4 qt (8 pt) = 1 gallon (gal).

EXERCISE 4-11 **QUICK CHECK**

Solve the following conversions:
1. ½ lb = _____ oz
2. 1 Tbsp = _____ drams
3. ¼ lb = _____ oz
4. ¹⁄₂₅₀ gr = _____ mg
5. 7 drams = _____ mL
6. 65 mg = _____ gr
7. 100 mg = _____ gr
8. 120 mg = _____ gr
9. 1.3 gr xxivss— = _____ mg
10. 1 oz = _____ drams

Avoirdupois System

The **avoirdupois system** is another type of measurement that originated in England. The avoirdupois is the common system of commerce. It is through the avoirdupois that items are purchased and sold by the ounce and pound. The avoirdupois system is similar to the apothecary system because it also uses grains, ounces, and pounds for weights. Table 4-5 shows the common avoirdupois weights and volumes.

AVOIRDUPOIS MEASUREMENTS

1. Dry weights use pounds (lb), ounces (oz), and grains (gr).
2. Liquid volumes use fluid ounces (fl oz), pints (pt), and gallons (gal).

EXERCISE 4-12 **QUICK CHECK**

Volumes
1. 1 fl dram = _____ mL
2. 8 oz = _____ cup(s) or _____ mL
3. 1 gal = _____ cup(s) or _____ mL
4. 5 mL = _____ tsp
5. 30 mL = _____ tsp or _____ Tbsp

Weights
6. 1 gr = _____ mg
7. 1 kg = _____ g or _____ mg
8. gr viiiss— = _____
9. 1000 mcg = _____ mg
10. 1 g = _____ mg

PRACTICE QUIZ #3

1. 5 mL = _____ tsp
2. 15 mL = _____ Tbsp
3. 30 mL = _____ tsp
4. 1 dram = _____ mL
5. 1 L = _____ mL
6. 454 g = _____ lb
7. 4.4 lb = _____ kg
8. 3000 mcg = _____ mg
9. 450 g = _____ mg
10. 25 kg = _____ mg
11. 50 mL = _____ tsp
12. 1.5 L = _____ mL
13. 3 lb = _____ kg
14. 25 lb = _____ oz
15. 2.25 mcg = _____ mg
16. 240 mL = _____ oz
17. 2 pints = _____ quarts
18. 1 gallon = _____ pints
19. ¼ L = _____ mL
20. 500 mL = _____ L
21. gr i = _____ mg
22. gr ¹⁄₁₅₀ = _____ mg
23. 30 g = _____ gr
24. 2% HC cream = _____ g
25. 9000 mg = _____ g
26. 0900 = _____
27. 2110 = _____
28. 1320 = _____
29. 2350 = _____
30. 2:30 PM = _____
31. 1100 AM = _____
32. 9:25 PM = _____
33. 4:10 AM = _____
34. 6 PM = _____
35. ix = _____
36. viii = _____
37. LX = _____
38. IV = _____
39. XC = _____
40. XXX = _____

Important Differences among Systems

You should know how metric system units vary from other units of measure such as ounces and grains. Most of the time they convert easily, but sometimes there are variances, making conversions between measurement systems approximate in these instances. Because the metric system is the approved system of measurement used in pharmacies, it is the measurement system you should use when preparing a compounded drug. However, you will see differences among manufacturers' products and their weights. For example, some manufacturers consider 473 mL to equal a pint, whereas others consider 480 mL to equal a pint. The rule is to follow the metric system because it is the approved system of measurement for pharmacy in the United States. Refer to Table 4-6 for a comparison of measurements between the apothecary, metric, and household systems of measurement.

TABLE 4-6 Apothecary/Metric/Household Conversions

Apothecary volume	Apothecary weight	Metric volume	Metric weight	Common household
1	1	30 mL	30 g	2 Tbsp
4	4	15 mL	15 g	1 Tbsp
2	2	7.5 mL	7.5 g	½ Tbsp
1	gr 60	4 mL	4 g	1 Tbsp
½	gr 30	2 mL	2 g	½ Tbsp

BOX 4-2 TIME SCHEDULE (PHARMACY ABBREVIATIONS)

bid = 2 times daily
q12h = every 12 hours
tid = 3 times daily
q8h = every 8 hours
qid = 4 times daily
q6h = every 6 hours

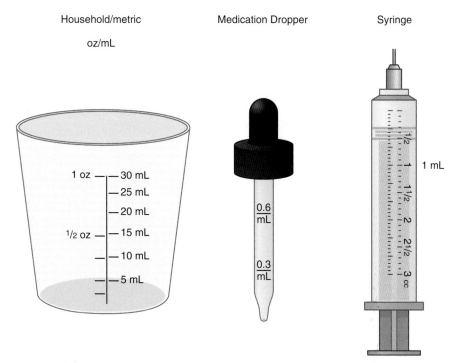

FIGURE 4-3 Common devices used for measuring liquid medications.

For the following examples, the orders will be written in standard abbreviations that indicate the frequency a medication is to be given. Refer to Box 4-2.

Oral Syringes and Injections

When filling prescription orders for liquids, for pediatric patients and those who cannot take solid dosages, you may need to provide an oral syringe with the prescription (Figure 4-3). In the case of injectable medications there may be several possible syringe sizes that can be used to withdraw the correct volume of solution. However, the syringe should never contain more than five times the volume of medication to be administered for accuracy.

Pediatric and Geriatric Dosing

Many prescriptions are filled daily for children, and it is important that the parent understand how much medicine to give the child. When the strength needed cannot be measured with a teaspoon or is an odd amount, you must use droppers. The pharmacist, not the technician, should show the parent of the patient how to measure the correct amount. Senior citizens must be careful in taking the correct amount of medication. For oral liquids, dosing devices with large boldface calibrations may help the geriatric patient see the correct amount. Many of these types of dosing devices are sold over the counter.

EXAMPLE 4-15

Order: docusate sodium 20 mg bid
    In stock: docusate sodium 4 mg/mL

1. How many milliliters are needed per dose?
    4 mg/mL = 20 mg/x = 5 mL
2. How many milliliters are needed per day?
    5 mL × 2 (bid) = 10 mL
3. How many doses can be taken from the 8-oz bottle? 240 mL (8 oz)/5 mL (per dose) = 48 doses

EXAMPLE 4-16

You receive an order for carbamazepine suspension 250 mg tid.
    In stock: carbamazepine 100 mg/5 mL bottle of 100 mL.

1. How many milliliters are needed per dose? 12.5 mL
2. How many milliliters are needed per day? 37.5 mL
3. How many doses can be taken from the 100-mL bottle? 8 doses

When preparing IVs and other parenteral medications you will need to calculate the correct dose based on the weight of the patient; this is especially true of infants, children, and senior citizens. Chemotherapy medications are often based on the body surface area of the patient. Always check your calculations at least three times before asking a pharmacist to check them. Below are examples of the most common methods of performing calculations. There are other formulas that can be used, such as Clark's rule and Young's rule. Although these are not commonly employed by technicians to perform calculations, the formulas will be outlined under the section Calculating Body Surface Area (BSA).

CALCULATING THE PROPER DOSE

All official compendia, drug references, and drug manufacturers provide proper dosing regimens based on kilograms; it is necessary to convert pounds into kilograms. Because most persons do not know their weight in kilograms, they will provide their weight in pounds. The pharmacy technician will need to convert the patient's weight from pounds to kilograms. It is important to remember that there are 2.2 lb per kilogram.

$$2.2 \text{ lb} = 1 \text{ kg}$$

and

$$1 \text{ kg} = 0.45 \text{ lb}$$

Tech Note!

This is how to remember kilogram conversion: Your weight is more than cut in half when measured in kilograms (2.2 lb = 1 kg). If you weighed 200 lb, you would weigh 90.0 kg.

To determine the number of kilograms in 1 lb, divide kilograms by 2.2 lb, which is seen in this example: 5 lb/2.2 lb/kg = 20.45 kg.

On the other hand, to calculate the number of pounds there are in 1 kg, multiply the number of kilograms by 2.2 lb/kg, as seen in the following: 55 kg × 2.2 lb/kg = 121 lb.

EXERCISE 4-13 QUICK CHECK

1. Dose ordered: 125 mg/kg/dose (q24h). Patient weighs 175 lb.
   How many g per day?
2. Dose ordered: 55 mg/kg/day (q8h). Patient weighs 48 lb.
   How many mg per dose?
3. Dose ordered: 220 mg/kg/dose (q12h). Patient weighs 141 lb.
   How many g per day?
4. Dose ordered: 1.12 mg/kg/day (q6h). Patient weighs 98 lb.
   How many mg per dose?
5. Dose ordered: 25 mg/kg/dose (q8h). Patient weighs 25 lb.
   How many g per dose?

CALCULATING PEDIATRIC DOSAGE

Pediatrics refers to the practice of medicine in children from childbirth until adolescence. This range of ages is subdivided into various groups:

- Neonates: newborn child from birth to 1 month
- Infant: 1 month to 1 year
- Early childhood: 1 year through 5 years
- Late childhood: 6 years through 12 years
- Adolescence: 13 years through 17 years

Pediatric dosages can be calculated using a proportion in the following format:

$$\text{mg of drug/kg of weight} = \text{mg of drug given to patient/patient's weight in kg}$$

EXAMPLE 4-17

The pharmacy receives an order for a baby girl weighing 7 lb.
The order calls for 20 mg/kg/dose.
This means that for every kilogram the child weighs, she should receive 20 mg of medication.
To solve the dosage, first find her weight in kg using ratio proportion:

$$2.2 \text{ lb}/1 \text{ kg} = 7 \text{ lb}/x \text{ kg}$$

$$x = 3.18 \text{ kg}$$

Now multiply the weight in kilograms by the recommended dosage.

$$20 \text{ mg} \times 3.18 \text{ kg} \times 1 \text{ dose} = 63.6 \text{ mg/dose}$$

Tech Note!

When rounding off numbers, complete all of the calculations first, and then round off at the end of the calculations if instructed to do so by the pharmacist. If you round off at each step, your answer will not be as accurate.

EXERCISE 4-14 **QUICK CHECK**

1. Patient: length 20 inches; weight 5 lb; dose 75 mg/m^2.
   A. What is the BSA in m^2?
   B. What is the mg per dose?
2. Patient: length 60 inches; weight 85 kg; dose 200 mg/m^2.
   A. What is the BSA in m^2?
   B. What is the mg per dose?
3. Patient: length 65 inches; weight 150 lb; dose 25 g/m^2.
   A. What is the BSA in m^2?
   B. What is the g per dose?

CALCULATING BODY SURFACE AREA (BSA)

The body surface area (BSA) method of calculating a patient's dose results in the most accurate dose because it is based upon both the height and the weight of the patient. Body surface area calculations are extremely important when calculating chemotherapeutic and pediatric doses. To calculate the body surface area of a patient, you need to know both the patient's weight (pounds or kilograms) and the patient's height (inches or centimeters) and be able to use a nomogram. A nomogram is a table used to determine a patient's body surface area. To determine the person's correct body surface area you use a straight-edge ruler to draw a straight line from the height of the patient to the weight of the patient on the nomogram. This line intersects at a point on the body surface area scale that will indicate the patient's body surface area. Based on this measurement you can determine the amount of drug to be used according to the following proportion:

$$\frac{\text{Body surface of patient} \left(\text{in m}^2\right)}{1.72 \text{ m}^2 \text{ (average adult body surface area)}} \times \text{Adult dose} = \text{Approximate dose for patient}$$

OTHER METHODS OF CALCULATING PEDIATRIC DOSES

There are two other methods that have been used in the past to calculate pediatric doses. Clark's rule uses the patient's weight as the basis for calculating the dose while Young's rule uses the patient's age as the criterion in calculating the patient's dose. Neither of these methods is as accurate as using body surface area.

Clark's rule:

$$\text{Weight of the child in lb}/150 \times \text{Adult dose} = \text{Child's dose}$$

Compared to Young's rule, Clark's rule is preferred because it is more accurate to use the child's weight than the child's age.

Young's rule:

$$\text{Child's age in years}/(\text{Child's age} + 12) \times \text{Adult dose} = \text{Child's dose}$$

GERIATRIC PATIENTS

Geriatric medicine is the field of medicine that encompasses the management of illness or disability in the elderly. A major consideration in the dosing of elderly patients is kidney function because reduced kidney function results in reduced drug elimination, increased drug accumulation, and possible toxic drug levels and adverse effects. Similar to the pediatric patient, renal clearance is extremely important when using specific drugs in the elderly population.

Tech Note!

Here is a hint for determining drops. Remember drops are written as *gtt*. Amounts differ between dropper sizes. About 60 drops are in 5 mL (cc). Also, drops can be intended for drip rates. The number of drops per milliliter depends on the tubing size of the administration kit.

EXERCISE 4-15 QUICK CHECK

1. Order: 2 L TPN to run at 150 mL/hr.
   A. How many hours will this solution last?
2. Order: 1500 mL of 20 mEq KCl for 12 hr. The tubing size is 20 gtt/mL.
   A. How many mL per hour?
   B. How many drops per minute will be delivered?
3. Order: 500-mL solution to run over 24 hr.
   A. How many mL per hour?
4. Order: 1000-mL solution to run over 18 hr.
   A. How many mL per hour?
5. Order: 2.5-L solution to run over 20 hr. The tubing size is 25 gtt/mL.
   A. How many mL per hour?
   B. How many drops per minute will be delivered?

Drip Rates

Hospital pharmacy technicians deliver a 24-hour supply of intravenous solutions to nursing stations daily. Large-volume parenterals (LVP) contain more than 250 mL of solution while small-volume parenterals (SVP) contain 100 mL or less. Most intravenous piggybacks are small-volume parenterals that are given over 30 to 60 minutes. Large-volume parenterals for continuous intravenous administration are "hung" at the patient's bedside and are allowed to drip slowly into a vein either by gravity or through a pump. They need to be given at a slow rate because veins can only handle a small volume at a given time. Both large- and small-volume parenterals allow the intravenous solution to be infused at a constant rate. In either case, the physician determines infusion rate in terms of milliliters per minute, drops per minute, or amount of drug (milligrams, units, or milliequivalents) per hour. In both LVP and SVP situations, the pharmacy technician must be able to calculate the volume needed to last over a certain amount of time, or he or she may need to calculate how much longer a currently hanging intravenous solution will last (Figure 4-4). Depending on the order received, the technician must be able to convert the numbers to determine this information. This ultimately will determine the amount of intravenous solution to be prepared that will have a duration of 24 hours.

These calculations involve determining the following:

1. The right amount of drug that is to be given over time
2. The amount of drug needed to last a certain time
3. The amount of time left until an IV is empty

Basic conversions are as follows:

Time: 1 hour = 60 minutes
24 hours = 1 day

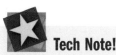

Tech Note!

Technicians and pharmacists do not determine the size of the tubing. This is predetermined by the doctor's orders to the nurse.

These calculations are affected by the size of tubing used to deliver the medication. We will use a common drop factor (drops/milliliter) to determine the volume. The drop factor is given on each set of tubing. If you have a tubing set that states 10 gtt/mL, this is the drop factor and will be used to determine the rate. Various drop factors are available: 10, 20, 25, 50, 60, and 100 gtt/mL. A drop factor (DF) of 50 gtt/mL is often referred to as a microdrip or microdrop administration kit.

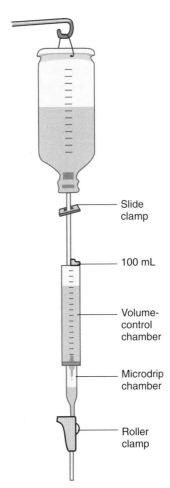

Slide clamp

100 mL

Volume-control chamber

Microdrip chamber

Roller clamp

FIGURE 4-4 Large-volume IV drip with smaller piggyback attached to tubing on pump.

EXAMPLE 4-18 CALCULATING DRIP RATES

You receive an order for a 2-L bag to be given over 24 hours. Your tubing delivers 15 gtt/mL. What are the drops per minute? To find this out, prepare the problem.
    Steps involved in determining drops per minute:

1. What is the drop factor?

$$15 \text{ gtt/mL}$$

2. What will be the milliliters per hour?

$$2000 \text{ mL/24 hr} = 83.33 \text{ mL/hr} \ (24 \text{ hr/day})$$

3. What will be the milliliters per minute?

$$83.33 \text{ mL/60 min} = 1.38 \text{ mL/min} \ (60 \text{ min/hr})$$

4. What will be the drops per minute?

$$1.38 \text{ mL/min} \times 15 \text{ gtt/mL (DF)} = 20.8 \text{ gtt/min or } 21 \text{ gtt/min}$$

(Please note that when expressing gtt/min the number is rounded upward to the nearest minute whether the answer is 20.1 gtt/min or 20.9 gtt/min.)

EXERCISE 4-16 **QUICK CHECK**

1. Aminophylline 500 mg in 1000 mL over 24 hours. The drip rate is 25 gtt/mL.
   A. What is the flow rate in drops/minute?
   B. How many mL would be delivered per hour?

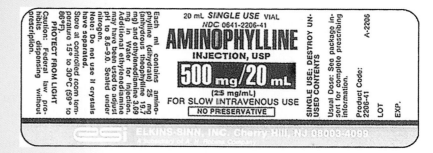

2. Heparin 20,000 units in 1 L over 24 hours. The drip rate is 50 gtt/mL.
   A. What is the flow rate in drops/minute?
   B. How many mL would be delivered per hour?

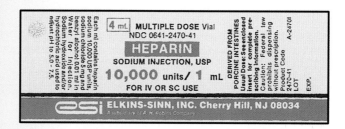

3. Heparin 100 units per 500 mL. Runs at 10 mL per hour.
   A. How many units will be delivered per hour?
   B. How many units will be delivered per min?

EXAMPLE 4-19 **DETERMINING VOLUME BASED ON DROP FACTOR (DF)**

A 3-L total parenteral nutrition bag is being administered to the patient over 24 hours. The tubing size delivers 15 gtt/mL.

1. How many milliliters per hour will be delivered?

   Determine milliliters/hour: 3000 mL/24 hr = 125 mL/hr

2. How many milliliters per minute are being delivered to the patient?

   Determine milliliters/minute: 125 mL/hr ÷ 60 min = 2.08 mL/min

3. How many drops per minute will be delivered?

   Determine drops/minute: 2.08 gtt/min × 15 gtt/min (DF) = 31.2 gtt/min or 32 gtt/min

EXAMPLE 4-20

How many drops per minute would an IV deliver to a patient receiving 40 mL/hr using a 20 gtt/mL set?
   Determine the milliliters/minute:

   40 mL/hr = 60 min = 0.666 mL/min

Tech Note!

A large-volume bag can hang for a maximum of 24 hours before it must be changed to prevent microbial growth, according to *USP*.

Determine the drops/minute:

$$0.666 \text{ mL/min} \times 20 \text{ gtt/mL (DF)} = 13.33 \text{ or } 14 \text{ gtt/min}$$

Dilution

The pharmacy often receives a prescription for a liquid or solid medication that is not available commercially in the strength prescribed by the physician. Often the commercial strength is greater than the prescribed strength. In this situation, the pharmacist or pharmacy technician must **dilute** the commercially available product to a lower strength. In this process, a pharmaceutical preparation is diluted through the addition of a diluent or **solvent** to the desired strength. The **diluent** (solvent) is an inert substance that does not have a concentration, or in other words has a concentration of 0%. The diluent adds either volume or mass to the preparation.

The concentration or strength of a substance can be expressed in three different ways. The most common expression is percent (%). In the practice of pharmacy, percent can be expressed in the following three ways: weight/weight (w/w%), weight/volume (w/v%), and volume/volume (v/v%). Weight/weight % (w/w%) is defined as the number of grams of solute dissolved in 100 g of final product. Weight/volume % (w/v%) is described as the number of grams of solute dissolved in 100 mL of solution. Volume/volume % is defined as the number of milliliters of solute dissolved in 100 mL of solution.

A second method of expressing the strength of a substance is using ratio strength. Often ratio strength is used to designate the concentration of weak solutions or liquid preparations. For example, a 1:1000 ratio strength is interpreted as the following: for solids in solids = 1 g of solute in 1000 g of solid preparation; for solids in liquids = 1 g of solid in 1000 mL of solution; and for volumes in volumes = 1 mL of solute in 1000 mL of solution.

A third method of designating strength is using fractions such as mg/mL. To convert percentage strength to mg/mL, multiply the percentage strength, expressed as a whole number, by 10. For example, convert 5% (w/v) to mg/mL:

$$5 \text{ mg/mL} \times 10 = 50 \text{ mg/mL}$$

To convert ratio strength to mg/mL, divide the ratio strength by 1000. For example, convert 1:20,000 (w/v) to mg/mL:

$$20,000/1000 = 1 \text{ mg/20 mL}$$

To convert product strength expressed as grams per liter (g/L), convert the numerator to milligrams and divide by the number of milliliters in the denominator. For example, convert a product concentration of 1 g per 100 mL:

$$1000 \text{ mg/100 mL} = 10 \text{ mg/mL}$$

During the dilution process, we begin with a substance with an initial weight (IW) or volume (IV) of a particular concentration (IS). We add a diluent to our initial product to prepare a substance that has a final weight (FW) or final volume (FV) of a final concentration (FS). This process can be expressed mathematically as:

$$(\text{IS})(\text{IW or IV}) = (\text{FS})(\text{FW or FV})$$

One must have three of the four variables to perform this calculation. The amount of diluent needed can be calculated by using the following equation:

$$(\text{FW or FV}) - (\text{IW or IV}) = \text{Amount of diluent}$$

There are several things to remember when using strengths: First, when ratio strengths are given, convert them to percentage strengths. Second, reduce all proportions to their lowest terms before performing the calculations. Third, the initial strength will always be greater than the final strength in a dilution problem, Finally, the final weight or final volume will be greater than the initial weight or **volume**.

EXERCISE 4-17 QUICK CHECK

Solve the following dilution problems:

1. How many grams of amino acid are in 500 mL of 8.5% solution?
2. You have dissolved 170 g in 1 L of water; what is the percentage strength of the solution formed?
3. If 200 mL of a 20% (w/v) solution is diluted to 1 L, what will be the percentage strength (w/v)?
4. How many milliliters of water must be added to 150 mL of a 25% (w/v) stock solution of sodium chloride to prepare a 0.9% (w/v) sodium chloride solution?
5. How many milliliters of a 1:50 (w/v) boric acid solution can be prepared from 500 mL of a 10% (w/v) boric acid solution?
6. A pharmacist has weighed 3 g of coal tar and given it to the technician to compound a 1% ointment. What will be the final weight of the correctly compounded prescription?
7. The order calls for 120 mL of a 10% magnesium sulfate solution and you have a 25% magnesium sulfate solution. How many milliliters of the 25% solution will you use?
8. You are asked to prepare 50 mL of a 1:100 rifampin suspension and you have in stock a 1:20 rifampin suspension. How many milliliters of the 1:20 suspension will you need?
9. The pharmacist receives a prescription for 100 mL of a 30% hydrochloric acid solution. The pharmacy carries a 90% hydrochloric acid solution. How many milliliters of the concentrated solution are needed to fill the prescription?
10. A stock bottle of Lugol's solution contains 4 ounces from the original pint bottle. The technician is able to make four 8-ounce bottles of a more dilute 4% solution. What was the original percentage strength of Lugol's solution?

Alligation

Alligation is a method by which we may calculate the number of parts of two or more ingredients of a given strength when they are mixed to prepare a mixture of a desired strength that you do not have in stock. A final proportion allows us to calculate the relative parts of each strength. To make this strength, you need to use two other strengths to attain the correct strength. For example, if a doctor orders 20% KCl but you only have 10% and 50% KCl on hand, calculate the amount of each solution needed to attain a 20% solution. You can do this using any two strengths as long as only one is less concentrated than the final solution. This means that you cannot make a 20% solution from a 5% solution and a 10% solution because both are less than the needed amount. However, you can make a 10% solution from a 5% and a 70% solution. Also, water is another element you might use as one of the solutions. The percentage of water is considered 0%. We will begin by working with these numbers.

Problem: You have in stock a 70% solution and a 20% solution. How much of each do you need to create 1 L of 40% solution?

This is as simple as tic-tac-toe; following these basic rules:

1. Draw a tic-tac-toe board.

2. Place your desired strength in the middle square.

    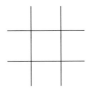

3. Put your higher-strength solution in the top left square.

    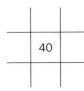

4. Put your lower-strength solution in the bottom left square. If you are using water, you will place a zero in this square because water has a concentration of zero.

70		
	40	
20		

5. Determine the difference between the numbers in the top left and middle squares, and place this new number in the bottom right square. Do the same with the bottom left number, and place this result in the top right square. Both of these numbers are assigned the unit "parts."

70		20	40 – 20 = 20
	40		
20		30	70 – 40 = 30

6. Create a fraction by adding the two new numbers (top and bottom right squares) together for a common denominator. Place the top right number over the denominator and do the same for the bottom right number.

70		20
	40	
20		30

    $$\frac{20}{20 + 30} \qquad \frac{30}{20 + 30}$$

7. Divide each fraction, and then multiply by the total volume you need.

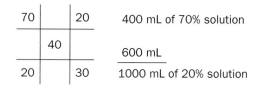

$$\frac{20}{50} \times 1000\ mL = 400\ mL$$

$$\frac{30}{50} \times 1000\ mL = 600\ mL$$

8. Check your answer by adding the two parts. They should equal the total volume.

70		20	400 mL of 70% solution
	40		600 mL
20		30	1000 mL of 20% solution

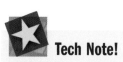

Tech Note!

Do not read your answer diagonally. Read your answer horizontally!

Answer: 400 mL of the 70% solution and 600 mL of the 20% solution will prepare a 1-L solution of 40%.

EXERCISE 4-18 QUICK CHECK

1. Order: prepare 500 mL of 20% KCl from your stock of 5% and 70% KCl.
    How many mL of each solution do you need?
2. Order: compound a 2.5% solution from a 10% stock solution and water for a total volume of 8 oz.
    How many mL of each solution do you need?
3. Order: prepare 1 L of 5% KCl from 50% KCl and sterile water.
    How many mL of each solution do you need?

PRACTICE QUIZ #4

1. 25 oz = _____ mL
2. 125 lb = _____ kg
3. 120 mL = _____ cups
4. 2000 mg = _____ g
5. 0900 = _____ o'clock
6. 1 dram = _____ mL
7. 3 L = _____ mL
8. 1.5 L = _____ mL
9. ⅛ L = _____ mL
10. 11:00 AM = _____
11. 125 lb = _____ kg
12. 1320 = _____ o'clock
13. 15 mL = _____ tbsp
14. 1 gallon = _____ Tbsp
15. 2 pints = _____ quarts
16. ½₀₀ gr = _____ mg
17. 2:30 PM = _____
18. 22,500 mcg = _____ g
19. 25,000 units/2 mL = _____ units/mL
20. 2110 = _____ o'clock

21. 30 lb = _____ kg
22. 2350 = _____ o'clock
23. 240 mL = _____ oz
24. 25 kg = _____ g
25. 25 lb = _____ oz
26. 1.5 g/10 mL = _____ mg/mL
27. 3000 mcg = _____ mg
28. 30 g = _____ grains
29. 60 mL = _____ tsp
30. 42 kg = _____ lb
31. 4:10 AM = _____
32. 4.4 lb = _____ kg
33. 450 g = _____ mg
34. 908 g = _____ kg
35. 1:1000 = _____ g/_____ mL
36. 49 kg = _____ lb
37. 3.375 g/100 mL = _____ mg/5 mL
38. 6 PM = _____
39. 10:25 PM = _____
40. gr ⅟₁₅₀ = _____ mg
41. 15 mL = _____ tsp
42. gr i = _____ mg
43. ix = _____
44. 8 tbsp = _____ mL
45. 50 g/100 mL = _____ mg/mL
46. 2.25 mcg = _____ mg
47. XXX = _____
48. 5 lb = _____ kg
49. 0.02 g = _____ mg
50. viii = _____
51. You receive an order for gentamicin 90 mg: You have a vial of 40 mg/mL. How many milliliters do you need to fill a one-time dose?
52. You must fill enough liquid Prozac 20 mg/5 mL for the following dosing: 10 mg daily × 30 days. How many milliliters do you need to fill this order?
53. Your pharmacy has Neosporin ointment on sale at 15% off the price of $2.95 per tube. How much will the customer save?
54. You have a pediatric order requesting amoxicillin 9 mg/kg/dose. If the child weighs 90 lb, how many milligrams and milliliters will the child receive per dose?
55. You receive an order for digoxin tablets 0.25 mg daily. You only have 0.125 mg in stock. How many tablets per dose will the patient need to take?
56. You have an order for 1 L of $D_{10}W$ with 20% KCl to run at 100 mL/hr. How many hours will this bag last?
57. You have an order for aminophylline drip 500 mL to run over 24 hr with a drop factor of 25 gtt/min. How many gtt/min will run?
58. You have an order to make a 1-L solution of a 30% solution: In stock you have 10% and 50% KCl. How much of each will you need to prepare 1 L?
59. You need to mix magic mouthwash that has a ratio of 1:1:1. Using diphenhydramine, Maalox, and lidocaine, how much of each do you need to make 8 oz? Give your answer in milliliters.
60. An order for a baby requires 15 mg/kg/day to be given 3 times daily. If the child weighs 25 lb how much will each dose be?
61. A pharmacy receives an order for 280 mL of a 5% salicylic acid solution. How much salicylic acid powder is needed to make the solution?
62. The pharmacist has weighed 15 g of coal tar and given it to the technician with the instructions to compound a 1% ointment. What will be the final weight of the correctly compounded prescription?

63. The pharmacy has 300 mL of a 50% solution; 200 mL is added to this solution to decrease the concentration. How many grams of active ingredient would there be in 4 ounces of this diluted solution?
64. If 5 grams is dissolved in 100 mL of solution, what is the percentage of the solution?
65. You dilute 100 mL of 5% solution to 500 mL. What is the percent strength?

DO YOU REMEMBER THESE KEY POINTS?

- How to convert Roman numerals to Arabic numbers
- How to convert the 24-hour clock to the 12-hour clock
- The methods to convert fractions, ratios, decimals, and percentages to each other
- The importance of using ratios and proportions in pharmacy calculations
- The primary system used in pharmacy is the metric system
- How to convert between units of measurement for weight and volume in the metric system
- The basic measurements of the metric, apothecary, and avoirdupois systems
- Drip rates of intravenous solutions can be expressed either as mL/hr or as gtt/min
- How to determine the duration of an intravenous solution
- Dilution is the process by which an inert substance is added to a preparation in which the final product has a lower concentration than the original product
- Alligation is a method to compound a substance when given two strengths to prepare a third strength
- All measurements must have units and it is important to label them correctly while performing calculations and on medication labels to avoid possible errors
- Double-checking calculations is important before preparing medications

TEST QUESTIONS

Convert the following units into percentages.

1. $\frac{1}{5}$ _____
2. 0.25 _____
3. $\frac{10}{25}$ _____
4. 2.275 _____

Convert the following fractions of grains into milligrams.

5. $\frac{1}{300}$ gr _____
6. $\frac{1}{150}$ gr _____

Write the Arabic numbers in Roman numerals and the Roman numerals in Arabic numbers.

7. 20
8. 50
9. 100
10. 59
11. 2
12. CXL
13. XC
14. XXXIV

15. XIX
16. VIII

Convert the following metric units into the units indicated to the right.

17. 5 cc = ___ tsp
18. 1 mcg = ___ mg
19. 15 cc = ___ tsp
20. 1000 mg = ___ g
21. 30 mL = ___ tsp
22. 900 mL = ___ oz
23. 1000 mL = ___ L
24. 0.25 L = ___ mL
25. 2 kg = ___ lb
26. 0.25 mg = ___ mcg

Solve the following drug orders. Be sure to show your work. Use the following conversions.

bid = 2 times daily
tid = 3 times daily
qid = 4 times daily
PO = orally/by mouth
IV = intravenous

27. You receive the following order: cimetidine 300 mg tab qid × 30 days. You have cimetidine 150 mg in stock. How many tablets will you need to fill this order?
28. Make a tobramycin IV 60 mg every tid in D_5W 50 mL. You have tobramycin 40 mg/mL in 2-mL vials. How much will you need in milliliters?
29. Make a vancomycin IV 750 mg every bid in D_5W 250 mL. You have vancomycin 1 g per 20-mL vial. How much will you take from the 1-g vial?
30. Make a 10% NS solution 1 L. You have 5% and 50% NS bags only. How much of each solution will it take to make a 10% NS 1-L bag?
31. Prepare 0.5 L of a 30% amino acid solution. You have 70% amino acids and sterile water in stock. How much of each solution is required to prepare a 30% solution?
32. Convert the following ratios into grams per milliliter.
  A. 1:10
  B. 2:100
  C. 1:1000
  D. 100:100
  E. 100:100,000
  F. 2:10,000
33. Prepare 5 mL of a 1:1000 epinephrine solution. You have 1:1000 mL stock solution. What will be the amount of epinephrine (in milligrams) in 5 mL?
34. Dispense ibuprofen liquid 40 mg/kg per day; give qid. You have ibuprofen liquid 100 mg/5 mL in stock. How much will this patient receive per dose if the patient's weight is 10 lb? How much liquid is needed to fill a 7-day supply?
35. 500 mL of heparin is to be given over 20 hours. The tubing size delivers 10 gtt/mL. How many drops per minute are being delivered to the patient?
36. What is the percentage of a 1:25 (w/v) solution?
37. You add 40 g of salicylic acid to white petrolatum to make a total of 800 g. What is the percent strength?
38. What is the initial strength of a solution that is made by adding 200 mL of purified water to make 600 mL of a 25% solution?
39. If you dilute 60 mL of a 30% solution to 480 mL, what is the percentage strength of the new solution?
40. How many milliliters of pure alcohol (w/v) are required to make 480 mL of a solution containing 30% alcohol?

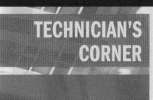

TECHNICIAN'S CORNER

A compounding order comes to the pharmacy with the following directions:

Gentamicin 15 mg/mL; dispense 5 mL ii gtt os bid

You have a 5-mL bottle of gentamicin ophthalmic drops 40 mg/mL in stock. You must decrease the concentration from 40 mg/mL to 15 mg/mL using sterile water.

BIBLIOGRAPHY

Gray Morris D: *Calculate with confidence*, ed 5, St Louis, 2010, Elsevier.
Mizner JJ: *Mosby's review for the Pharmacy Technician Certification Examination*, ed 2, St Louis, 2010, Elsevier.

5

Dosage Forms, Routes of Administration and Drug Classifications, Drug Abbreviations, and Medical Terminology

Objectives

UPON COMPLETING THIS CHAPTER, YOU SHOULD BE ABLE TO DO THE FOLLOWING:

- List at least three reasons why certain drugs need to be given by certain routes.

- Discuss the different components of medications and explain how a drug's composition affects its bioavailability and pharmacological effectiveness.

- List the most common routes and dosage forms of drugs.

- List three different common drugs and their storage requirements.

- Describe why additives are necessary in the production of medications.

- Define the common abbreviations for extended-release agents.

- List both pros and cons for the various routes of administration described in this chapter.

- Explain the difference between pharmacokinetics and pharmacodynamics.

- List and explain the absorption, distribution, metabolism, and excretion of drugs in the body.

- Define half-life and describe factors that influence it.

- Define first pass as it relates to metabolism and explain why it is important in drug delivery.

- Define the bioequivalence of drugs and its relationship to the Orange Book.

- List both pros and cons for controlled-release agents.

- Explain how pH plays a part in the reactivity of drug administration.

- Demonstrate the ability to translate abbreviations for dosage forms and routes of administration.

- List the types of medications along with their classification.

- List the segments that make up medical terms and provide examples of each.

- Define medical terminology abbreviations.

TERMS AND DEFINITIONS

Absorption *The taking in of nutrients and drugs from food and liquids*

Behind-the-counter *Nonprescription drugs that are kept behind the pharmacy counter and may have limited amounts sold or require the permission of a pharmacist to purchase*

Bioavailability *The degree to which a drug or other substance becomes available to the target tissue after administration*

Bioequivalence *The relationship between two drugs that have the same dosage and dosage form and that have similar bioavailability. Generic versions of a medication must show bioequivalence to the innovator product as a requirement of drug approval.*

Distribution *The location of a medication throughout blood, organs, and tissues after administration*

Excretion *The final elimination of a drug or other substance from the body via normal body processes, such as kidney elimination (urine), biliary excretion (bile to stool), sweat, respirations, or saliva*

Half-life *1. The amount of time it takes a chemical to be decreased by one half. 2. The time required for half the amount of a substance, such as a drug in a living system, to be eliminated or disintegrated by natural processes. 3. The time required for the concentration of a substance in a body fluid (blood plasma) to decrease by half*

Instill *To place into; instillation instructions are commonly used for ophthalmic or otic drugs, as examples*

Legend drugs *Drugs that require a prescription*

Metabolism *The processes by which the body breaks down or converts medications to active or inactive substances. The primary site of drug* *metabolism in humans is the liver; however, select drugs are metabolized through other processes.*

Over-the-counter (OTC) *Medications that can be purchased without a prescription*

Parenteral medication *Medication administered by injection or topically that bypasses the gastrointestinal system*

Pharmacokinetics *The study of the absorption, metabolism, distribution, and excretion of drugs*

TERMS AND ABBREVIATIONS

Dosage form	Abbreviation/ term	Main routes of administration (ROA)	Abbreviation
Buccal tablet or film	buccal	Indwelling urinary catheter	Foley
Capsule	Cap	Gastrostomy tube	GT
Chewable tablet	chew tab	Inhalant	INH
Diluent	Dil	Injection	INJ
Elixir	Elix	Intradermal	ID
Enema	enema	Intramuscular	IM
Enteric-coated tablet	EC tab	Intrathecal	IT
		Intravenous	IV
Gel cap	Cap	Intraperitoneal	IP
Liquid	Liq	Intravenous piggyback	IVPB
Lotion	Lot		
Lozenge	Loz	Nasogastric	NG
Metered dose inhaler	MDI	Nasogastric tube	NGT
		Right eye	OD
Mixture	Mix	Left eye	OS
Ointment	ung, oint	Both eyes	OU
Patch, transdermal	patch, TD	Orally, by mouth	PO
Powder	pwdr	Rectal, per rectum	PR
Solution	sol, soln	Small bowel feeding tube	SBFT
Spray	Spry		
Suppository	Supp	Subcutaneous	Subcut
Suspension	Susp	Vaginal, per vaginal	PV
Syrup	Syr	Sublingual	SL
Tablet	Tab	Topical	TOP
Tincture	Tinc		
Troche	troche		
Vaginal cream	vag cr		
Vaginal tablet	vag tab		

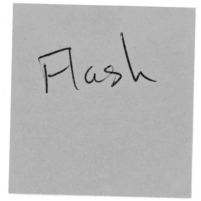

Introduction

For a technician to become proficient, it is necessary to interpret orders correctly. Although it may be true that many doctors' handwriting is referred to as "chicken scratch," it is the responsibility of the pharmacy to interpret and clarify orders if necessary. Many of the abbreviations that are used in prescribing medication look very much alike. For instance, mg (milligram) can look much like mcg (microgram) when written quickly. In this chapter we explore the common abbreviations seen in pharmacy as they apply to dosage forms and routes of administration. In addition to learning the many different types of dosage forms that are available and the reasons why they are necessary, we will discuss the pharmacokinetics related to the manufacturing of dosage forms. In addition, we will present a brief overview of the segments used to compose medical terms. We will cover medical and drug abbreviations as well.

Where Did Pharmacy Abbreviations Originate?

Much of the terminology in pharmacy and medicine comes from the Latin and Greek languages. Because pharmacy began in Europe, most of the abbreviations have their origins in a foreign language. The use of Latin and Greek has continued into the twenty-first century with little change. Although these abbreviations tend to be confusing at first, they serve an important function. For example, if each pharmacy used its own terminology, it would be virtually impossible for one pharmacy to fill another pharmacy's prescriptions. Therefore the medical community uses terms in Latin and Greek. These terms serve as a universal language that all medical doctors, nurses, pharmacists, technicians, and other medical personnel can understand. However, the ability to clarify doctors' orders is still a real dilemma in the United States. The number of errors caused by doctors' poor handwriting and by inaccurate transcribing of orders by pharmacists and technicians is of great concern (Chapter 14). Correct interpretation of doctors' orders by pharmacy staff is obviously extremely important. Interpreting orders can be a time-consuming function of filling prescriptions, and most patients want their medications quickly. This time pressure leaves the pharmacy staff little time to confer or call doctors' offices for every unclear order; however, clarification must occur if errors are to be avoided. The pharmacy technician must be careful to write the various abbreviations as neatly as possible because other technicians and pharmacists will be reading your writing. Scrolls, stylized, or fancy lettering can easily be misinterpreted. The pharmacy technician must learn all of the dosage forms and their abbreviations to decipher doctors' orders.

Do Not Use List

Because of the concern over drug errors that have occurred from the misinterpretation of medication orders, both the Institute for Safe Medication Practices (ISMP) and The Joint Commission (TJC) have provided a "Do Not Use List" that outlines the most common misread abbreviations. To reduce the number of mistakes, all practitioners have been informed that these abbreviations should be avoided. In this chapter these specific abbreviations have been included in the Terms and Abbreviations list at the start of the chapter in order to inform prospective technicians of those terms when they are encountered. However, these abbreviations should be avoided and instead spelled out in full. The "Do Not Use List" from TJC is provided in Table 5-1 and the list from ISMP is provided in Table 5-2, which addresses all the areas that influence drug errors.

Dosing Instructions

Dosing times are also abbreviated on prescriptions. Although many abbreviations are listed as "Do Not Use" per recommendations of both TJC and ISMP, they will be seen in many orders. In addition, many pharmacy computers are programmed to accept these abbreviations.

TABLE 5-1 TJC Official "Do Not Use" List*

Do Not Use	Potential Problem	Use Instead
U (unit)	Mistaken for "O" (zero), the number "4" (four) or "cc"	Write "unit"
IU (International Unit)	Mistaken for IV (intravenous) or the number 10 (ten)	Write "International Unit"
Q.D., QD, q.d., qd (daily)	Mistaken for each other	Write "daily"
Q.O.D., QOD, q.o.d, qod (every other day)	Period after the Q mistaken for "I" and the "O" mistaken for "I"	Write "every other day"
Trailing zero (X.0 mg)†	Decimal point is missed	Write X mg
Lack of leading zero (.X mg)		Write 0.X mg
MS	Can mean morphine sulfate or	Write "morphine sulfate"
MSO4 and MgSO4	magnesium sulfate	Write "magnesium sulfate"
	Confused for one another	

*Applies to all orders and all medication-related documentation that is handwritten (including free-text computer entry) or on pre-printed forms.

†**Exception:** A "trailing zero" may be used only where required to demonstrate the level of precision of the value being reported, such as for laboratory results, imaging studies that report size of lesions, or catheter/tube sizes. It may not be used in medication orders or other medication-related documentation.

TABLE 5-2 ISMP Error-Prone Abbreviations, Symbols, and Dosage Designations

Abbreviations	Intended Meaning	Misinterpretation	Correction
µg	Microgram	Mistaken as "mg"	Use "mcg"
AD, AS, AU	Right ear, left ear, each ear	Mistaken as OD, OS, OU (right eye, left eye, each eye)	Use "right ear," "left ear," or "each ear"
OD, OS, OU	Right eye, left eye, each eye	Mistaken as AD, AS, AU (right ear, left ear, each ear)	Use "right eye," "left eye," or "each eye"
BT	Bedtime	Mistaken as "BID" (twice daily)	Use "bedtime"
cc	Cubic centimeters	Mistaken as "u" (units)	Use "mL"
D/C	Discharge or discontinue	Premature discontinuation of medications if D/C (intended to mean "discharge") has been misinterpreted as "discontinued" when followed by a list of discharge medications	Use "discharge" and "discontinue"
IJ	Injection	Mistaken as "IV" or "intrajugular"	Use "injection"
IN	Intranasal	Mistaken as "IM" or "IV"	Use "intranasal" or "NAS"
HS	Half-strength	Mistaken as bedtime	Use "half-strength" or "bedtime"
hs	At bedtime, hours of sleep	Mistaken as half-strength	
IU*	International unit	Mistaken as IV (intravenous) or 10 (ten)	Use "units"
o.d. or OD	Once daily	Mistaken as "right eye" (OD-oculus dexter), leading to oral liquid medications administered in the eye	Use "daily"
OJ	Orange juice	Mistaken as OD or OS (right or left eye); drugs meant to be diluted in orange juice may be given in the eye	Use "orange juice"

Continued

TABLE 5-2 ISMP Error-Prone Abbreviations, Symbols, and Dosage Designations—cont'd

Abbreviations	Intended Meaning	Misinterpretation	Correction
Per os	By mouth, orally	The "os" can be mistaken as "left eye" (OS-oculus sinister)	Use "PO," "by mouth," or "orally"
q.d. or QD*	Every day	Mistaken as q.i.d., especially if the period after the "q" or the tail of the "q" is misunderstood as an "i"	Use "daily"
qhs	Nightly at bedtime	Mistaken as "qhr" or every hour	Use "nightly"
qn	Nightly or at bedtime	Mistaken as "qh" (every hour)	Use "nightly" or "at bedtime"
q.o.d. or QOD*	Every other day	Mistaken as "q.d." (daily) or "q.i.d. (four times daily) if the "o" is poorly written	Use "every other day"
q1d	Daily	Mistaken as q.i.d. (four times daily)	Use "daily"
q6PM, etc.	Every evening at 6 PM	Mistaken as every 6 hours	Use "daily at 6 PM" or "6 PM daily"
subcut	Subcutaneous	subcut mistaken as SL (sublingual); subcut mistaken as "5 every;" the "q" in "sub q" has been mistaken as "every" (e.g., a heparin dose ordered "sub q 2 hours before surgery" misunderstood as every 2 hours before surgery)	Use "subcut" or "subcutaneously"
ss	Sliding scale (insulin) or ½ (apothecary)	Mistaken as "55"	Spell out "sliding scale;" use "one-half" or "½"
SSRI	Sliding scale regular insulin	Mistaken as selective-serotonin reuptake inhibitor	Spell out "sliding scale (insulin)"
SSI	Sliding scale insulin	Mistaken as Strong Solution of Iodine (Lugol's)	
i/d	One daily	Mistaken as "tid"	Use "1 daily"
TIW or tiw	3 times a week	Mistaken as "3 times a day" or "twice in a week"	Use "3 times weekly"
U or u*	Unit	Mistaken as the number 0 or 4, causing a 10-fold overdose or greater (e.g., 4U seen as "40" or 4u seen as "44"); mistaken as "cc" so dose given in volume instead of units (e.g., 4u seen as 4cc)	Use "unit"
UD	As directed ("ut dictum")	Mistaken as unit dose (e.g., diltiazem 125 mg IV infusion "UD" misinterpreted as meaning to give the entire infusion as a unit [bolus] dose)	Use "as directed"

TABLE 5-2 ISMP Error-Prone Abbreviations, Symbols, and Dosage Designations—cont'd

Dose Designations and Other Information	Intended Meaning	Misinterpretation	Correction
Trailing zero after decimal point (e.g., 1.0 mg)*	1 mg	Mistaken as 10 mg if the decimal point is not seen	Do not use trailing zeros for doses expressed in whole numbers
No leading zero before a decimal point (e.g., .5 mg)*	0.5 mg	Mistaken as 5 mg if the decimal point is not seen	Use zero before a decimal point when the dose is less than a whole unit
Drug name and dose run together (especially problematic for drug names that end in "l" such as Inderal40 mg; Tegretol300 mg)	Inderal 40 mg Tegretol 300 mg	Mistaken as Inderal 140 mg Mistaken as Tegretol 1300 mg	Place adequate space between the drug name, dose, and unit of measure
Numerical dose and unit of measure run together (e.g., 10 mg, 100 mL)	10 mg 100 mL	The "m" is sometimes mistaken as a zero or two zeros, risking a 10- to 100-fold overdose	Place adequate space between the dose and unit of measure
Abbreviations such as mg. or mL. with a period following the abbreviation	mg mL	The period is unnecessary and could be mistaken as the number 1 if written poorly	Use mg, mL, etc. without a terminal period
Large doses without properly placed commas (e.g., 100000 units; 1000000 units)	100,000 units 1,000,000 units	100000 has been mistaken as 10,000 or 1,000,000; 1000000 has been mistaken as 100,000	Use commas for dosing units at or above 1,000, or use words such as 100 "thousand" or 1 "million" to improve readability

Drug Name Abbreviations	Intended Meaning	Misinterpretation	Correction
ARA A	vidarabine	Mistaken as cytarabine (ARA C)	Use complete drug name
AZT	zidovudine (Retrovir)	Mistaken as azathioprine or aztreonam	Use complete drug name
CPZ	Compazine (prochlorperazine)	Mistaken as chlorpromazine	Use complete drug name
DPT	Demerol-Phenergan-Thorazine	Mistaken as diphtheria-pertussis-tetanus (vaccine)	Use complete drug name
DTO	Diluted tincture of opium, or deodorized tincture of opium (Paregoric)	Mistaken as tincture of opium	Use complete drug name
HCl	hydrochloric acid or hydrochloride	Mistaken as potassium chloride (The "H" is misinterpreted as "K")	Use complete drug name unless expressed as a salt of a drug
HCT	hydrocortisone	Mistaken as hydrochlorothiazide	Use complete drug name
HCTZ	hydrochlorothiazide	Mistaken as hydrocortisone (seen as HCT250 mg)	Use complete drug name
MgSO$_4$*	magnesium sulfate	Mistaken as morphine sulfate	Use complete drug name
MS, MSO$_4$*	morphine sulfate	Mistaken as magnesium sulfate	Use complete drug name
MTX	methotrexate	Mistaken as mitoxantrone	Use complete drug name

Continued

TABLE 5-2 ISMP Error-Prone Abbreviations, Symbols, and Dosage Designations—cont'd

Drug Name Abbreviations	Intended Meaning	Misinterpretation	Correction
PCA	procainamide	Mistaken as patient controlled analgesia	Use complete drug name
PTU	propylthiouracil	Mistaken as mercaptopurine	Use complete drug name
T3	Tylenol with codeine No. 3	Mistaken as liothyronine	Use complete drug name
TAC	triamcinolone	Mistaken as tetracaine, Adrenalin, cocaine	Use complete drug name
TNK	TNKase	Mistaken as "TPA"	Use complete drug name
$ZnSO_4$	zinc sulfate	Mistaken as morphine sulfate	Use complete drug name

Stemmed Drug Names	Intended Meaning	Misinterpretation	Correction
"Nitro" drip	nitroglycerin infusion	Mistaken as sodium nitroprusside infusion	Use complete drug name
"Norflox"	norfloxacin	Mistaken as Norflex	Use complete drug name
"IV Vanc"	intravenous vancomycin	Mistaken as Invanz	Use complete drug name

Symbols	Intended Meaning	Misinterpretation	Correction
	Dram	Symbol for dram mistaken as "3"	Use the metric system
	Minim	Symbol for minim mistaken as "mL"	
x3d	For 3 days	Mistaken as "3 doses"	Use "for 3 days"
> and <	Greater than and less than	Mistaken as opposite of intended; mistakenly use incorrect symbol; "<10" mistaken as "40"	Use "greater than" or "less than"
/ (slash mark)	Separates two doses or indicates "per"	Mistaken as the number 1 (e.g., "25 units/10 units" misread as "25 units and 110" units)	Use "per" rather than a slash mark to separate doses
@	At	Mistaken as "2"	Use "at"
&	And	Mistaken as "2"	Use "and"
+	Plus or and	Mistaken as "4"	Use "and"
°	Hour	Mistaken as a zero (e.g., q2° seen as q 20)	Use "hr," "h," or "hour"

*These abbreviations are included on The Joint Commission's "minimum list" of dangerous abbreviations, acronyms, and symbols that must be included on an organization's "Do Not Use" list, effective January 1, 2004. Visit www.jointcommission.org for more information about this Joint Commission requirement.

Classifications of Medications

Classifications of medication serve to place drugs into groups. Although many medications are used for reasons other than their intended purpose, it is important to know the body system a medication is intended to affect. Each drug can be further broken down into groupings based on pharmacology, intent of use, route of use, or mechanism by which the drug affects its intended body system. Various classifications and attributes of drug therapy will be discussed later in this chapter. In Table 5-3 a generalized list is given to familiarize oneself with the various drug classifications that are available and the body system with which each classification is associated. Each type of medication may have several dosage forms, giving the consumer or physician a choice in how they are administered. For consumers, the choice may be based on which dosage form is easier to take or it may be based on cost. For a physician, the best way to administer medications may be based on how rapidly the medication is needed by the patient.

TABLE 5-3 General Classifications of Medications

Body System	Drug Classification
Gastrointestinal tract	Antacids, H_2-antagonists, proton pump inhibitors, antiemetics, laxatives, antidiarrheals, vitamins, dietary minerals
Blood and blood-forming products	Anticoagulants, antiplatelets, thrombolytics, antihemorrhagics
Cardiovascular system	Antihypertensives, diuretics, vasodilators, beta-blockers, calcium channel blockers, ACE inhibitors, angiotensin II receptor antagonists, antihyperlipidemics
Skin	Emollients, antipruritics, antipsoriatics, medicated dressings
Reproductive system	Hormonal contraceptives, fertility agents, sex hormones
Endocrine system	Hypothalamic-pituitary hormones, corticosteroids, sex hormones, thyroid hormones, antithyroid agents, antidiabetics
Infections, infestations	Antibiotics, antivirals, vaccines, antifungals, antiparasitics
Malignant disease	Anticancer agents
Immune disease	Immunomodulators
Muscles, bones, and joints	Anabolic steroids, nonsteroidal antiinflammatory drugs (NSAIDs), antirheumatics, corticosteroids, muscle relaxants, bisphosphonates
Brain and nervous system	Anesthetics, analgesics, anticonvulsants, antidepressants, antiparkinsonian drugs, antipsychotics, stimulants
Respiratory system	Decongestants, bronchodilators, cough medications, H_1-antagonists
Other	Radiopharmaceuticals, contrast media, antidotes

Different Types of Drug Sales

There are currently three classifications of drugs that describe their availability to consumers. **Over-the-counter** (OTC) drugs are commonly used and may be purchased without a prescription. **Legend drugs** are those that require a prescription from a prescriber before they can be used and are often denoted as "Rx." **Behind-the-counter** (BTC) drugs are those that do not require a prescription but are kept in the pharmacy; their sales are limited by quantity or may require pharmacist approval.

Dosage Forms

A dosage form refers to the means by which a drug is available for use or the vehicle by which the drug is delivered. With individual packaging the dosage form is given on the package. For example, the form may be a tablet or capsule. However, many types of tablets and capsules exist. Tablets are available in a wide variety of shapes and sizes. For example, they may be scored or unscored (Figure 5-1) or they may be coated or uncoated (Figure 5-2). Much of what determines the dosage form of a medication is determined by the effectiveness of the drug. For instance, heparin (an anticoagulant) is available only in parenteral (intravenous [IV] or subcutaneous [subcut]) form because it becomes ineffective when taken orally as a result of its interaction with stomach acids. Manufacturers prepare certain medications with the ability to release the active ingredient over an extended period. This allows the patient to take the medication less often, which increases compliance. Another consideration is given to the person

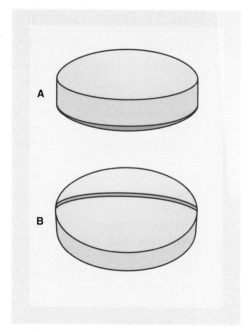

FIGURE 5-1 A, Unscored tablet. **B,** Scored tablet.

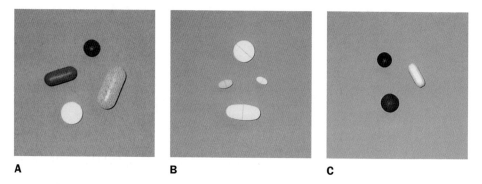

FIGURE 5-2 A, Plain tablets. **B,** Scored tablets. **C,** Enteric-coated tablets.

taking the drug. This includes age and condition of the person. If the prescription of acetaminophen (Tylenol) is intended for a child, that dosage form should be available in liquid if at all possible for ease of administration. The following list of dosage forms gives a brief explanation of their differences. All the different forms can be divided into three major categories that are composed of subcategories:

1. Solids: tablets, chewable tablets, enteric-coated tablets, extended-release agents, capsules, caplets, lozenges, troches, implant capsules, patches
2. Liquids: syrups, elixirs, sprays, inhalant solutions, emulsions, suspensions, solutions, and enemas
3. Semisolids: creams, lotions, ointments, powders, gelatins, suppositories, inhalant powders

Many of the top-selling drugs are available in several different dosage forms. Different dosage forms give more options to the consumer; however, the selection of a dosage form also depends on whether the drug will still be effective in a different form. Of the top 200 best-selling drugs, the ones that are available in at least 3 different dosage forms are given in Table 5-4. It is always important to know what dosage form is being requested because each form is dosed in different strengths, depending on the drug's reactive properties and the most suit-

TABLE 5-4 25 Top Selling Generic Drugs with Multiple Dosage Forms

25 Common drugs offered in multiple dosage forms	Tablet	Chewable Tablet	Capsule	Caplet	Solution	Gel Caps	Suspension	Syrup	Elixir	Injectable	Topical patch	Aerosol	Suppositories or Rectal Form	Topical Dosage Forms
Acetaminophen	X	X		X	X	X		X	X				X	
Acetaminophen/codeine	X						X			X			X	
Albuterol	X				X			X				X		
Amoxicillin	X	X	X				X							
Carbamazepine	X	X					X			X				
Clindamycin			X		X					X				X
Diazepam	X				X					X			X	
Digoxin	X		X						X	X				
Diltiazem	X		X							X				
Diphenhydramine	X		X		X			X	X	X				X
Erythromycin	X	X	X					X		X				X
Furosemide	X				X					X				
Guaifenesin	X		X		X			X						
Hydrocortisone					X					X			X	X
Hydroxyzine	X		X				X	X		X				
Ibuprofen	X		X		X		X			X				
Metaproterenol	X				X			X				X		
Nitroglycerin	X		X							X	X	X		
Phenobarbital	X		X						X	X				
Phenytoin	X		X				X			X				
Potassium chloride	X	X			X					X				
Prednisone	X							X	X					
Promethazine	X							X		X			X	
Ranitidine	X		X		X			X		X				
Risperidone	X				X					X				

Tech Note!

Remember that in order to substitute a different dosage form for the one ordered, the prescriber must give permission. The pharmacist must call the prescriber and explain the reason for the change.

able form for the consumer. For example, if erythromycin tablets are ordered for a young child, the pharmacist may need to call the doctor to request either chewable tablets or an oral suspension.

SOLIDS

Solid agents can be contained in various packages and when administered enterally can be given orally, rectally, or sublingually. When we think of solids, we normally consider medications given by oral or rectal routes, rather than parenteral routes. Parenteral is a term used to describe a medication that is usually given by injection into a vein, skin, or muscle. The following brief descriptions explain the wide variety of solids available.

Tablets/Caplets

Hundreds of types of tablets are available that range in size, shape, color, thickness, and composition. The most common type of tablet contains some type of filler. These fillers are composed of inert substances (no active ingredient) that serve to fill space or cover the tablet (sugar coatings). Sugar coatings improve taste and color or hide unpleasant odors. Finally, certain additives may be used to improve the absorption and/or distribution throughout the body. Some tablets are made to be administered sublingually (under the tongue) or vaginally. Also, some tablets are available in a scored form to allow the dosage to be cut in half if needed. Chewable tablets are convenient for persons who have difficulty swallowing tablets and for children who are unable to swallow large tablets. Other tablets are enteric-coated to help protect the drug through the acidic environment of the stomach until it reaches the more alkaline intestine. In other cases, the protective covering may delay the release of the drug while it travels through the stomach so that it will not irritate the stomach or become inactive. Orally disintegrating tablets (ODTs) may be dissolved in the mouth without water, easing administration for those with difficulty swallowing medication. Caplet dosage forms are related closely to tablets, but they are smooth-sided and are therefore easier to swallow. The word caplet refers to the shape of the tablet. Tablets are often identified by shape, color, and imprint codes, which are determined by the manufacturer.

Many medications have extended-release forms and regular forms. You must know which form the doctor has ordered. Abbreviations for agents that release medication over different periods of time and in different quantities are as follows:

Tech Note!

Dosage forms that are especially made to release over time should not be crushed or broken into pieces. This would alter the release process. Some companies have their own unique names for extended-release agents. For example, Theo-24 is a theophylline agent that is released over 24 hours, which is why the company has named it Theo-24 because it is taken every 24 hours.

CD	Controlled-diffusion
CR	Continuous/controlled-release
CRT	Controlled-release tablet
IR	Immediate-release*
LA	Long-acting*
ODT	Orally disintegrating tablet
SA	Sustained-action*
SR	Sustained/slow-release*
TD	Time-delay
TR	Time-release
XL	Extra-long*
XR	Extended-release*

*Also available in capsule forms.

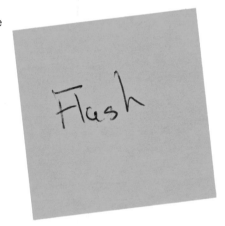

Capsules

Capsules are composed of a gelatin container. Capsules can have a hard or a soft outer shell. The shells of hard capsules are composed of sugar, gelatin, and water. Their color is determined by the manufacturer and is used primarily for identification, along with the capsule imprint coding. Another type of capsule is the Pulvule, which is shaped slightly different for identification purposes. Spansules are capsules that can be pulled apart to sprinkle the medication onto food for children, making it easier to administer; the medication inside a spansule is specially coated to slow the dissolving rate so the medicine can be delivered at a time (dependent on the coating) after the capsule contents are consumed. The medicine inside a spansule should not be crushed or chewed. Soft-gelatin capsules (gel caps) cannot be pulled apart, and often hold medications in liquid form. Because of the many capsule sizes available, they can be produced to administer medication in many ways. For example, as seen in Figure 5-3, these capsules can even hold a small capsule or tablet inside. The reason behind this manufacturing decision is to determine the best absorption and distribution of the medication. Caplets are not capsules; they are simply tablets that have a shape similar to a capsule; the shape may ease swallowing. More medications are being prepared as caplets to ensure that they are tamper proof. Figure 5-4 shows more shapes and sizes of capsules.

Capsule Sizes. Capsules are available in different sizes, as seen in Figure 5-5. They vary in color, transparency, and identifying marks. The larger half of the capsule is known as the body, and the shorter half is known as the cap. Many

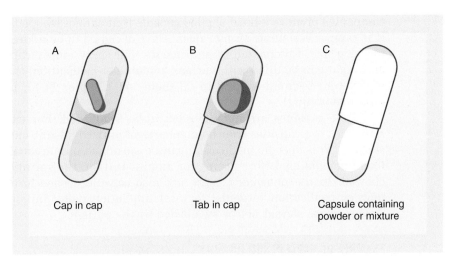

FIGURE 5-3 Different types of capsules.

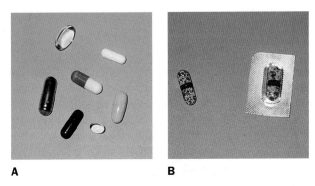

FIGURE 5-4 Types of capsules. **A,** Capsules. **B,** Extended-release capsules.

Number	Quantity	Example
000	1.37 mL	
00	0.95 mL	
0	0.68 mL	
1	0.5 mL	
2	0.37 mL	
3	0.3 mL	
4	0.2 mL	
5	0.13 mL	

FIGURE 5-5 Different sizes of capsules. Eight sizes are available; each holds a specific volume, and each holds a specific amount of medication. The size numbers are 5, 4, 3, 2, 1, 0, 00, 000—5 being the smallest and 000 being the largest. (From Clayton B, Stock Y: *Basic pharmacology for nurses*, ed 12, St Louis, 2003, Elsevier.)

companies produce a hard-shelled capsule that cannot be opened, ensuring that it is tamper resistant. Many capsules are designed to be taken orally and swallowed whole. Compounding pharmacies will carry empty capsules of varying sizes that can be filled with various amounts of medication; there are a variety of different techniques used to fill them (see Chapter 11 for more information on compounding).

Some capsules are not intended to be swallowed. For example, Topamax Sprinkles are capsules that hold spheres of anticonvulsant medicine inside the capsule. This specific medication can be sprinkled onto a small amount of soft food immediately before dosing for administration; the sprinkles should not be chewed. In the pharmacy, there are also capsule dosage forms that hold dry powder medication intended for oral inhalation using inhaler devices; these dosage forms should not be swallowed by the patient.

EXAMPLE OF CAPLETS AND CAPSULES

Acetaminophen caplets (Tylenol; OTC), hydroxyzine pamoate capsules (Vistaril; Rx)

Lozenges/Troches

Lozenges and troches are other forms of tablets that are not intended to be swallowed but to dissolve in the mouth, which releases the medication more slowly. The medications in lozenges and troches are often aimed at local action in the mouth and/or throat. Many cough drops come in this type of dose form. Lozenges are similar to hard candy. Troche sizes vary, some are larger than normal-size tablets and are flat; they usually have a chalky consistency in order to dissolve in the mouth. Clotrimazole troches are normally administered buccally (in the cheek) and left to dissolve, whereas most lozenges are allowed to be dissolved in the mouth.

EXAMPLE OF LOZENGES AND TROCHES

cetylpyridinium chloride-lozenge (Cepacol; OTC); clotrimazole troche (Mycelex; RX)

BIOMATERIALS

Biomaterials are polymers (long chains of hydrocarbons) that combine with or encapsulate a drug; the drug is then released in a predetermined predictable way. The dosage form of these drugs can be capsules, tablets, or implants. Both pH and solubility can activate the drug (see Chapter 31) and release its contents over a period of anywhere from 12 hours (e.g., cold medicine) to several years (e.g., Norplant implant). These drugs are able to treat conditions without overdosing or underdosing the patient, and they also promote compliance (patient adherence). These dosage forms help maintain a steady concentration of drug dosing within the accepted therapeutic range/window for the drug. The therapeutic window is essentially a range of concentrations where a drug is determined to be effective with minimal toxicity to most patients. The top concentration of the range is the maximum concentration for most patients to limit toxicity and the lowest concentration is that below which the drug is not therapeutically effective for most patients. There are three different components that determine the rate of release of these agents:

1. Water-insoluble agents (for example, ethyl cellulose)
2. pH-dependent agents (for example, sodium alginate)
3. pH-independent agents (for example, hydroxypropyl methylcellulose)

Another consideration of these medications is they are more expensive to manufacture and that cost is passed along to the consumer.

Implants

Implants are sterile, solid dosage forms that consist of drugs and rate-controlling excipients, and they are usually intended for insertion (implantation) into a body cavity or under the skin. Some implants are biosoluble, meaning they degrade within the body over time, while others are not and must be removed after a specified length of time. Many drug-containing implants are actually classified by the FDA as medical devices, rather than drugs; examples include implantable orthopedic antibiotic beads and various drug-eluting stents for arteries in the heart. There are some implants, however, that are regulated as prescription drugs. Some popular examples of implants include Zoladex subcutaneous implant (used for a variety of conditions, including prostate cancer), Gliadel Wafer (delivers chemotherapy directly to brain tumor site), and Implanon, a subdermal contraceptive rod (provides birth control that lasts for up to 3 years).

Transdermal Patches

Transdermal patches are solid pieces of material that hold a specific amount of medication to be released into the skin and absorbed into the bloodstream over time. Patches are convenient dosage forms because they are administered easily and eliminate possible upset stomach. Anginal medication such as transdermal nitroglycerin patches can be placed on the chest once daily. Some motion sickness patches (e.g., Transderm-Scōp) can be applied and left in place for up to 3 days. Fentanyl (Duragesic), a chronic pain medication, is a transdermal patch with a 3-day delivery time (Figure 5-6). Nicotine patches help with smoking cessation, and most are found over-the-counter (OTC). There are many estrogen-containing transdermal patches suited for hormone replacement therapy or prevention of osteoporosis; most are changed once or twice weekly.

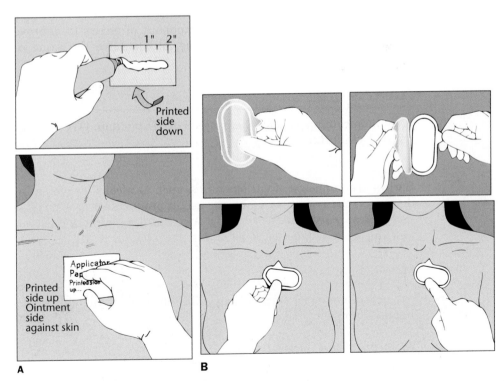

FIGURE 5-6 A, Example of nitroglycerin ointment patch. **B,** Example of a transdermal patch. (From Clayton B, Stock Y: *Basic pharmacology for nurses*, ed 14, St Louis, 2007, Elsevier.)

Tech Alert!

Never carelessly discard a medication patch in the trash. The medication present on an unprotected discarded patch could potentially penetrate the skin of a young child or pet. The best approach is to wrap and discard the patch in such a way that a child or pet would not be able to grasp it. One recommendation is that the patch be folded onto itself to cover the adhesive area; then place the patch in a pouch or baggie and discard it away from the reach of children or pets.

EXAMPLE OF TOPICAL PATCHES

nitroglycerin patches (Nitro-Dur; Rx), scopolamine transdermal patches (Transderm Scop; Rx), fentanyl patch (Duragesic; Rx)

LIQUIDS

Liquids are composed of various solutions. Traditional names for these dosage forms relate to the types of liquid with which the medication is mixed. Depending on the type of taste, speed of action, or route of administration intended, a physician can choose the best agent for the job. Liquids can be administered by many routes, which makes them a popular choice for drug delivery. For example, enemas are liquid-filled bottles with a dispensing top that can be placed into the rectum to administer the solution into the lower intestine. Other sterile liquids are used in eye and ear products, which are used to treat a variety of conditions. Solutions also can be used topically to treat skin conditions. The following examples show the various types of liquids available.

Syrups

Syrups are sugar-based solutions that have medication dissolved into them. The sugar improves the taste of the drug. Syrups tend to be thicker (more viscous) than water.

EXAMPLE OF SYRUPS

prednisolone syrup (Prelone; OTC), metaproterenol syrup (Alupent; Rx)

Elixirs

Elixirs are clear, sweetened solutions that contain dissolved medication in a base of water and alcohol (hydroalcoholic base). Drugs that are formulated as elixirs usually require alcohol as a solvent for the drug to be placed into solution. Sweeteners are a necessary component of elixirs to improve the taste of the alcoholic mixtures. Unlike syrups, elixirs have the same consistency as water.

EXAMPLE OF ELIXIRS

brompheniramine/pseudoephedrine elixir (Dimetapp; OTC), theophylline elixir (Elixophyllin; Rx)

Sprays

Sprays are composed of various bases, such as alcohol or water, in a pump-type dispenser. Sprays are available for use in products such as nasal decongestants and topical sunscreens. A nitroglycerin translingual spray also is available for use under the tongue for relief of anginal pain.

EXAMPLE OF SPRAYS

oxymetazoline nasal spray (Afrin; OTC), nitroglycerin sublingual spray (Nitrolingual Pumpspray; Rx)

Inhalants and Aerosols

Certain patient populations need to have their medications delivered directly to the source of inflammation, such as the bronchial tree. Because these areas are so small, the medication particles must be extremely fine to reach these areas effectively. Inhaler agents are available in a variety of forms, but all must be

Tech Note!

Most inhalants are propelled by the use of various gases. In the past, most propellants contained chlorofluorocarbons (CFCs), which have been found to destroy the ozone. As the ozone layer is destroyed, ultraviolet light is allowed to enter the atmosphere at levels that are known to cause skin cancer. Consequently, since 1980 the use of propellants containing CFCs has been banned and guidelines have been adopted to use other types of propellants. The replacements for chlorofluorocarbons must not harm the environment or alter or destroy the medication.

able to be inhaled easily into the lungs. Common devices of this type, available OTC, are vaporizers and humidifiers that distribute medications by adding agents to a container located on the device. In the hospital, respiratory therapists use nebulizers to give breathing treatments to patients, but patients also can use nebulizers at home if they, or their caregivers, are trained in their use. Inhaled anesthetics are solutions that are inhaled; they are administered during surgery by an anesthesiologist. Many of the prescribed inhalants contain drugs that treat asthma and allergies. Some devices are called metered dose inhalers (MDIs) and dispense a specific amount of drug with each puff or inhalation (Figure 5-7, *A*); the other common type of medication inhaler is a dry powder inhaler. Some aerosols are used to deliver medication into the nasal passages, whereas others are inhaled orally into the respiratory tract. For orally inhaled agents, although the sizes of the particles are extremely small, unless the patient uses this device correctly much of the drug is swallowed rather than inhaled into the lungs where it is needed. Many physicians encourage the use of an AeroChamber or other spacers (Figure 5-7, *B*) along with traditional metered dose inhalers. These allow the patient to take a breath of medication without worrying about poor timing and coordination, which would result in loss of medication. The chamber holds the medication until each puff can be inhaled. Dry powder inhalers can be easier to administer because the patient prepares the medication before inhalation, allowing the patient to focus on proper breathing and administration technique.

EXAMPLE OF AEROSOL AND MDIs

Epinephrine aerosol (Primatene Mist; Rx/OTC), albuterol metered dose inhaler (Alupent; Rx)

Emulsions

An emulsion is a mixture of two or more unblendable liquids; in an emulsion one liquid is dispersed throughout the other. They are fairly unstable; emulsifiers are often added to improve stability and dispersion. A mixture of water and oil may be used with an emulsifier to bind the two together. Many different types of emulsifiers are used, depending on what medication the manufacturer is preparing. A classic example of an emulsion from your kitchen is simple vinaigrette; vinaigrettes quickly separate unless shaken continually. In pharmacy, calamine lotion is a classic topical emulsion purchased over-the-counter (OTC). Propofol injections and intravenous lipid infusions are prescription medications

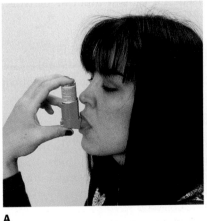
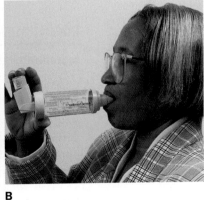

A   **B**

FIGURE 5-7 A, Inhaler. **B,** Inhaler attached to an AeroChamber (also known as a spacer). (From Potter PA, Perry AG: *Fundamentals of nursing*, ed 7, St Louis, 2009, Elsevier.)

Tech Note!

An emulsifier is a substance that binds oil to a water base. An emulsifier binds to both substances and holds them together. For example, take a look at mayonnaise. Mayonnaise is composed of oil and water and uses egg yolks as an emulsifier, which allows the product to form a smooth consistency. Oil can have water as a base; in some cases, water is contained in an oil base. Although most emulsions are used topically, a few parenteral emulsion agents can be given, such as lipids (also known as fat), which are used for nutritional parenteral feedings. Various types of emulsion preparations can be administered topically, orally, and even parenterally.

Tech Note!

It is always important to shake oral suspensions well before using. However care must be taken with injectable suspensions, because some drugs, including many biologic medicines, will be inactivated with vigorous shaking. Always follow the manufacturer's directions for handling. For example, some types of insulin suspensions should be rolled, not shaken. This is to avoid the destruction of the proteins that would result from shaking.

that are emulsions stabilized with ingredients such as soybean oil and egg lecithin.

EXAMPLE OF EMULSIONS

propofol (Diprivan; Rx), intravenous lipid emulsion (Intralipid; Rx)

Suspensions

Suspensions are liquid dosage forms that have very small solid particles suspended in the base solution. Certain active ingredients are found to be unstable when dissolved in a solution but are stable in a suspension form. Suspensions, like syrups and other oral solutions, can be used orally by children and seniors because the patients can take the medication more easily. Oral suspensions should have a "Shake Well" ancillary label that is easily visible on the front of the bottle and in the directions; if the product is prepared (reconstituted) in the pharmacy, proper adherence to the directions for mixing and placement of the date of expiration ("use by" date) on the label or auxiliary label are very important. Suspension dosage forms are also formulated to be used topically, in the eye, ear, rectally, and even parenterally.

EXAMPLE OF SUSPENSIONS

prednisolone ophthalmic suspension (Pred Forte; Rx), amoxicillin suspension (Trimox; Rx), ibuprofen suspension (Children's Motrin; OTC)

Enemas

Enemas may be administered for two different reasons—retention or evacuation. Retention enemas are used to deliver medication to the body in a manner that bypasses the stomach. Conditions such as ulcerative colitis (inflammation of the intestines) can be treated with antiinflammatory agents in this manner. A rectal diazepam gel (Diastat) is available (for certain patients) for the immediate treatment of seizures. The most common reason for enemas, however, is to evacuate the lower intestine for a variety of reasons, such as preprocedural care (for example, to prepare for surgeries or examinations involving the intestine) or for women about to give birth. Evacuation enemas can be administered from prefilled squeeze bottles. Some enemas are available OTC that are used strictly for the relief of constipation. However, because of the dramatic effects of enemas, physicians usually do not recommend these as the first line of treatment for constipation. Enemas are manufactured in a water base, which is faster acting than an oil base. The typical amount of time for an evacuation enema to be effective is less than 10 minutes.

EXAMPLE OF ENEMAS

mesalamine enema (Rowasa; Rx) sodium biphosphate enema (Fleet enema; OTC)

SEMISOLIDS

Semisolid agents are different in their composition from liquids or solids. Although they contain solids and liquids, they normally are intended for topical application. Examples include creams, lotions, ointments, gels, pastes, and suppositories.

Creams

Creams usually have medications in a base that is part oil and part water and is intended for topical or local use. When an emulsifier is added, the water and oil will remain combined. Creams are massaged easily into the skin and do not leave a heavy, oily residue. Creams can be formulated to be used vaginally or in the rectum, taking into account the sensitive tissues to which they will be applied.

EXAMPLE OF CREAMS

hydrocortisone cream 1% (Cortaid; OTC), betamethasone cream 0.05% (Diprolene; Rx)

Lotions

Lotions are thinner than creams because their base contains more water. They penetrate well into the skin and do not leave an oily residue after application.

EXAMPLE OF LOTIONS

hydrocortisone 1% lotion (Eczema medicated lotion; OTC), hydrocortisone lotion 2.5% (Rx)

Ointments

Ointments contain medication in a glycol or oil base, such as petrolatum. Ointments can effectively cover the skin's surface while repelling moisture. Ointments can be used rectally or topically, and can be formulated and sterilized for use in the eye as an ophthalmic agent.

EXAMPLE OF OINTMENTS

bacitracin/neomycin/polymyxin ointment (Neosporin; OTC), erythromycin ophthalmic ointment (Roymicin; Rx)

Gels

Gels contain medication in a viscous (thick) liquid that easily penetrates the skin and does not leave a residue. Many sunscreens are available in this dosage form. Medications for various skin conditions are available in gels as well.

EXAMPLE OF GELS

naftifine gel (Naftine; Rx), benzocaine (Orajel; OTC)

Pastes

Pastes contain a lesser amount of liquid base than solids. They are used for topical application and are able to absorb secretions, unlike other topical agents.

EXAMPLE OF PASTES

amlexanox paste (Apthasol; Rx), zinc oxide paste (Desitin; OTC)

Suppositories

Suppositories can be used rectally and vaginally. They have several advantages over other dosage forms. Rectal suppositories bypass the stomach, which is important if the patient has nausea and vomiting. They can relieve these symptoms without requiring an injection, which is much more invasive. They also are good for relief of constipation. Rectal antiinflammatory suppositories can be used to help treat inflammatory bowel conditions. Vaginal suppositories are used mostly to treat localized conditions of the vaginal area tissues, including yeast infections and atrophy related to menopause.

EXAMPLE OF SUPPOSITORIES

promethazine suppositories (Phenergan; Rx), miconazole vaginal suppositories (Monistat 3; OTC), bisacodyl suppositories (Dulcolax; OTC)

Powders

Powders do not fit neatly into the category of semisolids. Powders are solids, yet they are packaged in some forms that allow them to be sprayed similar to liquid dosage forms, or inhaled (see inhalants). Therefore topical powders have been included in the semisolids section. One of the main uses of topical powders involves decreasing the amount of wetness of an area. Most antifungal foot agents are available in powdered forms to keep the area as dry as possible, decreasing the ability of the fungus to thrive. Powders also can be spread over a wide area if needed.

EXAMPLE OF POWDERS

Tolnaftate powder (Desenex spray; OTC), nystatin powder (Mycostatin topical, Rx)

Injectables

Injectables normally are used for rapid response, although diabetic patients may use long-acting insulins along with short-acting insulins. Table 15-6 lists commonly used insulins. The onset of action of many injectable drugs takes only a few minutes, as opposed to the possible 45 minutes that oral medications can take to become effective. Although diabetic persons are the most common users of injectable drugs outside the hospital setting, other types of injectables used in the home are anticoagulants (e.g., subcutaneous heparins) and certain injectables for multiple sclerosis patients. Inside the hospital, many oral medications are available in injectable form, and some are only available in injectable form. Technicians need to pay close attention to store injectables in the correct manner and environment. Storage temperatures range from room temperature to refrigerated. Some injectables, such as phytonadione (AquaMEPHYTON; vitamin K), must be kept in a light-protected ampule and should be stored at room temperature. Other injectables need to be stored in light-protected bags after being reconstituted into an IV bag, such as ciprofloxacin. Glass containers are packaged securely to protect them from breakage. Ampules are made of glass (Figure 5-8, *B*). Ampules can range in volume from 0.5 to 50 mL. When opening these various sizes of ampules, use the techniques outlined in Chapter 12. Many vials are in plastic and glass containers (Figure 5-8, *A*) and range in size from 1 to 100 mL. Other medications that are available in intravenous form are premade IV bags and those prepared by a technician. Another form of vial is the ADD-Vantage vial, which keeps the medication separate from the diluent until it is time to reconstitute. This saves waste when using an expensive drug that has a short shelf life after preparation (Figure 5-9 gives instructions on mixing). Other types of containers include premade, large-volume IV fluids and IV piggyback drugs (Figure 5-10).

EXAMPLE OF INJECTABLES

furosemide vial (Lasix; Rx, light protected), interferon beta-1a pre-filled syringe (Avonex; Rx)

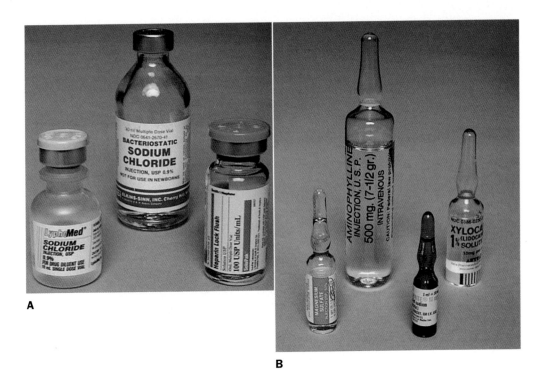

FIGURE 5-8 **A,** Medication in vials. **B,** Medication in ampules.

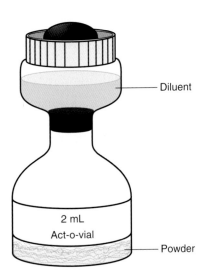

FIGURE 5-9 This type of vial is called Add-A-Vial or Mix-O-Vial. The advantage of this type of medication dosage form is its longer shelf life. *1,* First remove the sterile cap. *2,* The powder is below, and the sterile diluent is on top of the vial. The vial is divided by a rubber stopper in the middle. *3,* Push the plunger down, forcing the stopper to fall into the bottom of the vial. This allows the diluent to mix with the powder. Shake well. Once dissolved, the medication is ready to be used.

Although many other types of dosage forms can be made by manufacturers or by compounding pharmacies, the various types covered in this chapter are the most commonly seen in the pharmacy. Because medications in the pharmacy are stocked according to their different dosage forms, it is important for the student technician to be familiar with all dosage forms to quickly locate a medication. Table 5-5 lists the most common dosage forms and their routes of

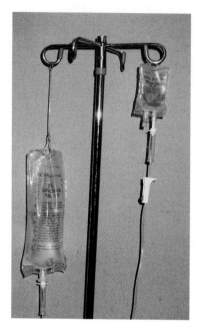

FIGURE 5-10 On the left is a large-volume IV. On the right is an IV piggyback.

administration. The advantages and disadvantages of each type of route of administration determine the doctor's final decision as to what type of agent the patient should receive. The following sections describe each route of administration and list the pros and cons of each.

Routes of Administration

BY MOUTH, OR ORAL

A positive aspect of taking tablets or capsules or any agent by mouth (PO) is the convenience of the drug for the patient. Most oral medications can be kept readily available throughout the day in a handy bottle. Tablets and capsules do not need to be measured, which increases their ease of use, and most oral forms are much less expensive than other alternatives. Some oral medications are systemic, which means they are absorbed and dispersed throughout the body, while others are not absorbed and act locally in the gastrointestinal tract once swallowed. Oral administration is also one of the safer ways to give medication, because if too much is given there may be time to react before the drug begins to work. The disadvantage of these drugs is that they do not work as quickly as parenteral medications; they take anywhere from 30 minutes to 1 hour to become active. This can be important, for instance, if the medication is intended for pain relief. Also, some drugs cannot be taken orally because they are not as effective. This complication is due to the acid pH of the stomach, which breaks down some substances before absorption and makes certain medications of little use.

SUBLINGUAL AND BUCCAL AGENTS

Although not many medications are available at this time in the form of sublingual (SL) or buccal (BUC) agents, the few that are commonly used are effective. Nitroglycerin is the most commonly used sublingual tablet that treats anginal attacks. Angina is a common heart ailment that affects millions of persons, with symptoms that include shortness of breath and pain in and around the chest

TABLE 5-5 Common Abbreviations Used with Dosage Forms

Abbreviation	Route of Administration	Specific Site of Action	Dosage Forms
PO	Oral	Absorbed into bloodstream	Tablet Capsule Solution Syrup Suspension Powder Elixir Tincture Troche
SL	Sublingual	Under the tongue	Tablet Sprays
BUC	Buccal	In the cheek	Lozenge/troche
PR	Per rectum	Rectum	Suppository Solution Enema Ointment
IV	Intravenous	In the vein	Solution/suspension
IM	Intramuscular	In the muscle	Solution/suspension
IT	Intrathecal	In the space surrounding spinal cord	Solution
IA	Intraarterial	In the artery	Solution
TOP	Epicutaneous or percutaneous	On the skin surface	Ointment Cream Paste Powder Spray Solution Lotion
	Transdermal	On the skin surface for delivery through the skin	Patch Disk
NAS	Intranasal	Nose	Solution Spray Inhalant
INH	Inhalant	Mouth	Solution Aerosol
PV	Per vagina	Vagina	Solution Ointment Foam Gel Suppository Sponge
Urethral	Urethral	Urethra	Solution Suppository

cavity. Nitroglycerin sublingual tablets (placed under the tongue) bypass the long passage through the gastrointestinal system and are absorbed readily into the bloodstream. This accelerates its action to a few minutes as opposed to the longer time requirement of oral agents (Figure 5-11, *A*). Buccal agents are another type of uncommon dosage form. Buccal tablets are placed between the gums and cheek, where the medication penetrates the mouth lining and then enters the bloodstream (Figure 5-11, *B*).

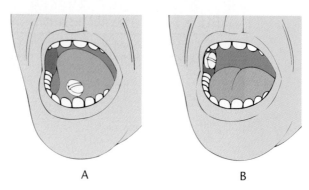

A   B

FIGURE 5-11 A, Sublingual tablet placement. **B,** Buccal tablet placement. (From Clayton B, Stock Y: *Basic pharmacology for nurses*, ed 14, St Louis, 2007, Elsevier.)

RAPIDLY DISINTEGRATING ORAL TABLETS

Some drugs are available in a newer dosage form that quickly disintegrates when taken orally and may be administered with or without water. This dosage form allows ease of administration for people who do not take larger sized tablets easily, or for those with conditions such as nausea and vomiting where taking a tablet may induce vomiting. Examples of orally disintegrating tablets (ODTs) include agents such as ondansetron (Zofran ODT) for nausea/vomiting, clonazepam orally disintegrating tablets for seizures, donepezil (Aricept ODT) for dementia, and rizatriptan (Maxalt ODT) for migraines.

RECTAL AGENTS

Rectal (PR) agents are used for many different reasons; for example, if a person is vomiting and cannot take oral medications, either suppositories or rectal suspensions can be used to treat the patient's condition. Different preparations are available, depending on the result desired. To reduce inflammation, ointments or creams can be used in addition to suppositories; these types of drugs work locally rather than systemically. However, for treating nausea/vomiting or motion sickness, a systemic-acting suppository can be used. Other agents include rectal solutions that also are used locally for various reasons, usually to clear the intestines of fecal material. The downside is that most persons do not feel comfortable using the rectal dosage forms. Also, depending on the drug and the retention time by the patient, the actual amount of drug absorbed may not be as predictable when compared with medications taken orally.

TOPICAL AGENTS

Many different preparations of topical (TOP) treatments are available. The effects of topical preparations range from systemic to localized (e.g., for rashes). The skin is the largest organ of the body because of its large surface area. The skin has many portals through which drugs can pass into the body. Openings include sweat glands, hair follicles, and other small openings in the pores of the skin. Many topical agents fight skin infections, reduce inflammation, and protect the skin from the ultraviolet rays of the sun. Topical agents work at the site of action, which makes them effective for localized use. In addition, manufacturers have created topical treatments that work systemically, such as medications for angina, blood pressure, hormonal replacement, motion sickness, and smoking cessation. These are prepared in a variety of dosage forms, from ointments to patches or small disks that can be applied to the skin. The medication is absorbed through the pores into the bloodstream, where it begins to work. An advantage of topical agents is the ease of application for the patient. Many topical medications act rapidly at the site of application to relieve itching or inflammation.

Patches can be worn all day, which increases patient compliance because the patient does not have to remember to take the medication at various times during the day. In fact, some patches, such as those for motion sickness, can be applied and left in place for days. The negative aspect of topical drugs is that they may cause skin irritation or may not be adequately absorbed transdermally; therefore many agents cannot be given by this route of administration. Because patches are generally more expensive to produce than other dosage forms, these medications tend to be more costly than their counterpart oral dosage forms.

PARENTERAL: INTRAVENOUS, INTRAVENOUS PIGGYBACK, INTRAMUSCULAR, AND SUBCUTANEOUS AGENTS

The word parenteral is Greek in origin and means "side of intestine" or "outside the intestine". A wide range of parenteral dosages and administration sites are available. The most common **parenteral medications** are given intravenously (IV), into the veins; intramuscularly (IM), into the muscles; or subcutaneously (subcut), under the skin. Very small–gauge needles are used, and the lengths depend on the sites being injected. Parenteral administration has clear benefits, such as the speed of action and completeness of dosing. Parenteral medications such as insulin have allowed millions of persons who suffer from diabetes to inject themselves daily, thus allowing them to maintain normal and productive lives. In addition, many parenteral drugs work faster than those given by the oral route. This is important for emergency situations, for patients who are unconscious or combative, or for patients who are unable to swallow. Also, smaller doses may be needed because of the high bioavailability of the agents injected. The disadvantage of parenteral drugs as a group is the increased risk of infection, since the techniques for administration are invasive. Any drug injection must be done using as sterile a technique as possible to avoid introducing any microbes into the body. Also, any injection is much more expensive than other routes of administration because of the required preparation and administration by trained personnel. Another disadvantage is that, because injectable drugs work quickly, once the drug is injected there is little or no time to alter its availability if an unintended dose is given or if an untoward reaction occurs.

EYE/EAR/NOSE (OPHTHALMIC, OTIC, NASAL)

Large assortments of agents are used for treating various conditions affecting the eyes, nose, and ears. A consideration one must remember when preparing and filling prescriptions for agents that treat the ear or eye is that doctors often use eye solutions to treat ear conditions; however, because the eye is sterile, ear solutions cannot be used to treat eye conditions. Therefore all ophthalmic drugs (eye preparations) are sterile. Otic drugs (ear preparations) are not necessarily always sterile because many otic agents treat the ear canal and do not typically penetrate a sterile environment. The pharmacy technician may prepare ophthalmic drugs in a laminar flow hood using aseptic technique (see Chapter 12). One must remember that all ophthalmic drugs need to be kept sterile. For the eye, ear, and nose there are different types of agents used, including ointments, solutions, and suspensions. Most treatments of the ear are for fighting an infection or removing earwax buildup. Most nasal sprays are used to treat symptoms of colds and allergies, whereas eye treatments are typically used for infections, inflammation, and conditions such as glaucoma (increased pressure of the eye). These types of dosage forms are effective at a specific site rather than involving the whole body. They can be administered with ease because of the small package size of the drug. Instructions for eye and ear preparations should use the word "**instill**" rather than "take" or "put." The main disadvantage of these drugs is that solutions used for the eye, if not kept sterile, can introduce bacteria into the area being treated. Also, ophthalmic drugs do not last as long as other treatments because of blinking of the eye and tearing, which wash the medication away from the site. Therefore dosing times may be frequent. In addition, most ophthalmic ointments make it hard to see clearly.

INHALANTS

Many persons suffer from lung diseases and use inhalants (INH) to treat their conditions. There are two types of inhalers: those that use a propellant to push the drug to the lungs, and those that use dry powder to release the medication as the patient takes a deep, fast breath. The dry powder inhalers may be a dry powder tube inhaler, a powder disk inhaler, or a single-dose dry powder disk inhaler. The choice of inhaler depends on its convenience for the patient as well as the medication needed. Some agents open the passageways to the lungs (e.g., bronchodilators), and some can be used to reduce inflammation (e.g., corticosteroids).

A positive aspect of inhalants is that most are available in handheld units and are convenient for carrying. The onset of action for short-acting bronchodilators, for example, is quick and can make an extreme difference in a person's ability to breathe comfortably. The disadvantage is that if not used properly little, if any, of the drug is able to reach the lungs. Breathing in as the inhaler is activated is important, and it may be necessary to shake some inhalers before drug administration. Dry powder inhalants are small and convenient to carry, do not require coordination of breathing at the exact time of medication release, and are not shaken before use, although some models do require cocking the device. Respiratory solutions that are packaged in unit dose ampules or vials are used to deliver a specific amount of drug per treatment with the use of a nebulizer.

INJECTABLE (LONG-ACTING)

An assortment of long-acting parenteral drugs is available that can be used in place of daily dosing. Examples include the use of medroxyprogesterone acetate (Depo-Provera, Depo-subcut Provera 104) for birth control, which must be injected every 3 months. Other parenteral long-acting medications include haloperidol decanoate, which is used monthly for the treatment of schizophrenia, and leuprolide acetate injection suspension (e.g., Lupron depot), which is injected either once monthly or once every 3 months for various hormonal disorders. The technician should note that long-acting depot injectable products are never to be given intravenously.

MISCELLANEOUS ROUTES

Other common routes of administration include vaginal or urethral dosage forms. These forms are suppositories, creams, ointments, foams, gels, and various inserts, such as rings. These types of delivery systems are used for treatment of infections and inflammation and, in the case of vaginal foams or rings, for local or systemic birth control, respectively. Although there are clear advantages in using these agents, such as bypassing a systemic effect for some medications and affecting the specific site only, they are not necessarily applied easily and can be uncomfortable.

Other Considerations: Form and Function

Dosage forms are created based on the results from many clinical trials that investigate the **pharmacokinetics** of the medication or the function of the drug in experiments.

PHARMACOKINETICS VS. PHARMACODYNAMICS

Pharmacokinetics is an all-inclusive word that represents many different components concerning the actions of the body on a drug, as opposed to pharmacodynamics (to be discussed later), which describes the effects the drug has on the body. For example, from the time a person takes a tablet, various considerations are examined, such as levels of drug in the blood and tissues, the absorption or movement of the drug throughout the body, and the overall distribution, metabolism, and excretion of the drug. This includes the reaction of the drug with other drugs to determine changes that may occur in the course of the drug's time in the body. As these components are tested and refined, the eventual result is a dosage form that is tailor-made to work at its optimal level, while always keeping patient adherence in mind. Patient adherence is the level at which patients will or will not take their scheduled drugs. If a manufacturer can make a drug that can be taken once daily rather than several times a day, the odds increase that the patient will take the medication as directed.

The following section describes the overall pharmacokinetics or life of the drug in the body. Absorption, distribution, metabolism, and excretion (ADME) will be discussed, as well as half-life, bioavailability, and bioequivalence. All information concerning the pharmacokinetics of a drug and its relation to the proper dosing and use of the drug is listed in several reference books (see Chapter 6) and official drug package inserts.

ABSORPTION

Medications are made specifically to pass through natural body barriers such as the skin, stomach, intestines, blood-brain barrier (surrounding the brain), and other membranous tissues. How well the drug passes through these barriers is one factor that determines its ultimate **absorption**, distribution, and effectiveness. Some considerations include whether the barrier is a lipid base (fatty) or not. Membranes surrounding organs, such as the intestine, have a variety of proteins and other structures implanted in a membranous protective structure that act as carriers for drug transport or as receptor sites. Important chemicals and drugs are able to pass a lock-and-key mechanism by latching onto receptive sites that allow the chemical or drug to pass into the organ to reach the final site of action intended for the drug. Figure 5-12 shows an example of this action.

DISTRIBUTION

After the systemic absorption of a medication, the medication is distributed throughout the body from the bloodstream into tissues, membranes, and ultimately organs of the body. Therefore **distribution** is the location of a medication throughout blood, organs, and tissues after administration and absorption. For some medications, the distribution of the drug in the blood is measured at certain times throughout the day to keep track of medication concentrations and to ensure therapeutic effectiveness. Clearance (the volume of plasma from which the drug is removed per unit of time) may also be determined from the changes in blood concentrations within the dosing interval. Not all systems are affected equally by the drugs administered, with some areas not allowing drugs to infiltrate as rapidly as other areas. The distribution of a drug is therefore not necessarily equal throughout the entire body. For example, the blood-brain barrier is a built-in system that functions to keep harmful chemicals away from the brain. Certain medications have to be made that can cross this barrier in order to help treat diseases. Likewise, many medications that may penetrate the blood-brain barrier can cause unwanted side effects, such as hypertension. These are just a

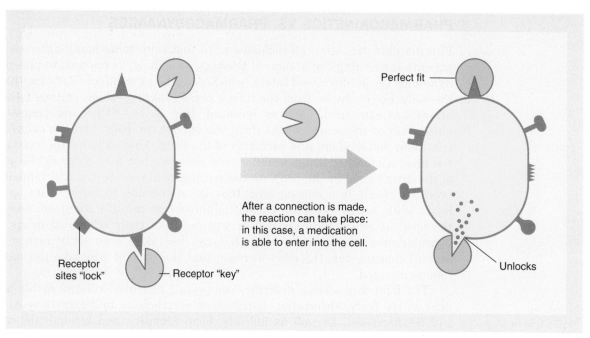

FIGURE 5-12 Lock-and-key mechanism allowing absorption to take place in a cell. These common reactions take place naturally throughout the body. Only after the correct receptor makes a connection with the matching receptor site will the cell allow a reaction to take place. Medications often mimic this natural mechanism.

BOX 5-1 IONIZATION

Weak acid in weak base is less ionized = transported more rapidly into lipid membranes

Weak base in weak acid is less ionized = transported more rapidly into lipid membranes

few of the hurdles drug companies must contend with when creating new medications. Morphine cannot cross the blood-brain barrier, whereas fentanyl can do so easily; therefore fentanyl has a faster acting capability. Also, most drugs are either weak acids or weak bases (see Chemistry, Chapter 31), which influences many of their pharmacokinetic characteristics, including their distribution to various body fluids and tissues (Box 5-1).

Protein binding is another important factor related to drug distribution. Most drugs will bind to blood proteins to some degree. Warfarin (a "blood thinner" or anticoagulant) and phenytoin (an anticonvulsant) are examples of types of drugs where alterations in protein binding can become clinically important to the amount of drug available for distribution and therapeutic effect. If a patient is treated with warfarin in concert with phenytoin, the drugs will compete for protein binding sites and the level of free (unbound) warfarin may increase to an unsafe level.

METABOLISM

Drug **metabolism** is the biochemical modification or degradation of drugs in the body. As the drug is being distributed throughout the body, some of the drug reenters the bloodstream and ultimately is transferred to the liver, where most drug metabolism takes place. Metabolism changes the chemical structure of the original drug. Certain agents such as pro-drugs can be altered in the liver to produce the active agent, or a drug can be made less toxic or ineffective. Some drugs can pass directly from the gastrointestinal tract to the liver, where the strength of the active ingredient is reduced before it enters the bloodstream. This alters the amount of available drug at the site where it is needed. There are other drugs that do not undergo any change at all and are excreted from the body in the same form in which they were introduced. Different influences can alter metabolism, such as age, gender, genetics, diet, and other chemicals ingested.

Most of the final metabolism of a drug takes place in the liver. This is the final processing center of the body that extracts toxins and unwanted chemicals and forwards them to the excretion process (such as the kidneys). The liver works hard, but has a limit to the amount it can process in a given time. Persons suffering from any type of liver damage must be monitored closely when taking various medications to ensure that toxic levels are not present in the liver.

EXCRETION/ELIMINATION

Excretion is the last phase of a drug's life in the body. Although excretion usually is associated with urination, it is important to know that there are many ways that a drug can be excreted from the body. In addition to excretion via the kidneys, drugs also may be expelled via the feces, exhalation, sweat glands, and even breast milk in women who are lactating. Urination and bowel movements are by far the most common methods of excretion. Remember that drugs that are not eliminated properly may accumulate in the body and can lead to toxicity. Less common routes of excretion, such as through breast milk, must be considered when a doctor prescribes a drug, although not all drugs are tested by the manufacturer for excretion into breast milk; therefore the doctor must use his or her judgment on the use of these agents.

BIOAVAILABILITY

Bioavailability is the proportion of the drug that is delivered to its destination and is available to the site of action for which it was intended. Different drugs clear in different ways and at different times. This is an important consideration when prescribing drugs and determining drug dosing intervals. Drugs that are intended for certain organs or tissues in the body must pass many different obstacles, such as the destructive actions of stomach acids. An intravenous (IV) injection has a bioavailability of 100%, but bioavailability varies for other routes of administration such as intramuscular (IM), subcutaneous (subcut), topical, and oral (PO). Many orally administered drugs travel to the liver and a proportion of the dose is metabolized before the drug has a chance to be distributed; this is called the "first pass" effect and it lowers the drug's final bioavailability. Drugs that experience a first pass effect are given in higher doses than their injectable counterparts. Certain oral medications do not experience this effect and have good bioavailability from oral or injectable routes. Intravenous agents bypass the first pass phenomenon because they enter directly into the bloodstream.

HALF-LIFE

Half-life refers to the time it takes the body to break down and excrete one half of the drug. To be more precise, it is the time taken for the plasma concentration of the drug to decrease by 50%. Of course, just monitoring the drug's plasma level is not the only factor that should be considered when determining half-life (e.g., muscle, fat, and tissue should be taken into account). After approximately 4 half-lives, elimination is 94% complete. For example, if a person takes a medication that has a half-life of 10 hours, this means that in

10 hours one half of the drug will be eliminated, and in another 10 hours another one half of the remaining drug will be eliminated. This is an important factor in the creation of all drugs because this information tells the manufacturer how long it takes the body to rid itself of the drug, and helps to determine proper intervals for dosing. If a person takes too much medication or takes doses too close together, the drug can accumulate, which can be dangerous to the patient.

BIOEQUIVALENCE

Bioequivalence is the comparison between drugs from different manufacturers or from the same manufacturer but different batches (lots). This is an important aspect of a drug because patients assume that every tablet they take is exactly the same as the one before and that all are the exact strength as listed on the label. Generic drug manufacturers strive to achieve the same equivalence as brand name manufacturers so that they can compete with the original manufacturer. A reference source that can be used to determine whether the generic drug is rated as bioequivalent to the brand name drug is the *Orange Book*. This book lists the approved drug products with therapeutic equivalence and evaluations.

The Use of Excipients

All medications are prepared with additives (excipients) for many different reasons, as shown in Table 5-6. These additives include coloring for better appearance of the product and flavorings to disguise taste and/or smell. Many times fillers are used to increase the size of the medication because there may be such a small amount of drug that it otherwise would be hard, if not impossible, to handle. Many different types of preservatives are available; each prevents certain microbes from affecting the drug. These preservatives prolong the shelf life after the patient obtains and opens the drug product. Other types of additives include those that either increase the dispersal rate of the drug once it reaches the intestines or decrease the rate of distribution of the medication. Again, many components that are involved in the preparation of dosage forms are added to improve the product for the patient's convenience. Patients are more likely to take medication once or twice daily as opposed to multiple times per day.

Some patients may be allergic to an ingredient, such as dyes, or may have conditions in which certain ingredients should be avoided. For example, patients with diabetes may be instructed to purchase drug products that are sugar-free or alcohol-free. Patients with phenylketonuria may need to avoid products containing aspartame as a sweetener. Certain products may be available in the form required, while others may not. For patients who need alternative ingredients, a compounding pharmacy may be able to prepare the same drug containing ingredients that are tolerated by the patient.

Manufactured Products

After learning how many different routes of administration there are and the dosage forms used, you may think that is all there is. The ever-changing world of drug manufacturing has made available many different choices and has turned a simple compressed powder, known as a tablet, into an intricate, complicated, and highly structured format. A tablet is not just a tablet, nor a capsule merely a capsule. As seen in Table 5-7, there are many different types of dosage forms depending on the desired effect of the drug in question. All manufactured types of dosage forms must be approved by the Food and Drug Administration

TABLE 5-6 Description of Additives

Type of Additive	Example of Chemical	Reason
Weak salt acid/base	Hydrochloric acid and sodium hydroxide (base)	Helps dissolve drug easier once it arrives in gastrointestinal system.
Preservative	Parabens	Increases shelf life.
Sweetener	Sucrose	Improves taste.
Flavoring	Cherry	Improves taste.
Coloring	Yellow dye no. 5	Improves visual appearance.
Buffer	Sodium acetate	Adjusts pH.
Antifungal	Benzoic acid	Prevents fungal growth.
Base	Petrolatum	Is a common component to which medication is added for ointments and creams.
Filler	Starch, powdered cellulose	Increases size of dosage form.

TABLE 5-7 Description of Dosage Forms

Dosage Form	Types	Result
Oral tablet	Layered	Slow release
	Film-coated	Protects against stomach acid
	Extended-release	Releases medication slowly
	Compressed	Hard dissolves slower; soft dissolves faster
Coated tablet	Sugar added and colored	Protects drug; covers taste
	Caplet	Hard, capsule-shaped tablet
	Colored	Appearance
	Gel	Smaller than a capsule, easier to swallow
	Enteric-coated	Delayed release; easier to swallow
	Dissolving	Dissolves in mouth on contact
Sublingual/buccal	Soft compressed	Dissolve in mouth
Chewable tablet		Chewed
Capsule	Gelatin cover	Allows for pharmacy-compounded agents; easy to swallow
	Spansule	Capsule holds small pellets or beads
	Pulvule	Manufacturer prepared (bullet shaped)
	Dry fill	Filled with powder
Hard gelatin		Filled with a tablet inside
		Filled with pellets
		Filled with another capsule
Soft gelatin	Wet fill	Filled with a liquid
		Filled with paste
Injectable vial	Multiple-dose vial	May be used more than once
	Single-dose vial	Must be discarded after one use
	ADD-Vantage vial	Rubber stopper is pushed, releasing diluents into powder product

(see Chapter 2). Approval of a drug product includes the constant testing of the product from batch to batch to ensure continuity of the medication. Injectable dosage forms are discussed further in Chapter 12. Pharmacies that provide compounded products must comply with the standards of the *United States Pharmacopoeia* or *National Formulary* monographs.

TABLE 5-8 Examples of Storage Requirements

Medication	Location	Considerations
Suppository	Drug shelf or refrigerator	Intended to melt at body temperature
Latanoprost	Refrigerator	Stored in refrigerator (2-8° C) until opened; may be kept up to 6 weeks at room temperature after opening
Metronidazole IV	At room temperature	Stored at 15-30° C and protected from light
Vaccines such as Hib, HepA, HepB, human papillomavirus, DTaP, DT, Td, Tdap, influenza, MMR, meningococcal, pneumococcal, rotavirus	Refrigerator	Kept in refrigerator (2-8° C)
Vaccines such as MMR, MMRV, varicella-zoster	Freezer	Kept in freezer (−15° C)
Insulin mixtures containing regular insulin and NPH, including combination formulations	Room temperature	Stored for 1 month at room temperature Stored for 3 months refrigerated (2-8° C)
Insulin, regular mixed with sterile water or sodium chloride	Room temperature	Must be used within 24 hr
Insulin aspart or combination aspart, NPH (e.g., NovoLog 70/30 FlexPen)	Room temperature	Stored for 14 days (below 30° C)
Penicillin IV	Drug shelf or refrigerator	Must be stored in refrigerator after reconstitution
Mannitol	At room temperature	Mannitol crystallizes at room temperature; do not use crystallized drug; drug must be warmed before using if crystals are present

Packaging and Storage Requirements

Medications are packaged according to manufacturers' specifications to ensure the effectiveness and shelf life of the drug. It is important for technicians to learn the various storage requirements of medications. Medications that have specific storage requirements will be clearly marked on the container or box in which they are packaged. Certain medications arrive in dry ice and must be unpacked and stored immediately at the proper temperature indicated. When the outside of a box is labeled "refrigerate or keep frozen," the contents should never be left at room temperature, because this can cause the medication to become unusable. Listed in Table 5-8 are some examples of storage requirements for various drugs, along with special considerations. All medications have a package insert that describes the storage and stability of the drug. Technicians should become familiar with this type of information. In addition to manufacturer storage requirements, repackaging medications have their own guidelines, which have been instituted by the FDA and can be found in Chapter 11.

Medical Terminology

Another aspect of working with patients is the ability to understand medical terminology. Just as many medication names are derived from the Greek and Latin languages, so are all medical terms. In this chapter we will cover the basics of medical terminology. A description of the segments of medical terms along with terms associated with each body system will be covered. Medical terms consist of segments or word parts. In combination they describe all conditions and anatomy known. In Table 5-9 a sample of abbreviations used in the medical field is given.

TABLE 5-9 Abbreviations for Conditions or Body Systems

Abbreviation	Meaning
ADHD	Attention deficit hyperactivity disorder
ADR	Adverse drug reaction
AIDS	Acquired immunodeficiency syndrome
BBB	Blood-brain barrier
BUN	Blood urea nitrogen
CABG	Coronary artery bypass graft
CAD	Coronary artery disease
CBC	Complete blood count
CCU	Coronary care unit
CHD	Coronary heart disease
CHF	Congestive heart failure
COPD	Chronic obstructive pulmonary disease
CVD	Cardiovascular disease
DNR	Do not resuscitate
DOA	Dead on arrival
DOB	Date of birth
DVT	Deep vein thrombosis
DX	Diagnosis
ED	Emergency department
EEG	Electroencephalogram
EENT	Eye, ear, nose, and throat
EKG	Electrocardiogram
ER	Emergency room
FX	Fracture
GERD	Gastroesophageal reflux disease
HBP	High blood pressure
HIV	Human immunodeficiency virus
HPV	Human papillomavirus
HTN	Hypertension
IDDM	Insulin-dependent diabetes mellitus
ICU	Intensive care unit
KVO	Keep vein open
LBP	Low blood pressure
LBP	Lower back pain
LLL	Left lower lobe
MI	Myocardial infarction
MRI	Magnetic resonance imaging
N & V	Nausea and vomiting
NICU	Neonatal intensive care unit
NIDDM	Non-insulin–dependent diabetes mellitus
NPO	Nothing by mouth
OBGYN	Obstetrics and gynecology
OR	Operating room
PPN	Peripheral parenteral nutrition
PT	Prothrombin time
RLS	Restless leg syndrome
SARS	Severe acute respiratory syndrome
SBO	Small bowel obstruction
SOB	Shortness of breath
TKO	To keep open
TPN	Total parenteral nutrition
TX	Treatment
UNG	Ointment
UTI	Urinary tract infection
WBC	White blood cell count

It is important to know the basics of how medical terminology applies to various conditions. Terms and drugs fit together like a hand and glove. There are four segments of word parts.

1. The prefix
2. The suffix
3. The root word
4. The combining form

When combining these word segments, there are only a few rules to follow as seen in Box 5-2. A list of common prefixes, suffixes, and root words with their combining forms is given in Table 5-10.

Although this chapter mentioned many competencies in which a technician must be proficient, most of what you will learn will occur while you are employed. However, it is important to always keep learning, because this will promote both self-development and advancement in your profession. New dosage forms are always being invented both for convenience and to achieve the best results. Staying current on the new trends can be accomplished by additional reading, continuing education, and on-the-job training.

BOX 5-2 OVERVIEW OF WORD PARTS OF MEDICAL TERMINOLOGY

Example of how a word is formed:

1. Prefix: placed before each combining form
   Example: peri- (around)
2. Suffix: placed after the combining form
   Example: -itis (inflammation)
3. The root word of the term
   Example: cardia (heart)
4. The combining form
   Example: cardi/o
   Read the term from right to left
   Put them together: pericarditis (i.e., inflammation around the heart)

Rules
1. Terms can be 1 to 4 combinations.
2. Read right to left.
3. There can be multiple terms that define the same word part.
4. If the combining form has 2 vowels (e.g., i, o) and the suffix begins with a vowel, drop the "o."

TABLE 5-10 Common Body System Word Segments

Prefixes	
a-	away from, without
hyper-	above, fast, elevated
hypo-	below, slow, low
post-	after
brady-	slow
tachy-	fast
poly-	many
sub-	under, less than, below
peri-	around, surrounding
pre-	before
dys-	painful or disordered

TABLE 5-10 **Common Body System Word Segments—cont'd**

Suffixes

-al	pertaining to
-itis	inflammation
-ology	study of
-ologist	specialist
-ectomy	removal
-otomy	opening
-algia	pain
-megaly	enlargement
-necrosis	tissue death
-sclerosis	hardening
-stenosis	narrowing
-plasty	repair
-gram	picture or record
-scopy	visual exam
-rrhage	excessive flow
-rrhea	flow or discharge
-rrhexis	rupture
-pnea	breathing

Colors

cyan/o	Blue
leuk/o	White
rubi/o	Red
melan/o	Black

Cardiovascular System

cardi/o	heart
angi/o, vas/o	blood vessel
arteri/o	artery
phlebo	vein
hem/o	blood
capill/o	capillaries

Digestive and Hepatic Systems

gastr/o	stomach
stomat/o	mouth
enter/o	relating to the intestine
col/o, colon/o	large intestine
proct/o, rect/o	anus or rectum
hepat/o	liver
cholecyst/o	gallbladder
pancreat/o	pancreas

Eyes

opt/i	eyes
ophthalm/o	eyes
ir/i, ir/o	iris
phac/o, phak/o	retina

Ears

acous/o, ot/o	ears or hearing
pinn/i	sound

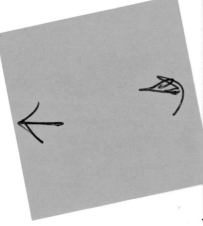

Continued

TABLE 5-10 Common Body System Word Segments—cont'd

myring/o	middle ear
tympan/o	membrane of middle ear, eardrum
labyrinth/o	inner ear

Endocrine System

adren/o	adrenal glands
gonad/o	gonads (male, female)
parathyroid/o	parathyroid gland
pinea/o	pineal gland
pituit/o	pituitary glands
thym/o	thymus
thyr/o, thyroid/o	thyroid gland

Integumentary/Skin System

cutan/o	skin
dermat/o, derm/o	skin
seb/o	sebaceous glands
hidr/o	sweat glands
pil/i, pil/o	hair
onych/o	nails

Nervous System

neur/o	nerves
encephal/o	brain
myel/o	spinal cord
mening/o	membranes covering spinal cord and brain

Reproductive System

pen/i, phall/i	penis
orch/o, test/i	testicles
oophor/o	ovaries
salping/o	fallopian tubes
hyster/o	uterus
placent/o	placenta

Respiratory System

nas/o	nose
sinus/o	sinus
rhino	nose
pharyng/o	pharynx
laryng/o	larynx
trache/o	trachea
bronchi/o	bronchi
aveol/o	alveoli

Musculoskeletal System

myo	muscle
oste/o	bones
myel/o	bone marrow
chondr/o	cartilage
arthro	joints
ligament/o	ligaments
burs/o	bursa

TABLE 5-10 Common Body System Word Segments—cont'd

Urinary System

nephr/o	kidneys
pyel/o	pelvis or kidney
ur/o, urin/o	urine
ureter/o	ureters
cyst/o	bladder
urethr/o	urethra

DO YOU REMEMBER THESE KEY POINTS?

- Various routes of administration
- Terms and definitions relating to pharmacokinetics
- Abbreviations for the routes of administration
- Reasons why different routes are used to administer drugs
- Forms and functions of medications
- Food and Drug Administration guidelines for proper manufacturing practices
- Types of additives used in manufacturing dosage forms and the reasons for their use
- How different dosage forms affect pharmacokinetics
- The importance of the half-life of a drug
- Storage requirements of medications
- Common medical terms and abbreviations
- Segments of medical terms
- Drug abbreviations

REVIEW QUESTIONS

Multiple choice questions

1. Why are sublingual tablets better for relieving anginal attacks than traditional tablets?
   A. They are smaller.
   B. They bypass the stomach, entering the bloodstream for quicker relief.
   C. They are cheaper.
   D. Both A and C are correct.

2. Why do manufacturers make dosage forms that are effective over a longer time?
   A. To cut down on the cost of making the drug
   B. To save time preparing each dose
   C. To enable the patient to take the medication less often
   D. To meet Food and Drug Administration standards

3. Preservatives are often added to medications to:
   A. Increase their shelf life
   B. Decrease the possibility of contamination
   C. Reduce the cost of manufacturing large amounts of the drug
   D. Both A and B

4. Often, parenteral medications are used because:
   A. They work fast
   B. They bypass the acidic secretions of the stomach
   C. The patient is unable to take medication by mouth
   D. All of the above

5. The definition of pharmacokinetics can be best described as:
   A. The study of the action of drugs in the body
   B. The appropriate dosing of a drug
   C. The pharmacy aspect of a drug
   D. The testing of a drug

6. An advantage of taking medications orally is/are:
   A. Lower cost
   B. Easier to administer than other routes
   C. Less chance of infection with oral dosage forms
   D. All of the above

7. The organ that performs most of the metabolism of a drug is:
   A. The kidney
   B. The blood
   C. The stomach
   D. The liver

8. If a drug has a half-life of 20 hours, this would mean that:
   A. Half of the drug would be eliminated from the body in the first 20 hours, followed by the second half in 20 more hours
   B. The drug will only last half as long as needed
   C. The drug will lose half its strength in half of 20 hours
   D. The drug will lose half its strength in 20 hours, followed by half of the remaining strength in the following 20 hours, and so forth

9. Of the body areas listed, which one is not a common route for excretion?
   A. Intestines
   B. Kidneys
   C. Mouth
   D. Skin

10. Dyes and sugars are used in preparing medications to:
    A. Improve appearance and taste
    B. Improve taste and shelf life
    C. Improve sales
    D. All of the above

11. Which of the following medications is available in capsule form?
    A. Flagyl
    B. Tegretol
    C. Diltiazem
    D. Lasix

12. Which of the following medications is available as an injectable form?
    A. Aspirin
    B. Albuterol
    C. Amoxicillin
    D. Ampicillin

13. Which of the following medications is available as a patch?
    A. Nitroglycerin
    B. Digoxin
    C. Guaifenesin
    D. Diphenhydramine

14. Which of the following terms means nose?
    A. Rhino
    B. Naso
    C. Pharyngo
    D. Both A and B

15. Which of the following term/s mean/s muscle?

A. Myelo

B. Myo

C. Mucuso

D. Both A and B

True/False

If the statement is false, then change it to make it true.

_____ **1.** Medications for the ear also can be used for the eye.

_____ **2.** Depending on the type of rectal medication given, the medication can work systemically or locally.

_____ **3.** Parenteral drugs are used only in emergency departments.

_____ **4.** A bioequivalent generic drug means it is equivalent to the brand name drug for effectiveness.

_____ **5.** Phenol is used in making drugs because of its taste properties.

_____ **6.** Fungal and bacterial contamination can occur if medications are not stored properly.

_____ **7.** Some medications require tests to determine whether the liver is eliminating them from the body appropriately.

_____ **8.** Ophthalmic medications can be delivered in lenses.

_____ **9.** Capsules can be manufactured to hold smaller capsules or tablets.

_____ **10.** Pharmacy technicians are not responsible for making errors if the doctor's handwriting is illegible.

_____ **11.** Duragesic, nitroglycerin, and scopolamine are examples of medications that are available in topical forms.

_____ **12.** A person suffering from inflammation of the middle ear would have tympanitis.

_____ **13.** A person with a rapid heart rate would have bradycardia.

_____ **14.** One symptom of rhinitis is a runny nose.

_____ **15.** Salpingo-oophorectomy describes the surgical removal of all female sex organs.

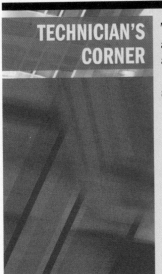

TECHNICIAN'S CORNER

The following examples list the proper way to transcribe orders along with an example of a prescription order for that route. Using these as a guideline, answer the question at the end of this Technician's Corner.

Remember that physicians should not use many of these abbreviations; still, they may write in upper or lower case letters for these orders.

1. Oral routes, written PO
   PO = by mouth, orally
2. Rectal routes, written PR
   PR = per rectal, rectally
3. Topically, written TOP
   TOP = to be applied to the surface of the skin
4. Parenteral drugs; written either IV, IM, or ID
   IV = intravenous
   IM = intramuscular
   ID = intradermal

Continued

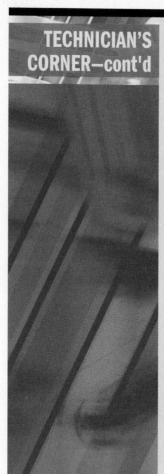

TECHNICIAN'S CORNER—cont'd

Question

A patient brings in a prescription. Transcribe this order into lay person's terms, and list any auxiliary labels that should be adhered to the prescription. Finally, list any questions that you may have about the order. Who would you ask?

Exercise: Determine the appropriate medical term for each of the conditions listed below:

1. Hardening of the arteries
2. Visual exam of the joints
3. Pain in the muscle
4. Inflammation of the brain
5. Inflammation of the bone and muscle
6. Painful menstruation
7. Surgical repair of a muscle
8. Abnormally low heart rhythm
9. Enlarged heart
10. Inflammation of the skin
11. Inflammation of the nasal cavity
12. Inflammation of the kidney
13. Abnormal narrowing of the arteries
14. Abnormal hardening of the arteries
15. Repair of the arteries
16. Rapid heart rate
17. Opening in the trachea
18. Painful breathing
19. Condition of a bluish color
20. Study of kidneys

BIBLIOGRAPHY

Ansel HC, Allen LV, Popovich NG: *Ansel's Pharmaceutical dosage forms and drug delivery systems*, ed 8, Baltimore, 2004, Lippincott Williams & Wilkins.

Brown M, Mulholland J: *Drug calculations*, ed 8, St Louis, 2007, Elsevier.

Drug facts and comparisons, ed 63, St Louis, 2009, Wolters Kluwer Health.

Gray Morris D: *Calculate with confidence*, ed 5, St Louis, 2009, Elsevier.

Potter PA, Perry AG: *Fundamentals of nursing*, ed 7, St Louis, 2008, Elsevier.

WEBSITES

Immunization Action Coalition p3049. (Technical reviewed by CDC 2007). Vaccine Handling Tips. (Referenced 8/24/09). www.vaccineinformation.org

Medscape website. Monograph-Insulins General Statement. (Referenced 8/24/09). www.medscape.com/druginfo/monoinfobyid?cid=med&drugid=5218&drugname=Humulin+R+Inj&monotype=genstatement&monoid=382933&mononame=Insulins%20General%20Statement&print=1

Orange book information. (Referenced 3/15/009). www.fda.gov/cder/ob

Wisniewski, RN, Carol Holquist, RPh. USPHS. The absence of a trade name does not equal a generic drug. 10/10/2005. (Referenced 4/3/09). www.drugtopics.com

Drug Information References

Objectives

UPON COMPLETING THIS CHAPTER, YOU SHOULD BE ABLE TO DO THE FOLLOWING:

- Demonstrate the appropriate way to research drugs and other information from reference books, journals, and electronic resources.

- Demonstrate the appropriate way to reference drugs and other information from the Internet.

- Describe the information contained in the following references:
  American Drug Index
  American Hospital Formulary Service Drug Information
  *Approved Drug Products with Therapeutic Equivalence
    Evaluations* (otherwise known as the *"Orange Book"*)
  Clinical Pharmacology
  Drug Facts and Comparisons or *e-Facts*
  Drug Topics Red Book
  Goodman & Gilman's The Pharmacological Basis of Therapeutics
  Handbook of Nonprescription Drugs
  Ident-A-Drug Handbook
  Martindale's The Complete Drug Reference
  Micromedex
  Physicians' Desk Reference
  *Remington's Pharmaceutical Sciences: The Science and Practice
    of Pharmacy*
  Trissel's Handbook on Injectable Drugs
  United States Pharmacist's Pharmacopeia
  United States Pharmacopeia National Formulary

- Explain the specialized reference books necessary in hospital pharmacy.

- List other types of reference materials in addition to books.

- Explain the importance of journals and newsmagazines as they pertain to pharmacy and continuing education.

- Describe how to find reputable websites for referencing.

- Demonstrate how to identify medications through reference books or electronic sources.

TERMS AND DEFINITIONS

Brand/trade name *Trademark of a drug or device held by the originating manufacturing company*

Chemical structure *The shape of molecules and their location to one another in a given compound*

Drug classification *Categorization based on various characteristics, including the chemical structure of a drug, the action of a drug, and/or the therapeutic or anatomical use of a drug*

Formulary *A list of preferred drugs to be stocked by the pharmacy; also a list of drugs covered by an insurance company*

Generic name *Name assigned to a medication or nonproprietary name of a drug*

Non-formulary *A list of drugs that are not normally stocked by the pharmacy; these drugs may not be covered by an insurance company unless specific conditions are met*

Package insert *The official prescribing information for a prescription drug; medication information sheet provided by the manufacturer that includes side effects, dosage forms, indications, and other important information*

Introduction

Drug information reference books are some of the most important tools that are used in pharmacy. Doctors, nurses, and other health care professionals call the pharmacy daily to ask questions concerning various medications. Pharmacists rely on credible, accurate, and up-to-date reference resources to help give the correct information to others. Although a few of the books in pharmacy are highly technical, most give basic information on drugs. Knowing which book to choose for referencing and how to access the information is an important skill for pharmacists and technicians. This chapter covers the references that are more commonly used in a pharmacy. In addition, other types of referencing materials that can be of help specifically to the technician are listed.

Understanding the Correct Way to Reference

Before you begin to look for information, take these key points into consideration. First, what exactly is the purpose of your search? What is the question that needs to be answered? Do you need to know the generic drug name

Tech Note!

Technically, all generic drug names are spelled in lower case letters as opposed to trade or brand names, which are capitalized: for example, atenolol (generic) and Tenormin (brand).

Tech Note!

Generic drug names do not typically begin with J or W because those letters do not exist in the languages of many countries outside of the United States that use generic drugs. Trade names can reflect the drug's primary characteristics or use but cannot imply a cure of a specific part of the body.

only, the drug's interactions and classification, or even perhaps the drug's appearance? Let us begin with the process of drug development, manufacturing, and naming drugs to learn the importance of each one of these components.

When a new drug is in the experimentation phase, the creators or the company give the drug a generic or investigational drug name based on its chemical attributes; the name also prepares the drug for recognition during future marketing after approval. Later, when the drug is approved through the Food and Drug Administration, a monograph, or official label, is created to include important findings, such as side effects that were reported during clinical trials.

The **classification** of a drug is important because it places the drug into proper categories based on its chemical structure, its mechanism of action, its anatomical function, and/or its therapeutic use. Many times, drugs within the same class act in similar ways. This information can assist the prescriber and pharmacist in knowing the expected therapeutic effect as well as possible adverse reactions.

The indication lists the main conditions for which the chemical is used. A contraindications list is also an important part of a drug monograph. This list identifies types of persons who should not be given the medication. Reasons may range from certain serious drug-drug interactions to conditions that conflict with the action of the drug. After all the studies have been done and the data have been analyzed, contraindications may still be discovered in post-market use and will be updated in the drug's monograph. It is always helpful to ensure that you are viewing the most recent information regarding a drug. The last date of update will be listed directly on the official product labeling.

The founding company also assigns the chemical name (derived from the **chemical structure**), generic name, and **trade name**, which are also found in the product's official label. Many times generic names are closely related to the chemical name of the drug, but not always. The drug's trade name may be related to the function or main use of the drug (Box 6-1). Examples of **generic names** can be seen in Box 6-2.

BOX 6-1 EXAMPLES OF TRADE DRUG NAMES THAT INDICATE THE FUNCTION OF THE DRUG

Lopressor
 For hypertension; conveys lowering blood pressure
Lotensin
 For hypertension; conveys lowering blood pressure
Lipitor
 Lowers blood lipids (cholesterol); conveys treatment of lipids
Neurontin
 Treats conditions affecting the neurons (nerves); conveys treatment of nerves
Restoril
 Treats insomnia; conveys restfulness
Wellbutrin
 Treats depression; conveys wellness
Celexa
 Treats depression; conveys celebration, wellness
Viagra
 Treats erectile dysfunction; conveys vigor, vitality

BOX 6-2 EXAMPLES OF SIMILAR ENDINGS OF GENERIC DRUG NAMES

Beta-blockers end in *-olol* (these agents are primarily used to treat high blood pressure [HBP]):
  atenolol (Tenormin)
  betaxolol (Kerlone)
  pindolol (Visken)
  nadolol (Corgard)
  timolol (Blocadren)

ACE inhibitors end in *-pril* (these agents are primarily used to treat HBP):
  captopril (Capoten)
  enalapril (Vasotec)
  lisinopril (Prinivil, Zestril)
  moexipril (Univasc)
  trandolapril (Mavik)

Calcium channel blockers end in *-dipine* (these agents are primarily used to treat HBP and heart rhythm disorders):
  amlodipine (Norvasc)
  isradipine (DynaCirc)
  nicardipine (Cardene SR)
  nifedipine (Procardia XL, Adalat CC)
  nisoldipine (Sular)

Penicillins end in *-cillin* (these agents are used to treat infections):
  ampicillin (found as a component in Unasyn)
  amoxicillin (Amoxil, also a component of Augmentin)
  dicloxacillin (no trade names available; generic only)
  penicillin G benzathine (Bicillin L-A)
  penicillin VK (no trade names available; generic only)
  ticarcillin (found as a component of Timentin)

References Used in Pharmacy

In addition to being familiar with the official label of a product, technicians also must be at ease using basic drug and pharmacy references in the pharmacy. Good references have a section on how to use the text, or online "help" sections to aid the reader in the use of computerized resources. If possible, it is helpful for the technician to be familiar with performing a reference search before it is required. Knowing how to use the reference properly allows the technician to find the correct information in a timely manner. In this way, the technician can assist the pharmacist in locating the correct information.

Although many different types of reference materials are available, this chapter describes only the most common types seen in a pharmacy setting. Many reference materials are available to technicians and pharmacists in a variety of formats, and it should be noted that online interfaces such as *Micromedex* and *Clinical Pharmacology* are more and more prevalent in the pharmacy setting. The following examples of commonly used reference materials are normally available in more than one form. All of the books can be found at online booksellers such as amazon.com. At the end of each description is a list of available products.

DRUG FACTS AND COMPARISONS

Drug Facts and Comparisons is one of the most often used books by pharmacists. This reference book was first published in 1946 and was created for quick and accurate reference and drug comparison. Because of its vital information and

TABLE 6-1 Sections in *Drug Facts and Comparisons*

Sections in Order of Reference	Contents of Each Section	Specific Information
Section 1	Index	Generic and trade names
Section 2	Keeping up	Orphan, investigational, and temporary listings
Section 3	Drug monographs	14 chapters of drug descriptions
Section 4	Drug identification	More than 250 drugs shown in color
Section 5	Appendix	Dosage calculations and list of manufacturers

TABLE 6-2 Sections of *Physicians' Desk Reference*

Sections in Order of Reference	Contents of Each Section	Specific Information
Section 1	Manufacturer indexing	Lists addresses and phone numbers
Section 2	Generic and trade names	Serves as an index for referencing manufacturers
Section 3	Product category index	Lists products by classification or method of action
Section 4	Product identification guide	Drugs shown in color
Section 5	Product information	Most FDA*-approved drugs
Section 6	Diagnostic product information	Information on drug products used as diagnostic agents
Miscellaneous section	Miscellaneous information	List of drug information centers, key to controlled substances, key for FDA pregnancy ratings, U.S. FDA telephone directory, and poison control centers

FDA, Food and Drug Administration.

the ease of use, it is a very popular pharmacy reference. *Drug Facts and Comparisons* has five sections, as shown in Table 6-1.

At the front of each classification section is extensive information on various aspects of the class of drugs. Included under each drug listing are indications for use. Also, a chart lists all of the dosage strengths, dosage forms, sizes, and manufacturers. Most pharmacies carry the unbound book to allow for monthly updates. *Drug Facts and Comparisons* answers many basic questions for the pharmacist. It is available in hardback, loose-leaf hardback, pocket-sized, or electronic subscription (Facts and Comparison eAnswers). An example of how to locate information on either over-the-counter (OTC) or prescription (Rx) drugs is provided in Box 6-3.

PHYSICIANS' DESK REFERENCE

The *Physicians' Desk Reference (PDR)* is a popular reference found in most doctors' offices and pharmacies. The *PDR* has been in publication for more than 50 years. The *PDR* has six sections, as shown in Table 6-2.

Each drug referenced in the *PDR* has a complete description, including its chemical structure and study results. This book is a compilation of package inserts (official labels) provided by manufacturers who have paid a fee for inclusion into the reference; not all package inserts are available. Package inserts can be hard to read. Although most pharmacies have a *PDR*, physicians are the

BOX 6-3 EXAMPLE OF INFORMATION IN *DRUG FACTS AND COMPARISONS*

Omeprazole

OTC	Prilosec OTC (mfg)	Time-delayed release: 20 mg	14 s, 28 s, 42 s
Rx	Omeprazole (various)	Capsules, delayed release; 10 mg	30 s, 100 s
Rx	Prilosec (mfg)		1000 s and 30 s

The solid line between drugs indicates the drugs are of different strength and/or equivalency. A broken line between drugs indicates that the drugs are equivalent; therefore they can be used interchangeably.

Looking Up Information Under Trade Name:

Prilosec (located in the back of the book under index)
  A. Generic name: given next to Prilosec, the trade name
  B. Manufacturer: in parentheses under or next to name of drug within the table
  C. Dosage forms: given in the middle of the table
  D. Strengths: given in the middle of table
  E. Package quantities available: given to the right
  F. OTC and/or Rx: located to the far left of the drug name
  G. Patient information and auxiliary label: located under monograph (see iv.)
      i. Under the table will be sections on indications, administration, and dosage.
      ii. Overall information on proton pump inhibitors (top of page: classification of drug) will be given under the monograph that is located at the beginning of the section, after the monograph on histamine H_2-antagonists.
      iii. Under the monograph the conditions treated by these types of agents will be listed including pharmacokinetics, contraindications, warnings, precautions, drug interactions, adverse reactions, overdosage, and patient information.
      iv. Under patient information, you can find information on what type of auxiliary label should be used on a prescription bottle.

Looking Up Information Under Generic Name:
Alprazolam
  A. Trade name: listed at the heading of the table
  B. Classification: at the top of the page
  C. Manufacturer: in parentheses under or next to name of drug within the table
  D. Dosage forms: given in the middle of the table
  E. Strengths: given in the middle of the table
  F. Package quantities available: given to the right
  G. Schedule: located to the far left of the drug name (Notice that there is no OTC or Rx listed; this is because all scheduled drugs are Rx.)
  H. Patient information pertaining to drinking alcohol or taking other CNS depressants: located under the benzodiazepines monograph

primary users, and again the *PDR* lists only Food and Drug Administration–approved drugs that the manufacturers choose to send for inclusion. This book is not as important in a pharmacy setting as it is in a physician's office. The *PDR* does contain useful drug manufacturer contact information such as addresses and phone numbers. However, manufacturer information is now available in many other online drug information subscription programs. The *PDR* is available in hardback and CD-ROM. Online subscription is free to prescribers.

DRUG TOPICS RED BOOK

One of the longest published reference guides is *Drug Topics Red Book*. This book is a good source of information pertaining to average and wholesale drug

TABLE 6-3 Sections in *Drug Topics Red Book*

Sections in Order of Reference	Contents of Each Section	Specific Information
Section 1	Emergency information	Lists addresses and phone numbers
Section 2	Clinical reference guide	Quick guide listings such as for sugar-free and alcohol-free products, sulfite-containing drugs, and drugs that cannot be crushed
Section 3	Practice management and professional development	Disease management programs, listed in alphabetical order with addresses and phone numbers
Section 4	Pharmacy and health care organizations	Lists 25 major organizations including ASHP,* NABP, and American Association of Colleges of Pharmacy; no technician organizations listed
Section 5	Drug reimbursement information	Lists State Aid Drug Assistance programs for all states; lists Medicaid upper limit prices and billing rules
Section 6	Manufacturer/wholesaler information	Lists addresses and phone numbers for manufacturers, wholesalers, OBRA '90 participating manufacturers (by identification number), and returned goods policies
Section 7	Product identification	Color photos of limited drugs; also includes list of look-a-like, sound-a-like drug names
Section 8	Prescription product listings	Contains *Orange Book,* which lists generic drug, manufacturer, National Drug Code, average wholesale price, direct price, and *Orange Book* code
Section 9	Over-the-counter/nondrug products listing	Lists drugs by generic name or trademark name and contains health-related item, universal product code, National Drug Code, average wholesale price, and suggested retail price
Section 10	Complementary/herbal product referencing	Short listing of popular herbal remedies along with a listing of those that may be contraindicated, require supervision by medical personnel, and have adverse interactions, followed by a list of both scientific and common herbal names

*ASHP, American Society of Health-System Pharmacists; *NABP,* National Association of Boards of Pharmacy; *OBRA '90,* Omnibus Budget Reconciliation Act of 1990.

costs and prices. The *New Red Book* has 10 sections, as outlined in Table 6-3. Community pharmacies, rather than hospital pharmacies, are more likely to use this book.

Red Book contains valuable information in the form of quick referencing charts that technicians can use, such as drugs that should not be crushed, drugs that are sugar-free and alcohol-free, and drugs excreted in breast milk. In addition, *Red Book* includes convenient tables showing pharmacy calculations and dosing instructions converted into Spanish. Although *Red Book* has an extraordinary amount of information, it is not an easy book to reference without knowing the abbreviations for the drug sections (Table 6-4). An added feature of *Red Book* is a listing of all nontraditional doctor of pharmacy (PharmD) programs, along with requirements and current enrollment numbers. This is information that few, if any other, books contain. This book is available in soft-covered and CD-ROM formats.

APPROVED DRUG PRODUCTS WITH THERAPEUTIC EQUIVALENCE EVALUATIONS: *"ORANGE BOOK"*

The *"Orange Book"* is a comprehensive listing of approved drug products with therapeutic equivalence evaluations that is provided by the U.S. Food and Drug Administration. This is the book to use for determination of whether a generic

TABLE 6-4 Abbreviations in *Drug Topics Red Book*

Abbreviations	Definitions	What Information Is Given
AWP	Average wholesale price	Average price wholesalers charge pharmacy
NDC	National Drug Code	Identifies each drug by number
OBC	*Orange Book* code	Gives therapeutic equivalence
DP	Direct price	Price for purchasing from manufacturer
NCPDP	National Council for Prescription Drug Programs	Standard billing units, such as milliliter and milligram
HRI	Health-related item	Nonmedication item required to treat patient (e.g., crutches, gauze, tape, or lancets)
UPC	Universal product code	Similar to National Drug Code for drug items

drug is the same as a brand drug. Other information includes discontinued drug products, orphan product designations, and approval lists. Information searches can be accessed by several different means: active ingredient, patent number, proprietary name, applicant holder, or application number. The *Orange Book* publication is updated annually. Frequent updates are made to the online version and it can be accessed free of charge.

AMERICAN HOSPITAL FORMULARY SERVICE DRUG INFORMATION

Used mainly by hospitals, *American Hospital Formulary Service Drug Information (AHFS DI)* provides drug monographs that list drug information, including the following:

- Uses and off-label uses
- Specific dosage and administration information
- Drug interactions
- Adverse reactions
- Acute toxicity
- Preparations, chemistry, and stability
- Mechanism of action
- Spectrum and resistance for antibiotics
- Pharmacology
- Pharmacokinetics
- Laboratory and test references

This information is derived from experts in the fields of medicine, pharmacy, and management, through an independent editorial review process. This book is available in hardback, electronic, and a mobile application version.

UNITED STATES PHARMACOPEIA–NATIONAL FORMULARY (USP–NF)

The *USP–NF* provides access to official standards of the FDA. It is a guide for the specifications—tests, procedures, and acceptance criteria—required for pharmaceutical manufacturing and quality control. This book aids compliance with standards and lists new product development and approvals. It is available in hardback, CD, or online with a subscription.

UNITED STATES PHARMACISTS' PHARMACOPEIA

United States Pharmacists' Pharmacopeia is a comprehensive compilation of information on compounding products and ingredients and their safety as well as products used to treat specific medical conditions. Also included are the most recent sterile preparation guidelines for *USP*, the most common **non-formulary** agents, veterinary compounding, dietary supplements, and laws pertaining to compounding. This book is available in hardback or online with a subscription.

CLINICAL PHARMACOLOGY AND OTHER GOLD STANDARD/ELSEVIER PRODUCTS

Clinical Pharmacology is an electronic drug compendium commonly encountered in retail and health system pharmacy settings. Similar to *Drug Facts and Comparisons,* the reference is very popular because of its ease of use and quick access to needed information. The information can be provided to the pharmacy or health system via online, intranet, CD-ROM, or mobile applications. The reference can be used by physicians, pharmacists, nurses, and other allied health professionals. Similar to the American Society of Health-System Pharmacists (ASHP) and *Micromedex DRUGDEX, Clinical Pharmacology* is an officially recognized compendium by the Centers for Medicare & Medicaid Services (CMS) because of its extensive amount of drug information, including off-label drug uses supported by clinical evidence. Data are continuously updated, making this reference a very timely resource for current drug information. *Gold Standard / Elsevier* also has a complement of other products that can be bundled to the subscription to enhance the base compendia product. The following are examples of the various types of information available:

- Comprehensive drug details, including pharmacology, pharmacokinetics, contraindications, boxed warnings, precautions, Pregnancy Category, breast-feeding, indications and dosage for all populations, off-label uses, and adverse events
- FDA-approved drugs and "How Supplied" data for generic, trade name, prescription, and nonprescription products; drug product images are included
- Drug product comparison reports
- International listing of drugs: Global Drug Name Index
- Drug interactions (available in professional and consumer-friendly reports)
- Identification of drug products: Drug IDentifier (includes, e.g., imprint codes, colors, shapes, scoring, and images)
- Consumer medication information: MedCounselor sheets
- Herbals and dietary supplements, including multivitamin and nutritional product listings
- IV compatibility report
- Integrated drug product data, including clinical decision support and pricing modules: Alchemy
- Toxicology and poisoning management: ToxED
- Material safety data sheets: ToxED

A screen shot of a *Clinical Pharmacology* drug monograph can be seen in Figure 6-1.

IDENT-A-DRUG

Ident-A-Drug lists tablet and capsule identifications. Most tablets and capsules have a code or number stamped onto them by the manufacturer for identification purposes. *Ident-A-Drug* includes more than 7000 listings. The drugs are not

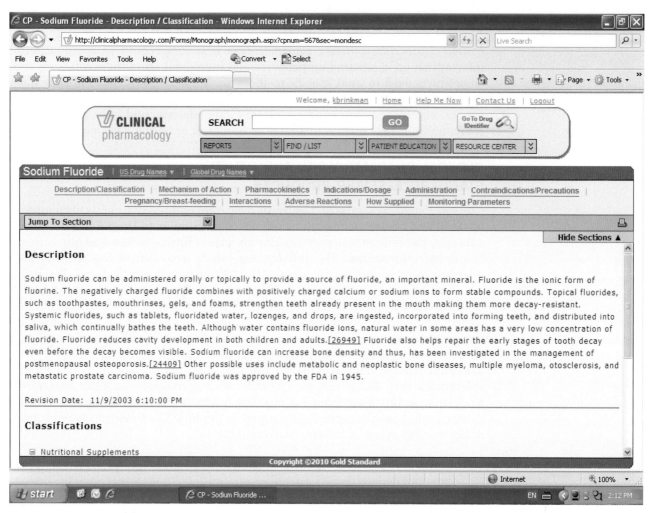

FIGURE 6-1 Screen shot from *Clinical Pharmacology* showing a drug monograph.

listed by pictures but by identifiable codes, colors, and shapes as well as whether the tablet is available scored. Once these characteristics are identified, the book provides the name of the manufacturer, generic and brand names, strength, and use of the drug. *Micromedex's* IDENTIDEX and *Clinical Pharmacology's* Drug IDentifier are also useful resources that are currently available in many pharmacies (both hospital and retail). *Micromedex* is an online interface that has pictures to aid in identifying drugs quickly and accurately. This type of referencing is very helpful when patients do not know the name of the drug they are taking but have a capsule or tablet of the drug to use as a reference. Emergency departments often encounter a patient who has overdosed on an unknown drug. If one tablet or capsule is brought in with the patient, the pharmacy probably can identify the drug using the *Ident-A-Drug* book, *Micromedex's* IDENTIDEX, or *Clinical Pharmacology's* Drug IDentifier (Figure 6-2). Although some books such as *Drug Facts and Comparisons* do have some pictures of tablets and capsules, these are not extensive and are not the first choice to use in identifying a drug. *Ident-A-Drug* is available as a soft cover book, mobile application, and online with a subscription.

MICROMEDEX HEALTHCARE SERIES

Micromedex Healthcare Evidence and Clinical Xpert provides an online and mobile application that can be used by physicians, pharmacists, and nurses

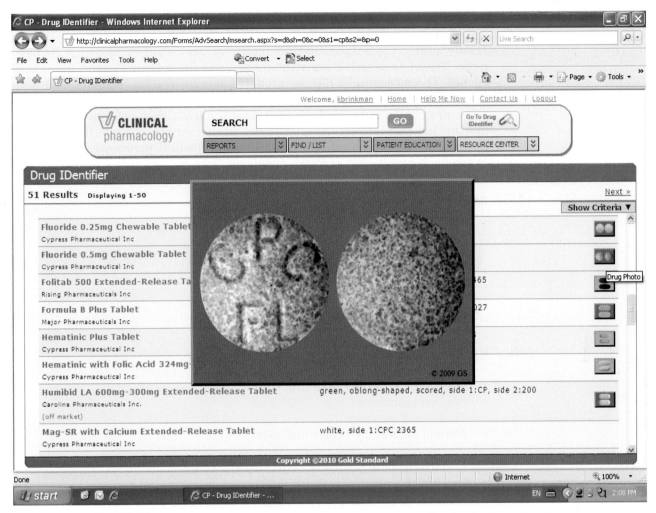

FIGURE 6-2 Screen shot from *Clinical Pharmacology* showing a pill using the Drug IDentifier.

within a health care facility. The information is provided through several different software programs that can be purchased. Examples of the various types of information available are listed below with the specific software programs.

- Comprehensive drug details: DRUGDEX
- FDA-approved drugs: *PDR*
- International drugs: Index Nominum
- Drug interactions: DRUG-REAX
- Identification of capsules and tablets: IDENTIDEX
- Dosing information and parenteral nutrition solutions for infants: NeoFax
- Pharmacokinetics calculators: KINETIDEX
- Proper drug usage and precautions: DrugNotes
- Drug information for more educated patients: Detailed Drug Information for the Consumer
- Drug pricing: ReadyPrice
- Herbals, supplements, and alternative therapies: AltMedDex
- Formulary management for hospitals: Formulary Advisor
- Monographs for P&T evaluations: P&T QUIK
- Manage medication reconciliation throughout the hospital workflow: Clinical Xpert Medication Reconciliation
- Verify IV compatibility: IV INDEX
- Material safety data sheets: Pharmaceutical MSDS

TRISSEL'S HANDBOOK ON INJECTABLE DRUGS

Mostly used in the hospital setting, the *Handbook on Injectable Drugs* by Lawrence Trissel is a well-known reference used for information on parenteral agents. The monographs discuss products, administration, stability, and compatibility with infusion solutions and other drugs. Although technicians cannot relay information from this book to doctors or nurses, they can find the information and have it ready for the pharmacist. In this way, they can facilitate a rapid response from the pharmacy to the necessary medical personnel. This book is available in hardback, CD-ROM, mobile application, and online formats.*

AMERICAN DRUG INDEX

This book contains listings for more than 22,000 drugs, both prescription and OTC. Information includes the following:

- Manufacturer names
- Pronunciation of drugs
- Active ingredients
- Dosage forms
- Strengths
- Packaging and uses
- Drugs that should not be crushed or chewed
- Look-alike or sound-alike drugs
- Storage requirements for *USP* drugs
- Trademark glossary
- Normal laboratory values and more

It is available in hardback or CD-ROM formats.

GOODMAN & GILMAN'S THE PHARMACOLOGICAL BASIS OF THERAPEUTICS

The following is a list of some of the information provided in this publication:

- Pharmacokinetics and pharmacodynamics
- Drug transport/drug transporters
- Drug metabolism pharmacogenomics
- Principles of therapeutics in all areas of the body system

This book is available in hardback format or as an online subscription.

HANDBOOK OF NONPRESCRIPTION DRUGS BY APHA

This reference provides self-care options for the following:

- Nonprescription medications
- Nutritional supplements
- Medical foods
- Complementary and alternative therapies
- Nondrug and preventive measures for self-treatable disorders
- Complementary and alternative medicine

---

*Many online drug compendia, including *Clinical Pharmacology* and *Micromedex*, have incorporated the online Trissel's databases into their product offerings.

- FDA-approved dosing information and evidence-based research on efficacy and safety considerations of nonprescription, herbal, and homeopathic medications

This book is available in hardback or e-book (downloaded textbook onto computer) formats.

MARTINDALE'S THE COMPLETE DRUG REFERENCE

Martindale's The Complete Drug Reference provides information on drugs in clinical use worldwide, as well as the following:

- Selected investigational and veterinary drugs
- Herbal and complementary medicines
- Pharmaceutical excipients
- Vitamins and nutritional agents
- Vaccines
- Radiopharmaceuticals
- Contrast media and diagnostic agents
- Medicinal gases
- Drugs of abuse and recreational drugs
- Toxic substances
- Disinfectants
- Pesticides

It is available in hardback or CD-ROM format.

REMINGTON'S PHARMACEUTICAL SCIENCES: THE SCIENCE AND PRACTICE OF PHARMACY

This book covers the entire scope of pharmacy—from the history of pharmacy and ethics to the specifics of industrial pharmacy and pharmacy practice. The following specific areas are included:

- Manifestations and pathophysiology of diseases
- Immunology
- Disease state management
- Specialization in pharmacy practice
- Professional communication
- Various aspects of patient care

It is available in hardback format.

PEDIATRIC DOSAGE HANDBOOK (LEXI-COMP)

This book provides information on suggested current dosages for pediatric patients.

GERIATRIC DOSAGE HANDBOOK (LEXI-COMP)

This book provides information on suggested current dosages for geriatric patients.

In addition to these well-known books, there are many specialty reference books such as those covering information on drugs in pregnancy and breastfeeding, psychotropic medications, and antibiotics. Many pharmacies have a wide range of these types of reference books available (Table 6-5).

TABLE 6-5 Main Attributes of Various References

Reference Book	Publisher	Available in	Updated
Drug Facts and Comparisons	Wolters Kluwer Health	Hardbound book	Yearly
		Loose-leaf book	Monthly
		Electronic	Current updates
		Mobile application	Current updates
Physicians' Desk Reference	Thomson Healthcare	Hardbound book	Yearly
		Mobile application	Current updates
Drug Topics Red Book	Medical Economics	Softbound book	Yearly and monthly
Orange Book	FDA	Electronic	Current updates
USP–NF	U.S. Pharmacopeia	3-volume hardbound	Monthly
		Online	Current updates
		CD	Monthly
Ident-A-Drug	Therapeutic Research Faculty	Softbound book	Monthly
		Online	Current updates
		Mobile application	Current updates
Goodman & Gilman's The Pharmacological Basis of Therapeutics	McGraw-Hill	Hardbound	Every 5 years
		Electronic	Current updates cut/paste
		Mobile application	With electronic subscription
Remington's Pharmaceutical Sciences: The Science and Practice of Pharmacy	Lippincott Williams & Wilkins	Hardbound	Every 5 years
United States Pharmacopeia	USP	Hardbound	Yearly
Drug Information	ASHP	Softbound	Yearly
American Hospital Formulary		Electronic	Current updates
Trissel's Handbook on Injectable Drugs	ASHP	Hardbound	Yearly
Pediatric Dosage Handbook	Lexi-Comp	Hardbound	Yearly
	APhA	Softbound	Yearly
Geriatric Dosage Handbook	Lexi-Comp	Hardbound	Yearly
	APhA	Softbound	Yearly

Pocket-Sized Reference Books

Technicians traditionally have not carried pocket versions of drug books. However, as roles expand at work, the pharmacy technician needs to have his or her own reference books. Some manufacturers produce small pocket versions of trade/generic name drug books, but the drugs listed often are limited to their drug line only. It is becoming more important for technicians to carry a good pocket guide not only of trade and generic names but also of drug classifications, indications, and side effects. Before purchasing a pocket guide, technicians should examine a variety of different guides to determine the one that is most pertinent to their job. One of the best books to keep is one in which a drug can be looked up by trade or brand name without having to check the index. The cost of these pocket handbooks ranges between $20 and $40. The disadvantage is that they are softbound and will need to be updated yearly to incorporate new drugs or discontinued ones. The advantage is that most of the drugs remain the same over time.

Electronic Referencing

Handheld devices such as personal digital assistants and cell phones incorporating wireless Internet access are becoming more popular and economical. One can download an assortment of drug guides and other reference materials onto a handheld device for easy access. These devices are small enough to be carried in a coat pocket or purse. However, many of these devices are more expensive ways to obtain reference materials. As technology advances, the prices of these handheld devices will decrease, making them more affordable. There are several companies that offer short-term trial periods of their product before purchasing, while others offer a limited amount of information for free. One example is Epocrates (www.epocrates.com), which offers a basic free drug information package that can be downloaded onto your personal computer or handheld device. The following information is included:

- Trade and generic name reference
- Classification
- Indications
- Interactions
- Dosing
- Pill identification

Drug information is also available in CD-ROM format; CD-ROMs may accompany drug books or can be purchased alone. These products generally must be purchased quarterly or annually to maintain currency.

THE INTERNET

Referencing should not be limited to books alone. The Internet has a lot of information; however, it is up to the reader to determine whether the information is reliable and accurate. Finding websites at universities and through publishing companies is a good way to look for information. Accessing personal websites may give you a person's perspective but may not provide medically sound information. A list of reputable websites for news concerning medications is provided at the end of this chapter.

Pharmacy organizations have websites on the Internet, and many have weekly news boards that reference important information concerning pharmacy. Because pharmacy is constantly evolving, much of the information cannot be included in journals. The news links are listed on the website. There are also many databases with up-to-date information and links (Table 6-6). This is a valuable tool used to keep members updated with accurate information. Also, these association sites have links to other pharmacy sites that may be of interest. Pharmacy associations also may offer Internet links where the user can have questions answered by other members.

Many websites provide continuing education in the form of online exams and live continuing education (CE) courses. For the online CE courses, sometimes the information can be downloaded and studied before taking the exam online; other online courses require live participation. Once completed, the certificate for the course is mailed, e-mailed, or provided online to you of CE certificates should be filed for reference when obtaining recertification. Many times these CE courses are offered free of charge, and although a certain amount of CE units are required for recertification, there is no limit to the number of CE courses you may take. Upon completion of the CE exam, you receive notification of your score and a certificate can be printed and filed in your records as a recertification reference. For more information on continuing education sources, see Chapter 3.

Journals and Newsmagazines

Nearly every pharmacy subscribes to journals and newsmagazines that pertain to pharmacy. These can be informative to the pharmacy technician. When a technician becomes nationally certified, he or she must complete continuing

TABLE 6-6 Online Websites and Databases

Websites	Name of Organization or Site	Type of Information
www.cdc.gov	Centers for Disease Control and Prevention	Current health issues
www.cms.gov	Centers for Medicare & Medicaid Services	Reimbursement information
www.drugs.com	Online database	Trade/generic names, drug interactions, and pill identifier
www.drugTopics.com	Online information	Up-to-date medical news and pharmacy issues
www.FDA.gov	Food and Drug Administration	Drug, food, and cosmetics safety information
www.fda.gov/drugs/default.htm	Food and Drug Administration, drug evaluation and research development	Links to: *Orange Book, MedWatch, NDC Directory,* and new drug approvals
www.Health.NIH.gov	National Institutes of Health	Health issues and studies
www.MayoClinic.com	MayoClinic	Information on conditions and diseases, lifestyle health issues
www.medicare.gov/pdphome.asp	U.S. Department of Health and Human Services	Information on Medicare Part D, formulary index
www.medlineplus.gov	National Library of Medicine database	Health and drug information, medical dictionary and encyclopedia
www.medscape.com	Online database	Information on diseases; links to medical journals and CE courses
www.PDRhealth.com	*Physicians' Desktop Reference* online	Information on both legend and OTC drugs, herbs, interactions' database; information on conditions and diseases
www.Rxlist.com	Online database	Both prescription and OTC drug information
www.webmd.com	Online database	Up-to-date health topics, conditions, and diseases and drug information
http://dailymed.nlm.nih.gov/dailymed/about.cfm	Online database	Includes package inserts for over 5000 drugs available in U.S.

education units and may at some point use these journals for completing some, if not all, of the necessary units. Journals offer continuing education at a reasonable cost; in addition, they allow the technician to stay current on the most recent drugs that are being developed. Journals and newsletters may be published monthly, bimonthly, quarterly, or even weekly. They contain articles on new drugs, technicians, the future of pharmacy, and various legislative changes that may be taking place. The information they can provide regarding the field of pharmacy can be beneficial. Many different journals, newsletters, and magazines are available. Other journals that technicians may not see in the pharmacy setting are those written by pharmacy technician associations. These journals are geared specifically toward technician issues. Table 6-7 provides a sample of the types of journals and pharmacy magazines available.

Additional Types of Information

In addition to large desktop books, pocket handbooks, journals, and the Internet, other sources of information can keep you current and on the cutting edge as a pharmacy technician. For examples of additional references geared toward technicians and health care workers, see Table 6-8. Another way to attain new drug information is to join an association. Membership can be rewarding and

TABLE 6-7 Types of Journals and Pharmacy Magazines Available

Newsmagazine	Journal Name	Published	Continuing Education Included	Website	Association
AAPT*		6 times yearly	Yes	www.pharmacytechnician.com	Yes
Computer Talk		6 times yearly	No	www.computertalk.com	No
Hospital Pharmacy		Monthly	Yes	www.hospitalpharmacyjournal.com	No
Drug Topics		Monthly	Yes	www.drugtopics.com	No
Today's Technician		6 times yearly	Yes	www.pharmacytechnician.org	Yes
Pharmacy Times		Monthly	Yes	www.pharmacytimes.com	No
Pharmacy Today (JAPhA)		Monthly	Yes	www.pharmacytoday.org	No
The Script		Monthly	No	www.pharmacy.ca.gov	No
U.S. Pharmacist		Monthly	Yes	www.uspharmacist.com	No
	AJHP	Twice monthly	Yes	www.ashp.org	Yes
	Journal of Pharmacy Technology	6 times yearly	Yes	www.jpharmtechnol.com	No

*AAPT, American Association of Pharmacy Technicians; AJHP, American Journal of Health-System Pharmacy.

TABLE 6-8 Additional Reference Books That Technicians May Find Helpful in Understanding Various Aspects of Health Care

Name	Useful Information
Gray Morris D: *Calculate with confidence,* ed 6, St Louis, 2010, Elsevier ISBN 978-0-323-05629-8	Math calculations for all types of dosage forms
Potter PA, Perry AG: *Fundamentals of nursing,* ed 7, St Louis, 2009, Elsevier ISBN 978-0-323-06784-3	How nurses approach patients In-depth information on disease states
Mosby's dictionary of medicine, nursing and health professions, ed 8, St Louis, 2009, Elsevier ISBN 978-0-323-04937-5 ISBN 0-323-01214-0	Anatomical diagrams along with definitions
Gerdin J: *Health careers today,* ed 4, St Louis, 2007, Elsevier ISBN 978-0-323-04474-5	Good description of more than 45 vocations in medical field Gives technician a better understanding of health fields
Elkin MK, Perry AG, Potter PA: *Nursing interventions & clinical skills,* ed 4, St Louis, 2008, Elsevier ISBN 978-0-323-04458-5	In-depth information on disease states

can serve as a good source of information and a way to network. Currently, the associations listed in Box 6-4 provide continuing education and information for technicians; their websites are also included in Box 6-4.

All of these organizations offer a great way to stay current on new drugs, devices, and current and future pharmacy issues. In addition, they usually offer a vehicle to order pharmacy technician certification review books and other reference books, sometimes at a reduced membership rate. These reference books can be found on their websites or at their bookstores (this information may be found at their seminars). The information and support they can provide is limited only by how much they are used. Also, many pharmacist associations, such as the American Society of Health-Systems Pharmacists and American

BOX 6-4 PHARMACY ASSOCIATIONS* THAT PROVIDE CONTINUING EDUCATION AND INFORMATION

National Pharmacy Technicians Association
    www.pharmacytechnician.org
American Association of Pharmacy Technicians
    www.pharmacytechnician.com
American Society of Health-System Pharmacists
    www.ashp.org
American Pharmacists Association
    www.pharmacists.com

*For additional associations look in the *Red Book* under Associations or search the web under Pharmacy Associations.

Tech Note!

Before you join an association, check out its website for information on the level of involvement of the association with its technician members. Many associations do not have a technician division or offer continuing education classes specifically for technicians. Most, but not all, have yearly seminars and a bimonthly journal containing continuing education and other useful information pertaining specifically to technicians. Becoming familiar with the various conditions of patients and understanding the terminology are essential for becoming a competent pharmacy technician. Table 6-8 lists good books that represent various aspects of health care. All health care workers should constantly pursue the acquisition of new information.

Pharmacists Association and their chapters, have specific divisions for pharmacy technicians, providing technicians with additional sources for learning new information. You must inquire about your local pharmacy associations to determine what they offer. Some technician divisions are active in supplying continuing education courses to technicians and host various functions for networking and unifying pharmacy technicians from different types of pharmacies. For more information on all associations, refer to Chapter 3.

Seminars and continuing education dinners, provided by pharmacy associations, are sometimes sponsored by drug companies and are another good source of information on drug topics, new drugs, and fulfilling continuing education requirements. You do not need to be a member of an association to attend, but the cost usually is lower for members. Although seminars normally are held once or twice yearly, depending on the association that is presenting the seminar, continuing education dinners may be hosted monthly by the local chapter of an association. At seminars, many of the technician classes include math, aseptic technique, the future of pharmacy technicians, law updates, and more. Monthly continuing education dinners or events usually have a limited amount of space available and, depending on the drug company sponsoring the event, there may be a speaker and a meal for a low cost or (more rarely) no cost. These costs usually are predetermined by the chapter of the association. All of these seminar classes and continuing education dinners can be used toward continuing education credit for pharmacy technicians.

Considerations When Choosing a Reference

At times, technicians may need to use a reference for obtaining information on a drug or for billing purposes. Knowing the proper book to reference is important not only for finding the correct information but also for saving time and avoiding frustration.

The references listed previously are large reference books that are provided for the staff in the pharmacy. Some online subscription contracts in the pharmacy may have codes that allow you individual access to use the reference at home; check with your employer. If you choose to buy your own reference books or online subscriptions for home use or pocket versions for use at work, you should consider some basics. If your main use of the reference will be to determine generic and trade names, indications, and side effects, then a reference such as *Drug Facts and Comparisons* is a good choice. As pharmacies update their reference books, you might be able to obtain a free copy of some print references. Some pharmacies who subscribe to electronic resources also receive complementary access for their employees' use at home; check with your

Tech Note!

If a technician needs to find a drug price and manufacturer for a drug such as Tenormin and its generic version, a book such as *PDR* is not helpful because the drugs are listed by manufacturer and the reference does not give prices. *Drug Facts and Comparisons* references drugs by trade or generic name but also does not list any prices. *Red Book* is an excellent source to find drug prices using the trade name. It provides prices for the trade name and generic equivalents.

employer. Also, check bookstores on the Internet for the previous year's edition of a desired resource. Older editions can be sold at a reduced price and may contain most of the information you require. However, you should consider the need to have updated information, as drug information changes very quickly. You might check other book companies for similar information. Many reference books contain the same type of information as *Drug Facts and Comparisons*. Another consideration may be the size of the reference book. For instance, although *Drug Facts and Comparisons* is a complete and up-to-date book, it is large and will not fit in your pocket for easy access; however, a pocket version is available. Other publishers also offer pocket versions of their references, including mobile versions for various technical devices.

Avoid books that only reference drug names one way (e.g., only trade or generic names) because their use can become time-consuming. Most drugs have many names depending on the drug company that manufactures them. If you are going to keep the book at home or in your office, you might be looking for a larger book. If your space is limited, you may be more interested in a handbook. Remember that smaller books will contain less information or will have harder-to-read print. If you are going to purchase a reference book at a bookstore, take a wide variety of drug names with you to reference in the store. If the book has all the drugs you are looking for and is easy to read, you will use the book more often. In Table 6-8 are additional reference books that are informative for the pharmacy technician. These range from information on various topics in the medical field to those resources that help you practice pharmacy calculations.

DO YOU REMEMBER THESE KEY POINTS?

- The major sources of information that a technician most often uses in pharmacy
- The benefits of joining a pharmacy association
- Why continuing education is important for pharmacy technicians
- The key attributes of each of the books explained in this chapter
- Other sources available to technicians in addition to books, journals, and magazines
- The types of information that a pharmacy technician should keep current
- The difference between organizations and associations outlined in this chapter

REVIEW QUESTIONS

Multiple choice questions

1. Which of the books listed provides package inserts from manufacturers?
   A. *Drug Facts and Comparisons*
   B. *Goodman & Gilman's The Pharmacological Basis of Therapeutics*
   C. *Red Book*
   D. *Physicians' Desk Reference*

2. Which book(s) listed below is (are) the best source for locating manufacturer addresses?
   A. *Red Book*
   B. *Physicians' Desk Reference*
   C. *Goodman & Gilman's The Pharmacological Basis of Therapeutics*
   D. *Drug Facts and Comparisons*
   E. Answers A, B, and D

3. If you need to find the average wholesale price (AWP) of a drug, the best source to look in is:

A. *American Drug Index*
B. *Drug Facts and Comparisons*
C. *Red Book*
D. A journal

4. The book that is available both hardbound and loose-leaf to allow for monthly updates is:

A. *Drug Facts and Comparisons*
B. *Red Book*
C. *Goodman & Gilman's The Pharmacological Basis of Therapeutics*
D. None of the above

5. The most widely used reference book in pharmacy is:

A. *Goodman & Gilman's The Pharmacological Basis of Therapeutics*
B. The dictionary
C. *Remington's Pharmaceutical Sciences: The Science and Practice of Pharmacy*
D. *Drug Facts and Comparisons*

6. The oldest pharmacy technician association is:

A. NPTA
B. AAPT
C. CPhT
D. None of the above

7. If you need to identify a specific tablet or capsule only by the markings, color, and shape, you will look in:

A. *Drug Facts and Comparisons;* loose-leaf version
B. *Ident-A-Drug*
C. *American Drug Index*
D. *Red Book*

8. The positive aspects of purchasing a pocket version of a drug handbook include all of the following except:

A. Pocket versions can be easily transported
B. The price of a pocket version is less expensive than a large version
C. The information in a pocket version is always the most recent
D. The information in a pocket version is fairly equal to the information of the larger version

9. One alternative to buying books is to:

A. Wait until the pharmacy is going to discard an old version
B. Check for lower prices as a member of an association
C. Use the Internet for information and read journals that your pharmacy provides for employees
D. Both A and C

10. All of the following books are updated at least yearly except:

A. *Drug Facts and Comparisons*
B. *Red Book*
C. *Goodman & Gilman's The Pharmacological Basis of Therapeutics*
D. *Physicians' Desk Reference*

11. E-courses offer the following except:

A. Live CE courses
B. Written exam materials that can be downloaded and studied before taking the exam
C. Exams that need to be read online and taken
D. CE courses that can be mailed to your home address so you can take the exam at home and return your answers by mail

12. Which of the following statements is true concerning online CE courses?
    A. They must be taken within their expiration date.
    B. They can only be taken by certified technicians and pharmacists.
    C. They are always offered for a fee.
    D. All of the above are true.

13. All of the following information can be found in the *Drug Facts and Comparisons (F&C)* book except:
    A. Schedule of a narcotic
    B. Storage and stability
    C. Patient information
    D. All of the above information can be found

14. Information about pharmacy associations can be found:
    A. Online
    B. In journals
    C. In the *Red Book*
    D. Both A and C

15. All of the following can be found on free downloaded materials from epocrates except:
    A. Contraindications
    B. Herbals
    C. Pill identification
    D. Both B and C

True/False

If a statement is false, then change it to make it true.

1. Classification and indication are identical.
2. If a drug is contraindicated, it is not available in the United States.
3. Monographs for a specific drug are produced after the experimentation phase and after approval from the Food and Drug Administration.
4. A Palm Pilot is a device that allows referencing materials to be downloaded for individual use.
5. Technicians can take continuing education courses only through pharmacists' journals.
6. The Internet has information that is incorrect and should not be used as a source.
7. Technicians do not need to use reference materials in a pharmacy.
8. Many pharmacy associations have technician divisions for members.
9. One of the best reasons to join and become involved in an association is to network.
10. Technicians are not expected to stay up-to-date with current medications or pharmacy trends.
11. 1 CE unit is given per 1 hour of training.
12. No more than 20 units of CE may be taken in any 2-year period.
13. Technicians are not allowed to take pharmacists' CE courses; they must take CE courses especially approved for technicians.
14. All pharmacy associations have a pharmacy technician division.
15. Complementary/herbal information can be found in the *Drug Topics Red Book.*

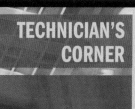

TECHNICIAN'S CORNER

A patient arrives at the pharmacy holding one capsule of medication that he or she needs to have refilled. The patient wants to know the price of the medication and whether it is available as a liquid. The capsule is white and has the markings "Watson 369" on one side and "5 mg" on the opposite side. What is this drug, and what is its intended use? Also list the average wholesale price, National Drug Code, and dosage forms.

BIBLIOGRAPHY

Berardi RR, et al: *Handbook of nonprescription drugs*, ed 14, Washington, DC, 2004, American Pharmacists Association.

Berardi M, et al: *Handbook of nonprescription drugs*, ed 15. Washington DC, American Pharmacists Association, 2006.

Billups NF, Billups SM: *American drug index 2009*, St. Louis, 2008, Wolters Kluwer Health.

Billups, Norman. *American drug index*. Ed. Norman Billups. 53. Philadelphia: Lippincott Williams & Wilkins, 2008.

Drug facts and comparisons, ed 60, St Louis, 2005, Wolters Kluwer Health.

Drug facts and Comparisons, ed 63. St Louis, 2008, Wolters Kluwer Health.

Drug topics red book, ed 109, Montvale, NJ, 2005, Thomson.

Gennaro A: *Remington's pharmaceutical sciences: the science and practice of pharmacy*, ed 18, Easton, Pa, 1995, Mack.

Gennaro A: *Remington's pharmaceutical sciences: the science and practice of pharmacy*, ed 18. Easton, 1995, Mack.

Hardman JG, Limbird LE, editors: *Goodman & Gilman's the pharmaceutical basis of therapeutics*, ed 11, New York, 2005, McGraw-Hill Professional.

Hardman JG, Limbird LE: *The Pharmaceutical basis of therapeutics*. Goodman and Gilman. 11. New York, 2005, McGraw-Hill Professional.

Jellin J, ed. *Ident-a-drug reference: for tablet and capsule identification*, Stockton, Calif, 2008, Therapeutic Research Faculty.

Reuters, Thomson: *Red book*, ed 113. Motvale, 2009, Physicians' Desk Reference.

Trissel L: *Handbook on injectable drugs*, ed 14, Elk Grove Village, Ill, 2006, American Academy of Pediatrics.

Trissel, Lawrence: *Handbook on injectable drugs*, ed 15. Elk Grove Village, Ill, 2009, American Society of Health-System.

US pharmacopoeia, ed 30, Rockville, Md, 2006, US Pharmacopeial Convention.

WEBSITES

Orange Book: Approved Drug Products with Therapeutic Equivalence Evaluations. July 2009. www.fda.gov/cder/ob

Drug names. www.webmd.com

Drugs@FDA Database. July 8, 2009. www.fda.gov/Drugs/InformationOnDrugs/ucm135821.htm

Gold Standard Clinical Pharmacology, http://clinicalpharmacology.com

Ipaktchian S. The Name Game. Igor: Naming and Branding Agency. The Patriot Ledger, Stanford Medicine Magazine. Stanford School of Medicine. June 7, 2005.

Micromedex Information. www.micromedex.com/products/hcs/

7

Prescription Processing

Objectives

UPON COMPLETING THIS CHAPTER, YOU SHOULD BE ABLE TO DO THE FOLLOWING:

■ Describe the responsibilities of a technician filling prescriptions within a community setting.

■ List the necessary information required for prescriptions and labels.

■ Demonstrate the ability to prioritize the filling of prescriptions.

■ Differentiate filling methods between controlled substances and non–controlled substances.

■ Describe laws pertaining to the technician's responsibilities when filling prescriptions.

■ List the 10 steps of carefully filling a medication order.

■ Differentiate between inpatient and outpatient information requirements.

■ List the types of automated machines used in filling prescriptions.

■ Explain the steps of reducing medication errors.

■ List the 5 rights of a patient in regard to medication safety.

Adjudication *Computerized billing*

Automated dispensing system (ADS) *Computerized, automated machines that hold a supply of various medications that can be accessed by authorized individuals to fill prescriptions in the community or institutional pharmacy setting; also used to obtain point-of-care patient medications in an institutional setting*

Auxiliary label *An adhesive label that is attached to a container with specific instructions or information pertaining to the medication inside*

Closed door pharmacy *A pharmacy that fills and delivers medications prescribed by institutions such as long-term care facilities; these pharmacies may also provide mail-order prescriptions; closed pharmacies are not open to the public*

Community pharmacy *Also known as an outpatient or retail pharmacy; pharmacies that serve patients in their communities; consumers can walk in and purchase a prescription or OTC drug*

E-Prescribing *Electronically sent prescription that is transmitted from the prescriber's computer or mobile device directly to the pharmacy*

Institutional pharmacy *A pharmacy in a hospital or institutional setting; this type of pharmacy may or may not provide retail services*

Non-formulary *A list of drugs that are not normally stocked by the pharmacy; these drugs may not be covered by an insurance company unless specific conditions are met*

Rx *Latin abbreviation for "recipe," meaning "to take"; it is commonly used to mean "prescription" and is often found as a symbol on the header of a prescription*

Script *A common slang term describing a medical prescription*

Sig *From the Latin "signa," which means "to write"; medication directions written on a prescription that describe how a medication should be taken or used*

Introduction

Filling a prescription is one of the most important and commonly performed duties of a pharmacy technician, regardless of the setting. The act of transcribing physicians' writing into lay terms sometimes can be frustrating, if not impossible. However, with time and experience, a good technician can determine easily whether he or she can process a prescription quickly or if assistance from the pharmacist is needed. Often the pharmacist cannot decipher the physician's writing either. In this case, the pharmacist is responsible for contacting the physician and asking for clarification of the prescription, also known as the **script.** Whether a technician is working in an institutional pharmacy, community pharmacy, or closed door pharmacy, the process of reading and documenting a physician's orders is similar.

This chapter first explores the various methods by which a prescription can arrive in a pharmacy and the fundamentals of reading a prescription. Skills required of technicians within a **community pharmacy** are more comprehensively covered in this chapter. Community pharmacies are retail pharmacies such as CVS, Walgreens, and those located in supermarkets. There are more retail pharmacies than any other type of pharmacy. **Closed door pharmacies** provide medications to institutions and long-term care facilities and/or to patients at home via mail service. They typically process a prescription similar to a retail pharmacy although they may package prescriptions differently for each type of setting. More information on closed door pharmacies can be found in Chapter 3. An overview of **institutional pharmacy** prescription processing is covered more thoroughly in Chapter 10. Institutional pharmacies are located inside facilities such as hospitals, prisons, and other institutions. Typically medications are filled for 24 hours. This chapter explores understanding and translating, filling, and filing a prescription; in addition, methods of resolving discrepancies in a script are also discussed. This chapter also describes the most common types of medication errors and suggests ways the technician can avoid some of the typical pitfalls. As with any skill, practice makes perfect. This chapter also provides exercises to practice competencies of common prescription discrepancies. For more information on medication errors see Chapter 14.

Processing a Prescription: A Step-by-Step Approach

Five basic steps are required for filling a prescription within a community pharmacy. Four of these steps relate directly to the technician; the fifth pertains directly to the pharmacist. Although these steps may seem simple, they require complete focus and concentration. Within each step are several important points to remember that have been outlined in this chapter. The five steps include the following:

1. Receiving the prescription
2. Translating the prescription
3. Entering information into the computer system
4. Filling the prescription
5. Providing patient consultation

RECEIVING THE PRESCRIPTION

Tech Note!

Prescriptions may be faxed to a pharmacy. However, it is a good idea for the pharmacist to know the prescriber who will be faxing prescriptions, because forgery is more likely to occur otherwise.

A prescription can arrive in a pharmacy by various methods. A prescription can be in the form of a written order that is on a conventional prescription pad listing the physician's information (Figure 7-1). A prescription can be carried into the pharmacy or be faxed from the physician's office to the pharmacy. Computer-generated prescriptions, with electronic transmission online or via mobile devices, are becoming common as well. Box 7-1 outlines the various methods used to transmit prescriptions to the pharmacy.

Prescription Information

Community Pharmacy Setting. If the order is written by a physician or other authorized person, it usually is delivered to the pharmacy by the patient. Therefore the person at the "take-in" counter handles the prescription initially. This is usually the clerk or technician. This person must ensure that the correct information is listed on the prescription. Box 7-2 lists the typical patient information needed to fill a prescription in the community setting. Additional information such as address, phone number, and birth date (if not provided by the prescriber) may need to be provided by the patient so that the computer system can be updated. The pharmacist normally obtains information on any over-the-counter (OTC) and herbal medications the patient may be using. This is important information to obtain because of the possibility of drug interactions. Additional information, such as allergies and current medical conditions, is also entered into the database for future reference.

Joe Smith MD(lic#2346)Rebecca ThomasDO(lic#99432)

Robert Mitchell MD(lic#51012), Richard Lane MD(LIC#56603)

Arizona Medical Group
12 Cactus Ave, Phoenix AZ
800-800-1111

For: Timothy Ladd   Date August 14, 2011

Address: 643 Palm Tree Ct, Phoenix, AZ

Rx *Soma 350mg tabs # 100*

     Take 1 tab tid prn pain

       ○ May substitute
       ○ DAW

      Refills: 0

                        Signature: *Joe Smith MD*

FIGURE 7-1 Example of physician's prescription.

In large retail companies the intake technician may scan the prescription and the patient's insurance card. If the coverage is Medicare, then Medicare Part A and B cards should be scanned separately from the Part D card and patient identification. This information is then available to be displayed on the monitor in case there is a billing error or question on identity. If the patient is a member of a health maintenance organization (HMO) or other managed care organization (MCO), the patient must provide his or her medical record number, unless it is already on file from a previous prescription. Some plans do not offer prescription coverage. For a prescriber, the Drug Enforcement Administration (DEA) number is required if a controlled drug is being dispensed. In addition, a controlled drug prescription must be written in indelible ink. A federal law implemented in 2008 required that all written prescriptions for covered outpatient drugs that are financed by Medicaid be written on tamper-resistant prescriptions, irrespective of whether the script is for controlled substances. Several states are also instituting such requirements for all prescriptions, except those that are transmitted electronically or within institutional settings. See Chapter 2 for more information on verification of DEA numbers.

Institutional Setting. In a hospital or inpatient setting, prescriptions are referred to as medication orders, and the information required on these orders differs from that required for outpatient prescriptions. If the physician or prescriber is employed by or considered approved staff by the hospital, the license number and DEA number are on file. Therefore it is not necessary for the prescriber to provide this information on the medication order or controlled drug order for use within the institution. Box 7-3 shows the information that is required for institutional prescriptions.

Most medications are provided from the pharmacy to fill the prescriber's orders for a 24-hour period. For example, for a multivitamin given as 1 tablet orally once daily, the pharmacy will load 1 multivitamin into the patient's

Tech Note!

An order written in the chart of a hospital patient is considered a legal prescription once signed by the prescriber.

BOX 7-1 COMMONLY FOLLOWED RULES FOR TAKING PRESCRIPTIONS

Call-in

Calling in a prescription can be done by a physician, nurse, or physician's assistant (as designated by the physician). When called in, the pharmacist transcribes the verbal order onto a blank prescription pad. Technicians should be aware of the specific rules of their state for taking verbal prescriptions. Taking a prescription over the phone must be done only by a registered pharmacist, or (depending upon the state) by a pharmacist intern or technician under the direct supervision of the pharmacist.

Fax

Faxed prescriptions are mostly used by hospitals, and are becoming more common in community pharmacies. Schedule II medication prescriptions, if faxed, must be followed by a written prescription received at the pharmacy within 7 days (per federal law). Faxed copies of prescriptions can be sent by a ward clerk in the hospital or from a physician's office. A faxed prescription must be on the physician's office letterhead to prevent fraudulent prescriptions. This letterhead often includes the names and license numbers of all prescribing physicians in the office as well as the address, phone number, and fax number.

Walk-in

Most prescriptions in a community pharmacy are taken into a pharmacy by the patient, by a relative, or perhaps by a friend. In hospitals, discharge orders usually are sent to the inpatient pharmacy via a pneumatic tube system or are hand-delivered by staff. In an outpatient dispensing pharmacy of a hospital, prescriptions are handled in the same manner as prescriptions received in a community pharmacy (see Chapter 10).

E-Prescribing

Sending prescriptions electronically is becoming more popular because of the increasing focus on error prevention. Physicians can enter their prescribing information either from a computer or (in some cases) from handheld electronic devices. The electronic prescription is transmitted directly to the pharmacy department where a pharmacist can review the order before processing. A list of pharmacies that accept E-prescriptions can be found online at www.learnaboutEprescriptions.com. However, E-prescribing at this time does not allow controlled drugs to be prescribed because of the current restrictions of federal law. These restrictions may change in time; the Drug Enforcement Administration (DEA) has been working with the U.S. Congress since 2007 to reform controlled substance regulations to allow for safe and secure E-prescription of controlled substances.

The following are some benefits of using E-prescribing:

- Saves money
- Incentives given by insurance companies
- Free prescribing software for prescribers offered as incentive
- Saves time
- Prescriber can send authorization, including prior authorizations, from any place or at any time
- More information available to prescriber on generic alternatives, formulary status, interactions during the E-prescribing process, rather than after the prescription is given to the pharmacy
- Refill requests approved faster
- Drug errors reduced
- Clear instructions and the lack of personal handwriting make it easier for pharmacy to interpret

The following are some barriers for E-prescribing:

- Use of proper software by pharmacy to ensure patient privacy
- Must adhere to all state and federal standards
- Must meet all requirements of HIPAA standards

BOX 7-2 REQUIRED PATIENT INFORMATION IN A COMMUNITY SETTING

Patient Information:
- Name
- Phone number and address
- Insurance information, if applicable
- Date of birth
- Picture ID for controlled substances (per pharmacy protocol)
- Allergies
- Other drugs taken (This information must be provided by the patient, and would include over-the-counter drugs, dietary supplements, and medications filled at other pharmacies.)
- Medical conditions (e.g., diabetes, hypertension, asthma). The entry of medical condition or other personal health data is often considered an optional data entry item; the technician should refer to applicable state laws and employer policy. The information is often helpful, if the patient provides it, because it allows for appropriate screening of drug-condition precautions.
- HIPAA compliance handout/signature

Provider's Information:
- Name
- Phone number and address
- Provider's license number (This may be required by state law.)
- Provider's Drug Enforcement Administration number, if applicable

Prescription Information:
- Name of medication
- Strength
- Dosage form
- Route of administration
- Quantity
- Sig (directions for taking or using)
- Refill information
- Provider's signature
- Date written
- Dispense As Written (DAW): prescriber desires brand name drug rather than generic version of drug

Tech Note!

Patients may be obtaining medications from other pharmacy locations or may be receiving treatment elsewhere for other conditions. Because of this, it is important to ask patients about their current conditions and all medications they are taking. In this way the pharmacist can counsel the patient on any interactions that may occur between the new medications and other concurrent medications.

medication tray every 24 hours and will continue this practice until the physician changes or discontinues the order. For injectable or intravenous medications, the pharmacy will also fill limited quantities and provide them to the patient's care area, usually for the next 24 hours. Exceptions to the daily fill practice are orders for antibiotics, which usually have an automatic stop date after a duration of treatment for the patient's condition, unless the prescriber specifies different orders.

TRANSLATION OF AN ORDER

When reading an order that is difficult to decipher, make sure you look at the entire order. For instance, what is the name of the clinic or office from which the order originated? Can you decipher the strength or dose? What is the route of administration? How often is the medication being ordered? What is the dosage form? Are there refills? If it is still difficult to decipher the name of the medication but you determine the strength is 0.125 mg and the medication is to be taken daily, this information limits the types of possible medications and the name of the medication may become apparent. In other cases, there will be too

BOX 7-3 REQUIRED PATIENT INFORMATION IN AN INSTITUTIONAL SETTING

Patient Information:
- Patient's name
- Medical record number
- Room number
- Allergies
- Height
- Weight (In many patients, such as pediatric, geriatric, and oncology patients, the height and weight of the patient are needed for dosage calculations.)
- Age or date of birth
- Laboratory parameters (important for drug monitoring or dose calculations)
- Diagnosis or suspected diagnosis

Prescriber Information:
- Covering physician's name
- Primary physician's name (may be different than covering physician)

Prescription Order Information:
- Name of medication
- Strength
- Route of administration
- Dosage form
- Sig (including frequency of administration and duration of treatment in some cases)
- Physician's signature
- Date and time order written or when order is to begin

Other Important Information, Usually Available from Medical Chart or Nursing Staff:
- Scheduled procedures
- Prognosis

Tech Note!

When you ask someone to decipher a drug name or instruction, do not share your interpretation with the person. This inadvertently can make that person see the prescription the same way you are seeing it. Simply ask, "What does this look like to you?" If the answer matches yours, then you have an unbiased opinion. However, if you are not sure, ask the pharmacist to contact the physician to confirm the prescription.

Tech Note!

More and more hospitals are using preprinted prescription order sets for certain disease conditions. The physician merely needs to indicate the correct drug, strength, dosage form and amount, and other orders for the individual patient, and then sign the script. The sets help ensure that quality management standards are met, and the preprinted format limits errors in order interpretation. Also, many physician's offices are E-prescribing prescriptions to the pharmacy from computers located in the exam room or from handheld devices. As physicians begin to move into the increasingly paperless world of prescriptions, the hope is that illegible handwriting will soon be a thing of the past.

many possibilities that fit the information that is available; it is best to request clarification of the order to avoid a medication error. There are many look-alike, sound-alike medications with similar dosing. Ultimately, if you are in doubt, ask another person such as the pharmacist.

When to Ask for Help

When a job relies on reading another person's handwriting and the handwriting is poor, it is common to need assistance in interpreting the writing. However, each person filling prescriptions is under intense pressure to fill them quickly, and this can lead to "guessing" at an order and then filling it. The following example is to help you feel comfortable in asking for help.

ENTERING THE INFORMATION INTO THE DATABASE

Community Setting

The way in which prescriptions enter the pharmacy will determine the processing of the medication. If the order is received by telephone, the pharmacist must translate the verbal order into a written order by using a prescription pad, and then it can be processed. If a hard copy is received, the order is interpreted and entered into the computer. (Figure 7-2). In a community pharmacy setting, the technician usually enters the prescription orders. The computerized label is checked against the prescription after it is filled. Two labels are always discharged from the printer; one is placed on the vial for dispensing, and the

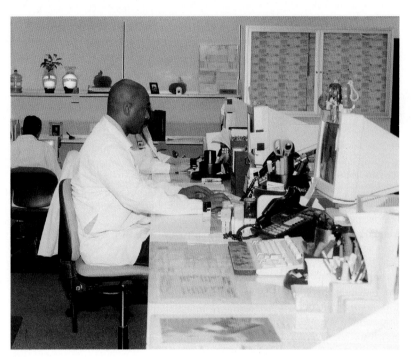

FIGURE 7-2 Technicians may enter information into the computer system in many pharmacy settings.

other is positioned on the back of the original prescription. Additional portions of the script label can be placed on a clipboard that is signed by the patient during medication pickup. This clipboard signature can be used both for reimbursement and for consultation documentation. The pharmacist and technician (in many states) must initial both copies. If the pharmacy uses electronic prescription pickup, the patient will sign an electronic signature device. Most pharmacies today copy (scan) prescriptions to the computer for verification. If a change must be made, the pharmacist can access the terminal easily and make the change to the order. At the time of consultation, the pharmacist has an additional opportunity to determine other medications the patient may be taking.

Institutional Setting

In a hospital, prescription data can be entered into the computer by either a pharmacist or a technician. Depending on the protocol for a hospital, the pharmacist may enter medication orders into the computer and the technician fills the order. In a hospital, there are multiple orders sent upon the admission of a patient and throughout the patient's hospital stay. Because all orders have to be verified by a pharmacist, it saves time if the pharmacist inputs the order and the technician fills the order. Computer systems allow the technician to enter medications and flag them for the pharmacist to check. This must be done before a label is created. Therefore, if the pharmacist enters the order, he or she only has to check the technician's work (pulled medications) once rather than twice— after the technician enters the order and after the technician fills it. In addition, most computers have an integrated system that alerts the person entering prescriptions of a serious drug interaction or other potential problems based on the patient's specific health information, including diagnosis and reported laboratory tests . A technician cannot handle interaction problems; a pharmacist must initiate a phone call to the physician or charge nurse to obtain an order change if necessary.

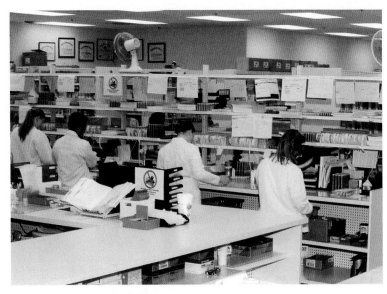

FIGURE 7-3 Technicians filling prescriptions.

FILLING THE PRESCRIPTION IN A COMMUNITY SETTING

After the prescription label is prepared, it is matched with the original order and sent to the counter for filling (Figure 7-3). Filling may occur using an automated dispensing system. Again, the technician (in most settings) receives the order. From the beginning, it is important that the technician pay close attention to the prescription he or she is filling because this is where many mistakes can be avoided. Following these 10 important steps may prevent the technician from making a grievous error:

1. Verify that all necessary information is on the prescription.
2. Pull the appropriate medication from the shelf.
3. Measure or count the necessary amount of the medication. If counted by the automated system (e.g., Baker Cells), then recount, especially controlled substances.*
4. Fill the vial with the medication, taking care not to touch the medication.
5. Ensure that the lid is the appropriate type (e.g., childproof) and is affixed properly onto the vial.
6. Apply the labels onto the vial and back of the prescription.
7. Place the technician's initials on the bottom right-hand side of all labels printed.
8. Apply any necessary auxiliary labels to the vial.
9. Place the medication and stock bottle on top of the original prescription.
10. Pass the medication onto the pharmacist for final inspection. Usually the pharmacist on duty logs on the computer with his or her initials, which will appear on the prescription label.

1. Verifying the Prescription

Although prescribers use many different types of prescription pads, the information is basically the same. Ensuring that all parts of the prescription have been

Tech Note!

If the prescription order seems incorrect, it probably is. Ask for assistance from your pharmacist if you cannot identify the problem.

---

*If available, check the medication item against the verification information (e.g., image, imprint, shape); in the pharmacy system; many large retail pharmacies have this information available and require this step in their protocols for prescription filling.

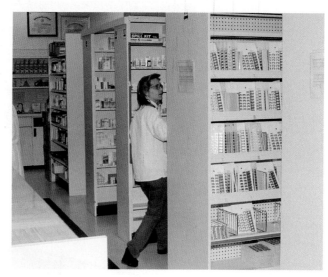

FIGURE 7-4 Pulling medication from the shelf.

Tech Note!

When checking the dosage form, do not make assumptions. To assume that a spansule is the same as a capsule is easy (they look similar); however, they are different dosage forms.

Tech Note!

To prevent grabbing the wrong bottle, keep medications separated from each other on the counter when filling prescriptions. Fill only one prescription at a time.

filled out is the first step in processing the prescription. When the label is passed along with the original prescription, it must be checked many times before it ever reaches the patient. The technician should hold the original prescription next to the label and check for any apparent errors or discrepancies. Look at the name of the drug, strength or dose, dosage form, route of administration, amount, and the **sig** (directions). Make sure all information matches. For direction abbreviations, see Chapter 5.

2. Pulling the Correct Medication

You will leave the counter to get the medication from the shelf (Figure 7-4). When doing this, make sure that you take the label with you for two reasons:

1. You do not forget the name of the medication for which you are looking (which is a time-saving action).
2. Once the bottle of medication is found, compare the label information to the bottle, checking the name, strength, dosage form, and National Drug Code.

3 and 4. Counting and Filling the Medication

After the technician locates the medication, removes it from the shelf, and returns to the counter, the prescription is filled.

Again, you should check your label and prescription against the medication bottle for accuracy. If the order is for a bottle of 100, check to make sure that the manufacturer's package size matches your order. For example, many times bottles hold different amounts. Although there are various ways to count medications, many pharmacies still use counting trays (count in multiples of 5), and then the medication is poured into the vial (Figure 7-5). A device that uses a beam of light is also used to count medications. As the light is broken, the digital counter adds another tablet or capsule on the monitor. Digital counters also can weigh the tablets or capsules as you pour them into the vial. The medication label is scanned into the scale's electronic system; the machine can then calibrate the amount of tablets or capsules based on their weight. An example of this type of digital counter is the Torbal DRX-300. Larger semiautomated or automated machines such as the Baker Cell system are used to verify and fill orders in fast-paced pharmacies. Dispensing systems are discussed later in this chapter.

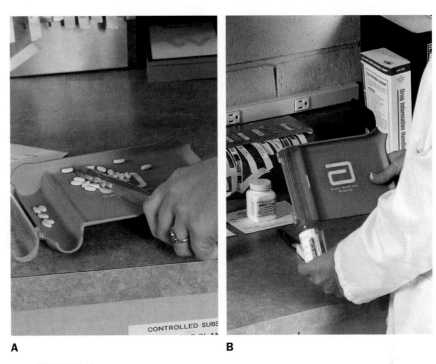

A   B

FIGURE 7-5 Technician counting and pouring tablets into medication vial.

TABLE 7-1 Exceptions for Safety Lids*

Drug	Dispensed Without Safety Lid	Reason
Nitroglycerin	Never has a safety lid	For emergencies
Isosorbide SL (sublingual)	May be dispensed without a safety lid	For emergencies
All other medications	Doctor's request documented on prescription or patient's request documented in computer or in hard copy	Any conditions

*Refer to the Poison Control Act of 1970 for all exceptions.

5. Prescription Lids

Once the vial is filled with the medication, the appropriate lid is applied to the vial. As the average human life expectancy increases, there is a growing segment of the population that is older than 70 years. Two of the problems that accompany aging are decreasing dexterity and strength. As most of us have experienced, there are safety lids that even Godzilla cannot remove! Not surprisingly, many older patients do not wish to have childproof safety lids on their medication. By law, the pharmacy must use safety lids in all cases except for a selected few. These cases are outlined in Table 7-1.

If the patient or his or her physician has requested no childproof caps, then the cap can be replaced with a snap-on lid. Many pharmacies (depending on regulation) require the patient to sign the back of the prescription or a release form requesting a non-childproof cap. This information is then listed on the patient information in the computer for future reference.

6. Applying the Label

When labeling a bottle, you must be professional and always provide a quality job. Do not place a torn label or place the label crookedly on a medication bottle.

If the label rips, print a new one. No one wants to believe that the prescription was filled in a rush, but rather with care and concern. When filling a prescription for a full bottle, such as cough syrup, you can place the label over the label of the existing bottle, making sure the lot number and expiration date are not covered. If the medication has to be counted or measured, pour the medication into an appropriate-sized bottle.

Sometimes labels must be reduced in size because of lengthy directions. For example, a tapering dose of prednisone is a typical challenge, but it is possible to fit these labels onto a vial or dose-pack even if you must use a vial that is larger than normal to accommodate the label. Carefully cut the label so that it will not be apparent to the patient. Also, the label must not cover any important print. In addition, **auxiliary labels**, when required, must be placed onto the bottle so that the patient can read the instructions easily. Many computer systems have a labeling system that allows the following information to be printed on one sheet:

- The prescription label
- A duplicate copy to be placed on the original hard copy
- Billing information
- Auxiliary labels

Once a prescription is entered into the computer system, the instructions and necessary information are printed on labels. Most labels contain preprinted information that is required by law, which consists of the following:

- Name, address, and phone number of pharmacy
- A prescription number, given automatically by the computer
- Patient name
- Drug name, strength or dose, and dosage form
- Manufacturer's name
- Instructions for use
- Date filled
- Refill information
- Prescriber
- Expiration date
- May also contain name or initials of pharmacist

7. Technician's Initials

All orders filled by a technician should be initialed by the technician as the prescriptions are filled, per state law. This is important for several reasons. The pharmacist who will give the final approval now knows that the prescription is filled. If the pharmacist has any questions, he or she knows whom to ask. Finally, if there is an error, the technician can be notified and learn from that error. In addition, the pharmacist must always sign off and approve the prescription or refill after completion. Some computer systems have the pharmacist's initials printed on the label, which is acceptable to most state boards of pharmacy.

8. Auxiliary Labels

All necessary auxiliary labels must adhere to the vial in a neat manner (Figure 7-6). These labels are normally printed along with the label, aiding the technician. However, it is still important to know what medications need special auxiliary labels because not all pharmacies have this ability. If many auxiliary labels are being printed, it is necessary to choose the most important ones that can fit easily on the medication bottle. Care should be taken not to conceal any instructions, lot number, or expiration date.

Tech Note!

All controlled substance prescription labels must have the following statement: "CAUTION: Federal law prohibits the transfer of this drug to any person other than the patient for whom it was prescribed."

Tech Note!

Prescription labels must bear the legend "federal law prohibits dispensing without a prescription."

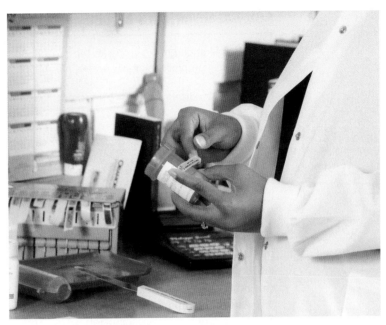

FIGURE 7-6 Applying an auxiliary label.

TABLE 7-2 Commonly Used Auxiliary Labels for Side Effects

Medication	Most Common Auxiliary Label
Contraceptives	Take as directed.
Nonsteroidal antiinflammatory drugs	May cause dizziness/drowsiness. Take with food.
Narcotics	Do not drink alcohol, and/or drinking may increase the effects of the drug.
Macrolide antibiotics	Take on an empty stomach. Take with plenty of water.
All antibiotics	Take until gone.
Sulfa antibiotics	May cause sensitivity to light. Take on an empty stomach. Take with plenty of water.
Warfarin	Do not take aspirin unless prescribed.

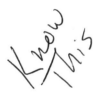

To realize which medications require an auxiliary label, the technician must know the classification of the drug, interactions, and side effects. Remembering a few common rules will help with the most general auxiliary labels (Table 7-2). For the most part, it takes time and experience to learn which auxiliary labels are important for various medications. However, it is ultimately up to the pharmacist to choose and approve the labels to place on the prescription bottle. Be sure to read auxiliary labels before adhering them to the bottle, because many different instructions are colored the same and may appear similar.

9 and 10. Pharmacist's Final Inspection

The last step in filling prescriptions is placing the filled vial, along with the medication container taken from the shelf, on top of the original prescription and passing it to the pharmacist for final inspection. The technician should give the order one final inspection to ensure that the patient's name on the prescription matches the label and that all other information is correct.

BOX 7-4 ADVANTAGES OF A COMPUTER DISPENSING SYSTEM

Increases speed of medication processing	As the prescription is entered into the computer system, the information is transferred to the dispensing system.
Reduces medication errors	The proper number of tablets or capsules is then dispensed into a container, and the correct drug product is verified.
Helps manage and track inventory	Medication can be scanned to keep accurate count of inventory. Daily printouts can be used by a technician or pharmacist to help the inventory technician keep the correct amount of drug on the shelf.

Only then should you pass the medication to the pharmacist and begin filling the next order.

Another important aspect of filling a prescription is to remember not to fill more than one prescription at a time; this is an invitation for error. You can pull several orders and give each a double-check for accuracy, but it is important to clearly separate them from the prescription you are currently filling.

If a new stock bottle is opened to fill an order, mark it across the front with an X (in pen) to alert fellow employees that it is not a full bottle. Do not cover the drug name, strength, National Drug Code, or expiration date with the mark. When the bottle is returned to stock, the next person pulling the bottle will know it is a partial bottle. If a full bottle is needed, he or she will choose an unmarked one. The overall time that a prescription is in the hands of the pharmacy technician is not long, which is why it is so important to make each moment count when trying to fill a prescription flawlessly.

Community Dispensing Systems

Many chain pharmacies are using **automated dispensing systems (ADS)** for three primary reasons: to reduce errors, to increase productivity, and to manage inventory (Box 7-4). Because of new laws that require pharmacies to decrease medication errors, pharmacies are converting rapidly to these types of systems.

Automated systems can now visually identify all the information on a label through a bar code located on the side of the prescription label. They also show the filler an image of the medication inside the container so it can be verified at the time of filling. Only after the authentication of the medication identification does the dispenser release the proper medication into the vial. When the dispenser needs to be filled, the technician will pull more medication and again the medication bottle will need to be scanned to ensure the correct drug has been selected; then the technician can fill the dispenser. As medications are added and used, the automated system keeps track of the inventory. New stock can be ordered in a timely manner so that the pharmacy will always have some of the medication readily available.

FILLING ORDERS IN AN INSTITUTIONAL SETTING

Institutional pharmacies do not follow the same steps as outpatient pharmacies for filling medication orders. Orders in this type of setting are sent via hospital order forms or done electronically, and involve a much wider range of medications. In addition, medication is provided for 24-hour periods. For complete information on steps involved in filling institutional orders, see Chapter 10, Hospital Pharmacy.

Computer Dispensing Systems

Another type of prescription filler besides the traditional pharmacist or technician is the emerging automated computer system. New and improved versions become available every year. Pharmacy personnel must become comfortable with manipulating these devices because they are here to stay. Several versions of dispensing systems are available: those made for filling outpatient prescriptions and those for hospitals, nursing care facilities, and large mail-order companies. Because of the many differences between types of pharmacy settings and because each pharmacy has different requirements, computer systems must be individualized according to the needs of the pharmacy. Therefore most manufacturers of automated systems offer various components to fit the specific needs of each pharmacy.

Inpatient Dispensing Systems

Most hospitals use some type of computerized dispensing system because it is important that medication be continually available for acute needs. Although many inpatient pharmacies are open 24 hours a day, 7 days a week, staffing is limited throughout the night, and computer dispensing systems can help reduce staffing needs. Medical personnel such as physicians or nurses should be able to access approved stock medications. Another major use of automation in hospital systems is to regulate controlled substances and track their movement. Accurate recording of the use and disposition of controlled substances is required by regulatory agencies, and medication dispensing systems help facilitate this reconciliation process. For more information on hospital automated dispensing systems, see Chapter 10.

Examples of inpatient and outpatient dispensing systems follow:

Manufacturer	Type of System	Function
Amerisource	MedSelect	Hospital
McKesson	Loop Distribution	Outpatient
Omnicell	MedGuard	Hospital
	Workflow Rx	Outpatient
Parata	RDS (robotic dispensing system)	Outpatient
Pyxis	ADS (automated dispensing system)	Hospital

THE 5 RIGHTS OF MEDICATION SAFETY

When a technician accepts the job of filling a patient's prescription, it is very important to always remember the basic rights of a patient in regards to medication safety. A helpful outlook is to think of yourself as the recipient of the medication that is being prepared. You would want extreme care taken in filling your own medication; strive to do the same for others. Checking the prescription at least three times during the filling process helps to ensure accuracy. In addition to always treating patients with respect and ensuring their right to confidentiality, the rights of a patient to medication safety are as follows:

1. The right patient
2. The right drug
3. The right dose
4. The right route
5. The right time

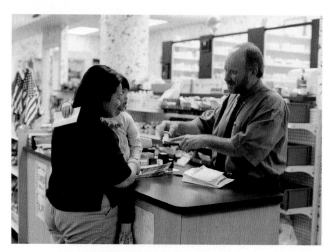

FIGURE 7-7 Patient consultation.

PHARMACIST CONSULTATIONS: WHEN AND WHO NEEDS THEM

As the patient's medication is entered into the computer system, one of the functions of pharmacy tracking is to determine whether it is a new prescription or a refill. First-time prescriptions are typically flagged in some manner that will alert the pharmacist. If flagging is not automatic, it is the responsibility of the individual pharmacist to check the computer system for this information. If the prescription is new, a sticker is placed on the medication bag, indicating to the technician or clerk that the patient requires an offer of consultation. The federal law is that with all new prescriptions or changes in an existing prescription, a patient receiving Medicaid coverage must be offered consultation. The patient can refuse consultation, but consultation must be offered per the Omnibus Reconciliation Act of 1990 (see Chapter 2). At this time, the pharmacist checks the patient's records to determine whether there are any potential drug or food interactions; then the pharmacist provides the patient with instructions for the proper use of the medication and describes possible side effects of the drug. At this time, the patient can also ask questions or address concerns specific to the medication (Figure 7-7). While federal law specifically addresses requirements related to those patients reimbursed by Medicaid, many states have passed regulations to mandate verbal, written, or both types of counseling to patients with each new prescription or refill. As with OBRA '90, the patient has the right to refuse verbal consultation.

Miscellaneous Orders

COMMUNITY SETTING

Unlike first-time prescriptions, transferring of prescriptions and receipt of authorization of refills can be performed by technicians, clerks, and pharmacy interns over the phone, as outlined in the following sections. Although these guidelines are enacted federally, statewide regulations may be more strict, and each pharmacy may have different employee protocols. To determine your state regulations, access your state board of pharmacy website.

DAILY HARD-COPY PRINTING (QUEUE)

Prescription labels are printed early in the morning and rechecked throughout the day. The morning pharmacy personnel should attempt to print the entire batch of labels before noon, if possible. Since a majority of patients drop off new scripts in the morning and pick them up in the afternoon, printing the queue of scripts in the morning can assist pharmacy personnel employed later in the day. Medication errors and stress will be reduced if employees do not have to search for labels and fill prescriptions at the last minute. It also gives the morning crew more time to resolve any issues with refills, insurance, or physician calls that might occur.

Refills

Tech Note!

The pharmacy technician should note on the patient's file whether the script was faxed or called in and at what time. Then when the patient contacts the pharmacy to locate his or her medication, other personnel on duty will know how to locate the information.

A pharmacy technician may phone a prescriber's office and receive authorization for a prescription refill. When a patient calls in a prescription refill or a request is faxed, the following information is normally required. However, if the patient does not provide the following information, the prescription information can be accessed from the computer by the patient's last name.

1. Patient's name
2. Patient's home phone number
3. Prescription number
4. Name of the medication, strength, dosage form, and quantity
5. Patient's date of birth (often needed for the physician to verify patient identity)
6. Last date filled
7. Contact information for the pharmacy

ZERO REFILL REORDERS

Many pharmacies have an additional phone number intended for patients desiring to fill prescriptions that have no refills remaining. Typically, the patient should allow 2 days to obtain proper authorization from the prescriber. Technicians are qualified to perform this task under the pharmacist's direction.

TRANSFERS

A pharmacist may transfer a previously filled prescription from one pharmacy to another. Most state boards of pharmacy prefer to allow transfers of a prescription to occur only one time; however, federal law stipulates that controlled substances may be transferred only one time. Always be aware of your board of pharmacy regulations. In general the following rules apply:

- A pharmacy technician may assist the pharmacist in the transfer of a prescription.
- Under the supervision of the pharmacist, the technician may fax a copy of the prescription to another pharmacy. The pharmacist directs the technician on what information is needed from the receiving or transferring pharmacy.
- Notation needs to be made both in the patient profile and on the original script that the prescription has been transferred. This will allow the pharmacy to direct the patient to the location of his or her prescription. When the prescription has been transferred, the original number of pills needs to be reported with the remaining number of pills. For example, Lipitor #100 with 3 refills is a total of 400 tablets. If the patient can only obtain a 30-day supply per month and has filled the script for 3 months, the patient has used 90 pills. The patient thus has 310 pills remaining on the script. This number needs to be reported, not that the patient has 9 refills of 30 pills remaining.

REFILLING AUTOMATED DISPENSING SYSTEM (ADS) MACHINES

Often the technician is responsible for refilling the ADS machines, under the direction and supervision of the pharmacist. Care must be taken to:

1. Guarantee that the right drug is being dispensed into the right dispenser (hopper).
2. Make certain that the NDC number of the hopper matches the NDC numbers for the stock used (e.g., sometimes generic medications change and the tabs/caps are different in color or shape).
3. Verify that the hoppers for the tabs/caps are the correct size (e.g., if too big, 3 to 4 tabs/caps are dispensed at once; if too small, tabs/caps cannot pass through the opening).
4. Ensure that the hoppers are kept clean. Failure to clean the hoppers can lead to mistakes in the counting of tabs/caps.

Filing Prescriptions

After the prescription is filled, the hard copy (i.e., original prescription) is filed for future reference. There are three methods for filing prescriptions (outlined in Table 7-3). If the order is received via e-mail, the script is saved in the computer bank as a hard copy. Federal law states that all prescriptions must be kept on file for a period of at least 2 years, although each state may increase this time. Check your state's board of pharmacy for this information. Filing is done by using the prescription number. On the back of the prescription is a copy of the label used on the dispensed drug, along with the initials of the technician and pharmacist who filled the order. In addition, some states require that all controlled substances (schedules III and IV) that are filled together or with other prescriptions must be stamped with a red "C" 1 inch from the top and on the right-hand side of the prescription label, to make it easier to find. The location of the stamp may differ depending on state law. All schedule II medications must be filed separately; they cannot be sent electronically or by fax, except in emergencies, in which case they must be followed with a hard copy on a tamper-proof C-II prescription form. For an example of a tamper-proof form, see Chapter 2.

Complete filing guidelines are discussed in Chapter 2. Usually, all prescriptions are filed at the end of the day. They are filed in small packets (usually grouped in hundreds) that are marked clearly on the outside with the date for easy reference. These are kept on the pharmacy premises. In addition to the hard copy, the computer-scanned copy indicates whether a drug is a controlled substance and lists all the other information required by federal and state regulations. At the end of the workday, electronic backup copies are usually made of all the orders in the system in case of a computer malfunction.

TABLE 7-3 Filing Prescriptions

System	Drawer I	Drawer II	Drawer III
1	C-II separate	C-III, C-IV, C-V	All other prescriptions
2	C-II separate	C-III, C-IV, C-V,* and all prescription drugs	
3	C-II, C-III, C-IV, C-V*		All other prescriptions

*If any C-III, C-IV, or C-V controlled drugs are kept with non–controlled drugs (system 2) or mixed with C-II drugs (system 3), they must be stamped with a red "C" for easy identification. All records must be kept on site for no less than 2 years. Many states, however, have longer requirements for keeping records; remember that the strictest law is the one that must be followed. When taking inventory, one must have exact counts of C-II substances at all times.

EARLY FILLS

A prescription can be filled early if the patient has a good reason; for example, the patient is going on vacation for an extended time, or the patient lost his or her medication. In these cases, the pharmacy may be able to obtain preapproval from the insurance company to fill the prescription early. Many insurance prescription plans allow for one early refill per medication, per calendar year. A portion of the cost of the drug may be paid to the pharmacy by the insurance company with the balance being paid when the original refill date arrives.

Medication Pickup

Patients can wait for their prescription, have it delivered, or pick it up another day. Many pharmacies provide an automated call service to patients to remind them their prescriptions are ready. Pharmacies have an established time for all prescriptions to be returned to stock (RTS) if not picked up, and this may range from a few days to several weeks. After this time, the medication will need to be reprocessed and the patient will have to wait. All pharmacies have a designated boundary around the counter to promote customer privacy both when dropping off or picking up prescriptions and when asking or receiving patient consultation; specific requirements for pharmacies are established in individual state board of pharmacy regulations. Other patients must stand at a distance and wait to be called to the counter; this promotes adherence to Health Insurance Portability and Accountability Act (HIPAA) regulations (see Chapter 2). Occasionally, a patient has a relative obtain a prescription. For these cases, making a note in the computer that lists the person or persons who are authorized to pick up another person's prescription is required. Regardless of who obtains the prescription, it is important to ensure that the right person gets the right medication. Therefore check all identification against the prescription before releasing the medication; in addition, the person picking up the medication must sign for it. In the case of a controlled substance, if the person picking up the medication is not the patient, that person must show identification to the clerk or technician and sign for it. All third-party prescriptions must have the signature of the receiver. Also, the pharmacy may require the purchaser to provide identification when picking up a controlled substance prescription.

Billing Patients

The billing portion of processing a prescription varies depending on the patient's insurance coverage, if any. If the person does not have coverage, there is no additional paperwork because the patient simply has to pay full price for the prescription. Many pharmacies have specials and/or coupons for discounted prices on new prescriptions that can be used at the time of purchase. Most persons have some type of drug coverage so their final price will be dependent upon the information obtained from their insurance card. Each type of insurance has its own limitations and conditions. Each pharmacy is responsible for contacting the coverage program for reimbursement. For more information on the types of insurance and the new Medicare (Part D) medication plan, see Chapter 13.

When the patient first drops off his or her prescription, the insurance company is billed before the medication is filled through a process called online **adjudication**. The patient's insurance card should be thoroughly checked. Some of the data that the technician must be able to locate on insurance cards are the Benefit International Identification Number (BIN #), which electronically identifies the insurance carrier; the Processor Control Number (PCN #), which identifies the plan; the ID number; the group number; and the person code (see Chapter 13). If there are any problems with the billing process, the pharmacy will contact the patient. For example, a wrong person code, a wrong date of birth, or the need for prior authorizations are types of problems that may occur. Prescriptions for **non-formulary** drugs need to be resolved by the pharmacist, who contacts the physician and requests a change to a similar formulary drug. Non-formulary drugs are those medications not approved by drug coverage plans, unless a prior authorization or approved exception occurs. Insurance termination and change of plan/co-pay issues must be investigated by the patient.

Changing Trends

Interpreting and transcribing prescriptions, producing labels, and filling and checking prescriptions are the "meat and potatoes" of the pharmacy business. Laws such as the Omnibus Budget Reconciliation Act of 1990 require that consultations be given to select patients. The increasing age of the American population has changed the primary focus of the pharmacist from filling prescriptions to interacting and consulting with patients and prescribers. Because of this nationwide change, the technician has been placed on the front line. This responsibility requires the technician to fill prescriptions as quickly and with the same accuracy as a pharmacist. Technicians also must know their limitations at all times. In addition to these capabilities, many technicians are in charge of the billing process and must be skilled in both understanding the policies and procedures of their pharmacy and processing various types of insurance claims. Patients expect perfection and proper billing practices when it comes to their medications. This weight clearly falls on the pharmacist in charge, per pharmacy law, although technicians may also be held accountable (see Chapter 2). This responsibility should never be taken lightly and it requires continuing education in all areas of pharmacy practice.

DO YOU REMEMBER THESE KEY POINTS?

- The various ways a prescription can be submitted to the pharmacy for processing
- The steps involved in filling a prescription
- Who can call in a prescription
- Who can transfer a prescription from one pharmacy to another
- The differences between information on inpatient and outpatient prescriptions
- The type of patient information needed in different pharmacy settings
- The importance of knowing when and why to ask for help from a pharmacist
- The number of times a pharmacy technician should check a prescription while filling the order
- The necessary authorization to use snap-on caps rather than childproof caps
- The auxiliary labels needed for the medications outlined in this chapter
- Why computer dispensing systems are used
- The rights of a patient in regard to medication safety
- When patient consultations are done and who is authorized to do them
- How to process refills
- Requirements of filing prescriptions (hard copies)
- Requirements for patients or family members picking up medication from the pharmacy

REVIEW QUESTIONS

Multiple choice questions

1. Of the alternatives listed, which are acceptable ways of receiving all prescriptions except C-II medications?
   A. In person (walk-in)
   B. Called in
   C. Electronically
   D. All of the above

2. When filling a prescription, the best times to check for errors are:
   A. When the order is first received, during filling, and after filling
   B. While filling the order, after filling, and when handing the order to the patient
   C. When checking the original order against the label, against the stock bottle before filling, and before filling the vial and affixing the labeling
   D. Before applying the label, before applying the auxiliary labels, and before giving it to the pharmacist

3. Of the information listed, which is vital information needed from a patient before filling his or her prescription?
   A. Full name
   B. Allergies
   C. Prescription insurance information
   D. All of the above

4. When in doubt about the directions on a prescription, it is best to:
   A. Call the physician's office immediately
   B. Try your best to decipher the order
   C. Ask the pharmacist for help
   D. Ask a pharmacy clerk for help with interpretation

5. Of the reasons listed, which is (are) the main reason(s) for using automated dispensing systems in a community pharmacy?
   A. To increase the accuracy of filling prescriptions
   B. To help control inventory
   C. To decrease the time it takes to fill an order
   D. All of the above

6. What information is not needed from a prescriber on a prescription order?
   A. Directions
   B. Refills
   C. Manufacturer
   D. Date written

7. Which of the medications listed does not require a safety lid?
   A. Warfarin tablets
   B. Amoxicillin suspension
   C. Nitroglycerin sublingual tablets
   D. All of the above

8. Of the information listed, which is not necessary on a prescription label?
   A. Date filled
   B. Expiration date
   C. Prescriber
   D. Patient's home address

9. Which one of the rights listed is considered one of The 5 Rights of Medication Safety?
   A. The right to the correct drug
   B. The right to the correct price
   C. The right to a similar drug alternative
   D. The right to the correct strength

10. Of the following basic steps required in filling a prescription, which is the responsibility of the technician?
A. Filling the prescription
B. Translating the prescription
C. Consulting the patient
D. Entering the information into the database

11. Which one of the following persons cannot send verbal medication orders to the pharmacy?
A. Ward clerk
B. Nurse
C. Physician's assistant
D. All of the above can send verbal orders to the pharmacy

12. Which of the following methods of filling prescriptions is not valid?
A. C-II separate, C-III to C-V and all other prescriptions filled together
B. C-II to C-V separate, all other prescriptions filled together
C. All prescriptions filled together
D. C-II through C-V separate, all other prescriptions filled together

13. What steps should NOT be done when filling medications?
A. Triple-check your order.
B. Place label on straight.
C. Conceal both the NDC and expiration date.
D. Flag order for consultation if necessary.

14. A prescription can be transferred ____ times.
A. Zero
B. 1
C. 2
D. As many times as necessary

15. An outpatient dispensing system uses what type of visual double-check of drug information?
A. It views the medication and double-checks the order.
B. It uses information contained on a bar code.
C. It uses information contained on the prescription.
D. Both A and C are correct.

True/False

If the statement is false, then change it to make it true.

_____ **1.** Insurance information for billing purposes should be processed when prescriptions are picked up.

_____ **2.** New prescriptions can be called in or taken into a pharmacy by the patient for filling.

_____ **3.** When prescriptions are written by a physician for a patient in the hospital, it is not necessary for the order to be presented on a prescription pad.

_____ **4.** Technicians regularly enter hospital orders and may call the physician for additional information.

_____ **5.** All prescriptions must have safety lids per federal law.

_____ **6.** Most pharmacy labeling programs print a second label to be placed on the back of the hard-copy prescription.

_____ **7.** Technicians need to sign their initials or last name on all prescription labels before passing them to the pharmacist for a final check.

_____ **8.** Antibiotics typically receive an auxiliary label "Take until gone" to ensure that the patient finishes the course of antibiotic treatment.

_____ **9.** The Omnibus Budget Reconciliation Act of 1990 ensures that technicians can handle drugs.

_____ **10.** Technicians cannot take prescription orders over the phone.

_____ **11.** Prescriptions are often taken by pharmacy clerks in retail pharmacy.

_____ **12.** Electronic prescriptions must be translated into written form by the pharmacist before they are filled.

_____ **13.** An order written in the chart of a hospital patient is considered a legal prescription once signed by the prescriber.

_____ **14.** Only the patient can pick up his or her medications from a pharmacy.

_____ **15.** All pharmacies are required to have automated dispensing systems according to the rules and regulations of each state's board of pharmacy.

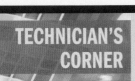

TECHNICIAN'S CORNER You fill a prescription with the wrong medication. The error is not recognized until later that evening when the prescriptions are being filed. What do you do?

BIBLIOGRAPHY

Nielsen J: *Handbook of federal drug law*, ed 2, Philadelphia, 1992, Lippincott Williams & Wilkins.

8

Over-the-Counter Medications

Objectives

UPON COMPLETING THIS CHAPTER, YOU SHOULD BE ABLE TO DO THE FOLLOWING:

- Describe why over-the-counter (OTC) medications are popular.

- List considerations concerning the use of OTC drugs.

- List the three categories used by the Food and Drug Administration for designating a medication as an OTC drug.

- Describe Food and Drug Administration regulations concerning the manufacture of OTC drugs.

- Explain the steps involved in medication becoming categorized as over-the-counter.

- List a minimum of five conditions treated with OTC drugs.

- Define behind-the-counter medication and explain how its status differs from OTC items.

- Explain why special considerations must be given to both geriatric and pediatric patients in the selection of OTC drugs.

Analgesic *A drug that relieves pain by reducing the perception of pain*

Antiinflammatory *A drug that reduces swelling, redness, and pain and that promotes healing*

Antipyretic *A drug that reduces fever.*

Antiseptic *A substance that slows or stops the growth of microorganisms on surfaces such as the skin*

Antitussive *A drug that can decrease the coughing reflex of the central nervous system*

ASA *Acetylsalicylic acid (aspirin)*

Behind-the-counter *Those medications that do not require a prescription but are kept under control; the use and/or amount of the medication is monitored by pharmacy*

Bulk forming *Fiber used to treat constipation or induce a feeling of fullness to decrease appetite*

Expectorant *Chemical that aids in the removal of mucous secretions from the respiratory system; loosens and thins sputum and bronchial secretions for ease of expectoration*

OTC *Over-the-counter; medications that do not require a prescription and may be purchased by customers at any retail outlet*

ROA *Route of administration*

Introduction

If you walk into a shopping center or your corner drugstore, you will see the massive number of **over-the-counter** (OTC) medications that are available for personal use (Figure 8-1). No prescriptions are necessary and no questions need to be answered to attain these drugs. In fact, most consumers show little, if any, consideration before purchasing several different OTC drugs to keep at home for themselves or their family. One could say that just as certain food staples are kept on hand in the kitchen, so have certain OTC medications become common staples of home medicine cabinets. For example, a basic shopping list might include items such as flour, sugar, eggs, acetaminophen (Tylenol), cough syrup, and ibuprofen (Motrin).

Since the mid-1980s there has been a sharp increase in the number of OTC drugs available to consumers. The following statistics give useful data on the use and sales of OTC items, the reduction in health care costs possible from the use of OTC drugs, and the future of OTC medications:

- U.S. retail sales of over-the-counter (OTC) medicines in 2008 (excluding Wal-Mart) were $16.8 billion (The Nielsen Company, 2009).
- Since 1976, 84 ingredients, dosages, or indications have made the "switch" from prescription to OTC status. Additionally, 15 medications were introduced during that time directly to the OTC market without having been prescription medicines first (Consumer Healthcare Products Association [CHPA], 2009).
- Consumer use of OTC heartburn medications is estimated to save the U.S. health care system $757 million annually, and saves the average consumer

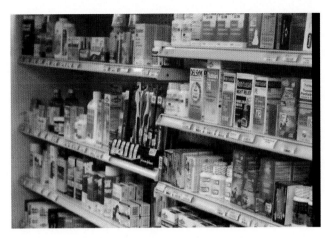

FIGURE 8-1 More than 100,000 OTC products exist from different combinations of only 1000 ingredients. (CPHA, 2001)

$174 annually; 94% of consumers report satisfaction with available OTC heartburn remedies (CHPA and The Nielsen Company, 2009).

- In 2008, prescription drug sales (retail and mail order) accounted for $253.6 billion from January '08 through December '08 (National Association of Chain Drug Stores [NACDS], 2008; www.nacds.org/wmspage.cfm?parm1=6531).
- Of the 3.54 billion scripts dispensed, traditional chain stores had the highest percentage of prescriptions (NACDS, 2008).

In this chapter common OTC medications will be explored as well as geriatric and pediatric considerations in the use of OTC drugs. Common dosage forms will be discussed along with the reasons people buy their own medications. This chapter will give an overall look into the use of OTC medications and the FDA regulations that pertain to them.

Obviously, OTC medications will continue to become available to consumers, and this means that it is increasingly important for consumers to learn about appropriate dosages and proper use of these medications. Although federal law requires that pharmacists counsel patients receiving new prescriptions, OTC medications do not fall into this category, unless a prescription is written for the over-the-counter item. However, when counseling a patient, the pharmacist should ask what OTC medications the patient is taking; then the pharmacist can inform the patient which types of OTC drugs should be avoided. The ability to buy drugs off the shelf can translate into substantial savings for consumers. This is only one of the many reasons why individuals want to buy their own medications. Drug companies know that customers want more drugs available to them. The following three reasons explain why consumers use OTC products:

1. Consumers want to save money, and OTC medications are generally less expensive than prescription drugs. In addition, further cost savings are incurred when physicians' appointments are not needed, which involve the cost of the office visit and missed time at work.
2. Consumers want to be involved in their own treatment; OTC medications give them this capability.
3. OTC medications are more easily obtainable than prescriptions because the many stores that carry OTC medications usually have longer hours than traditional pharmacies.

See Table 8-1 for common brands of over-the-counter medications.

When patients decide to treat themselves by purchasing OTC medications, however, important factors should be taken into account. First, there are a wide variety of drugs from which to choose. Therefore correctly identifying the cause of the symptom or problem is the first step. If the self-diagnosis is wrong, the OTC medication may mask the underlying condition from which the person is suffering. For example, if a person suffers from diarrhea and purchases an antidiarrheal medication, the diarrhea may cease for a short time, but the underlying cause could be something more serious that may need to be diagnosed by a physician. Ultimately, this can cost the person more money, or worse. Many hospital stays have been attributed to patients' misuse of drugs, both OTC and prescription. Most persons have not been trained to scrutinize OTC medications. This includes checking the drugs at home regularly for expiration dates. Another overlooked aspect of buying OTC drugs is tampering, because these drugs are readily accessible. Previously, several persons were the victims of someone who tampered with Tylenol. Since that time, manufacturers have taken steps to assure consumers that their medications are safe by adding tamper-proof wrapping. Consumers should check for any tampering before purchase. Although there is only a slight risk, it is possible for someone to tamper with the product.

Many OTC medications list specific age groups that should avoid the medication. Thus parents should consult with their pediatrician before giving children any OTC medication, especially any child younger than 4 years. In addition to these considerations, children with colds may develop ear infections and other conditions that warrant seeing a pediatrician for an appropriate prescription medication. Below are some important considerations that consumers should address before buying and using OTC medications:

- Various OTC medications have identical ingredients; however, consumers often purchase a more expensive name brand, not realizing that they are obtaining the same medication as the less expensive generic form.
- Manufacturers may swap "like ingredients." The label will show the ingredient change or reformulation. Consumers often overlook this because they do not read labels carefully, if at all. Consequently, consumers may be unaware that they are using a different formulation than they used previously.
- The person who is on a special diet, has allergies, has diabetes, or who is taking other medications that may interact with OTC drugs should use caution in selecting an OTC product.
- One should take extra care when purchasing medication for infants or young children; consumers should know and follow guidelines on the safety of agents based on the child's age. This includes topical agents.
- When trying a new agent, one should watch carefully for any adverse reactions that may occur.
- Many, if not most, OTC and prescription medications cannot be taken if one is pregnant or nursing; persons who are pregnant or breast-feeding should always get professional advice before taking an OTC product.

Three FDA Categories Concerning Classification of Over-the-Counter Drugs

In general, those medicines classified as OTC medications by the FDA have the following characteristics:

- Their benefits outweigh their risks.
- The potential for misuse and abuse is low.

TABLE 8-1 Common Over-the-Counter Brand Preparations

Brand Name	Generic Name	Classification
Fever/Pain Product		
Tylenol	acetaminophen	Antipyretic/analgesic
Fever/Pain/Inflammation Products		
Bayer	aspirin	NSAID,* analgesic
Motrin, Advil	ibuprofen	NSAID, antipyretic/analgesic
Excedrin	aspirin/caffeine/acetaminophen	NSAID (migraines)
Sleep Aid		
Benadryl	diphenhydramine	Histamine blocker, sedative, antihistamine
Cold/Cough Products		
Robitussin	guaifenesin	Expectorant
Benylin	guaifenesin/dextromethorphan	Expectorant/antitussive
Benadryl	diphenhydramine	Antihistamine
Sudafed†	pseudoephedrine	Decongestant
Nasal Products		
Neo-Synephrine	phenylephrine	Decongestant
Privine	naphazoline	Decongestant
Eye (Ophthalmic) Product		
VasoClear	naphazoline	Eye decongestant
Sore Throat Products		
Sucrets	dyclonine	Analgesic
Chloraseptic	benzocaine	Topical anesthetic
Stomach Products		
Pepcid AC	famotidine	H_2-antagonist
Prilosec OTC	omeprazole	Proton pump inhibitor
Zantac 75 or Zantac 150	ranitidine	H_2-antagonist
Tagamet HB	cimetidine	H_2-antagonist
Milk of Magnesia	magnesium hydroxide	Antacid, laxative
Tums	calcium carbonate	Antacid/calcium carbonate supplement
Prevacid 24 hour	lansoprazole	Proton pump inhibitor
Intestinal Products		
Metamucil	psyllium	Fiber
Imodium A-D	loperamide	Antidiarrheal
Anticonstipation Products		
Senokot	senna extract	Laxative
Dulcolax	bisacodyl	Laxative
Miscellaneous Products		
Compound W	salicylic acid	Keratolytic (warts/corns)
Calamine	calamine	Antipruritic
Tinactin	tolnaftate	Antifungal
Lotrimin	clotrimazole	Antifungal
Monistat	miconazole	Antifungal
Anusol-HC	hydrocortisone	Antihemorrhoidal

*NSAID, Nonsteroidal antiinflammatory drug.
†Pseudoephedrine does not require a prescription but it is a behind-the-counter drug.

- Consumers can use them for self-diagnosed conditions.
- They can be adequately labeled for proper use.
- Health practitioners are not needed for the safe and effective use of the product.

Although OTC medications may seem harmless, they can be deadly if taken inappropriately or if the person has an allergic reaction. One may experience additional side effects from OTC medications, such as interactions with prescription medications. Before OTC medications are allowed to enter the market, the Food and Drug Administration (FDA) classifies them during data review according to one of the following three categories. Obviously, only if the proposed medication falls under the first category (category I) would it eventually become available to the consumer.

- Category I: Generally Recognized as Safe and Effective (GRASE) for the claimed therapeutic indication
- Category II: Not GRASE
- Category III: Cannot determine if GRASE; additional data must be acquired to determine whether the drug is safe and effective

Food and Drug Administration Regulations

To determine into what category proposed OTC drugs fall, the FDA regulates five major areas concerning the safety of OTC medications. The following five areas are explored individually:

1. Purity
2. Potency
3. Bioavailability
4. Efficacy
5. Safety and toxicity

PURITY

The purity of a product represents the lack of contamination from environmental factors of the chemical (drug) contained in the product. Any food, drug, or product that contains any avoidable, added, poisonous, or deleterious substance is unsafe and is considered adulterated. Few agents are pure because many medications are prepared on a large scale and dust particles are present in the mix. A certain amount of dust is allowed by government standards. Purity also is affected by other additives, such as those listed in Box 8-1. Various ingredients are used in the preparation of medications to make the appropriate dosage

BOX 8-1 TYPES OF PRODUCT ADDITIVES

Fillers	Enable manufacturers to make tablets or capsules large enough to ingest
Dyes	Used to color tablets and coatings for more aesthetic appearance
Solvents	Mixtures used along with chemical agents as a dissolvent
Buffers	Used to adjust the pH of a medication
Waxes	Used to mold various medications, such as suppositories

BOX 8-2 MEDICATIONS MEASURED IN UNITS (REQUIRES A PRESCRIPTION)

Heparin	25,000 units/mL
Insulin	100 units/mL
Injectable penicillin	100,000 units/mL

forms, to alter drug absorption characteristics, and to make medications taste better.

POTENCY

The potency of a medication refers to the strength of the drug. This measurement is done by chemical analysis and is measured in grams (g), milligrams (mg), micrograms (mcg), or milliequivalents (mEq), as examples. If the drug cannot be measured in a laboratory by such analytical methods, then it is tested on research animals, and the strength of the drug is measured in units based on biological activity. Examples of these medications are shown in Box 8-2.

BIOAVAILABILITY

Bioavailability is the percentage and rate of a drug that is absorbed and transported to the site of action. Because of variances in absorption, the amount of drug that is able to enter the bloodstream can differ. This can be caused by the specific properties of the drug that are the responsibility of the manufacturer. Although the main ingredient may be exactly the same, many times the inert, or inactive, agents in the drug differ. Also the type of dosage form is important; for example, oral medications are low in solubility or have slow absorption properties that also affect the overall bioavailability. This is due to the drug having to pass through the gastrointestinal tract, liver, and intestines. The variance in bioavailability is important in order to provide proper treatment. In addition, the patient's personal medical history, genetics, age, and gender as well as concurrent medications being taken have an effect on bioavailability. The total bioavailability is measured by the concentration of the drug in the blood or tissue at a specific time of administration.

EFFICACY

Efficacy is the ability of the drug to produce the desired effect(s) in the body for the intended use. Clinical trials of the drug, which include the use of a placebo, are conducted to judge the effectiveness. Many variances may affect the end result. These variances may be caused by other influences on a person, such as unknown health conditions, age, weight, lifestyle, gender, and genetics.

SAFETY AND TOXICITY

Safety and toxicity represent opposite effects of the drug being studied. After the drug is administered to test subjects, the number of adverse or undesirable effects is recorded. Laboratory animals often are used as test subjects in the beginning stages of trials, and it is sometimes impossible to know what effects might occur in human beings. In later years of drug studies, published results include the effects of drugs on pregnancy and other outside influences that cannot be replicated in a laboratory. All drugs can be toxic if not taken correctly. The difference between dosages that produce toxic effects and those that produce desirable effects is documented. This difference is referred to as the "margin of safety." If a dose of a drug falls into the margin of safety, it is considered a "therapeutic dose." Even so, before a drug is considered safe, the potential for adverse effects must be compared with the benefits.

There are certain instances when a seemingly subtherapeutic dose may be given to achieve a therapeutic response in an individual patient. Because each person is unique, the side effects or potency may not follow the scientific findings. Although these instances may occur, they are not commonly encountered.

How a Prescription Drug Becomes an Over-the-Counter Drug

There are several entities that may request a prescription drug to be classified as an OTC drug. These include the manufacturer, health care organizations, and consumer groups. The reasons range from financial savings in health care costs for consumers to potential increased profits for manufacturers from more widespread sales. One of the main considerations the FDA must make is whether there is enough information proving the medication is safely taken without a health care provider's prescription and oversight of treatment. Another factor that should be considered is whether the consumer can self-medicate correctly and safely with the drug by following the medication's instructions.

The amount of research that occurs before releasing a new OTC drug is extensive. The FDA must approve all new drugs entering the marketplace and has strict guidelines in place. The same standards of safety and effectiveness that are placed on legend drugs (those requiring a prescription) also are used to approve OTC drugs. The FDA uses three phases of testing as criteria for minimum standards of a new product or of a product that is going to be marketed as an OTC drug, as shown in Box 8-3.

BOX 8-3   FOOD AND DRUG ADMINISTRATION PHASES OF OVER-THE-COUNTER DRUG APPROVAL

Phase 1: Advisors evaluate the agent in question with regard to whether it is safe and effective when taken by the consumer/patient. They also review labeling appropriateness, including dosage instructions, therapeutic indications, and warnings about side effects and misuse of the medication. Upon the decision of the evaluators, the ingredients will be placed into one of the following categories:

- Category I: generally recognized as safe and effective for the claimed therapeutic indication
- Category II: not generally recognized as safe and effective or unacceptable indications
- Category III: insufficient data available to permit final classification

Phase 2: A review is done by the FDA regarding the ingredients and intended use of the product in question. The review includes the class of drug based on panel findings. In addition, the public is able to provide comments and be informed of any new findings that may have resulted since the first evaluation. All of this information is taken into consideration and the agency then publishes their conclusions in the *Federal Register* as a tentative monograph. Once this is completed, there is a designated waiting time in which any objections to the findings should be registered. If there are objections they are presented before a hearing with the Commissioner of the FDA.

Phase 3: The final phase is when the monograph is finally published. The monograph lists conditions in which the OTC drug product is generally recognized as safe and effective.

Drug companies must perform comprehensive studies on the drug's labeling to determine whether consumers can easily and safely take the medication in question. In addition, for those drugs where the dosage is lower than a prescription dose, studies must be conducted to evaluate the effectiveness of the drug at the lower dosage. A monograph is information about a drug that includes descriptive information about clinical trials, all side effects of the agent, appropriate dosing based on symptoms/disease state, and all types of reported interactions. Additional information must be provided for those medications that may be used for children.

If the agent meets all the criteria, it is approved as an OTC medication. If the agent is approved already as a prescription drug and the manufacturer wants it to be offered also as an OTC drug, it does not require further testing. However, the drug does need to be considered safe enough to self-administer before it is marketed as OTC. Many drugs that are sold OTC are also marketed as legend drugs. The difference is often the strength of the drug, and the indications for use. For instance, ibuprofen is available OTC in 200-mg tablets for the relief of fever or mild pain or inflammation; however, if 400, 600, or 800 mg is needed, a prescription (or Rx) is required, as these dosages are often needed for more complicated conditions. See Table 8-2 for a list of common differences between OTC and Rx (prescription) medications.

Although there are approximately 100,000 OTC products on the market today (see fda.gov), only 1000 active ingredients are approved.[1] This list

TABLE 8-2 OTC Versus Rx Medications

Brand	Generic	Strength	FDA Class
Tagamet HB	Cimetidine	200 mg	OTC
	Cimetidine	300, 400, 800 mg	Rx
Pepcid AC	Famotidine	10, 20 mg (max strength)	OTC
	Famotidine	20, 40 mg; other dosage forms and strengths	Rx
Prilosec OTC	Omeprazole	20 mg tab	OTC
Prilosec	Omeprazole	10, 20, 40 mg cap; 2.5 and 10 mg granules for oral suspension	Rx
Motrin IB, Advil, and various manufacturers	Ibuprofen	100, 200 mg tab; 100 mg/5 mL, 100 mg/2.5 mL suspension; 40 mg/mL infant drops	OTC
Motrin and others	Ibuprofen	400, 600, 800 mg tab	Rx
Aleve, Midol Extended Relief	Naproxen sodium	200 mg	OTC
Naprosyn, Naprelan controlled release	Naproxen	250, 375, 500, and 750 mg tab; 125 mg/5 mL suspension	Rx
Anaprox, Anaprox DS	Naproxen sodium	275, 550 mg	Rx
Zantac 75, Zantac 150	Ranitidine	75, 150 mg	OTC
Zantac, Zantac Efferdose	Ranitidine	150, 300 tab; 25 or 150 mg efferdose; 75 mg/5 mL syrup and all other dosage forms and strengths	OTC
Axid AR	Nizatidine	75 mg tab	OTC
Axid	Nizatidine	150, 300 mg tab; 15 mg/mL liquid	Rx
Imodium A-D caplets	Loperamide	2 mg tab; 1 mg/mL, 1 mg/5 mL, 1 mg/7.5 mL liquids	OTC
	Loperamide	2 mg cap	Rx
Dramamine, Calm-X, Triptone	Dimenhydrinate	50 mg tab; 12.5 mg/4 mL and 12.5 mg/5 mL liquid	OTC
Dramamine	Dimenhydrinate	15.62 mg/5 mL liquid	Rx
Antivert	Meclizine	12.5, 25 mg tab	OTC
	Meclizine	50 mg tab, 25 mg cap	Rx

undoubtedly will continue to grow; it gives a sense of how OTC drugs are manufactured and combined to give the customer many more choices of products than ever before.

Conditions Treated with Over-the-Counter Drugs

As stated previously, thousands of OTC medications are available when you consider the brands, generic versions, combinations, various strengths, and dosage forms. Table 8-3 lists some of the most common OTC medications, the symptoms they treat, and the most popular routes of administration. As new medications enter the market as OTC drugs, the routes of administration from which consumers can choose will increase. For example, many analgesics are becoming available as topical patches, and many sore throat remedies are being produced as chewing gum.

ANALGESICS AND ANTIPYRETICS

Analgesic and **antipyretic** agents help reduce or relieve pain (analgesic) and fever (antipyretic). Acetylsalicylic acid, abbreviated ASA and usually known by the more common generic name aspirin, has added effectiveness as an anti-inflammatory agent. Aspirin also decreases the clotting ability of platelets; therefore it also is used as prophylaxis to decrease the risk of blood clotting in heart disease and stroke. Examples are shown in Table 8-4.

TABLE 8-3 Common Types of Over-the-Counter Products*

Type of Drug	Symptom Treated	Route of Administration
Analgesics	Pain	Orally, topically, rectally
Antiinflammatories	Inflammation/arthritis pain	Orally
Antipyretics	Fever	Orally, rectally
Antiarthritics	Joint pain/inflammation	Orally, topically
Antihistamines	Allergies/sneezing	Orally, inhalation
Decongestants	Congestion	Orally
Headache products	Pain	Orally
Sleep aids	Insomnia	Orally
Expectorants	Productive cough	Orally
Cough suppressants	Dry cough	Orally, inhalation
Colds/flu	Inflammation	Orally, inhalation
Sore throat products	Pain	Orally
Sunscreens	Preventive sun barrier	Topically
Sunburn products	Pain/inflammation	Topically
Antacids	Indigestion	Orally
Antidiarrheals	Diarrhea	Orally, rectally
Laxatives	Constipation	Orally, rectally
Antiacne products	Pimples	Topically
Antibiotics	Prevent infections	Topically
Antifungals	Dry, flaking skin and pain caused by fungus	Topically
Cold sore preparations	Painful canker sores	Topically
Wart removal products	Skin growth	Topically

*Other topical over-the-counter products are listed later in this chapter under skin care products.

TABLE 8-4 Analgesics and Antipyretic Products

Condition	Product	Dosage Forms*
Fever/pain	Acetaminophen (Tylenol)	Tab, cap, liq
Fever/pain	Aspirin (Bayer, Alka-Seltzer)	Tab, cap, powder
Fever/pain	Ibuprofen (Motrin)	Tab, cap, liq
Pain/arthritis	Capsaicin (Zostrix)	Top

*cap, Capsule; liq, liquid; supp, suppository; tab, tablet; top, topical.

Tech Note!

Reye's syndrome is a rare condition that can affect children and teenagers who have an active case of certain viral illnesses, such as chickenpox or influenza, and consume aspirin products. The symptoms include vomiting, lethargy, delirium, and coma. Permanent brain damage can occur, and the infection can be fatal. Although the percentage of fatalities is less than 20%, it is safer to prevent the possibility of such adverse effects by avoiding the use of aspirin in such patients.

Tech Note!

Activated charcoal can be used to treat an overdose of aspirin or acetaminophen. It decreases the absorption of these drugs when given quickly after overdose. Because overdose of aspirin or acetaminophen can be life-threatening, patients should immediately seek emergency help (call 911 or go to the emergency department) and should not self-treat an overdose.

Common Patient Information

Children and teenagers should avoid taking aspirin for chickenpox or flu symptoms without consulting a physician because aspirin has been associated with Reye's syndrome.

Interactions between Aspirin and Other Agents. Aspirin has many interactions that are important to note because they can result in adverse effects for the patient. Table 8-5 provides a list of common interactions between various types of medications and aspirin. Interactions are not necessarily dangerous, but they can alter the effects of one of the two agents being taken concurrently. Many times, patients do not familiarize themselves with these types of interactions, which is why patient consultation is important. If a patient ever asks for advice from a technician or clerk, he or she must be referred to the pharmacist. Technicians must know these interactions so that they can alert the pharmacist if they notice a possible interaction with the patient's prescriptions or medication orders.

TABLE 8-5 Examples of Common and Important Interactions between Aspirin and Other Medications

Drug	Common Use of Drugs	Results of Drug-Aspirin Interactions
Alcohol	Lifestyle choice: how often and how much is ingested	May increase bleeding and risk of gastrointestinal ulcer
Anticoagulants	To reduce possibility of blood clots	May prolong or increase bleeding
Carbonic anhydrase inhibitors (diuretics)	To decrease edema (fluid buildup)	Aspirin toxicity may occur
Methotrexate	To treat certain skin conditions/cancer	Methotrexate effects may be increased and excretion decreased
NSAIDs*	To treat inflammation, pain, fever	Antiplatelet effects of aspirin may be decreased; may increase gastric side effects
Sulfonylureas/insulin	To lower glucose level (diabetes)	Aspirin may further lower blood glucose level
Valproic acid	To treat seizures	Displaces valproic acid from binding sites in blood, increasing potency of valproic acid

*NSAID, Nonsteroidal antiinflammatory drug.

TABLE 8-6 Headache Products

Condition	Product	Dosage Forms
Headache/ migraine	Aspirin/caffeine/acetaminophen combination (Excedrin)	Tablet
	Aspirin/calcium carbonate combination (Bayer Women's Aspirin Plus Calcium)	Caplet
	Acetaminophen/caffeine combination (Excedrin Tension Headache [aspirin free])	Caplet

TABLE 8-7 Antiinflammatory Products

Condition	Product	Dosage Forms*
Inflammation/pain	Ibuprofen (Motrin, Advil)	Tab, susp, infant drops
	Naproxen sodium (Aleve)	Tab
	Ketoprofen (Orudis KT)	Tab, cap

*cap, Capsule; susp, suspension; tab, tablet.

Headache Products. Depending on the severity of a headache, one can try many of the OTC medications. Those agents listed under analgesics are used mostly for pain. Some agents contain other additives, such as caffeine, that can help treat more severe headaches (Table 8-6). However, if a person suffers regularly from headaches such as migraines, a prescription drug is usually required.

ANTIINFLAMMATORIES

OTC agents that treat inflammation are referred to as nonsteroidal **antiinflammatory** drugs (NSAIDs). They reduce pain by decreasing inflammation of soft tissue (e.g., muscle strain). Nonsteroidal antiinflammatory drugs also are used as antipyretic and analgesics, as seen in Table 8-7.

Common Patient Information
Do not take this medication if you are allergic to aspirin. Antiinflammatory drugs may cause drowsiness and may upset the stomach. Take them with food or milk. Do not take these medications if you are in the last trimester of pregnancy.

ALLERGY AND COLD AGENTS

Decongestants (Table 8-8) and antihistamines (Table 8-9) are available for the relief of the symptoms of the common cold and allergies. These agents promote drying of mucous membranes and opening of airways. Allergies require antihistamine agents.

Decongestants
Decongestants are indicated for stuffiness and congestion of the nasal passages and sinuses. Because they cause vasoconstriction, decongestants act to open these passages and allow the release of mucus, thus reducing congestion. Decongestants used for chest congestion permit the coughing up (expectoration) of phlegm. Decongestants used topically through nasal application have limited

Tech Note!

Decongestants can interact with antidepressants. Patients using certain antidepressants and those with heart conditions should not use decongestant agents without the knowledge and approval of their physician.

TABLE 8-8 Decongestant Products

Condition	Product	Dosage Forms*
Common cold/ allergies	Oxymetazoline (Afrin)	Nasal spray
	Phenylephrine (Neo-Synephrine)	Nasal spray
	Normal saline (Ocean)	Nasal spray
Common cold	Pseudoephedrine† (Sudafed)	Tab, cap, liq
	Clemastine (Tavist)	Tab, liq

*cap, Capsule; liq, liquid; tab, tablet.
†Pseudoephedrine (Sudafed) is a decongestant and is less likely to cause drowsiness. Pseudoephedrine is used exclusively as a decongestant, not for allergies.

TABLE 8-9 Oral Antihistamine Products*

Condition	Product	Dosage Forms†
Rhinitis, common cold	Chlorpheniramine (Chlor-Trimeton)	Tab, cap
Rhinitis, pruritus	Diphenhydramine (Benadryl)	Tab, cap, liq
Allergic rhinitis	Loratadine (Claritin)	Tab, gel cap, chewable tablet, liq

*These agents also are available in many combinations with agents that treat cough, fever, and pain.
†cap, Capsule; liq, liquid; tab, tablet.

absorption, but good activity to open nasal passages. Decongestants are available in prescription and OTC preparations.

Common Patient Information. Decongestants may cause high blood pressure, headaches, and insomnia. They should not be taken concurrently with a monoamine oxidase inhibitor (MAOI) antidepressant agent.

Antihistamines

Antihistamines are used when the patient exhibits allergic symptoms, including pruritus (itching), hives, sneezing, and runny eyes. Their action is to block histamine (H_1-receptors), which causes allergic reactions. Many different types of these agents are available OTC. First-generation agents include diphenhydramine (Benadryl) and chlorpheniramine (Chlor-Trimeton). Cetirizine (Zyrtec) is considered a low-sedating antihistamine because it causes slightly less drowsiness than older generation agents. Loratadine (Claritin) is available as well and does not typically cause drowsiness. Persons suffering from severe allergies may require prescription medications. For mild allergies, the antihistamines available are normally effective.

Common Patient Information. Certain antihistamines may cause drowsiness. Because these agents act on the central nervous system, alcohol will intensify the effects of drowsiness and should be avoided.

SLEEP AIDS

Many persons suffer from insomnia. Almost all OTC medications used to treat insomnia are a form of diphenhydramine; some products also contain acetaminophen or magnesium salicylate to assist with nighttime pain relief (Table 8-10). These agents can be used for transient insomnia, which is considered a short-term sleeping problem (non-chronic).

TABLE 8-10 Antiinsomnia Products

Product	Dosage Forms*
Diphenhydramine (Benadryl)	Tab, caplet, liq
Diphenhydramine citrate/acetaminophen (Excedrin PM)	Tab, caplet
Doxylamine succinate (Unisom Nighttime Sleep Aid)	Tab

*liq, Liquid; tab, tablet.

TABLE 8-11 Cold and Cough Products

Condition	Product	Dosage Forms*
Congested cough	Guaifenesin/pseudoephedrine (Robitussin PE)	Tab, liq, syr
	Guaifenesin (Robitussin)	Tab, cap, syr
Dry cough	Guaifenesin/dextromethorphan (Robitussin DM)	Liq, syr

*cap, Capsule; liq, liquid; syr, syrup; tab, tablet.

TABLE 8-12 Sore Throat Products

Condition	Product	Dosage Forms
Sore throat	Benzocaine (Chloraseptic)	Lozenges, spray
	Dyclonine (no brand)	Lozenges
	Benzocaine (Cepacol)	Lozenges

Common Patient Information
Sleep aids may cause drowsiness. Avoid alcoholic beverages while taking these medications. If you are taking sedatives or tranquilizers, do not take sleep aids without consulting a physician. Do not use these products if you have asthma, glaucoma, emphysema, or an enlarged prostate. For chronic insomnia, consult a physician.

COUGH MEDICINES

The cold and flu section of the pharmacy is one of the largest; many manufacturers offer the same type of ingredients in different proportions (Table 8-11). For congested coughs, **expectorants** can help expectorate phlegm. For dry, non–phlegm-producing coughs, an **antitussive** agent is commonly used to reduce the coughing.

Common Patient Information
If you are taking sedatives or tranquilizers, do not take cough medicines without consulting a physician.

SORE THROAT PRODUCTS

Sore, scratchy, and dry throats usually arise from a cold or flu. They can be treated with many different agents available as OTC medications (Table 8-12). If a sore throat continues without relief for more than 2 days, one should see a physician to rule out an infection. A sore throat can be a symptom of a streptococcal bacterial infection, also known as strep throat. Strep throat should be treated with antibiotics. However, while the patient is taking antibiotics, he or

TABLE 8-13 Stomach Products/Antacids

Condition	Product	Dosage Forms*
Heartburn	Cimetidine (Tagamet HB)	Tab, liq
	Ranitidine (Zantac 75)	Tab
	Famotidine (Pepcid AC)	Tab
	Nizatidine (Axid AR)	Tab
	Omeprazole (Prilosec OTC)	Tab
Antacids	Calcium carbonate (Tums)	Chewable tab
	Aluminum hydroxide/magnesium hydroxide/ simethicone (Mylanta)	Tab, liq, gel cap

*liq, Liquid; *tab*, tablet.

Tech Note!

Chronic pain in the stomach or chronic heartburn symptoms may be an ulcer caused by *Helicobacter pylori,* which is a bacterium that can cause the symptoms of heartburn. If the problem persists for more than 2 weeks, it is better to seek advice for a possible underlying problem.

Tech Note!

Gas can be painful and embarrassing but is not life-threatening; simethicone can provide over-the-counter relief. Diarrhea and constipation can have severe outcomes if they are not controlled. For example, infants can die of dehydration because of excess loss of electrolytes through watery stools. In extreme cases, constipation can cause rupture of the bowel, which requires surgery to repair; however, such occurrences are very rare. Psyllium is the only agent that can be used for helping both constipation or diarrhea because it works as a bulk-forming agent. Psyllium has been noted to moderately reduce levels of bad cholesterol.

she also may relieve throat pain with various syrups and sprays. The components typically used in these products include menthol, alcohol, and topical anesthetics, such as benzocaine.

Common Patient Information
Do not exceed recommended dosages.

STOMACH REMEDIES/ANTACIDS

Several classes of OTC medications are used to treat the common upset stomach (Table 8-13). Histamine$_2$-antagonists (H$_2$-antagonists) are used to reduce acid secretion, which helps to decrease what is commonly known as heartburn or acid reflux. Proton pump inhibitors work differently than H$_2$-antagonists to relieve acid secretions. Although both work directly on the lining of the stomach, they each target different receptors. Antacid agents are used to balance the pH level in the stomach, which ultimately helps decrease heartburn. Each medication is effective in its own way.

Common Patient Information
Antacids are for short-term relief of heartburn. If problems persist, see your physician. Antacids may be taken without regard to meals. Occasional side effects can include constipation, diarrhea, and stomach cramps. Drug-drug interactions are more likely when taking antacids. For example, calcium antacid products may decrease the absorption and effectiveness of certain antibiotics, such as tetracyclines or quinolone class agents, or of levothyroxine (a thyroid hormone). Antacids can interfere with the absorption of certain medicines that require an acidic pH of the stomach for proper absorption, such as oral antifungal drugs and certain medicines for the treatment of human immunodeficiency virus (HIV) infection.

INTESTINAL REMEDIES

Remedies for intestinal discomfort and pain resulting from constipation, diarrhea, or gas (flatulence) are listed in Table 8-14. Laxatives and stool softeners are commonly purchased to ease bowel movements. For diarrhea, anticholinergic agents are effective because they dry mucous membranes; a **bulk-forming** fiber such as psyllium powder absorbs excess water, creating bulk in the intestinal tract. Loperamide works well for immediate results, but should not be taken in certain circumstances. Psyllium (Metamucil) is a good natural choice that many

TABLE 8-14 **Intestinal Products**

Condition	Product	Dosage Forms*
Constipation	Combination stimulant (Ex-Lax)	Tab, chew tab
Stool softener	Docusate sodium (Colace)	Gel cap, liq
Diarrhea	Loperamide (Imodium A-D)	Tab, cap, liq
Flatulence	Simethicone (Mylicon, Gas-X)	Tab, chew tab, liq
Irregular bowels	Psyllium (Metamucil)	Powder for suspension

*cap, Capsule or caplet; liq, liquid; tab, tablet.

TABLE 8-15 **Over-The-Counter Skin Products**

Dosage Forms*	Indications
Creams	Dry, scaling, pruritic areas; thickened areas; infections
Ointment	Dry, scaling, pruritic areas; thickened areas; infections
Lotions/gels	Hairy areas, lesions that ooze, wet areas; infections
Sprays	Acute weeping lesions; infections

*Creams, lotions, and gels are absorbed through the skin; ointments and sprays remain on top of the skin to prevent moisture from evaporating.

physicians recommend, because the fiber adds bulk to the stool, making it less watery. For the treatment of gas, simethicone (Gas-X) is the most commonly used agent. Beano, which contains the enzyme alpha-galactosidase, is ingested along with foods that contain gas-producing carbohydrates. Beano neutralizes the production of gas, which is created as a by-product from bacteria that reside in the intestines as foods are digested.

Common Patient Information
Do not use laxatives in the presence of abdominal pain, nausea, or vomiting. Do not use laxatives longer than 1 week. Loperamide may cause drowsiness or dizziness and may cause dry mouth.

SKIN REMEDIES

There are several OTC agents that are available to treat a variety of skin conditions (Table 8-15). Minor cuts and scrapes can be treated by topical agents that work as an antiinfective, such as Neosporin. Acne, common among teenagers, is treated primarily by benzoyl peroxide to dehydrate pimples. Hives can occur as an allergic reaction and are treated by antihistamines or by topical hydrocortisone. Athlete's foot or jock itch is a fungal condition that can be treated by several types of nonprescription topical antifungals in a variety of dosage forms. A viral infection causing common warts can be treated effectively with salicylic acid and other topical agents. A list of commonly found remedies is in Table 8-16.

Geriatric and Pediatric Considerations

As the population ages and lives longer, the number of older people buying OTC medications increases. Compared to legend drugs, there are more OTC drugs available in different dosage forms, strengths, and combinations. The choices are staggering and the health risk is high. As people age their metabolism changes. In general, the speed of drug clearance slows and the risk of drug-drug

TABLE 8-16 Common Agents Used to Treat a Variety of Conditions

Skin Condition	OTC Product	Trade Name	Dosage Form
Cuts/scrapes	Bacitracin	Bacitracin	Ointment
	Neomycin	Neomycin	Ointment
	Polymyxin B sulfate, neomycin, bacitracin	Neosporin	Ointment, cream
Acne	Benzoyl peroxide	Clearasil Max Strength	Cream
		Oxy 10 cover	Cream
		Oxy 5	Lotion
		Clean & Clear	Lotion
Hives, inflammation	Diphenhydramine	Benadryl	Lotion, cream
	Hydrocortisone		Cream, ointment
Athlete's foot	Miconazole	Lotrimin AF, Zeasorb-AF	Powder
	Tolnaftate	Tinactin	Liquid, powder, aerosol, cream
	Terbinafine	Lamisil	Cream, topical solution
Warts	Salicylic acid	Freezone	Liquid
		Compound W	Gel, liquid
		Wart-Off	Solution

interactions increases because many elderly take prescription drugs on a daily basis for conditions related to age and illness. Many senior citizens buy their medications OTC because of a lack of insurance benefits and may choose the wrong medication; many times an appropriate medication is not available in OTC form. Table 8-17 lists general changes in the body as we age and the effect of those changes on drug response.

Infants and children are at risk for receiving an inappropriate medication, the wrong dose, or the wrong drug product for their age. Older labeling on OTC products stated that children under the age of 2 years should not receive the product without the consent of a physician. Most products are dosed based on the age and weight of the child. However, since a parent does not need a prescription to obtain these medications, they have been used in excess many times. Many parents have difficulty measuring the proper dose of medicine for their child. Others may misuse the product. For example, diphenhydramine, a well-known antihistamine, is often given inappropriately to help children sleep rather than for its intended purpose. New labeling states no child under the age of 4 years may be given this medication and that the drug must be dosed by a physician if the child is between 4 and 6 years of age. Although some medications still can be given to children older than age 2, there are new restrictions being imposed. Parents should read all of the labeling information carefully before purchasing OTC drugs, and make sure they understand the directions for use. It is especially important not to choose products with the same active ingredients, as inadvertent drug overdose may occur if the child receives the drug from multiple sources. Consulting with the pharmacist or the physician is very important so that any drug-drug or drug-food interactions can be detected. Also, preexisting conditions may have a profound effect on the metabolism of a drug. A child is still growing and changing through adolescence. Medication should always be dosed not only according to age but also according to the weight of the child.

TABLE 8-17 Effects Drugs Have on an Aging Body

	What Changes	Effects	What to Do
Weight	As people age body fat increases	This affects amount of medication you can take and how long it takes to metabolize.	Consult your physician before taking any OTC medications and ask what strength and dosing you should take.
Lifestyle	Alcohol intake	Alcohol and certain OTCs can cause adverse effects.	Just as legend drugs have interactions with alcohol, so do OTCs. Consult your physician to see if it is okay to take a specific OTC drug.
Memory	Memory decreases	Forgetting to avoid certain OTCs or not taking them as prescribed can lead to overdosing or drug interactions.	There are cards you can keep in your wallet listing all your medications, time of dosing, strength, etc. There are a wide variety of pill dispensers available that are marked with day of the week as a reminder.
Existing medications	Many OTCs can counteract effectiveness of your prescription drugs or may contain same ingredients as other OTCs you are taking	OTCs can increase or decrease potency of your normal medications.	Make sure you have provided pharmacy a list of all OTCs, including herbals, vitamins, and minerals. Have pharmacy assess for possible drug-drug or drug-food interactions before purchasing OTCs.
Health history	Certain OTCs should not be taken with preexisting conditions	May worsen health or counteract medications taken to manage care.	Make sure your physician or pharmacist knows your allergies and preexisting conditions so correct OTC can be recommended.

Behind-the-Counter Drugs

There are several countries that have a third class of drugs that are referred to as **behind-the-counter** (BTC). Both Canada and England allow consumers to purchase certain medications without a prescription, but under the care of a pharmacist. The drugs are considered safe enough to use without the prescriber's supervision. In Canada since 1995 pharmacies have sold various medications such as Polysporin eye/ear drops, EpiPen, and even Tylenol with Codeine #1 with only the counseling of a pharmacist. In the United States, the FDA is faced with the conflict of having BTC drugs as a third category, in addition to OTC and legend drug categories. The American Medical Association (AMA) is opposed to BTC agents, claiming patients need the diagnosis and care of a trained physician. On the other hand, many consumer groups and drug manufacturers are supportive of this new category. Drug companies have attempted to lobby for the BTC drug category in the past but it has been declined by the FDA. One concern is who will be responsible for reimbursement of the pharmacist's consultation time. Currently unless the medication is a prescription, the pharmacy cannot bill for dispensing fees. Therefore at this time the United States does not have a third category, although the debate continues and many entities believe there will be a BTC category at some point in time.

TABLE 8-18 Current BTC Medications

Brand	Generic	Conditions
Sudafed	Pseudoephedrine	Log book containing purchaser's name, address, identification, and signature; date and time of sale; name and quantity of product sold Limited amount may be purchased in 1 day and 1 month
Various brands of cold medicines	Ephedrine	Same as above
Plan B	Levonorgestrel (a progestin)	Person must be older than 18 in most states

There are certain drugs that are kept behind-the-counter here in the United States. Although they are referred to as BTC drugs, the drugs do not belong to an official "class" of drugs under the FDA. In 1998, an emergency contraceptive, Preven, was able to be purchased without a prescription (Preven is now off-market); then in 1999 Plan B, another emergency contraceptive, was approved by the FDA for BTC status. Under the DEA's 2005 Combat Methamphetamine Epidemic Act (Chapter 2), any products containing pseudoephedrine and ephedrine must be kept behind the pharmacy counter. There are strict provisions for the sale of the types of agents listed in Table 8-18.

DO YOU REMEMBER THESE KEY POINTS?

- The responsibility of the patient to know the type of OTC product that he or she is taking
- The problems associated with more drugs becoming categorized OTC
- Guidelines regulated by the FDA for a legend drug to become an OTC product
- Guidelines regulated by the FDA for the manufacturing practices of OTC products
- Terms and definitions associated with OTC products
- Reasons consumers desire to diagnose and treat themselves
- The difference between generic and trade name drugs
- The three categories of OTC products
- The main interactions between aspirin products and other medications

REVIEW QUESTIONS

Multiple choice questions

1. All of the medications listed are H_2-antagonists EXCEPT:
   A. Cimetidine (Tagamet)
   B. Famotidine (Pepcid)
   C. Loperamide (Imodium)
   D. Ranitidine (Zantac)

2. Which of the following is NOT regulated by the Food and Drug Administration?
   A. Purity
   B. Bioavailability
   C. Color and texture
   D. Potency

3. Children under the age of _____ do NOT have recommended dosages listed on over-the-counter products.
   A. 1 year
   B. 2 years
   C. 4 years
   D. 5 years

4. Fillers are used to:
   A. Make the drug taste better
   B. Change the pH
   C. Change the shape
   D. Make the tablet larger

5. The best definition for the word *efficacy* is:
   A. The ethical use of drugs
   B. The ability of a drug to produce the desired chemical change in a person
   C. The laboratory-testing phase of a drug to determine its effectiveness
   D. The results seen in a person's illness

6. Two major over-the-counter agents for use as nasal decongestants are:
   A. Oxymetazoline and acetaminophen
   B. Oxymetazoline and phenylephrine
   C. Phenylephrine and dyclonine
   D. Dyclonine and pseudoephedrine

7. New restrictions prohibit use of nonprescription diphenhydramine under the age of:
   A. 1 year
   B. 2 years
   C. 4 years
   D. 6 years

8. Which of the following drugs cannot be used as an antiinflammatory?
   A. Aspirin
   B. Ibuprofen (Advil)
   C. Acetaminophen (Tylenol)
   D. Naproxen sodium (Anaprox)

9. The over-the-counter product most commonly used as an antihistamine is:
   A. Aspirin
   B. Ibuprofen
   C. Diphenhydramine
   D. Chlorpheniramine

10. The following consideration(s) must be given with respect to children:
    A. Metabolism
    B. Child's weight
    C. Child's age
    D. All of the above

11. Senior citizens may encounter the following problems:
    A. Preexisting conditions and current illnesses
    B. Changing metabolism and current medications
    C. Lifestyle and mental state changes
    D. All of the above

12. OTC agents such as Tums and Milk of Magnesia can decrease the effectiveness of:
    A. Quinolones
    B. Tetracyclines
    C. Vitamins
    D. Both A and B

13. OTC ibuprofen is used for:
  A. Fever
  B. Inflammation
  C. Pain
  D. All of the above

14. What is the main ingredient in expectorant OTC medications?
  A. Guaifenesin
  B. Diphenhydramine
  C. Naphazoline
  D. None of the above

True/False

If a statement is false, then change it to make it true.

_____ **1.** Drug manufacturers can swap or replace "like ingredients" without specifically notifying the public.

_____ **2.** Analgesic OTCs are available in oral, rectal, and topical dosage forms.

_____ **3.** All antibiotics are by prescription only.

_____ **4.** Aspirin should not be taken with NSAIDs.

_____ **5.** Antipyretics lower fever.

_____ **6.** Analgesics reduce swelling.

_____ **7.** Cold sores and warts are treated with the same medication.

_____ **8.** OTC laxatives should not be used more than 3 weeks.

_____ **9.** Metamucil controls diarrhea and lowers levels of bad cholesterol.

_____ **10.** The most used over-the-counter agent for acne is tetracycline.

_____ **11.** All OTCs should be listed along with current prescription medications in the pharmacy database.

_____ **12.** All OTC medications for children contain instructions for usage based on both age and weight.

_____ **13.** Diphenhydramine is a medication intended to induce sleep in children.

_____ **14.** The consumption of alcohol is safe in OTC medications, unlike prescription drugs.

_____ **15.** Aspirin should not be given to children because of the possibility of Reye's syndrome.

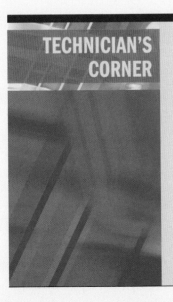

TECHNICIAN'S CORNER

1. A patient comes into the pharmacy asking for a drug that is sold over-the-counter but can only remember the name of the ingredient—benzoyl.
   How do you answer this question?
   Where is this product found?

2. A woman arrives at the pharmacy with a toddler. She asks what type of stool softener to use for her constipated and cranky baby.
   How do you answer this question?
   What will you tell the woman?

3. A patient approaches the pharmacy counter carrying two bottles of cough syrup, guaifenesin/pseudoephedrine (Robitussin PE) and guaifenesin/dextromethorphan (Robitussin DM). She wants to know the difference between them.
   How do you answer this question?
   At what point would you ask the pharmacist for help?

REFERENCE

1. Sorial S: *California society of health-system pharmacists seminar*, Oct 22, 2005.

BIBLIOGRAPHY

Barkauskas Violet, et al: *Health & physical assessment*, ed 3, St Louis, 2002, Mosby.
Drug facts and comparisons, ed 63, St Louis, 2010, Lippincott Williams & Wilkins.
Gerdin Judith: *Health careers today*, ed 4, St Louis, 2010, Elsevier.

WEBSITES

American Association of Retired Persons: Using meds wisely: over-the-counter drug fact labels. Retrieved 8/2009, from www.aarp.org/health/usingmeds/health/usingmeds//l

Consumer Healthcare Products Association. OTC facts and figures. Retrieved 8/2009, from www.chpa-info.org/ChpaPortal/ForConsumers/Drug_Facts_Label/

Consumers Health Education Center: OTC fast facts. Retrieved 8/2009, from www.OTCsafety.org

Kids' Cold Medicines: New Guidelines. WebMD.2009 www.chpa-info.org/pressroom/OTC_FactsFigures.aspx
www.webmd.com/cold-and-flu/cold-guide/kids-cold-medicines-new-guidelines

OTC Facts and Figures. 9/2009. www.chpa-info.org/pressroom/OTC_FactsFigures.aspx

Small Business Assistance: Frequently Asked Questions on the Regulatory Process of Over-the-Counter (OTC) Drugs. FDA 2009. www.fda.gov/Drugs/DevelopmentApprovalProcess/SmallBusinessAssistance/ucm069917.htm

WEBSITES

www.bemedwise.org
www.aarp.org
www.chpa-info.org
www.heall.com
www.medic8.com/healthguide/search.htm

Complementary and Alternative Medicine

Objectives

UPON COMPLETING THIS CHAPTER, YOU SHOULD BE ABLE TO DO THE FOLLOWING:

- Define the term alternative medicine.

- Differentiate between Eastern and Western medicine.

- Describe why alternative medicine has become popular.

- Discuss the goals and treatments discussed by the National Center for Complementary and Alternative Medicine (NCCAM).

- Discuss the goals and treatments discussed by the BioTherapeutics, Education & Research (BTER) Foundation.

- Explain what is meant by the placebo effect.

- Describe the following treatments and the belief systems of each:
  Acupressure/acupuncture
  Ancient Chinese medicine
  Aromatherapy
  Art therapy
  Ayurveda
  Biofeedback
  Chiropractic manipulation
  Crystal healing
  Herbal remedies
  Homeopathy
  Spiritual healing

- Identify common herbal preparations and describe their typical uses.

- Describe the use of maggots in wound care.

- Describe the use of leeches in medical therapy.

Antiemetic *Agent that stops nausea and vomiting*

Antihypertensive *Agent that decreases blood pressure*

Ayurveda *A holistic traditional medical system originating in India; in the system the prevention of disease is emphasized*

Chiropractic *Manual manipulation of the joints and muscles*

Diagnosis *A physician's recognition of a condition or disease based on its outward signs and symptoms and/or confirming tests or procedures*

Herb *Any nonwoody (herbaceous) plant that is valued for its aromatic, medicinal, flavorful, or other properties*

Homeopathy *A system of therapy based on the belief that dilutions of medicinal substances that cause a specific symptom can be used to treat an illness that yields the same symptoms; homeopathic remedies are regulated by the FDA under the Food, Drug, and Cosmetic Act.*

Placebo *Inert compound believed by the patient to be an active agent*

Prophylaxis *To prevent disease*

Synthetic medicine *Medication made in a laboratory from chemical processes*

AGENTS COVERED IN THIS CHAPTER

Common Name	Species	Common Name	Species
Aloe vera	*Aloe vera* (family Liliaceae)	Ginseng	*Panax quinquefolius*
Black cohosh	*Cimicifuga racemosa*	Goldenseal	*Hydrastis canadensis*
Chamomile	*Matricaria recutita*	Hawthorn	*Crataegus laevigata*
Feverfew	*Tanacetum parthenium*	Milk thistle	*Silybum marianum*
Garlic	*Allium sativum*	Purple coneflower	*Echinacea purpurea*
Ginger	*Zingiber officinale*	St. John's wort	*Hypericum perforatum*
Ginkgo	*Ginkgo biloba*	Valerian	*Valeriana officinalis*

Introduction

This chapter covers the current views on complementary and alternative medicine (CAM) in the United States, including the origins of various nontraditional therapies from Eastern and Western cultures. This chapter also explores the reasons why nontraditional therapies have become popular and how they are being integrated into traditional medicine. An in-depth review of herbal remedies is presented using examples of top-selling herbs such as ginkgo, feverfew, and ginseng. Common uses and known interactions of these herbs are explained. In addition, the placebo effect is discussed.

Physicians are prescribing herbal medications for conditions such as sleeplessness and forgetfulness. It is common practice for physicians and pharmacists to ask patients what herbal medications they are taking in order to determine any drug-drug interactions that may occur with traditional medications. Although some of the treatments outlined in this chapter are not necessarily effective or appropriate, nevertheless they are here to stay. Therefore it is important that technicians have a working knowledge of these types of alternative treatments. This chapter outlines considerations concerning traditional medicine and its herbal counterparts. The 12 most popular alternative treatments are discussed.

What Is Alternative Medicine?

To determine the meaning and scope of alternative medicine, one first must define traditional medicine. Traditional medical treatment includes medication prescribed by physicians, consisting of common agents or treatments for medical conditions. This includes physician visits, possibly followed by radiographic examinations, laboratory tests, or other tests to enable the physician to make a correct **diagnosis**. Traditional medicine involves the use of legend (prescription) and over-the-counter (OTC) medications. Follow-up visits ensure the success of the treatment and regular visits monitor the patient's condition.

The alternative approach might consist of visits to a **chiropractor**, **homeopathic** physician, or other practitioner, followed by treatments used within those specific areas of study. These treatments might include herbs, acupuncture, acupressure, or yoga. Many alternative approaches have been in existence for thousands of years, whereas traditional medicine has existed for only a few hundred years. Nevertheless, traditional medicine is the standard for the Western world today.

Alternative medicine has been viewed as ineffective, ancient, and more closely related to superstition than "real" medicine. Many alternative treatments were considered as extreme measures taken only by those who have lost all hope of recovery using traditional methods. The more controversial types of nontraditional medicine and therapies became labeled "alternative medicine" and were grouped with ancient remedies such as ayurveda and Chinese medicine. Other controversial therapies include treatments such as hydrotherapy and crystal, spiritual, and magnetic healing. However, alternative medicine now is making a comeback. Why? This chapter answers this question and explains the considerations one must give to both traditional medicine and complementary and alternative medicine.

Overview of Eastern versus Western Medicine

Eastern medicine includes treatments originating from eastern Asia, India, Japan, and other Far East and Middle East countries. Over the centuries, advancements made from each of these cultures have helped lay the foundation for Western medicine. As medicinal knowledge was gathered over the ages, it was transcribed and translated into other languages and was subjected to further experimentation. European scientists added their own herbal remedies to the growing list of herbal treatments made from varieties of plants indigenous to their terrain.

With the invention of the first microscopes in the late 1500s through the 1600s, scientists had new pathways of exploration during the golden age of microbiology (see Chapter 30). Illnesses that were once believed to be caused by evil spirits now were identified as microbial diseases. As science advanced through the age of antimicrobial therapy in the twentieth century, it was possible to produce medicines that could effect a predetermined specific action within the body. The term "magic bullet" identifies specific medications that target only specific organs or cells within the body, and that would provide a perfect cure for a disease without risk of side effects. The quest for such treatments is the cornerstone of Western medicine today and will continue to be in the future. One must not forget that Western medicine has been influenced by thousands of years of experimentation gathered from many different cultures.

Western medicine has omitted all cultural superstition and has relied on scientific methods to prove effective treatments. Yet some of the most powerful drugs have originated from ancient herbal remedies or are derived from the plants used in those remedies. For example, many cardiac glycosides from various plant extracts have been used in ancient cultures worldwide for various purposes, including digitalis (foxglove), first mentioned in the writings of Welsh physicians in the thirteenth century. Today digoxin is one of the most prescribed heart medications in the geriatric community. Digoxin is derived from the *Digitalis* species and cannot be manufactured synthetically. Digoxin helps the heart beat in slow yet strong beats and is used to treat many persons who have congestive heart failure. Plant derivatives used in Western medicine include quinine for malaria, psyllium for high cholesterol and bowel regularity, and reserpine for high blood pressure. Homeopathy (discussed later in this chapter) was practiced first in the late 1700s when diseases were treated with dilutions of herbal medications that caused symptoms of the same illness when given to healthy persons. Homeopathy is based on "like treating like" in disease versus medication.

Trends toward Alternatives

For thousands of years, practitioners of Eastern philosophy considered the whole person when making a proper diagnosis and plan of treatment. This holistic approach included the person's diet, dreams, and even smell. According to the World Health Organization, alternative medicine now is estimated to be used by more than 70% of the world's population. Most of the countries that use alternative medicine are developing countries. These cultures use herbs as their main form of treatment because they cannot afford or obtain traditional medicine. There is also a strong belief system in place that continues from generation to generation.

Starting in the 1980s, Eastern medicine, specifically herbal remedies, became popular in the Western world. Because herbs are not considered a form of traditional medical treatment, they became grouped with all types of nontraditional remedies that were considered ineffective, including crystals and aromatherapy, hydrotherapy, and sound therapy. However, during the past 2 decades, many of these nontraditional methods of treatment have become commonplace in the Western world. Consumers spend millions of dollars annually on alternative treatments. Until recently, most traditional practitioners have discounted all types of nontraditional or alternative medicine. However, if there is no basis of truth to any of these alternative medicines, then why is the interest in CAM increasing in the United States?

Because of current lifestyles, stresses, and emerging diseases, persons are becoming aware that traditional medicine has its limitations. As one ages, one's body experiences more age-related problems, such as diabetes, dementia, and strokes. As new medicines are produced by drug manufacturers, the risk of side effects and the rising cost of drugs can prompt a person to try alternative medicine. Also, many manufacturers of herbal remedies and other therapies claim their products can increase a person's life span with good health. This claim is sometimes enough for consumers to try these therapies. Another reason alternatives to traditional medicine are becoming more popular is that many times they claim to treat extreme illnesses. A person diagnosed with a cancer for which there is no current medication or therapy available may seek alternatives as a last resort for treatment.

Organizations Related to Alternative Medicine

In the 1990s alternative therapies were a topic of discussion within the traditional medical community. As medical practitioners researched the types of treatments used by their patients, it was necessary to assemble a list of all types of known alternative treatments. The National Center for Complementary and Alternative Medicine (NCCAM) was formed in the early 1990s to address these issues. The three main goals of the NCCAM are to perform research on alternative treatments, train individuals who are interested in learning techniques, and provide the consumer with information on the various types of therapies available. NCCAM has identified and classified various therapies and continues to receive funding from the U.S. government for more research. More than half of the medical schools in the United States currently are offering classes on alternative medicine. Areas of study include dietary supplement therapy (such as vitamins and minerals), herbal medicine, acupuncture, and homeopathy.

The term complementary is used concurrently with alternative because nontraditional therapies have found a place alongside traditional medicine. Therefore the term complementary and alternative medicine (CAM) is an accurate description of how these two forms of treatment are being used together. More physicians, nurse practitioners, and other health care providers are suggesting herbal treatments and nondrug alternatives in place of, or concurrently with, traditional treatments. Nondrug alternatives may include techniques such as biofeedback, massage, and meditation. Self-hypnosis has been found clinically to reduce surgical pain in patients. Acupuncture has been used in hospitals to provide pain relief to adolescent patients. Table 9-1 lists types of complementary therapies.

Another source for information on nontraditional treatments can be found through the BioTherapeutics, Education & Research Foundation, known as the BTER Foundation. This organization began as a nonprofit charity in 2003. It is dedicated to "The BeTERment of health, by supporting patient care, education and research in Biotherapy and symbiotic medicine." Areas of interest include the following:

- Maggot therapy
- Leech therapy
- Honeybee therapy
- Ichthyotherapy (fish)
- Pet therapy
- Phage therapy (bacteria)
- Helminthic therapy (worms)

These treatments are funded by individual contributions and grants. They have educational links that provide specifics on the various topics of therapy. In the following paragraphs, a brief description of both maggot therapy and leech therapy and their history will be given. For a quick overview of all the areas of study listed under the BTER Foundation website, see Table 9-2.

MAGGOT THERAPY

Maggot debridement therapy (MDT) is a therapy that has been used since the sixteenth century. Throughout time maggots were known to have a dramatic effect on wound healing. During the Civil War it was noticed that soldiers whose damaged limbs were infected with maggots healed faster than soldiers with non-infected damaged limbs. Maggot therapy became popular enough in the United States during the 1930s and 1940s that hundreds of hospitals used this type of therapy rather than the current treatments of the time. However, as

TABLE 9-1 Twelve Alternative Treatments

Type of Treatment	Description of Alternative Treatment
Acupressure	Acupressure is based on the same principles as acupuncture. Instead of using needles to unblock the pathways carrying energy, the practitioner uses his or her hands to apply pressure to specific points on the body.
Acupuncture	Acupuncture is based on the meridians in the body. These lines are believed to carry energy to specific parts of the body. When they become blocked, illness or pain can occur. The practitioner relieves blocked pathways with the use of needles.
Aromatherapy	Using the nasal senses, various blends of fragrances result in relief of certain ailments. Herbs and perfumes are used. Mostly oils are used because they are considered more healing than the whole plant or portions of plants.
Art therapy	Art therapy is based on psychoanalysis and how the mind can manifest specific images. These images then can be expressed in drawings or paintings, hopefully stimulating enlightenment. Then the patient can work on the problem through feedback.
Ayurveda	Ayurveda is based on the spiritual side of the body and all that affects the body, including the environment, emotional stability, and physical health. Practitioners find ways to change what is necessary to enable the patient to be more in tune with the world. This includes various postures, meditation, and massage. Changing habits is a large part of this treatment.
Biofeedback	Biofeedback is a learned technique that enables self-control of various physiological responses of the body. This includes voluntary systems and involuntary systems of the body. A practitioner teaches it only until the patient is proficient in using the technique.
Chinese medicine	Chinese medicine is based on the body spirits of the yin (meaning man) and yang (meaning woman) that are acknowledged as having similar elements yet that are different in order. Therefore each is treated differently. Diagnosis is based on the person's dreams, tastes, sensations, smell, and other senses. Various types of treatments are used, including herbal remedies and acupuncture.
Chiropractic	Chiropractic treatment is based on the belief that the realignment of the body, specifically the spine, can remedy certain conditions. Periodic adjustments usually are required to align the spine and various joints throughout the body. In this way, pressure or pain is relieved.
Crystal healing	Continual use of various stones and gems is required to produce healing. Practitioners of crystal healing place specific stones on parts of the body for certain lengths of time to withdraw disease. Patients are taught which types of stone can be used for their healing abilities.
Herbal remedies	Medicinal purposes of herbs have been learned through historical literature and by word of mouth. Trial and error are the main guidelines of herbal treatments if used without consultation from an authority, such as a practitioner who has a legitimate degree in herbal use. Currently, many herbal agents are being tested, and testimonials of side effects and interactions are being compiled for reference.
Homeopathy	Homeopathy is the traditional belief that "like cures like." Various types of toxins are mixed in extreme dilutions to the point at which they are often undetectable by scientific means. This minute amount of the same disease from which the patient is suffering allows the patient's body to fight the illness.
Spiritual healing	In the belief system of spiritual healing, the patient's treatment is attained through prayer of the practitioner and patient. The practitioner claims to be a pathway for divine intervention. Recovery is instantaneous, and no follow-up visits are necessary.

TABLE 9-2 BTER Foundation Research Areas

Type of Treatment	Also Known As	Information about Treatment	Sources for More Information
Maggots	Larva therapy	Debridement of dead tissue; use of live fly larvae for cleaning wounds that have not responded to typical antibiotic treatment	www.post-gazette.com/ pg/04195/345382.stm
Hirudotherapy	Leech therapy	Used to treat venous diseases such as thrombophlebitis, hematomas They remove stagnant blood that accumulates in reattached limbs through their saliva, which contains vasodilators, anticoagulants, and anesthetics	http://biotherapy.md.huji.ac.il/
Apitherapy	Honeybee therapy	Honeybee venom has shown antiinflammatory effects that can be used for conditions such as rheumatoid arthritis and some neurological conditions such as multiple sclerosis Treatment given as a subcutaneous injection	The American Apitherapy Society, Inc., www.apitherapy.org
Ichthyotherapy	Fish therapy	Use of specific fish to treat skin conditions such as psoriasis; fish consume scales of psoriasis	www.psoriasisfishcure.com/
Pet therapy	Seeing eye dogs; pet therapy; sniffer dogs	Seeing eye dogs: animals to assist the blind Pet therapy: animals that provide comfort and companionship for those who suffer from depression or loneliness Sniffer dogs: used in detecting cancers in humans by odor that emanates from cancer cells, such as melanoma (skin cancer)	www.deltasociety.org/Page.aspx?pid=183
Phage therapy	Microbial therapy	Phages (viruses) are used to infect and kill bacteria such as *Enterococci, Escherichia coli, Staphylococci,* and *Mycobacterium tuberculosis* when traditional antibiotics do not work.	www.phagetherpy.com
Helminthic therapy	Intestinal parasitic worms	Treatment for inflammatory bowel disease and other hypersensitivity disorders; *Tinea suix* (pig whipworm) used to treat Crohn's colitis.	Hunter, McKay: Helminths as therapeutic agents for inflammatory bowel disease, *Aliment-Pharmacol-Ther* 19(2):167-177, 2004 (Jan 15)

antibiotics were further developed physicians treated infections with stronger antibiotics, and while maggot treatments were still used MDT was saved for those rare cases in which treatments or antibiotics were ineffective. Since then, additional clinical and scientific studies have been conducted and have established that maggot therapy is still a very useful treatment.

Maggots are fly larvae, and there are three specific species that can be used medicinally. Only those maggots with specific life cycles are used, the most common being *Phaenicia sericata,* the green blowfly. They have three primary uses, including cleaning and disinfecting wounds and accelerating wound healing. They are used on patients who have undergone amputations, replacing costly surgical techniques used to clean the large wound. The therapy entails placing maggots on the wound, which is then wrapped. The maggots will eat only the dead tissue in the affected area, growing from 1 to 2 mm up to 1 cm over several days. They are then washed off the wound site. The cost of treatment is half that of traditional treatment. The maggots are stored at room temperature in the pharmacy. Currently there are more than 20 countries that use MDT to treat thousands of patients.

LEECH THERAPY

Leeches have been used throughout the ages for various reasons. The most popular use in history was for bloodletting (see Chapter 1) in Egypt, Europe, and other countries. It was believed they could cure obesity, hemorrhoids, headaches, and even mental illness. They were so popular for these conditions that they were even farmed at one point to keep up with the demand. As knowledge of human physiology and treatments progressed, the use of leeches fell out of favor because they had no real medicinal application for any of these conditions. It was not until the mid-1980s that scientists reexamined the chemical attributes of these small creatures for their use in postsurgical treatments.

Persons who have undergone either reconstructive or plastic surgery, particularly for skin grafting or reattachment techniques and microsurgery, are at risk for venous congestion—blood clotting and stagnating within the veins. If this occurs, oxygen and nutrients cannot travel to their intended sites and the tissue will ultimately die. Compared to leeches, there are no manmade medicines that can safely or as effectively treat patients with this condition. Within the saliva of leeches there are several chemicals that are useful in specific cases. Leeches have a natural anticoagulant called hirudin, a vasodilator called prostaglandin that reduces swelling, and a chemical anesthetic that numbs the area where the leeches feed. The prevention of blood clotting in the local area allows for good nutrient supply to the affected area and permits healing to occur. In addition, a bacterium located in the stomach of leeches *(Aeromonas hydrophila)* digests blood and produces an antibacterial substance, which kills dangerous bacteria that cause tissue necrosis.

As repulsive as these creatures seem, they do miraculous work and they are extremely inexpensive compared with common medications and treatments. Prices range from $5 to $7 each, far less than the cost of medicine, and leeches double the success rate of transplanted tissue. A leech therapy session can cost just $75.00, not counting personnel time for their care and application. Other conditions are now becoming popular for the investigational use of leeches, including for certain dermatological and ophthalmological conditions, cardiovascular disease, inflammation of the middle ear, and osteoarthritis of the knee. Leeches have many positive attributes: they work specifically at the site of action rather than having a systemic effect, they are easy to place at the site of action, and they fall off the site once they have finished feeding (usually in 30 minutes). However, there are a few possible side effects that must be considered. They can cause excessive blood loss to the point where a blood transfusion is necessary,

BOX 9-1 UGLY MEDICINE

Leeches

Patient's feelings about the use of leeches range from repulsion to amazement. Most will describe the attachment of the leeches as painless. Other testimonials describe the leech attachment sensation as being similar to a mosquito bite, while others claim it is as painful as a wasp bite. Patients state they feel something similar to a caterpillar without legs on their skin. A rhythmic pulling sensation may be noticeable for a few minutes at the start of treatment. The pain and sensation vary greatly among patients and may be influenced by their personal feelings about leeches. It appears that the more patients focus on the initial attachment of the leeches, the higher they rate their pain level. For this reason the patient is encouraged to focus on something other than the leech therapy. Some people do not want to look at the leeches at all, but this is encouraged after they have attached so the patient can notify the physician or nurse when the leeches detach. There is normally pruritus at the site for a few days after treatment, and a small three-pronged scar that fades in time is common (see www.leeches.biz/safety-adverse-effects.htm).

Maggots

Wormy, squirmy fly larvae crawling under your bandages is the feeling many patients may have with maggot therapy. The flies used are not your average housefly but disinfected maggots grown in a laboratory. Most patients begrudgingly will accept the therapy because it is so effective, but it can be hard to handle emotionally. For wounds that are close to nerves, analgesics may need to be administered to lessen the pain as the maggots scratch and poke at the dead tissue. Also antianxiety medications can be given to patients before initiating treatment. To watch a video about a patient's personal treatment with maggots, go to: www.youtube.com/watch?v=bAY7OKp6D7w.

---

patients may have an allergic reaction or become infected, and there is the possibility for a leech to be lost in body openings. Leeches are specially ordered from the medicinal leech farm for time of use and are usually overseen by the pharmacy department; they are stored in specialized solutions or gels in the refrigerator. See Box 9-1 for a description of patients' experiences with leech therapy.

Both maggots and leeches from select companies have been FDA-approved as medical devices. Their use in treatments has become so popular that many insurance companies now reimburse maggot and leech therapies.

Ancient Chinese Medicine

For more than 4000 years, Chinese medicine has been a well-known art based on years of trial and error. Although herbal remedies might come to mind readily when the topic of Chinese medicine is discussed, it involves much more than the use of herbaceous plant parts. The heart of Chinese practice is yin and yang, which represent male and female entities, respectively. The ancient Chinese belief contends that although men and women are made of the same substances, their spirits are different, and therefore appropriate treatment is different. Female spirits are believed to be darker in color, which coincides with the earth, whereas male spirits are lighter in color, similar to the color of the sky.

Practitioners conduct an examination by asking the patient about dreams, strange tastes, or smells experienced. Also, a visual examination of the skin and voice tone is performed. Once the diagnosis is completed, the practitioner may prescribe the necessary treatment that could include a variety of herbs, minerals, and/or vegetables. Herbs are used extensively in Chinese medicine and can treat more than one ailment at a time. For example, goldenseal may be used for headaches, allergies, and infections concurrently. Also, various herbal plants

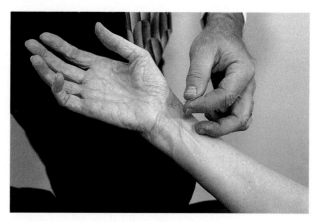

FIGURE 9-1 Acupuncture. (From Potter PA, Perry AG: *Fundamentals of nursing*, ed 7, St Louis, 2009, Elsevier.)

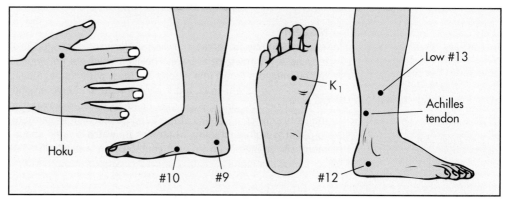

FIGURE 9-2 Acupressure points. (From Potter PA, Perry AG: *Fundamentals of nursing*, ed 5, St Louis, 2001, Elsevier.)

have the ability to work for or against a specific physiological condition, such as raising or lowering blood pressure levels, depending on the person's condition. Herbs and other remedies are used in Chinese medicine to cure the body of the original illness as well as a **prophylaxis**. Chinese medicine is still in use today; many health care providers, including pharmacists, take classes based on Chinese knowledge of herbs and their medicinal uses.

ACUPUNCTURE

Acupuncture has been used for thousands of years with extensive studies in the Eastern and Western world. Acupuncture is used for conditions such as chronic pain, depression, addiction, and other ailments. Acupuncture is based on the Chinese belief that the body is made of energy channels. When these channels become blocked, sickness may result. The use of needles at specific points throughout the body is thought to release these channels, bringing the body into harmony once again (Figure 9-1).

ACUPRESSURE

Acupressure is closely related to acupuncture because it also uses specific energy points across the body. Instead of using needles, pressure is applied by hand to the specific point to unblock the channels. Insurance companies are beginning to pay for acupuncture and acupressure treatment if recommended by a physician for the treatment of pain. Acupressure classes are available, teaching the person how to perform the technique on his or her own body (Figure 9-2).

Additional Forms of Complementary and Alternative Medicine

ART THERAPY

Art therapy became popular in psychology in the late 1960s. Psychiatrists asked patients who were mentally disturbed or traumatized to draw their feelings on paper if they were unable to discuss problems verbally. Such therapy was a way for patients to express themselves, relieve anxiety, and begin the road to recovery. Art therapy can be used for simple stress relief therapy or as therapeutic treatment for persons suffering from life-threatening illnesses, such as cancer. Patients may gather in groups or individually with a practitioner who guides them through the techniques of mental and visual awareness concerning their disease state or condition. This type of therapy is intended to supplement counseling.

Art therapy is used extensively in children with autism or other psychological conditions and now is used for many types of treatment in adults as well. Various forms of expression include painting, working with clay, making facial masks, and making batik. A master's degree is offered in this area of study through various colleges. Other art therapies include music, poetry, drama, and dance. The National Coalition of Creative Arts Therapies Association offers information on these types of therapies and schools for training.

AYURVEDA

Ayurveda is an ancient Indian approach to medicine still practiced today. Dating back thousands of years, ayurveda is based on the person knowing the spiritual self. This knowledge encompasses the body and all that affects it. With an insight into the various effects of outside influences on the body's spirit, it is possible to make assumptions. One can predict whether something will have a positive effect or negative effect on the body. For example, certain colors, sounds, clothing, and other environmental stimuli are taken into consideration. The types of food and herbs that are consumed also play a role in the overall health of the person. These assumptions are then applied to physical and spiritual activities of the ill person. Based on the type of personality of the subject, the practitioners suggest ways to alter food and/or lifestyle to cure and prevent illnesses. This form of treatment exists today in many parts of the world. Medical schools teaching this approach are located in India. Courses in Indian medicine also are offered in various medical schools in the United States.

BIOFEEDBACK

Biofeedback has existed for approximately 50 years and has proved to be effective for treatment of stress, hypertension, and other conditions. Biofeedback uses the patient's mental ability to alter their own vital signs such as blood pressure, heart rate, and even gastrointestinal activity. The body is divided into two types of movement—voluntary and involuntary. Voluntary movements include the musculoskeletal system and involve purposeful actions such as walking, sitting, standing, and bending. Persons have control over these functions daily; therefore adjusting behavior does not take much conscious effort. However, with biofeedback one also is taught how to mentally access and alter involuntary body functions, such as heart beat, breathing, and digestion. These functions do not normally require conscious thought.

Biofeedback usually is taught by an instructor who uses electrical leads that provide a readout of data. Patients are connected to monitors that allow them

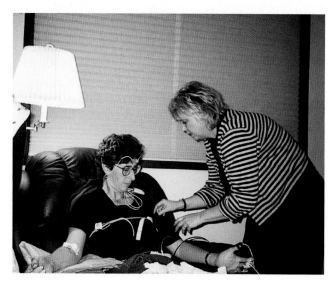

FIGURE 9-3 Biofeedback. Example of electrode placement. (From Potter PA, Perry AG: *Fundamentals of nursing*, ed 5, St Louis, 2001, Elsevier.)

to see what their bodies are experiencing. A monitor can show the activity of a specific organ. For example, the instructor might have the patient alter the heart rate to a certain level through concentration. When that level is reached, a new level is set. Gradually, the person is able to adjust body functions as needed without the use of a monitor. Biofeedback is a way of connecting the mind to the body. Patients need to practice these techniques frequently to achieve their full benefit. Biofeedback is used as an alternative to medication for conditions such as anxiety, low back pain, neuromuscular dysfunction, and tension headaches. Biofeedback therapy is partially reimbursed by many insurance companies with a physician's approval. Once the technique of biofeedback is perfected, it can be done at any time without supervision (Figure 9-3).

CHIROPRACTIC THERAPY

Chiropractic therapy is an orthopedic approach to treating pain resulting from misalignment of the bones. Chiropractic therapy began in the late 1800s when it was believed to have cured deafness in a man after his back popped into correct alignment. Certain changes in the skeletal structure are believed to interfere with the nervous system and other organ systems. The treatment given to a patient by a chiropractic physician is referred to as manipulation. Treatment can include hands-on adjustments of the spine or joints and application of massage and heat therapy. Research has proved that some forms of manipulation can be helpful, specifically manipulation of the lower back. Although use of chiropractic therapy is increasing, various forms of treatment are controversial. Some physicians promote the use of manipulation of certain parts of the skeletal structure, whereas other physicians believe it may be harmful. This is especially true when chiropractors manipulate skeletal structures to cure infections or treat conditions such as hearing loss or diabetes.

Skepticism about the ability of manipulation to treat many common illnesses abounds, and studies are being conducted to determine exactly which therapy works and why it is effective. Practitioners must attend an accredited school to attain the degree Doctor of Chiropractic (DC). Many insurance companies cover chiropractic treatment based on scientific evidence and referrals from a physician such as an orthopedic physician. Chiropractic therapy usually takes many sessions of treatment.

Pharmacist's Perspective
BY SUSAN WONG PharmD

Educate Yourself about Complementary and Alternative Medicine and Health

Many questions arise when discussing a person's health. What is health? Some may believe that it is not getting sick, in other words, staying well. Others may think it is fixing something that has gone wrong or broken. Still others believe it is maintaining overall happiness and balance. All of these play an important role in being healthy. How to do this is another story. The four important steps follow:

1. A patient or customer must become a good self-observer.
2. A patient or customer must learn to recognize that he or she has control of lifestyle and choices.
3. A patient or customer must make lifestyle changes or other changes as necessary.
4. A patient or customer must follow the results of changes, as well as document and communicate them with the health care provider.

Your role as a pharmacy technician may be as a bridge of information between the pharmacist and the patient to help the patient become or stay healthy.

To do any and all of these things, one first must understand what makes a person tick. Over many centuries, different philosophies have developed that address health. Native Americans chewed on willow leaves for relief from pain or swelling. In Europe, this eventually led to the discovery and concentration of the active component salicin and, with the help of some chemistry, the development of acetylsalicylic acid (aspirin). In Chinese medicine, a practitioner prescribes a tailored mixture or formula to cure pain and restore balance, or one can use one of the patent medicines (ready-made formulas for a general condition). Many Eastern philosophies incorporate emotional, mental, and spiritual balance into the equation. Unfortunately, how these remedies and philosophies interact may not always be clear. That is why it is important to educate oneself and communicate to others; especially important is the communication between a patient and the health care provider.

In the world of drugs, herbs, and nutritional supplements, it is important to clearly distinguish between the types of treatments. Understand how each of these single or multiple agents can affect a particular situation before they are used. Sometimes one therapy may counteract another or actually may augment the effects of another. This may be good or bad depending on the person's situation and overall health. Patients should keep a diary of what has been used, what they are currently using (if anything), and any questions they may have. Patients should keep track of how they feel and what may have caused it, including any prescription drugs, OTC drugs, herbs, or supplements, and should tell the health care provider exactly what they are using. The patient must let the medical physician, pharmacist, chiropractor, herbalist, nutritionist, or anyone who is involved in the patient's health and well-being know what he or she is taking. Health care providers may not know exactly how some substances interact, but they will find out for the patient before they recommend a product's use.

In Western medicine, drugs are highly refined chemicals (of plant and synthetic origin) that are taken for a specific purpose or endpoint. They have been studied extensively and documented in the scientific literature. These drugs are available mostly as single-agent pills or capsules. Multiple-agent compounds are designed to work together on one symptom or to tackle many symptoms. There are many new ways for medicines to enter the body, such as injections or shots; skin patches; creams, lotions, and ointments; inhalers; suppositories when the patient cannot swallow or suffers from nausea and vomiting; drops for eyes, ears, and nose; and drops or liquid to swallow. All of these dosage forms have developed in the last 10 to 50 years and are designed to get the medicine to exactly where it is needed. More targeted therapy allows a smaller effective dose with a reduced risk for side effects.

Just because a drug can be bought OTC does not mean that it is the best thing to use. For example, the asthma inhalers that can be purchased OTC certainly work but can cause some serious side effects in persons with a heart condition or anxiety. The patient should always consult the pharmacist if he or she is uncertain. Also important is that the patient obtain the right kind of drug in the right form and that the patient knows why, when, and how to use it.

For herbs, a similar situation exists in which there are single-agent herbs and multiple-agent formulas that work for different ailments. Fortunately, most are available in an oral form that can be swallowed or taken as a tea or infusion. Unfortunately, compared to medicinal drugs, herbal supplements are not regulated as closely in the United States. Medical drugs are tested much more rigorously and take longer to reach the market. However, herbs have been used for centuries, even millennia, to heal and cure patients when used correctly. The patient must be aware of the exact genus and species of herb to ensure the right effect. Similarly named herbs can have different effects. Be aware of the source of the active agents, for example,

Continued

roots, leaves, berries, or tree bark. Also of importance for some herbs is when they are harvested: spring and fall harvests may have different chemical characteristics. Always be aware of the labels. Read labels and learn exactly how and when to take herbs. Use reputable sources and standardized extracts (standardized to known active ingredients) when buying herbs.

Food and dietary supplements are similar to herbs in that they are much less regulated than drugs. We know we need certain foods, vitamins, and minerals to survive—too much or too little can affect health adversely. Different diets can rob patients of certain essential nutrients, so it is best for the patient to check with the physician/consultant before starting a diet. Most persons who follow a well-balanced diet do not need additional supplements. Others who may have chosen certain vegetarian diets or weight loss diets may be missing some nutrients and need supplements. Remember that different types or amounts of exercise can affect one's diet and nutrient needs.

For example, osteoporosis can occur in men but most commonly occurs in women. A well-balanced diet with plenty of exercise can help prevent long-term detrimental effects. Some persons take calcium supplements to augment their bone and mineral stores. The normal recommended daily allowance for calcium in adults is about 1200 mg. By taking calcium supplements of 1000 to 1500 mg per day, a healthy adult can avoid detrimental bone loss. Recently, an innovative supplement was introduced to the market that is not a pill but a chocolate-flavored chew. It provides 500 mg of calcium, just like old-fashioned oyster shell calcium, but in a candy-like form. Sounds good, doesn't it? The fine print for the product shows that a tiny amount of vitamin K has been added. For persons who are receiving a closely monitored blood-thinning agent, such as warfarin to prevent strokes, taking this calcium product could be very harmful. Even this very small amount of vitamin K can counteract the positive effects of a blood-thinning agent and place a patient at risk for blood clots.

Green tea also has high amounts of vitamin K that can counteract blood-thinning agents such as warfarin. As persons age and engage in more healthy behaviors, they should pay close attention to what they take and how it is administered; otherwise, they could be doing more harm than good.

In today's medicine, we really do not know how the Western philosophy of treating illness and promoting health interacts with the Eastern philosophy. A few terms to consider follow:

- Allopathy—a system of medical practice employing all measures that have proven value in the treatment of disease
- Homeopathy—a system of medical practice that treats a disease by the administration of minute doses of a remedy that would in healthy persons produce symptoms similar to those of the disease

- Vegetarianism—the theory or practice of consuming a diet consisting of vegetables, fruits, grains, nuts, and sometimes limited animal products (e.g., milk, cheese, and eggs)
- Nutriceuticals/nutritional supplementation—whole foods, vitamins, minerals, enzymes, amino acids, phytochemicals, and other natural resources that are designed for use in the immune system, the inner healing force
- Herbal or botanical medicine—plants or plant substances that are used for medicinal purposes or crude drugs of vegetable origin used for the treatment of disease states, often of chronic nature, or to attain or maintain a condition of improved health
- Phytotherapy—the use of vegetable drugs in medicine
- Aromatherapy—the treatment of medical conditions with the aromatic essential oils of fragrant herbs
- Ayurveda—a holistic medical system that covers all aspects of health and well-being (physical, emotional, mental, and spiritual). Ayurveda includes methods of healing from diet, herbs, exercise, and lifestyle regimens such as yoga and meditation and is based on a person's dominant *dosha,* one of three body/personality types
- Traditional Chinese medicine—a system of acupuncture, herbs, and diet based on the parallelism and synchronicity of events in the inner and outer world of the human organism; it is based on a person's Tao (one of five archetypes that symbolize human character or personality types), the five organ networks and their climates, and finally the balance (yin/yang) between qi (the life force), blood (governing the tissue), and moisture (governing the internal environment)

Lastly, age, gender, and body type can affect how a body responds to what is put in it. Well-known in Western medicine is that pediatric (birth to 18 years old) and older patients (60 to 65 years and older) tolerate medications differently because of natural metabolic changes. Lifestyle issues such as smoking and alcohol use also affect responses to medicines. Medication doses are adjusted according to these factors and to the desired endpoints. It might be safe to infer that these changes may have similar effects when using Eastern medicines and therapies as well. Patients must be careful before starting any new therapies and must consult experts if necessary.

All patients must monitor any and all agents they put into their bodies. Patients need to educate themselves about health and how they choose to maintain it. Patients should always inform their health care providers of any herbal remedies they are taking. This decreases the probability of a drug-drug or drug-food interaction. ▪

Herbal Medicine

Although herbal remedies have been in existence for thousands of years (see Chapter 1), this basic therapy has gained renewed popularity during the past decade. The herbal remedy market is expected to grow even more in the coming years because of many factors, such as the increasing age of the population and the rising costs associated with traditional health care and medications. The technician must know various interactions between legend drugs, OTC drugs, and herbal remedies. Most persons believe that it is not important to notify their physician or pharmacist that they are taking herbal medications because they believe these medications to be natural and therefore not harmful. However, there are many documented reports of harmful interactions between natural products, legend drugs, and OTC medications (Table 9-3).

TABLE 9-3 Examples of Herbal-Drug Interactions

Herbal Drug	Drug	Interaction
Black cohosh	Estrogens, esterified	May increase estrogen activity.
Echinacea	Ketoconazole	May have additive hepatoxic effects.
	Tacrolimus	May decrease effects of tacrolimus.
Feverfew	NSAIDs	Ibuprofen: may increase risk of bleeding.
		Indomethacin: may decrease effects of feverfew.
	Heparin	May have additive effects.
	Warfarin	May increase risk of bleeding.
Garlic	Chlorzoxazone	May decrease effectiveness of chlorzoxazone.
	Nimodipine	May increase antihypertensive effect.
	Quinapril	May increase antihypertensive effect.
	Reserpine	May have increased antihypertensive effects.
	Terazosin	May decrease effects of terazosin.
Ginkgo biloba	NSAIDs	May increase risk of bleeding.
	Chlorothiazide	May increase blood pressure.
	Clopidogrel	May increase risk of bleeding.
	Ethosuximide	May decrease effectiveness of ethosuximide blood concentrations.
	Imipramine	May decrease seizure threshold.
	Warfarin	May increase risk of bleeding.
Ginseng	Digoxin	May increase serum digoxin levels.
	Estrogen, esterified	May increase hormonal effects.
	Nimodipine	May worsen hypertension.
	Oxymorphone	May decrease opioid analgesic effectiveness.
	Quinapril	May worsen hypertension.
	Terazosin	May decrease effectiveness of terazosin.
	Tolazamide	May increase risk of hypoglycemia.
	Tolbutamide	May increase risk of hypoglycemia.
	Warfarin	May decrease effectiveness of warfarin.
Kava kava	Alprazolam	May increase effects of benzodiazepines.
	Chlorzoxazone	May increase CNS depression.
	Buspirone	May increase sedation.
	Levodopa	May decrease effects of levodopa.
	Pimozide	May increase dopamine antagonist effects.
	Sulfinpyrazone	May increase risk of bleeding.
	Thiothixene	May increase CNS depression.

Continued

TABLE 9-3 Examples of Herbal-Drug Interactions—cont'd

Herbal Drug	Drug	Interaction
Ma huang (ephedra)	Chlorthiazide	May decrease hypotensive effect of chlorothiazide.
	Isoproterenol	May increase CNS stimulation.
	Nisoldipine	May decrease effectiveness of nisoldipine.
St. John's wort	Amoxapine	May increase risk of serotonin syndrome.
	Chlorpropamide	May increase risk of hypoglycemia.
	Cyclosporine	May decrease cyclosporine effectiveness.
	Dapsone	May decrease dapsone blood concentration.
	Desipramine	May increase desipramine's pharmacological effects and risk of toxicity.
	Duloxetine	May increase adverse effects.
	Estrogen, esterified	May decrease levels of esterified estrogens.
	Fluoxetine	May increase fluoxetine's pharmacological effects and risk of toxicity.
	Imipramine	May increase imipramine's pharmacological effects and risk of toxicity.
	Lamivudine and many antiviral drugs for HIV	May decrease blood concentration and effectiveness in treating HIV.
	Methocarbamol	May increase CNS depression.
	Oxytetracycline	May increase risk of photosensitivity.
	Paroxetine	May increase paroxetine's pharmacological effects and risk of toxicity.
	Piroxicam	May increase risk of phototoxicity.
	Quinine	May decrease quinine levels.
	Reserpine	May increase CNS depression.
	Sulfisoxazole	May cause photosensitization.
	Theophylline	May decrease metabolism of theophylline.
	Tolbutamide	May increase risk of hypoglycemia.
	Venlafaxine	May increase sedative-hypnotic effect of venlafaxine.
	Warfarin	May increase risk of bleeding.
	Yohimbine	May increase risk of hypertensive crises.

Many of the drugs used in traditional medicine today are medications originally derived from plant sources. The main difference is that extensive testing and documentation have preceded their use. Through testing, specific chemicals have been isolated in many herbal plants. Those chemicals that have proven effectiveness against certain conditions then are made **synthetically** in a laboratory if possible, to help ensure quality manufacturing from batch to batch. Therefore most American medicine discovered from plants does not incorporate the whole plant or even part of the plant. Herbs and herbal supplements are subjected to the regulations enforced by the Food and Drug Administration. However, the Food and Drug Administration does not regulate herbs in the same way as drugs because they are considered a dietary supplement.

This section discusses some of the more popular herbs and precautions to take before self-administration. Because many herbs have been used in different cultures for thousands of years, they often have many different names. For example, *Echinacea* is also known as black sampson, sampson root, narrow-leafed purple coneflower, and red sunflower. Table 9-4 lists common uses and cautionary notes for the herbal treatments listed.

HERBAL TREATMENTS

Aloe vera, from the plant called aloe, is one of the most popular herbal agents. Many different species are used to produce topical agents to treat minor burns, acne, and various skin irritations. If taken internally, aloe works as a laxative

TABLE 9-4 Common Uses and Cautionary Notes for Herbals

Herb	Species	Various Uses	Caution
Black cohosh	*Cimicifuga racemosa**	Menopause, premenstrual syndrome	Should not be used if pregnant. May cause liver toxicity.
Chamomile	*Matricaria recutita**	Gastrointestinal upset, skin conditions	Should not be used if pregnant. Safe if used in small quantities and short term.
Feverfew	*Tanacetum parthenium*	Migraine	Should not be used if pregnant.
Garlic	*Allium sativum*	Antiinfective, antibiotic	Safe if used in small quantities.
Ginger	*Zingiber officinale*	Motion sickness, nausea	Safe if used in small quantities.
Ginkgo	*Ginkgo biloba*	Increases circulation	Should not be used if pregnant.
Ginseng	*Panax quinquefolius*	Stress relief	Safe if used in small quantities.
Goldenseal	*Hydrastis canadensis*	Urinary tract infections	Should not be used if pregnant or if hypertensive problems exist.
Hawthorn	*Crataegus laevigata*	Chest pain, increases blood flow	Studies are not complete.
Milk thistle	*Silybum marianum*	Common cold	Studies are not complete because of the many different species and parts of herbaceous plant used.
Purple coneflower	*Echinacea purpurea*	Liver health	Safe if used in small quantities.
St. John's wort	*Hypericum perforatum*	Antidepressant	Safe if used in small quantities.
Valerian	*Valeriana officinalis*	Sleep aid	Safe if used in small quantities.

*Various species are used; some side effects may differ depending on species.

and also is used for bleeding ulcers. Dosage forms are gels, powder, capsules, tonic, and juice. Pregnant women should not take aloe internally.

Black cohosh (Figure 9-4) *(Cimicifuga racemosa),* from the family Ranunculaceae, is used primarily for hot flashes associated with menopause. Other indications are rheumatism and cough; black cohosh also can be used as an insect repellent (called bugbane). Although short-term studies have concluded that black cohosh is safe, cetain studies have shown that liver toxicity may occur. Therefore a cautionary statement must be contained within the label of this agent. No extensive scientific studies have been done on this herb. One must not confuse black cohosh with similar sounding herbs, such as blue or white cohosh. These are not used for the same purpose and have different interactions with other medications.

Chamomile is from the family Asteraceae (Compositae) and has more than 20,000 known species. The species *Matricaria recutita* is used for motion sickness, flatulence, and gastrointestinal disturbances. In the topical form, chamomile is used for open ulcers, hemorrhoids, and other inflammatory conditions of the skin. When taken orally, chamomile has been documented to cause emesis, and if used topically, one should keep the medication away from the eyes because it can cause irritation. Oral chamomile is contraindicated in pregnancy and (because of lack of testing) during lactation. Chamomile also has been reported to worsen asthma attacks. Chamomile has several interactions with anticoagulants, benzodiazepines, and central nervous system depressants. Most of these interactions can cause an additive effect of the medication if taken with chamomile.

Feverfew also is derived from the family Asteraceae. The species *Tanacetum parthenium* is used for many different ailments including fever, headaches,

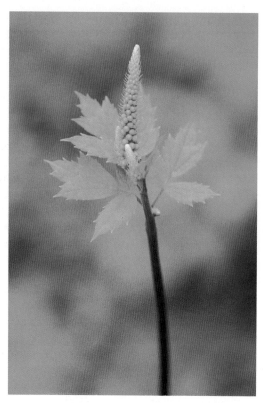

FIGURE 9-4 Black cohosh. (Courtesy Martin Wall Photography, 2011.)

gastrointestinal upset, arthritis, and asthma; its primary use is in the prevention of migraines. Feverfew can be used in topical and oral forms. In the oral form, feverfew is known to cause irritation of the mouth and tongue and a variety of gastrointestinal disturbances such as nausea, vomiting, and diarrhea. Side effects, such as increased bleeding, have been reported when feverfew is taken with anticoagulants. Nonsteroidal antiinflammatory drugs may decrease the effects of feverfew.

Garlic (Figure 9-5) is from the family Amaryllidaceae (Liliaceae) and is most well-known as a common herb used in most kitchens in America. Although it is known for its wonderful flavor, it has purported medicinal uses as well. The species *Allium sativum* has several uses that range from stress relief to an anticancer agent. Some persons use garlic to treat high blood pressure, colds and flu, and for overall wellness. Although garlic is safe most of the time, it is important not to overmedicate because it has been reported to cause adverse side effects such as heartburn, gastrointestinal burning, and even destruction of normal intestinal flora. (Normal flora of the gut are necessary for digestion of food and some vitamin absorption.) Garlic should not be used medicinally when one is taking anticoagulants because it may increase the risk of bleeding. Garlic should not be taken by persons with diabetes because it may interact with ongoing medication therapy, such as insulin or hypoglycemic agents. Persons suffering from gastrointestinal disorders should be cautioned of possible interactions with garlic use.

Ginger is from the family Zingiberaceae, known as the ginger family, and has 1000 species. The species *Zingiber officinale* is known for its **antiemetic** and antivertigo properties and is used in gastrointestinal upset and other gastrointestinal conditions, including bleeding, flatulence, stomachache, diarrhea, and more severe conditions such as malaria and cholera. Like garlic, ginger has been shown to have interactions with anticoagulants, producing possible increased

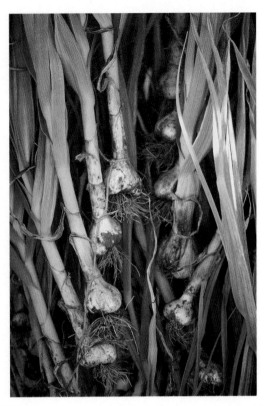

FIGURE 9-5 Garlic. (Courtesy Martin Wall Photography, 2011.)

bleeding risks. Ginger also may interact with gastrointestinal medication such as H_2-antagonists (ranitidine) and proton pump inhibitors (omeprazole). Use of barbiturates with ginger may increase the effects of such agents. Ginger also may affect blood pressure medication, cardiac drugs, and diabetic agents.

Ginkgo biloba is the only remaining species of the family Ginkgoaceae and sometimes is referred to as a living fossil. Its most popular use is to treat poor circulation, but it also can be employed to treat asthma, and less frequently to regulate blood pressure, improve liver function, increase memory, and treat heart disease. Some drug interactions include increased bleeding when taken with anticoagulants and increased blood pressure when taken with antihypertensive medications. Persons suffering from bleeding disorders, epilepsy, or infertility should avoid ginkgo. Many medicinal herbs are made from different parts of a plant; therefore it is important to know what part of the plant is used for which type of condition. Primarily, the ginkgo leaf is used as the medicinal agent, but seeds are also available. Studies have not shown their effectiveness, but raw seeds are known to be dangerous if taken orally.

Ginseng is from the family Araliaceae. The ginseng species *Panax quinquefolius* is used widely for overall wellness, including strengthening the immune system. Ginseng also is used for other ailments such as inflammation and depression, and as a diuretic. Drug interactions of ginseng include decreased effectiveness of anticoagulants and altered effectiveness of some cardiac agents, diuretics, diabetic agents, and antidepressants.

Goldenseal is from the family Ranunculaceae, known as the buttercup family. The species *Hydrastis canadensis,* when taken orally, is used for gastrointestinal conditions, inflammatory conditions, and painful menstruation. Topically, goldenseal has been used for dandruff, eczema, and pruritic rashes. Goldenseal has been reported to have interactions with H_2-antagonists

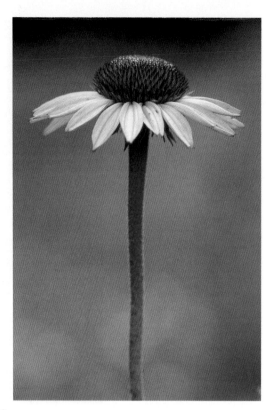

FIGURE 9-6 Purple coneflower. (Courtesy Martin Wall Photography, 2011.)

(ranitidine), blood pressure medications, anticoagulants, and central nervous system sedating drugs.

Hawthorn is available in many different preparations depending on the part of the plant used; however, all are members of the family Rosaceae (the rose family). The species *Crataegus laevigata* is used mostly to increase blood circulation and improve heart conditions, although studies have not proved its effectiveness conclusively. However, hawthorn has been reported to have possible interactions with various cardiac agents such as vasodilators, antiarrhythmics, antianginal agents, and antihypertensive drugs. Hawthorn also may interact with central nervous system depressants.

Echinacea (purple coneflower, Figure 9-6) is in the family Asteraceae or Compositae, depending on the species used. The species *Echinacea purpurea* is typically utilized to treat colds and infections and to strengthen the immune system. Therefore persons taking any type of immunosuppressive agents should be aware that *Echinacea* might alter the effects of such agents. In addition, persons with diabetes and any persons who have a condition that involves the immune system should not take *Echinacea* because this herb may negatively impact their condition.

Milk thistle is from the family of Asteraceae or Compositae. The species *Silybum marianum* is used primarily for liver conditions. Like several other herbs, various parts of the plant are used. The effect varies depending on what part is used. Unlike many other herbs, milk thistle does not have any reported major contraindications.

St. John's wort is part of the Clusiaceae family. Wort means "flower" in Old English, not to be confused with wart, which is a viral growth on the skin. More literature has been written on the effectiveness of this herb than on many others. Some of its uses include improvement of mild depression. However, St. John's wort has been shown to interact with other herbs that increase sedation, such as valerian. St. John's wort has many documented serious interactions with medications such as antianginal agents, antidepressants, HIV medications, anticoagulants, and medications used during organ transplant procedures.

Valerian is from the family Valerianaceae. The species *Valeriana officinalis* is used mostly for sleeplessness and depression. Because of its strong ability to induce sleepiness, it should not be taken with alcohol, barbiturates, benzodiazepines, or any other sedative type of medication. Valerian may increase the effects of such drugs and/or their side effects.

Knowledge of the family name of the herb is important in case of possible unwanted interactions or reactions. For instance, if someone is allergic to corn, then any herbal drug from the same family may cause an allergic response. Therefore that person should avoid all herbs from this family. Several herbal books can be referenced to determine the family of an herb. Knowing the species of the herb is also important because species can vary even if they are closely related. Some studies have been completed on only one of many species of herbs used to prepare herbal supplements.

Use of correct or safe dosages is difficult because the ingredients of each batch of herbs can vary widely. Therefore the strength of each tablet or capsule may fluctuate from one production lot to another. The time of harvesting, the parts and concentrations of the plants used, and the consistency in the method of preparation can alter the effectiveness of herbal supplements.

HERBAL PREPARATIONS

How herbs are prepared can determine the strength of the active ingredients. Herbs that are brewed for teas are usually more potent than those prepared in capsule form. Teas can be prepared by various methods. Infusions are made by pouring hot water onto herbs and letting them brew (steep) for a few minutes. Decoctions are herbs that are simmered over heat in water for 15 to 20 minutes, and cold infusions are left to soak in cold water over many hours. Various methods are suggested depending on the type of herb being prepared (Table 9-5). Medical schools are including studies of herbal remedies because of their

TABLE 9-5 Herbal Preparations

Dosage Form	Route of Administration	Ingredients	Use, Strength, Onset of Action
Syrups, diluted; tinctures	Internal	Alcohol, glycerin	Usually this is a potent form.
Tablets, capsules	Internal	Powdered	Slower to act; these are broken down in stomach.
Teas	Internal	Syrups, sweeteners	Better tasting when sweeteners added; teas are stronger than tablets or capsules.
Aromatic solutions, baths	External	Scented water	Used to treat skin conditions and burns.
Oils	External	Extracted oil from herbs	Used for sore muscles and skin conditions.
Compresses, salves	External	Made from teas, salves from herbal oils	A cloth soaked in herbal tea is applied to skin site; used for conditions such as bruises and cramps.

prevalence and possible benefits when used correctly along with traditional medicine.

Homeopathy

Homeopathy, translated from Greek, simply means "like suffering." The premise of homeopathy is the belief that "like cures like." Homeopathy also is referred to as the law of similars. The belief is that if a small amount of the substance that caused a person's disease or condition is consumed, it will enable the body to fight the disease. In the late 1700s homeopathy was made well-known by Samuel Hahnemann, a German physician. After ingesting a small amount of quinine, he exhibited symptoms of malaria, the disease that quinine cured. Over time he perfected the necessary minute amount of agent that was needed to instigate a cure rather than disease. Homeopathy was first used in the United States in the 1800s, and was a popular treatment. Although homeopathy has remained a well-accepted form of treatment in parts of Europe, it became an alternative treatment in the United States. Homeopathy, however, has regained some popularity over the last decade along with all other forms of alternative medicine.

Thousands of homeopathic remedies are available, but only one correct remedy for each illness; therefore homeopathic physicians must know what will work for the patient. Unlike herbs and other alternative treatments, the FDA oversees the manufacturing of homeopathic drugs. Under the guidelines of the FDA a homeopathic drug must meet standards for strength, quality, purity, and other parameters established in the *Homeopathic Pharmacopeia,* which contains monographs on ingredients used in homeopathic treatment. All homeopathic agents must be manufactured using good manufacturing practice (GMP) although there are a few exceptions because of the nature of certain ingredients. Specific guidelines include the following:

- Expiration dates may be exempt.
- Testing and release for distribution: Homeopathic agents are exempt from laboratory studies to determine the identity and strength of each active ingredient before being released for distribution.

In addition, if the homeopathic drug is a prescription it must contain the same labeling as indicated for prescription drugs ("Caution: Federal law prohibits dispensing without a prescription"). If sold over-the-counter, the agent must comply with the general labeling provisions for OTC drugs (e.g., indications for use, warnings, directions for use).

Although more medical schools are offering classes on homeopathic medicine, it is still somewhat controversial in the traditional medical community.

All drugs are prepared following guidelines in the *Homeopathic Pharmacopoeia* of the United States. Many of the remedies include herbal treatments. The process of preparing homeopathic agents involves blending and condensing the main ingredients, followed by diluting the active ingredients, and finally preparing the dosage form. The dilution of these active ingredients renders a trace amount of the agent that can equal as little as 1 part per million. Many times this minute amount is so small that it cannot be detected by chemical analysis.

More information on homeopathic medicine can be obtained from the National Center for Homeopathy. Although most homeopathic agents are available OTC, there are homeopathic practitioners who can oversee treatments. Various credentials are available, such as Diplomate of Homeopathic Academy of Naturopathic Physicians (DHANP), Diplomate of Homeotherapeutics (DHt), and Certified in Classical Homeopathy (CCH).

The Placebo Effect

One must consider the effectiveness of **placebo** drugs when discussing nontraditional medication. A placebo is an inert substance, meaning it contains no active ingredients. Therefore a placebo's ability to help a patient recover from illness or to decrease pain is based on the power of the patient's belief that the medication was effective (placebo effect). Many persons believe so strongly in certain remedies or therapies that it is difficult to determine whether the therapy or the belief of the patient is the likely cure. Through extensive double-blind tests, more information is becoming available regarding whether various treatments and herbal medications are truly effective. Double-blind studies are conducted in which the patient and the treating physician are not informed whether the patient is receiving the investigational drug or a placebo (inert drug). In this way the patient's or physician's bias cannot influence the findings, which should provide a clearer picture as to whether the drug is working or whether positive results are caused by the placebo effect.

DO YOU REMEMBER THESE KEY POINTS?

- The difference between Eastern and Western beliefs concerning medicine and healing
- Why alternative medicine is becoming more popular
- The responsibilities of the National Center for Complementary and Alternative Medicine concerning alternative medicine
- How the placebo effect influences the healing process
- The names of major alternative therapies and descriptions of how they are effective
- The current regulations pertaining to herbal remedies
- How individuals feel about informing their physicians about taking herbal medicines
- The main uses for the herbal medications covered
- How different dosage forms of herbal medications are used when prepared in different forms
- How homeopathy originated and the belief systems behind it
- The uses of maggots and leeches in wound treatment
- The uses of other nontraditional biotherapeutics

REVIEW QUESTIONS

Multiple choice questions

1. Of the following statements regarding biofeedback, which is NOT true?
   A. It is used to treat low back pain.
   B. Treatment may be covered partially by insurance companies.
   C. The patient is able to adjust his or her body functions to a degree.
   D. It must be used with supervision from a biofeedback therapist.

2. Chamomile most likely would be used to:
   A. Treat an upset stomach
   B. Relieve stress
   C. Increase circulation
   D. All of the above

3. Art therapy is often used for all of the following conditions or patients EXCEPT:
   A. Persons with severe illnesses
   B. Children with autism
   C. Persons who have a difficult time communicating
   D. Persons with an artistic ability

4. Homeopathy is known as the law of similars, which can be best described as:
   A. Taking a similar drug that works but at a much reduced cost
   B. Taking a drug that is similar to legend drugs but does not require a prescription
   C. Taking a drug that causes the same illness as the one you are trying to cure
   D. Taking a drug that causes a similar reaction to traditional agents

5. The herb that is known to increase circulation and memory is:
   A. Garlic
   B. Goldenseal
   C. Ginger
   D. *Ginkgo biloba*

6. Which of the remedies listed is regulated by the Food and Drug Administration?
   A. Herbal agents
   B. Homeopathic agents
   C. Healing gemstones
   D. Acupuncture

7. The most common use of *Echinacea purpurea* is:
   A. As an immune builder
   B. To treat gastrointestinal conditions
   C. To treat skin conditions
   D. As an antioxidant

8. *Silybum marianum* is known commonly as _____ and is used most commonly to treat _____.
   A. Ginger, motion sickness
   B. St. John's wort, depression
   C. Milk thistle, liver and spleen conditions
   D. Garlic, infections

9. Garlic has been shown to:
   A. Interact with anticoagulants
   B. Increase flatulence
   C. Affect blood pressure medication
   D. Both A and C

10. The one drug classification that has unwanted interactions with many herbal drugs is:
   A. Antiulcer agents
   B. Anticoagulants
   C. Vitamins
   D. Heart medications

11. Bee venom is used to treat:
   A. Bee stings
   B. Rheumatoid arthritis
   C. Neurological conditions
   D. Both C and D

12. Which of the following statements is NOT true concerning the use of leeches?
   A. All species of maggots can be used.
   B. The larvae range in size from 1 to 2 mm.
   C. The most common larva is the blue blowfly.
   D. When done feeding, they are simply washed off the wound site.

13. Of the indications for maggots which is NOT true?
A. They are used for cleaning the wound.
B. They disinfect the wound.
C. They accelerate healing.
D. They have a strong anticoagulant chemical.

14. The FDA has approved the following treatment(s):
A. Maggots
B. Herbal treatments
C. Leeches
D. Both A and C

15. Which of the following statements is true concerning leeches?
A. They have a natural anticoagulant.
B. They have a natural anesthetic.
C. They have a natural vasodilator.
D. All of the above are true of leeches.

True/False

If a statement is false, then change it to make it true.

_____ **1.** Acupuncture is used in hospitals within the United States to help relieve pain.

_____ **2.** *Ginkgo biloba* is the last remaining species of the Ginkgoaceae family.

_____ **3.** Ayurveda is an old Chinese form of medicine no longer in use.

_____ **4.** Chinese philosophy relies on the belief of spiritual healing.

_____ **5.** Herbal drugs are safe because they are natural.

_____ **6.** Ingesting herbal tea is less potent than taking tablets or capsules.

_____ **7.** Acupressure uses the same techniques as acupuncture.

_____ **8.** The main purpose of the National Center for Complementary and Alternative Medicine is to inform the public about herbal remedies.

_____ **9.** The terms *alternative* medicine and *nontraditional* medicine describe all forms of treatments other than the commonly used methods of Western physicians.

_____ **10.** When taking any herbal agent, it is important to know the species name in case of possible allergic reactions to the specific species.

_____ **11.** Phage therapy involves infecting bacteria with viruses that only kill the microbe, leaving human cells alone.

_____ **12.** Ichthyotherapy is also known as insect therapy.

_____ **13.** Hirudotherapy is also known as leech therapy.

_____ **14.** Apitherapy is also known as bee therapy.

_____ **15.** Maggot therapy is still not used in more than one or two countries as a treatment in place of traditional methods.

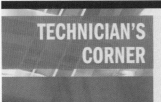

TECHNICIAN'S CORNER

1. A customer enters your pharmacy and inquires about which herbal remedies are effective for colds. What should you tell the customer?
2. An elderly customer suffering from the flu asks you if it is okay to take garlic tablets with her warfarin. What do you know about drug interactions (if any) between these two agents, and what should you tell the customer?

BIBLIOGRAPHY

Freeman LW: *Mosby's complementary & alternative medicine*, ed 2, St Louis, 2004, Elsevier.

Loecher B: Altshul O'Donnell. *Women's choices in natural healing*, Pennsylvania, 1998, Rodale Press.

Potter P, Perry A: *Fundamentals of nursing*, ed 5, St Louis, 2009, Mosby.

Skidmore Linda: *Mosby's handbook of herbs & natural supplements*, ed 4, Philadelphia, 2009, Elsevier Health Sciences.

WEBSITES REFERENCED

Biotherapeutics Education & Research Foundation (BTER) Website. Referenced 9/09. www.bterfoundation.org

CPG Sec. 400.400 Conditions Under Which Homeopathic Drugs May Be Marketed (CPG 7132.15). FDA Inspections, Compliance, Enforcement, and Criminal Investigations. Reference 9/2009.

Mahady GB et al: United States Pharmacopeia review of the black cohosh case reports of hepatotoxicity. Referenced 9/2009.Menopause.2008 July-Aug:15 (4 Pt1): 628-38. www.ncbi.nlm.nih.gov/pubmed/18340277

Rubin R: USA Today. Health and Behavior. Maggots and Leeches: Good Medicine. 2008. Referenced 8/09. www.usatoday.com/news/health/2004-07-07-leeches-maggots_x.htm

10

Hospital Pharmacy

Objectives

UPON COMPLETING THIS CHAPTER, YOU SHOULD BE ABLE TO DO THE FOLLOWING:

- Define the most common tasks performed by hospital pharmacy technicians.

- Identify hospital units according to their specialty.

- Explain the functions of various hospital pharmacies.

- List the patient information required for processing orders.

- Describe the functions of satellite pharmacies.

- Recognize the differences in floor stock depending on the area of the hospital.

- List special unit services and the type of stock they require.

- Explain the reasons for stock rotation, PAR levels, and ordering practices.

- Describe how ADS machines help to maintain PAR levels, increase speed, and control inventory.

- Describe the differences between horizontal and vertical laminar flow hoods.

- Explain the increased use of glove boxes as it relates to *USP <797>*.

- Describe how CPOE systems are used in medication ordering.

- List the types of medications used on crash carts and the areas where they are stocked.

- Explain the use of investigational drugs in a hospital setting.

- List three types of purchasing systems used in pharmacy.

Aseptic technique *The procedures used to eliminate the possibility of a drug becoming contaminated with microbes or particles*

Automated dispensing system(s) (ADS) *Computerized cabinets that control inventory on nursing floors, in emergency departments, and in surgical suites and other patient care areas*

Computerized physician order entry (CPOE) *Computerized order entry*

Crash carts *Also known as code carts. A moveable cart containing trays of medications, administration sets, oxygen, and other materials that are used in life-threatening situations such as cardiac arrest*

Electronic medication administration record (E-MAR) *Medication orders that are transcribed listing drug, strength, dose, dosage form and dosing time. Nurses record time and their initials of when the dose was given*

Formulary *A list of drugs that have been approved for use in hospitals by the pharmacy and therapeutics' committee of the institution and become the standard stock carried by the pharmacy and other departments*

Institutional pharmacy *Hospital pharmacy*

Investigational drug *A drug that has not been approved by the FDA for marketing but is in clinical trials; can also pertain to an FDA-approved drug that is seeking a new indication for use*

NKA *No known allergies*

NKDA *No known drug allergy*

Non-formulary medications *Drugs that are not approved for use within the institution unless specific exceptions are filed and accepted by the institutional protocols*

PAR *Periodic automatic replenishment*

Prn *Latin term (pro re nata) meaning "as needed"*

Protocol *A set of standards and guidelines within which a facility operates*

Pyxis *An automated dispensing system often used in hospitals*

Satellite pharmacy *A smaller pharmacy located in a hospital away from the central pharmacy*

Stat order *A medication order that must be filled as soon as possible, usually within 5 to 15 minutes*

SureMed *An automated dispensing system often used in hospitals*

The Joint Commission (TJC) *An independent nonprofit organization that accredits hospitals and other health care organizations in the United States. Accreditation is required in order to accept Medicare and Medicaid payment*

Unit dose *Individual pre-packaged medications used for one dose.*

United States Pharmacopeia <797> (USP <797>) *Guidelines enforceable for the safe preparation of sterile products*

Introduction

Probably one of the most challenging settings in which a pharmacy technician can be employed is in a hospital pharmacy, also known as the **inpatient pharmacy.** The dynamics of this environment can be exhilarating and exhausting, depending on the circumstances. Because there are fewer hospital pharmacies than community pharmacies, there are fewer job openings for pharmacy technicians in hospitals. However, as a result of the current changes in the pharmacist's role within the hospital setting, the number of highly skilled technicians needed has increased. Pharmacists once prepared all intravenous antibiotics, chemotherapy drugs, and large-volume parenteral medications in addition to other inpatient tasks. Because of the increase in patient volume and the need for pharmacy interventions and evaluations as they pertain to patient profiles, today's pharmacists do not have time to perform many of the important tasks they did in the past. Technicians have assumed control of these tasks, which include preparing intravenous medications, loading patient medication drawers, and entering patient data into the pharmacy computer systems. This chapter will outline the daily tasks of a pharmacy technician, list the various areas or departments of a hospital that require medication supply from the pharmacy, and describe **The Joint Commission (TJC)** standards relevant to pharmacy and medication use. As the health care industry continues to change and improve, so will the vital roles required of pharmacy technicians as they strive to provide improved health care services.

Types of Hospitals

Depending on the function of the hospital (facility), patient populations vary. The size of a hospital may be thought of as the number of beds available for patient use. Many small cities or towns may have small facilities with a bed capacity of 50 or less. Larger urban areas have facilities that can range from 50 beds to more than 250 beds. Other factors that differentiate hospitals from one another are their capabilities for diagnosis, surgery, and outpatient services. For instance, many hospitals do not have computed tomography (CT) scanners, which are large and expensive; patients needing computed tomography scans are sent to another hospital to have procedures performed or diagnostic examinations done.

Another important difference between hospitals is the organization of their pharmacies. Many older hospitals may have one central inpatient pharmacy that is responsible for supplying the entire hospital and all clinics. Larger hospitals or those with specialized areas may have a central pharmacy and smaller **satellite pharmacies** located at various points throughout the facility. For instance, a large teaching facility may have specialized areas of treatment such as pediatrics, burn units, intensive care units, and cancer units. Because of the large volume and specialty of the medications needed for these areas, these units may have small pharmacies that stock specific medications; this practice can accelerate the distribution of commonly used medications.

Hospitals are funded by various entities. Health insurance companies and Medicare pay for services in many institutions; others are funded by donation, for example, Shriners Hospitals for Children. These institutions treat children who cannot afford treatment in mainstream hospitals. Other institutions are managed completely by the government, for example, state mental institutions. Listed in Table 10-1 are hospital facilities and types of pharmacy layouts.

Hospital Pharmacy Standards and Procedures

POLICIES AND PROCEDURES

All pharmacies have a policies and procedures (P & P) handbook—policies outline the rules of the facility and procedures explain how, when, and/or why the policies are to be executed, in other words the protocol of the facility. These

TABLE 10-1 **Example of Various Sizes and Types of Hospitals**

Types of Hospitals	Bed Capacity	Usually One Pharmacy	Central Pharmacy and Satellites	Each Pharmacy Independent from One Another	Type of Care Given
Small	25-50	X			Limited, minor surgeries; critical care is temporary
Medium-sized	50-100	X			Most surgeries, a coronary care unit and an intensive care unit
Large	100	X	X	X	Treats most conditions; physical therapy, intensive care unit, coronary care unit; may have specialty areas such as burn or pediatric units
Teaching	100	X	X	X	Covers all conditions and has specialty areas for teaching purposes; trains medical physicians and other health care providers
Institutional	10-100	X		X	Care ranges from treating severe emergencies to continuing treatment but also may include triage to a larger facility that specializes in a particular area; found in institutions such as prisons and mental facilities
Convalescent or long-term care	100	X			Depending on type of convalescent home, level of care given may vary; some patients are sent to a hospital for surgery and recovery, and then are sent back to their main resident home

Tech Note!

All pharmacy employees are responsible for knowing the policies and procedures (P & P) of the pharmacy in which they are employed. During your externship, be sure to familiarize yourself with the specific rules and regulations of the pharmacy by reading the materials contained in the P & P binder.

rules apply to all pharmacy employees. For example, information contained in the P & P binder concerns daily work routines and responsibilities, benefits, protocols for emergency situations, mandatory training, and other important and useful information. Technicians should be familiar with the P & P handbook of their facility.

HOSPITAL PROTOCOL

Protocol also defines the guidelines within the hospital setting, such as the **formulary** (medications that are approved for use) and **non-formulary** medications (those not approved). These rules must be enforced and updated constantly. A committee composed of pharmacists, physicians, nurses, other health care workers, and administrators meets on a routine basis to discuss appropriate changes to the protocol. The purpose of the committee is to choose the best medicine for patients at the best cost. A drug education coordinator is a pharmacist who helps educate the health care providers about the changes in protocol

Tech Note!

The abbreviation **NKA** means no known allergies, while the abbreviation **NKDA** indicates no known drug allergies. Both of these abbreviations are used in pharmacy and by hospital personnel. Allergy information and any other previous history of a serious adverse drug event must be entered into the computer system before any medications can be released to the nursing floors; this information includes any specific allergies to foods, dyes, preservatives, or inactive ingredients, because these allergies may also pertain to medications. The proper recording of this information helps to ensure that no preventable allergic or untoward reactions take place in the patient.

concerning drug coverage and also assists the hospital pharmacy in implementing these changes. Not all hospitals have the extra help needed to perform these duties; sometimes the tasks of the drug education coordinator may be part of the job description of staff pharmacists or the pharmacy manager.

HOSPITAL STANDARDS

All hospitals must meet federal and state guidelines if they are to be reimbursed for patients who have Medicare or Medicaid insurance coverage. Various agencies, such as the U.S. Department of Health and Human Services, ensure that hospitals meet all standards of safe operation. Each state's board of pharmacy may inspect pharmacies to guarantee that all personnel are working within legal guidelines. The board has the authority to fine, and even close, any pharmacy noncompliant with current laws.

The following are some of the agencies that govern the operations of hospitals:

- **The Joint Commission (TJC).** Hospitals pay a fee for TJC accreditation. This inspection is completed every 3 years and is conducted over a 2-day period. The Joint Commission inspects only hospital pharmacies, not community pharmacies, as well as the entire hospital.
- Health Care Financing Administration (HCFA). Programs include Medicare, Medicaid, and the Health Insurance Portability and Accountability Act (see Chapter 13).
- Department of Health and Human Services (HHS). This department is the primary agency that protects the health of the American people and also provides services. This agency includes more than 300 programs and is linked to the Health Care Financing Administration and Medicare and Medicaid standards.
- State board of pharmacy (BOP). Each state's BOP develops, implements, and enforces pharmacy practice standards in that state for the purpose of protecting the public.

Hospital Orders

FLOW OF ORDERS

When a physician visits a patient in the hospital and writes medication orders for the patient, the orders are equivalent to a prescription. Figure 10-1 illustrates a visual representation of the flow of orders. The order is written on a physician's order sheet and is placed in the patient's chart (Figure 10-2). The chart is a record that contains all of the medical orders written by medical staff, along with nursing assessments and notes, medication administration records, lab results and other vital information regarding the patient's admission. The chart remains in the patient care area where the patient is admitted. The unit clerk or nurse periodically checks all records for new orders that need to be sent to various areas of the hospital. These include dietary restrictions to be sent to the dietary department, laboratory test requests to be sent to the laboratory, and orders for medications to be sent to the pharmacy. The physician, nurse, or unit clerk must include all the necessary information on the patient's admitting record and subsequent medication orders to ensure that the orders are filled correctly. This includes the patient's full name, date of birth, medical record number, room number, diagnosis, weight, and, of course, drug allergies.

Some hospital pharmacies are not open 24 hours a day or on weekends or holidays, while others are open all day, 365 days of the year. For those that are not staffed by pharmacy personnel at all times, there are contingent policies and

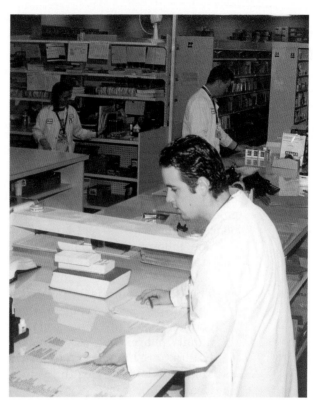

FIGURE 10-1 The flow of orders. As orders arrive, they are entered into the computer. If an order is unclear or if there is a question, the pharmacist contacts the physician.

UNIVERSITY HOSPITAL AND MEDICAL CENTER

PHYSICIAN ORDER SHEET

Patient name: *Jonathan Simmons*
Medical Record Number: *88454959 - 2*
Physician: *Dr. Cynthia Gardella*

Medication or Patient Treatment

- Press firmly using a ball point pen
- White copy remains in patient record. Fax copy to pharmacy
- Do not enter antibiotics or TPN orders on this sheet

Date	Time	
6/23/2011	10²⁰ A	V.O. Dr. Gardella → C. Kipton, RN
		Percocet 5mg. tabs
		ĩ ĩ po Q 4 hrs for pain
		C. Kipton, RN 10²² A

FIGURE 10-2 Example of a physician's order. Note the medical record number in place of a prescription number. Also, the patient's room number and allergies should be listed (not shown). (From Elkin MK, Perry AG, Potter PA: *Nursing interventions and clinical skills*, ed 4, St Louis, 2007, Elsevier.)

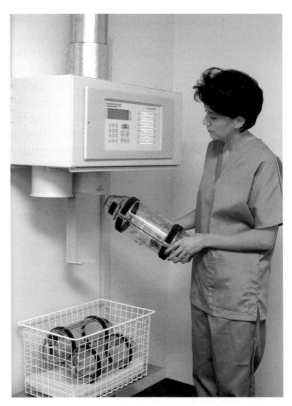

FIGURE 10-3 Pneumatic tube system. A pneumatic tube system is used to transport orders to the pharmacy and medications to hospital floors. (Courtesy of Swisslog Healthcare Solutions, 2011.)

regulations that allow specific nursing personnel to have limited inpatient pharmacy access to obtain needed medications. In other facilities, an "on-call" pharmacist may provide the necessary services in times of less than full operation. Still other pharmacies may have off-site pharmacies that will provide courier services to deliver needed orders.

Various methods are used to send orders to the pharmacy. One device is a pneumatic tube system that allows a person to send orders and other small items by way of an air-propelled tube. In this system, cylindrical canisters can carry intravenous bags and other medications to the hospital floor (Figure 10-3). A disadvantage of this system is that the tube can get jammed easily or by accident be sent to the incorrect department. Also, fragile items, such as those encased in glass; controlled substances; expensive medications; or protein-derived medications should not be sent via the pneumatic tube system because they can break during the rough ride or become lost in the system. Another way of receiving orders is via fax machine. Although the fax machine is an effective way to send orders to the pharmacy quickly, often the quality of the fax can cause a delay in filling the order. Pharmacists need to verify all unreadable orders over the phone or have the order faxed again. **Computerized physician order entry (CPOE)** is a new technology being implemented that sends the medication order electronically to the pharmacy.

Other methods of obtaining physicians' orders include the use of staff to deliver the orders to the pharmacy. This normally is done when a system breaks down, such as the pneumatic tube system, or if the facility is extremely small.

Once the orders are received in the pharmacy, they need to be processed in the same way that a regular prescription is processed. However, instead of using the name, address, and phone number for identification, the pharmacy uses the patient's medical record number. Even though this method is the primary way patients are identified, all information, including name and room number, should always be verified against the order. In this way, errors are decreased, especially when two patients with the same last name are on the same floor. The pharmacy uses name alert stickers that are placed on the patient's drawer and medication when two patients have the same last name and are on the same floor. Many computer systems also have name alert functions to help distinguish between patients with similar identifying characteristics.

Most computer systems allow pharmacy technicians to enter the patient's medical record number and drug orders. In many hospitals the pharmacist enters the order because if the information is entered by the technician, it must be checked by the pharmacist to ensure accuracy before a label is released. Many pharmacists believe that the work is doubled if the technician enters an order and then the pharmacist must reread and approve the order. As the orders are signed off, labels are produced from a printer that has the patient's name, medical record number, and room number along with the medication information. The name of the drug, strength, dosage form, route of administration, dose, quantity and dosing interval are included on printed labels. Because the labels are being produced continually, the technician usually pulls them off the printer and fills the order from the unit dose (UD) pick station. A variety of medication and dosage forms are always kept in stock for starter doses and for medications not stocked in automated dispensing systems (ADS).

Patient drug labels are usually placed on small plastic baggies so that medications can be checked visibly against the label by the pharmacist before they are placed in a pneumatic tube or taken to the patient's floor. Some orders that are sent to pharmacy have "at once" (stat) or "as soon as possible" (ASAP) stamped or written on the order. These orders need to be filled immediately because they are ordered in this manner only when an emergency situation exists. If the order has any discrepancies it is the pharmacist's responsibility to contact either the nurse or the physician caring for the patient. Once the orders have been cleared they are then entered, verified, and sent.

Standing orders are written protocols for drugs or treatment that are to be used in a specific situation. For example, if a procedure is to be performed, a preprinted order with the list of medications to be administered is on file for the physician to use. This saves the physician from having to write the same order each time he or she performs the procedure. This includes orders for **prn** (as-needed) drugs that can be given in case the patient needs additional medication. A standing order may have a variety of prn medications with dosage forms, routes of administration, and dosing times that only needs the physician's checkmark and signature.

POINT OF ENTRY (POE)

The published reports from many drug error prevention studies are responsible for a complete revamping of order entry. According to the 2006 Institute of Medicine report *Preventing Medication Errors,* it was estimated that 1.5 million preventable medication errors occur annually in the United States alone. Many of these errors were found to be preventable. One major change that could counteract errors would be the implementation of electronic systems that can quickly and clearly transfer patient information to and from the pharmacy. **Point of entry** systems provide electronic access to medical information and drug information data and allow physicians, nurses, and pharmacists to directly communicate to one another, limiting errors of transcription. Systems used include computerized physician order entry, IV smart pumps for infusible medications, computerized adverse drug event monitoring (CADM), and bar code point of entry (BPOE) medication systems. These systems are a technological step above the previous systems called computer on wheels (COWs), which are computers on stands that are located at the bedside of the patient. These new systems are mainly used in specialty units such as ICUs, where it is important that the nurse stay in close proximity to the patient. However, their abilities are limited because they do not have bar code reading abilities and are much larger than handheld devices.

COMPUTERIZED PHYSICIAN ORDER ENTRY (CPOE)

Although this technology is still in its infancy and is not used in every hospital, it is becoming more popular because it eliminates the need to decipher physicians' handwriting and the order is sent safely to the pharmacy for processing via computer entry. It is estimated that approximately 27% of hospitals use CPOE (Health Information Management System Society, 2007). Medication orders can be clearly identified, and the computer systems check new medications against current medications for interactions or contraindications. If there is a possibility of an interaction, the computer will show an alert icon on the screen and the order cannot proceed until the problem is resolved. The systems may also check for proper dosage selection based on patient parameters and diagnoses. Physicians can enter all lab results, dietary requirements, medications, and special notes in the computer, therefore having all the patients' information accessible to them at one time. Medication orders are sent directly to the pharmacy, eliminating the possibility of a lost order.

BAR CODE POINT OF ENTRY (BPOE)

Nurses are now electronically connected to the pharmacy ordering process through the use of bar codes. The nurse can ensure accuracy of medication dosages at the patient's bedside before any medications are given. Each unit dosed medication is bar coded and can be scanned with a handheld device. Information is linked to pharmacy and to **electronic medication administration record** (E-MAR) systems. The nurse is alerted to any special notes or warnings as each dose is verified for the patient. If there is any discrepancy between the current orders and the medications sent for the patient, it is detected by the scanner and the nurse is alerted to the specific problem. For example: A medication is sent to the floor for administration, the nurse scans the tablet's bar code, and the BPOE system informs the nurse that the order has been discontinued. An error has been averted.

Orders are sent to the nurse in "real time" on the nurse's handheld device, along with any notes. Once the order is sent to the nurse, it must be verified before administration. If there is a discrepancy, the nurse is able to send a note to the pharmacy for clarification. This constant communication between nursing and pharmacy ultimately benefits patient care. The interaction between the nurse and the E-MAR is useful because the patient's vital signs and other chart notes can be entered from the bedside directly onto the E-MAR. For example, the patient's blood pressure, respiration rate, and pain levels can be entered. The nurse's ability to check on dosages at the patient's bedside helps to ensure the five rights of medication safety (see Chapter 7), reduces the time required for charting, and creates less paperwork, so the nurse can spend more time attending to the patient.

COMPUTERIZED ADVERSE DRUG EVENT MONITORING (CADM)

These are computerized systems that detect and monitor adverse drug events. Although pharmacy has used this type of system for years, it is now being integrated into the CPOE and electronic health record (EHR). This allows for a more comprehensive health care practice.

The overall change using these new systems is not without problems. Pharmacy must make sure all medications are bar coded for identification, and the information in the computer must accurately reflect the way the dosage form is to be given. Usual workflow of personnel is often impacted and must be adjusted to accommodate the new technologies. Training pharmacists, physicians, and nurses to use these electronic systems is a large task and must be continually analyzed for accuracy and interactions between systems already in place. Most people find major changes in their daily routine very hard to accept; therefore it is important to implement a system that is not too difficult to use. More hospitals are implementing these systems as new versions are being developed for ease of use and accuracy.

Responsibilities of an Institutional Technician

Pharmacy technicians must have many skills in today's pharmacy; because the roles of pharmacists are continually expanding, so must the roles of the pharmacy technician. Because pharmacists have more interaction with the proper dosing of medications and implementation of formulary, the pharmacy technician completes many of the daily tasks that otherwise would require a pharmacist. The inpatient pharmacy has many different functions that depend mostly on the size of the hospital and number of pharmacies in operation. Many hospitals have 24-hour pharmacies. Technicians need to be flexible to work all shifts, including holidays. They also need to be multifunctional because there are usually half as many technicians and pharmacists employed during night and weekend shifts in most hospital pharmacies. However, the patient load may remain the same or even increase during these times. Therefore it is essential that the technician be able to perform all of the functions necessary for all shifts.

Table 10-2 outlines some of the more common pharmacy job descriptions. Because hospital pharmacies need to be staffed year-round, it is important to have employees who can function in all areas. As a technician learns more skills throughout the pharmacy, he or she becomes more valuable.

PATIENT CASSETTE DRAWERS

One of the most long-standing daily tasks of a technician is loading the patient cassette drawer from a pick station. These stations within the pharmacy can be quite extensive in size depending upon the hospital needs. All unit dosed (UD) medications are arranged in order by generic name and are located in sections that separate solid oral dosage forms, liquids, suppositories, and other miscellaneous types of medication containers. Even though pick stations can hold many medications, there are patients that may require medications that must be taken from the normal stock area, such as injectable dosage forms.

Once the starter dose has been sent to the floor, the medications that will be needed for the next day must be loaded in a cassette drawer. The technician will read the daily medication record printed each morning and fill the necessary medications into the cassettes. Normally, routine medications are placed in these drawers in the front while as-needed (prn) doses are put in the back separated by a divider. Routine medications are those that are taken on a schedule every day, whereas prn medications are those that can be taken only if needed. For example, most acetaminophen (Tylenol) is ordered as-needed for headache or fever.

The patient cassette drawers are held in large push carts so they may be delivered to the floor each day. All medications are delivered to the patient floors using two carts that are rotated daily. Before the patients' drawers are loaded with the next 24-hour supply, all previous medications should be emptied from the drawer. This is to decrease the possibility of errors. Many hospitals use both

TABLE 10-2 Common Job Descriptions

Technician Responsibilities	Description
IV room	Prepares all parenteral intravenous preparations, including large-volume drips and parenteral nutrition; prepares drugs that are under investigational trial and logs these special medications in appropriate manner as required by law.
Chemotherapy	Prepares cytotoxic agents and other medications that may accompany these agents.
Controlled substances	Gathers all controlled substance inventory sheets from all areas of hospital; technician also may fill and deliver all controlled substances; pharmacist is required to verify pharmacy inventory daily.
Patient medication	Fills medication drawers on a pharmacy cart that will deliver filling medications to all hospital patients; also may deliver carts to all patient areas and restock any floor stock medications; if hospital uses an automated medication dispensing system instead, technician will need to fill this unit on all floors; fills prescriptions for patients who will be discharged on an as-needed basis.
Preparation of medication	Fills unit-dosing bulk medications; compounds drugs such as for ointments, creams, and solutions.
Filling requisitions	Fills all requisitions sent to pharmacy; stocks inventory; orders pharmacy stock; controls narcotics inventory, and audits narcotics if required; transports medications throughout hospital facility.
Inventory	Orders all medications and supplies for pharmacy; also may order specialty items for other areas of hospital; handles all returns and recalled items that need to be sent back to manufacturer; responsible for handling all invoices and for putting all stock in appropriate bins; rotates stock, performs nursing floor inspections, and inspects other pharmacy supply areas for outdated drugs and inventory levels; restocks these areas if necessary; this may include the operating room, postoperative area, preoperative area, and other sterile areas.
Discharge pharmacy	Fills prescription orders as patients are discharged from hospital; medications are sent to the floor for patients, or patients may come to the pharmacy window to pick up medications.
Satellite pharmacy	May be responsible for all tasks related to a small, isolated pharmacy, such as answering phones, ordering and putting away stock, preparing parenteral medications, transcribing, pulling all medication orders, and making deliveries to nursing stations.
Miscellaneous duties	Ability to work in all areas of the pharmacy as needed; answers phones, trains new technicians and pharmacist interns; works on a team with other technicians, clerks, and pharmacists.

patient cassette drawers and automated dispensing systems (discussed in next section). Commonly used medications are stocked in the automated machines while specialty or uncommon medication dosages are loaded in the cassettes.

Another type of automated system used by large hospital pharmacies is the robot-dispensing machine. This machine uses mechanical arms to scan bar codes on each unit dosed medication to identify the correct dose. (Dose information is fed into the machine by computer input from the pharmacist or technician.) The machine fills each patient's medication cassette with 99% accuracy as the cassette moves along a conveyer belt. Once the medication is filled, the cassette is delivered by the technician, who will return the previous day's cassette for the next day's filling.

Although some hospitals still use solely the patient cassette system, more facilities are implementing automated dispensing systems and robotics. These systems accelerate delivery of medication to the patient and also help to ensure accuracy. Automated floor dispensing systems used in hospital settings include

Pyxis and **SureMed**. Both Pyxis and SureMed are machines that are preloaded with a variety of commonly used medications located on the nursing floor. The pharmacist needs only to enter the order and verify it; then the nurse can retrieve the medication on the patient's floor by using a thermal fingerprint for access. Although these systems seem to replace the need for technicians, they require constant filling and updating of new medications daily. Technicians now are trained properly to use these sophisticated dispensing systems to fill patient prescriptions and to complete many other pharmacy duties.

PREPARING UNIT DOSE MEDICATIONS

Another important daily task technicians perform is the preparation of unit dose medications that are not available from the manufacturer or stocked by the pharmacy. Although there are many premade unit dose containers available from manufacturers, not all drugs are available in UD form. In other cases, the hospital may prefer to make their own unit dose packaging because it can be less expensive and the hospital can make specific amounts to lessen waste.

Technicians are responsible for determining which medications need to be made based on the utilization of stock by patients, documenting all necessary information per protocol, and preparing the doses. The final check is done by the pharmacist. Bulk bottles of medication are pulled from stock shelves and made into UD oral syringes and other dosage forms. There are many different types of methods and machines that can aid in their preparation (see Chapter 11). Only those medications that are used on a regular basis are made into UDs. For uncommon medication orders or dosage strengths, the technician must prepare individual dosages as a patient need arises.

Unit Dose Liquids

In the past, bulk liquid items were sent to the floor for several days' use. For example, if a physician ordered Mylanta 15 mL 5 times daily, the pharmacy would send an 8-oz bottle that would stay on the patient's floor until empty. This minimized the need to place several UD cups in a small cassette drawer. As a result of new standards implemented to decrease drug errors (see Chapter 14), The Joint Commission now requires hospitals to make all medications patient-dose specific. This requires every liquid dose to be prepared in a unit dose package and labeled before sending it to the patient's room. A hospital may have a separate room dedicated for preparing all the oral liquid medications and use oral syringes to prepare each dose. Other pharmacies may make all their own unit dose cups from their bulk stock; this would be done by a technician following repackaging guidelines outlined in Chapter 11. If unit dose cups are made, this increases the need to prepare each oral dose in an oral dose syringe.

CONTROLLED SUBSTANCES

Description

The task of counting, dispensing, and tracking controlled substances is a critical job that requires perfection. Many hospitals utilize pharmacy technicians to restock and fill narcotics for the entire hospital. Within each hospital unit that stocks controlled substances, two nurses must conduct an actual count at the change of every shift. Therefore all controlled substances are counted 2 or 3 times daily depending on the length of a nursing shift. One nurse counts the controlled substances while the other nurse confirms the count on the controlled substance sheet or on the automated dispensing system (ADS) record. If the narcotics are documented on paper, the count is transferred to a new inventory sheet each morning, and the last day's sheet is sent to the pharmacy for filing. **Periodic automatic replenishment (PAR)** levels are written at the top of the controlled substance sheets and list the amounts of medications that should be kept on the floor at all times. Often the technician is responsible for retrieving these sheets daily from all units and beginning assessment of how many controlled substances of various sizes and strengths must be provided to keep the unit at or close to its PAR level. If ADS machines are used a PAR list is generated daily that records the current count of narcotics. Narcotics that are not being used may be returned to the pharmacy at the time of delivery.

In the pharmacy, controlled substances normally are kept in a locked room or vault, which may be under surveillance. All written records must be in pen, and all inventories must be ultimately verified by a registered pharmacist.

For narcotic deliveries or returns, no counter signature is required because the ADS unit will keep track of all added or deleted stock. This takes the place of the counter signature. All additions or deletions are documented by the ADS machine, which shows who opened the cabinet, when the cabinet was opened, and in what drawer the additions or deletions were made. The technician must count first, then add or remove items, and then recount afterwards. Only one type of narcotic dose form is allowed per drawer container. The stock is put into the ADS and a receipt is printed. This verification receipt is then taken to the pharmacy and kept in the narcotic count area. All narcotics must be checked by a pharmacist before leaving the pharmacy and a counter signature will be needed when returning stock to the narcotic cabinet along with the receipt from the ADS machine.

Duties

Each hospital has its own system for delivering controlled substances, but one of the most important aspects is to keep the controlled substances nonidentifiable. For example, those hospitals without an ADS system might place controlled substances in brown paper bags that are stapled shut; most persons would never know that controlled substances are being delivered in this type of container. Even so, the pharmacy technician should never let these controlled substances out of sight when delivering them throughout the hospital. Other hospitals may have lock boxes for their narcotic delivery. After the technician has confirmed the pharmacy-controlled substances' count for the day, he or she must sign out each drug onto a dispensing sheet that is used to deliver the controlled substances, which is confirmed by the pharmacist. A pharmacist must verify all final counts, and monthly or bimonthly inventories are taken depending on state regulations.

All controlled substances are signed into the nursing department by adding them onto the controlled substances' sheet. The addition or return of stock must be observed by the pharmacy technician and the nurse. All controlled substances then must be countersigned onto or off the pharmacy inventory sheet by both the technician and the nurse. The actual counting of the current levels of controlled substances should be performed by the nurse and pharmacy technician to verify all existing controlled substances before adding additional ones into stock. In addition to delivering controlled substances, the technician may be asked by the nurse to return certain substances to the pharmacy. The same validation system is used to enter onto the pharmacy inventory sheet those drugs that are to be returned to the pharmacy. Only registered nurses, not licensed practical nurses, can sign in controlled substances.

An ADS machine verifies the count as the technician enters the narcotic to be added. An electronic record is maintained that includes the time the drawer was accessed, the name of the person accessing the drawer, the count before opening the drawer, the amount added or deleted, and the final count.

Upon return to the pharmacy, all controlled substances must be signed back into the pharmacy stock. This normally is done by a technician and verified by a pharmacist. One of the most important parts of this job is to verify that all numbers are correct. The pharmacist must never sign in controlled substances without first visually counting the existing and returned stock.

Narcotics are normally filed in stock under their generic name and by their schedule. All controlled substances are confined in the same area. Binders may be used to keep inventory of each drug. As stock is removed, the amount is taken off the inventory sheet and the remainder must be counted and correct. Certain scheduled drugs are also stored in a refrigerator, and in the pharmacy a small refrigerator is often kept within the locked room or vault for this purpose. Nursing units have a lock box in their medication refrigerator for scheduled drugs.

DAILY IV PREPARATION DUTIES

At the beginning of the day and evening shifts, all intravenous labels representing all current orders are printed from the computer system. Throughout the day, intravenous medication information is added or deleted as new medication orders arrive in the pharmacy. All changes in intravenous medication information are kept updated by the technician and the pharmacist who work in the intravenous room. Normally, while the technician labels all premade intravenous antibiotics and other intravenous medications, the pharmacist answers the phones and enters new and changed orders. Pharmacists are also responsible for contacting the nurse or physician if there is a problem with an order. For example, if an order is sent to the pharmacy for ampicillin/sulbactam (Unasyn) and the patient has an allergy to penicillin, the pharmacist contacts the physician and asks the physician to substitute this antibiotic with one that will not cause an allergic reaction in the patient.

Orders in an inpatient pharmacy are affected by the time of day. For example, in the early morning there may be several preoperative (pre-op) medications ordered and later in the morning postoperative (post-op) medications may be ordered for surgical patients. Also, more diagnostic exams are performed in the morning or afternoon hours than in the evening. Medications that are required for these diagnostic tests must usually be sent by pharmacy.

The pharmacy technician is responsible for stocking the intravenous room with all of the supplies needed for the day. The technician also must make sure that the work area stays clean. Usually the same technician prepares all intravenous medications, and then at the end of the shift, he or she delivers them to the nursing floors. When the intravenous medications are delivered to the nursing stations, the unused intravenous medications are returned to the pharmacy. If they have not expired, they are placed in the refrigerator or back into stock for future use; otherwise, they are logged and wasted. Because each intravenous preparation must be registered and justified, most pharmacies keep a binder or book in which information about all wasted intravenous preparations is written. The technician must remember that it is important to complete all tasks before the end of the shift and to replace all stock items as much as possible for the next shift.

Aseptic Technique
Aseptic technique is a method to prevent contamination of an object by microorganisms. The use of this technique is important in preparing all intravenous medications, intravenous nutrition solutions, chemotherapy products, and compounded ophthalmic medications. All technicians must be tested periodically on the proper guidelines of aseptic technique, which usually is done by management at the yearly evaluation. Samples normally are taken from a newly prepared parenteral medication and are sent to the laboratory for testing, or kits may be used to test on site. This testing is completed to ensure that microbial contamination is not present in medications that must be sterile. To learn more about bacteria and harmful microbes, see Chapter 30.

USP <797>

All facilities dispensing sterile products must now meet enforceable regulations according to the ***United States Pharmacopeia (USP <797>)***. Previously these were guidelines that were suggested for the preparation of all sterile products, but they were not enforced. As a result of the increase in drug contamination and medication errors, a higher rating was given to these guidelines, and they are now enforced through The Joint Commission on-site visits as a part of TJC standards. Aseptic technique and *USP <797>* regulations are discussed in detail in Chapter 12.

IV TECH

Description

An IV tech is responsible for the preparation of various parenteral medications. This includes antibiotics; large-volume drips such as heparin, aminophylline, and potassium infusions; and other parenteral medication orders. Some hospital pharmacies are responsible only for the large volumes of intravenous medications that need to be prepared with special additives; the nurses on the floor maintain a floor stock of premade, large-volume bags that can be supplied by central supply or by the pharmacy. Typical antibiotics and other IV admixtures can be prepared in a horizontal laminar flow hood after donning proper attire consisting of gloves, gown, cap, and shoe covers. Many hospitals cannot convert their compounding areas to *USP <797>* standards; therefore they have begun to contract out their bulk of IVs to *USP <797>* certified compounding pharmacies. The policies vary from hospital to hospital.

Horizontal laminar flow hoods are cabinets that direct filtered air horizontally toward the opening of the cabinet, which provides a sterile environment for preparing parenteral medications (Figure 10-4). There are other types of hoods, such as partially covered vertical hoods and biological safety cabinets (BSCs). Each type meets specific requirements within the environment. For more information on flow hoods and their uses, see Chapter 12.

CHEMOTHERAPY PREPARATION

Description

The hospital technician may be responsible for preparing chemotherapeutic medications. The same aseptic techniques are used in preventing contamination when preparing any parenteral medication. However, a few differences between the intravenous and chemotherapy environments should be noted.

A horizontal flow hood is used for preparing nonchemotherapeutic intravenous medications. When working inside the horizontal flow hood, the orientation of the hands must not block the airflow. This means that hands cannot be moved behind the vial, needle, or intravenous bag. In addition, there is only one high-efficiency particulate air (HEPA) filter located at the back of the hood.

Class II vertical flow hoods (partially open-front) are used to prepare chemotherapeutic agents (Figure 10-5). The air is pulled down toward the tabletop filter, from the ceiling of the hood that contains the first HEPA filter. The chemotherapy hood does not allow the air to leave the container compartment; instead, the air is recycled through a second HEPA filter that removes any particulate matter before the air is recirculated into the work environment. The flow of air vertically helps protect the person preparing the agents from unwanted exposure. To maintain sufficient airflow, hands should not move over or above the items in the vertical flow hood. In addition, technicians must wear a gown, cap, shoe covers, and double gloves (latex or nonlatex) or special chemical-safe gloves (nitrile or neoprene rubber and polyurethane) within a class II vertical flow hood.

Tech Alert!

Safe practices recommend that gloves used to prepare chemotherapeutic agents should not be worn more than 30 minutes. Hands must always be washed before and after removal of gloves. In addition, gloves should be worn when handling or performing inventory of chemotherapeutic agents.

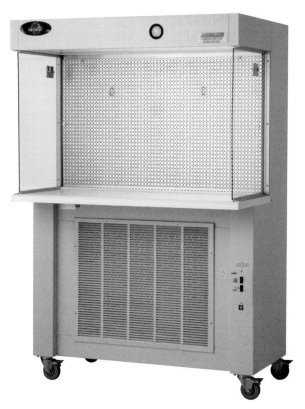

FIGURE 10-4 Airegard 301 (Horizontal Laminar Flowhood Clean Bench). (Courtesy of NuAire, Inc., 2011.)

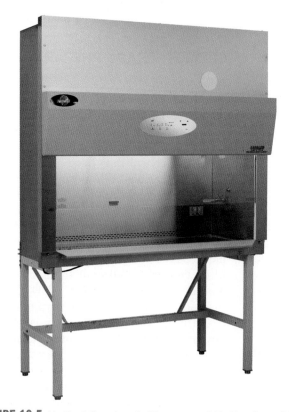

FIGURE 10-5 Vertical flow hood. (Courtesy of NuAire, Inc., 2011.)

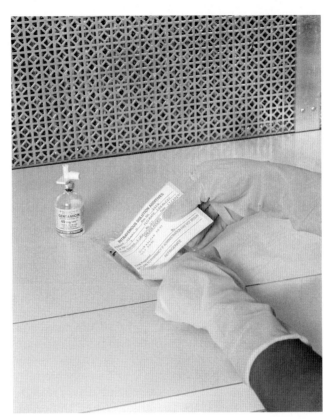

FIGURE 10-6 Proper placement of labels on parenteral solutions.

Tech Alert!

Gloves must be surface cleaned before wiping down the final preparation, placing the label on the preparation, and moving the preparation to the pass-through area for removal from the sterile parenteral preparation room. The inner pair of gloves (used when preparing chemotherapeutic agents) is used to affix labels and place the agent into a sealable containment bag for transport and must be done within the BSC. In addition, a new pair of gloves must be donned before handling the completed preparation, to avoid any unwanted exposure to the agent by yourself or others.

LABELING

Description

The proper placement of labels is important to ensure visibility of the parenteral solution and contents (Figure 10-6). All labels must be placed squarely onto the medication and should be clear and easy to read.

The technician must initial all medications even if the label is being placed on a premade bag. Before intravenous piggybacks and drips are delivered to the appropriate floors, the pharmacist must check each medication and countersign with his or her initials. Labels usually contain the same type of information regardless of the facility. In addition to labeling parenteral medications, the technician must be aware of additional information, such as medications that need to be placed in light-protected bags and those requiring refrigeration. The technician must know the storage requirements and the stability of the medications he or she prepares.

All drugs must be labeled before they leave the pharmacy. The required parts of a label include the patient's name, patient's medical record number and room number, name of the drug, strength of the medication, name of the solution with which the medication was mixed, and the rate of infusion. The pharmacy technician must check this information several times before he or she applies the label to the medication. Additional information contained on a label includes the time the dose should be given, the date, and the expiration date. Expiration dates are important because many intravenous preparations are returned to stock if not expired. Many pharmacies use the Julian date. This is the day of the year that does not take into account the month. For instance, if the day is February 1, the Julian date is 32 because it is the 32nd day of the year (January has 31 days plus February 1 equals 32). Determination of the expiration date from the Julian date is much easier because it is not necessary to remember how many days are in a particular month. When IVs are delivered to the floor the technician checks the remaining IVs for unused medications. If the IV was not used it is picked up by the pharmacy at the time of the daily IV delivery and returned to stock for later use. Those that have expired will be logged into a logbook. The IV will be emptied (normally into the sink, unless the drug is a potential environmental hazard or biohazard) and the Viaflex bag disposed in the garbage. Viaflex bags are made of flexible polyvinyl chloride (PVC). The technician should always be familiar with the disposal regulations of the facility before emptying any medications into sewage systems.

INVENTORY CONTROL TECHNICIAN

Description

Most hospitals have a technician who is in charge of maintaining stock levels and completing the special ordering of medications. The technician who orders the stock is responsible for the actual ordering, billing, and restocking of the pharmacy shelves; however, it takes a group effort in the pharmacy to maintain stock levels and avoid having to borrow items from another hospital or special-order them at a higher cost. Many methods of keeping stock at necessary levels are available. Before today's electronic stocking methods were employed, a hospital pharmacy had ordering cards that were used to reorder stock when it was low. Each person was responsible for pulling the card (normally kept with the medications) and placing it in a designated area where the inventory technician could place the order. When the order arrived, the card was put back into the box along with the new stock. The electronic stocking method typically used today employs a handheld device that reads bar codes for electronic ordering. In this case, the inventory technician must check visually to see what medications need to be ordered. A third method of stocking requires each item to be tagged with a manufacturer's sticker as it arrives in the pharmacy. Stickers are provided by the manufacturer and must be affixed to each item before it is placed on the shelf. This sticker lists the stock number of the medication along with the price. When an item needs to be reordered, the sticker is taken off the container and placed on an ordering sheet; it is then entered into an electronic device for transmission by phone or by online ordering.

Medications, devices, and other pharmacy supplies are available from various sources:

- Prime vendors are large distributors of various medications and retail products to pharmacies. A contract outlining cost, delivery dates, return policies, and payment schedule is made between the pharmacy and the distributor, usually requiring the pharmacy to order medications through their specific company. Even with the additional percentage fee that is added for this type of supplier, there can be a substantial savings to the pharmacy. Examples of prime vendors include AmerisourceBergen, McKesson, Total Pharmacy Supply, and Cardinal Health.
- Wholesalers are companies that stock a variety of drug manufacturers' medications and normally have a "just-in-time" turnaround for ordered drugs. This means the drugs ordered today will arrive tomorrow. This type of ordering is very useful in pharmacies where space is limited for overstock items or the medication is needed by the next day. There is an additional percentage fee that is added onto the shipments but the additional fees can be offset by ordering in bulk, resulting in a substantial savings overall. Examples include HD Smith, Anda, and Cardinal Health.
- Direct manufacturer ordering may be used under certain circumstances. For example, a group of pharmacies may join a group purchasing organization

(GPO) that contracts with the manufacturer for better pricing. The contract is usually based on the quantity ordered and includes specific return policies and conditions. Other reasons for directly ordering from manufacturers include the following: the wholesaler and/or prime vendor does not stock the drug or the drug is not available from the normal source at the time of ordering; the medication may only be available to select patients who meet certain treatment parameters (for example, FDA regulations or investigational protocols). In this case, the manufacturer records and verifies the information before sending the medication for the specific patient. Examples of drug manufacturers include Abbott Laboratories, Bristol-Myers Squibb Co., Janssen Pharmaceuticals, Inc., and Upsher-Smith Laboratories, Inc.

Duties

Every day the pharmacy depletes some of its stock of drugs and supplies. Although pharmacies have different systems of ordering the medications, most orders normally are placed using a computer. Depending on the location of the warehouse or manufacturer, the turnaround time for the shipment may vary. For example, a medication whose supplier is thousands of miles away must be ordered earlier than a medication from the pharmacy's warehouse (which usually takes less than 24 hours). Knowing the right time to order medications is a skill that pharmacy technicians must acquire; it is crucial to keep the pharmacy completely stocked with necessary medications.

When the shipment arrives, all included medications and supplies must be verified against the inventory list; initialing and writing "received" on each invoice are important. Some medications are back-ordered; these items are currently not in stock from the manufacturer but will be sent as soon as they are available. If the medication is one that cannot be left out of stock for any amount of time, it may be necessary to borrow from another pharmacy. This can be done by calling a pharmacist at a neighboring hospital and asking whether that pharmacy has enough to share. A loan/borrow sheet is filled out, and either a taxi or a hospital courier normally is sent to carry the medication from one location to the other. After the original ordered stock arrives, replacements for the borrowed items are then returned to the lending pharmacy.

Placing stock onto the shelves is another important duty of the pharmacy technician; it is the point at which the stock is rotated. Placing medications with later expiration dates farthest back on the shelf ensures that the medications with the earliest expiration dates will be used first. The inventory technician is also responsible for returning damaged items and expired agents and handling recall items following the manufacturer's guidelines. Timing is probably one of the most important aspects of keeping inventory at a constant level. The technician can order appropriately if he or she learns the pharmacy protocol for ordering, compensates for items that take longer to ship, and considers upcoming holidays. Patient load directly relates to the types of medications to be ordered as well. It is a well-known fact that during the winter months hospitals have more patients because more people become ill this time of year. The elderly are especially at risk. Also, certain hospitals have primary functions such as burn centers, rehabilitation, or specific surgeries and their specialties influence the overall increase in the use of medications specific to those patient needs.

Supplying Specialty Areas

In several areas of a hospital the pharmacy must maintain a PAR level of medications. Technicians must recognize each of the abbreviations representing the units and clinics that require medication from the pharmacy. Box 10-1 provides a list of each major area of a hospital. The supplies kept on hand in these units are referred to as floor stock. The technician must be fully aware of the types of

BOX 10-1 EXAMPLES OF PRIMARY UNITS AND AREAS THAT REQUIRE MEDICATION FROM PHARMACY

CCU	Coronary care unit
CLINICS	Patients may visit a clinic to be seen by a physician, physician's assistant, or nurse practitioner
ED or ER	Emergency department; area of hospital where patients can receive emergency care with physicians and nurses on staff 24 hours a day
ICU	Intensive care unit
L&D	Labor and delivery; unit where mother goes through labor and delivers a baby
MED-SURG	Medical unit for patients who have undergone surgery or who may be under observation
NICU	Neonatal intensive care unit; can also stand for neurological intensive care unit
NSY	Nursery; unit where babies are taken for care and observation by nurses
OB/GYN	Obstetrics/gynecology; unit that takes care of expectant mothers or those who have just given birth
ONCOLOGY	Unit that takes care of patients with cancer
OR	Operating room
ORTHO	Orthopedics unit; takes care of patients who may need treatment or surgery on bones or joints
PACU	Postanesthesia care unit
PED	Pediatrics; unit for children younger than age 14 years
POST-OP	Unit where patient is kept after an operation or procedure
PRE-OP	Unit where patient is kept before an operation or procedure
UROLOGY	Unit that takes care of patients who may need treatment, surgery, or procedures on the urinary system

medications used in each of these areas because each unit, ward, or clinic has its own special stock. Because of the special needs of each area, many pharmacies have special forms that are preprinted with complete descriptions of commonly used drugs. This helps to decrease the incidence of stock being sent to the wrong areas within the hospital. The pharmacy normally receives the supply ordering forms from the specialty areas daily. Although they are not a high-priority task, these orders should be filled before the end of the day. In addition, the technician may need to deliver the medications and check various areas of the hospital for any outdated medications. This task should be done monthly, preferably before the end of the month. Outdated medications normally can be returned to the pharmacy if they will expire within 3 months. Expired medications may be returned to the manufacturer for credit (most manufacturers accept returned expired medications in batches of 100) or they may be taken by an independent company and destroyed in a proper manner. This depends on the contract between the hospital and the manufacturer. Also, some hospitals contract an outside company that specializes in drug inventory to visit the pharmacy periodically and document all expired medications before they are destroyed.

Each department—such as pre-op, post-op, the operating room, wards, and clinics—is stocked with specific medications depending on the type of services it provides. Because of the many different areas throughout a hospital, the pharmacy must stock a wide variety of medications in different dosage forms. Therefore the pharmacy technician must have a good understanding of which medications are appropriate for each department. Departments such as the

BOX 10-2 EXAMPLES OF HOSPITAL CODES*

- Code red: Fire
- Code blue: Medical emergency—adult
- Code white: Medical emergency—pediatric
- Code pink: Infant abduction
- Code purple: Child abduction
- Code yellow: Bomb threat
- Code gray: Combative person
- Code silver: Person with a weapon and/or hostage situation
- Code orange: Hazardous material spill/release
- Code triage internal: An internal disaster
- Code triage external: An external disaster

*Codes vary among hospitals.

Tech Alert!

When refilling a crash cart, NEVER assume that the unused drugs left inside the tray are correct. A prime example is the common error between pediatric and adult strengths of lidocaine. Epinephrine is always stocked on a crash cart. Both strengths are packaged in prefilled syringes and appear similar in appearance. *Note the dosages of pediatric (1:100,000 [0.01 mg/mL]) and adult-strength (1:10,000 [0.1 mg/mL]) epinephrine. Placement of adult-dose epinephrine in pediatric trays is a common error. If an adult dose of the medication was filled into a pediatric tray, this could cause death rather than save a life. Always remove all medications and start anew. Following the prepared list, check all the strengths of the medications and the expiration dates.*

emergency department, operating room, and intensive care unit stock many drugs in injectable form and a wide variety of oral and injectable controlled substances. Pediatrics uses many of the same medications that are used in the other departments, except in lower doses, as well as medications that are in special pediatric dosage forms. The labor and delivery department stocks injectables and other drugs used for labor, contractions, and cesarean births. The tasks of collecting and filling all floor stock medications are part of the daily routine of a technician. As always, it is necessary that all orders be verified and initialed by a pharmacist before they can be delivered to the correct departments unless the tech-check-tech process is approved under hospital protocol (see Chapter 3).

Another important pharmacy task is the refilling of **crash carts**. These are trays used by all areas of the hospital. They contain only injectable medications used for a code (respiratory distress) situation. Each hospital has a set of codes, listed in Box 10-2. It is the responsibility of each employee to know the hospital's code names. The naming of the code varies from hospital to hospital. Table 10-3 lists examples of the types of commonly used injectable drugs. Pharmacy stocks extra trays in case of a stat call for another tray. The three types of trays are adult, pediatric, and neonatal. Each type of tray contains a different strength of drug. When a tray has been used, the pharmacy technician will take a new tray, retrieve the used tray, and refill the missing contents. Also at this time the technician checks expiration dates on all medications. These dates are listed on a preprinted form. All crash cart medications should always be placed in the tray in the same order. The familiar order enhances the ability of the nurses or physicians to quickly grab a needed medication. If all crash carts were in a different order, the nurse would have to search for the life-saving medication. As always, it is necessary that all orders be verified and initialed by a pharmacist before they can be delivered to the correct departments. All crash carts are wrapped in a disposable cover and assigned a lock, which is broken at the time of use. Each lock is imprinted with a number controlled by pharmacy, and the location of every crash cart is documented.

Nonclinical Areas Stocked by the Pharmacy

Nonclinical areas of a hospital can include areas that a patient never sees or those areas that are used as temporary patient care areas. Some examples of these special areas of the hospital, along with the types of medications that the pharmacy may be responsible for ordering and stocking, are included in Box 10-3.

TABLE 10-3 Commonly Used Crash Cart Medications and Their Classification

Medications	Classification	Common Dosage Forms Stored on Cart
Adenosine	Antiarrhythmic	Vial
Amiodarone	Antiarrhythmic	Ampule, vial
Atropine sulfate	Anticholinergic	PFS*
Calcium chloride	Electrolyte	PFS
Dextrose 50%	Carbohydrate	PFS
Dextrose	Carbohydrate	IV solution bags[†]
Digoxin	Cardiac glycoside	Ampule
Dobutamine	Vasopressor	Vial
Dopamine	Vasopressor	Vial, IV bag[†]
Enalaprilat	ACE inhibitor	Vial
Epinephrine	Vasopressor	PFS
Furosemide	Loop diuretic	Vial
Glucagon	Glucose-elevating agent	Vial
Heparin	Anticoagulant	IV bag,[†] vial
Lidocaine	Antiarrhythmic	PFS, IV bag[†]
Magnesium sulfate	Electrolyte	Vial
Mannitol	Osmotic diuretic	Vial, IV bag[†]
Metoprolol	Beta-blocker	Ampule
Naloxone	Narcotic antagonist	Ampule
Nitroglycerin	Antianginal	Vial
Nitroprusside	Antihypertensive	Vial
Norepinephrine	Vasopressor	Ampule
Procainamide	Antiarrhythmic	Vial
Propranolol	Beta-blocker	Vial
Sodium bicarbonate	Alkalinizing agent	PFS
Sodium chloride	Electrolyte	Vial, also IV solution bags[†]
Vasopressin	Vasopressor	Vial
Verapamil	Calcium channel blocker	Vial

*ACE, Angiotensin converting enzyme; PFS, prefilled syringe; IV, intravenous.
[†]Bags of medications may be kept in different drawer than the medication tray.

BOX 10-3 SPECIAL DEPARTMENTS STOCKED BY THE PHARMACY

Anesthesia	Physicians or nurse anesthesiologists who administer medications used before and throughout surgery
Respiratory	Therapists who administer breathing treatments to hospitalized or clinic patients
Injection clinic	Nurses administer adult and pediatric immunizations and also may perform allergy skin tests
Radiology or imaging department	Technicians and physicians may administer dyes for imaging and may need to use a medication cart (known as crash cart) for adverse reactions or incidents

Central Supply

Another area that stocks supplies for the hospital is central supply. Usually boxes of large-volume IV drips and mixtures are kept here as well as dressing, tubing, and instruments used by various departments. Pharmacy orders stock normally on a daily basis from central supply. The type of stock ordered includes sterile water and various strengths of solutions such as premade potassium

Tech Note!

Clearly identifying yourself as a technician when answering the phone immediately lets callers know whether or not you can help them. This information prevents the caller from having to repeat a possibly lengthy question.

common question asked of the pharmacy is, "Where are the medications that I ordered?" Any pharmacy technician can answer this question by simply accessing the computer system to see whether the medication was sent or by checking the orders that have not yet been entered. The technician can also check the ADS machine to see if the stock is empty; this can be done from the main pharmacy ADS machine. However, all other questions should be referred to the pharmacist. As a result of new technology, many facilities no longer rely on phone calls at all. Instead, an instant message may be sent over the computer to the pharmacy for a missing medication. The technician can look into the ADS machine to see if the stock is empty and fill the missing medication. The technician can then communicate (via computer) with the nurse that the order is being processed.

Stat and ASAP Orders

Medication orders that need to be filled within minutes are referred to as **stat** orders. When the pharmacy receives a stat order, it should take precedence over all other orders. Normally, a stat order can be filled in 5 to 15 minutes, depending on the preparation time required for the medication. Some stat orders can be filled quickly using stock off the shelf, whereas others may require special preparation, such as the mixing of an intravenous preparation. When this happens, the medication is made as quickly as possible using proper aseptic technique. Stat orders are those that literally can mean the difference between life and death; they must be taken seriously. If possible, a stat order should be hand-delivered to ensure that it arrives at the correct destination safely and quickly.

An **ASAP** order is not normally as urgent as a stat order. However, these orders should be put in front of the new orders to ensure fast processing by the pharmacist.

Specialty Tasks

In addition to the previously outlined tasks that technicians commonly perform, there are additional duties that require the skills of a technician. These duties include assisting with clinical duties and anticoagulant therapy tasks. Some hospitals that have nuclear medication pharmacies are using technicians to prepare these medications. These agents may be used in diagnostic procedures. As the role of the pharmacy continues to change, so will the tasks of the pharmacy technician. (For other types of jobs pertaining to technicians, refer to Chapter 3.)

Investigational Drugs/Biological Therapies

An investigational drug is an agent not yet approved by the FDA for use. After a drug has finished pre–human testing and the results are positive, the next phase involves treating a patient. The drug company must apply for permission through the FDA. The application is referred to as an Investigational New Drug (IND) application. The FDA must approve the use (through clinical trials) of an investigational drug to ensure the patient would not be exposed to high risks. If the drug is approved, patients can apply to participate in a clinical trial. Under certain circumstances the clinical trial may be performed in the hospital.

There are many reasons people want to participate in a clinical trial. Common reasons include they have exhausted all other currently approved treatments or they believe the investigational drug will be more effective than what they are currently using. Others may want to participate in the study to promote the future development of medicine.

It is common for hospitals to treat patients with investigational drugs. Depending on the hospital this practice may be more or less common. The Joint Commission regulations must be met as well. There are strict protocols for ordering, storing, inventory, and final disposal of the drug(s). All investigational drugs are delivered to the central pharmacy where they are signed in by the pharmacist and stored separately from other drugs. Each drug has a logbook that must contain the following information:

- Drug name
- Drug strength
- Unit size
- Protocol title and numbers
- Principal investigator
- Manufacturer's lot number
- Identification
- Date dispensed
- Units and/or doses dispensed
- Stock balance
- Pharmacist's initials

Once the study is complete the remaining drugs are to be returned to the sponsor along with the log records. Copies of the records are to be kept by the pharmacy under "closed studies."

Technicians play a role in all aspects of hospital pharmacy. As most hospitals also have an outpatient pharmacy and/or discharge pharmacy within the facility, technicians are utilized as well. The technician that has experience in many different settings will have a broader knowledge base about pharmacy practice and normally is always in demand.

DO YOU REMEMBER THESE KEY POINTS?

- Duties of a pharmacy technician, including the areas described in this chapter
- How often medications are supplied to nursing units using a cart-filling method
- Steps in and frequency of filling automated medication dispensing systems
- The difference between a centralized pharmacy and a satellite pharmacy
- Duties involved in ordering and maintaining the stock levels of the pharmacy
- Hospital areas that the pharmacy stocks
- Specialty areas of the hospital for which the pharmacy stocks or orders medication
- Abbreviations of units/departments located within a hospital and the types of service they provide
- What PAR levels are and who is responsible for maintaining them
- Different types of hospitals, what differentiates them from one another, and how that affects the overall service that they may provide
- Which agencies monitor hospitals, including pharmacies within the hospital
- The various ways that orders are processed by the pharmacy
- How ADS machines function in the hospital setting and how they are stocked
- How POE systems are being implemented to reduce drug errors

REVIEW QUESTIONS

Multiple choice questions

1. P & P binders contain information pertaining to all of the following EXCEPT:
   A. Employees' weekly schedule
   B. Emergency situations
   C. Training
   D. Daily work routines

2. The Joint Commission is an agency that inspects and accredits:
   A. Hospitals
   B. Hospital pharmacies
   C. Pharmacists
   D. Both A and B

3. Hospital orders contain which of the following information?
   A. Laboratory orders
   B. Dietary restrictions
   C. Medication orders
   D. All of the above

4. All of the following information is necessary on a physician's order EXCEPT:
   A. Patient's name
   B. Patient's room number
   C. Patient's next of kin
   D. Patient's medical record number

5. Hospital technicians must be available to:
   A. Work various shifts
   B. Work weekends
   C. Fill different jobs per operational needs
   D. All of the above

6. Technicians have all of the following responsibilities EXCEPT:
   A. Printing intravenous labels before filling them
   B. Preparing antibiotics
   C. Discontinuing intravenous medications per physician's orders
   D. Contacting the physician for order clarification

7. By law, which of the following tasks cannot be done by a technician?
   A. Ordering pharmacy stock
   B. Filling chemotherapy orders
   C. Filling controlled substance orders for schedule III to V medications
   D. Final checking and signing off of orders

8. Which statement is false concerning the use of investigational drugs?
   A. An IND application must be filed with the FDA before the clinical study.
   B. All investigational drugs must be disposed on-site at the hospital where the study has taken place.
   C. A logbook containing all required information on the investigational drug must be maintained by the pharmacy.
   D. Clinical trials with investigational drugs is the last phase before a drug is approved by the FDA.

9. Technicians can answer which of the following questions over the phone?
   A. Generic or trade name of the drug
   B. Whether or not the drug is in stock
   C. If the drug order has been filled and sent to the floor
   D. All of the above

10. The differences between intravenous therapy and chemotherapy parenteral preparation include all of the following EXCEPT:
    A. The type of flow hood used
    B. Hand placement
    C. Size of the hood
    D. Aseptic technique

11. The main reason for using ADS machines is to:
A. Allow for ease of filling
B. Keep track of stock levels
C. Enforce accuracy of dosing
D. Both C and D

12. CPOE systems are used to:
A. Provide clear, concise orders
B. Save on stock
C. Increase speed
D. All of the above

13. Stat orders should be filled within:
A. 5 minutes
B. 15 minutes
C. 20 minutes
D. 30 minutes

14. Which of the following drugs is NOT kept on a crash cart?
A. Epinephrine
B. Sodium bicarbonate
C. Nitroprusside
D. Ampicillin

15. Under the tech-check-tech regulations, technicians
A. Must be audited continually
B. Can check (technician filled) floor stock
C. Can check (technician filled) medication cassettes
D. Must have specialized training before checking-off technicians

True/False

If the statement is false, then change it to make it true.

_____ **1.** Protocol is policy that is set by the pharmacist on duty.

_____ **2.** Hospitals must meet state and federal guidelines if they are to be reimbursed.

_____ **3.** Orders written by physicians in a hospital setting are not the same as prescriptions.

_____ **4.** Medications normally are placed in see-through plastic containers for security reasons only.

_____ **5.** Only pharmacists can fill orders that are received from the hospital floors.

_____ **6.** Technicians need to use aseptic technique only in the chemotherapy hood.

_____ **7.** A PAR level refers to the location and capabilities of the pharmacy within the hospital.

_____ **8.** All units within a hospital have the same floor stock to treat patients.

_____ **9.** Technicians cannot answer any questions that nurses direct to the pharmacy.

_____ **10.** It is best to identify yourself as a technician when first answering the phone.

_____ **11.** Nursing floors would order their tubing from central supply rather than the pharmacy.

_____ **12.** Pharmacy may order more common drugs from central supply on a daily basis.

_____ **13.** The central ADS computer is located in the pharmacy department.

_____ **14.** Only a pharmacist has the authority to deliver narcotics to nursing floors.

_____ **15.** Both POE and CPOE work in the same way with respect to drug ordering.

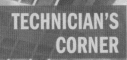

TECHNICIAN'S CORNER

While in the pharmacy, you get an order for Ms. Jeni Gilbert. Only her name and her room number are written on the order. The order is for ceftriaxone 1 g q6h. This is not the appropriate dosing regimen for this medication.

What information must you have before you can process this order? What actions should you take concerning the wrong dosing times for this medication?

BIBLIOGRAPHY

Ansel H, Allen L, Popovich N: *Pharmaceutical dosage forms and drug delivery systems*, ed 8, Baltimore, 2004, Lippincott Williams & Wilkins.

Elkin M, Perry A, Potter P: *Nursing interventions & clinical skills*, ed 4, St Louis, 2008, Elsevier.

United States Pharmacopeia; <797> Pharmaceutical Compounding-Sterile Preparations. Revision Bulletin, 2008.

WEBSITES

www.hhs.gov
www.redcross.org/
www.vchca.org/mc/medstaff/formularies/HIGHRiskMeds2005.pdf
www.psqh.com Patient Safety & Quality Healthcare ©2007 by Lionheart Publishing, Inc.
www.ashp.org/DocLibrary/Policy/IDS/ReceiptandControl.aspx
www.research.uci.edu/ora/hrpp/investigational.htm#Control

11

Repackaging and Compounding

Objectives

UPON COMPLETING THIS CHAPTER, YOU SHOULD BE ABLE TO DO THE FOLLOWING:

- List the steps in the repackaging of medications.

- List five reasons pharmacies often repackage bulk medications into unit dose packages.

- Describe the proper handling of medications during repackaging.

- Describe the way in which ointments or creams should be packed into jars.

- Demonstrate how to complete a repacking logbook with the necessary information.

- Explain the calculations used to determine "beyond-use" date when repackaging.

- List the common reasons for using unit dose medications.

- Describe the types of containers used for repackaged and compounded medications.

- Define terms used in compounding procedures.

- List the common reasons why patients need compounded medications.

- Describe the equipment used in compounding drugs.

- Explain the considerations that must be given to storage and stability of compounded products.

- Differentiate between types of scales used to weigh compounds.

- Demonstrate how to complete a compounding sheet with the necessary information.
- Explain the correct methods in the preparation and cleanup of compounding areas.
- Demonstrate compounding procedures.
- Describe the types of dosage forms compounded for animal use.

TERMS AND DEFINITIONS

Blister pack *Container usually made of plastic that holds a single-dose tablet or capsule*

Bubble pack *A preformed card with depressions that can hold medications; they are sealed with a foil card backboard*

Calibration *The markings on a measuring device*

Compounding *The act of mixing, reconstituting, and packaging a drug*

Cream *A hydrophilic base*

Elixir *A base solution that is a mixture of alcohol and water*

Emulsification *To make into an emulsion, or bind together*

Excipient *Inert substance added to a drug to form a suitable consistency for dosing*

FDA *Food and Drug Administration*

Good manufacturing practices (GMP) *Federal guidelines that must be followed by all entities that prepare and package medication or medical devices*

Homogeneous *A uniformed composition throughout the medication mixture*

Hydrophilic *Water loving; any substance that easily mixes in water*

Hydrophobic *Water hating; any substance that does not mix or dissolve in water*

Mortar and pestle *A bowl and rounded knob used to grind substances into fine powder or to mix liquids*

Ointment *A hydrophobic product such as petroleum jelly*

Oleaginous base *Ingredient used in compounding that does not dissolve in water*

Periodic automatic replacement (PAR) *A minimum set amount of stock that needs to be kept on hand*

Punch method *Manual filling of capsules with powdered medication that has been premeasured*

Reconstitution *To mix a liquid and a powder to form a suspension or solution*

Repackaging *The act of reducing the amount of medication taken from a bulk bottle; unit dosing is a form of repackaging*

Solute *The ingredient that is dissolved into a solution*

Solution *A water base in which the ingredient or ingredients dissolve completely*

Solvent *The greater part of a solution that dissolves a solute*

Strip pack *A strip of heat-sealed packets each holding one tablet or capsule used in the repackaging process*

Suspension *A solution in which the powder does not dissolve into the base and must be shaken before use*

Syrup *A sugar-based liquid*
Triturate *To grind or crush powder such as a tablet into fine particles*
Troche *A flat disklike tablet that dissolves between the gum and cheek*
Unit dose *A single dose of a drug*

Introduction

There are several different types of pharmacy settings, each stocking specific types of medications and dosage forms that best suit their functions. **Repackaging** medications is a method used by pharmacies to provide a specific service to their patients. Often bulk containers of medication are repackaged into single dose containers. For example, a bottle of #100 aspirin 81-mg tablets can be packaged into 100 individual containers; one dose is referred to as a **unit dose.** Hospitals use unit dose containers; they order them from the manufacturer and make their own when necessary. These include **unit dose blister packs** or **strip packs and liquid cups** that contain one medication for one dose. Nursing and home health care facilities may use a **bubble pack** (i.e., punch cards), which may contain one to several tablets/capsules for dosing several days of medication. Proper procedures must be followed when repackaging medications; this includes accuracy, technique, and documentation.

Compounding is common in hospital and community pharmacies. Specialized **compounding** pharmacies are equipped to prepare a wide assortment of solutions, ointments, creams, suppositories, or other drug delivery systems. Compounding pharmacies also prepare medications in various dosage forms and strengths for animals. Although the types of products compounded may differ, many of the same rules apply for medications compounded for both humans and animals. This chapter discusses the equipment and storage/stability capacity necessary for compounding medications as well as the formulas used, documentation needed, and skills required by technicians when repackaging and compounding products. Unit dose packaging is discussed first; non–sterile compounding and sterile compounding are discussed later in the chapter.

Repackaging

By using unit dose medications, a hospital saves a substantial amount of money per patient. Although packaging guidelines are not exactly the same between pharmacies and manufacturers, both entities must use good manufacturing practices. **Good manufacturing practices (GMP)** are Food and Drug Administration (FDA) guidelines designed to guarantee safe and effective products for the consumer.

The following list has five reasons that a pharmacy repackages a bulk drug into unit dose medications:

1. Certain drugs cannot be purchased from a manufacturer in prepackaged unit dose strips. The pharmacy personnel must make their own unit dose.
2. The cost of unit dosing certain medications may be less expensive when done by the hospital than if purchased from a manufacturer.

TABLE 11-1 Examples of Good Manufacturing Practice Guidelines

Item	Guidelines
Drugs and labels	All medications must be checked by a registered pharmacist
Equipment	In good condition and clean
Expiration date	6 months or one fourth of time of manufacturer's expiration date, whichever is less (recently updated to maximum of 1 year of manufacturer's expiration date or, if manufacturer's date is less than 1 year, then that date may be given)
	Bulk container must not have been previously opened
Package	Appropriate for the drug
Preparation	Not more than one item prepared at a time
Records	All items repackaged are logged for reference

3. Because of the packaging, speed and efficiency are increased because of the pharmacy's ability to immediately prepare the exact amount of medication needed without having to order and wait for the drugs to arrive.
4. Because of the label on each dose of drug, the chance of errors is decreased.
5. If unit dose medication is not used, it can be returned to stock and used for another patient at a later time.

Examples of GMP guidelines that the technician and pharmacist should follow when preparing unit dose medications are listed in Table 11-1. The types of packages used in pharmacy must be considered before repackaging. Some medications are degraded upon exposure to sunlight. These products must be packaged in amber-colored bottles or vials. A sample of the types of containers used in repackaging is listed in Table 11-2. Each type of container holds specific amounts and types of medications (Figure 11-1). Liquids normally are placed in glass or plastic bottles or plastic or foil cups. Tablets and capsules usually are placed in **blister packs** or **strip packs** (Figure 11-2).

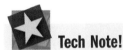

Tech Note!

It is common practice to use only amber-colored containers to avoid possible degradation of medication, although clear unit dose packs are available.

REPACKAGING EQUIPMENT

Types of unit dosing equipment vary depending on the amounts of drugs that are repackaged. For large pharmacies that supply many patient medications, automated packaging machines may be used. They not only fill the unit dose containers but also may generate labels for the drugs and apply them to the containers as they pass through the machine (Figure 11-3). Other types of equipment are much less high-tech; a technician can manually place each tablet or capsule into the individual blister pack and then apply the label. Although this type of repackaging is considered nonsterile, the technician should carefully use appropriate aseptic techniques to keep the process of preparing medications as clean as possible.

REPACKAGING TECHNIQUES

Non–sterile technique is required for repacking medications. Technicians need to use the following garments, techniques, and equipment:

- Wear lab coat.
- Pull hair back.
- Wash hands.

TABLE 11-2 Unit Dose Containers

Type of Container	Medication Types	Volume/Size
Plastic cups	Liquids, suspensions	5, 10, 15, 30 mL
Syringes	Parenterals, oral liquids, transdermal gels	0.5, 1, 3, 5, 10, 15, 20, 30, 60 mL
Oral syringes	Liquids	1, 3, 5, 10 mL
Heat-sealed strip packs	Tablets, capsules, troches	1 unit dose
Amber blister packs	Tablets, capsules	1 unit dose
Various sizes of bubble packs	Tablets, capsules, troches	1 to 3 medications
Amber glass	Liquids	5, 10, 25, 30 mL
Applicators	Suppositories, creams, ointments	1 application
Foil cups	Liquids, suspensions	5, 10, 30 mL
Plastic suppository shells	Suppositories	1- to 5-g sizes in different colors

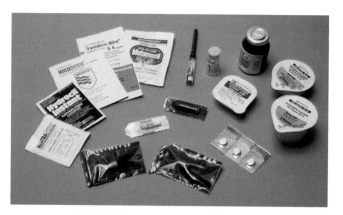

FIGURE 11-1 Sample of containers.

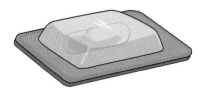

FIGURE 11-2 A sample blister pack container.

- Wear face mask when applicable
- Wear gloves if the tablets or capsules will be touched.
- Use pill counting tray and spatula if the tablets will be dispensed from the tray.

All equipment should be kept clean and in good condition at all times. The process of repackaging should take place in a designated area of the pharmacy, away from high-traffic areas. This reduces airflow over the medication, which may cause contamination. If the technician is using manual methods to load medications into blister packs, it is important that the technician wears gloves

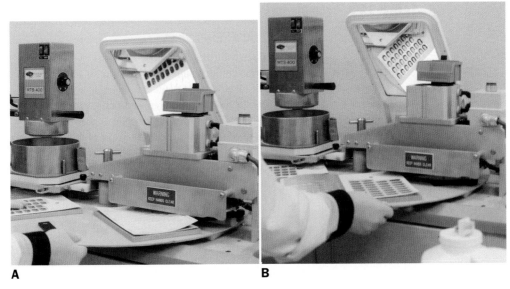

A   **B**

FIGURE 11-3 A technician is responsible for the proper preparation and labeling of all repackaged medications. **A,** The empty medication card is rotated under the hopper, where the medication is placed into the card. The medication card is then rotated to the heating element, where the seal is made to enclose each tablet. **B,** The technician uses a mirror to verify that each sheet is filled completely.

 Tech Note!

To reduce cross-contamination of patients' prescriptions, pill counting trays should be cleaned after each use. If residue is left behind on the pill counter and the next patient is allergic to the previously counted medication, it is possible for that patient to have an allergic reaction. When chemotherapy medication is counted, a tray marked specifically for counting chemotherapy should be used to avoid cross-contamination. All trays are cleaned with alcohol prep pads.

after washing his or her hands. If pill trays are used to guide tablets or capsules into their containers, the tray should be washed with alcohol after each use. The preparation required to repackage medications is simple. If tablets or capsules are to be unit dosed, it is important to have enough packages and labels ready for use. In addition to these supplies, keeping medications separate from one another is important. Only one item at a time should be prepared because leaving multiple drugs on a countertop leads to errors. Keeping the area clean and well organized not only helps avoid contamination of drugs but also reduces the chance of errors.

DOCUMENTATION

Keeping track of the products that you are repackaging is one of the major steps that must not be overlooked. Just as manufacturers must document all drugs they have packaged, so must pharmacy. For instance, if a manufacturer recalled a drug that had been repackaged, it is important to have an accurate count of how many unit doses were made and an identifying mark (lot number) on each of them. Therefore documentation for repackaged drugs must have the information shown in Table 11-3. Table 11-4 provides examples of how the drug manufacturers' names normally are abbreviated. It is important to enter as much information as possible on the record's form as well as on the medication container. Usually a separate binder is used for repackaging record keeping. Figure 11-4 shows a sample of the type of unit dosing log record used.

LABELING AND CHECKING REPACKAGED MEDICATIONS

Common dosage forms of drugs that normally are repackaged in a pharmacy include oral medications such as tablets, capsules, and liquids. Tablets may be cut in half and repackaged per facility protocol.

Many different types of computer labeling programs are used to generate unit dose labels in the pharmacy. The pharmacy technician is responsible for

TABLE 11-3 Example of Unit Dose Record Log Sheet Information*

Item	Description
Date	Date that drug is made, which includes day, month, and year
Drug	Drug name, usually by generic and then brand name if indicated on log sheet
Dosage form	Tablet, capsule, spansule, troche, suspension, elixir, solution
Manufacturer	Manufacturer of drug, usually abbreviated
Manufacturer's lot number	Control number located on side of label or on bottom of bottle
Manufacturer's expiration date	Located with lot number; remember that if date indicates only month and year, drug is good through end of month
Pharmacy lot number	Each item repackaged in pharmacy is given a number consecutive to previous batch prepared
Pharmacy beyond-use date	Calculate new expiration date, which is 6 months or one fourth of time of manufacturer's expiration date, whichever is less
Technician	Must initial logbook entry
Pharmacist	Each item made must be checked off by a pharmacist

*The information on the label of the unit dose item is much less than what is required in the logbook, but it is just as important. The following are the components necessary on a typical unit dose label: name of drug; generic name; trade name (trade name commonly given for the easy identification of the proper medication); strength; dosage form; pharmacy lot number; pharmacy expiration date.

TABLE 11-4 Examples of Manufacturer Abbreviation Codes

Manufacturer	Code	Manufacturer	Code
3M Pharmaceuticals	3MP	Johnson & Johnson	JJ
Abbott Laboratories	ABB	Lederle	LED
A H Robins	ROB	Marion Merrell Dow	MMD
AstraZeneca	AZN	Mead Johnson Nutritionals	M/J
Barr Laboratories	BRR	Merck & Co	MSD
Bausch & Lomb	B-L	Novartis Pharmaceuticals	NVR
Bayer Pharmaceuticals Corp	BYR	Novo Nordisk	NNP
Boehringer Ingelheim	B-I	Novopharm	NOV
Burroughs Wellcome	BW	Parke-Davis	P-D
Ciba Pharmaceuticals	CIB	Pfizer Pharmaceuticals	FD
Colgate Oral Pharmaceuticals	COP	Pharmacia & Upjohn	UPJ
Dey LP	DEY	Procter & Gamble	PG
DuPont Pharmaceuticals	DUP	Purdue Pharma	PUR
Econo Med Pharmaceuticals	ECO	Roche Laboratories	ORC
Eli Lilly and Company	LY	Roxane Laboratories	ROX
Endo Pharmaceuticals	END	Rugby Laboratories	RUG
Eon Laboratories	EON	Sandoz	SAN
Fujiswawa Pharmaceutical	FUJ	SmithKline Beecham Pharmaceuticals	SKF
G & W Laboratories	G&W	Taro Pharmaceuticals	TRO
Geigy Pharmaceuticals	GEI	Teva Pharmaceuticals	TEV
Geneva Pharmaceuticals	GG	Upsher Smith Laboratories	UPS
GlaxoWellcome	GLX	Wyeth-Ayerst	WY
Hoechst Marion Roussel	HMR	Zenith Goldline Pharmaceuticals	Z/G
ICN Pharmaceuticals	ICN		

	Date	Drug (generic)	Strength	Dosage form	Amount	MFG	MFG lot#	MFG exp date	Pharmacy expiration date	Pharmacy lot #	Tech	RPH
1	2/11/2011	aspirin	81mg	tab	100	Bayer	JGH405	7/15/2012	Jun-11	A1001	LP	TG
2	2/12/2011	perphenazine	2mg	tab	100	Schering	XYZ124	12/1/2012	Jul-11	A1002	TK	DS
3												
4												
5												
6												
7												
8												
9												

FIGURE 11-4 Sample of a unit dose log record.

Tech Alert!

PAR levels are set amounts of drugs or equipment that must be kept in stock at all times. All departments have PAR levels. Stock is normally ordered on preprinted sheets that list the PAR level and have a space for entering the amount of medication needed to generate the PAR level.

determining which drugs are needed to replenish the pharmacy stock according to **periodic automatic replacement** (PAR) levels and then preparing the necessary medications. Technicians must calculate the correct beyond-use date, document the essential components of the drug, generate the labels, fill the medication, and apply the label neatly on the container. Finally, the pharmacist checks the completed work to ensure that the label, drug, and logging of the medication are correct.

In specific situations a technician who has received specialized training may check another technician's work; this is referred to as tech-check-tech. Certain states have allowed pharmacy technicians to check the work of other technicians. This is limited to checking repackaged unit doses, floor stock, and patient medication drawers. Even if your state has approved the use of the tech-check-tech process, each pharmacy can choose whether to adopt the process and provide the necessary training (see Chapter 3).

STORAGE AND STABILITY

The U.S. Food and Drug Administration (FDA) is responsible for providing guidelines for all manufacturers that package medications. Expiration dates are determined on the basis of tests conducted by manufacturers and the FDA; however, these rules do not apply to medications repackaged in a hospital setting for individual patient use. The beyond-use dates assigned to repackaged products are established according to *United States Pharmacopeia (USP)* guidelines. Items repackaged for use within a hospital or for a specific patient's use cannot be mass-produced. Only drug manufacturing companies following FDA guidelines are in the business of mass production.

EXPIRATION DATES VERSUS BEYOND-USE DATING

Assigning the beyond-use date for a repackaged medication is a simple yet important process. There is an important distinction between "expiration" dates and "beyond-use" dates. Expiration dates are assigned by the manufacturer, whereas beyond-use dates are given by pharmacy when repackaging or compounding medications. Once a bulk bottle is opened and the medication repackaged, the manufacturer's expiration date is no longer valid. The correct drug life is determined by calculating the new expiration date from the bulk medication. One common way of dating drugs is to set the expiration date at the end of the month. For example, when you are preparing a label for a drug that you have determined will expire at the end of September 2010, you would write 9/10. This means the drug is effective through the month of September. Because regulations change concerning appropriate beyond-use dating, two methods are outlined in this chapter; the specific requirements of your state will dictate which method should be used. This information should be outlined in each facility's policies and procedures manual.

Method 1

The life of a repackaged drug is 6 months or one fourth of the manufacturer's expiration date, whichever is less. The manufacturer's expiration date gives the exact amount of time the drug is in date. To find the new beyond-use date, use the date provided on the medication container, determine the number of months the drug is effective, and then divide by 4. Example 11-1 shows this calculation for proper dating.

EXAMPLE 11-1 EXPIRATION DATING (6-MONTH VERSION)

Acetaminophen 500-mg tablets
Today's date: August 2010
Per manufacturer, the medication expires in December 2013
Calculation: 8/10 to 12/13 = 3 years × 12 months = 36 months/4 = 9 months
You may give this drug only 6 months until expiration, or until 2/11.

Method 2

The repackaged medication can be given a maximum of 1 year drug life as long as it does not exceed the safety margin given by the drug company. For example: if a drug has a 5-year shelf life, expiration must not extend past 1 year. This 1-year expiration date can only be given if supported by proper documentation showing the drug company followed all safety and stability criteria mandated by the FDA (see Chapter 2). See Example 11-2 for calculations.

EXAMPLE 11-2 BEYOND-USE DATING (1-YEAR VERSION)

Cimetidine 300-mg tablet
Today's date: August 2010
Expires in August 2014
Calculation: 8/10 to 8/14 is 4 years × 12 months = 48 months/4 = 12 months
You may give this drug a 1-year beyond-use date maximum; it would expire in 8/11.

Tech Alert!

Proper repacking techniques are paramount during the preparation of unit dose medications. Gloves must be worn, and the pill counting tray/device should be cleaned between uses to avoid cross-contamination.

Compounding

HISTORY

The art of compounding dates back more than 4000 years, beginning with medicinal mixtures using plants, animals, and minerals. Historians have found recipes for various treatments engraved onto ancient scrolls dating back to 1500 BC, and **mortar and pestles** have been unearthed dating back to the early Egyptian and Roman societies. Even throughout recent civilization, pharmacists compounded each prescription individually. In the United States the first pharmacopoeia was published in 1820 and listed more than 80% of the prescriptions that were made; all were compounded products at that time. As the pharmaceutical business grew, more drugs were manufactured in common dosages by drug companies, decreasing the number of products that needed to be compounded by the pharmacy. It was not until the late 1990s that compounding once again became popular (USP Bulletin, Compounding Pharmacies at the Fonefront of

BOX 11-1 WHY COMPOUND MEDICATIONS?

There are several reasons medications need to be compounded by pharmacy, including the following:

- The medication is no longer manufactured by the drug company.
- The patient is allergic to a preservative, dye, or other additive in the normal drug.
- A specialized dosage or strength is needed for a patient with unique needs (for example, an infant or a patient with diabetes).
- Combining several medications will increase patient compliance.
- The patient cannot ingest the normal dosage form.
- The medication requires flavorings and/or additives to make it more palatable for patients, most often children.

Personalized Medicine. Spring 2007, volume 96 no. 4). The common dosages made by drug manufacturers cannot be used by everyone; advancements in the knowledge of pharmacodynamics necessitate the availability of individualizing medication dosages for some persons.

Premade dosages do not necessarily treat everyone; each person is different because of other concurrent conditions or physiological factors that affect the drug being prescribed. This is evident in pediatrics, where dosages must be calculated and provided based on the weight of the child, because the metabolic rate of children is quite different than that of adults. Another need is for dosages that are much easier for a child to take. Examples of these dosage forms include popsicles and lozenges that deliver medications. Hospice patients, who may not be able to swallow oral medications or have injections, require a different dosage form that is not available by a manufacturer. A list of reasons for compounding medications is given in Box 11-1. Persons who would benefit with a combination drug that is not already packaged can have a combination drug made specifically for them. For example, women who are menopausal can have medications made specific to their hormonal needs.

NON–STERILE COMPOUNDING

Non–sterile compounding consists of compounding two or more medications in a nonsterile environment; it does not mean the final product is not sterile. Certain medications must be sterile, such as ophthalmics and other agents, depending on the area or condition that is being treated. The FDA requires that compounded products adhere to the *United States Pharmacopeia–National Formulary (USP–NF) <795>* standards although they do not specifically regulate compounding. Although each state board of pharmacy regulates compounding pharmacies, many states require pharmacists to comply with *USP–NF <795>* standards. Other standards that must be followed involve the quality and stability of ingredients, the policies and procedures used during preparation, the equipment required, and the quality control and documentation guidelines that must be followed (per board of pharmacy). Aseptic technique is discussed in-depth in Chapter 12. Box 11-2 lists the types of dosage forms that can be compounded under *USP–NF <795>*.

Most community pharmacies do not have the staff, the wide variety of supplies, or the time to prepare the various dosage forms and medication strengths. For this type of task there are compounding pharmacies that specialize in this area. However, there are still basic types of compounding that the average technician will encounter even if the technician works in institutional settings and community pharmacies. Compounding standards, common preparations

BOX 11-2 EXAMPLES OF DOSAGE FORMS THAT CAN BE COMPOUNDED

Topicals
- Creams
- Gels, jellies
- Ointments
- Pastes
- Sticks

Oral Liquids
- Elixirs
- Solutions
- Suspensions
- Syrups
- Tinctures

Oral Solids
- Capsules
- Lollipops
- Lozenges
- Popsicles
- Tablets
- Troches
- Effervescent tablets

Suppositories
- Rectal
- Urethral
- Vaginal

prepared in most pharmacies, and types of items prepared in specialized compounding pharmacies will be discussed.

COMPOUNDING AREA

When setting up a compounding area there are certain criteria that should be met per *USP <795> (Compounding Standards)*. Although the compounding area and its supplies can be located within a pharmacy, it should be away from areas where normal prescription processing, chemicals, dust, or open boxes are located. The compounding surface area should be smooth and in good condition and provide good lighting. Overhanging shelves or any ledges should not be located over the workspace because dust can accumulate in these spaces. There should be a sink located close to the compounding site for hand washing and cleaning. All surfaces of the area should be cleaned between compounding product(s) as well at the beginning and at the end of the day (when in use) to avoid cross-contamination. The temperature and humidity should be monitored to avoid decomposition of chemicals.

EQUIPMENT

Pharmacies have a large amount of equipment on hand to perform their daily functions. Types of equipment include personal protective wear, measuring and weighing devices, an assortment of containers, and labels. The minimum required equipment list is provided by each state board of pharmacy (see your state's requirements), although there are additional types of equipment that pharmacies may want to stock for preparing products. This determination is normally made on the basis of the amounts and types of nonsterile products that the pharmacy provides. Table 11-5 lists common types of equipment necessary in a compounding area. Various types of compounding equipment that are required for specific uses are discussed in the following paragraphs.

Personal Protective Equipment

Compounding in the pharmacy requires many different pieces of equipment. Personal protective equipment is used to ensure the sterility of the product as well as to protect the technician from spills while working. The following are considered necessary personal protective equipment:

- Gloves
- Goggles

TABLE 11-5 Examples Of Compounding Equipment

Equipment	Use
Autoclave	For sterilization
Balance	Class A balance, torsion digital balance
Beakers	1, 5, 10, 20, 50, 100, 500, 1000 mL
Blender	Electric
Capsule molds	For making multiple capsules
Containers	Spray bottles, ointment tubes, plastic jars, vials, bottles, stick containers, ophthalmic containers
Crimpers	For sealing tubes and glass bottles
Disposable weighing devices	Papers (glycerin), boats (plastic)
Droppers	Sterile and nonsterile
Filters	0.5 and 0.2 micrometers
Foil wraps	For wrapping suppositories
Funnels	For transferring liquids
Glass stirring rods	For stirring/mixing liquids
Glass tile	For mixing ingredients
Graduated cylinders	For performing various measurements
Heat gun	For sealing packages
Hot plate	For melting ingredients
Magnetic stir plate	Automatically stirs for long periods of time
Magnetic stirrers	Used in beaker to stir contents
Metal measuring scoop	For transferring powders to scale
Molds	Capsules, tablets, lozenges, troches, suppositories, popsicles, lollipops
Mortar and pestle	Glass, porcelain
Paper sheets 12 × 12	For levigation and mixing ingredients
Pipettes	For adding minute amounts of liquids: 50 micrograms (mcg) to 1 mL
Refrigerator	For storage
Rubber grippers	For removing glass from hot plates
Sieves	For removing particles
Sink	For washing all equipment
Solvents	For cleaning surface area of compounding room
Spatulas	For moving and mixing ingredients
Thermometers	For ingredients that must be prepared at a certain temperature
Tongs	For removing hot contents
Vertical flow hood	For preparing compounds that require aseptic environment
Wash bottle	For rinsing
Weights	Brass weights used on class A balance

- Gown
- Hair cover
- Lab coat
- Mask
- Shoe covers

Measuring Devices

Graduated cylinders (Figure 11-5) are available in various sizes (from 1 mL to 1 L), types (e.g., glass and plastic), and shapes (e.g., conical and cylindrical) to measure liquids (Table 11-6). Other types of measuring instruments can range

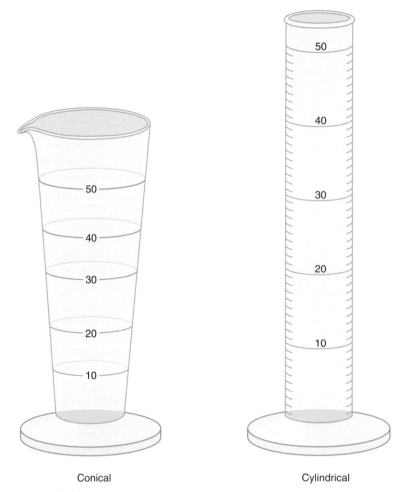

Conical   Cylindrical

FIGURE 11-5 Graduated cylinders are used for liquid measurement.

TABLE 11-6 Types of Graduated Cylinders

Type	Use
Glass	Used for hot liquids or liquids not compatible with plastic devices
Plastic	Used for cold liquids
Cylindrical shapes	Used to measure liquids more accurately
Conical shapes	Wider platform is more stable when measuring viscous liquids and easier to mix solutions; however, because sides flare outward, reading meniscus is more difficult

from syringes (for small volumes) and pipettes (for very minute volumes) to large automated measuring machines. These electronic machines, ointment mills, and capsule-filling machines are used in compounding pharmacies to prepare large amounts of medications. Capsule-filling machines normally fill anywhere from 100 to 300 capsules at one time.

Mixing Equipment
Various sizes of mortars and pestles (e.g., glass and porcelain) are necessary depending on the types of ingredients to be prepared (Figure 11-6). Various spatula types include metal and plastic (Table 11-7).

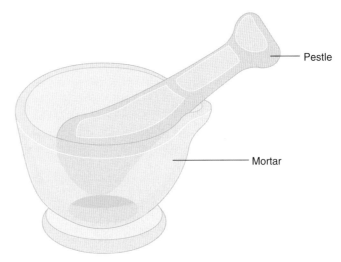

FIGURE 11-6 Mortars and pestles are used to crush solids. Both glass and porcelain types are used in compounding.

TABLE 11-7 Types of Compounding Mixing Equipment

Mortar and Pestles	
Glass	Used for preparing liquids such as solutions and suspensions and for mixing oily or staining materials
Porcelain	Used for blending powders and pulverizing soft aggregates or crystals
Spatulas	
Plastic	Used on mixtures that may react with metal
Metal	Used for mixing ointments or creams and handling dry chemicals
Long: >6 inches	Used for ointments or creams and powder blends for capsules
Short: ≤6 inches	Used in handling dry chemicals

Weighing Equipment

One of the most expensive pieces of equipment is the balance or scale used to weigh powders. Scales differ in their range of weight and style. A class III balance (Figure 11-7, *A*) is a torsion balance. This type of scale uses a counterbalance (weights) to determine the weight of the substance being measured, and is referred to as a mechanical scale (required by most states' BOPs). This type of scale has special weights that are labeled in a range of milligrams and grams (Figure 11-7, *B*). Weights used on this type of scale should be stored in a hardshelled container. Another style of balance is the electronic balance (class II) that has a digital readout of the weight. No weights are used with this balance; instead, the calibrations are electronic; this balance can weigh heavier substances than the class III balance, as shown in the following comparison:

Digital balance/class II: capacity 100 g; readable to 0.0001 g; example, Sartoris GD503

Digital balance/class II; capacity 200 g; readable to 0.01 g; example, PCE-LSM200

Class III balance: capacity 60 g; sensitivity to 2 mg; example, DRX-3 Torbal

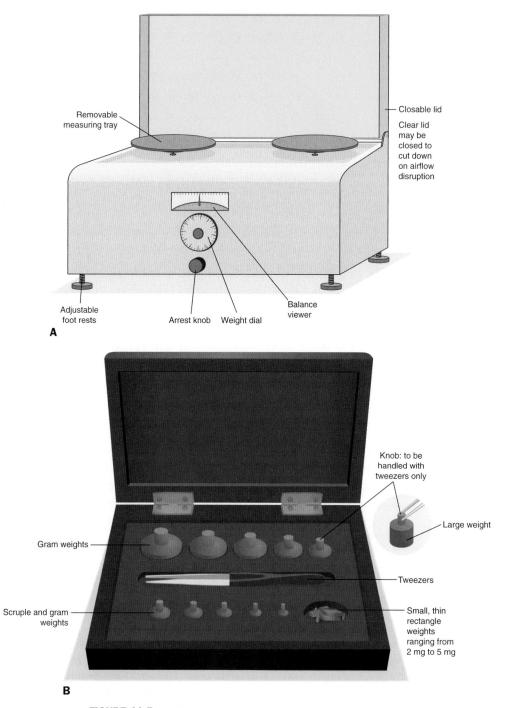

FIGURE 11-7 A, Class A balance. **B,** Pharmaceutical weights.

Appropriate care and cleaning of these sensitive instruments are the responsibility of the person using them and should be performed before, during, and after use.

ADDITIONAL SUPPLIES

Mold Forms

Various suppository molds can be used to prepare suppositories. These include the traditional metal molds in which cavity openings range from 1 to 2.5 g. Dif-

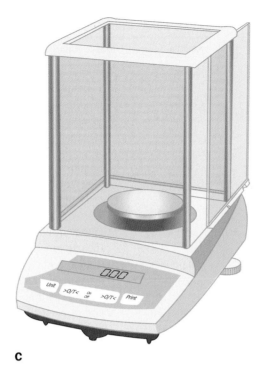

c

FIGURE 11-7, cont'd **C,** Analytical balance.

ferent mold sizes (6 to 100) allow for different amounts of suppositories to be prepared. The molds are held together by nuts and screws while the ingredients solidify. Other options are hard rubber molds; similar to the metal molds, hard rubber molds are held together by screws that are loosened when the suppositories are solid. Flexible rubber molds in strips that can be placed in the refrigerator, if necessary, are also available. Because strips of molds are used, the exact amount of suppositories can be removed for filling a prescription while the remainder can be left in the refrigerator for the next order.

Other items besides equipment used in compounding medications are **excipients;** these are inert substances added to a drug to form a suitable consistency for dosing. Various chemicals are used to alter the pH and solubility of medications as required, and a wide variety of medications are used, including those in crystalline forms, which are used as the active ingredient in the compounded dosage form.

Excipients

There is a wide range of excipients (additives) that can be used in the preparation of medications to achieve the required consistency, effectiveness, and functional properties. These are used in a variety of dosage forms such as liquids, suspensions, tablets and capsules, and coatings. Table 11-8 gives a list of the common additives.

Taste

Flavorings are often added to medications to mask the bad taste of the ingredients. There are four basic tastes that the tongue recognizes: sweet, sour, salty, and bitter. Masking the taste becomes more difficult as the distaste increases. Flavorings such as saccharin impart a bitter taste followed by a sweet taste, whereas sucrose gives an immediate sweet taste. Sucrose flavorings are the most commonly used because of this property. Preservatives can alter the properties of flavorings, causing different results in taste. Many of the flavorings have a

TABLE 11-8 Common Additives

Additive	Description
Gums	Naturally occurring plant derivatives that are water-soluble. They provide a variety of properties, including gelling, thickening, and film-forming.
Coatings	Surrounding layer of polymeric material that coat a tablet, capsule, or pellet. This is done to change color; protect active ingredient from moisture, light, pH of stomach; avoid bad taste or odor when taken by mouth. Film coatings can provide functional properties that enable creation of a sustained or delayed release dosage form.
Disintegrants	Added to a tablet or capsule blend to help break up compacted mass when put into a fluid environment. Especially important for rapid-release agents.
Lubricants	Additive for powder blend to prevent compacted powder mass from sticking to equipment during process of making tablets or capsules.
Suspending agents	Insoluble particles that are dispersed in a liquid; act by increasing the viscosity of the liquid vehicle. This reduces rate of sedimentation of particles in a suspension.
Plasticizers	Blend of plasticizers in acrylic emulsion coatings. They have a wide variety of functional properties (retarding drug release) and allow for flexibility in coating.
Emulsifying agents	Maintains dispersion of finely divided liquid droplets in a liquid vehicle. Made from two or more immiscible liquids, such as water and oil, and can be liquid or semisolid (creams and lotions).

TABLE 11-9 Common Flavor Additives for Taste*

Classification of Drugs	Flavorings That Are Best Suited for Use
Antibiotics	Citrus flavors, cherry, pineapple, orange, berry, banana, strawberry-vanilla, banana-vanilla, lemon custard, fruit cinnamon
Antihistamines	Cherry, cinnamon, grape, lime, peach-orange, raspberry, root beer, wild cherry, apricot
Barbiturates	Lime, orange, banana-vanilla, banana-pineapple, peach-orange, root beer
Decongestants and expectorants	Cherry, lemon, loganberry, gooseberry, orange-peach, apricot, strawberry, pineapple, raspberry, tangerine, custard-mint-strawberry
Electrolytes	Cherry, grape, lemon-lime, raspberry, wild cherry
Geriatrics	Black currant, grenadine-strawberry, lime, root beer, wild strawberry

*Additional flavorings include menthol, monosodium glutamate, peppermint oil, spearmint oil, and wintergreen.

color additive; for those that do not, dyes can be used, although they are not absolutely necessary. Colors should match the flavor; for example, cherry flavor should be colored red. Each recipe will indicate which flavorings and/or colors can be mixed into the compounded product. Examples of the types of agents used as flavorings when compounding antibiotics, antihistamines, barbiturates, decongestants, and electrolytes are shown in Table 11-9. Considerations must always be given to the stability and solubility of the additives. Also patient aller-

BOX 11-3 COMPETENCIES

To decrease the probability of errors and to maximize the quality of the preparation there are several steps that should be taken, including the following:

1. Identify the proper equipment needed to prepare the medication.
2. Wear the proper gear.
3. Wash hands appropriately.
4. Clean the compounding area and necessary equipment with antibacterial solvent.
5. Assemble all necessary materials before beginning the compounding process.
6. Perform all necessary calculations to determine the amounts of ingredients necessary.
7. Determine the intended use, safety, and legal limitations of the prescription to be compounded.
8. Compound only one preparation at a time.
9. Compound the preparation following the prescription or formula (recipe).
10. Assess weight variation, consistency of mixture, color, odor, clarity, and pH of preparation.
11. Determine the beyond-use dating for the product prepared.
12. Complete log sheet and add notation to describe the appearance of the formulation.
13. Label the prescription container to include all required information.
14. Immediately clean and store all equipment used.
15. Thoroughly clean surface areas.

Before compounding, be sure your state allows compounding by a pharmacy technician. If you have any questions on how to prepare a product, ask the pharmacist at the beginning of the compounding process, not in the middle.

gies must be checked before preparation. Children's medications are often flavored with similar types of flavors that are found in candy and drinks.

Non–Sterile Compounding and Techniques

PERSONAL PREPARATION

Before beginning the compounding process, the technician should tie back long hair and wear a lab coat and gloves to reduce contamination of the product. In addition to these personal considerations, a technician who is sick or has any open wounds should not make any compounding products. For commonly compounded items, a recipe book or formula cards listing compounds, their weights, and step-by-step instructions are used by pharmacists and technicians. To decrease the possibility of errors when compounding, there are several skills in which the pharmacy technician should be competent (Box 11-3).

WEIGHING TECHNIQUES

Using a class A balance begins by gathering the necessary ingredients and supplies, such as glycerin paper or weighing boats and weights. There are adjustable legs on the balance to level it on the compounding surface, if necessary. Each balance also has an arrest knob that is used to lock the scale in place, which reduces the possibility of damage to the balance. There are six steps in the proper setup of a balance; each step is critical to obtain the proper weight of a substance. These steps are listed in Box 11-4. Inside the container that holds the weights is a pair of tweezers for grasping the brass or metal weights. Use of tweezers prevents hand oils from being transferred to the surface of the metal. Oils can corrode the metal, altering the exact weight. Pharmacy balances are

BOX 11-4 INSTRUCTIONS FOR USING A CLASS A BALANCE

1. The balance must be steadied on the counter. Every balance has adjustable legs; they are used to level the balance before beginning.
2. Lightweight papers then are added to both sides of the balance to protect the weighing plates and to hold the substance being weighed.
3. The balance must be "zeroed out" to prevent the paper from being included in the weight of the drug.
4. At this point, the counter-weight can be placed on the right side of the balance.
5. Once the weight is in place, the balance must be set to the proper weight.
6. The substance to be measured then can be placed on the opposite plate until the two plates balance.

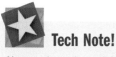

Tech Note!

Always place the weights on the right side of the balance. This is done to ensure continuity of measurement.

very sensitive. Regardless of the substance that you are weighing, it is important to keep airflow around the balance to a minimum. Even the motion of a person walking by can set the balance into a rocking motion, making calibration difficult. Pharmacy balances have a glass lid that can be used to impede air currents while weighing compounds. As the balance reaches equilibration, it is important to add less and less substance to the balance. One way of doing this is to use a spatula and pick up a small amount of substance; then lightly tap the side of the spatula (from behind the substance) to flick on a few granules at a time. This technique is easier with powders than with other substances. Compounding is time-consuming. It is important to always strive for accuracy. Thus you must take your time. Rushing to prepare a compound is a recipe for disaster.

MEASURING LIQUIDS

Measuring liquids requires a few simple steps to ensure the proper volume. Because of the water molecules clinging to the sides of a container (called capillary action), the amount of liquid appears to be more than the actual amount. When reading the calibrations of a beaker or graduate you must have the liquid at eye level. You must read the graduated cylinder at the bottom of the liquid line, also known as the meniscus, as shown in Figure 11-8.

When choosing a vehicle in which to measure your liquids, remember that it is best to choose the container size closest to the volume required because the calibrations are more accurate than in larger containers. For maximum accuracy in measuring liquids use the 20% rule; choose a graduate no less than 20% of the capacity of a graduate. For example, if 80 mL of solution is needed, use a 100-mL graduate (20%); if a 250-mL graduate is used (over 32%), the measurement is not accurate. In some cases two measuring graduates are used to attain an accurate volume, or in the case of extremely small amounts, a syringe is used.

Depending on the type of product being prepared, different techniques are required. For each type of compounded product, there are specific steps that must be carefully followed as well as appropriate labeling. Pharmacy technicians often prepare compounded products and should be familiar with the behavior of each type of additive as well as the final product.

PREPARING SOLUTIONS

When preparing solutions, you must understand the major parts of the liquid: the **solvent** is the larger part of the overall **solution**, the **solute** is the ingredient or agent used within the solvent, and the solution is the final dosage form that results from the solute and solvent being combined. Most solutions are simply mixed by adding the solute to the solvent in portions for proper mixing or by adding two solutions together. One of the most important techniques of

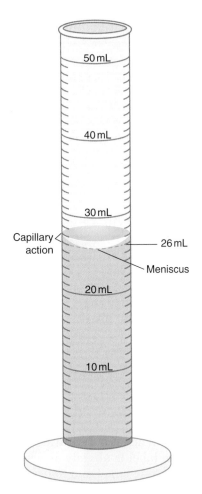

FIGURE 11-8 The meniscus is the level at which liquids are measured and recorded. For accuracy always have the container at eye level when determining the volume.

mixing solutions is to measure carefully and mix thoroughly. Solutions are prepared in all types of pharmacy settings. Always check the final solution for any possible precipitation or discoloration, which indicates an inappropriate concentration or mixture of ingredients.

Solubility

A drug's solubility will dictate the type of dosage form that needs to be prepared. For example, if it is water-soluble then a **syrup** or solution can be prepared; however, if it is insoluble then an **elixir**, a **suspension**, or possibly an emulsion can be made. The pH affects the solubility of a drug as well, and in this case buffers may be used to maintain the correct solubility characteristics. Buffers are solutions that resist pH changes when either acids or bases are added to the solution. Factors that affect solubility characteristics are listed in Box 11-5.

RECONSTITUTING PREMADE SUSPENSIONS

The only type of compounding that may be done away from the compounding area is the **reconstitution** of premade oral suspensions. Reconstituting involves mixing a diluent (liquid) into a powder to form a solution or suspension. These products are simple to prepare and do not need to be logged or labeled in the same manner as compounded products.

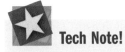

Tech Note!

When orders indicate a solution to be a specific strength with instruction to "qs" the solution to a final volume, this means that the solution is to yield a final volume and final strength exactly as ordered by the physician.

BOX 11-5 SOLUBILITY CHARACTERISTICS

1. Small particles dissolve faster than large particles.
2. Stirring increases the dissolution rate.
3. The more soluble the drug, the faster it dissolves.
4. Viscous liquids decrease dissolution rates.
5. Increased temperature normally increases dissolution rate.
6. Mixing an electrolyte with a non-electrolyte drug can either increase or decrease the dissolution rate.

TABLE 11-10 Common Auxiliary Labels Placed on Medication Containers

Dosage Form	Type of Auxiliary Label
Suspensions	SHAKE WELL
Ophthalmic preparations	FOR THE EYE
Otic preparations	FOR THE EAR
Ointments, creams, lotions	FOR TOPICAL USE;
	FOR EXTERNAL USE ONLY
Suppositories	FOR RECTAL USE;
	FOR VAGINAL USE
Patches	APPLY TO SKIN

When reconstituting prepackaged drugs such as an amoxicillin suspension, the label is already attached to the product. All the technician must do is read the side panel and follow the directions indicating the proper amount of sterile water (SW) to be mixed with the powder. The expiration dating that must be applied to the product after reconstitution is marked clearly on the side of the medication and is effective as soon as the suspension is mixed. Therefore, after mixing the drug, the technician should write the expiration date on the front of the label. In addition to this patient information, any necessary auxiliary labels must be attached. Table 11-10 lists common auxiliary labels.

Suspensions are different from solutions because they mix a **hydrophobic** (not water-soluble) ingredient into a **hydrophilic** (water-soluble) solution. When reconstituting a suspension, if the manufacturer suggests 110 mL of distilled water to be mixed with the powder in the bottle, you should add only half of the water (or another partial amount as the manufacturer directs) at first. This allows the powder to mix with the water in enough free space within the bottle; this reduces the volume within the bottle and makes it easier to mix in the remaining amount. The powdered ingredient is suspended in sterile water after mixing. Therefore all suspensions must be shaken well before each use to mix the powder evenly, which then can deliver the proper amount of medication. Many antibiotics, but not all, must be refrigerated after mixing.

SOLIDS: TABLETS, CAPSULES, AND LOZENGES

Tablets, capsules, and lozenges can be compounded by pharmacy technicians. Advantages for the use of these preparations include that the medication is custom-made for each patient's specific needs. Molds are used for forming these types of oral dosage forms. A product can be made accurately using careful measuring, weighing, and mixing procedures. As you can imagine, this technique is slow and arduous; therefore the technician's ability in preparing these dosage

BOX 11-6 TABLET ADDITIVES

Diluent bases: These can be combined to increase the firmness of the tablet.
  Dextrose
  Lactose
  Mannitol
  Sucrose
For drugs that react chemically with sugars, the following can be added:
  Bentonite
  Calcium carbonate
  Calcium phosphate
  Kaolin
Liquids can be added to moisten and mold powder:
  Mixture of alcohol and water in different percentages (50% to 80% alcohol): Alcohol accelerates drying, and water causes sugar to dissolve and bind the tablet. If the ingredients dissolve in water quickly, then adding water can be omitted.

forms requires great skill and experience. Pharmacies can provide individualized strengths and dosage forms to meet the needs of the patient. Molded tablets can be prepared using a tablet **triturate** mold. Compressed tablets are made using a pellet press or single-punch tablet-making machine. Tablets by far are the most common dosage form used because of their ease of administration: they can be taken orally, sublingually, or as a buccal dose, or they can be prepared similar to troches and wafers.

Molded Tablets

Molded tablets disintegrate quickly when they are exposed to moisture. Because molded tablets are small they are limited to substances that require a smaller dose. Ingredients used in preparing molded tablets require a base and additional additives to the active drug; types of additives are listed in Box 11-6.

Tablet Molds. Tablet molds are made of metal and consist of a top plate (i.e., cavity plate) that has holes and a bottom plate (i.e., peg plate) that has pegs. Capacities for tablet molds can range from 60 to 100 mg.

Steps Necessary for Preparation of Molded Tablets. Because molds have a fixed volume, they must be **calibrated** (Box 11-7). This is because each base used in preparing a molded tablet has a different density, which will change the capacity of each hole in the mold plate. The procedure used in compounding molded tablets is listed in Box 11-8.

Compressed Tablets and Lozenges

For preparing tablets or lozenges a single-punch tablet press can be used to make one dose at a time or a metal punch press can be employed to make multiple doses. These presses are available in a variety of sizes to make various strengths of tablets or lozenges. Types of lozenges include hard or soft, and tablets can be chewable, effervescent, or disintegrating. The metal punch press is composed of two parts; the bottom has a small cavity in one end of the tube; the top has a rod that pushes through the cavity. The rod does not extend totally through the cavity; instead, it leaves a small gap. The punch fits into the press. As the handle is depressed and then released, the rod moves in and out of the bottom piece. To make a compressed tablet follow the steps outlined in the following section.

BOX 11-7 CALIBRATING THE MOLD

1. Tablets that contain only a powder base are made first. Weigh the entire batch and then average the weight per tablet.
2. Determine the average weight of only the active drug; fill a few cavities in the mold and average the weight per tablet.
3. The quantity of the total prescription is divided by the average weight of each tablet's active ingredient. This gives the percentage of the cavity volume that is needed by the active drug.
4. Subtract the percentage in step 3 from 100%; this equals the volume (%) available for the base.
5. Use percentages of both the active drug in the cavity and the base in the cavity to calculate the amount of base and drug to weigh. (For example, if the mold holds 10 cavities, with each cavity holding 100 mg, then 1000 mg of mixture will be needed to fill the entire mold.) From this calculation, the base and drug to weigh can be calculated. (For example, multiply 1000 by the two different percentages from steps 3 and 4.)
6. Between 5% and 10% excess mixture is normally prepared to allow for powder loss and any variance in the capacity of the molds.

BOX 11-8 COMPOUNDING PROCEDURE FOR MOLDED TABLETS

1. Prepare the powder mixture using proper techniques for that specific recipe; then sift the mixture through an 80- to 100-mesh sieve.
2. Moisten the mix (alcohol/water) until it has the consistency of Playdough.
3. Place the cavity plate on either an ointment tile or a glass plate.
4. Take the molded form and press into the cavity plate using a hard rubber spatula.
5. Apply sufficient pressure onto each cavity to make sure all cavities are filled equally and fully.
6. Inspect the cavity plate to ensure all cavities are filled to capacity (there should be very little mixture left unused).
7. Align the cavity plate onto the peg plate and then slowly press down evenly onto the peg plate.
8. The cavity plate will fall, having pushed out the tablets onto the pegs.
9. Leave the tablets on the pegs until dried.

To view video visit http://pharmlabs.unc.edu/labs/tablets/videos.htm.

Making a Tablet. The following steps are used in making a compressed tablet:

1. Place the powder into the bottom piece.
2. Depress the handle and then release. The powders are compressed and will occupy the gap left in the press.
3. Let the tablets harden; then remove them from the punch press.

Compounding Capsules. Various sizes of capsules are kept in stock for these types of preparations. An advantage of capsules is a masked taste, and they are easier to swallow than tablets. After the proper proportions are prepared, the powder is then blocked. Using a steel spatula the powder is gathered and compressed onto a flat surface, making it easier to fill the capsule using the **punch** method. The body (i.e., the larger part of the capsule) is punched, attached to the end (i.e., the smaller part of the capsule), and then weighed to make sure each capsule is filled with the same amount of drug. The error rate is calculated by recording each capsule weight and determining the average weight. Following

TABLE 11-11 Capsule Sizes

Number	Approximate Amount Contained (mg)	Example
000	1000	
00	750	
0	500	
1	400	
2	300	
3	200	
4	150	
5	100	

quality control measures from *USP <795>*, capsules, powders, lozenges, and tablets must not weigh less than 90% or more than 110% of the calculated weight for each unit.

In larger pharmacies automated capsule-filling machines can quickly and accurately fill various capsule sizes, saving the pharmacy staff hours of compounding and allowing them to fill other orders or more difficult mixtures. The punch method is used when preparing smaller quantities of capsules. Capsules are composed of vegetables or gelatin materials. Great care must be taken to accurately load the capsule.

Other solids include mini-tabs (mostly used for pediatric patients), troches, and lozenges. **Troches** and lozenges are larger than tablets and are intended to dissolve slowly in the mouth. Troches often are placed in the cheek (buccal) for administration. Table 11-11 shows the sizes of capsules and the quantity of medication each one holds.

Lozenges. **Lozenges** are made by molding or by compression and have several advantages. They are normally made with flavors to enhance their taste. They also can be used as buccal tablets that are absorbed through the buccal lining of the mouth when the appropriate ingredients are used. Children have a much easier time taking gummy-type lozenges than other dosage forms since they mimic candy. Lozenges either dissolve or disintegrate slowly in the mouth.

The following traditional drugs are used to make lozenges:

- Phenol
- Sodium phenolate
- Benzocaine
- Cetylpyridinium chloride
- May also contain: anesthetics, antimicrobials, antitussives, antiemetics, and decongestants

Molding mixtures are used to prepare different types of lozenges and may contain the following ingredients:

- Sugars to form a hard lozenge
- Polyethylene glycol (PEG) to form a soft lozenge
- Gelatin to form a chewable lozenge

Hard Lozenges. Hard lozenges can be made into the traditional round shape or manufactured to look like a lollipop or sucker. A combination of sugars is mixed with other ingredients and the medication, which is then poured into a mold and allowed to cool before removal. When heating the various ingredients together, great care must be taken in monitoring the temperature, moisture content, and pH of the final product.

Considerations in preparing hard lozenges include the following:

- Drugs that may degrade in high heat cannot be made into hard lozenges.
- The dosage form needs a low moisture content, between 0.5% and 1.5%.
- Certain syrups cannot be stirred until a specific temperature is reached.
- Between 55% and 65% sucrose and between 35% and 45% corn syrup must be used to avoid grainy consistency.
- If acidic flavorings are used, this lowers the pH; calcium carbonate, sodium bicarbonate, or magnesium hydroxide must be used to raise the pH to 5 or 6.

Hard Lozenge Formula*
1. Drug: 2 g
2. Powdered sugar: 84 g
3. Corn syrup: 32 g
4. Water: 48 mL
5. Mint extract: 2 mL

Soft Lozenges. Soft lozenges can be made relatively quickly and then colored and flavored. They can be chewed or dissolve in the mouth. Ingredients used include polyethylene glycol (PEG) 1000 or 1450, chocolate, or a sugar/acacia base. Lozenges can be hand-rolled and cut into pieces or poured while warm into a plastic troche mold. After the mold cools, a spatula is used to level the excess solution; using a hair blow-dryer will give a smooth appearance.

Softeners are mixed and heated to 50° C; mixtures may include the following ingredients:

- Acacia gel: used to add texture and smoothness
- Silica gel: used as a suspending agent, keeping materials from settling to the bottom of the mold
- Flavoring
- Food extracts
- Syrup flavor concentrates
- Volatile oils
- Sweeteners
- 9 parts NutraSweet and 1 part saccharin

Soft Lozenge Formula
1. Drug: 1 g
2. PEG: 10 g
3. Aspartame: 20 packets
4. Mint extract: 1 mL
5. Color: qs

---

*Use food color to confirm adequate mixing in lab.

Chewable Lozenges. Gummy-type lozenges are made primarily for children. The formulations consist of glycerinated gelatin and water. Fruit flavoring is used to sweeten the ingredients and disguise the taste of glycerin, which is very acidic. After the ingredients are combined they are heated at a low heat until a fluid forms, which is then poured into preshaped gummy molds and cooled.

Chewable Lozenges Formula
1. Drug: 0.5 g
2. Glycerin: 70 mL
3. Gelatin: 18 g
4. Water: 12 mL
5. Methylparabenzamide: 0.4 g
6. Flavoring oil: 3 to 4 gtt
7. Color: qs

SEMISOLIDS: OINTMENTS, STICKS, AND SUPPOSITORIES

Ointments, pastes, and creams each have different consistencies depending on the amount of solids used. Pastes have more solids in them than ointments and creams. **Creams** are semisolid emulsions that are similar to ointments but they are opaque instead of translucent. All three final forms have smooth consistencies. The classifications of ointments are listed in Box 11-9. Semisolids are prepared in all types of pharmacy settings. It is important to mix all ingredients in the right order, following the recipe completely for uniformity.

Medication Sticks

Medication sticks provide another way of administering medication. Agents such as antibiotics, local anesthetics, sunscreens, antivirals, and oncological drugs can be manufactured as medication sticks and applied directly to the site on the body that needs treatment. They can also be applied to certain epidermal sites for a systemic effect (i.e., affecting the whole body).

Various waxes are used to make either hard or soft sticks and are dependent on specific blends and temperatures to achieve the desired consistency. Additional ingredients—such as resins, polymers, oils, and gels—determine the texture and appearance (i.e., clear or opaque [cloudy]) of the finished product.

When combining two or more ingredients that have different ranges of melting points, melt the ingredients sequentially from highest to lowest melting point. This practice will prevent overheating as the temperature is reduced on the hot plate.

Filling Ointment Jars

The appropriate size container should be selected; these range in size from $\frac{1}{4}$ ounce to 1 pound. Using a small spatula, pack the ointment carefully into the bottom and sides of the container and then fill the center. The jar can be tapped to release any trapped bubbles. The final step is to top off the jar, smoothing the ointment level at the top. For melted ointments, pour the ointment into the jar while still warm, let the ointment solidify, and then smooth off the top by using a heated metal spatula.

Filling Ointment Tubes

Ointment tubes are available in different sizes. For choosing the appropriate size, first roll the ointment (on glassine paper) into a cylinder slightly smaller than the circumference and length of the tube. Before placing the roll into the back of the tube, take off the cap to release the displaced air when the ointment is inserted. Place both the ointment and the rolling paper into the tube; then

BOX 11-9 CLASSIFICATIONS OF OINTMENT BASES

Absorption Bases: Properties include the following: absorb water; highly compatible with medications; increased stability to heat; greasy; most are not washable. Examples:
- Hydrophilic (water-loving) petrolatum bases (USP)
- Petrolatum mixed with cholesterol (Aquaphor)

Emulsion Bases: Properties include the following: insoluble in water; not washable unless mixed with water-in-oil (w/o) base; subject to water loss; washable and nongreasy when in an oil-in-water (o/w) base; more prone to mold growth unless a preservative is added. Examples:
- Lanolin
- USP (water/oil)
- Hydrophilic ointment
- USP (oil/water)
- Vanishing creams (oil/water)

Oleaginous Bases: Properties include the following: insoluble in water; good compatibility with a variety of medications; difficult to remove from clothing and skin; difficult to determine the amount of medication released upon application. The types of bases are listed below.
- Petrolatum (Vasoline)
  - Consistency can be altered by adding mineral oil or white wax
  - Will not absorb much water unless mixed with cholesterol
  - Stable bases that mix well with most substances
  - All bases are greasy
  - Melting point between 38° and 60° C
- Jelene (Plastibase)
  - Mixture of hydrocarbons in both liquid and wax types
  - Jellylike consistency
  - Able to withstand a wider range of temperatures before melting
  - Release medication faster than petrolatum base
- Silicones
  - Polymers of silicon and oxygen
  - Protect skin from moisture

Water-Soluble Bases: Properties include the following: will both absorb and dissolve in water; are nongreasy and therefore washable; are not susceptible to mold or microbial growth; the color of the base can change in the presence of certain drugs unless cetyl alcohol is added. Example:
- Polyethylene Glycols aka: Carbowaxes: Consistency dependent on molecular weight, which is noted by a number; the increasing number relates to the solidity of the agent. Carbowax 300 is a liquid at room temperature whereas 1540 is a solid.

cover the end of the tube with a spatula and carefully pull out the paper, leaving the ointment inside the tube. Fold the end of the tube over twice, use crimpers to seal the end of the tube, and label the product.

Soft Sticks

Soft sticks can be clear or opaque; they spread the medication evenly when applied, they soften at body temperature, and they do not leave a residue on the skin after application.

Ingredients used in soft sticks:

- Waxes
- Polymers
- Oils
- Gels
- Petrolatum

- Cocoa butter
- Polyethylene glycol (PEG)

Formulations

Soft Opaque Stick Formulation
1. White beeswax: 30 g
2. Cetyl alcohol: 8 g
3. Cocoa butter: 6 g
4. Carnauba wax: 1 g
5. Castor oil (tasteless): 2 mL
6. Aquabase T: 20 g
7. Petrolatum: 13.5 g
8. Perfume: 0.9 mL
9. Preservative: 0.1 g
10. Butyl stearate: 5 mg
11. Active drug: qs

Soft Clear Stick Formulation (e.g., analgesic stick: methyl salicylate is active ingredient for topical pain relief)
1. Sodium stearate: 13%
2. Methyl salicylate: 35%
3. Menthol: 15%
4. Propylene glycol: 25%
5. Water: 12%

Hard sticks contain crystalline powders that are held together either by heat or by a binding agent. This type of stick must be moistened before it becomes active and will leave a white residue when applied.

Hard Stick Formulation (e.g., styptic stick: stops bleeding from minor cuts, such as razor cuts)
1. Ammonium chloride: 7 g
2. Aluminum sulfate: 27 g
3. Ferric sulfate: 40 g
4. Copper sulfate: 26 g

The following are additional types of ingredients that can be used in sticks:

- Lubricants:
  - Paraffin
  - Castor oil
  - Corn oil
  - Cottonseed oil
  - Oleic oil
  - Peanut oil
  - Soybean oil
  - PEG 300 or 400
- Skin care additives:
  - Vitamin A
  - Vitamin E
- Sun protection agents:
  - Zinc oxide
  - *p*-Aminobenzoic acid (PABA)

Sizes and styles of applicators differ depending on their intended use. Lip balms are prepared in small cylindrical-shaped plastic applicators. To fill the applicators without leaving an indentation in the top (caused by the cooling process), follow these steps:

1. Turn the base of the applicator two full turns to raise the bale (the bottom platform).
2. Slightly overfill the tube with the base. Do this when the mixture has cooled as much as possible to avoid shrinkage.
3. Top the base by pressing a warm spatula on the top of the base to cover any hole that may have appeared during the cooling process.
4. Turn the base of the applicator downward and place the cap on top.

Suppositories

Several sizes and shapes of suppositories are used to administer medications to vaginal, rectal, and urethral areas; suppositories are made with either solutions or ointments. There are three different ways to prepare suppositories: hand-rolling, compression, and fusion-molding. The various bases used in suppositories serve two purposes: they provide a medium that can carry the medication to the site of absorption and they allow the medication to be released over different lengths of time. Common bases used are listed in the following sections.

Oleaginous Bases. Cocoa butter or synthetic triglycerides can be used because they remain solid at room and body temperatures and melt at warm temperatures. However, care must be taken when heating suppositories made with cocoa butter. If a suppository is heated above 35° C (95° F) its properties will change, and it will not keep a solid form when temperatures rise to 30° C (77° F). The synthetic triglycerides are more stable, although they are more expensive. Stepan, the manufacturer of Wecobee, makes several bases from coconut oil with a temperature range from 33.9° C up to 40.5° C, depending on which formula is used. Other triglyceride products by different manufacturers include Dehydag, Hydro-Kote, Suppocire, and Witepsol. Because of the temperature range at which suppositories will melt, they should be stored in a cool place or the refrigerator.

Water-Soluble Bases. Polyethylene glycol (PEG) polymers or glycerinated gelatins can be used in the manufacturing of suppositories. These types of ingredients dissolve in body fluids and are not as dependent on temperature; therefore they can be stored at room temperature. PEG polymers are a popular choice because of their properties: they are nonirritating, they can be used to make suppositories either by molding or by compression, and they have a wide melting point range. Different weights of PEG bases are normally mixed together or with another base to form different levels of solidity and dissolving lengths. The combinations include the following:

- PEG 1450 (30%) and PEG 8000 (70%)
- PEG 1000 (75%) and PEG 3350 (25%)
- PEG 1450 (2.3 g) and silica gel (25 mg)
- PEG 300 (60%) and PEG 8000 (40%)

Glycerinated Gelatins. These are often used for vaginal suppositories and have a wide range of additives, such as zinc oxide and boric acid. Their properties include an ability to disperse slowly in mucous secretions; they are translucent and gelatinous solids. They must be kept in a cool place because they will decompose in humid environments. If they are to be kept for an extended period of time, preservatives are added, such as methylparaben, propylparaben, or a combination of both. They should be dipped in water before administration to activate the gelatin.

Preparing Suppositories

Using Molds. If suppository molds are used, they must be kept at room temperature because the rapid cooling of refrigeration can cause the suppositories to break. The formulation should be poured into each mold cavity in a steady and consistent manner to prevent a layered appearance. Also, pouring the ingredients just before they reach their congealing point will allow for a solid suppository. If they are poured too soon (after heating) they can produce a hole in the top of the suppository; this is due to contraction. Hard molds such as metal or rubber require a lubricant, which will aid in removal of suppositories. A light coat of vegetable oil spray before pouring the mixture can be used for this purpose.

When filling molds, pour to the top of each one; filling slightly over the mold is also permissible because the excess can be removed with a heated metal spatula. A black light (used to improve visualization) is used to fill suppository shells (unit dose) to ensure the ingredients are filled to the proper line. These shells may be filled either by pouring or by using a syringe, which limits spillage and allows better control over the volume filled. It is important to be very careful when removing suppositories; the two halves should not be pried apart; instead, they should be pushed away from one another by placing the top of the screws on the table and pushing down on the mold (Figure 11-9).

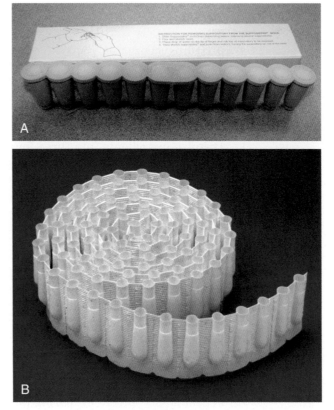

FIGURE 11-9 Suppository molds can be used as well as hand-rolled method. **A,** Suppository molds prepared in the pharmacy. **B,** Suppository packaging. (Courtesy of Total Pharmacy Supply, Inc., © 2011.)

Using Hand-Rolling Method. Another way of preparing only a few suppositories is to roll them by hand. For this method cocoa butter is used as a base because it does not have to be melted. Triturate the grated cocoa butter along with the active ingredient in a mortar. Form a ball-like shape using the palm of your hands; then roll the suppository into a cylinder using a large spatula or a small flat board on a pill tile. The cylinder is cut into suppository segments, which are then rolled on one end to form a conical shape.

Packaging Suppositories. If plastic shells are not used then it is necessary to wrap each suppository separately, using foil wrappers that are available in different sizes and colors.

NASAL PREPARATIONS: OINTMENTS, SUSPENSIONS, GELS, AND SOLUTIONS

Nasal preparations can be compounded into dosage forms such as jellies, gels, and ointments that can be administered as topical agents (e.g., ointments, gels, jellies), sprays (e.g., solutions), drops (e.g., solutions, suspensions), or nasal inhalers (e.g., volatiles). Excipients used include buffers, preservatives, tonicity adjusting agents, gelling agents, and antioxidants, all of which must be nonirritating. These are the same types of agents that are used in ophthalmic formulations. They are quickly absorbed into the bloodstream for rapid onset of activity.

Common preservatives used in nasal products include the following:

- Benzalkonium chloride
- Benzethonium chloride
- Phenylmercuric acetate
- Phenylmercuric nitrate
- Thimerosal
- *p*-Hydroxybenzoates

The preparation method for each type of dosage form begins with accurate measuring and weighing of each ingredient.

Preparing Solution
1. Dissolve ingredients into three fourths of the total amount of sterile water (SW) for injection to be used; mix well.
2. qs the SW to the total volume required.
3. Determine pH, clarity, and other quality control factors from a sample of solution.
4. Filter through a sterile 0.2-micrometer filter into a sterile nasal container.
5. Package and label.

Preparing Suspensions
1. Repeat steps 1 through 3 under "Preparing Solution."
2. Package in an appropriate container for autoclaving.
3. Autoclave, cool, and then label (this step is optional depending on the recipe).
4. Choose a random sample to check for quality of product (e.g., sterility, pH).
5. Package and label; shake well before using.

Preparing Ointments
1. Repeat step 1 under "Preparing Solution."
2. Sterilize each ingredient using an appropriate method.
3. Mix each of the ingredients with the sterile vehicle.
4. Perform quality control on a sample of the mixture.
5. Package and label; for topical use only.

Preparing Gels

1. Repeat step 1 under "Preparing Solution."
2. Filter through a 0.2-micrometer filter into a sterile container.
3. Add the (sterilized) gelling agent and mix well.
4. Add SW for injection to volume/weight and mix well.
5. Perform quality assurance (QA) on sample.
6. Package and label; for topical use only.

Beyond-use dating should be no more than 14 days (refrigerated) for agents that contain water formulations. Other (nonaqueous) formulations normally have beyond-use dating that is no more than one fourth of the manufacturer dating or 6 months, whichever is less. All other formulations have a recommended beyond-use dating of 30 days or the end of therapy, whichever comes first.

Packaging

The types of containers used for compounded products must be appropriate. The container must protect the contents and have a child-resistant cap (if applicable), the appropriate label, and auxiliary label(s). Once mixed to the proper concentration, all products are filled into the appropriately sized container. This should be done neatly to avoid waste. Containers vary in size and in manufactured materials, depending on the circumstances in which the drug is used (Table 11-12). Containers used to package compounded products include glass and plastic bottles, syringes, dropper bottles, and jars of various sizes. There are a variety of capsule sizes used to hold medications and suppository molds for rectal preparations.

Syringes sometimes are used to prepare oral, vaginal, or parenteral compounds. Once the drug is loaded into the barrel of the syringe, a cap is placed over the top to keep the contents inside. For those items that should not be injected, an oral syringe or other syringe to which a needle cannot be attached should be used; using an oral/nonparenteral syringe will alleviate dosage administration errors.

Certain containers do not have childproof caps or lids; therefore the patient must be instructed by the pharmacist to keep these types of containers out of the reach of children. The following are some examples of these types of containers:

*   Syringes
*   Cream or ointment jars
*   Dropper bottles
*   Ointment tubes

Tech Alert!

Ophthalmic, inhalant, otic, and nasal preparations carry a high risk of cross-contamination if used by more than one patient. Never share these agents.

Tech Note!

Read all instructions before beginning to compound materials. Make sure that all the ingredients are available to avoid a delay in product preparation. Also, it is important to reorder stock after ingredients are depleted so that the ingredients are available for the next prescription.

TABLE 11-12 Types of Containers/Sealants and Dosage Forms They Contain

Container/Sealant	Dosage Forms
Foil paper	Suppositories
Polystyrene	Use for solids in bottles and jars
Metal tubes	Ointments and semisolids
Amber bottles	Tablets, capsules, liquids
Heat-sealed strips*	Tablets, capsules
Amber blister packs*	Tablets, capsules

*For institutional use only.

TABLE 11-13 *USP <795>* Guidelines

Solids and nonaqueous liquids	Medications prepared from commercial dosage forms; one fourth of remaining expiration date of commercial product or 6 months maximum
Solids and nonaqueous liquids	Medications prepared from bulk ingredients; up to 6 months
Water-containing formulations	Medications prepared from ingredients in a solid form; up to 14 days when stored in refrigerator
All other formulations	Up to 30 days or intended duration of therapy, whichever comes first

Stability

Several factors affect the stability of a drug. The amount of light, air, temperature, and even pH alter the longevity of a drug. Legally, the date given to a pharmacy-prepared product cannot be longer than any of the ingredients in the product. The pharmacist or the pharmacy technician must find the appropriate expiration date from the manufacturer's literature if it is not already provided. In addition to this reference, many compounding books contain calculations that determine appropriate expiration dates. Prepared recipes contain all necessary information. The beyond-use date of a preparation is set from the time of compounding, not from the time when the medication is dispensed. If there is no literature to determine the beyond-use date, *USP <795>* has provided guidelines that can be used (Table 11-13) to set the appropriate dating.

Documentation

Just as in repackaging, documentation of compounded medications is important. By keeping accurate records the integrity of the product dispensed is ensured, and falls within FDA guidelines for quality assurance. Although protocol varies between pharmacy settings, most compounding ingredients and steps are put into a recipe format for the person preparing the medication. Along with the recipe, document the information shown in Box 11-10. In addition to the compounding log sheet, pharmacies are required to have material safety data sheets (MSDS) either in hard copy or as electronically accessible forms for all chemicals and drug substances. If, however, commercial products are used in preparing the medication, the package insert may be used.

Once the label is affixed to the container, all necessary auxiliary labels are then chosen. Many auxiliary labels not only instruct the patient in the intended use of the product but also indicate the appropriate storage requirements. In addition, some labels allow for expiration dates to be added.

Safety

All chemicals should be safely stored inside cabinets or behind shelf brackets to avoid spillage. Several additives can be harmful if they are inhaled or come into contact with eyes or skin. Every pharmacy has an MSDS binder with information regarding all chemical products and how to handle spillage or contact. It is important to know where the MSDS binder is kept within the pharmacy department.

Cleaning up excess ingredients appropriately is important; the method of cleaning and disposing of agents or any equipment used depends on the type of agents used. Hazardous chemicals must be discarded properly according to pharmacy protocol. Nonhazardous chemicals can normally be discarded in a

BOX 11-10 INFORMATION NECESSARY ON COMPOUNDING LOG SHEET AND MEDICATION LABEL

Log Sheet Information
- Date prepared
- Names of ingredients
- Manufacturer of each ingredient
- Lot number and expiration date of each ingredient (this includes sterile water container, if used)
- Amount or weight of each ingredient
- Dosage form of each ingredient
- Pharmacy lot number assigned
- Pharmacy beyond-use date assigned
- Technician's initials
- Pharmacist's initials
- Date dispensed
- Patient's name and medical record number
- Documents are kept on the pharmacy premises for no less than 3 years from the time the medication was prepared

Medication Label Information
- Name of patient and medical record number
- Date
- Drug name
- Drug strength
- Physician
- Sig: directions
- Pharmacy lot number and expiration date
- Initials of both technician and pharmacist

regular trash container. Any glass or needles must be placed in a sharps container.

Sterile Compounding

Sterile compounding is performed for most parenteral medications that are administered intravenously (IV), intramuscularly (IM), intrathecally (IT), subcutaneously (SubQ), intradermally (ID), or intranasally, or by otic or ophthalmic routes of administration. The primary characteristic of these agents is that they are sterile upon completion of compounding. This means they are free from any contamination such as microbial growth, pyrogens, and particulate matter. Pyrogens are the by-products of living microorganisms. Any particles larger than 50 micrometers can be seen with the unaided eye; for those particles much smaller than 50 micrometers, a filter must be used to capture any particulates. Although hospital pharmacies can prepare dosage forms other than parenteral medications such as ophthalmics, specialty items are commonplace in a compounding pharmacy.

There are advantages to typical parenteral medications, such as they work quickly in emergency situations in which the patient either is unconscious or is unable to take oral medication. Disadvantages include the higher cost of these drugs, the risk of infection, and the need for a skilled nurse or other trained person for their administration.

The equipment and supplies used in preparing sterile products include laminar flow hoods, glove boxes, filters, sterile solutions, needles, syringes, and a skilled person to prepare the agent using aseptic technique (see Chapter 12).

Ophthalmic Agents

There are several types of dosage forms that can be prepared for the treatment of various eye conditions. These include eye solutions, suspensions, and ointments. All ophthalmic agents that are purchased over-the-counter are sterile, and any eye agents that are compounded must also be sterile in the final container. Preservatives are used to ensure sterility once the container is opened.

Just as pH and stability are major factors in compounding medications, they are also important when compounding eye formulas. The pH of both blood and tears is 7.4; therefore ophthalmic agents should be prepared with this pH goal in mind. However, ophthalmic agents usually have a pH that ranges from 6.5 to 8.5. Although pH 7.4 is the optimum goal, sometimes this is impossible to attain because of other factors, such as stability or therapeutic activity of the drug. The tears of the eye do act similar to a buffer and can adjust the pH of a substance applied to the eye(s). Because tears have this ability, the pH can range from 4.5 to 11.5 if necessary, because the eyes will try to compensate. Other factors such as the viscosity and tonicity of the formulation also can influence the overall pH. All of these factors need to be controlled to maintain a safe pH while following *USP <797>* regulations covering sterile compounding procedures.

Ophthalmic agents must be made in a laminar flow hood using aseptic technique (see Chapter 12) and packaged in sterile containers. Solutions may require 0.2-micrometer filtration to remove any particles before packaging; suspensions cannot be filtered because the necessary particles would be removed by the filter; and ointments must have each ingredient sterilized separately and then added using aseptic technique. The properties of each type of ophthalmic agent are listed below:

- **Solutions:** These sterile ophthalmic agents are prepared especially for the eye environment. Most solutions are dispensed in eye dropper bottles that hold approximately 15 mL and are dosed in drops (gtt). An example of a compounded ophthalmic solution is given in Example 11-3. This compound can be prepared in the lab setting.
- **Suspensions:** These formulations contain small solid particles. The recommended size of the particles should not exceed 10 micrometers to avoid eye irritation. Suspensions must be shaken before use.
- **Ointments:** These agents have an ointment base consisting of an oil and white petrolatum that melt at body temperature. They must be nonirritating; they should not contain any large particles that could aggravate the eye upon application. They tend to last longer in the eye than suspensions and do not wash away with tears. Blurred vision is common after application; therefore they may be prescribed at bedtime. Small ointment tubes are normally used that hold approximately 3.5 g of drug.

The following additives are commonly used in ophthalmic agents:

- Sodium chloride
- Benzalkonium chloride (preservative)
- Sterile water for injection
- Boric acid USP
- Polyvinyl alcohol (increases viscosity)
- Povidone-iodine
- Chlorobutanol (preservative)
- Polysorbate (wetting agent)

★ Tech Note!

Parenteral refers to administering a dosage for systemic effect outside of the enteral routes (i.e., orally, sublingually, rectally). Most commonly, the term refers to those medications given by injection or intravenously, but it can also include intraperitoneal drugs. By the nature of their route of administration, most parenteral dosage forms must be sterile.

EXAMPLE 11-3

Cefazolin Super Eye Drops

50 mg/mL: 10 mL
(After lab discard product safely)

Ingredients/Supplies

Cefazolin 500 mg #1 vial
Artificial tears 15-mL bottle
Sodium chloride 0.9% for injection 10 mL
5-micrometer filter needle #1

Procedure

Prepare in a laminar flow hood using aseptic technique:
1. Remove 7.2 mL of the artificial tears from the 15-mL bottle using a syringe and needle; discard syringe.
2. Reconstitute the 500-mg vial of cefazolin with 2 mL of 0.9% sodium chloride (preservative free).
3. Draw the reconstituted cefazolin into a syringe; using a 5-micrometer filter needle, inject 2.2 mL (500 mg) into the artificial tears bottle (10-mL total volume).
4. Shake well.

Log Sheet for Cefazolin Super Eye Drops 50 mg/mL

Date prepared: 3/4/11
Amount prepared: 10 mL

Drug Name	Manufacturer	Mfg log #	Mfg exp Date	Amount Used
Cefazolin 500 mg	UDL	ZZ109	6/12	1 vial
Artificial tears	BL	49087211	1/12	7.8 mL
0.9% NaCl for injection	UDL	009342	8/13	2 mL

Storage: Refrigerate
Stability: 28 days
Pharmacy Lot # 99456
Prepared by: May Atkinson
RPh: Paul Rodriquez
Apply copy of label here.

Tech Alert!

You can use an ophthalmic preparation in the ear but never an otic preparation in the eye. The eye will become infected if a nonsterile solution is placed into it, or if a sterile otic medication is not formulated for the proper osmotic content or pH required for use in the eye.

Bells Compounding Pharmacy
21 Star Street.
Your City,State,Zip,Phone

Cefazolin Super Eye Drops 50mg/mL   Qty: 10mL
  Rx#99432
For: Janet Jones   Dr. J. James

Apply 1 drop to each eye twice daily

Beyond use date: 4/8/11   Refills 0
Date Prepared: 3/4/11

FOR THE EYE ONLY
REFRIGERATE

Compounding Professionalism

Pharmaceutical eloquence is the special use of finishing technique to give the final product a professional look. Great care must be taken when topping off jars of creams and ointments. By holding the spatula very straight across the top of the ingredients and slowly turning the container, the top will achieve a smooth appearance. Then slowly lift the spatula as you are turning to leave a small curl in the center of the cream/ointment.

Regulatory and Quality Control

The repackaging and compounding of pharmaceutical products are subject to regulatory control. The manner in which the medication is packaged affects both the product inside the package and the user's compliance with following the physician's orders for taking the medication. Many medications can degrade with UV light exposure; therefore they must be placed in amber-colored containers to protect the medication. Storage is another consideration that must be given to the prepared product within a specific type of container. All labeling requirements must be followed or the prescription is considered misbranded. Under the FDA Modernization Act of 1997 the following restrictions were placed on pharmacies:

- Compounded drugs may be made in limited quantities.
- The compounded products must be made from approved ingredients that meet manufacturing and safety standards.
- The drug product must not be identified by the FDA as a product that presents demonstrable difficulties for compounding in terms of safety or effectiveness.

Chemotherapeutic Agents

Special consideration must be given when preparing chemotherapeutic agents. Parenteral products or compounded creams, for example, should be prepared only in a safe environment, such as a vertical flow barrier-hood (see Chapter 12). Patients who cannot swallow tablets and capsules must have their medications prepared in other dosage forms, such as various solutions or transdermal delivery systems. When patients are self-administering chemotherapy medications, they should always follow proper guidelines to limit unwanted exposure, and they should be instructed in proper disposal so that others will not be exposed to the chemotherapeutic agent. Pharmacy preparation and clean-up must be done slowly and carefully and the proper documentation should be completed.

Veterinary Medications

Many pet owners must medicate their animals. Administering oral medications to a pet can be difficult. Many delivery systems have been developed to avoid forcing a tablet down the throat of an animal. For example, dog treats can be made that have the medication mixed into the treat; other forms of dosing include liquids and transdermal routes of administration. Sticks can be prepared to administer antibiotics to the inside of the ear; liquids poured onto a pet's food reduce the stress on both the animal and the owner. Labeling requirements for compounded veterinary products are listed in Box 11-11.

Compounding pharmacies provide many more choices for patients to administer their medications in the appropriate strength and dosage form to their pets, as shown in Table 11-14.

BOX 11-11 LABELING REQUIREMENTS FOR ANIMAL PRESCRIPTIONS

1. Name and address of the veterinarian
2. Active ingredient or ingredients
3. Date dispensed and expiration date
4. Name of pet
5. Directions for use specified by the practitioner and the class/species or identification of the animal
6. Dosage
7. Frequency
8. Route of administration
9. Duration of therapy
10. Any warnings and side effects must be given by the veterinarian and/or pharmacist to ensure safety
11. Name and address of the dispenser (pharmacy/pharmacist)
12. Prescription number
13. Date filled

TABLE 11-14 Pet Dosage Forms and Flavorings

Treats	Chewable flavored (beef, chicken, turkey) tablets for oral doses
Sticks	Transdermal gel applicators used for topical administration
Miniature tablets	Extremely small tablets; easy to put into food
Beads and pellets	Biodegradable dosage forms used in chemotherapeutic and other compounded agents

Compounding

Compounding medications requires skill and the ability to focus intently on the task at hand. Virtually all pharmacies will compound products to some degree. Technicians prepare these products using great care and pharmaceutical eloquence. This can only be accomplished through practice and perseverance. Specialized compounding pharmacies are becoming more popular as a result of the special needs of more people. These pharmacies can offer the consumer alternate routes of administration, better tasting medication, and an array of dosage forms to specifically suit each person's need. In addition, because of the wide variety of species, sizes, weights, and breeds of animals, many veterinary medications are custom-made. Formulations have been prepared to treat animals ranging in size from birds to whales. This industry will undoubtedly increase in popularity as a result of the special service they provide.

PERSONNEL TRAINING

Pharmacy programs must include supportive personnel (technicians) with adequate training to perform the necessary functions of compounding. To build and maintain a high skill level, training programs should be offered on a periodic basis. Instructions on compounding should include the following:

- Calculations
- Compounding equipment
- Dosage forms
- Interpretation of symbols
- Literature

- Safety
- Techniques

These programs may include watching instructional videos or observation and dialog between instructor and personnel. The instruction should also include either a written test or a quality control test of finished preparations. The highest level of competency in compounding procedures will be ensured if pharmacies provide initial training followed by recurrent training in methods, regulations, and techniques of compounding. In this way the pharmacy is providing the customer the highest product quality.

Compounding Calculations

Although many formulas are already documented in a compounding recipe book, there are situations where the final product may need to be prepared in a different strength or volume than that listed in the recipe, or products of different strengths may need to be used to prepare a final percent solution. In this case the pharmacist or technician will need to perform calculations to attain the correct weights and/or volumes for the final product. The following sections discuss calculation procedures for reducing or enlarging formulas, determining partial dosage units, changing stock solutions, mixing products of different strengths, performing solubility expressions, and converting units to weights. Remember: 1 mg = 1 mL can be used in conversion calculations, as shown in the following orders.

REDUCING OR ENLARGING FORMULAS

Enlarging a formula:
  Recipe: 100 mL of 2 g of ibuprofen gel
  How much ibuprofen powder is required to prepare 240 mL of gel?

$$2/100 = X/240 = 4.8 \text{ g of ibuprofen powder is needed}$$

Reducing a formula:
  Recipe: 100 mL of 2 g of ibuprofen gel
  How much ibuprofen powder is required to prepare 40 mL of gel?

$$2/10 = X/40 = 0.8 \text{ g of ibuprofen powder is needed}$$

Reducing a formula:
  Recipe: 100 mL of 5 mg/mL drug D
  Ingredients:
- Drug D 50-mg tablets #10
- Sterile water for injection 4 mL
- Artificial banana flavoring 3 mL
- Simple syrup (with suspending agent) mixture qs to 100 mL

To decrease this recipe to 35 mL of drug D 5 mg/mL suspension:

Take the total volume ordered (35 mL) and divide by the amount you have in the recipe (100); this will give you the final percentage to alter the formula. Then multiply each ingredient by this amount (0.35):

$$35/100 = 0.35\% \text{ of the original formula is needed}$$

To determine the new amount of each ingredient, multiply each ingredient by 0.35%:

Drug D: 10 tablets × 0.35 = 3.5 tablets

Sterile water: 4 mL × 0.35 = 1.4 mL

Banana flavoring: 3 mL × 0.35 = 1.05 mL

Sterile water for injection: qs to 35 mL

DETERMINING PARTIAL DOSAGE UNITS

Recipe: Mixture M, the original formula, calls for 125 mg of drug M
Drug M (capsule) 125 mg (5 capsules at 25 mg each)
Ora-Plus 60 mL
Ora-Sweet qs 120 mL
Using 25 mg of drug M capsules, determine the amount needed to make 120 mg:

120 mL is needed (can be written 120 mg/25 mg = 4.8 caps)

Then:

1. Empty 5 capsules onto weighing boat or paper, and weigh.
2. Determine how many grams you will need to remove.
   a. If the weight of 5 capsules is 1.6 g:

4.8 cap/5 cap = 0.96 × 1.6 g = 1.536 g is needed

3. Remove 0.064 g of drug M.

CHANGING STOCK SOLUTIONS

Prepare three 15-mL bottles of medicated solution with 0.01% ingredient A.
In stock: 17% ingredient A
How much of the 17% ingredient A will be used to prepare the three bottles of
   solution S?
   NOTE: 0.01% final strength needed = 0.01 g/100 mL; ingredient A = 17% =
   17 g/100 mL.

15 mL × 3 = 45 mL total volume to be prepared

45 mL × 0.01 g/100 mL = 0.0045 g needed

0.0045 g/x mL = 17 g/100 mL = 0.026 mL of ingredient A is needed

MIXING PRODUCTS OF DIFFERENT STRENGTHS

Order: 120 g of 0.1% ointment O
In stock: 1 oz of 0.1% ointment O base
½ oz of 0.15% ointment O base
2.5 oz of 0.005% ointment O base
If these three ingredients are mixed together, how much of ointment powder
   drug O must be added to prepare the prescription?
   NOTE: To calculate the percentage of each ingredient needed, divide each
   percentage by 100 (shown in parentheses); to convert the final answer
   from milligrams to grams, divide the answer by 1000 mg/g (shown in
   parentheses).

0.001 g (0.1/100) × 120 = 120 mg is ordered

$$0.001\,g\,(0.1/100) \times 30\,(1\,oz) = 0.03\,g \text{ or } 30\,mg\,(0.03\,g \times 1000\,mg/g)$$

$$0.0015\,g\,(0.15/100) \times 15\,(\tfrac{1}{2}\,oz) = 22.5\,mg\,(0.0225\,g \times 1000\,mg/g)$$

$$0.00005\,g\,(0.005/100) \times 75\,(2.5\,oz) = 3.8\,mg\,(0.0038\,g \times 1000\,mg/g)$$

Total amount = 56.3 mg

120 mg − 56.3 mg (3 other ingredients) = 63.7 mg of additional powder O is needed

PERFORMING SOLUBILITY EXPRESSIONS

Order: An order is received for 150 mL of drug X to be prepared in a 1:15 solution.
How much drug X will be required to fill this order?

$$1/15 = x/150 = 10\,g \text{ of drug X is needed}$$

Measure 10 g of powder X and qs to 150 mL

CONVERTING UNITS TO WEIGHTS

Order: 150,000 units of drug N per gram of ointment; quantity: 60 g to be dispensed.
How much of drug N should be weighed (based on 4400 [USP] units/mg)?

$$150,000 \text{ units/g} \times 60\,g = 9,000,000 \text{ units are needed}$$

$$9,000,000 \text{ units}/4400 \text{ units/mg} = 2.045\,g \text{ are required}$$

DO YOU REMEMBER THESE KEY POINTS?

- The proper steps to follow when repackaging medication
- The documentation necessary for repackaged and compounded products
- The proper steps to follow when compounding a product
- Types of additives that are used to improve taste and appearance of oral solutions
- The various types of scales that are used in compounding
- How expiration dates are determined when repackaging
- Why pharmacies repackage products
- The various types of equipment used in packaging medications
- The sizes of capsules used in compounding
- How ointments, suppositories, nasal sprays, and other dosage forms are prepared
- Information required on labels
- GMP used when preparing compounded products
- Common auxiliary labels used on compounded products
- The various types of containers used in compounding products
- The various types of equipment necessary for compounding
- Regulations pertaining to compounding pharmacies on limits of quantities
- The use of compounded products for animals

REVIEW QUESTIONS

Multiple choice questions

1. Of the answers listed, which is NOT a common reason for repackaging medication?
   A. Cost-effectiveness
   B. More competitive against other hospitals
   C. Reusable
   D. Reduction of errors

2. The best description of the guidelines for assigning an expiration date to a repackaged drug is:
   A. Half of the manufacturer's expiration date
   B. Less than the manufacturer's date
   C. One fourth of the manufacturer's expiration date or 6 years, whichever is less
   D. One sixth of the manufacturer's expiration date or 6 months, whichever is less

3. To grind or crush powders into fine particles using a mortar and pestle best describes:
   A. Trituration
   B. Levigation
   C. Mixing
   D. Stirring

4. Using the 6-month expiration dating method, determine the expiration date of a drug to be unit dosed that has a manufacturer's expiration date of 7/11. If today's date is 6/10, the drug will expire in:
   A. 9/10
   B. 7/10
   C. 12/10
   D. 3/11

5. Of the information listed, which is NOT required to be entered into a repack logbook?
   A. The date the drug was made
   B. The patient's name
   C. The initials of the pharmacist
   D. The pharmacy lot number

6. The type of balance(s) that can weigh 10 g of powder accurately is(are):
   A. Class A
   B. Class B
   C. Both A and B
   D. None of the above

7. The type of mortar and pestle that is best used for grinding coarse granules into a fine powder is(are):
   A. Glass
   B. Porcelain
   C. China
   D. All of the above

8. A meniscus is best described as:
   A. A beaker filled with a small amount of water
   B. Water molecules attaching to the sides of a container
   C. A container used to measure very small amounts of liquid
   D. The lowest level of liquid, which is the point that should be used to assign a measurement

9. The arrest knob on a balance is used to:
   A. Measure the weight of a compound
   B. Balance the feet of the balance
   C. Adjust the balance's weights
   D. Lock the balance

10. Emulsification is a process that binds_____additives with solutes.
    A. Alcohol
    B. Hydrophilic
    C. Hydrophobic
    D. None of the above

11. When repackaging medications, which type of container can hold more than 1 dose?
    A. Blister pack
    B. Strip pack
    C. Bubble pack
    D. Both A and B

12. When preparing non–sterile compounds, it is NOT necessary for the technician to:
    A. Wash his or her hands
    B. Wear goggles
    C. Wear gloves
    D. Keep his or her hair tied back

13. What type of medication can be compounded for animal use?
    A. Tiny tablets
    B. Transdermal sticks
    C. Transdermal patches
    D. Both A and B

14. According to the FDA regulatory guidelines for compounding pharmacies, they are NOT allowed to:
    A. Advertise their compounding products
    B. Prepare large quantities of compounded product
    C. Prepare transdermal medications
    D. None of the above

15. Medication sticks can be used for all of the following treatments EXCEPT:
    A. Burns
    B. Sores
    C. Infections
    D. All of the above

16. Which agent would constitute an oleaginous base?
    A. A greasy base
    B. A water base
    C. An alcohol base
    D. A lotion base

17. Which of the factors listed below has(have) an effect on the longevity of a drug?
    A. pH
    B. Light
    C. Temperature
    D. All the factors listed can alter the longevity of a drug

18. Beyond-use dating differs from expiration dates because:
    A. Beyond-use dating is used when compounding only and expiration dates are used for repackaging
    B. Beyond-use dating is used when repackaging or compounded products whereas only manufacturers use expiration dates
    C. Expiration dates are used only for medications whereas beyond-use dating applies to all additives
    D. None of the above

19. The two functions of a suppository base are:
    A. To provide a sterile environment for the drug and a safe method of administration
    B. To provide an easy way to prepare the medication and to lengthen the stability of the drug
    C. To control the release of the active drug and to provide a sterile environment for the drug
    D. To provide a vehicle for the medication that can control delivery of the drug

20. Excipients are:
    A. Buffers
    B. Base solutions
    C. Preservatives
    D. All of the above

True/False

If the statement is false, then change it to make it true.

_____ 1. Good manufacturing practices are a set of hospital standards on the practices of compounding medications.

_____ 2. If gloves are worn for repackaging, washing hands is not necessary.

_____ 3. A unit dose medication delivers only one dose of a drug.

_____ 4. When compounding, it is always better to place the weights on the same side of the scale.

_____ 5. Spatulas commonly are used for mixing and for loading compounds into jars.

_____ 6. Most pharmacies have recipe books for compounded products.

_____ 7. When compounding, it is not necessary to document the expiration date of all ingredients.

_____ 8. All mortars and pestles are used for the same purpose.

_____ 9. Tapping a jar of cream or ointment eliminates smoothing out the top of the compounded product.

_____ 10. A bulk bottle refers to a compounded or repackaged product made in a pharmacy.

_____ 11. Pharmaceutical eloquence should be used when preparing all compounded products.

_____ 12. A prescription is not necessary to prepare medications for animals.

_____ 13. The FDA Modernization Act of 1997 governs the actions of compounding pharmacies.

_____ 14. Bubble packs are used in all types of pharmacies.

_____ 15. Water does not have an expiration date and does not need to be documented on compounding log records.

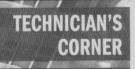

TECHNICIAN'S CORNER

You receive an order for 2.5% hydrocortisone cream in 50 g. You have 2.5% hydrocortisone powder and Dermabase in stock.

What is the strength of the hydrocortisone used (in grams)?
How much Dermabase do you need to equal a total volume of 50 g?
What documentation is required for these items?
What would you place on the label (include auxiliary labels needed)?

BIBLIOGRAPHY

Allen L: *The art, science, and technology of pharmaceutical compounding*, Washington, 2002, American Pharmaceutical Association.

Allen L. USP <795> Pharmaceutical Compounding-Nonsterile Preparations. *Secundum Artem* Current and Practical Compounding Information for the Pharmacist. Volume 13, Number 4 (ACPE No. 748-000-05-001-H01)

Ansel H, Allen L, and Popovich N: *Pharmaceutical dosage forms and drug delivery systems*, ed 8, Baltimore, 2004, Lippincott Williams & Wilkins.

Leon S, et al: *Comprehensive pharmacy review*, ed 7, Baltimore, 2009, Lippincott Williams & Wilkins.

WEBSITES REFERENCED

Allen L Jr: Secundum Artem. Volume 5 Number 1. Compounding Oral Liquids. Referenced 8/09. www.paddocklabs.com/forms/secundum/volume_3_1.pdf

ASHP Technical Assistance Bulletin on Compounding Nonsterile Products in Pharmacies. 1994. Page 73. Referenced 8/09. www.ashp.org/DocLibrary/BestPractices/CompoundingNonsterile.aspx

Excipients Category List. Referenced 8/09. www.pformulate.com/labclass/categories.htm

Pharmaceutics and Compounding Laboratory. UNC School of Pharmacy. Compounding Lab Exercises. Referenced 8/09. http://pharmlabs.unc.edu/index.htm

Report: Limited FDA Survey of Compounding Drug Products. Referenced 8/09. www.fda.gov/Drugs/GuidanceComplianceRegulatoryInformation/PharmacyCompounding/ucm155725.htm. Page updated 6/09.

Artem S: Volume 7 Number 1. Compounding Nasal Preparations. Referenced 8/09. www.paddocklabs.com/images/PadSec7-1.pdf

Artem S: Volume 14 Number 1. Compounding Rectal Dosage Forms-Part II. Referenced 8/09. www.paddocklabs.com/forms/secundum/Volume14.4.pdf

Spies A: CE: Compounding: The Practice of Pharmacy or a Liability Risk? Drug Topics, July 15, 2002. http://pharmlabs.unc.edu/

The Pharmaceutics and Compounding Laboratory. Pharmaceutical Solutions III. Ophthalmic solutions. Referenced 8/09. http://pharmlabs.unc.edu/labs/ophthalmics/objectives.htm

USP & Compounding. Compounding Pharmacy Resources. Referenced 8/09. www.usp.org/pdf/EN/distributors/compounding.pdf

Wedgewood Pharmacy. Veterinary Dosage Forms. 2009. Referenced 8/09. www.wedgewoodpharmacy.com/dosage forms Veterinary Dosage Forms

12
Aseptic Technique

Objectives

UPON COMPLETING THIS CHAPTER, YOU SHOULD BE ABLE TO DO
THE FOLLOWING:

- List the sizes of syringes and needles used in the pharmacy setting.

- Describe how often hoods must be inspected.

- Describe how to properly care for laminar flow hoods.

- Explain the use of aseptic technique within a horizontal flow hood.

- List the types of stock used within an intravenous room.

- Explain the differences between total parenteral nutrition and peripheral parenteral nutrition.

- Describe how to properly dispose of needles, vials, and cytotoxic supplies.

- Describe how to prepare and transport medications in syringes.

- List the medications that must be placed in glass containers.

- Describe aseptic technique within a vertical flow hood.

- List various containers used in the laminar flow hood.

- Explain the anatomy of a syringe and needle.

- Describe five medication delivery systems.

- Demonstrate the five steps of preparing medications from ampules.

- List the main components of *USP <797>* regulations.

- Explain the history of *USP <797>*.

- List the three risk levels of drug preparation determined by *USP <797>*.

- Define the terms used under *USP <797>*.
- Demonstrate how to manipulate a needle and syringe.
- Demonstrate the steps in reconstituting a parenteral powder.
- Demonstrate the procedures in preparing the IV hood for use.

TERMS AND DEFINITIONS

Aseptic technique *The procedures used to eliminate the possibility of a drug becoming contaminated with microbes or particles*

Clean room *As it pertains to pharmacy, a contained and controlled environment within the pharmacy that has a low level of environmental pollutants such as dust, airborne microbes, aerosol particles, and chemical vapors; the clean room is used for preparing sterile medication products*

Compounded sterile products (CSPs) *Preparations prepared in a sterile environment using nonsterile ingredients or devices that must be sterilized before administration*

Gauge *The size of the needle opening*

Horizontal laminar flow hood *Environment for the preparation of sterile products where air originating from the back of the hood moves forward across the hood and into the room*

Hyperalimentation *Parenteral nutrition for persons who are unable to eat solids or liquids*

Laminar flow hood *Environment for the preparation of sterile products*

Nosocomial infection *An infection that is obtained after being admitted into an institution*

Parenteral medication *Medication that bypasses the digestive system but is intended for systemic action; the term parenteral most commonly describes medications given by injection, such as intravenously or intramuscularly*

Peripheral parenteral *Injection of a medication into the veins located on the periphery of the body, instead of a central vein or artery*

Precipitate *To separate from solution or suspension*

Reconstitute *To add a diluent such as saline or sterile water to a powder*

Standard operating procedures (SOPs) *Written guidelines and criteria that list specific steps for various competencies*

Standard Precautions (i.e., Universal Precautions) *A set of standards that lowers the possibility of contamination and lowers the risk of transmission of infectious disease; used throughout a health care facility, including to prepare medications*

Total parenteral nutrition *Large-volume intravenous nutrition administered through a central vein (e.g., subclavian vein), which allows for a higher concentration of solutions*

Vertical laminar flow hood *Environment for the preparation of chemotherapeutic and hazardous agents where air originating from the roof of the hood moves downward (over the agent) and is captured in a vent located on the floor of the hood*

Introduction

Proper preparation of parenteral medications is one of the most crucial responsibilities of the hospital pharmacy technician. Preparation of all parenteral medications in a manner that reduces the possibility of contamination is important. This is possible only through the proper manipulation of materials used within the appropriate hood. Various sizes and types of hoods are available; all are capable of excluding bacteria and other unwanted particulates if the technician uses proper aseptic technique.

The pharmacy technician may prepare sterile products in pharmacy settings such as home health services and long-term care facilities. This chapter predominantly focuses on the technician working in a hospital pharmacy. A description of *United States Pharmacopeia (USP) <797>* regulations is explored as well as policies established by other organizations to monitor compliance in the sterile preparation of compounding products. Wider varieties of parenteral medications are used in the hospital than in any other setting. Within the hospital, the pharmacy technician may be responsible for many daily tasks related to compounding sterile products. Each skill has its own set of guidelines that are outlined within the three risk levels of *USP <797>*.

This chapter explores several types of parenteral medications, including the terminology and equipment commonly associated with medications as well as the various methods used in their preparation. One must understand many important aspects of sterile preparation of medications before an order can be filled, including type of drug to be prepared, equipment used, sterilization steps per *USP <797>*, expiration dates, storage, and proper disposal of equipment. These are the technician's responsibilities; in addition, technicians must be competent in understanding drug abbreviations and calculations that may be required to prepare medications. These are all important competencies of a pharmacy technician.

Terminology Used in Pharmacy

There are solutions, medications, and supplies that may be required when preparing sterile products. The terms used to identify these items often are abbreviated in physicians' orders and on supply lists. Pharmacy technicians need to understand these terms and abbreviations in order to interpret orders and fill stock levels in the IV room. Box 12-1 lists some of the most common terms and abbreviations used for intravenous supplies.

Standard Precautions of a Health Care Worker

When working in a hospital setting all employees must comply with the policies of Standard Precautions. To prevent the dissemination of highly contagious disease, hospitals usually require an employee to receive both tuberculosis (TB) testing and an immunization against influenza annually. Standard Precautions are practices employed to prevent the transmission of infection and contamination; they are based on the principle that all blood, body fluids, secretions, excretions (except sweat), nonintact skin, and mucous membranes may contain infectious agents. Based on the anticipated exposure to potentially infectious substances, each area within the hospital has specific guidelines (located in the policies and procedures manual) that employees are expected to meet, including hand washing, orderliness, and cleanliness. Pharmacy does not supply blood or blood products. However, pharmacy personnel must participate in training

BOX 12-1 ABBREVIATIONS AND DESCRIPTIONS OF PHARMACY STOCK

Types of Containers Used for Preparing Parenteral Medications; Description of Container and/or Contents

Amp	Ampule; 1- to 50-mL glass container
Vial	0.5- to 100-mL glass or plastic container with a stopper
MDV	Multidose vial; holds multiple doses of medication
SDV	Single dose vial; holds one dose of medication
Flexible bag	Plastic container (empty or filled with various fluids ranging from 50 to 3000 mL)

Common Types of Solutions Used/Ordered for Parenteral Agents

Diluent	Agent used to dilute medications; can be sterile water, normal saline (NS), or others
D_5NS	5% dextrose in normal saline
$D_{10}NS$	10% dextrose in normal saline
NS	Normal saline; has a concentration of 0.9% sodium chloride
0.45NaCl	One-half normal saline; has a concentration 0.45% sodium chloride
LR	Lactated Ringer's solution; isotonic solution containing sodium, potassium, calcium, acetate, and chloride
¼ NS	One fourth normal saline (concentration 0.225% sodium chloride)
$D_5 ½ NS$	5% dextrose and 0.45% normal saline contained in the same bag of solution
SW	Sterile water; usually used to reconstitute other medications
D_5W	5% dextrose in water
$D_{10}W$	10% dextrose in water

Routes of Administration for Parenteral Agents

IV	Intravenous; into the vein
IV push	Into the vein directly from a syringe
IM	Intramuscular; into the muscle
ID	Intradermal injection up to 1 mL into the upper layers of the skin
SubQ	Subcutaneous; under the skin
IT	Intrathecal; into a sheath (hollow tube) such as the lumbar sheath located at the base of the spine

Miscellaneous Terms Used Concerning Parenteral Medications

On call	Physician wants dose to be ready when he or she decides to give the medication; most anesthesiologists order on-call preoperative medications
NPO	Nothing by mouth
Pre-op	Medication to be given before surgery (examples, sedative or antiemetic)
Post-op	Medication to be given after surgery (examples, pain control, antiemetic)
prn	Medication is to be given as needed
qs	Quantity sufficient; adding enough diluent or medication to attain the correct amount needed
Drip or infusion	An intravenous bag that is infused over a specified amount of time but is not given IV push

sessions regarding bloodborne pathogens so that they not only understand various aspects of contamination but also are aware of ways to prevent exposure and transmission of infections. For example, training includes the interpretation of room signs that indicate patient isolation (e.g., droplet or contact isolation) and the precautions and procedures that should be followed if access to these rooms is necessary.

Other hospital-wide standards include the following:

- Employees are not to use patient restrooms; only use employee restrooms.
- Medication refrigerators/freezers may only hold medications; they should not be used for storage of food or drink.
- Eating is prohibited in any drug preparation or patient care areas.

The following are examples of procedures specific to pharmacy:

- All injectable drugs and other sterile products must be made in a "clean room" under laminar flow hoods.
- Laminar flow hoods are recertified every 6 months by an independent contractor.
- Routine maintenance of the hoods includes cleaning all work surfaces and prefilters.
- All inspections are to be kept on file in the pharmacy department.

Supplies

Before discussing the actual techniques required to prepare injections, intravenous drips, chemotherapy, and other sterile products, the types of supplies and equipment necessary for these processes should be explained. Different types of equipment are available for IV preparation depending on the amount or volumes that are to be prepared. For instance, many different types of automated pumps automatically fill intravenous bags and other sterile containers. These pumps range in complexity and cost. For example, if large multiadditive automated machines are rented by the pharmacy then only the tubing required for that specific pump needs to be purchased. Small pumps, such as Baxa's Repeater pump, are used to administer smaller reconstituting volumes into a single dose vial (SDV) or larger volumes into multidose vials (MDVs). In addition, a wide variety of supplies used in the clean room must be kept in stock for daily use. For this reason, it is a necessity for the technician to inventory these supplies and reorder stock on a daily basis, anticipating stock needed for the next day. Table 12-1 lists common supplies stocked by pharmacy clean rooms.

SYRINGES

Syringes used in the pharmacy are available in eight basic sizes: 0.5, 1, 3, 5, 10, 20, 30, and 60 mL. As the size of the syringe increases, the accuracy decreases (Figure 12-1 illustrates the anatomy of a syringe). For parenteral products, it is necessary to obtain the exact amount of drug ordered. Syringe tips are available in two types. A tension-type syringe has a 1-mL volume. In this case the needle is attached by friction only, as seen in Figure 12-2, *A*. This type of syringe can be used for withdrawing insulin and other medications that require volumes equal to or less than 1 mL. However, tension-type tips cannot be used when preparing chemotherapy doses because of the risk of the needle detaching from the syringe and causing a spill or a possible needle stick to the technician. All other sizes of syringes hold their needles in place by a lock mechanism, commonly referred to as a Luer-Lok (Figure 12-2, *B*). This ensures a safe seal for the withdrawal of medication.

Most syringes are made of plastic and must be discarded after one use. Glass syringes rarely are used in the pharmacy, although they can be used when a patient has an allergy to plastics. Glass syringes, unlike plastic syringes, can be sterilized and reused.

Another type of syringe is a Tubex or Carpuject, as seen in Figure 12-3. These system cartridges can hold a variety of medications and are available in 0.5-mL up to 3-mL volumes. The bottom of the cartridge is screwed into the

TABLE 12-1 Commonly Used Intravenous Room Supplies

Supplies	Common Description
70% isopropyl alcohol	Antiseptic for cleaning hood
Alcohol pads	Alcohol on pads for convenience
Ampule breaker	Plastic device; one end smaller for small ampules, other end for larger ampules; helps to prevent crushing glass or cutting oneself when opening ampules
Filter needles	Needle includes a filter; it eliminates glass from entering final solution when drawing from an ampule
Filter straws	Used for withdrawing medication from ampules
Filters	Used for specific medications to trap particles 5 to 0.22 μm from entering IV fluids
Male/female adapter	Universal size; fits a syringe on each end for mixing two contents
Syringe needles	Most common bore sizes used in pharmacy are 16 to 20 gauge
Syringe caps	A sterile cap used to prevent contamination of syringes during transportation out of pharmacy
Syringes	Instrument that holds between 0.5 and 60 mL for administration of medications
Transfer needles	A needle on both ends used to transfer a vial to a bottle
Tubing for pumps	Tubing is specific for manufacturer's machine
Tubing transfer sets	Blood transfer sets; used to transfer large containers into empty containers
Mini-spike	Large-bore spike that is pushed into vial with a syringe attachment at other end
Forceps	Instruments that lock; used to obstruct tubing while transferring medications

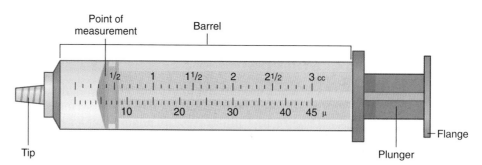

FIGURE 12-1 Anatomy of a syringe. As the syringe decreases in size, the calibrations (volume markers) become larger, allowing a more accurate dosage.

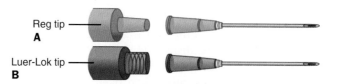

FIGURE 12-2 Two types of syringes. **A,** Regular tip syringe. The regular tip is held in place by pressure, as seen in the 1-mL syringe. **B,** The Luer-Lok syringe has spirals to secure the needle, as seen on a larger 3-mL syringe. (From Potter PA, Perry AG: *Fundamentals of nursing,* ed 5, St Louis, 2001, Elsevier.)

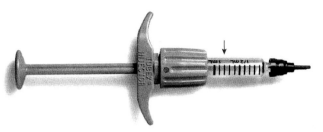

FIGURE 12-3 Tubex holders are intended to be reused. They hold the disposable Tubex or Carpuject cartridges. Each cartridge is prelabeled with the medication name, strength, volume, and concentration. The pharmacy stocks holders and cartridges.

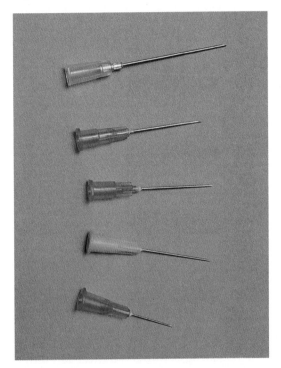

FIGURE 12-4 Needle sizes shown are (from top to bottom) 19, 20, 21, 23, and 25 gauge. Technicians may use a 19-gauge needle for small volumes such as 1 mL or less. Larger gauges (not shown) include 18 and 16 gauge for larger volumes. (From Potter PA, Perry AG: *Fundamentals of nursing*, ed 7, St Louis, 2009, Mosby.)

system's syringe holder. The syringe cartridge holders for these systems are reusable and normally are dispensed to the nursing units by the pharmacy upon request. The Tubex or Carpuject cartridge is discarded after use; if desired, the holders may be autoclaved for sterility.

NEEDLES

Needles are made of aluminum or stainless steel. Needles are available in many different **gauges** (sizes) and lengths. Higher gauged needles, such as those ranging between 20 and 25 gauge, are used by nurses to administer injections. The nurse determines which gauge and needle length to use depending on the injection site. In the pharmacy needles are used to draw solutions into a syringe, not to administer medications to patients. A limited number of needle gauges are available in the pharmacy, and the lower gauge needles make drawing medications easier. The most common needle sizes used for preparing intravenous medications are 19, 18, and 16 gauge, which are used to draw solutions from vials or other containers (Figure 12-4). The length of these needles is

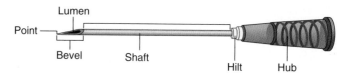

FIGURE 12-5 Anatomy of a needle.

normally 1 to 1.5 inches. The gauge (size) number of a needle is inversely proportional to the bore (opening) size of the needle. This means that as the bore size increases, the gauge decreases. For example, a 25-gauge needle has a much smaller opening than a 19-gauge needle. In addition, as the bore size increases, the risk of coring the vial's rubber stopper increases. The bore size refers to the circumference of the needle opening; as this increases so does the probability of coring or cutting out a piece of rubber from the vial's rubber stopper. When a vial is cored, a chunk of rubber is dislodged and may fall into the vial. To avoid coring, the bevel edge should face upward. If coring does occur, a filter needle must be used to prevent the piece of cored rubber from entering the parenteral solution. No part of a needle below the hub should be touched (Figure 12-5). The point and shaft must remain sterile.

FILTERS

Different types and sizes of filters can be used when preparing parenteral medications. Filters are located within the hub of the needle or spike, depending on the type being used. Typical filter sizes are 10, 5, 1, and 0.45 micrometer (µm); the smallest filter is 0.22 micrometer, which removes all unwanted particles from the solution. If it is necessary to use a filter needle, the technician must follow manufacturer's guidelines regarding filter needles suggested for the specific medication. Some medications should never be filtered, because filtering would remove active drug from the solution. Another type of filter is the filter straw. This strawlike needle can withdraw a larger amount of solution quickly, sifting it through a filter located in the hub of the needle. The filter straw often is used to remove any fine particles of glass from an ampule. The filter straw must be replaced with a normal needle before pushing the medication into the final container. Types of filters and other materials used in the IV room are illustrated in Figure 12-6.

STOCK LEVELS

All of the items stored in the intravenous room of the pharmacy must be kept in stock and above their minimum levels at all times. Before and after each shift, the intravenous technician is responsible for reordering and restocking the clean room for the next shift. Many intravenous supplies can be ordered from the central supply area of the hospital and will arrive by the next shift. However, in cases in which the manufacturer or a centralized distribution center is located off site, delivery can take from 2 days to 1 week. Therefore to ensure that required pharmacy stock is always on hand the technician must be knowledgeable in delivery options.

Many intravenous antibiotics are available in premade bulk packs; for example, 12 or 24 packs are frozen in boxes. Although they are convenient, they are more expensive than those prepared by technicians. Most of the time, technicians prepare the IVs needed throughout the week. Certain intravenous medications can be frozen in either IV solutions or syringes, but each bag must be marked with the date of reconstitution, beyond-use date, concentration/strength,

Tech Note!

Never use an unmarked reconstituted vial, because the amount of diluent is unknown. Instead, discard unmarked reconstituted vials. Frozen parenteral products must be thawed slowly using either a cool bath or a thawing platform. They should never be placed in hot water or in a microwave oven. Once such medications are thawed, they must be marked with the new expiration date per literature or manufacturer guidelines.

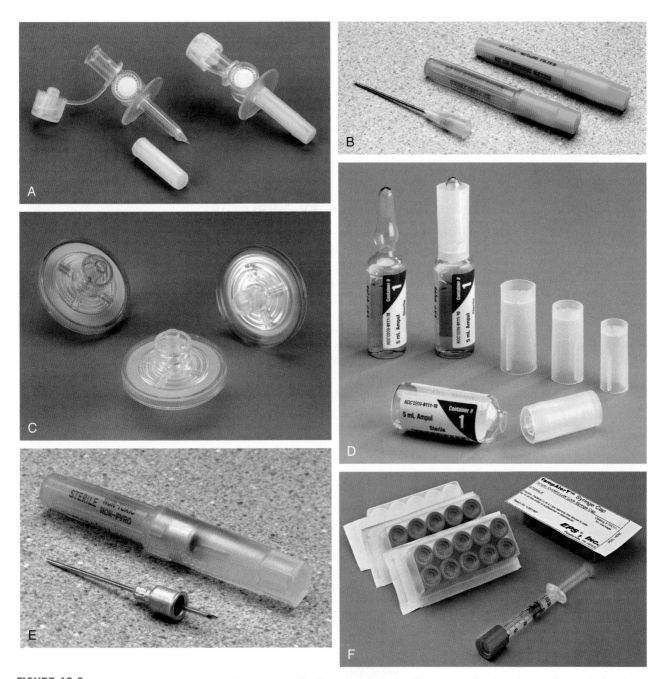

FIGURE 12-6 A, Mini-spikes used in multidose vials. **B,** Filter needles. **C,** Filter sizes. **D,** Ampules and ampule breakers. **E,** Transfer needle. **F,** Syringe and caps. (Images courtesy of Medi-Dose, Inc./EPS, Inc., © 2010.)

and the preparer's initials. The expiration dates for frozen, refrigerated, or room temperature products are determined by using the manufacturer's information, known stability data, and other pharmaceutical specialty publications and research. Large, temperature-controlled refrigerators may be used to store thawed intravenous medications. Antibiotics and other medications that are in multiple dose vials can be stored in the refrigerator after opening, sometimes for days, and used as determined by *USP* guidelines for multiple dose vials. All of these items should be visually checked each day for stock levels and outdates.

Routes of Administration (ROA)

Because prepared solutions differ in their volumes and/or concentrations, understanding the routes of administration is important. For example, if a dose of ceftriaxone 1 g is to be given IM, it is normally divided into two syringes for the nurse to inject into each side of the hip area. There are several areas on the body where injections can be given. The route of administration of each type of medication must be denoted on the label. This will be discussed later in the chapter.

Medication Delivery Systems

Many different types of containers are used to deliver medications. Such containers are developed to be stable and easy to use. In addition, because many medications are not premade for final use by the manufacturer and must be prepared in the pharmacy, it is important to determine if the medication would have to be discarded (i.e., wasted) if not administered to the patient in a timely manner. For example, once a medication is **reconstituted**, it must be used within a certain time or it expires, resulting in lost revenue for the pharmacy. Sometimes the drug may not be given to the patient for whom it was prepared; the physician may have decided to use a medication of a different dose, type, volume, and solution. This type of waste only adds to the high costs of health care. There are systems that can be used to eliminate waste, such as the ADD-Vantage system. Although these systems are expensive, they can be beneficial by reducing waste, and ultimately adding cost efficiency. These systems as well as others are discussed later.

PIGGYBACK CONTAINERS

Flexible bags and bottles are the two main types of piggyback containers. Most IV bags are made of polyvinyl chloride (PVC), which consists of several flexible layers of plastics. Other types of IV bags are made with non-PVC materials such as ethylene vinyl acetate (EVA). The EVA bags are not as flexible as PVC bags. Piggyback IVs are intended to be placed on top of a primary IV using tubing connection sets such as that shown in Figure 12-7. Containers can be purchased prefilled with solutions or may be empty and filled with a custom-made intravenous solution. The sizes and types of piggyback containers and solutions vary

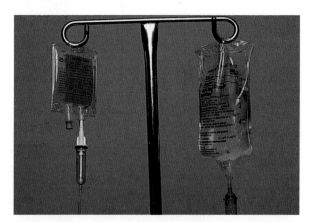

FIGURE 12-7 This gravity pump system intravenous piggyback setup shows a 100-mL Viaflex container *(left)* piggybacked to a large-volume 1-L IV *(right)*. (From Potter PA, Perry AG: *Fundamentals of nursing*, ed 5, St Louis, 2001, Elsevier.)

from 50 to 250 mL. Examples of specialized containers used for medication dispensing include large- and small-volume drips, syringe pumps, and miscellaneous dispensing systems. Many controlled substances also are prepared in such systems and are dispensed to the nursing floor after being documented according to established procedures for controlled substances.

Large- and Small-Volume Drips

Large-volume drips include Viaflex bags in 500-mL and 1-, 2-, and 3-L volumes. Volumes greater than 1 L are often reserved for use with parenteral nutritional formulas. Bottles are also available in various sizes, ranging from 500 mL to 1 L. These can deliver a variety of fluids, including parenteral nutrition. Parenteral nutrition is a combination of essential nutrients that is administered through a drip system for several hours or up to 24 hours. Parenteral nutrition solutions will be discussed later in this chapter. Small-volume piggyback containers and solutions are available in 50-, 100-, 150-, and 250-mL volumes. Small-volume drips can be piggybacked onto large-volume drips. All Viaflex bags have a 10% overfill of solution. To attain an accurate final concentration of drug, some mixtures require that a volume of base solution equal to the volume of medication being added, plus the solution overfill, be removed during the mixing process. This type of procedure usually occurs with critical care medication drips where small changes in drug concentration may greatly influence the dosage given to the patient and the subsequent patient response.

BURETROL SYSTEMS

A Buretrol (also Volutrol system) is a tubular drip chamber with its own flow regulator located below it. It holds up to 150 mL of IV fluids. It is located between the bag of IV fluids and the patient's IV catheter set. Buretrols can either be added to the peripheral line tubing or be built into the peripheral line tubing; both of these types are available in minidrip or maxidrip. This system allows the nurse to administer small amounts of medication over a predetermined period. They are commonly used for pediatric patients. An example of a Buretrol is given in Figure 12-8.

Tech Note!

All dosage forms of controlled substances that are delivered to nursing floors must be signed out of the pharmacy stock and into the floor stock of the receiving station. Documents registering controlled substances should be kept up to date, and all controlled substances should be counted at the end of every shift to account for all narcotic use or waste.

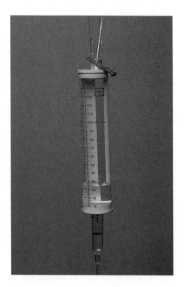

FIGURE 12-8 Volutrol drip systems are used mostly for pediatric patients. Nurses prepare these. (From Potter PA, Perry AG: *Fundamentals of nursing*, ed 5, St Louis, 2001, Elsevier.)

CONTINUOUS ANALGESIC DELIVERY SYSTEMS

Patients who require analgesics after major surgery or those persons who are in hospice normally have their medications prepared in the pharmacy. Within the hospital setting, nursing stations stock various strengths of controlled substances intended to relieve extreme pain. Depending on the physician's order, the nurse can prepare intramuscular or IV push doses from the controlled substances cabinet.

When a patient is in severe pain, physicians often order analgesic medications such as morphine or fentanyl (both C-II) on a schedule (for example, every 6 or 8 hours). When this strength of analgesic is given in larger doses to patients who have no history of opioid use, the initial effects of the medication may be extreme, causing side effects that include nausea, vomiting, and in some cases difficulty breathing. Toward the end of the 6 or 8 hours, some patients are once again suffering from pain and waiting for the next dose to be administered. To provide a more constant degree of comfort and to limit unwanted side effects, some patients may be given either an implantable port or a catheter system attached to a portable electronic pump system, which administers a steady flow of analgesics that controls the patient's pain more effectively. These pumps are used to dispense controlled substances at a specific rate of infusion. There are two types of portable electronic pumps that can be used to deliver controlled substances—a syringe system or a cassette system. Technicians may prepare either syringes or cassettes that are placed into a pump that automatically delivers the medication over a predetermined time. These pumps can be programmed for short or long durations to deliver medication, not to exceed a 24-hour period. These devices are especially effective for those patients who require constant pain control or patients who are discharged home with this type of medication. Another type of dispensing system that uses syringes relies on gravity for delivering the solution. The syringes are placed in a freestanding IV pump system on wheels; these are used only in the hospital.

PATIENT-CONTROLLED ANALGESIA (PCA) SYRINGE SYSTEM

Patient-controlled analgesia is a method of administration that allows the patient to control the rate at which the drug is delivered for the relief of pain. The PCA pump holds a syringe of pain medication that is attached to the IV line and is regulated by a computerized device that automatically dispenses the medication. The pump may be programmed to deliver a small, constant dose of pain medicine, and the patient has the option of receiving additional doses (bolus) if necessary. This is done by depressing a button attached to a line located on the machine. The boluses are preset for amount and frequency; even if the patient presses the button many times, he or she will receive only the predetermined amount of drug. For example, if the dose is set at 1 mg/mL with dosing intervals every 6 minutes and a 1-hour lockout dose of 10 mg, regardless of how many times the patient presses the button within 6 minutes he or she will receive only 1 dose. The 1-hour lockout limits medication administration to a total dose of 10 mg in 1 hour. This safeguards the patient from overdosing. The PCA syringe device is normally used in a hospital setting for acute postoperative pain control. Children ages 7 years and older can typically use this pump device independently once they are familiar with it. Young or debilitated patients need assistance from a nurse or caregiver to receive their dosing. Many manufacturers provide prefilled PCA syringes that may be used directly from the packaging in these pumps. Alternatively, pharmacy technicians (using aseptic technique in a horizontal flow hood) can also prepare the syringes for PCA pumps. Each syringe must be labeled, capped, and checked by the pharmacist before delivery. When the pharmacy technician is ready to have a prepared medication inspected by the pharmacist, he or she should include the finished product along with the syringe, opioid analgesic container, and the diluent used in its preparation.

PCA Syringe Systems

The following are some examples of PCA syringe system manufacturers:

- Medfusion: www.smiths-medical.com/brands/medfusion/
- SYNDEO PCA Syringe Pump: www.baxter.com/
- Crono PCA 50: http://intrapump.com/crono_pca_50.html

PATIENT-CONTROLLED ANALGESIA (PCA) CASSETTE SYSTEM

Cassette pumps are another type of PCA that can be used at home. The programmed pumps work similarly to the syringe pumps in that they are preset for dosage administration. Additional boluses may be programmed into the pump per physician's orders and cannot be altered by the patient. A bolus is a predetermined amount of drug that can be administered by the patient at one time when pain intensifies. The cassettes are available in various sizes, such as 50- or 100-mL volumes; pharmacy may prepare the cassettes. They have a short piece of tubing with a Luer-Lok that can be connected to a 60-mL syringe that is used to load the proper amount of solution. Priming the line (tubing) is required after the cassette is filled. To prime a line, the tubing is allowed to fill with solution so there is no air in the tubing; then it is secured with a twist cap. This is usually done by pharmacy at the time the medication is prepared. Figure 12-9 shows examples of both types of PCA devices.

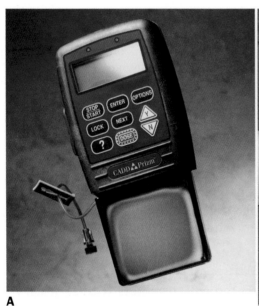

A

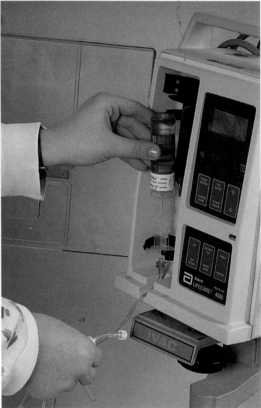

B

FIGURE 12-9 **A,** Controlled analgesia device pump. **B,** Patient-controlled analgesia pump.

PCA Cassette Systems

The following are some examples of PCA cassette system manufacturers:

- CADD pumps: www.smiths-medical.com/brands/cadd/
- LMA e-PainCare System: www.lmana.com/pain-management/e-paincare.php
- Solace: www.solacepainrelief.com/

VIALS

There are two different types of vials; those that are intended for immediate use are referred to as single dose vials (SDVs) and those that can be used more than once are called multidose vials (MDVs). Because they are not discarded after one use, MDVs contain preservatives. Volumes for SDVs and MDVs range from 1 mL up to 100 mL and may contain either solution for withdrawal or powder for reconstitution. When an MDV solution is used, the date the vial was opened must be written on the label along with the initials of the person who opened the vial. Reconstituting a medication is the addition of a diluent, such as sterile water, to convert the medication into solution form. If an antibiotic MDV portion has been used, the following information must be denoted on the vial: the date the vial was opened, the date the vial expires, the diluent used (if applicable), the concentration (e.g., mg/mL), and the technician's initials. Bulk vials can be reconstituted in varying concentrations per manufacturer instructions to provide multiple IV bags for future use. For example, cefazolin 10 g bulk vial can be reconstituted with 45 mL of sterile water, which provides a final concentration of 1 g per 5 mL. This will supply 10, 1-g bags of cefazolin that can be used immediately or be refrigerated or frozen for later use. Beyond-use dates differ between frozen and refrigerated medications. Many antibiotics are available in bulk containers.

Specialized types of vials, such as the ADD-Vantage system (Figure 12-10), can be placed onto a small piggyback solution via an adapter; these are not mixed with the solution until immediately before administration. The pharmacy technician is responsible for the proper attachment of the vial to the proper solution, but the nurse is responsible for breaking the adapter seal between the vial and the piggyback and mixing the powdered drug with the solution. Because the medication does not mix with the solution until the seal is broken, the IV can be returned to the pharmacy if it is not used. This greatly reduces the amount of wasted medication.

A controlled-release infusion system (CRIS) is another type of delivery system in which the vial is reconstituted (mixed) but is not added to the piggyback. At the time of administration, the vial is attached to a special port on the side of the tubing set that allows the medication to enter the piggyback, where it then is delivered through the IV tubing.

Aseptic Technique

When preparing **compounded sterile products (CSPs)**, aseptic techniques must be used. Normally, nurses do not have the advantage of using a laminar flow hood; however, they still need to use strict aseptic technique and must sometimes prepare products for immediate use. **Aseptic technique** is directly associated with Universal Precautions. Universal Precautions are guidelines followed by all health care workers when exposure to body fluids or blood products is likely. These precautions involve washing hands and donning gloves and gowns (i.e., personal protective equipment) when in the presence of any body fluids. Similarly, aseptic technique is used when preparing both hazardous and nonhazardous products. Products that have been tested and shown to cause adverse or toxic effects in humans are classified as hazardous. Examples of these

Tech Note!

When adding a diluent to a powder it is important to read the instructions on the vial for reconstitution volumes. The final concentrations of many medications depend on both the volume of the diluent and the volume of the powder. For example, cefazolin 10 g powder and 45 mL of sterile water yield 10 g/50 mL; the cefazolin powder is responsible for the additional 5 mL of volume. Each manufacturer will indicate how much diluent to use along with the final concentration.

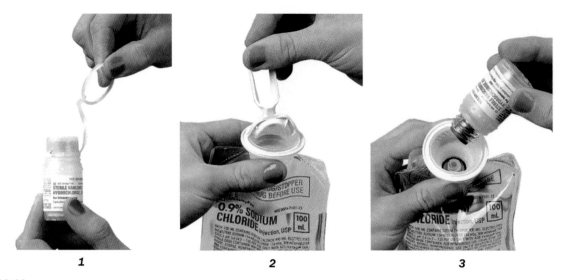

1   *2*   *3*

FIGURE 12-10 ADD-Vantage system: To prepare IV, follow the three steps listed. *1,* Remove the vial top. *2,* Pull up flange, removing the seal on the intravenous bag. *3,* Screw the vial into the port. Do not break the seal between vial and bag.

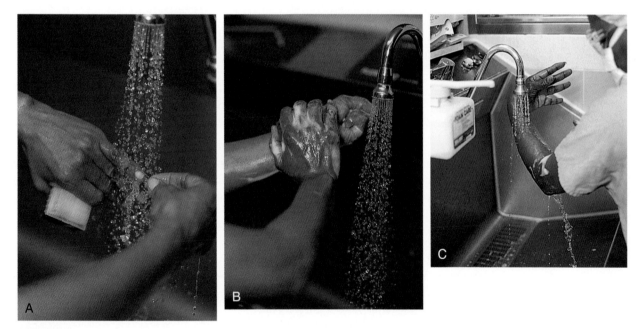

FIGURE 12-11 Proper hand washing technique. (From Potter PA, Perry AG: *Fundamentals of nursing,* ed 5, St Louis, 2001, Elsevier.)

types of medications include chemotherapeutic agents, radioactive compounds, and various hazardous chemicals such as phenol and glacial acetic acid. These precautions are used to keep contamination from occurring by a product or to a product. For pharmacy technicians, the importance of using aseptic technique cannot be stressed enough. A medication that contains any microbes or unwanted debris can cause a dangerous infection, or even death, when it is administered to a patient. Steps used in aseptic technique begin with hand hygiene (as shown in Figure 12-11) followed by proper donning of gloves (Figure 12-12) and gown, cleaning of the flow hood, and finally preparation of the parenteral medication. Each of these steps will be outlined and illustrated for clarity. Box 12-2 lists the preparation required by personnel using aseptic technique; except for donning of the surgical facemask immediately before entering the hood, all of these steps

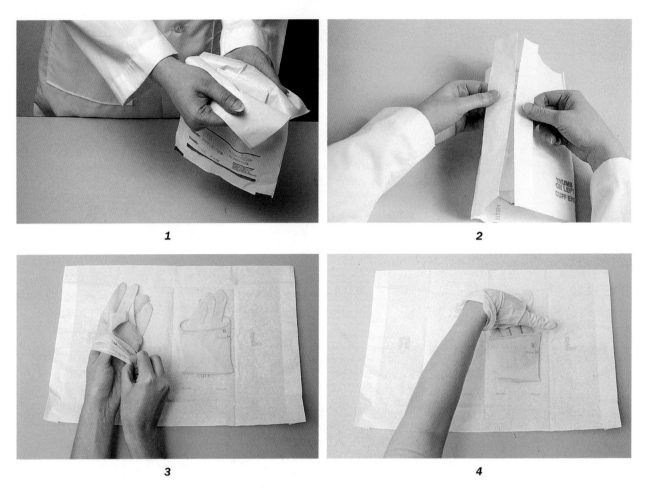

FIGURE 12-12 Steps for proper sterile gloving. *1,* Open glove packet. *2,* Open glove cover without touching gloves. *3,* Holding cuff of glove, pull glove over hand. *4,* Slide gloved hand under the cuff of the second glove. Carefully pull on glove. (From Elkin MK, Perry AG, Potter PA: *Nursing interventions and clinical skills,* ed 4, St Louis, 2007, Elsevier.)

BOX 12-2 PERSONNEL PREPARATION*

1. Do not wear jewelry in the hood. This includes artificial nails, because of microbial growth around or underneath the nails.
2. Tie back long hair away from the face.
3. Wash hands before entering the intravenous area (see Figure 12-11).*
   a. Wash hands, fingernails, wrists, and arms to the elbows with antimicrobial soap and hot water.
   b. Wash for at least 15 seconds but no more than 90 seconds.
   c. Dry hands with hand towels that do not shed.
   d. Use foot pedal to turn off water.
4. Don the following garb:
   a. Lab coat or cover that reaches the knee
   b. Head cover
   c. Foot covers
   d. Beard or sideburn cover (if applicable)
   e. Gloves: should be powder free; clean periodically with 70% isopropyl alcohol

*Procedure for the proper sanitation of hands is found in Appendix F.

Tech Alert!

Did you know that all rooms are highly contaminated with microscopic debris such as dust? Droplets from sneezing can attach themselves to dust particles and remain in the air for weeks. If these contaminants become part of a medication that is intended for intravenous use, they can cause infections, or worse. The intravenous route is the most dangerous to a patient because it bypasses our most protective barrier (i.e., the skin) and directly enters the bloodstream.

should be completed outside the clean room. When leaving the IV area, the hair cover, gloves, and facemask must be removed. Other considerations include preparation of the rooms and equipment that are used in preparing sterile products. Accuracy in performing calculations and measuring medications is paramount, and all calculations and measurements should be double-checked and must be verified by a pharmacist. Both drug errors and breaches of aseptic technique are discussed under *United States Pharmacopeia's USP <797>* regulations. They are discussed next.

USP <797>

The *United States Pharmacopeia (USP)* is responsible for providing safety guidelines for the preparation of parenteral and other sterile medications. In the 1970s, because of the dramatic increase in **nosocomial infections,** the National Coordinating Committee on Large Volume Parenterals (NCCLVP) provided guidelines for the preparation of parenterals. Nosocomial infections are infections that originate in a hospital (the term health care–acquired infections is usually used today to describe nosocomial infections). Later in the 1980s the effort of NCCLVP was replaced by several other organizations as they began to establish standards for pharmacists and technicians in the safe preparation of parenterals. These organizations included the American Society of Health-System Pharmacists (ASHP), the National Association of Boards of Pharmacy (NABP), and the United States Pharmacopeia (USP). Through the 1990s both recommendations and guidelines were written for safe standards by these organizations but they were not monitored or enforced. In the mid-1990s it was determined through health system surveys that very few pharmacies followed these standards explicitly. For example, most pharmacies did not perform quality assurance checks or solution tests on a regular basis for prepared parenterals and many did not provide education and training for personnel on a periodic basis. In addition, various IV medications were reported contaminated with bacteria because of poor aseptic technique. The reports of patient harm from improper medications being prepared by pharmacy continued through the 1990s.

Beginning in 2004 the *USP <797>* regulations were written with the intent that it would be an enforceable standard. The *USP <797>* standards are to be met by all practice settings where sterile products are compounded. USP, ASHP, and The Joint Commission outlined a timeline for total compliance, realizing it would take time to adhere to all of the changes mandated. Pharmacies and other areas that prepare sterile products must research, create, and document their **standard operating procedures (SOPs)** for *USP <797>* regulations. There are three major sections to *USP <797>:*

1. Responsibilities of personnel: The risk levels of classification of compounded sterile products
2. Verification: Accuracy and sterility of compounded sterile products
3. Training: Individual training and continued evaluation of personnel with respect to compounded products, including both quality and control of the preparation environment

Furthermore, *USP <797>* requires standard operating procedures (SOPs) that include automated systems used in compounding procedures, storing sterile products, and assigning expiration dates, to maintain both quality and control even after the parenteral medication leaves the pharmacy. Other areas that are under *USP <797>* include any medication prepared by nurses, physicians, or other practitioners intended for patient use regardless of the setting. The types of products include diagnostics, nutrients, irrigations, radiopharmaceuticals, and otic and ophthalmic solutions. Additionally, patient or

TABLE 12-2 Terms/Abbreviations Used in Pharmacy

Terms	Definition
Ante area	An area in which all preparations for IV admixture are gathered, including labels, gowning, and drug materials
Beyond-use date (BUD)	The date or time a drug or material can no longer be used; drug is ineffective after this date
Biological safety cabinet (BSC)	A cabinet that has a HEPA filter for laminar airflow
Buffer area	An area in which hoods are kept and IV preparation takes place
Clean room	A space where microbial containment is kept at a specific level of safety to ensure a certain level of cleanliness
Compounding aseptic isolator (CAI)	An isolator cabinet designed to contain all contaminants; prevents contaminants from escaping IVs and being transferred to surrounding area
Critical site	An area exposed to air or touch, such as vial, needle, or ampule
Direct compounding area (DCA)	A critical area within the hood (ISO Class 5) where areas are exposed to filtered air; also known as "first air"
First air	The air from the HEPA filter that passes over materials; this air is contaminant free
Hazardous drugs	Drugs that have been proven to have dangerous effects during animal or human testing; they may cause cancer or harm to certain organs or to pregnant women
Media-fill test	A test performed on compounded products to ensure no contamination has taken place during preparation phase
Multiple dose container/vial (MDV)	A vial or container that can be used for more than one admixture; MDV normally contains preservatives; the maximum dating is 28 days unless specified by manufacturer
Negative pressure room	A room in which air flows into the room and away from adjacent rooms, which results in positive pressure in the room
Positive pressure room	A room in which air flows out of or toward adjacent rooms, which results in a lower pressure in the room
Primary engineering control (PEC)	A practice in which an ISO Class 5 system is in place that provides safety for admixtures; this includes laminar flow hood, glove boxes, vertical flow hoods, or compounding aseptic isolators
Single dose container/vial (SDV)	A vial or container that can only be used once

caregiver training, patient monitoring, and adverse event reporting (see Chapter 14) must be maintained. There are many terms and abbreviations used in describing areas of the pharmacy where aseptic technique is used. These are defined in Table 12-2.

Risk Levels

The *USP <797>* has identified three risk levels (low, medium, high) that are based on various criteria; these are outlined in Table 12-3. Additional requirements include the amount of space between the hood areas and sink and the storage location of products. For more information on standards of *USP <797>*, visit www.usp.org.

TABLE 12-3 *USP <797>* Risk Levels

Low risk: uses a Class 100 laminar flow hood; sterile ingredients/devices; only syringe transfer used for measuring/mixing no more than 3 products	Medium risk: all low risk plus no broad-spectrum antibiotic present even over "x" days; complex aseptic technique manipulations; multiple doses in 1 container for multiple patients or multiple doses for 1 patient	High risk: all low/medium risk plus sterile products compounded from nonsterile ingredients; use of nonsterile device before terminal sterilization; sterile ingredients, components, or devices exposed to air quality; Class 100 hood if opened or partially used and not adequately preserved
Batch doses that have preservatives	Batch doses; no preservatives	Preparation of nonsterile medications
	Reconstituted doses; no preservatives	95% purity of ingredients
Ampule extraction using filter needles	Preparation of IVs that contain more than one additive and evacuate air; kept at room temperature over several days	IV preparations reconstituted from nonsterile powder that will be terminally sterilized
		Compounded bladed irrigations
Manually prepared TPN with only three ingredients	TPN prepared by a compounder	Parenteral nutrition

Low Risk Level 1. This risk level encompasses medications and procedures used to prepare sterile products, including sterile medications, needles, and syringes; sterile technique; and use of a Class 5 hood. The technique necessitates performing only minimal manipulations within the hood. This is the most common type of IV preparation performed. Technicians must wear gown, gloves, cap, and mask during manipulation; these items of clothing are typically referred to as personal protective equipment, and must be provided by the facility. The technician must verify all ingredients and instructions and visually inspect the solution after preparation. Each person's knowledge of aseptic technique and proper manipulations must be monitored and verified annually. An annual media-fill test must be done for each person compounding products in the hood. Safety measures include proper testing and certification of the hood.

Medium Risk Level 2. This risk level encompasses bulk compounding; this includes multiple IVs prepared for several patients or multiple compounded products to be used for one patient over several days. This would include preparing **hyperalimentation** to be used over 1 week. Many manipulations must be performed while in the hood. The requirements include all those listed for level 1 plus additional guidelines. A more in-depth evaluation must be performed, including a more stringent media-fill test to be conducted annually. This is done by performing a systematic evaluation of manipulations to determine that a sterile product has been prepared.

High Risk Level 3. Risk level 3 includes all the requirements of levels 1 and 2, plus additional guidelines. The types of products that this level encompasses are those that are susceptible to contamination because of the preparation of nonsterile products and/or delayed sterilization. An example would be the preparation of a morphine and bupivacaine solution from a bulk powder (nonsterile) for use in an intrathecal pump. The requirements for this level include semiannual certification of aseptic compounding. Technicians must demonstrate they can prepare such a product and ensure its sterility. In addition, any batches over 25 units require pyrogen testing to be performed. This is to verify that the batch is free of any contamination.

EDUCATION AND TRAINING

Both pharmacists and technicians must be able to show competency in compounding. Before compounding is permitted, the pharmacist and technician must complete video/written and practical instruction followed by a media-fill test and a written exam. Training and testing must be repeated annually for low and medium risk levels and semiannually for high risk level.

Although persons who prepare sterile products must receive training on standards of sterile compounding, those instructions will differ depending on the amount and type of manipulations they perform. Normally physicians, nurses, and emergency medical technicians (EMTs) will only prepare low risk products. Pharmacy technicians and pharmacists must be instructed on all standards if they are to prepare all types of sterile products. For example, an IV technician may only need risk level 2 training whereas technicians that prepare chemotherapy or hyperalimentation will need training for high risk level 3 preparations. Several steps must be accomplished in order for proper training to be completed. By viewing *ASHP Aseptic Technique and Proper Compounding* instructional videos that can be found at: (www.ashp.org/Import/membercenter/Technicians/Training.aspx), technicians can learn safe handling of sterile products. In addition, aseptic technique verification services, such as Valiteq Products, provide training packets for various risk levels. Both ASHP and Valiteq have compounding manuals that can be used throughout the training period. Valiteq includes media-fill tests (Box 12-3) and a written exam as well as a visual check-off list for observation of the preparer. Once the preparation is complete, the growth medium is incubated according to set requirements and tested at various times for any observation of abnormal growth. No growth is acceptable for a passing score. A 90% passing score is required on the written test and practical observation in the hood. These check-offs must be completed and passed before the technician is permitted to prepare sterile products. Personnel who fail any of the tests must repeat instruction and reevaluation. Checklists are often made by pharmacies to document the evaluation of the person compounding. A sample form (Figure 12-13) lists the standards required

---

BOX 12-3 MEDIA-FILL TESTS

What is a media-fill test?
A microbial growth medium such as a trypticase soy broth (TSB) solution is substituted for the actual drug to simulate the admixture compounding technique. After using the TSB, the final container is incubated (20° to 35° C for 14 days) and then checked for turbidity; if positive, it confirms the presence of microbial contaminants.

How often are media-fill tests done?
Per *USP* <797> regulations a media-fill test must be completed at the time of hire, and then (at minimum) yearly for low and medium risk compounding levels and twice a year for high risk compounding levels.

Under what conditions is a media-fill test performed?
It is suggested that the test should be done in a manner to mimic a real case scenario; for example, at the end of the day when the preparer is tired or at stressful work times during the day.

What happens if the test results are positive?
The written policies for the pharmacy include steps that should be taken for positive test results; they include retraining in aseptic techniques with a mentor and then repeating the media-fill test. If the test results are positive again, then it is suggested that the clean room and hoods be tested for any contamination. All results should be documented.

COMPOUNDING EVALUATION CHECKLIST
(circle answer)

No jewelry	YES	NO	N/A
Hair tied back	YES	NO	N/A
All calculations done prior	YES	NO	N/A
All products gathered prior	YES	NO	N/A
Washes hands appropriately	YES	NO	N/A
Gowns appropriately	YES	NO	N/A
Cleans hood 70% isopropyl alcohol	YES	NO	N/A
Cleans hood appropriately	YES	NO	N/A
Puts all items into the hood properly	YES	NO	N/A
Uses aseptic manipulation in the hood	YES	NO	N/A
Works within 6" radius of hood	YES	NO	N/A
If left the hood, sterilizes gloves prior to re-entering	YES	NO	N/A
Checked label 3 times	YES	NO	N/A
Uses proper equipment while in the hood	YES	NO	N/A
Uses foil cover on port after adding medication	YES	NO	N/A
Checks final product for color, clarity	YES	NO	N/A
Places label properly on product	YES	NO	N/A
Label is correct	YES	NO	N/A
Calculations are correct	YES	NO	N/A
Expiration date given	YES	NO	N/A
Signature of preparer signed	YES	NO	N/A
Disposes of vial and used packages appropriately	YES	NO	N/A
Cleans hood after use	YES	NO	N/A
Did not spill any contents	YES	NO	N/A
Did not break airflow	YES	NO	N/A
Checked for any particulates in diluted solution	YES	NO	N/A

Name _____   Date_____Time _____

Evaluator _____

Comments:_____

FIGURE 12-13 Compounding evaluation checklist.

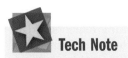

Tech Note

The final product must always be checked for color, clarity, or evidence of precipitation.

of personnel who prepare sterile products. An observer must rate each standard while preparations are being compounded to ensure compliance.

REQUIREMENTS FOR COMPOUNDING

It is required that all personnel who prepare parenteral medications must be trained and monitored for compliance with techniques on a periodic basis. This includes ensuring that the drug ingredients, containers, labeling, and equipment are correct. Products must be stored according to manufacturer guidelines or other scientific findings (to be discussed later). Pharmacists must determine the risk level of each type of preparation as well. Although *USP <797>* outlines risk, the standards do not rate every type of manipulation; the standards outline basic guidelines. The determination of which level applies to additional types of manipulations must be made by the pharmacist on an individual basis. The hoods and clean room as well as the pharmacy rooms adjacent to these

TABLE 12-4 *USP* Air Standards Based on 0.5-μm Particle Size

BSC or Room	Description	Number of Particles/m²	Area in Pharmacy	Required Testing for Compliance
ISO 8	Class 100,000	3,520,000	Nonhazardous room	Checked every 12 months
ISO 7	Class 10,000	352,000	Clean room (i.e., buffer room and anteroom)	Checked every 12 months
ISO 6	Class 1000	35,200	Anteroom	Checked every 6 months
ISO 5	Class 100	3,520	IV hood	Checked every 6 months

BOX 12-4   ENVIRONMENT TERMINOLOGY

Clean or buffer room—space adjacent to the PEC room where sterile preparation takes place

Anteroom—space adjacent to the clean or buffer room

Primary engineering control (PEC)—space or hood where sterile preparation takes place

Biological safety cabinet (BSA)—a hood that should be used for hazardous sterile preparation within the clean room

Laminar airflow workspace (LAFW)—a hood that should be used for nonhazardous sterile preparation within the clean room

Compounding aseptic isolator (CAI)—a Class III glove box that can have either negative or positive air pressure

Compounding aseptic containment isolator (CACI)—another type of Class III CAI glove box that exhausts 100% of the air through a HEPA filter; to be used for preparation of hazardous medications; may also have either negative or positive air pressure

Air lock—a space of separation between two different air pressures; may be a pass-through chamber or room; a door must be present to prevent loss of pressure in the higher pressured room

Air pressure—can be either positive or negative; positive air pressure environments may only be used for nonhazardous sterile preparation; negative air pressure environments can be used to prepare both nonhazardous and hazardous sterile preparations

rooms must be within the guidelines of *USP <797>*. It is essential that any contamination be kept away from these areas. The guidelines for air standards in IV areas and individual hoods are listed in Table 12-4.

IV ENVIRONMENT

Most pharmacies can easily meet the educational and training aspects of *USP <797>;* however, this is not true of the new regulations related to the areas where these products are prepared. Each type of environment within the pharmacy is required to meet minimum standards pertaining to particle size and quantity. According to studies conducted by *USP,* using a **laminar flow hood** in an open room is no safer than preparing products on a countertop. This has been one of the greatest changes in pharmacy. As a result of the enormous expense required to create these new areas, many hospitals now contract out to specialized pharmacies to prepare their sterile products. Those facilities that have been able to meet USP standards must also test the air on a periodic basis to ensure guidelines are met. The terms and definitions used to describe types of environments are listed in Box 12-4.

The **anteroom** is adjacent to the buffer room (or "**clean room**"). The minimum size of air particles allowed in the anteroom is 0.5 micrometers.

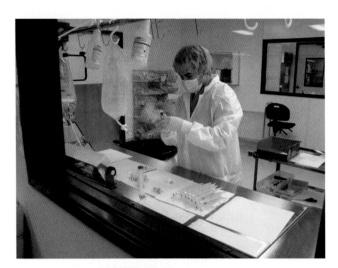

FIGURE 12-14 Clean room.

However, the "clean room," where the technician actually prepares sterile products, must meet more stringent requirements pertaining to air particulate size (Figure 12-14).

USP <797> also requires specific types of hoods to be used for compounding specific sterile products. Laminar flow hoods that only have positive (horizontal) airflow may be used to prepare nonhazardous medications (see Figure 10-4), whereas a negative (vertical) airflow environment may be used to prepare hazardous products per *USP* guidelines (see Figure 10-5). In addition, biological safety cabinets (BSCs) are totally enclosed environments that are available in either positive or negative airflow, or they may be switched between the two types of airflow (see Figure 10-7). All types of hoods have high-efficiency particulate airflow (HEPA) filters, although the way in which they expel the air differs. Proper use of these hoods requires additional training. The hoods must be verified/certified every 6 months to ensure their ability to filter contaminants. Both anterooms and clean rooms must be within standards. Assessments must be completed annually; any movement of the equipment requires additional inspection.

Pharmacies must use special equipment and chemicals to sterilize the room; specialty knowledge regarding the proper way to clean the room is also required. For example, hoods and surface areas must be cleaned and sterilized daily, the walls and floor weekly. SOPs must be written and studied, and evaluation exams taken by all who work in these areas.

STORAGE AND STABILITY

As the duration of time a compounded IV is exposed to room temperature increases, so does the risk of bacterial growth. In addition, refrigeration temperatures must be monitored at least once daily to ensure constant conditions. As required by risk level, there are guidelines for both temperature ranges and expiration dates of compounded medications (Table 12-5). The limits are for those products that are aseptically prepared but have not passed a sterility test. The limits do not apply to batches that have been tested. Products that have been tested for sterility may be given longer expiration dates. Storage requirements extend into training the patient and/or caretaker in the proper use and storage of compounded products as well. Monitoring and reporting any adverse events through the proper channels must be consistently performed and also documented.

TABLE 12-5 Storage Risk Levels: Temperature Ranges and Expiration Dates of Compounded Medications

Level of Risk	Room temperature: 20-25° C or 68-77° F	Refrigeration: 2-8° C or 36-46° F	Freezer: 5-10° C or 13-14° F
Low	48 hours	14 days	45 days
Medium	30 hours	7 days	45 days
High	24 hours	3 days	45 days

HOOD CLEANING AND MAINTENANCE

Airflow

Depending on the type of sterile product being prepared, there are three types of hoods used—**horizontal flow hoods**, **vertical flow hoods**, and glove boxes (i.e., biological safety cabinets [BSCs]). Laminar airflow workbenches (LAFWs) (i.e., hoods) are used for many types of parenteral or sterile product preparations. Horizontal hoods provide positive air pressure, moving the filtered air outwards toward the preparer. For chemotherapeutic agents, a vertical flow hood can be used because of the direction of the airflow and the specifications of the hood. A vertical flow hood provides negative air pressure, circulating the air through an additional HEPA filter and then through a vent away from the preparer. A vertical flow hood can be used to mix non–chemotherapeutic agents if needed; however, chemotherapeutic agents should never be mixed in a horizontal flow hood. Glove boxes are closed systems that use a HEPA filter and a sophisticated venting system. These provide the greatest amount of safety to the preparer because of the containment ability. With all systems, strict aseptic technique and care must be used because spillage can still occur on the surface of the IV bag or container and can cause contamination or unwanted exposure on removal from the hood.

In a horizontal flow hood, the outside airflow starts in the back of the hood, passes through a special filter, and circulates out toward the opening. This special filter is a high-efficiency particulate air (HEPA) filter that traps all particles larger than 0.2 micrometers. The sides of the hood and items within the hood create a disruption of airflow. For this reason, the technician must work 6 inches in from the sides and front of the hood. In addition, movement within the hood should be kept to a minimum to decrease disruption of airflow.

In a vertical flow hood, the concept is similar, although air cannot be released back into the room. For this reason, vertical hoods have a Plexiglas shield that separates the technician from the inside work surface. The air passes into the HEPA filter and then into the workspace area. The technician must not block the downward flow of air while working. A grid at the front of the tabletop draws in the air and filters it once again through a HEPA filter before it is released into the workspace area or is vented to the outside, depending on the type of venting system used. Both horizontal and vertical flow hoods must be turned on at least 30 minutes before use.

The biological safety cabinet (BSC) is also referred to as a glove box or barrier isolator; it is becoming the most popular type of hood for sterile preparation. This type of hood reduces the risk of contamination caused by accidental mishandling of drugs while compounding and decreases the number of environmental microbial contaminants, thus increasing the sterility of the prepared product. This ultimately protects patients from possible harmful medications. It also protects the person preparing the chemotherapeutic agent, because these medications can be harmful if inhaled or contacted by the skin. There are three

TABLE 12-6 HEPA Filtering System Standards

Class	Risk Levels	Safety Level	Filtering System
Class I	Low to moderate risk biologicals	Bio-safety level I	HEPA filters air before it is exhausted
Class II	Low to moderate risk biologicals	Bio-safety level II	HEPA filters exhaust air to room or to a facility exhaust system
Class III	High risk biologicals	Bio-safety level III	Containment of hazardous materials

BOX 12-5 DAILY CLEANING OF LAMINAR AIRFLOW WORKBENCH

1. Cleaning must be done daily in addition to between preparations when necessary.
2. Before cleaning the laminar flow hood, put on gown and gloves.
3. Inspect all surfaces for any crystallized solutions. Clean these with sterile water before continuing.
4. Moisten a 4 × 4-inch gauze or other disposable cloth or gauze with 70% isopropyl alcohol and wash the inside of the hood. This includes the sides and tabletop. DO NOT SPRAY THE AIR FILTER AT THE BACK OF THE HOOD.
5. Then, starting from the top right-hand side of the hood, wipe down, across the surface, and up to the top of the left-hand side of the hood.
6. Moving forward a few inches, repeat the motion in the opposite direction.
7. The side-to-side, back-to-front motion is essential for cleaning before use of the hood each day. In addition, clean the hood periodically throughout the course of the day to ensure a sterile environment.
8. Carefully clean the HEPA filter grid at the back of the hood. DO NOT SATURATE GAUZE WITH ISOPROPYL ALCOHOL WHEN CLEANING THE GRID. Clean the horizontal rod that is used for hanging IV bags.
9. Wipe the horizontal IV rod.
10. Document the daily cleaning in the logbook.

different levels and classifications of BSCs, as listed in Table 12-6. The air is redirected through a HEPA filter and uses an additional airflow system to help decontaminate the medication preparation. Daily monitoring of the pressure gauge, flow indicators, or alarms should be documented.

A BSC must be turned on at least 10 minutes before use. After the technician washes his or her hands and cleans the hood properly, the technician can place all of the necessary materials and medications needed inside a holding chamber. Using the attached gloves, the technician takes the materials from the sterile chamber and transfers them into the main hood. All products and supplies should be placed at least 4 inches inside the sash. At this point, the technician may prepare the medication. Any high-risk medication can be prepared in this type of hood. Inspections should be performed every 6 months. In an effort to comply with *USP <797>* guidelines, these types of hoods are becoming more common in pharmacies.

Cleaning and Maintaining Hoods

All hoods in the pharmacy must be thoroughly cleaned using the appropriate solvent and cleaning methods. Box 12-5 lists systematic instructions of how to clean a horizontal flow hood. Box 12-6 lists the instructions on how a vertical flow hood should be cleaned. Cleaning BSCs differs from cleaning horizontal and vertical flow hoods, as described in Box 12-7.

BOX 12-6 CLEANING THE VERTICAL FLOW HOOD

1. Cleaning should be done before each use. Let the hood run for at least 30 minutes.
2. Glove and gown before cleaning.
3. Wet a 4 × 4-inch gauze pad or other disposable cloth with 70% isopropyl alcohol and wipe the inside of the hood. This includes the back, sides, and tabletop. DO NOT SPRAY THE CEILING INSIDE THE VERTICAL HOOD BECAUSE THIS IS WHERE THE FILTERING SYSTEM IS LOCATED. Start on the (inside) back of the hood and wipe from the top right across to the left-hand side, drop down a few inches, and then wipe across the wall to the right-hand side. Continue this process until the back wall is wiped completely.
4. Then repeat the cleaning procedures, working from the top right-hand side, across the tabletop, and up the left side until the entire hood is done.
5. In addition to the sides, tabletop, and back of the vertical flow hood, you also should wash the inside of the Plexiglas protective shield and the horizontal IV rod.
6. Document daily cleaning in the logbook.

BOX 12-7 CLEANING THE BIOLOGICAL SAFETY CABINET

Biological safety cabinets are intended to operate 24 hours a day. They must be cleaned every 30 minutes while continuous compounding is taking place; otherwise, clean after spills or if any contamination is suspected. The placement of hands when cleaning BSCs is similar to that used when cleaning a vertical flow hood. However, instead of using gauze and isopropyl alcohol 70% to clean the cabinet, plastic-backed absorbent towels (nonshedding) are used with 70% ethanol (EtOH) in a 1:100 dilution of household bleach. These dilutions are called sterile alcohol by manufacturing companies that supply BSC materials.

1. Glove and gown before cleaning.
2. The cabinet blowers need to run for at least 30 minutes before entering if the hood is not operating.
3. Wipe the work surface with sterile water and soap if needed (the water must be sterile so the surface does not become contaminated).
4. Using an absorbent towel and solvent, clean the work surface, interior walls, the inside of the window, and the horizontal rod in the cabinet.
5. Using a towel, wipe from back-to-front and side-to-side.
6. Carefully clean the HEPA grills.
7. Dispose of towel in a biohazard bag when done.
8. Document the daily cleaning in the logbook.

HAND PLACEMENT

Regardless of which type of hood is used, the placement of the hands is one of the most important aspects to consider when preparing sterile medications. One should practice some simple yet important techniques. These techniques decrease the possibility of contamination and errors when preparing sterile products. Figure 12-15 outlines the necessary steps to take when working in the hood. When working in a horizontal hood you must not block the airflow at any time; this can be done by grabbing the vial/ampule by the front; avoid placing the hands/fingers right behind the top of the container. When holding up the vial/ampule keep fingers from blocking airflow. This technique takes time to perfect and should be practiced constantly until it becomes second-nature. When working in a vertical flow hood, avoid placing hands/fingers over the container, as this would break airflow. It is also important not to overload the hood with drugs and supplies. This can lead to a break in aseptic technique and increases the

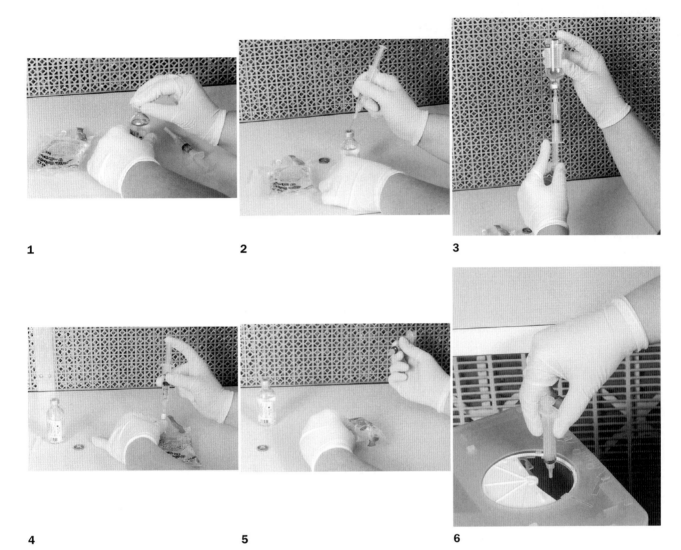

FIGURE 12-15 The six-step process of using aseptic technique in the hood is as follows: (1) Using alcohol, wipe the tops of the vials and the ports on the intravenous bags from back to front (wipe around the vial and bag rather than over or behind). (2) Place the needle bevel side up and push it into the rubber stopper of the vial. Preload the syringe with the necessary amount of air to replace solution. (3) Invert the vial and syringe 180 degrees. Push in the air from the syringe and pull out the solution. (4) After removing the syringe from the vial, insert the needle into the intravenous bag and inject the medication using a steady hand. (5) After injecting the intravenous bag with the medication, immediately flip the bag over. This decreases the possibility of forgetting which bags have been injected and which ones have not. (6) Never recap the used needles; instead, discard each syringe in a sharps container along with the uncapped needle after use. Syringes cannot be reused when changing from one drug to another. This decreases the chance of drug-to-drug contamination.

likelihood of drug errors. When using a BSC it is necessary to follow strict protocol in handling and transferring solutions. Guidelines for working inside a BSC are listed in Box 12-8.

DISPOSAL

Once the technician has finished using the hood area, he or she should clean all unused materials and discard any used products. To clean a horizontal flow hood, wipe down the surface with a 70% isopropyl alcohol swab and then allow the surface to air-dry. Dispose of all paper products in a trash bin; dispose of

BOX 12-8 BSC GUIDELINES FOR MEDICATION PREPARATION

1. Fill the syringe carefully to minimize air bubbles.
2. Expel air, liquid, and bubbles from the syringe vertically over a piece of 2 × 2-inch sterile gauze moistened with disinfectant.
3. To avoid transfer of infectious material to fingers, do not contaminate the needle hub when filling the syringe.
4. Wrap the needle and stopper in 2 × 2-inch gauze moistened with disinfectant when removing a needle from a vial.
5. Do not bend or recap needles from syringes. If you must recap or remove a contaminated needle from a syringe, use the one-handed scoop method.

Tech Note!

Always check the pharmacy protocol regarding the disposal of sharps containers. This information can be found in the policies and procedures handbook. Never place your hands into a sharps or hazardous waste container! This could result in a needle stick or exposure to a hazardous chemical.

Tech Note!

Always know the location of the cleanup kit for hazardous waste spills. In addition, take time to review the policies and procedures in case of a chemotherapy spill.

needles, syringes, and vials in a sharps container. Most sharps containers are made of heavy-duty plastic; they have a separate lid that can be locked into place on top of the container. There is a one-way opening in the lid for the disposal of needles and other sharps. Normally a 7-gallon size is used and is located outside the hood. When cleaning a vertical flow hood, discard needles, syringes, and vials in a small sharps container placed inside the hood area. Wrap all other materials to be discarded into the spill-proof pad and place inside a chemotherapeutic protective bag. This may be discarded in a special hazardous materials bin located outside the hood. All materials used in the BSC, including disposable needles and syringes, must be placed in appropriate sharps disposal containers and discarded as infectious waste. This is contained inside the hood area.

For all hoods, the last step is to clean the entire area with the proper alcohol solution as per the type of cabinet involved. Sharps containers are to be replaced when two-thirds full and must be picked up or delivered to an approved "red bag" or medical waste treatment site.

SPILLS

If a spill occurs in a horizontal flow hood, it may be cleaned using a gauze pad and 70% isopropyl alcohol. The gauze can be discarded in a regular trash bin. Always wear the proper protective equipment for the type of spill to be handled. If a small spill occurs in a vertical flow hood, it should be cleaned with sterile gauze and 70% isopropyl alcohol and discarded inside a chemotherapeutic protective bag. If a small spill occurs in a BSC, wipe up the spill with a disinfectant-soaked paper towel and then clean the surface with 70% isopropyl alcohol. The outer pair of gloves must be replaced after cleaning up a spill. Dispose of the materials in the appropriate container. For specific information on spill size and cleaning techniques, see the policies and procedures binder.

PARENTERAL ANTIBIOTICS AND SOLUTIONS

Manufacturers have suggested guidelines for dosing regimens and volumes of solutions that are followed by most physicians. As shown in Table 12-7, the manufacturer's guidelines are determined by which microbe is being attacked. Pharmacies have a chart that instructs the person preparing the medication as to the type and amount of diluent needed, the normal dosing times, and expiration dates. Antibiotics also differ in how they should be prepared and how long it takes the powder to dissolve in the diluent. Once the drug is reconstituted, the solution should be checked for color and clarity.

TABLE 12-7 Example of Suggested Dosing Times, Solutions, and Appropriate Volumes for Antibiotics

Generic Name	Trade Name	Common Dosing Regimens (in hours)	Common Solutions	Common Volumes
Ampicillin	Omnipen	q8-q6	NS*	Less than 1.5 g (50 mL), more than 1.5 g (100 mL)
Cefazolin	Ancef, Kefzol	q8-q6	D_5W or NS	Less than 2 g (50 mL), more than 2 g (100 mL)
Cefotaxime	Claforan	q6-q12	D_5W or NS	Less than 2 g (50 mL), more than 2 g (100 mL)
Ceftazidime	Fortaz	q8-q6	D_5W or NS	Less than 2 g (50 mL), more than 2 g (100 mL)
Ceftriaxone	Rocephin	q8-q24	D_5W or NS	Less than 2 g (50 mL), more than 2 g (100 mL)
Doxycycline	Vibramycin	q12	D_5W or NS	250 mL
Erythromycin	E-Mycin	q6-q24	NS	250 mL[†] (10 mg) or 500 mL[†] (20 mg) lidocaine
Gentamicin	Garamycin	q8-q18[†] based on glycoside levels	D_5W or NS	Less than 100 mg (50 mL), more than 100 mg (100 mL)
Imipenem- cilastatin	Primaxin	q6-q12	NS	Less than 500 mg (100 mL), more than 500 mg (250 mL)

*D_5W, 5% dextrose in water; *NS*, normal saline.
[†]Erythromycin stings when given intravenously; therefore it is commonly mixed with lidocaine to relieve the pain.
[†]See Chapter 25 for more on antibiotics.

Technique

When adding a diluent to a powder an equal amount of air must be removed from the vial or a positive pressure is created. This will cause pressure resistance in the syringe. For example, if you are adding 10 mL of diluent to a powder, push on the syringe until you feel a very slight resistance and then stop and withdraw an equal amount of air from the vial to relieve the positive pressure. Repeat this until all of the diluent has been added. To work with negative pressure, first withdraw air from the vial until you feel resistance and then allow the vial to pull diluent out of the syringe. Never let go of a syringe. This type of technique works well because there is less chance that a spill will occur.

Use of Ampules to Prepare Medications

Intravenous push or intramuscular medications can be prepared by the nurse at the nursing station or at the patient's bedside; however, the pharmacy does prepare some IV push and intramuscular medications. These agents are placed in a syringe and sealed with a syringe cap until it is time to administer the medication. One must follow five steps when preparing these syringes from ampules; the procedures differ from those followed when using a vial. These steps are outlined next and in Figure 12-16.

TECHNIQUE

When pulling solution from an ampule there is no positive or negative pressure because this is an open system. This means the container is open and able to allow air to enter it, replacing the missing volume of solution. However, it is important to remember to use a filter needle when transferring drug from an ampule because small pieces of the ampule may detach and fall into the solution when the ampule is broken. A filter needle may only be used for one draw (push

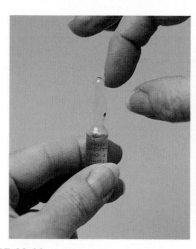 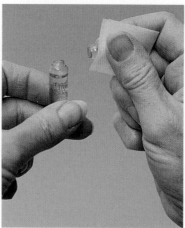 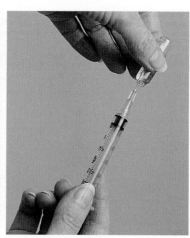

FIGURE 12-16 Proper manipulation of ampule: Ampule sizes range from 1- to 50-mL glass containers. For larger ampules, an ampule breaker is suggested. For smaller ampules, follow these steps: (1) Tap top of ampule to empty top of container. (2) Using an alcohol swab, wipe the neck of the ampule and snap open (away from you). (3) Tilt the ampule at an angle (the solution will not spill) and withdraw needed amount of drug using a filter needle. (4) Replace the filter needle with a regular needle and inject into solution; however, if sending the syringe, remove the needle and cap the end of the syringe. (5) Label container and place in proper location for pharmacist's inspection. (From Potter PA, Perry AG: *Fundamentals of nursing*, ed 5, St Louis, 2001, Elsevier.)

or pull); either it can be replaced by a regular needle before the drug is pushed into a piggyback or a regular needle can be used to withdraw the solution and then a filter needle can be used to push the filtered solution into the piggyback; otherwise, the glass that is trapped in the filter needle will be pushed into the final solution.

HYPERALIMENTATION

Hyperalimentation (also known as hyperals) are large volumes of parenteral nutrition solutions normally prepared for persons who cannot orally consume nutrition (i.e., they cannot eat). The following are some reasons for this inability to eat:

- Recent stomach or intestinal surgery
- Unconscious (coma)
- Various conditions that may adversely affect the gastrointestinal system.

Two main types of hyperalimentation are prepared in the pharmacy: **total parenteral nutrition (TPN)** and **peripheral parenteral nutrition (PPN).** In a hospital setting, after the initial hyperalimentation (hyperal) is prepared and hung, daily laboratory tests of electrolyte levels are drawn from the patient to determine necessary changes. For example, if a patient's potassium levels begin to drop, then the next hyperal will be altered to compensate for this decrease. In this way, the patient receives exactly the nutrients needed each day. Home health clinics and some hospitals prepare hyperalimentation solutions that last 1 week. If this is done the vitamin additive must be added daily to the hyperal because this is one limiting factor for the bag's 24-hour expiration. Electrolyte levels are tested weekly instead of daily. Some patients may receive this type of nutrition for many months. Figure 12-17 shows TPN connected to an automatic infusion pump system.

Many different protocols are used to prepare parenteral nutrition. The following is a list of typical solutions prepared in a hospital pharmacy. The large-volume components (e.g., protein, carbohydrates, and fats) are premixed and

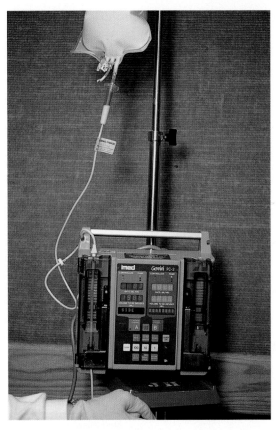

FIGURE 12-17 A total parenteral nutrition preparation connected to an infusion set. (From Elkin MK, Perry AG, Potter PA: *Nursing interventions and clinical skills*, ed 4, St Louis, 2007, Elsevier.)

Tech Note!

Some chemicals can precipitate other chemicals, creating solid flakes in the intravenous solution. Always check your intravenous bag for clarity after you finish preparing the solution.

ordered in cases from the manufacturer. Added to these solutions are the various electrolytes and other compatible medications requested by the patient's attending physician:

- TPN normally contains 50% dextrose, 10% amino acids, and 20% fat.
- Peripheral parenteral nutrition normally contains 25% dextrose, 10% amino acids, and 10% fat.
- Hyperals are prepared for neonates, children, and adults.

As a result of the regulations required by *USP <797>*, many pharmacies contract out their TPN/PPN orders to specialized compounding companies. Bags can range in volumes from 50 mL for neonates up to 3 L for adults. It is important to note that neonatal and pediatric additives differ in concentration from adult formulas and therefore great care must be taken when pulling the correct medication for preparation if your facility prepares these products.

Because of the range of concentrations of PPN solutions, they are administered differently than the higher concentration TPN solutions. TPN is administered intravenously via the subclavian vein and superior vena cava because of the higher concentration of nutrients. Patients must have a catheter surgically inserted for this procedure. PPN is administered via a peripheral vein, located either in the back of the hand or in another peripheral area in the upper extremity, and therefore is a less complicated procedure. Most facilities have a standard order to initiate patient hyperalimentation. The volume of hyperalimentation typically ranges from 2 to 3 L. The physician determines the rate of infusion over the course of 24 hours. Regardless of how many milliliters run per hour, the hyperalimentation must be changed at least every 24 hours to ensure the sterility of the solution. A standard rate of infusion is 100 mL/hour; therefore, 2400 mL may be used over the course of a day. Most hyperalimentation preparations are tailor-made for each patient. Figure 12-18 gives an example of a protocol order.

ELECTROLYTES AND ADDITIVES

All TPN contains dextrose and amino acids; both ingredients help to nourish the body. The metabolism of dextrose (i.e., sugar) provides calories and a quick energy source for the body, whereas amino acids are the essential components that the body uses to synthesize protein, needed enzymes, and other important molecules. In addition, lipids commonly are added to give the body the necessary fat needed for the synthesis of important cell components, such as cell walls. The rest of the additives are additional electrolytes such as those listed in Table 12-8. These components can be determined daily if the patient is in a hospital setting. Other medications—such as ranitidine, cimetidine, or famotidine (all histamine$_2$-antagonists)—that help patients with stomach problems also can be added to hyperalimentation. In addition to stomach medications, insulin often is added in quantities up to 100 units per bag. Only regular insulin is added to hyperalimentation preparations, because regular insulin is the only insulin product that may be given intravenously.

TABLE 12-8 Types of Parenteral Additives

Abbreviation	Definition of abbreviation	Concentration	Notes
KCl	Potassium chloride	2 mEq/mL	
KPO$_4$	Potassium phosphate	Potassium 2 mEq/mL; phosphate 3 mEq/mL	Always determine phosphate concentration first
CaGluconate	Calcium gluconate	0.465 mEq/mL	
MgSO$_4$	Magnesium sulfate	1 mg/mL	
KAc	Potassium acetate	2 mEq/mL	*Used to balance
NaAcetate	Sodium acetate	2 mEq/mL	*Used to balance
NaPO$_4$	Sodium phosphate	2 mEq/mL	
NaCl	Sodium chloride	2 mEq/mL	*Used to balance
Miscellaneous Additives			
MVI	Multivitamin		Both adult and pediatric dosing
MTE	Multiple trace elements		Both adult and pediatric dosing
Zn	Zinc		
Se	Selenium		
Regular insulin	Insulin		Can be added to TPN and PPN†

Other Nonsupplements Added to TPN or PPN Solutions		
Generic name	Trade name	Concentration
Ranitidine	Zantac	40 mg/mL
Famotidine	Pepcid	20 mg/mL
Cimetidine	Tagamet	150 mg/mL

*To balance means the pharmacist determines the amount to be added.
†PPN, Peripheral parenteral nutrition; TPN, total parenteral nutrition.

TPN ORDER SHEET

HOME HEALTH	DATE
PATIENT	ADDRESS

TPN FORMULA:

AMINO ACIDS: ☐ 5.5% ☐ 8.5% ☑ 10%	425 mL
☐ WITH STANDARD ELECTROLYTES	
DEXTROSE: ☐ 10% ☐ 20% ☐ 40% ☐ 50% ☑ 70% (check one)	357 mL
LIPIDS: ☐ 10% ☑ 20% FOR ALL-IN-ONE FORMULA	125 mL

FINAL VOLUME qsad STERILE WATER FOR INJECTION	400mL	1307 mL

Calcium Gluconate	0.465m Eq/mL	5	mEq
Magnesium Sulfate	4m Eq/mL	5	mEq
Potassium Acetate	2m Eq/mL		mEq
Potassium Chloride	2m Eq/mL		mEq
Potassium Phosphate	3m M/mL	22	mM
Sodium Acetate	2m Eq/mL		mEq
Sodium Chloride	4m Eq/mL	35	mEq
Sodium Phosphate	3m M/mL		mM
TRACE ELEMENTS CONCENTRATE	☐4 ☐5 ☐6		mL

Patient Additives:

☐ MVC 9 + 3 10 mL Daily

☐ HUMULIN-R _10_ u Daily

☐ FOLIC ACID _____mg _____times weekly

☐ VITAMIN K _____mg _____times weekly

☐ OTHER: _MVI 12 1.5mL/daily_

☐ OTHER: _____

Directions:

INFUSE: ☑ DAILY

☐ ____ TIMES WEEKLY

OTHER DIRECTIONS:

_____

_____

_____

_____

Rate: ☐ CYCLIC INFUSION: OVER ____ HOURS (TAPER UP AND DOWN) | ☐ CONTINUOUS INFUSION: AT ____ mL PER HOUR | ☑ STANDARD RATE: AT _110_ mL PER HOUR FOR _12_ HOURS

LAB ORDERS:

☐ STANDARD LAB ORDERS
SMAC-20, CO2, Mg+2 TWICE WEEKLY
CBC WITH AUTO DIFF WEEKLY
UNTIL STABLE, THEN:
SMAC-20, CO2, Mg+2 WEEKLY
CBC WITH AUTO DIFF MONTHLY

☐ OTHER: _____

_____

_____

VALIDATION:

_____

DOCTOR'S SIGNATURE

Print Name: _____

Office Address: _____

_____

Phone: _____

WHITE: Home Health   CANARY: Physician

FIGURE 12-18 Example of a total parenteral nutrition order.

TABLE 12-9 Additional Considerations for the Preparation of Drugs

Medication	Special instructions
Insulin	NS* or ½; must be placed in glass container
Amiodarone	D_5NS
Nitroglycerin	D_5NS or NS; must be placed in glass container
Ciprofloxacin	Protect from light
Lorazepam	Protect from light; stable longer in glass than in plastic

*D_5NS, 5% dextrose in normal saline; *NS*, normal saline.

HOME INFUSION PHARMACY

Patient A   Date: 03/26/2012
RX#37856

Amino*Acids 10%=425 mL Dextrose*70%=357 mL
Ster*Water=400 mL Lipids*20%=125 mL
MVI=10 ml/day *Additives per liter*
Sod*Chlor=35 mEq Pot*Phos=15 mM Calcium=
5 mEq Magnesium=5 mEq

Qty#   TPN 40–51GM Protein+Lipids
Infuse nightly 8pm to 8am thru IV PICC line via sigma
pump. *****Add 10 units Humulin-R to each bag just
prior to infusion***** **Note: contains TPN soln+lipids:
rate adjusted** Settings: rate=104 mL/hr
volume=1248 mL

REFRIGERATE

Expiration date: 04/01/07

FIGURE 12-19 Example of an intravenous medication label.

Tech Note!

Each type of medication has its own unique properties. For example, ceftazidime produces gas when reconstituted. Therefore, to prevent the solution from shooting out of the vial, the gas must be released first. This can be done by puncturing a needle into the vial to allow venting of the gas. Erythromycin powder, on the other hand, is difficult to dissolve into the diluent; therefore it is important to allow additional time when reconstituting erythromycin. Allow the vial to sit in the hood (and shake it occasionally) until the powder turns into a solution.

Compatibility Considerations of Parenteral Medications

Many different types of medications are prepared in a clean room. Some medications must be protected from light, whereas others must be kept in bottles (as discussed previously). Refer to Table 12-9 for additional considerations in the preparation of parenteral drugs. Special instructions regarding the preparation of many types of parenteral medications can be found in reference books located in intravenous rooms. The intravenous technician must become familiar with the idiosyncrasies of medications to ensure that all solutions he or she makes are effective and safe.

Components of a Label for Intravenous Medication

The final step in preparing parenteral medications is the application of the label. First, check the label against the medication and the physician's orders to ensure that the right medication is being given to the right patient. Although each pharmacy prepares its own label, all labels require the same minimum information. Figure 12-19 shows an example of a label for intravenous medication.

All labels produced for parenteral medications must be initialed by the technician who prepares them. A registered pharmacist is responsible for the final label inspection. Many pharmacy labels rely on the Julian date for determining the expiration date of the medication. If the medication is not used, perhaps because of a discontinued order, it is recycled for use on another patient. The Julian date is the actual consecutive day of the year. For example, January 1 is day 1, January 31 is day 31, and February 1 is day 32; the numbers then continue consecutively until day 365, which is December 31. Determining an expiration date is easier when using the Julian date instead of a traditional month/day/year system. However, if a computer system is used that relies on the calendar date, it should indicate the expiration date as well.

After the label has been applied, the intravenous preparations are left for the pharmacist to check along with the vial or container of medication used to make the intravenous preparation. Once this is completed, the intravenous preparations are loaded onto a cart or delivery vehicle that delivers them to their destinations. In a home health setting, a delivery service may be used to transport the medications to the patient's home. Within a hospital, this task normally is done by the technician. When the intravenous preparations are placed in the correct nursing unit, all unused intravenous preparations are obtained and are returned to the pharmacy for recycling. As long as the intravenous preparations are within their expiration dates and are kept at proper temperature, they can be used to fill new orders.

DO YOU REMEMBER THESE KEY POINTS?

- The major responsibilities of a hospital technician
- The types and sizes of syringes available in an intravenous room
- The parts of a syringe and needle
- The important aspects of aseptic technique and when they should be used
- How to determine the Julian date
- Different types of parenteral medications and when they are used
- Different equipment and supplies used in an intravenous area
- The types of solutions used to mix various antibiotics and parenteral medications
- The main routes of administration
- Ratings given to hoods and rooms within pharmacy
- Components of an IV label
- How to clean and set up supplies in a hood
- The various electrolytes used in preparing parenteral nutrition
- The three risk levels of *USP <797>*
- How to manipulate a needle and syringe
- How to reconstitute a powder
- The differences in air flow and safety between horizontal and vertical and BSCs
- Steps taken to discard materials from horizontal and vertical laminar flow hoods as well as BSC's
- Disposal techniques of hazardous materials

Multiple choice questions

1. Which of the skills listed is the *most* important aspect of preparing sterile products?
   A. Maintaining aseptic technique
   B. Working in a horizontal flow hood
   C. Using 70% isopropyl alcohol to disinfect the hood
   D. Donning scrubs, shoe covers, and facemask

2. A male/female adapter is used for which of the following reasons?
   A. To attach a needle to a syringe
   B. To attach syringes to tubing
   C. To attach syringes to syringes
   D. To attach two intravenous bags together

3. The smallest filter that can be used is a:
   A. Filter straw
   B. Filter needle
   C. 5-μm filter
   D. 0.22-μm filter

4. Complying with *USP <797>* regulations by using a microbial growth medium that is substituted for the actual drug to simulate admixture compounding is referred to as a:
   A. Media-Fill test
   B. Microbial test
   C. Sterility Solution test
   D. None of the above

5. Which of the following sizes of needles is NOT commonly used when preparing an IV medication?
   A. 16 gauge
   B. 18 gauge
   C. 19 gauge
   D. 25 gauge

6. Hands should always be washed or sanitized:
   A. When entering the intravenous room
   B. Before working in the horizontal flow hood
   C. Before working in a vertical flow hood
   D. All of the above

7. Laminar flow hoods should be cleaned:
   A. With 70% isopropyl alcohol
   B. At least 30 minutes before using
   C. At least once a day
   D. All of the above

8. Chemotherapeutic agents should be disposed of:
   A. In a plastic chemotherapy bag
   B. In a sharps container
   C. Only at the end of a shift
   D. By a biohazard team of professionals

9. HEPA stands for _____ and traps particles larger than:
   A. Heated environmental parenteral air filter, 2 μm
   B. High-environmental particulate air filter, 0.2 μm
   C. Horizontal-efficiency particulate air filter, 0.2 μm
   D. High-efficiency particulate air filter, 0.2 μm

10. You may find all of the following medications in a hyperalimentation preparation EXCEPT:
    A. Heparin
    B. Insulin
    C. Ranitidine
    D. Ampicillin

11. A room adjacent to the clean room must meet standards classified as:
A. ISO Class 5
B. ISO Class 6
C. ISO Class 8
D. ISO Class 10

12. First air refers to:
A. The air from the HEPA filter that passes over the materials
B. The first air that you breathe in the clean room
C. The air contained inside a vial
D. The first air inside a laminar flow hood

13. Low-risk IVs kept at refrigerated temperatures expire within:
A. 7 days
B. 14 days
C. 21 days
D. 30 days

14. BSCs should be inspected every:
A. Month
B. 3 months
C. 6 months
D. 12 months

15. SOP means:
A. Safe Operating Protocol
B. Safe Operations Policy
C. Standard Operating Policy
D. Standard Operating Procedure

True/False

If the statement is false, then change it to make it true.

_____ **1.** Intravenous stock ordering should be done weekly.

_____ **2.** *USP* <797> divides risk levels into 3 groups.

_____ **3.** Vials and intravenous bag ports should be wiped from front to back.

_____ **4.** Syringes normally are made of glass.

_____ **5.** Needles are made of aluminum or stainless steel.

_____ **6.** As the syringes increase in size, the calibration is less accurate.

_____ **7.** Laminar flow hoods should be checked monthly.

_____ **8.** You may recap syringes if they have been used only once.

_____ **9.** You must wear goggles when preparing chemotherapy agents.

_____ **10.** A sharps container must be replaced when it is full.

_____ **11.** BSCs are used to prepare chemotherapeutic agents.

_____ **12.** All hoods are cleaned and the waste disposed in the same manner.

_____ **13.** Both insulin and nitroglycerin IVs should be placed into a glass container.

_____ **14.** Horizontal flow hoods are not safe for the preparation of chemotherapeutic agents.

_____ **15.** It is safe to use a tension-tip syringe to prepare chemotherapeutic agents.

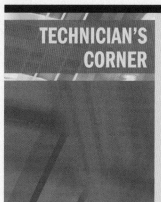

TECHNICIAN'S CORNER

The pharmacy receives an order for patient R. Jones.

Allergies: PCN, sulfa, morphine
Diagnosis: Sepsis, diabetes

Transcribe the following order into lay terms and determine whether any of the orders should be brought to the attention of a pharmacist; if so, explain why.

#1 Unasyn 3 g q6h in 100 mL NS
#2 Vancomycin 1 g in 100 mL D_5NS
#3 NPH insulin "rainbow coverage" or "sliding scale"

BIBLIOGRAPHY

NuAire Marketing Dept., Plymouth, Minn.

Ballington D: *Pharmacy practice for technicians*, ed 4, St Paul, 2009, EMC/Paradigm.

Baxa Corporation: USP <797> Training Requirements: A Case Study, 2006.

Elkin M, Perry A, Potter P: *Nursing interventions & clinical skills*, ed 3, St Louis, 2003, Elsevier.

Fred L, R.ph: *Manual for pharmacy technicians*, ed 3, Bethesda, 2005, American Society of Health-Systems Pharmacists.

ISMP Teleconference. Turning a New Chapter on IV Drug Compounding Safety: USP/NF Chapter <<797>> Volume 19, Number 9, pp 899-920, 2004. Wolters Kluwer Health Inc.

Potter P, Perry A: *Fundamentals of nursing*, ed 5, St Louis, 2004, Mosby.

WEBSITES

www.ncbi.nlm.nih.gov/pubmed/6798865?ordinalpos=1&itool=EntrezSystem2.PEntrez.Pubmed.Pubmed_ResultsPanel.Pubmed_DiscoveryPanel.Pubmed_Discovery_RA&linkpos=1&log$=relatedarticles&logdbfrom=pubmed

www.devicelink.com/pmpn/archive/02/04/005.html

www.pppmag.com/documents/V4N8/p2_4_5.pdf

http://my.clevelandclinic.org/services/pain_management/hic_patient-controlled_analgesia_pca_pump.aspx

www.microcln.com/PDF/CleaningandSanitizingProcedure.pdf

www.cdc.gov/OD/OHS/biosfty/bsc/BSC2000sec5.htm

ASHP Aseptic Technique and Proper Compounding instructional videos: www.ashp.org/Import/MEMBERCENTER/Technicians/Training.aspx

13

Pharmacy Stock and Billing

Teresa Hopper and Deby Harris

Objectives

UPON COMPLETING THIS CHAPTER, YOU SHOULD BE ABLE TO DO THE FOLLOWING:

- Explain the function of a drug formulary.

- List the primary types of insurance companies and describe how they manage drug coverage.

- Describe the differences between generic and trade drugs and explain how these differences affect cost to the patient and pharmacy.

- Differentiate between Medicaid and Medicare programs, including eligibility.

- Explain the use of Medigap plans and their limitations.

- List the five individual coverage plans offered by Medicare.

- Explain the process of third-party billing.

- Differentiate between HMO and PPO health care programs.

- Explain the purpose of workers' compensation.

- Indicate how to read a prescription drug card.

- Define the steps taken to handle recalled, returned, or expired medications.

- Summarize why and how prior authorization occurs and describe the pharmacy's responsibilities in attaining authorization.

- Describe three main ordering systems available in a pharmacy to keep stock levels constant.

- List the types of automated dispensing systems used in pharmacy.

TERMS AND DEFINITIONS

Adjudication *Electronic insurance billing for medication payment*

Average wholesale price (AWP) *The average price at which a drug is sold; the data are compiled from information provided from manufacturers, distributors, pharmacies. The AWP is often used in calculations related to medication reimbursement*

Closed formulary *In a closed formulary, medication use is tightly restricted to those medications provided within the formulary list. Medications that are NOT listed as preapproved drugs per the health plan provider or pharmacy benefits manager are not reimbursed except under extenuating circumstances and with proper documentation*

Co-pay *The portion of the prescription bill that the patient is responsible for paying*

Drug Topics Red Book *Reference book listing NDC numbers, manufacturers, and average wholesale pricing of drug products. Note that pharmacies often include this type of product and pricing information on their online database systems, which are provided by companies such as First DataBank and Gold Standard*

Drug utilization evaluation (DUE) or review (DUR) *The process by which pharmacists ensure proper medication utilization*

Formulary *A list of preapproved medications that are covered under a prescription plan or within an institution*

Health Insurance Portability and Accountability Act (HIPAA) *Federal guidelines for the protection of a patient's personal health information*

Material safety data sheets (MSDS) *Information sheets supplied to the pharmacy from the manufacturer of chemical products; data sheet for each product lists hazards of the product and procedures to follow if exposed to that product*

Medicare Modernization Act (MMA) *The enactment of prescription drug coverage provided for persons covered under Medicare; sets limitations on payments*

National Drug Code (NDC) *Ten-digit number given to all drugs for identification purposes. In health and drug databases, the NDC is represented as an 11-digit number, where placeholder zeros are inserted in the proper order within the code for the purpose of standardizing data transmissions*

National Provider Identifier (NPI) *Number assigned to any health care provider that is used for the purpose of standardizing health data transmissions*

Open formulary *A formulary list that is essentially unrestricted in the types of drug choices offered or that can be prescribed and reimbursed under the health provider plan or pharmacy benefit plan*

PAR *Periodic automatic replacement of stock levels to a certain number of allowed units*

Patient profile *A document listing necessary patient personal and health information including comprehensive information on the medications they are taking*

Pharmacy and therapeutics committee (P&T committee) *Medical staff composed of physicians and pharmacists who provide necessary information and advice to the institution or insurer on whether a drug should be added to a formulary*

POS *Point of sale or service; where the sale or service takes place*

Prior authorization *Insurance-required approval for a restricted, non-formulary, or noncovered medication before a prescription medication can be filled*

Trade, brand, or proprietary drug name *The name a company assigns for marketing and identification purposes to a commercial drug product; most brand names are trademarked and belong to originator products; the named products are often protected, for a time, by patents*

Treatment authorization request (TAR) *Similar to preauthorization form but is the process used for Medicare and Medicaid*

TYPES OF INSURANCE

HMO *Health maintenance organization*

Medicaid *Government-managed insurance program that supplements Medicare if the individual meets specific requirements. Provides health care services to low-income children, the elderly, blind, and those with disabilities*

Medicare *Government-managed insurance program composed of several coverage plans for health care services and supplies. Funded by both federal and state entities, individuals must meet specific requirements to be eligible. Individuals must be 65 years or older, or younger than 65 with long-term disabilities, or suffer from end-stage renal disease*

Medigap Plans *Supplemental insurance policies provided through private insurance companies to help cover costs not reimbursed by the Medicare plan, such as co-insurance, co-pays, and deductibles*

PPO *Preferred provider organization*

Workers' compensation *Government-required and government-enforced medical coverage for workers injured on the job, paid for by the employer. The programs are managed by each state in accordance with the state's workers' compensation laws*

Introduction

Everyone working in the pharmacy is responsible for maintaining the inventory stock. This is an essential part of the daily tasks of pharmacy staff. As stocks are depleted, it is important to order replacement inventories. Although there are many different systems available for ordering stock, the task of ordering can be delegated to a specific person within the pharmacy. It is then the responsibility of staff to inform the inventory control person of decreasing stock levels.

Along with ordering stock, pharmacy technicians help manage the third-party billing process. Proper knowledge of billing procedures is a skill that normally is learned over time as one works in the pharmacy. Because each pharmacy contracts to accept different insurance companies, the technician must become acquainted with the normal billing procedures of that particular pharmacy and its associated insurance companies. Common types of billing practices are covered in this chapter that may help you understand the proper information needed to file a claim for reimbursement.

In addition, this chapter introduces the pharmacy technician to basic information about the major types of insurance coverage. A firm knowledge of terminology and guidelines must be in place for proper ordering and billing practices. This chapter begins with a discussion of formulary and the necessary knowledge needed concerning insurance companies. Also discussed are pharmacy inventory, some major types of devices used to keep track of inventory, and ways to handle special obstacles as they occur.

Formulary and Drug Utilization

A formulary is analogous to a backbone. The **formulary** is a list that describes all the medications covered under a specific insurance plan. It may also offer alternative medications if the first choice is not covered. For medications to become part of a formulary, they must meet certain requirements such as effectiveness and cost. These are determined by pharmacists and physicians who are members of the **pharmacy and therapeutics committee** (P&T committee). Formularies are not the same at all institutional pharmacies or for all health plans. An institution can have an **"open" formulary,** which means any drug can be ordered and stocked for patient use, whereas a **"closed" formulary** places certain restrictions on the drugs that are ordered and can be used by patients.

Often retail pharmacies will stock a variety of medications to accommodate both their patients and the many different insurance companies for which they are contracted providers. Each insurance company will have its own formulary, with recommendations for therapeutic alternatives when a drug is not covered under a particular plan. Many insurance companies have a variety of prescription plans and formularies that coincide with the many different types of health plans they provide. An example of such a formulary (which is extensive) can be found at http://www.ghc.org/health_plans/pdf/Medicare/Comprehensive Formulary HMOPP010.pdf. A hospital or home health care pharmacy is more likely to have a "closed" formulary, or a specific list of drugs to be kept on hand and dispensed to the patients and health plans served by the pharmacy.

Drug utilization evaluation (DUE), formerly known as drug utilization review (DUR), is an important process in ensuring the correct drug is prescribed for a condition. Pharmacists must perform this function. They screen the medication order for potential problems such as drug-drug interactions, duplicate therapy, or other possible errors. This is done before dispensing the drug, which decreases the risk of the patient receiving the wrong treatment (see Pharmacist's Perspective).

Pharmacist's Perspective
BY SUSAN WONG PharmD

Drug Utilization and Formulary Selection Process

Today's health care is in crisis. Health insurance companies and plans come and go. Ownership and management of hospitals and pharmacy benefits are in a state of flux. One of the greatest contributors to this instability is increased drug costs. The last few years have seen double-digit increases in annual drug costs. The average life span of Americans has become longer as medicine has evolved and progressed. However, as we live longer, we need more medicines to treat our illnesses and keep us alive. Drug companies spend a great deal of time and money to develop and market their new drugs. They must recoup these investments during the patent life of a drug.

During the time in which a drug is under patent, its rights and exclusivity are under the sole ownership of usually one (and sometimes more than one) drug company. The company prices the new medicine in relation to its use, its costs over time, and its acceptability in the current market. Not until the patent expires and all efforts to lengthen the patent life have been exhausted will drug company competitors be allowed to manufacture a generic version of an originator drug. At that time, retail drug costs drop as a result of open competition.

In the past decade, there also has been an explosion of "me-too" drugs. These drugs are in the same or similar chemical classes and have the same or similar action, but have slight modifications in their chemical structures. These slight differences might affect the side effect profile of a drug or its half-life (length of activity), or the different chemical structures may not have any significant variations in action at all. The slight variation in chemical structure allows

Pharmacist's Perspective—cont'd

BY SUSAN WONG PharmD

the different drugs to be registered and licensed as separate drug entities within a drug class. Many of the drugs commonly used today for heart disease, hypertension, diabetes, hyperlipidemia, and others have brother or sister drugs that are in the same class (or family) and have the same action—hence the name "me-too" drugs.

All of these factors have necessitated the use of the formulary system for many organizations, such as insurance companies, health maintenance organizations, and others. A formulary is a list of medicines that are preferred agents and provides a way of managing the use of drugs so that they are the most cost-effective for a given organization. The goal for any health care organization is to use the right medicine in the right amount at the right time to achieve a favorable outcome (i.e., health). The formulary system employs a team of professionals to review all the possible medicines for a given use and their costs to an organization for an average patient, and then to encourage or regulate the use of a preferred agent or agents for a given class or type of drug. The formulary review process, through the pharmacy and therapeutics committee, also includes periodic reevaluations of medicines as new drugs enter the market or as problems arise with established drugs.

The next time you go to the supermarket and walk down the laundry soap aisle, notice how many types, sizes, colors, additives, and so on are on the shelves for laundry soap. Now I would be willing to guess that they all clean your clothes pretty well. Some have fresh scents, some have no scent, some have bleach alternatives, and some claim to save the colors in your clothes. Some may cost $5 and some may cost $15, but they all clean your clothes. You might buy the brand that cleans your clothes for the most economical price. Some folks may need certain brands or formulations because of allergies. Most will buy the bigger sizes (because they get more for their hard-earned cash). Choosing a preferred medicine for a formulary is a similar process (but a bit more scientific). If a patient has an allergy to, or has failed therapy with, the preferred agent the patient may need to use a nonformulary medicine. In this instance, the pharmacy may have to order a nonpreferred medicine on the formulary to meet the needs of the patient.

As a pharmacy technician, you may be involved with the recording or billing of medicine that a patient has received. Alternatively, you may be involved with procuring a medicine that is not on the formulary and is used infrequently. Accuracy is the key because the improper recording of a medicine can affect what a patient must pay for the medicines and the reimbursement your pharmacy employer receives from the patient's insurance plan. Accuracy also can affect your employer if you are involved in supply chain management or inventory/stocking of your supplies. It is crucial for all involved to use the medicines that do the job and are most cost-effective. This helps patients spend their health care dollars wisely. ∎

Many formulary drugs are generic versions of innovator (brand name) products. These drugs are as effective as the brand name drugs but are less expensive. A health plan or prescription plan committee composed of pharmacists, physicians, and other health care administrators reviews drugs that have been approved by the Food and Drug Administration (FDA) to ensure that they are cost-effective. In addition, consideration may be given to drug companies that bid or give rebates when their drug is chosen for a formulary. This decrease in price to the pharmacy ultimately saves money for both the insurance company and the patient. Although most insurance companies cover most of the cost of a generic drug, some do allow the patient to choose the brand name drug. However, if the patient selects the brand name drug, the patient must pay the difference in cost between the generic and brand name drugs and also may be responsible for any co-payment (co-pay) required. For example, if the normal **co-pay** is $5 per prescription and the patient chooses a brand name medication that costs $10 more than the generic equivalent, then the patient must pay $15. The dollar amount of a prescription also depends on orders such as dispense-as-written (DAW) drugs that require specialty codes. The three DAW codes that are most often used in the pharmacy setting are 0, 1, or 2. A DAW 0 indicates the physician authorizes a generic substitution and that the pharmacy dispense the generic drug to the patient. If a generic is not available the trade name product must be given; however, the DAW code must still be zero because this indicates that if a generic becomes available at a later date then the physician has given permission to the pharmacy to make the substitution. DAW 1 indicates dispense as written and is usually used by the physician to indicate that the trade or brand name medication is in some way medically necessary for the successful treatment of the patient. DAW 2 indicates that the physician has approved the generic substitution of the medication prescribed; however, the patient has insisted on receiving the brand name medication.

There are other DAW codes that are assigned very infrequently and should only be used under the permission and direction of the pharmacist. It is important to pay attention to the DAW codes and use the correct one. Insurance companies audit pharmacies; they specifically verify whether DAW 1 claims sent by the pharmacy have prescriptions in which the physician specifically indicates a brand name drug be dispensed. The selection of proper DAW codes is easy to overlook and can cause seemingly simple mistakes. If these mistakes are found in an audit, however, they can cause the reversal and repayment of hundreds to thousands of claims and may result in the insurance company terminating its contract with a pharmacy.

Each insurance company has different policies concerning payment. Finally, formularies are not permanent by any means. If and when new generic drugs are introduced, cost and other factors are reviewed again. Typically, the types of drugs not included on a formulary are new drugs, uncommon drugs, and extremely expensive drugs. However, if a non-formulary drug can be justified as a medically necessary substitution by the physician, it may be approved for reimbursement under the insurance plan.

Generic versus Trade Name Drugs

The terms **trade**, **brand**, and **proprietary** are used interchangeably to refer to the name of a drug product that was first patented and marketed by the owner or manufacturer. Another name for such a product is innovator product. After a certain amount of time passes, the patent expires. Eventually, other drug companies can apply for the right to produce the same drug product, although not all drugs will be available in generic form. For example, it is usually not advantageous to drug companies to make generic medications that are used by a small percentage of the population. Brand name drugs that are produced by noninnovator companies as an alternative to the innovator product are considered "generic." A common example in pharmacy is the many different generic brands of birth control pills. Although the FDA approves generic drugs as equivalent to the trade name drug, the drugs often have different appearances because of different manufacturing procedures. Brand name drugs generally have from 17 to 20 years (depending on a drug company's petition to the FDA) of protection before patents expire (CDER). Once generic competition is introduced, prices can drop 50% to 80%. Drug price competition and patent term restoration expedite the availability of less costly generic drugs by permitting the FDA to approve applications to market generic versions without repeating the research needed to prove them safe and effective. At the same time, the brand name companies can apply for up to 5 years of additional patent protection for the new medicines they developed or for a new indication of a medication to compensate for the time lost while their products were undergoing the FDA approval process.

Third-Party Billing

The term third-party billing refers to the portion of payment reimbursed by insurance companies. The three entities that are responsible for payment include the patient, the hospital or facility, and the insurance company. It is customary for the pharmacy to bill the insurance company on behalf of the patient. The patient is often responsible for meeting the co-payment or deductible at the time the medication is dispensed, and the pharmacy must collect the rest of the drug cost from the insurance based upon contracted rates and dispensing fees. A co-pay is a predetermined amount the patient always pays when a medication is dispensed, whereas a deductible is the amount of "out-of-pocket" cost the patient must pay before his or her insurance coverage is activated. Because there are so many different insurance companies, each with different billing requirements, it often takes more than 1 year for a technician to become proficient in third-party **adjudication**, or claim billing. This chapter begins by listing the primary types of insurance, followed by their common traits and the problems that may arise when processing medication claims.

POINT OF SALE (POS) BILLING

Pharmacies that send claims electronically to an insurance company participate in point of sale (POS) billing. Electronic billing is performed via a secure data and transactional network to ensure patient confidentiality. The insurance company verifies eligibility, identifies covered drugs, prices a claim, and returns a response to submitting pharmacies within seconds during the prescription processing functions. Examples of the types of pharmacy claims processed are listed in Table 13-1.

Types of Insurance

For billing purposes the technician must know the patient's type of insurance coverage. Understanding the policies and procedures of the many different insurance policies is nearly impossible, especially because their guidelines change regularly. Therefore this chapter covers the most basic information applied to the major types of billing. Technicians must be able to differentiate between different types of insurance, obtain the necessary insurance information from the insurance card, determine if the patient has prescription (Rx) coverage and who should be billed, and transmit the claim correctly. In general, the only time a technician needs to know what kind of insurance the patient has (i.e., HMO vs PPO) is when Medicare coverage is used. The following example lists the types of insurance plans or cards in use today:

- Pharmacy benefits card (has "Rx Yes" printed on it)
- Drug discount card
- Prescription coupon card—provided by drug manufacturers to patients; coupon cards are provided either as an incentive for the patient to try the drug or as an aid to patients who meet certain income requirements
- Medicare card
- Medicaid card
- Medicare Advantage card
- Medigap card
- Workers' compensation (no card is required)

HEALTH MAINTENANCE ORGANIZATION (HMO)

An **HMO** has specific features that distinguish it from traditional insurance programs. An HMO is an effective method of controlling health care costs. Aetna, Blue Cross, United Healthcare, PacifiCare, Champus Tricare Program, and Kaiser are just five examples of the many insurance companies that offer HMO coverage. Special features of HMOs include the following:

TABLE 13-1 Types of Insurance Claims

Entity	Specifics of Coverage
Part D Coverage	Many state governments play a substantial role in offering direct pharmaceutical assistance benefits to eligible residents. Most commonly, individual states have offered substantial subsidies to low- and moderate-income seniors. About half the states also include younger adults with disabilities among those who are eligible.
State Pharmaceutical Assistance Program (SPAP)	Enacted for patients who lack insurance coverage for medicines or who are not eligible for other government programs. By late 2008, at least 42 states had established or authorized some type of program to provide pharmaceutical coverage or assistance. The subsidy programs, often termed "SPAPs," use state funds to finance a portion of the costs, usually for a defined population that meets enrollment criteria.
340 B	Requires drug manufacturers that contract with Medicaid programs to provide discounts on "outpatient" drugs purchased by those covered under Medicaid.
AIDS Drug Assistance Program (ADAP)	Patients suffering from AIDS who earn less than a specified annual income may be provided lower cost on drug regimens. This varies per state.
Smoking Cessation Program	Program covers smoking cessation medications and even counseling under certain insurance plans; often provided as "add-on" services that patient must purchase in order to participate. There is currently limited availability of these types of plans in the United States.
Tuberculosis Control Program	Provides government coverage for medications necessary to treat tuberculosis.
Medicaid Fee-For-Service (FFS)	Mandatory medicaid coverage includes: 1. Low income families with children that receive cash assistance through the Temporary Assistance for Needy Families (TANF) program or 2. Those with assets and incomes meeting the requirements of the Aid to Families with Dependent Children (AFDC) program prior to the passage of the TANF welfare reform law 3. Persons receiving or who are eligible for Supplemental Security Income (SSI). 4. Pregnant woman and children with family income below a specific level. 5. Children that receive foster care and adoption assistance under the Social Security Act 6. Dual Eligible Medicare beneficiaries, also known as Qualified Medicare Beneficiaries (QMBs) Additional qualifications vary by state

1. Primary care physician: The insurance company allows or requires the patient to choose a primary physician to coordinate all of the patient's medical needs.
2. Independent physician association (IPA): The provider offers a discounted rate to the patient through the contract made with the insurance company. In return, the physician accepts a lower payment than normally is charged for the procedure performed. These are contracted providers; examples of contracted providers are certain hospitals, clinics, and medical groups.
3. Co-pay: The insurance company requires the patient to pay a predetermined amount for office visits, emergency department visits, and drugs, regardless of the final cost. The rate varies depending on the patient's coverage plan. The insurance company is responsible for the remainder of the cost.

What If Your Patient Has HMO Insurance?

If a patient has HMO insurance, the technician must obtain information from the patient such as address, date of birth, insurance number, and full name.

The technician will also need to obtain the patient's prescription insurance card and verify that the pharmacy is a contracted provider for that particular insurance company and group. The pharmacy bills the insurance company first, through online adjudication, and receives an authorization number as well as co-pay information for the patient. Adjudication is the processing of claims over a computerized system. If the insurance claim is rejected then the pharmacy will either have to troubleshoot the issues or have the patient pay full price for the medication. It is then the patient's responsibility to contact the insurance company and attempt to obtain reimbursement. The patient is responsible for the entire cost only if the insurance company denies coverage based on eligibility or authorization not received before service. HMOs may require **prior authorization** on certain medications per their formulary guidelines. State regulations regarding the types of forms used to approve such medications may vary.

PREFERRED PROVIDER ORGANIZATION (PPO)

The difference between HMOs and **PPOs** is that the patient usually pays more out-of-pocket expenses for PPOs. The benefit is that the patient can choose a physician from the insurance plan list of contracted providers or may choose to consult any specialty physician without primary care physician referrals. There are no requirements to choose a specific primary care physician.

Aetna, Blue Shield, Blue Cross, United Healthcare, State Farm Insurance, and others offer PPO plans. That is, some insurance companies offer both PPOs and HMOs. This is why it is important for the patient to choose the right insurance plan. Patients choosing a PPO may have a co-pay for their office visits; the PPO co-pay tends to be higher than an HMO co-pay, and PPOs may have a deductible (the amount that the patient must pay before the insurance company pays). The insurance then pays a certain percentage of the medical expenses and medication bills if the patient's claims meet the criteria (i.e., charges were incurred by a contracted provider and the service provided was within the allowed amount of the PPO). This helps control the cost to the insurance company because the patient pays everything that the insurance company does not pay.

What If Your Patient Has PPO Insurance?
You must determine whether the patient has medication coverage through the PPO plan. In addition, you must establish whether the patient pays the complete cost for the medication and then files for direct reimbursement, has a deductible, or has a co-pay. This is determined from the information on the patient's health insurance card as well as through the online billing process. A sample health insurance card is shown in Figure 13-1. After transmitting the information to the insurance provider, an approval code is sent to the pharmacy. If the patient has a co-pay or deductible then the insurance company should monitor the patient's obligation. If the patient must self-bill the insurance company for reimbursement, then the patient will need the receipt and its corresponding approval code to submit to the insurance company.

From the pharmacy perspective, the billing processes for an HMO and a PPO are similar. The difference is that if the patient has a PPO, he or she may have a deductible to meet before the cost share (such as a percentage) or co-pay becomes activated. Often patients forget they have a deductible to meet or they do not realize it resets at the beginning of the year. In addition, they forget that each family member must meet his or her own deductible before the insurance will pay that individual's portion. For example, for a family of four with a $1000 deductible, if mom receives $1000 of medical services, then the insurance will pay a portion of her medication for the remainder of the year. However, if the

```
┌─────────────────────────────────────────────────┐
│                 HOPPER HEALTH                     │
│  ───────────────────────────────────────────────│
│        HOSPITAL ADMISSIONS REQUIRE PRIOR APPROVAL │
│                                                   │
│   JOHN A DOE                                      │
│   YBC999999999  99                                │
│                                                   │
│   GROUP: 272550000001            75.00 EMER ROOM  │
│                                  20.00 OFFICE VISIT│
│                                                   │
│   BCBSKC  RX          1-800-228-1436              │
│                                                   │
│   BC PLAN: 240   BS PLAN: 740                     │
│     CUST SERV: 816-232-8396/800-822-2583          │
└─────────────────────────────────────────────────┘
```

FIGURE 13-1 Sample health insurance card.

daughter then needs medication, the mother must meet her daughter's $1000 deductible before the insurance will pay their portion of the daughter's medication.

DRUG DISCOUNT CARDS OR DRUG COUPON CARDS

Patients can obtain drug discount cards from a variety of sources. These do not offer insurance benefits but instead allow the patient to obtain medications at the contracted provider rate. For example if Aetna Health Insurance contracts with a pharmacy to pay the **average wholesale price** (AWP) –10% plus a $2.00 dispensing fee for a drug that would normally be sold at retail for AWP +15% plus a $5.00 dispensing fee, then the patient can obtain the medicine at the less expensive rate through a prescription discount card.

Drug manufacturers provide drug coupon cards to patients either as an incentive for the patient to take the drug or as an aid to patients who meet certain income requirements. Both types of cards are billed as a third-party claim in order for the pharmacy to receive reimbursement and the patient to receive his or her discount.

Government-Managed Insurance Programs

Programs such as Medicare and Medicaid are examples of state-managed and federal-managed medical insurance plans. Each employee in the United States pays the government a percentage of his or her income toward Medicare. A percentage of each state budget is applied toward Medicaid. Each plan has specific guidelines that must be followed precisely for patients to qualify for reimbursement.

HISTORY OF MEDICARE AND MEDICAID

Both Medicaid and Medicare were implemented in 1965. **Medicaid** provided health care services to low-income children, the elderly, the blind, and persons with disabilities. Until 1977 Medicaid was associated with the Social Security Administration. Later in 1986 coverage was expanded to infants of pregnant women with low income, and was state-regulated. Through the following years, many revisions were made, including increasing the eligibility age of children and covering certain persons who were disabled or unable to return to work. Medicaid is funded by both federal and state governments and the benefits vary widely. Each state is responsible for payment to health care providers. Participants must prove their income and financial resources are at or below national poverty levels. Although each state may vary in its scope of coverage, the state must provide a minimum level of benefits according to federal guidelines. The following benefits are included:

- Hospital inpatient services
- Outpatient services
- Physician services
- Skilled nursing care
- Home health care
- Laboratory services
- Radiology services

In 1966 more than 19 million people enrolled into the newly formed **Medicare** program. Coverage consisted of several parts as listed in Box 13-1. As of 1972 Medicare eligibility was extended to include persons older than age 65, persons younger than 65 with long-term disabilities, and persons suffering from end-stage renal disease (ESRD).

In 1987 both Medicare and Medicaid required health care providers to include patient privacy provisions if they were to participate in the government-sponsored programs. Medicare revised its coverage in 1988, implementing prescription drug benefits along with a cap on patient liability. In 1996 the **Health Insurance Portability and Accountability Act** (HIPAA) (linked to the Employee Retirement Income Security Act of 1974) provided new rules for improving portability (continuity) of coverage and simplified standards for electronic transactions, among other changes.

Also in 1997 Medicare implemented many changes, including the following:

- Expanded education; new information helped participants make a more informed choice regarding their health care.
- Developed five new payment systems for services, including:
  - Inpatient rehabilitation hospital or unit services
  - Skilled nursing facility services

BOX 13-1 MEDICARE COVERAGE TYPES

Part A: Covers institutional costs if the participant meets the criteria established by federal and state regulations.

Part B: Covers physician and other outpatient services, including diabetes testing, physical therapy, and other preventive costs.

Part C: Also known as Medicare Advantage; this is an optional plan to Parts A and B. This is a private plan that uses Medicare and must be equivalent to coverage provided by Parts A and B. Some Part C plans cover certain prescription drugs. A person should have either Part C or Medigap, because both will not be cumulative in coverage.

Part D: Medicare Part D specifically covers prescription drugs. The coverage is provided by individual private insurance plans that are overseen by Medicare. A monthly premium is paid and the plan chosen by the patient may have an annual deductible. Once the deductible is paid then the insurance plan will pay either all or some of the remaining costs, up to a maximum of $2700 (for 2009). After the $2700 maximum is reached, there is a gap in the coverage of drug costs and the patient must self-pay for prescriptions until $4350 out-of-pocket payments are reached (2009 limit). After the $4350 limit is attained, the participant pays only 5% of the drug costs and the remaining cost is covered by Medicare.

TABLE 13-2 Chronological Changes in Medicare/Medicaid Coverage

Year	Description
1965	Medicaid and Medicare were signed into law
1966	19 million people requested Medicare benefits
1972	Medicare expanded coverage to include persons younger than age 65 with low income and those with end-stage renal failure
1977	Medicaid and Medicare were placed under the control of the Social Security Administration
1980	Medigap was introduced to fill the gap that was present in Medicare coverage; patients could choose between 12 different Medigap plans
1986	Medicaid expanded coverage to include infants and pregnant women of low income
1987	Medicare and Medicaid payment was linked to OBRA87 and specifically addressed poor conditions of nursing homes
1988	Medicare introduced a prescription drug benefit plan
1990	OBRA90 required that all health care personnel participating in Medicare/Medicaid programs protect patient privacy; required patient consultation by pharmacists
1996	HIPAA implemented patient privacy rules for Medicare payment and provided electronic payment methods
1997	Medicare made several important changes expanding coverage and developed five new payment systems
1997	Both Medicare and Medicaid were placed under the control of the Health Care Financing Administration
2003	Medicare Modernization Act (MMA) provided drug discount cards to eligible persons
2003	Medicare Part D was introduced under MMA; provided subsidies for eligible persons to be implemented by 2006

- Home health services
- Hospital outpatient services and rehabilitation
- Expanded preventive benefits

A large change was made in 2003 with the **Medicare Modernization Act (MMA)** and the creation of prescription drug discount cards that allowed competition between health plans, benefiting participants. In 2006 Medicare Part D was enacted; this requires the federal government to provide subsidies to participants whose income is less than 150% of the federal poverty limit. Those with higher incomes would pay a greater share of drug costs as of 2007. Certain individuals may be covered under both Medicaid and Medicare and are known as "dual eligible"; Medicaid supplements Medicare coverage.

Many savings programs assist low-income participants with out-of-pocket health care costs. Each state has its own programs for assistance and may or may not include services such as home-delivered personal care and other community-based services for the disabled. A timeline is given in Table 13-2 that explains various changes in the coverage and events in both Medicare and Medicaid programs.

Medicare services were expanded in 1980 with the creation of the **Medigap** plan, also regulated by the federal government. The Medigap plan offers optional insurance policies that can be purchased via privately owned insurance companies. The plans are intended to fill the gap in the Medicare program coverage. However, if you have Medicare Part C, then Medigap cannot be used. There are

Tech Note!

In 1997 both Medicaid and Medicare were reorganized and became subsidiaries of the Health Care Financing Administration (HCFA).

12 different Medigap policies, labeled A through L. Most of the insurer plans do not differ significantly in their policies. Each person must purchase his or her own policy.

CURRENT USE OF MEDICARE/MEDICAID INSURANCE

Medicare

Medicare is a federally sponsored program for seniors, the disabled, and dialysis patients. Medicare functions much like an HMO and a PPO. The patient must see a provider who accepts Medicare, but the patient has a yearly deductible and a percentage share of cost. The share of cost is similar to a deductible and co-pay combined. The patient is responsible for paying a deductible up to a certain amount in a hospital setting. At present, Medicare pays outpatient costs with the exception of some diabetic supplies and equipment; however, Medicare Part B covers the costs of diabetic testing supplies and transplant drugs or dialysis medication. Major drug companies may offer drug programs to the elderly and the disabled that will provide medications to those who use specific products. Before 2006 Medicare did not offer any prescription drug coverage. That has changed and it is now called Medicare Part D.

Medicare Part D. As previously stated, Medicare is a health insurance program for persons 65 years of age and older, some disabled persons younger than age 65, and persons with end-stage renal disease (i.e., permanent kidney failure treated with dialysis or a transplant). Medicare Part D was intended to help certain persons with their prescription drug costs, but not everyone. The language of the plan and the multitude of medical insurance companies have made it increasingly difficult for a person to decide whether to enroll in Medicare Part D. This can only be determined by the specific needs of the patient; therefore there is no one best choice. It is important to note that each plan may vary considerably in specific coverage. At this time the maximum deductible for any plan cannot exceed $265 per year. The two types of coverage are basic and enhanced. Again, each has variable deductibles that apply. The basic coverage has a higher deductible than the enhanced coverage.

Other guidelines for seniors to consider when choosing the Medicare Part D plan can be found on the Medicare website at www.medicare.gov. Examples include the following:

1. Medicare drug plans benefit certain groups of persons, such as the following:
    a. Low-income families
    b. Those with Medigap coverage
    c. Those individuals who have more than $750 annually in drug costs
2. Those individuals with multiple prescriptions may benefit from this plan, but there are considerations that must be taken into account, such as the following:
    a. Certain prescriptions tend to insist on formulary drugs as opposed to non-formulary drugs.
3. Those individuals who are in good health or who spend less than $750 annually may benefit by waiting to find a drug plan, equivalent to Part D, through another insurance company.
4. Not all generic drugs are bioequivalent to the name brand. In addition, not all brand drugs are available in generic form. This can make a huge difference in the choice of drug for the patient.
5. Check the formulary of each plan. Note, however, that each plan can change in the future.
6. Ask about any restrictions on certain medications.

7. Determine if the insurance plan uses "step therapy." (This means that the drug company makes the patient take the most inexpensive drug first; if that drug is ineffective, then the insurance company approves the second most inexpensive drug and so on until an effective medication is found for the patient.)

As patients transition into Medicare Part D, they may experience the following:

1. The computer may indicate no coverage for the person.
2. There may be a change in medications.
3. Because of changing medications, the person may experience a change in health

What If Your Patient Has Medicare Insurance? Any changes in Medicare drug coverage will increase the number of consultations by the pharmacist, because pharmacists must explain different issues caused by a change in medications. In addition, persons may need to have their prescriptions filled at a different pharmacy. This is because of the time it takes to register the patient in the Medicare database. Pharmacies must apply for a **National Provider Identifier (NPI)** from the Centers for Medicare & Medicaid Services. All providers who bill electronically must use an NPI (Health Insurance Portability and Accountability Act regulation). Any pharmacist who provides services such as consultation and does not bill for this time under a pharmacy with an NPI will need his or her own NPI. The NPI number may be assigned either per person or per pharmacy depending on each state's laws. For example, in Nevada individual pharmacists must apply for an NPI number to process prescriptions covered by Medicare, whereas in California this number is assigned for each pharmacy. If a patient is not in the system yet and the physician has ordered a drug that is not covered, the pharmacist may call the physician for a substitute if possible, or the patient may pay out-of-pocket for the medication and try to be reimbursed when he or she is in the system.

An important "bottom line" approach to consider is this:

> The patient will be encouraged to receive generic drugs. Brand name drugs are often covered at a much higher cost if a generic is available, and this cost may be prohibitive enough to force many people into using the generic versions. Typically, brand name drugs are covered at the generic price and the patient is responsible for paying the difference. For a drug such as Zocor (generic name simvastatin), this difference in cost can be as much as $100. The overall use of generic drugs will increase greatly under Medicare Part D. This can make a huge difference to the patient because not all generic drugs are bioequivalent to the brand drug. Not all brand drugs are available in generic form. A bioequivalent generic drug has the same active ingredient and is equal in strength, bioavailability, and dose to a brand drug. Although generic drugs may be bioequivalent and have the same active ingredient as brand name drugs, they can contain different fillers that may alter their effectiveness. Many pharmacists, physicians, and other caregivers are concerned about the consequences of replacing drugs that are effective with less expensive (generic) drugs.

Many times pharmacists must explain the types of benefits, and there is little doubt that technicians will be a part of this situation. This is especially true for technicians who work at a pharmacy counter or who are in charge of billing. Many patients will need help from technicians regarding options that are available if their medications change or they have other problems with their insurance coverage. Technicians will need to keep themselves updated on any new changes in the system in order to help their patients. Technicians must have patience and communication skills to explain technical issues or terms such as coverage, formulary, generic availability, and so on into language understood by the patient.

There is open enrollment for Medicare plans each year from November 15 to December 31. This is when a patient can change plans. There is also a 6-month open enrollment for "Medigap" coverage. An example is given in Box 13-2.

Because different items are covered under different parts of the plan, it is important for the technician to obtain not only the Medicare Part D card (Figure 13-2) for pharmacy billing but also a copy of the Part A and Part B cards, in case other items (Box 13-3) are needed.

BOX 13-2 MEDIGAP COVERAGE

A patient has Medicare Part D prescription coverage. This particular hypothetical plan will typically pay for generic medications or brand name drugs with a yearly maximum payout of $1200. If the patient purchases $1200 in medication in the first 3 months of the year, the patient's insurance will not pay for any medication prescribed during the remainder of the year. At this point, the patient can apply for coverage for this "gap." This coverage can help pay the deductible or co-pay on Medicare Parts A, B, and D. The patient must determine if Medigap would be beneficial.

BOX 13-3 VARIOUS SUPPLIES COVERED BY MEDICARE

Typical supplies or prescriptions that may be covered under specific parts of Medicare insurance:

Blood glucose testing strips (Part B)
Lasix (generic only, Part D)
Hospital stay (Part A)
Heparin for home dialysis (Part B)
Lancets (Part B)
Insulin (Part D)

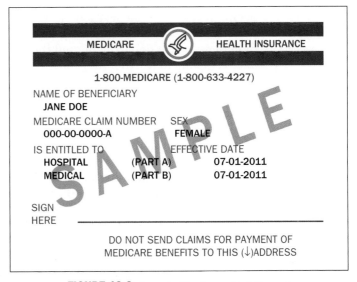

FIGURE 13-2 Sample Medicare Part D card.

Medicaid

Each state has its own Medicaid program for low-income residents. This also includes uninsured pregnant women and those with certain disabilities. Medicaid is funded by both the state and federal government. Depending on each state's level of unemployment and poverty they may receive matching funds from the federal government. Medicaid can be used with Medicare if the person qualifies. In addition, each state may have many different programs that help defer the cost of health care and medication. The following are the three major levels of coverage within the Medicaid system:

1. The patient may not be responsible for any cost.
2. Share of cost: In the share of cost level, the patient's plan requires that the patient pay a deductible (i.e., a specific dollar amount must be met before the insurance company pays). For instance, the patient may be responsible for the first $1000, but any remaining amount is paid by Medicaid.
3. Geographical managed care program: A geographical managed care plan allows patients to belong to a medical group with which Medicaid has a contractual agreement. This includes HMOs, thus allowing patients to have Medicaid benefits similar to benefits offered by HMOs. (Regulations of each state may vary.)

What If Your Patient Has Medicaid Insurance? You must know whether the patient has Medicaid benefits. If the patient is covered under Medicaid, you need a copy of the patient's insurance card. This card identifies the program under which the patient is covered. These plans include national programs as well. Each program differs in patient coverage

WORKERS' COMPENSATION

Workers' compensation is a type of insurance paid by employers to entirely cover injuries suffered by employees while on the job. Federal law requires employers with a certain number of employees to offer workers' compensation. Insurance coverage is provided by private insurance carriers.

Anyone who works for a company that pays into workers' compensation may be eligible to use this insurance if he or she has a work-related injury. The patient does not have to pay anything. Instead, claims are filed electronically or in hard copy to the insurance companies. If the patient arrives at the pharmacy with a workers' compensation claim, it is important to obtain billing information before dispensing medication, if possible. This may involve contacting the patient's employer, obtaining the billing information over the phone from the human resources department, and then calling the workers' compensation insurance company for further information. To avoid any billing errors, it is important to keep detailed notes regarding communication when processing workers' compensation claims. Be sure to include the name of the person who was consulted, the date of the consultation, and detailed notes about your conversation. It is also important to follow HIPAA guidelines. The only people who need to know that the patient is injured or ill are those in the human resources department. They do not need to be given a specific diagnosis from the pharmacy; they just need to provide the billing information.

Billing the Insurance Company

The information needed by insurance companies to process a claim from the pharmacy or to reimburse the patient is the same as the information required on a pharmacy label, plus date of birth, insurance group number, and identification number. All information must be verified before the medication is dis-

Tech Note!

Regardless of the patient's type of insurance, you should always treat people with respect. Take care to ensure the patient is treated with respect and receives superior service when handling prescription billing.

TABLE 13-3 Minimum Information Required by Insurance Companies

Required by Insurance Company	Reason
Patient's name	To verify insurance coverage
Date medication is filled	To process claim for reimbursement purposes: must be done within a specific time period determined by provider
Pharmacy name and address	To pay pharmacy
Medication prescribed	To verify whether drug is on the formulary and is covered
Dosage	To determine cost of medication
Date of birth	To verify medication is dispensed to correct patient
Identification number	To provide authorization of coverage

pensed. Once the patient's information has been entered into the pharmacy computer system, it is important to keep that information updated both for the pharmacy and for the insurance company (Table 13-3).

PRIOR AUTHORIZATION

Often an insurance company will pay for a medication only if a prior authorization is first received. Prior authorization is needed for a variety of reasons. Reasons include that the drug of choice is not formulary or the insurance company has determined less costly methods of treatment are available and requires that the patient use these first. There are two types of forms used: prior authorization forms or **treatment authorization request** (TAR) forms. Most insurance companies require a prior authorization form. The pharmacy typically does not contact the insurance company regarding prior authorization. If a third-party claim is rejected as "prior authorization required" then either the pharmacy contacts the patient's physician or the pharmacy directly notifies the physician's office. The physician's office then contacts the insurance company to request the prior authorization. Policies may vary depending on the insurance provider and the medication prescribed. For Medicare and Medicaid the TAR form is used, which requires the same information as forms used for standard insurance companies (Figure 13-3). The physician will often need to produce documentation explaining why a specific course of therapy is needed, such as the following: the patient tried the other therapies and they were ineffective; the patient has allergies to certain medications; the patient must undergo diagnostic tests that require the requested therapy. All of this information must be provided by the physician because the pharmacy does not have access to patient records. The insurance company will either approve or deny the authorization in 24 to 48 hours. Rarely does the insurance company or the physician alert the pharmacy when authorization has been approved; therefore the pharmacy should attempt to re-bill the claim in 48 to 72 hours. If the claim is still denied, then the pharmacy may need to contact the physician's office or the insurance company to determine if the authorization was submitted and if there is a special over-ride code needed in order to bill the claim. Regardless of whether the claim is approved or denied, the patient should be contacted within 3 days so he or she is not waiting for a medication that has been denied.

Each plan has its own formulary, limitations, and exclusions. In addition to these variances, each pharmacy has certain insurance types that it accepts or rejects. This means that if the pharmacy accepts the co-payment as payment in

Tech Note!

Authorization forms can be submitted electronically, along with any supporting documentation. This is due to the development of ePA modules, or electronic prior authorization modules, that are now available as well as the ability to send these documents through secure, HIPAA-compliant electronic channels.

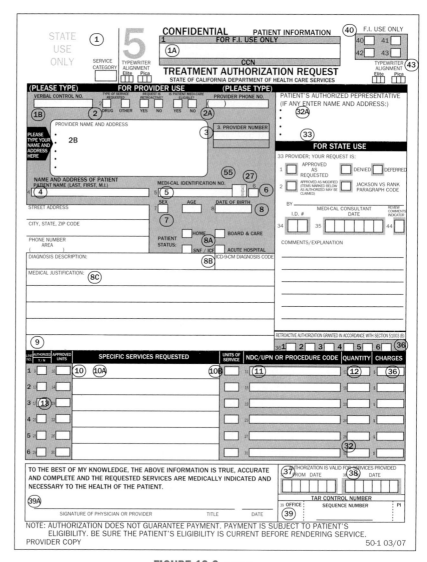

FIGURE 13-3 TAR form.

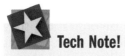

Tech Note!

Identify each insurance card as either a prescription discount card, prescription coupon card, or insurance card. For each card identify the payer and the BIN, PCN, group, and ID numbers.

full, the pharmacy will bill the insurance company for the cost of the medication. Otherwise, the pharmacy may not accept the insurance based on the limits of payment. Insurance cards have all of the information necessary to perform the billing process. For an explanation of the information contained on an insurance prescription card see Box 13-4.

PATIENT PROFILES

Each pharmacy has its own specific computer system, which details each **patient's profile**. Figure 13-4 shows an example of a pharmacy patient profile database. This profile must be kept updated for proper billing. Basic information that can be viewed on this computer system includes the following:

- Patient information:
  - Name
  - Date of birth
  - Address
  - Phone number

BOX 13-4 INFORMATION CONTAINED ON A PRESCRIPTION CARD

Each insurance card will have information regarding the coverage plan, patient's name, patient's identification number, and phone number of the insurance company. The basic information needed to bill a third-party claim is provided on the card. If there is any additional information that is needed, the insurance company or provider should be contacted.

- Pharmacy Benefit International Identification number (RxBIN)—Used much like an IP address to direct the claim to the correct third-party provider. All network pharmacy payers have an RxBIN.
- Pharmacy benefit Processor Control Number (PCN)—Some, but not all, network pharmacy payers use this number, labeled RxPCN for network pharmacy benefit routing along with the RxBIN. This number, if it is used, is required for specialized health care coverage plans such as those that begin with the letter U, W, X, or Y. For example, dental coverage plans are identified by a PCN identifier with the letter "W." This has been used increasingly in the past few years because of the greater number of plans available to patients.
- Prescription group number (Rx Grp #)—Directs the claim to the specific insurance benefits for that group. Groups are usually organized by collections of people who work for the same company or have similar benefits packages.
- Identification number (ID #)—Is a unique identification number that is specific to each member or member family group. Some insurance companies, such as Kaiser, issue an ID number to each person in the plan. Some issue one to the cardholder and each member of the family will have the same ID number.
- Person code—Each member of the family has the same ID number; however, an individual code is used to differentiate family members from one another. Often the cardholder, or the primary person on the insurance, will be person 00 or 01. The spouse or other insured adult will be person 01 or 02. The children covered under the plan will then be listed in numeric order according to their birth order.
- Date of birth (DOB)—Must match the date the insurance company has on file for each patient.
- Sex code—Must match gender filed by insurance company. The insurance company will also reject claims for drugs if the sex code is incorrect. For instance if the technician submits a claim stating that Mary Clein is a male and attempts to bill her insurance for Ortho Tri-Cyclen then the claim may be rejected by the insurance company because males are typically not prescribed birth control pills.

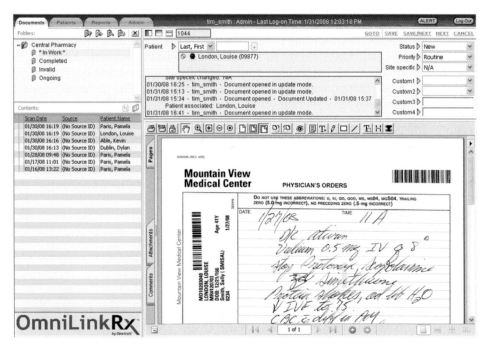

FIGURE 13-4 Computer patient profile using OmniLinkRx. (Courtesy of Omnicell, Inc., © 2010.)

- Gender
- Allergies
- Insurance provider's information: provider's phone number and insurance number (per hospital or institution policies)

If the information contains a mistake, the insurance claim may be rejected.

If the patient does not have insurance, he or she must pay full price for prescriptions. The cost of a prescription can vary greatly. Many pharmacies offer coupons on new prescriptions. The use of generic drugs can reduce the medication cost greatly.

If the patient has insurance, determining the guidelines of the program is of primary importance if the pharmacy is to receive reimbursement. The process by which all claims are processed over a computerized system is referred to as adjudication. The insurance determines the amount of coverage per medication based on various criteria such as the following:

1. Average wholesale price (AWP): The average wholesale price can be found in ***Drug Topics Red Book,*** or this information may be contained in a portion of the pharmacy database. Use the *Red Book* to determine the price of a medication based on the listed price. The *Red Book* provides monthly updates to keep the pharmacy current on price changes; online databases in the pharmacy often supply "real-time" updates to medication price changes.
2. Co-pay: The insurance company pays a certain amount of a patient's bill. The amount of co-pay depends on whether the patient uses an HMO, PPO, or a government-sponsored program. Processors—companies that work for insurance companies—are responsible for the approval of drug coverage, collection and processing of claims, and payment.

PROCESSING CLAIMS

When handling a patient's medication claim, the pharmacy technician may be responsible for using the insurance company claim form to relay the necessary patient information. Because each company needs their forms filled out entirely and correctly, the technician must know the specific needs of the company. There are universal claim forms as well that are used (Figure 13-5) in certain circumstances. Sometimes patients will arrive at the pharmacy with a claim form that the pharmacy needs to complete for reimbursement. Although claims can still be filed the traditional way (i.e., filling out a hard-copy form and mailing it), most pharmacies file claims electronically. The general types of information required may include the following:

Tech Note!

The NDC was developed by the FDA for the drug industry for identification purposes. The NDC is composed of three sections, each with a different meaning. The first set of numbers refers to the manufacturer; the second, the drug product; and the third, the trade package identification.

- Processor—typically the insurance company
- Member's identification number—can be either the assigned number specific to that patient or the Social Security number; however, fewer insurance companies are using Social Security numbers because of the potential for identity theft
- Group number (if applicable)
- Plan code (if applicable)
- Insurance carrier

CLAIM PROBLEMS

A prescription may not be covered for the insured patient for many reasons. For example, the **National Drug Code** (NDC) may not be covered. The NDC

Prescription Drug Claim Form   STANDARD CLAIM

INSTRUCTIONS:

■ In order to process your claim(s) in a timely manner, <u>you must provide all information requested below.</u>

■ We will send any reimbursement and/or communications to the address provided below, except if a confidential address is on file.

■ Please allow up to 21 days from the time you send this form until the time you receive the response to allow for mail time plus claims processing.

■ Please use a separate claim form <u>for each plan participant</u>.

■ Sing in the space provided. Your signature certifies that the information is correct and complete.

■ Please make a copy of all documents and receipts before you send them to Caremark. No documents will be returned.

■ Do not staple or tape receipts or attachments to this form!

INSURED INFORMATION REQUIRED:

Cardholder's Name: _____
                FIRST   MIDDLE   LAST

Street Address: _____

City: _____ State: ___ Zip: _____

RXGRP#: [ ][ ][ ][ ][ ][ ][ ]

ID #: [ ][ ][ ][ ][ ][ ][ ][ ]   Plan Participant ID Code: [ ][ ]

Employer/Company Name: _____

I certify that the information I have provided is correct and that the plan participant indicated below is elible for benefits. I have received the medicine described hereon and authorize release of all information contained on this claim form to Caremark and the plan administrator. I agree that any benefits payable hereunder for prescription drugs are not assignable and that any assignment thereof shall be void. I further represent that there has been no assignment of benefits hereunder.

CARDHOLDER'S SIGNATURE: _____

PLAN PARTICIPANT INFORMATION

Plan Participant Name: LAST [ ][ ][ ][ ][ ][ ][ ][ ][ ][ ][ ]   FIRST [ ][ ][ ][ ][ ][ ][ ][ ][ ]

Plan Participant's Relationship to Cardholder: Self [ ] Spouse [ ] Dependent [ ]

Date of Birth: [ ][ ][ ][ ][ ][ ]   Male: [ ] Female: [ ]

Check if Full-Time College Student _____

PHARMACY INFORMATION REQUIRED:

Pharmacy Name: _____   NABP #: [|][ ][ ][ ][ ]   Phone: [ ][ ][|][ ][|][ ][ ][ ]

Address: _____

City: _____ State: ___ Zip: [ ][ ][ ][ ]

PHARMACIST'S SIGNATURE: _____

PRESCRIPTION CLAM INFORMATION

If you are including all original receipts with the following information, it is not necessary to complete this section.
Exception: When submitting compound receipts, this section <u>must be completed</u>.

1 Ɽ#: [ ][ ][ ][ ][ ]   New or Refill (circle one)   Date Filled: MONTH [ ][ ] DAY [ ][ ] YEAR [ ][ ]   Quantity (ml., #tablets, gm., etc.) [ ][ ][ ]

Days Supply: [ ][ ]   Name of Medication: _____   Prescriber DEA# [ ][ ][ ][ ][ ][ ]

NDC#: [ ][ ][ ][ ][ ][ ][ ][ ][ ]   Form of Medication (capsules, cream, etc): _____

Drug Manufacturer: _____   Dosage (250 mg., etc.): _____   Is this a compound? Yes [ ] No [ ]

Prescription Cost: $[ ][ ][ ].[ ][ ]   Tax: $[ ][ ][ ].[ ][ ]   Total Cost: $[ ][ ][ ][ ]

2 Ɽ#: [ ][ ][ ][ ][ ]   New or Refill (circle one)   Date Filled: MONTH [ ][ ] DAY [ ][ ] YEAR [ ][ ]   Quantity (ml., #tablets, gm., etc.) [ ][ ][ ]

Days Supply: [ ][ ]   Name of Medication: _____   Prescriber DEA# [ ][ ][ ][ ][ ][ ]

NDC#: [ ][ ][ ][ ][ ][ ][ ][ ][ ]   Form of Medication (capsules, cream, etc): _____

Drug Manufacturer: _____   Dosage (250 mg., etc.): _____   Is this a compound? Yes [ ] No [ ]

Prescription Cost: $[ ][ ][ ].[ ][ ]   Tax: $[ ][ ][ ].[ ][ ]   Total Cost: $[ ][ ][ ][ ]

14089 11/04

FIGURE 13-5 Universal claim form.

number is organized into three sections: the labeler code, the product code, and the package code (Figure 13-6). All medications have an NDC number. When a prescription is not covered, it can be frustrating for both the patient and the technician, and even for the insurance company representative. Other common reasons that a prescription may not be covered are as follows:

• Coverage has expired.
• Coverage limits have been exceeded.
• Patient is trying to refill a prescription too early.
• The cardholder's information does not match the processor's information.

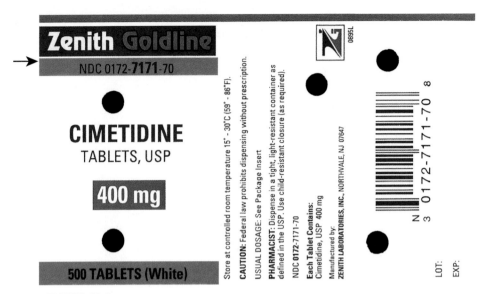

FIGURE 13-6 The arrow on the drug label shows the NDC code for this drug.

- The physician who wrote the prescription is not the patient's primary care physician.
- The prescription is requesting an invalid amount of medication; most insurance companies will only cover a 30-day supply.

COVERAGE EXPIRATION POLICY FOR DRUGS

If the patient has lost his or her coverage, the claim is rejected. Following the Health Insurance Portability and Accountability Act (HIPAA) regulations in 2003, the pharmacy does not have access to information regarding the reason for rejection and is disclosed only a termination date. Patients often are unaware of why coverage has been discontinued and may want the pharmacy to investigate. Pharmacy personnel are not permitted to call the patient's insurance carrier regarding these types of inquiries. Patient confidentiality would be breached, and legal action could result. The only recourse is to explain to the patient that he or she must contact the insurance company to resolve the issue. In the interim, the patient must pay full price for the medications. If there has been an error, reimbursement is made after the insurance company corrects the problem.

Limitation of Plan Exceeded
The term limitation of plan exceeded refers to a patient who has exhausted his or her pharmacy benefits for the specified time period or quantity limitation on a drug.

If a prescription requests a greater quantity of the drug than is allowed by the insurance plan, the plan limits are exceeded. For example, some government insurance plans limit the number of prescriptions that can be filled per month or per year. If the prescription is written for a specific quantity of medication that exceeds the maximum amount to be filled per day, the prescription is rejected and the patient must contact the insurance company for special permission to obtain the drug. Limit exceeded could also mean that the patient has met a yearly or lifetime benefit amount.

Some patients are exempt from these types of limitations because of their illness. These include persons who suffer from diabetes or those who have been diagnosed with human immunodeficiency virus (HIV) or acquired immunodeficiency syndrome (AIDS). Persons with diabetes mellitus require a continuous

Tech Note!

Only a pharmacist can contact the physician to request a change in medication.

refill of lancets and blood-testing strips to monitor their blood glucose levels. In addition, they must refill their insulin syringes monthly. In the case of persons being treated for human immunodeficiency virus or acquired immunodeficiency syndrome, the medication is expensive and these patients usually have to take many medications simultaneously. When a claim is rejected because the maximum limits of the insurance are exceeded, the technician must explain the problem to the patient. The patient is ultimately responsible for contacting the insurance company to dispute the problem.

Handling Non-formulary Drugs or Noncovered National Drug Codes

Formularies tend to be specific. This includes the decision of which drugs are included on the member's plan. These drugs are identified by their NDC, a code assigned to every drug in the United States. If the code submitted is not in the formulary, the claim is rejected by the insurance company. In pharmacy, these types of medications are referred to as non-formulary drugs. In this case, two options can be explored. First, the pharmacist can contact the physician and request that the prescription be changed to a drug that is covered under the patient's insurance plan. Second, the physician can submit a prior authorization form to the insurance company indicating why the patient must take the non-formulary drug. The type of prior authorization form varies depending on insurance company guidelines. Physicians normally complete and submit the prior authorization form for approval. This approval process can take up to 2 weeks. Therefore the patient can either purchase the medication for immediate use or wait to have the prescription filled after approval or rejection is given by the insurance company. If the patient pays upfront and the medication is approved, the patient is reimbursed by the insurance company after the pharmacist completes a reimbursement form for the patient. The form is sent to the insurance company to reimburse the patient for the covered drug cost.

FILLING A PRESCRIPTION TOO SOON

Patients attempt to have their prescriptions refilled when they still have medication remaining for several reasons. Most of the time it is not a problem to obtain a refill 1 week before the prescription's refill date; however, there are instances in which the patient may request a refill as early as 1 week after having the prescription filled. For example, the patient may be leaving the country for an extended time and wants to ensure that sufficient medication is available until he or she returns. Most insurance plans will allow extra refills in circumstances such as vacations or the occurrence of devastating events. For example, when hurricane Katrina devastated the southern United States, many insurance companies allowed early refills and replacement fills on prescriptions, and even permitted patients to be treated by physicians outside their medical plan. If the patient's insurance will not pay, the patient is responsible for the cost of the medication. Prescriptions normally are written for a 30-, 60-, or 90-day supply, depending on the condition being treated. Mail-order companies usually fill up to a 90-day supply for many chronically needed medications. Sometimes the amount of medication prescribed is limited because of safety or legal issues that surround the dispensing of a specific medication. Because certain medications are dangerous, they may not be prescribed for more than 30 days. Examples include DEA schedule II controlled substances and a specific drug called isotretinoin (acne medication), which has been linked to teratogenicity if given to pregnant women. Many insurance plans allow additional savings if refills are ordered via mail-order pharmacies that are on their list of participating pharmacies.

Sometimes a physician instructs the patient to increase the dosage, thus forcing the refill process before its allotted time. In this case a new prescription order must be submitted to the insurance company. In some cases the technician must contact the insurance company "help desk" to explain the circumstances of the prescription change. However, some insurance companies may require a direct response from the patient's physician before granting approval.

NON-IDENTIFICATION MATCH

Probably one of the most common problems is when the cardholder's information does not match the processor's information, thus resulting in a claim rejection. To determine whether this is the case, the technician should always recheck the information submitted to the insurance company. Items to double-check include the following:

- Health plan card number, identification number, and insurance number
- Patient's name, date of birth, and relationship to the insured person

The relationship of the patient to the cardholder is important because he or she may be a new spouse or adopted child or there may have been other significant changes. In this case the technician may be able to ask for a new insurance card for the member through the insurance help desk.

PHARMACY STOCK

Each pharmacy orders drugs that include formulary drugs and a limited amount of non-formulary or less commonly used drugs. The established level of medication stock kept on hand at any given time is referred to as the **periodic automatic replacement** (PAR) level. This is the minimum amount of medication that should be maintained in the pharmacy at any given time. Just as insurance billing has become a common task of pharmacy technicians, so has the responsibility of ordering medications. Different systems are available that can keep an updated inventory of medications and alert the technician when new stock must be ordered. This can be done several ways, such as at the POS, by order cards, or by handheld inventory computers. Because there are so many different types of systems in use today, this chapter explores the main characteristics of various systems and explains when and how stock arrives at the pharmacy. Also included is proper storage of all drugs. In addition, this chapter discusses how recalls are addressed and how returns are processed.

Although some pharmacies may contract out the job of processing returns and sending them to the manufacturer, this function is usually assigned to a pharmacy technician who is an employee of the pharmacy. Typically, an inventory technician is in charge of all aspects of ordering, restocking, and returning stock within the pharmacy.

Ordering Systems

Maintaining a periodic automatic replacement (PAR) level in the pharmacy is important for several reasons. Many manufacturers do not fill orders on the weekend or holidays. This means the pharmacy could deplete its stock during this time. The pharmacy may have to wait until the following delivery day to receive the necessary stock. This is serious if a patient cannot obtain an essential medication because the pharmacy is out of stock. Patients visiting a community pharmacy may be able to go elsewhere to have prescriptions filled, but hospitalized patients rely on the hospital pharmacy to stock medications.

In cases when stock will not arrive until the following Monday or Tuesday, the only recourse is to use an express-delivery company contracted by the pharmacy or to borrow the medication from another pharmacy. Express delivery can range from delivery of a medication by courier to air delivery of the medication.

In some cases pharmacies will even contact other stores in the area to "borrow" stock for patients. Of course this is done only in case of an emergency when all other options have been exhausted. Express delivery also is expensive and in many cases unnecessary if the pharmacy staff understands when to reorder a specific drug. Shipping time varies depending on the type of drug ordered. This is when pharmacy personnel must demonstrate their teamwork. It is improper and inappropriate to assume that medication ordering is another team member's responsibility.

SPECIAL ORDERS

When a pharmacy does not carry a medication (perhaps it is new or uncommon), it may be ordered from a drug wholesaler. It is important to know the length of time needed for the wholesaler to deliver a medication and to follow the order's progress. Special order prescriptions should be filed in a specific location within the pharmacy. The technician must check for special orders each time stock arrives. This will ensure that the patient is not waiting for a medication that was received by the pharmacy 1 week ago. In addition, if medication has not been delivered by the expected date, then the wholesaler should be contacted to determine if there is a back-order, ordering problem, or other issue. By notification of any ordering issues as soon as possible, patients will not have their therapy delayed any longer than necessary.

More pharmacies rely on computerized systems that are programmed to order medications. This is by far one of the best ways to maintain appropriate stock levels, although not all pharmacies have this system. Three main systems are discussed in this chapter, although there are many more types. All systems are similar to those discussed in the following sections.

BAR CODING

Most manufacturers identify their products with bar codes that can be scanned. This process accelerates the input of information because one pass of the bar code device identifies the drug, strength, dosage form, quantity, cost, package size, and any other information necessary to fill the medication or device. Pharmacies can use these bar codes as well. The medication is scanned at the register, identified as the point of sale, and electronically deleted from the computerized inventory list. When the in-stock quantity drops below the PAR level, it is reordered automatically. Other devices used to scan drugs are handheld components that identify the necessary drug information. The technician only needs to enter the quantity to be ordered. The information from this handheld set then is transferred to the main computer ordering system.

AUTOMATED DISPENSING SYSTEMS (ADS)

For the pharmacy to determine the necessary stock levels, there has to be a way to inventory the stock that is not on the stock shelves but is in use or in a different location. For example, automated dispensing systems (ADS) are used in community pharmacies to monitor the inventory as tablets and capsules are dispensed into a drug vial from a bulk bin. As the pills pass a beam of light, they automatically are removed from the inventory. An example of this type of system is a Baker Cell system. Systems of this type are being developed constantly, and they work similarly.

In the hospital, the pharmacy is responsible for supplying various clinics and nursing units with stock. To avoid a stock shortage, dispensing systems that link the nursing units to the pharmacy computer system allow the stock levels to be viewed at any time. Each time the nurse indicates the type and amount

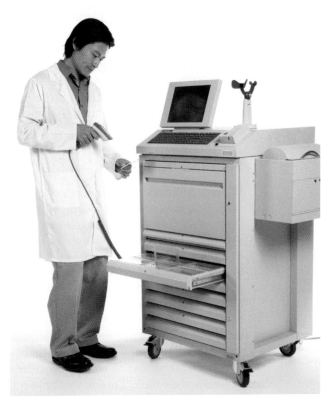

FIGURE 13-7 OmniRx. (Courtesy of Omnicell, Inc., © 2011.)

Tech Note!

Automated systems used in hospitals are being transitioned from nurses and pharmacy personnel entering personal codes to using fingerprint identification, therefore making it more difficult to misuse the system.

of drug taken from these drug cabinets, it is deducted from the current stock levels in the cabinet and this information then is transferred electronically to the pharmacy unit. Various reports can be generated from this centralized unit, which can provide an overall stock inventory for a specific drug. In addition to the inventory status, such units also monitor controlled substance use and inventory. All persons adding drugs to or taking drugs from the unit are identified, and a log is kept of all users. This also ensures the proper use of controlled substances and detects any discrepancies. Examples of these types of automated dispensing systems are hospital units such as Pyxis (see Chapter 7) and OmniRx (Figure 13-7) or Baker Cell systems.

MANUAL ORDERING

Although manual ordering is being eliminated slowly as the primary ordering technique, it is still important in the continued monitoring of stock levels. Some pharmacies still visually note that stock is getting low or use ordering cards that stay inside the medication box. These cards list the drug information, including the ordering number and the necessary PAR levels to aid the technician in ordering the proper amount. Employing the card system or simply writing down the right amount of stock to be ordered depends on the PAR levels or special orders.

More commonly, orders are processed electronically via the computer or handheld computers that transmit the order. The following list categorizes the drugs stocked by many pharmacies:

- Formulary: In a hospital pharmacy these drugs, normally stocked by the pharmacy, are approved by a P&T committee. In a retail pharmacy a specific formulary indicates which drugs are on the approved list of a patient's insurance company. Because there are many different insurance companies and thus many different formularies, retail pharmacies will stock a wide range of products.

- Fast mover: These drugs typically are kept in a separate area from the normal stock because of the high volume of use. These must be ordered in larger quantities, keeping the overstock in close proximity, or must be ordered more often.
- Slow mover: These drugs are prescribed regularly by a few physicians but are not commonly prescribed. They must be checked before ordering and periodically to ensure that the drugs are not close to expiring.
- Special orders: These are drugs typically used by only a few patients, but they may be important for proper treatment. It is easy to forget to order these drugs because of their infrequent use. Usually they are ordered at the time of use and some of these drugs may be non-formulary.
- Time of year: The drugs that are part of this category vary depending on the time of year. Many medications that are fast movers during a particular time of year may need their PAR levels raised during that period. For example, albuterol inhalers are normally fast movers in the spring when allergy symptoms increase and consequent asthma or respiratory tract symptoms. Antiviral medications used to treat influenza would be prescribed more often during the flu season, from fall to spring. All pharmacy staff must be aware of the types of medications used during different times of the year and understand how levels fluctuate.

Responding early when a medication trend is seen is a skill that takes time and experience. When stock begins to become depleted, it is everyone's responsibility to make sure that the stock is ordered.

NEW STOCK

Stock normally arrives daily (excluding weekends and holidays) to the pharmacy from different sources (except for central supply in a hospital setting which functions 7 days a week). For billing purposes, it is important that all stock be checked completely against the invoice when first received. See Box 13-5 for a step-by-step approach that should be used when receiving stock.

PROPER STORAGE

As stock arrives it is important to follow the manufacturer's requirements for storage. Certain medications must be frozen at temperatures between –20° and –10° C, refrigerated at temperatures between 2° and 8° C, or stored at room temperature. Light or humidity can also affect the stability of the medication; therefore care must be taken to protect stock from either light sources or excessive humidity. If these guidelines are not followed the medication is then compromised, rendering it unusable. Just as it is important to return unused stock to its proper location when it is being returned from the nursing floors (in hospital pharmacy), it is also essential that the pharmacy technician places new stock into their respective areas of storage as soon as possible. Chemicals such as phenol and other toxic materials are usually kept behind cabinet doors and low to the ground. It is not wise to leave these types of materials exposed to the public, because they are toxic. Read the packaging on all medications and follow the manufacturer's requirements for storage. Storing medications in the proper location is the responsibility of everyone working in pharmacy.

Tech Note!

You should not allow any medication into the pharmacy unless it is properly dated. That is, the expiration date should be sufficiently long to increase the likelihood that the drug will be used before it expires. Most pharmacies use a 3-month expiration time. This means that a drug that expires in 3 months or less may expire before use unless it is a fast mover. Drugs that are not expired and unlikely to be used may be returned to the manufacturer for a refund.

BOX 13-5 RECEIVING STOCK

1. Retrieve the manufacturer or warehouse invoice.
2. Account for all boxes. For example, if the invoice indicates there are five boxes, your first task is to verify that there are five boxes.
3. If any box is marked refrigerate or freeze, you must comply with the instructions immediately to avoid product damage.
4. All information must be checked against the invoice. For example, check the following:
   Name of drug
   Strength or dosage
   Dosage form
   Quantity
   Expiration date of product*
5. Compare the invoice with the order form to ensure that only the items requested were received.
6. Then sign and date the invoice and forward it for processing per pharmacy protocol.
7. Once the received order has been confirmed as correct, the technician may place the stock in the correct location, per pharmacy protocol. Rotating stock is another important priority. New stock typically has later expiration dates and should be placed behind the existing stock that expires sooner. All stock should be rotated in this manner to avoid accumulation of expired drugs, which may be used accidentally.
8. Finally, it is important to return inventory cards to the medication box for future use.

Inventory may not sound important. However, marking stock shelves clearly ultimately lessens the probability of drug errors. For example, if a drug is accidentally placed in a box intended for a different drug with a similar-sounding name, it may be used to fill a prescription for the sound-a-like drug and ultimately affect the patient's health and well-being.

*Checking the expiration date is important. Drugs that are used rarely and have short expiration dates may stay on the shelf and expire before use.

Returns

Medication is returned to the warehouse or manufacturer for four main reasons:

1. Drug recalls
    Class I: recalls for drugs that may pose serious threat to users' health or even death
    Class II: recalls for drugs that may cause a temporary health problem and have a low risk of creating a serious problem
    Class III: recalls for drugs that violate FDA regulations concerning container defects or have strange taste or color of contents
2. Damaged stock
3. Expired stock
4. Medication is about to expire; the pharmacy can return for credit or full price to the wholesaler if drug has at least a 9-month expiration date

Depending on the reason, certain documentation must accompany the medication. Pharmacy policies and procedures should list the steps involved for returns. Except for scheduled drugs that fall under the jurisdiction of the Drug Enforcement Administration (DEA) (see Chapter 2), most medications can be returned by the technician without a pharmacist's signature.

DRUG RECALLS

Manufacturers are required by law to recall any product that has been found to violate any of the following guidelines:

1. Labeling is wrong.
2. Product was not packaged or produced properly.
3. Drug batch was contaminated.
4. The FDA has required removal of the drug from the market as a result of safety risks.
5. Any other change occurs that causes the drug to fall outside the FDA or manufacturer's guidelines.

Recall notices may arrive at the pharmacy by mail or fax. Notices should identify the necessary information about the drug or device in question and describe the necessary steps to follow the recall procedure. This information includes the drug name and the reason it is being recalled. One of the most important pieces of information provided is the lot number of the drug. This is the key to identifying the recalled medication. Retail pharmacy corporations and hospitals often have detailed procedures and teams of persons who ensure the documentation, implementation, and completion of recall procedures, including final notification to the manufacturer and the FDA of the completion of removal of the recalled product. Upon receipt of the recall notification, pharmacy staff should immediately inspect and remove all stock from shelves, refrigerators, and freezers.

The pharmacy should place the recalled medication in a designated area or container for either return to the manufacturer or disposal in accordance with the recall notice. Technicians are responsible for checking all of the drug stock throughout the pharmacy and facility to ensure that the recalled drug is not in stock. If this is the case, the recall form is initialed to indicate that the item is not in stock. If pharmacy stock does include a drug with the recalled lot number, the pharmacist must be notified in case a patient has been issued one of these products. Prescribers also are notified by manufacturers and the FDA in the same manner as pharmacy. Any patient who may have been issued a recalled item should be notified by phone so that he or she may check the lot number of the drug or device. It is the responsibility of the prescriber to notify patients currently using a recalled medication or device if treatment is to be discontinued or altered. The pharmacy can help facilitate the patient's return or disposal of a recalled medication. A sample recall notification can be seen in Box 13-6.

DAMAGED STOCK

If you notice that some drugs were damaged en route to the pharmacy but you were not aware of damage at the time of delivery, it is not too late to return the damaged stock to the manufacturer. It may be necessary to first contact the manufacturer and obtain an approval code before the damaged goods are returned. The patient may also notice damaged stock. Sometimes EpiPen or Imitrex injections have bent needles, broken plungers, or other issues. In these cases the patient returns the medications and the pharmacy replaces the item. The pharmacy must then contact the manufacturer, who will send a replacement to the pharmacy directly and may or may not collect the damaged merchandise.

EXPIRED STOCK

Many pharmacies have a policy to pull any medication that will expire in 3 months or less. This ensures that there are no drugs on the shelves close to their

BOX 13-6 RECALL NOTIFICATION

April 7, 2004

URGENT EXPANDED DRUG RECALL NOTIFICATION—PATIENT LEVEL

Subject: DURAGESIC (fentanyl transdermal system) CII 75 mcg/hour, NDC #50458-035-05, Lot Control Numbers 0327192 (exp. 10/05), 0327193 (exp. 10/05), 0327294 (exp. 11/05), 0327295 (exp. 11/05), and 0330362 (exp. 12/05)

Dear Pharmacist:

Janssen Pharmaceutica Products, L.P., would like to inform you of an expanded recall to users of DURAGESIC (fentanyl transdermal system) CII 75 mcg/hour, NDC #50458-035-05, Lot Control Numbers 0327192 (exp. 10/05), 0327193 (exp. 10/05), 0327294 (exp. 11/05), 0327295 (exp. 11/05), and 0330362 (exp. 12/05). The company recalled one lot of DURAGESIC 75 mcg/hour patches (Control Number 0327192) in Feb 2004 after determining that a small percentage of patches in this lot might leak medication along one edge. Since then, a small number of patches with the same problem have been identified in one additional lot. As a precaution, the company is recalling four additional lots of 75 mcg/hour patches that were produced on the same manufacturing line during the same period.

Exposure to the leaked medication could result in inadvertent ingestion or an increased transdermal absorption of the opiate component fentanyl, leading to potentially life-threatening complications.

Conversely, leakage of medication could lead to inadequate dosing, resulting in treatment failure and/or opiate withdrawal.

Anyone who comes in contact with the leaked medication is advised to rinse exposed skin thoroughly with water only; soap should not be used.

Only control numbers listed above are included in this expanded recall. All other control numbers of DURAGESIC 75 mcg/hour patches and other dosage strengths are unaffected by the recall.

This corrective action and return policy are being made with the knowledge of the FDA (Food and Drug Administration) and the DEA (Drug Enforcement Administration).

Check your stock immediately. If you have any product with Lot Control Numbers 0327192 (exp. 10/05), 0327193 (exp. 10/05), 0327294 (exp. 11/05), 0327295 (exp. 11/05), and 0330362 (exp. 12/05), STOP the distribution of these lots immediately, fill out the included Business Reply Card indicating quantities to be returned, and promptly mail the card to: Universal Rx Solutions, 2084-900 M, Lake Industrial Court, PO Box 998-30012, Conyers, GA 30013-5758.* Once received, Universal Rx Solutions will send a DEA 222 form, instructions, and a mailing label to return the product. Please allow 2 to 3 weeks for the DEA 222 form and return kit to arrive.

It is very important that you fill in the requested information on the BRC and return it upon receipt, even if you do not have any of these lots, so that we can verify your receipt of this recall notification. Please order replacement merchandise using normal ordering procedures.

Wholesalers, in addition to completing the enclosed BRC, please also notify those to whom you have distributed these lots and request that they contact Universal Rx Solutions at 1-800-777-6565 and choose option 6 at the prompt. Do not copy your BRC or provide it to customers—a pharmacy specific BRC will be supplied to pharmacies directly from Universal Rx Solutions. Should customers call requesting information about return of product from affected lots, please direct them to contact Universal Rx Solutions at 1-800-777-6565.

Pharmacies, in addition to completing the enclosed BRC, please also notify immediately those patients to whom you have distributed these lots of DURAGESIC 75 mcg/hour patches (Control Numbers 0327192, 0327193, 0327294, 0327295, and 0330362) and request that they return their unused and unopened pouches from these lots directly to you. These lot numbers were distributed from December 15, 2003, through March 12, 2004. Please return the recalled items to: Universal Rx Solutions,* 2084-900 M, Lake Industrial Court, PO Box 998-30012, Conyers, GA 30013-5758. Please see detailed instructions below. Please call 1-800-777-6565 with questions regarding your product return. Do not return recalled product without obtaining a DEA 222 form from Universal Rx Solutions.

BOX 13-6 RECALL NOTIFICATION—cont'd

1. Patients will bring the unused DURAGESIC patches from recalled lots in unopened pouches back to pharmacies and receive replacement product.
   - Replacement of the same number of DURAGESIC 75 mcg/hour patches from recalled lots may or may not require an additional prescription. Note: In some states, a prescription is required for this substitution. We advise you to check with your state board of pharmacy, drug control division, to verify your local state laws and regulations and comply with them. Pharmacists will be requested to return the patches from the recalled lots to Universal Rx Solutions for a full refund. If DURAGESIC 75 mcg/hour patches from unaffected lots are not available, a suitable substitution should be made, e.g., using either a 50 mcg/hour patch and a 25 mcg/hour patch or three 25 mcg/hour patches. Note: It is anticipated that a new prescription will be required for substitution of other dosage strengths. We advise you to check with your state board of pharmacy, drug control division, to verify your local state laws and regulations and comply with them. Pharmacists are requested to return the patches from recalled lots along with DEA form 222 to Universal Rx Solutions for a full refund.
   - If the patches are returned to a pharmacy different than the original issuing pharmacy, a prescription is required for replacement.
2. Pharmacies should accept the unused and unopened pouches from patients and document receipt with a memo to the pharmacy's 222 file (system type, number received, reason [recall], patient, and date). If the receiving pharmacy is not the original issuing pharmacy, this should be noted in the memo. If the identity of the issuing pharmacy is known, it should be noted in the memo.
3. Pharmacies should store returned pouches in a manner consistent with how they store other CII drugs, taking appropriate safeguards against inadvertent redispensing.
4. Pharmacists should contact Universal Rx Solutions at 1-800-777-6565 and choose option 6 to obtain a 222 form and return kit.
   - The return kits will provide detailed instructions for returning product from recalled lots and will include pre-paid Fed-Ex labels. Please use the return kit labels and follow all directions included with the kit when making your return. Pharmacies will be reimbursed for product returned in accordance with this recall. This reimbursement will be made by credit memorandum (direct account) or check (indirect account) 4-6 weeks after receipt of product. Specific information to help you respond to questions from your patients is available at www.DURAGESIC.com or www.Janssen.com. Report adverse events and product defects relating to DURAGESIC to Janssen Pharmaceutica Products, L.P., at the contact number listed below or to the FDA MedWatch Program by phone (1-800-FDA-1088), by fax (1-800-FDA-0178), by mail (using postage-paid form to MedWatch, FDA, 5600 Fishers Lane, Rockville, MD 20852- 9787), or via www.accessdata.fda.gov/scripts/medwatch.

If you have additional questions regarding this product recall or require further assistance, please contact the Janssen Medical Services Contact Center at 1-800-Janssen (1-800-526-7736).

Please see attached Full Prescribing Information, including Boxed Warnings.

Sincerely,

Janssen Pharmaceutica Products, L.P.

*Universal Rx Solutions (USI) is committed to protect the privacy of consumers' health information, and to comply with applicable federal and state laws that protect the privacy and security of consumers' health information. USI policy establishes the basic requirements for the use or disclosure of consumers' protected health information, consistent with this commitment. See www.fda.gov/cder/drug/shortages/duragesic-Letter.pdf.

expiration date. Depending on the contract between the pharmacy and the manufacturer, it may be acceptable to return items as long as they can be bundled into a minimum package size rather than as partials. For instance, if the stock of cimetidine expires within 3 months, the manufacturer may allow it to be returned for full or partial credit if a box of 100 tablets can be returned at one time. Following manufacturer's guidelines for returns is important. Hazardous chemicals, including cytotoxic agents, must be repackaged carefully to avoid breakage during transport.

Pharmacy personnel can also pull and return slow moving stock that has 9 to 12 months before expiration; the pharmacy can receive credit from the wholesaler, who in turn may be able to resell the drug to another pharmacy. This only applies to unopened bottles and regulations vary according to the wholesaler's or manufacturer's specific operating policies.

Many pharmacies have a service that will process returns to drug companies for a percentage of the credits obtained. These companies visit the pharmacy at various times, ranging from once every 3 months to once a year, and complete all the paperwork and documentation for returning expired inventory.

AUTOMATED RETURN COMPANIES

There are companies that have the sole job of processing returns for hospitals, wholesalers, pharmacy chain stores, and independent retailers. They are responsible for all records, recalled items, and disposal of hazardous waste. Pharmacies contract with these companies for regular pickups; it is the pharmacy's responsibility to choose a licensed qualified business to perform these services.

NONRETURNABLE DRUGS AND THEIR DISPOSAL

Many items cannot be returned to manufacturers; the following are some examples of nonreturnable drugs: any drug that is reconstituted or compounded within the pharmacy; partially used bottles of medication; any drugs that have been repackaged by the pharmacy. These drugs, including most reconstituted agents such as amoxicillin suspension, can be discarded in the pharmacy garbage. They should not be allowed to infiltrate the water supply. In most cases, especially in chain pharmacies, the drugs are sent to a central location for destruction or returned to the manufacturer for credit.

Many agents must be disposed of carefully. Cytotoxic agents must be discarded in a specialized sharps container marked "hazardous waste." Nontoxic intravenous agents should be discarded in a standard sharps container marked for proper disposal. Controlled substances must be counted and co-signed by a pharmacist before they are destroyed. Before any scheduled medications are destroyed, the DEA must be contacted for specific instructions concerning their destruction. A pharmacist must always be present to co-sign for the disposal of controlled substances, and must return to the DEA required information concerning the disposal. The DEA issues a receipt for schedule II merchandise destroyed. This receipt must be kept for 5 years with the schedule II inventory.

Suppliers

When ordering stock for the pharmacy, the technician orders from a centralized warehouse that the pharmacy owns, from a wholesaler, or directly from the manufacturer.

Each of these suppliers has pros and cons. As seen in Table 13-4, the benefits of using wholesalers as opposed to dealing directly with the manufacturer differ mostly in the amount of stock that must be ordered and kept as overstock and

Tech Note!

Patients should be instructed in the proper disposal of unused medications. For many drugs, it is advisable to mix them with either coffee grounds or kitty litter and then place them in the garbage. Used transdermal patches and other novel dosage forms will need special care for disposal to prevent accidental exposures. Certain pharmacies allow patients to return to the pharmacy any expired or unused prescriptions found in their medicine cabinets. Check with your local pharmacy to see if this service is available. Medications should never be emptied into a toilet or a drain because then the drugs can infiltrate the water supply.

TABLE 13-4 **Difference in Ordering from Manufacturers, Wholesalers, and Warehouse Repackaging Plants**

Factors to Consider	Manufacturer	Wholesaler/Vendor Repackaging Plant	Warehouse
Supplier cost	No shipping fees	Lower per contract	Lowest cost
Supplier has electronic inventory control mechanism	No	Yes	Yes
Supplier able to stock large supplies when ordering	Yes	No	Yes
Supplier provides special delivery service	Varies by manufacturer	Yes	Yes
Supplier handles special orders	Yes	Some special orders must be done through manufacturer	Some special orders must be done through manufacturer

the difference in cost. The fourth column of Table 13-4 describes factors to consider when ordering medications from a warehouse; in this situation, the pharmaceutical company orders high volumes of drugs from the manufacturer and may repackage the medications into more suitable sizes for the ordering physician. This serves several purposes, such as easier handling, increased productivity, and lower cost. However, large-quantity bottles are hard to handle. They are more likely to be dropped, spilling the contents. Medications may be prepackaged in smaller, easy-to-handle containers to eliminate the bulkiness of the larger bottles. If the pharmacy warehouse prepackages common dosages, the labeling process will be faster. For example, sulfamethoxazole/trimethoprim (Septra, Bactrim) normally is ordered to be taken twice daily for 10 days or twice daily for 15 days. These tablets are prepackaged in bottles of 20 and 30, eliminating the time it takes to count out the proper amount at the pharmacy counter. The technician must check the label against the prescription to determine the appropriate drug and quantity, and then the prescription is ready to be inspected by the pharmacist and dispensed. Finally, because the volume of drugs is much higher than what a typical pharmacy can stock, pharmacies have contracts with these warehouses that save the pharmacy a substantial amount of money. This ultimately keeps the cost lower for the consumer.

Special Ordering Considerations

Special considerations must be given to a host of drugs ordered by pharmacy. Some of these include controlled substances, investigational drugs, cytotoxic drugs, and hazardous substances. Each of these types of medications requires special ordering, inventory, storage, handling, and return documentation. The DEA requires special forms to be completed for ordering schedule II controlled substances and for their return.

Investigational drugs typically have documentation that must be completed and returned to the manufacturer each time a medication is dispensed. Cytotoxic drugs do not need special documentation, but they should be handled with great care and placed in a safety cabinet according to manufacturer guidelines. Certain cytotoxic agents must be refrigerated and should be clearly marked to separate them from other agents. Most pharmacies stock certain chemicals that are considered hazardous. You must know where the **material safety data sheets** (MSDS) of your pharmacy are located in case of a spill. Agents such as phenol should be stored behind cabinet doors to protect persons from accidentally knocking the bottle off a shelf and inhaling the toxic fumes, or possibly contacting the agent.

Although many of the guidelines can be found in each pharmacy's policies and procedures manual, it is the responsibility of the pharmacy technician to be aware of these guidelines as well as both federal and state regulations. This requires continuous efforts in updating the most current regulations that apply to your pharmacy. Patients rely on the knowledge of the pharmacy technician, which is why competencies in the area of billing and inventory are extremely important in the daily functions of pharmacy.

DO YOU REMEMBER THESE KEY POINTS?

- Why pharmacy formularies are important
- The major types of insurance and the differences between them
- The differences between government-managed insurance programs
- The necessary information that patients must provide to the pharmacy for billing prescriptions to third parties
- The types of problems that often arise when processing insurance claims
- The importance of the National Drug Code and how to decipher it
- The responsibilities of a pharmacy technician concerning stock levels and ordering stock for the pharmacy
- Common types of automated dispensing systems and pharmacy settings in which they are used
- The steps that should be followed when receiving stock
- The parts of a health insurance card and their definitions
- The steps involved in billing insurance companies
- Reasons for returning stock to the manufacturer or supplier
- Who issues recalls and how they are addressed
- How to return expired or recalled stock
- The importance of storing stock at the appropriate temperature

REVIEW QUESTIONS

Multiple choice questions

1. Prescriptions can be filled for _____ days maximum with the authorization of the prescriber and health plan.
   A. 30
   B. 60
   C. 90
   D. All of the above

2. Medicare is a government-managed insurance program that covers all of the following EXCEPT:
   A. Senior citizens
   B. Patients using dialysis
   C. Children
   D. Persons who are disabled

3. Medicaid covers all of the following persons EXCEPT:
   A. Persons who are disabled
   B. Persons with low income
   C. Women who are pregnant
   D. Single working persons with above-average income

4. Geographical managed care can be best described as:
   A. A medical group that is covered under Medicare and works much like an HMO
   B. A program that belongs to a medical group covered by Medicare and works much like an HMO
   C. A program that belongs to a medical group covered by Medicaid and works much like an HMO
   D. An HMO program that covers general medical groups

5. Information required by insurance companies does not include:
   A. Date medication is filled
   B. Name of pharmacy filing the prescription
   C. Name and dosage form of drug
   D. Name of technician

6. Insurance claims that are transmitted electronically to the insurance provider are called:
   A. E-mail
   B. NDC claims
   C. Adjudication
   D. Co-pay

7. Of the automated systems listed, which is used most commonly to manage levels of controlled substances?
   A. Pyxis
   B. Baker Cell systems
   C. Bar coding
   D. Both A and C

8. Various types of agents ordered for a pharmacy may include:
   A. Formulary drugs
   B. Hazardous substances
   C. Cytotoxic drugs
   D. All of the above

9. The proper storage of medications is the responsibility of:
   A. The inventory technician
   B. The pharmacist in charge
   C. The technician
   D. Everyone working in the pharmacy

10. An inventory system that automatically orders stock as it is used is called:
    A. Pyxis
    B. POS
    C. MSDS
    D. Inventory cards

11. Reasons pharmacies return medications to manufacturers include all of the following EXCEPT:
    A. Merchandise has been damaged
    B. Patients return medications
    C. Medication is close to expiration date
    D. Drug has been recalled

12. When a workers' compensation claim arrives at the pharmacy, the technician must:
    A. Obtain permission from a government agency at a later time
    B. Obtain information from the patient's human resources department
    C. Collect payment from the patient, who then will be reimbursed from the insurance company
    D. Wait until payment is made by the insurance company before releasing the medication

13. Medicare Part B pays for all of the following supplies EXCEPT:
A. Diabetes supplies
B. Dialysis supplies
C. Transplant supplies
D. Postsurgical supplies

14. Third-party billing involves all of the following entities except:
A. The patient
B. The workplace
C. The pharmacy
D. The insurance company

15. Certain restrictions may apply to addictive or dangerous drugs when filling days' supply; these include all of the following EXCEPT:
A. Meperidine
B. Accutane
C. Insulin
D. Morphine

True/False

If a statement is false, then change it to make it true.

_____ **1.** Trade and generic drugs cost the pharmacy the same price.

_____ **2.** If a patient's drug claim is rejected by the insurance company, the technician may call the help desk and attempt to reactivate it.

_____ **3.** Periodic automatic replacement levels are levels of drugs that should be kept at a predetermined amount in the pharmacy.

_____ **4.** All drug recall notifications must be initiated by the Food and Drug Administration.

_____ **5.** The sole responsibility of the pharmacy inventory technician is to keep all drugs and pharmacy supplies in stock.

_____ **6.** Drug companies never allow pharmacies to return drugs.

_____ **7.** The only drug return that requires a pharmacist's signature is a controlled substances return.

_____ **8.** All hazardous substances should be kept behind cabinet doors for safety purposes.

_____ **9.** MSDS is defined as *medication safety drug sheets* and provides descriptions of drugs.

_____ **10.** Drugs that expire within 3 months may (in many cases) be pulled and returned to the manufacturer.

_____ **11.** Unused liquid medications can be discarded by pouring down the drain or toilet.

_____ **12.** The PCN number on a prescription card indicates which person is insured.

_____ **13.** All providers who bill electronically must use the NPI number.

_____ **14.** Prescription coupon cards are supplied to the patient by the pharmacy.

_____ **15.** PPOs offer more options for the patient in choosing a physician.

TECHNICIAN'S CORNER

The pharmacy technician accidentally fills the quinine stock box with quinidine. What is the difference between these two medicines? As a technician, what can you do to avoid confusion between these two drugs?

BIBLIOGRAPHY

[CDER] www.fda.gov/cder/about/smallbiz/patent_term.htm

[Consumer Reports] Prescription Drug coverage: Things to consider. www.medicare.gov/pdp-things-to-consider.asp#Coverage

Medicare overview. www.medicare.gov/MedicareEligibility/home

Drug Utilization and POS: www.ghsinc.com/pharmacy/pos

Medicaid Fee For Service: www.goldbamboo.com/lg.html?in=100002192162

State Pharmaceutical Assistance Program (SPAP) www.ncsl.org/PROGRAMS/HEALTH/drugaid.htm

www.deadiversion.usdoj.gov:80/pubs/manuals/pharm2/pharm_content.htm

http://money.cnn.com/retirement/guide/retirementliving_healthcare.moneymag/index11.htm

www.seniors-health-insurance.com/medicaid.php?source=google

State raise taxes for federal matching funds on Medicaid: www.healthimaging.com/index.php?option=com_articles&view=article&id=21635

Medicaid Mandatory Coverages: www.medicaidinformation.info/articles/55330/Medicaid-Coverage-Mandatory

WEBSITES

www.medicare.gov

www.ConsumerReports.org

www.Webmd.com

www.drugtopics.com

www.accesstobenefits.org

www.nlm.nih.gov

www.fda.gov

www.texmed.org

www.prescriptiondrugrecall.com/

www.purdue.edu/uns/insidepurdue/2008/080201_Cessation.html

CHAPTER

14

Medication Safety and Error Prevention

Objectives

UPON COMPLETING THIS CHAPTER YOU SHOULD BE ABLE TO DO THE FOLLOWING:

- List the most common types of errors made by technicians.

- List the organizations or groups where drug errors can be reported.

- Explain the necessity of reporting drug errors.

- List the most common drug errors caused by patients.

- Describe the guidelines that have been established and are monitored to prevent errors.

- List and describe four automated systems and explain how they prevent errors.

- Explore new ways that health care personnel can decrease drug errors.

American Society of Health-System Pharmacists (ASHP) *Association of pharmacists, pharmacy students, and technicians practicing in hospitals and health care systems, including home health care; ASHP has a long history of advocating patient safety and establishing best practices to improve medication use*

Automated dispensing systems (ADS) *Electronic systems used to dispense medications*

Institute for Healthcare Improvement (IHI) *A nonprofit organization committed to the improvement of health care by promoting promising concepts through safety, efficiency, and other patient-centered goals*

Institute for Safe Medication Practices (ISMP) *A nonprofit organization devoted entirely to promoting safe medication use and preventing medication errors. Gathers information on drug errors and suggests new safer standards to avoid such errors*

Institute of Medicine (IOM) *Established under the National Academies and a part of the National Academy of Science, this nonprofit organization provides scientifically informed analysis and guidance regarding health and health policy. Projects include studies of drug safety systems within the United States and recommendations for patient safety*

Medication error prevention *Methods used by pharmacy, medicine, nursing, and other allied health professionals to prevent medication errors*

MEDMARX *A national Internet-accessible database that hospitals and health care systems use to track adverse drug reactions and medication errors*

MedWatch *Program established by the FDA for reporting drug and medical product safety alerts and label changes; the program also provides a voluntary adverse event reporting system for medications, medical products, and devices*

National Coordinating Council for Medication Error Reporting and Prevention (NCC MERP) *Founded by the USP, this is an independent council of more than 25 organizations gathered to address interdisciplinary causes of medication errors and strategies for prevention*

Pharmacy Technician Certification Board (PTCB) *Offers national certification for pharmacy technicians in the United States*

Pharmacy Technician Educators Council (PTEC) *U.S. organization that promotes teachers' strategies and instructions for pharmacy technician education*

United States Pharmacopeia (USP) *Independent organization that strives to ensure the quality, safety, and benefit of medicines and dietary supplements by setting standards and certification processes*

Introduction

Drug errors are unacceptable in any situation involving medical treatment or medications, but the reality is that they will never disappear. It is a human trait that people make mistakes. At times, errors may not be realized before they cause harm. When discussing drug errors it is important to note that not all errors are harmful and not all are caused by pharmacy. Within this chapter, types and incidence of errors are discussed, and specific cases that unfortunately caused harm are presented. An attempt will be made to identify the common causes for many drug errors and ultimately the ways in which they can be avoided. Other topics discussed in this chapter include the process of drug error reporting (that is, when errors should be reported and whom should be contacted) and the importance of taking responsibility for your own medical treatment, which includes your medications.

Pharmacy technicians are at the forefront with regard to prevention of drug errors; ironically, they also can cause errors relatively easily. Many technicians have relied on the pharmacist to catch their mistakes, but this is not the correct approach to preventing medication errors. Just as technicians can make mistakes, so can pharmacists.

In 1999 the **Institute of Medicine** (IOM) prepared a report titled *To Err Is Human—Building a Better Health System*. The report provided a strategy for government, health care providers, industry, and consumers to use to prevent errors in health care. At the time the report was released, the statistics (based on various data from hospital admissions in New York, Colorado, and Utah) estimated that at least 44,000 people per year died because of medical errors; the numbers included errors made by physicians, nurses, and pharmacy staff. The data from the combined sources suggested that as many as 98,000 people per year died from medical errors. The reason these statistics seem so shocking is that most errors were never reported or addressed at an official level. The cost of these sometimes fatal errors is estimated at $8.8 billion a year. Studies reported by IOM "indicate that 400,000 preventable drug-related injuries occur each year in hospitals. Another 800,000 occur in long-term care settings, and roughly 530,000 occur just among Medicare recipients in outpatient clinics. The committee noted that these are likely underestimates."

What Constitutes an Error?

An error is any type of preventable mistake that is made, intentional or unintentional, regardless of whether it causes harm. Not all drug errors cause harm to the patient. For example, if a patient was dosed the right drug but in the wrong strength, the mistake may have been overlooked for a couple of doses before being detected and restarted at the correct dosage. An error also occurs when a medication (such as an antibiotic) is discontinued per physician's orders, but an additional dose is given to the patient after discontinuation. Another example of an error is when a patient receives a 300-mg dose of enteric-coated aspirin instead of a 325-mg dose of uncoated aspirin.

Patients themselves cause many drug errors when taking their own medications at home. They may take their medications at the wrong time, in the wrong amount, in the wrong combination, or with the improper technique of administration. It is difficult to know how many drug errors occur at home because they are not typically reported to anyone and may continue to occur unless realized by the physician or pharmacist or, even worse, manifested by an adverse drug event or reaction (ADE or ADR). These types of situations are part of the drug error dilemma and are taken very seriously by all involved in patient care. Beginning in 1993 the **American Society of Health-System Pharmacists** (ASHP) outlined the types of errors that occur in a hospital setting; these are listed in Table 14-1 with examples given for each type. Although the data were collected almost 20 years ago, the same errors are still being made.

The **National Coordinating Council for Medication Error Reporting and Prevention** (NCC MERP) has categorized specific types of errors and described the consequences of such errors (Table 14-2). Based on the information from the MERP database (http://cme.medscape.com/viewarticle/556487) that

TABLE 14-1 Common Hospital Pharmacy Errors (ASHP)

Error	Description
Prescribing error	Prescriber orders a medication that is incorrect (example: incorrect usage, dosage form, route, concentration, rate of infusion) or is selected incorrectly based on indications or contraindications (allergies, existing condition); medication reaches patient
Omission error	Failure to administer an ordered dose to a patient before next dose is due, without an apparent reason for omission or appropriate documentation (example: nurse forgets to give a dose to patient)
Wrong time error	Medication administered outside scheduled time frame; if facility allows plus or minus 30 min, dose is given outside of this variance (each facility sets their acceptable time frame for variances)
Unauthorized drug error	Medication administered to a patient from an unauthorized prescriber; physician not licensed in that state or not an authorized prescriber
Improper dose error	Patient administered a dose that is greater or less than prescribed amount (example: aspirin 325 mg is given instead of 500 mg)
Wrong dosage form	Medication administered in a dosage form other than what was ordered (example: capsule for tablet, ointment for cream)
Wrong drug preparation	Drug is incorrectly formulated (example: wrong calculations or wrong solution used for reconstitution) or manipulated (example: break in aseptic technique), and medication is administered to patient
Wrong administration	Drug is given using wrong procedure or technique (example: giving an IM dose as an IV dose or placing an ophthalmic solution in wrong eye)
Deteriorated drug error	Medication is administered that has expired or integrity of ingredients has been compromised (example: storing a drug at room temperature when it should be refrigerated)
Monitoring error	Failure to review a prescribed medication for proper regimen, appropriateness (example: not monitoring patient's response to prescribed medication), detection of problems in dosage (example: not recognizing side effects from drugs), or failure in using laboratory results to correctly adjust dose
Compliance error	Patient does not adhere to prescribed medication regimen (example: taking a q8h dose every 6 hr or stopping a medication before scheduled)

TABLE 14-2 MERP Error Categories

Category	Definition	Type of Resulting Error
A	Circumstances that have potential for causing errors	No error
B	Error occurred but did not reach patient	Error, No harm
C	Error reached patient but did not cause harm	Error, No harm
D	Error reached patient, did not cause harm, but needed monitoring or intervention to prove no harm resulted	Error, No harm
E	Error occurred that may have contributed to or resulted in temporary harm to patient and patient required intervention	Error, Harm
F	Error occurred that may have contributed to or resulted in temporary harm to patient and resulted in monitoring or hospitalization	Error, Harm
G	Error occurred that may have contributed to or resulted in temporary or permanent harm to patient	Error, Harm
H	Error occurred that may have contributed to or resulted in harm to patient and required hospitalization to sustain life	Error, Harm
I	Error occurred that may have contributed to or resulted in patient's death	Error, Death

compiles drug errors, the following were the top 10 medications related to health care professional errors in 2007:

1. Insulin
2. Morphine
3. Potassium chloride
4. Albuterol
5. Heparin
6. Vancomycin
7. Cefazolin
8. Acetaminophen
9. Warfarin
10. Furosemide

How Errors Occur

Errors are never intentional, but occur as a result of a series of circumstances or events. For example, during the communication between the physician's office and the pharmacy several factors could contribute to the creation of a medication error, including the following common causes:

- Ambiguous strength labeled on drug container or label
- Excessive workload of pharmacy personnel
- Failure to transcribe orders properly
- Illegible handwriting
- Inaccurate dosage calculation
- Inadequately trained personnel
- Labeling errors
- Look-alike, sound-alike drug names

Physicians' handwriting has long been known for its illegibility; reading drug names, strengths, and dosages can be very problematic. An alternative to a handwritten prescription is a new technology called E-prescribing. Prescriptions can be sent via computer or mobile device directly to the pharmacy where they can be easily and quickly interpreted. There are several software programs that facilitate E-prescribing. Although E-prescribing has been implemented in various medical institutions and physicians' offices, many physicians still handwrite their orders on prescription pads or order sheets. It is the responsibility of the pharmacy and nurses to interpret these prescriptions correctly. Sample case scenarios show the possible progression of an ultimate drug error:

SCENARIO #1: MISINTERPRETATION OF PHYSICIAN'S ORDERS

A prescription arrives in the pharmacy for digoxin 0.125 mg; because of the illegibility of the physician's handwriting it is transcribed inaccurately as 0.25 mg. The wrong medication strength is sent to the floor, where the nurse gives the patient the wrong dose.

SCENARIO #2: MISSED DOSE

A medication order arrives in the pharmacy and is processed correctly and sent to the patient. The nurse pulls the correct drug and dose but forgets to give it to the patient; therefore the patient misses a dose. Whether the nurse forgets to give the dose or the patient (at home) forgets to take the medication, this constitutes a medication error.

SCENARIO #3: WRONG PATIENT

A medication order arrives in the pharmacy and is processed and sent to the floor correctly, but the nurse gives the drug to the wrong patient.

SCENARIO #4: ADVERSE EFFECT

A patient takes an over-the-counter drug along with a prescription drug, and it causes an adverse or toxic effect because of a drug-drug interaction.

SCENARIO #5: NONCOMPLIANCE

A patient obtains his or her prescription at the local pharmacy and begins to take the medication; the prescription instructs the patient to take daily for 30 days. After 1 week the patient feels much better and stops taking the medication.

Where Errors Are Made

Errors are made everywhere. Most often they are reported in community and institutional pharmacies such as hospitals, although they occur in many different settings. The Medication Error Reporting and Prevention (MERP) organization tracks errors and their causes and has provided a list of five recommendations to avoid errors specifically in nonhospital settings. An example of some non–health care settings are listed in Box 14-1 along with the five recommendations from MERP.

Why Errors Occur

It is human nature to make errors; humans are not perfect. A person can look at the name and strength of a drug yet fail to register the correct information, substituting unintended information in its place. Errors can be created by

BOX 14-1 NON–HEALTH CARE SETTINGS

- Elementary and secondary schools
- Child day care centers
- Summer camps
- Adult day service centers (adult day care)
- Group homes for the developmentally disabled
- Assisted living/residential care
- Board and care homes
- Jails (city and county)
- Prisons (state and federal)

Recommendations from MERP
1. Develop written policies and procedures for personnel who administer medications.
2. Provide training to personnel who are responsible for medication management.
3. Ensure that controlled medications are stored properly to prevent theft and diversion.
4. Encourage personnel to report medication errors to appropriate drug error reporting program.
5. When a medication error occurs, evaluate possible causes in order to improve the facility's system for drug management and to prevent future errors.

focusing on more than one task at a time. People tend to filter out information even under normal circumstances. Think about the examples below of errors in everyday life and note whether any have ever happened to you:

- You pick up the phone to call a specific person and you call another instead.
- You leave to drive to school and you start to drive toward work.
- You read the words on a page of a textbook and although you read each word correctly you do not remember what you have just read.
- You reach for the correct spice on the kitchen shelf and you grab the wrong one because it was similar in size, shape, color, or labeling.

Even the most highly skilled person will occasionally make errors. You know what you want to do but your mind changes its focus and you follow the wrong information. This type of "automatic behavior" plays a role in the creation of errors. In addition, when repetitive actions are carried out daily, it is easy to become complacent and lose focus on the task at hand.

Both treating patients and supplying medications accurately are critical responsibilities, and it is expected that errors will be avoided. All health care workers strive to avoid errors on a daily basis, although this is an almost impossible task. The following are some examples of the daily obstructions encountered by pharmacy personnel:

- Stress, because of the number of orders that need to be processed
- Noise in the workplace that distracts focus from the medication ordered
- Multitasking: Doing two or more things at once, such as answering the phone and checking medications at the same time. This can distract attention away from the order.
- Medication names that sound alike
- Medications that look similar (e.g., colors, shapes, sizes, or a similar area where they are stored)
- Labels that look similar because of the same color and/or lettering
- Hard to read labels as a result of small print

The first response to an error is normally to blame rather than to explain the reasons behind such an occurrence. All health care workers are at risk of being found guilty of errors that are considered negligence according to federal and state laws. The case of a medical error reported in Colorado (Example 1) identifies the complexity of a drug error. A case that was highly publicized across the country (Example 2) clearly illustrates the need for well-educated and trained technicians.

EXAMPLE 1

Police charged three nurses with negligent homicide following an infant's death from a fatal overdose. A subsequent analysis (Smetzer & Cohen, 1998), however, uncovered a chain of numerous errors from the time of prescription to the time of injection. Police did not charge the physician who wrote the cryptic prescription or the pharmacist who misread the dosage. (Nursing error by Marc Green. Expanded version of Nursing error and human nature, *J Nurs Law* 9:37-44, 2004.)

EXAMPLE 2

On May 7, 2007, The Ohio State Board of Pharmacy revoked the license of a staff pharmacist at Rainbow Baby's and Children's Hospital in Cleveland after a 2-year-old patient (Emily) died as a result of a sodium overdose in a chemotherapy solution. The board concluded that the pharmacist did not follow proper hospital procedures regarding the supervision of a pharmacy technician who prepared the solutions. No disciplinary action was taken against the technician because Ohio does not license or register pharmacy technicians. The technician resigned in the aftermath of the incident. William Winsley, RPh, MS, executive director of the board, stated that both the pharmacist and the technician were experienced and had prepared intravenous and chemotherapy solutions many times. However, he said, "the pharmacist failed to adequately check the technician's work." The supervising pharmacist, who failed to notice the technician's mistake, lost his state license and pleaded no contest to involuntary manslaughter; he was sentenced to 6 months in jail and 6 months of house arrest (Radwan C: Pharmacy technicians face states' scrutiny, regulation, *Drug Topics,* Aug 25, 2009. Available at http://drugtopics.modernmedicine.com/drugtopics/Associations/Pharmacy-technicians-face-states-scrutiny-regulati/ArticleStandard/Article/detail/621364).

Emily's Law was passed in 2009 by the governor of the state of Ohio. This act requires all pharmacy technicians in the state to be of legal age, to have a high school diploma or equivalent, to pass a state and federal background check, and to pass a certifying competency examination approved by the board of pharmacy before being awarded technician status. The National Pharmacy Technician Association (NPTA) supports the legislation as a model for national and state standards. U.S. Representative Steve LaTourette proposed Emily's Act for U.S. congressional approval but it was rejected.

Look-Alike, Sound-Alike (LASA) Drugs

Each year the FDA reviews approximately 400 brand names for drugs before they are allowed to enter the market; the FDA rejects approximately 33% of the proposed drug names. Sometimes drug names change after the products are marketed and already on pharmacy shelves. For example, in 2005 when Amaryl (glimepiride) was confused with Reminyl (galantamine), the Reminyl name was subsequently changed to Razadyne. Before the change occurred, one person died.

In February 2008, the *USP* released its 8th annual MEDMARX data report, detailing evaluations made between January 1, 2003, and December 31, 2006, of more than 26,000 records from more than 670 health care facilities. Among LASA drug errors, 1.4% (384) caused harm to the patient. Of these, 64.4% originated at the pharmacy, with pharmacy technicians committing the initial error in 39% of the cases and pharmacists in 24% of the cases. Examples of LASA error pairs provided by the *United States Pharmacopeia* included Mellaril/Elavil, Paxil/Taxol, Prilosec/Prozac, and Celebrex/Celexa (Michele B. Kaufman, PharmD: *Formulary,* Feb 1, 2009. Available at http://formularyjournal.modernmedicine.com/formulary/Modern+Medicine+Now/Preventable-medication-errors-Look-alikesound-alike/ArticleStandard/Article/detail/579387).

The *USP* has listed 1400 look-alike and sound-alike drugs; the list can be accessed free of charge. Other sources available without charge include references from the **Institute for Safe Medication Practices** (ISMP) and The Joint Commission (TJC). The following list provides links to these sources:

USP: www.usp.org/hqi/similarProducts/choosy.html
ISMP: www.ismp.org/tools/confuseddrugnames.pdf
TJC: www.jointcommission.org/NR/rdonlyres/C92AAB3F-A9BD-431C-8628-11DD2D1D53CC/0/LASA.pdf

Examples of the names of similar sound-alike drugs are listed in Table 14-3.

TABLE 14-3 Commonly Confused Drug Names

Advicor	Advair
Amicar	Omacor
Amphotericin B lipid complex	Amphotericin B desoxycholate
Celebrex	Cerebyx
Clonidine	Clonazepam
Darvocet	Percocet
DiaBeta	Zebeta
Effexor XR	Effexor
Ephedrine	Epinephrine
Heparin	Hespan
Humulin (human insulin products)	Humalog (insulin lispro)
Hydromorphone INJ	Morphine INJ
Hydroxyzine	Hydrazaline
Lamisil	Lamictal
Lamivudine	Lamotrigine
Leukeran	Leucovorin
Lorazepam	Alprazolam
Metformin	Metronidazole
MS Contin	OxyContin
Mucinex	Mucomyst
Novolin (human insulin products)	Novolog (human insulin aspart)
Novolin 70/30 (70% isophane insulin [NPH] and 30% regular insulin INJ)	Novolog mix 70/30 (70% insulin aspart protamine suspension and 30% insulin aspart)
Opium tincture	Paregoric (camphorated opium tincture)
OxyContin CR	OxyContin IR
Prilosec	Prozac
Retrovir	Ritonavir
Roxanol (concentrated)	Morphine oral liquid (nonconcentrate)
Tizanidine	Tiagabine
Topamax	Toprol XL
Tramadol	Trazodone
Vinblastine	Vincristine
Wellbutrin SR	Wellbutrin XL
Zantac	Xanax
Zantac	Zyrtec
Zestril	Zyprexa
Zestril	Zetia
Zocor	Zyrtec
Zyprexa	Zyrtec

LOOK-ALIKE DRUG NAMES/TALL MAN LETTERING

The FDA has approved a list of name sets and ISMP has a list of look-alike drug name sets that would benefit from tall man lettering (not yet approved by the FDA). This change in the previous labels on drugs will help to discern between similar sounding drug names and their appearance. The *FDA-Approved list of Established Drug Names with Tall Man Letters* includes the following examples:

acetoHEXAMIDE—acetaZOLAMIDE
buPROPion—busPIRone

chlorproMAZINE—chlorproPAMIDE
clomiPHENE—clomiPRAMINE
cycloSPORINE—cycloSERINE
DAUNOrubicin—DOXOrubicin
dimenhyDRINATE—diphenhydrAMINE
DOBUTamine—DOPamine
glipiZIDE—glyBURIDE
hydrALAZINE—hydrOXYzine
medroxyPROGESTERone—methylPREDNISolone—methylTESTOSTERone
niCARdipine—NIFEdipine
predniSONE—prednisoLONE
sulfADIAZINE—sulfiSOXAZOLE
TOLAZamide—TOLBUTamide
vinBLAStine—vinCRIStine

For a list of ISMP additional drug names with tall man lettering and to view the FDA's list, visit www.ismp.org/tools/tallmanletters.pdf.

Drug Interactions as a Source of Error

The probability of drug-drug interactions is increased in seniors or severely ill patients because of the multiple medications they often receive. Seniors may have multiple conditions that are treated concurrently. In addition to the changes in metabolism that occur with aging, taking similar drugs that have the same side effects may increase the risk and/or the severity of adverse effects. Table 14-4 lists examples of drugs that should not be given concurrently.

WARFARIN (COUMADIN) INTERACTIONS

Coumarin anticoagulants such as warfarin have the potential for many interactions with drugs, food, and dietary or herbal supplements. Certain warfarin interactions can be deadly. Warfarin is given to prevent clots that can cause strokes or heart attacks; the prothrombin time (PT) and the International Normalized Ratio (INR) must be maintained at a specific level to ensure that blood clots do not form and the patient does not bleed internally. Regular blood tests are performed to check the PT/INR level of patients being administered warfarin. Special consideration is given to those patients receiving warfarin. Examples of common warfarin interactions are given in Table 14-5. Although warfarin has several drug-drug and drug-food interactions, many other drugs have potentially severe interactions.

TABLE 14-4 Examples of Drug-Drug Interactions

Drug	Drug	Result of Drug Interaction
ACE inhibitors	Spironolactone	Increased serum potassium levels
Ciprofloxacin	Multivitamin with minerals	Decreased effect of ciprofloxacin because minerals in multivitamin can decrease antibiotic absorption if taken at same time
Digoxin	Verapamil and amiodarone	Digoxin toxicity
Theophylline	Quinolones	Theophylline toxicity

TABLE 14-5 Example of Warfarin Interactions with Drugs, Supplements, and Foods

Drugs		
Warfarin	Aspirin	Possible increased risk of bleeding
Warfarin	Phenytoin	Increased phenytoin or warfarin levels
Warfarin	Quinolones	Increased chance of bleeding
Warfarin	Sulfa drugs	Increased chance of bleeding
Warfarin	Cimetidine	Increased chance of bleeding
Warfarin	Heparin	Increased chance of bleeding
Warfarin	Amiodarone	Increased chance of bleeding
Warfarin	NSAIDs	Increased chance of bleeding
Supplements		
Warfarin	Gingko biloba	Increased chance of bleeding
Warfarin	Vitamin K	Decreased activity of warfarin
Warfarin	Garlic	Increased chance of bleeding
Warfarin	Ginseng	Decreased activity of warfarin
Warfarin	St. John's wort	Decreased activity of warfarin
Foods		
Warfarin	Broccoli and other green vegetables or foods high in vitamin K	Decreased effect of warfarin
Warfarin	Soybean and canola oils	Altered effect of warfarin
Warfarin	Cranberry juice	Altered effect of warfarin

Errors in the Pharmacy

No one wants to make an error, but when it does happen, negative feelings and assumptions may emerge. For example, it may seem that the person who made the mistake is careless, lazy, or untrained. The fear of being suspended or terminated is a frightening event to consider; the reality that a patient suffered as a result of an error is horrible. Additional fears are the legal ramifications of lawsuits and possible public humiliation. All of these fears are in the back of the technician's mind along with the constant need to maintain the workflow.

In fact, a pharmacy can fill 1000 prescriptions correctly but if 1 error occurs, the pharmacy management will likely counsel the technician and pharmacist to "be more careful," thus placing the blame on these employees specifically. This fear of being reprimanded adds to the stress on the pharmacy staff. Many times there is no action taken to review the overall process of how the mistake occurred.

Many pharmacy organizations and entities such as **MedWatch**, The Joint Commission, ISMP, MERP, and others have uncovered the need to study errors in a much different light. First, the need for open error reporting without fear of retaliation is essential if the root causes of errors will ever be revealed. Pharmacy staff needs to know they will not be punished; instead, the error will be examined and new strategies may be established that make it more difficult for errors to occur. It is important to have tools that can be utilized for error prevention. Even then, human factor errors will occur, but the goal is to decrease them as much as possible through the knowledge of how they occur. MedWatch and other error-reporting agencies encourage reporting all types of errors by both health care workers and the public. A MedWatch report can be accessed via the Internet, making it a simple way to report an error. A sample of a Med-Watch form is shown in Chapter 2 (Figure 2-3).

Although drug errors do not necessarily cause dire consequences for all patients, there are many instances in which they do. In these cases the only adequate outcome is to identify the causes of the error and establish safeguards that will prevent the error from recurring. For grieving family and friends this is of little help, and for the person(s) responsible this is a life-changing event that can result in loss of license, penalty fines, and, in certain instances, incarceration. Examples of fatal errors are listed in the following section.

DOCUMENTED ERRORS

- At least 17 babies were given overdoses of heparin, and 1 baby died in a Corpus Christi, Texas, hospital in 2008.
- In 2001, Terry Smith lost his life in Jacksonville, Florida when a technician typed out the prescription label for methadone to be taken prn when it was supposed to be taken bid. Terry died two days later after taking 22 tablets for chronic neurological pain. (Kevin McCoy, *USA TODAY: http://www.usatoday.com/money/industries/health/2008-02-12-pharmacy-errors_N.htm*)

MEDICATION ERRORS THAT INVOLVE ALLERGIES

Although many people are aware of the medications to which they are allergic, many allergic reactions cannot be avoided before drug administration.

While allergic reactions are not always medication errors, many people can have an allergic reaction as a result of the physician not documenting or reviewing the patient's allergies before prescribing medications. In 1 study of more than 50 patients hospitalized because of allergic reactions to medications, contributing factors to the allergic events were reported and included the following:

- Physician not aware of allergy (41%).
- Physician did not believe the allergy was real (5%).
- Physician aware of allergy but felt the benefit outweighed the risk (4%).
- Physician not aware that the agent was in the same class of drugs (3%).

The primary reasons for allergy-related prescribing errors included workload and failure to review the patient's drug history and profile. However, on most occasions the physician was alerted about the allergies by a nurse or a pharmacist, with most errors being prevented by pharmacists (Jones A, Como J: *Assessment of medication errors that involved drug allergies at a university hospital,* 2003. Accessed at www.medscape.com/viewarticle/458863).

PARENTERAL ERRORS

The most frightening errors are those that take effect quickly and may not be easily reversed. This is the case for parenteral medications. There have been several cases of heparin and insulin overdoses (see scenarios under the section titled How Errors Occur). Heparin is of great concern because it is common to flush intravenous (IV) lines with Hep-Lock solutions, which may be confused with the similarly sized and labeled vials of much more concentrated heparin solutions. In the hospital setting many floors keep several different concentrations of heparin and the labels can be confusing because they are similar in appearance. Potassium chloride (KCl) solutions are also problematic. There have been several cases of patients dying from the administration of concentrated KCl injections by personnel who misunderstood the labeling; concentrated KCl should never be given undiluted. As a result of these errors, concentrated KCl has been pulled from nursing floors and is strictly regulated by the pharmacy, yet errors can still occur.

Other considerations are given when administering parenterals. Pharmacy technicians need to be aware of the range of normal dosages, and if an ordered dose is suspect they need to alert the pharmacist immediately. For example, a patient with diabetes has orders for several IVs, which are normally prepared in dextrose. This order should be suspect because of the patient's diabetic condition. The physician may not want the medication prepared in dextrose but instead may wish to use normal saline.

SUSTAINED RELEASED (SR) DOSAGE FORM ERRORS

The clear advantage to sustained released medications is the ability of the patient to take his or her medication once daily rather than several times a day. This improves patient compliance and can ultimately result in better health. Directions that the dosage is in sustained-release form are usually printed below the drug name on the manufacturer's label. If an SR medication is given in place of a regular dose, then adverse effects can occur, including death. In addition, if a patient is receiving nourishment through a feeding tube and an SR dose is crushed, it becomes an immediate release (IR) dose that is much higher in strength and can result in an adverse reaction. Many errors occur because of suffixes on drug products that are not clearly understood. According to a report from ISMP, suffixes such as LA, CR, CD, ER, XL, and SR on drug products do not provide a clear meaning to indicate release properties or dosing frequency. The *USP* defines two categories of modified release formulations: delayed and extended release. Delayed release denotes a formulation that has a coating to delay release of the drug until the product has passed through the stomach. Extended release denotes any formulation designed to deliver the dose over a longer interval than an immediate release product of the same drug. Because of the confusion of suffixes (i.e., the choice of a wrong suffix, the use of an unclear suffix, or the omission of a proper suffix during prescription or dispensing), one form of drug may be given in place of the proper drug product.

Errors Related to Patient Care

NOSOCOMIAL INFECTIONS

Hospital-acquired infections have plagued hospital settings for decades. It is estimated that approximately 2 million patients suffer from these infections annually and that they are responsible for 90,000 deaths (*Hospitals & Health Networks,* Oct 2008). There are several reasons for infections to occur. Nurses, physicians, or any medical staff who have patient contact should wash their hands both before and after contact. If medication is contaminated at any point, this can cause the patient great harm, including nosocomial infections. When a patient is discharged it is important to clean any areas that were contacted by the patient. All hospitals and other institutions have infection control specialists who are responsible for the training of staff and patients as well as the investigation of all cases of hospital-acquired infections (HAIs). However, the training from institution to institution varies widely. Using Universal Precautions (e.g., hand washing) is a necessity in all institutions.

HOME HEALTH CARE ERRORS

More patients are discharged home with instructions for self-administration of medications or with the help of visiting nurses. This is due to rising costs associated with hospital stays. However, receiving care in the home also carries the risk of improper dosing and contamination to IV sets that may ultimately cause infections. The home-infusion industry has grown to an $11 billion industry annually (Laura Landro, *Wall Street Journal,* Oct 15, 2008). Many elderly and disabled patients do not have coverage for infusion sets and supplies because Medicare only covers the cost of medication. Self-dosing errors can increase the risk of an adverse effect. Patients may try to use medical supplies intended for single use more than once to try to save costs; poor aseptic technique may increase the risk of infection.

Age-Related Errors

MEDICAL ERRORS AND THE ELDERLY

Tech Alert!

Expired and improperly stored medicines can result in unintended effects. Expired tetracycline may cause kidney damage. Aspirin is converted to acetic acid (causing aspirin deterioration and lack of efficacy) after prolonged storage in a high-moisture area such as the bathroom.

More people are living into their 80s and beyond. Life expectancy in the United States has risen from 49 years (1900) to 79 years in this last century. One fast-growing segment of the population is persons more than 100 years of age (National Institute on Aging, 2003). This is due to several reasons that include increased activity, better dietary intake, and improved health care. Medication plays an important role in the longevity of persons suffering from various conditions such as osteoporosis, cardiovascular disease, and diabetes. It is estimated that 2.2 million older Americans are taking some type of medication and receiving various treatments (www.medicinenet.com, Salynn Boyles). These include prescription drugs, vitamins, minerals, supplements, herbals, and over-the-counter agents. Seniors mix these agents on a daily basis, and as the amount of medications increases so does the possibility of drug-drug interactions. People tend to believe that any medication purchased over-the-counter is safe. This is a misconception, especially when these agents are mixed with prescription medications. Consideration must be given to drug-food interactions as well. In addition, many older adults may forget to take their medication or may double the dose. These common errors can result in underdosing or overdosing.

MEDICAL ERRORS AND PEDIATRIC PATIENTS

Most of the emergency room (ER) cases (more than 66%) relating to pediatric patients and medication are due to overdosing of prescription and OTC medications. Most overdoses are primarily a result of failure to store medications in a secure area out of reach of children. In the United States alone more than 71,000 children under the age of 19 years are taken to the ER for unintentional overdoses of drugs kept at home. Toddlers (2-year-olds) were most likely to experience poisoning (Carilion Clinic: *Home medications cause most accidental poisonings,* Aug 2009; available at www.carilionclinic.org/Carilion/P09833).

Pictograms and the use of plain language have been shown to decrease the possibility of parents dosing their children inappropriately. Many parents have problems reading and understanding dosage instructions. This is more prevalent in multicultural areas where English is a second language. In a study conducted in an urban public hospital emergency room, a control group (standard labeling information) and an intervention group (using pictograms and plain language) were studied. Both were given standard instructions by the medical staff. Results showed that parent nonadherence was lower in the intervention group (9.3%) as compared to the control group (38%) (L. Barclay, Medscape, Sept 2, 2008). FDA committees have also suggested the use of new labeling on certain over-the-counter medications to ensure that parents receive proper advice before administering medications to young children. New labels read: "Do not dose children under the age of 4 years." In addition, the new labels state that a physician should be consulted for children ages 4 to 6 years. This has changed from the previous guidelines of not dosing children less than 2 years old. These changes in labeling (voluntarily done by manufacturers) will hopefully decrease the number of parents who administer incorrect doses or dose their children at the wrong time. In some cases, parents do not use the medication for its intended purpose.

Children and infants are also at risk of drug errors in a hospital setting, with incorrect dosing being the most commonly reported error. Dosing errors include computation errors of dosage and dosing intervals. Children vary in weight, body surface area, and organ system maturity; all of these factors affect their ability to both metabolize and excrete medication. In addition, there are not many standardized dosing regimens for children available, which increases the probability of drug errors. Various causes identified for errors in hospital settings include the procedure or protocol was not followed, miscommunication, inaccurate or omitted transcription, improper documentation, drug distribution system error, computer entry error, and lack of system safeguards (Prevention of medication errors in the pediatric inpatient setting, *Pediatrics* 112(2):431-436, Aug 2003. Available at http://aappolicy.aappublications.org/cgi/content/full/pediatrics;112/2/431).

How to Stop Errors from Occurring

A PHARMACIST'S DAILY ROUTINE

Most pharmacies are located in the retail setting and most pharmacists are overworked on a daily basis. Many pharmacies fill as many as 300 to 400 prescriptions a day and have to address discrepancies in orders as well as counsel patients. In addition, pharmacists must check the work of technicians.

The limited time that a rushed pharmacist has to check technicians' work adds to the potential for errors. Another potentially dangerous situation is when the same pharmacists and technicians work together for a long time. After pharmacists have worked many years with the same technicians a bond of trust may develop and pharmacists may become complacent about checking the technicians' work, either not checking it at all or just quickly scanning the completed order.

COMPUTERIZED PRESCRIPTION ORDER ENTRY (CPOE)

There are many new systems in place that are working toward decreasing errors. Many physicians use E-prescribing from the physician's office to the pharmacy or computerized prescription order entry (CPOE) by the prescriber in institutional settings. The idea behind this type of ordering (i.e., electronic ordering) is that it circumvents having to decipher poor handwriting because orders are sent via a computer directly to the pharmacy. However, there are many physicians and institutions who have not yet accepted this type of ordering. It should be noted that even when using the CPOE system, errors can still be made; selecting the wrong drug or dose from drop-down menus is still possible. In addition, introducing new technology often results in the introduction of new types of potential errors. More insurance companies and government-funded plans are applying pressure on physicians to use E-prescribing in order to be eligible for bonus payments. However, adoption of the technology can be costly, and in some cases, state or federal laws have not allowed for full adoption of E-prescribing in all circumstances (for example, allowing the prescribing of

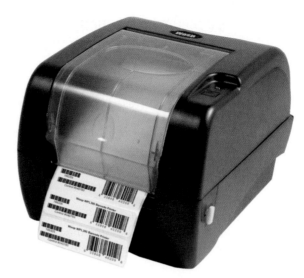

FIGURE 14-1 WPL305 desktop bar code printer. (Courtesy Wasp Barcode Technologies, © 2011.)

controlled substances). Data transmission standards must be agreed upon and adhered to by all technologies to ensure proper communication between devices and computer databases.

In hospitals and other inpatient institutions, the use of CPOE is becoming more popular along with bar coding methods (Figure 14-1). Bar codes provide the following three forms of identification of a drug:

- National Drug Code
- Lot number of the drug
- Expiration date of the drug

Although the overall risk of errors is decreased through the use of CPOE systems, they are not 100% error free. There are concerns about the lack of evaluation of their effectiveness because there are many different types being marketed. Potential dangers in certain CPOE systems include the following: the computerized software does not recognize discrepancies in prescribing between the outpatient medication regimen and the hospital treatment plan; many systems do not require prescribers to address computer alerts. (*Does computerized provider order entry reduce prescribing errors for hospital inpatients? A systematic review*. Available at www.jamia.org/cgi/content/full/16/5/613.)

The following are other concerns pertaining to CPOE systems:

- Ordering and administration: Misidentification of patients and patient variables (e.g., height and weight)
- Mismatch of drug orders to chemotherapy protocols or miscalculations*

The problems with these systems are due to new technology. It takes time to address the flaws, which may be why many hospitals are slow at implementing these new systems. Also, it is very time-consuming to electronically connect all the necessary personnel and still ensure that patient confidentiality is maintained. It also takes time to understand new steps in health care professional workflow. For example, after physicians see their patients, they can sit at a

*Error reduction in pediatric chemotherapy. Available at http://archpedi.ama-assn.org/cgi/reprint/160/5/495.pdf?ijkey=22818b58f60fb802b3176c790503ed87e863f708.

BOX 14-2 ORGANIZATIONS THAT TRACK ERRORS

- FDA's MedWatch
- Institute of Medicine (IOM)
- Institute for Safe Medication Practices (ISMP)
- National Coordinating Council for Medication Error Reporting and Prevention (NCC MERP)
- *United States Pharmacopeia (USP)* Medication Errors Reporting Program and MEDMARX
- The Joint Commission (TJC)

computer or use a handheld device to enter new or changed orders and send them directly to the pharmacy. Nurses may also enter additional nursing notes that are documented in the system.

Reporting Errors

The most important aspect of errors is the reporting process. In years past, the most common response to an error was to place blame on the person who caused the error and then tell the person to be more careful. This type of response was found to be nonproductive because most people will not report errors if they know they will be reprimanded. Also trying to "be more careful" does not give the person the tools necessary to avoid further errors. Therefore the emphasis towards finding ways to reduce errors has been found to be more productive. For this reason the tracking systems in place do not focus on blame but are more interested in how the error occurred. In this way, the reasons why an error occurred can be examined and constructive changes can be made and tracked. An example of the types of organizations that track errors in this way are listed in Box 14-2.

The FDA has a new agency, the Office of Postmarketing Drug Risk Assessment, that evaluates new brand names to prevent sound-alike drug names. They work with the drug companies in changing drug names if they sound too much alike.

ISMP tracks drug errors and works toward decreasing them through Medication Errors Reporting Prevention (MERP). This can be accessed via the Internet, where health care workers can report incidences of errors, near-errors, or hazardous conditions in the workplace. When reporting incidences, questions concerning how the error was discovered and recommendations for preventing recurrence of the error are included in the report. Specific incidences include the following:

Administering the wrong:
  Drug, dose, strength, route of administration, dosage form
Errors in:
  Prescribing medications
  Transcribing medications
  Dispensing medications
  Monitoring medications
  Performing calculations
  Preparing medications
MERP recommendations:
- **Medication error understanding:** Improves the collection, classification, and analysis of data linked to types, causes, and sources of error as well as the impact of errors on patients. Tracking medication errors

in a systematic manner and prioritizing reduction activities are also included.

- **Medication error reporting:** Increases awareness of reporting systems available, such as Medication Error Reporting Prevention (MERP), MEDMARX, and MedWatch (FDA). These programs maintain a classification system that identifies types of errors; the data obtained can then be used to analyze and report error statistics.
- **Medication error prevention:** With continuous research and reporting, areas can be identified where changes can be made to prevent future errors. This includes distinctive packaging, labeling, and nomenclature for drugs that are at high risk of errors.

Reporting can be done anonymously and voluntarily without fear of retribution. The MERP institute reviews all medication error reports, attempts to understand the reason(s) for errors, and works toward producing initiatives to educate and improve medication safety. The following five guidelines are used to share information with health care professionals about potentially dangerous events:

1. Knowledge
2. Analysis—the evaluation of data
3. Education
   a. Providing confidential consulting services to health care system to proactively evaluate medication systems
   b. Educational programs that include:
      i. Teleconferences on medications and issues
      ii. Patient resources (posters, pamphlets, videos, books, etc.)
   c. High drug alerts (newsletter) and potentially dangerous abbreviations.
4. Cooperation
   a. Working with other entities:
      i. Legislative and regulatory bodies
      ii. Health care practitioners
      iii. Health care institutions
      iv. Regulatory and accrediting agencies
      v. Pharmaceutical industry
5. Communication
   a. Bringing information to:
      i. Consumers
      ii. Employers
      iii. Health care providers
   b. Providing a voluntary reporting program

One of the areas of concern is the use of abbreviations. Many have been misinterpreted, which has resulted in drug errors. ISMP has provided a list of terms to be avoided (Table 5-2); they recommend that the term be spelled out completely.

The Joint Commission is another organization that helps institutions implement safety standards to decrease errors. They have outlined the following 5 areas for patient safety, each having 10 criteria:

1. **Leadership Process and Accountability: Summary**
   Leadership structure, individual accountability, policies and procedures (in all areas), and the managing of daily operations are identified. The institution is compliant with all laws and regulations. Leaders are educated about quality and are actively involved in setting quality and safety priorities. Both leaders and managers collaborate on quality and patient safety

activities (e.g., patient assessments, medication use systems). Organization provides a mechanism that is based on the safety of the patient as it relates to any type of drug research and/or organ transplant that may take place through data collection, analysis, and improvement.

2. **Competent and Capable Workforce: Summary**

   Personnel files contain credentials of all employees (e.g., education, training, licensure, work history, and copies of evaluations). Personnel job descriptions match their credentials. Proper training is given in areas including cardiopulmonary resuscitation (CPR), basic life support (BLS), infection prevention, and safety. Staff health and safety standards are met, and accurate patient records are reviewed and transferred to appropriate unit/nurse. Review of credentials, licensure, education, training, and competence of physicians. Review of nurses' ability to provide appropriate patient services based on their competence, license, training, and education. Review of credentials of other health professionals. Health care students within the institution must be adequately monitored, supervised, and oriented to patient safety.

3. **Safe Environment for Staff and Patients: Summary**

   Regular safety inspections of the building's environment (e.g., broken furniture, faulty equipment, missing signs) and fire safety measures (i.e., must work properly, exits not blocked). Water quality and electrical sources that are required 24 hours a day, 7 days a week work properly; alternate source plans in place to ensure the safety of patients. Proper use and maintenance of all biomedical equipment and biohazardous materials. Education, training, and certification (if applicable) of employees on infection prevention and control; includes proper disposal of needles and infectious wastes. Hand hygiene program with documented guidelines. Reduction of health care–associated infections through proper implementation of hand hygiene program and barrier techniques (e.g., gloves, masks, eye protection).

4. **Clinical Care of Patients: Summary**

   Patient's identification is checked before medication, blood products, treatments, or procedures are administered. Patients understand the risks, treatments, and procedures before giving consent. Medical and nursing assessments are documented in the patient's record in a reasonable time frame so treatment can take place as soon as possible. Laboratory and diagnostic services are available, reliable, and safe. Consent forms are completed for all treatments and/or procedures. Patient education and training are provided so that patients can participate in their own care (e.g., granting consent during hospitalization and learning proper medication use after discharge). All services (e.g., surgery, anesthesia, postsurgical unit) are appropriate to the patient needs.

5. **Improving Quality and Safety: Summary**

   There must be an adverse event reporting system and the system must be analyzed. Changes are made to increase patient safety based on causes of adverse events; these include medication errors, unanticipated death of a patient, surgery on the wrong patient or body part, and patient falls. High-risk patients are monitored (e.g., immunosuppressed, comatose, emergency care patients). Patient and staff satisfaction is monitored within the facility for improvement purposes. A complaint process is in place for both patients and family members. Staff understands how to improve processes by participation in improvement activities. Clinical outcomes are monitored and improved if necessary. Quality and safety information is communicated to staff via newsletters, reports, and posters, for example, to improve patient safety.

One of the primary responsibilities of The Joint Commission is to review documentation that tracks progress in each of these areas. For a comprehensive outline of the five safety standards visit www.jointcommission.org.

VERBAL ORDERING ERROR PREVENTION

MERP suggests verbal communication of prescriptions or medication orders should be limited to urgent situations in which immediate written or electronic communication is not feasible. Health care organizations should establish policies and procedures regarding verbal orders, including the following:

- Describe limitations or prohibitions on use of verbal orders
- Provide a mechanism to ensure validity/authenticity of the prescriber
- List the elements required for inclusion in a complete verbal order
- Describe situations in which verbal orders may be used
- List and define the individuals who may send and receive verbal orders

PARENTERAL MEDICATION ERROR PREVENTION

There have been many tragic outcomes from overdosing IV medications or administering the wrong drug (see scenarios under section titled How Errors Occur). The effects of an IV error are manifested very quickly and may not be reversed in time. A summit was held with ASHP, ISMP, The Infusion Nurses Society, the National Patient Safety Foundation, and The Joint Commission to propose strategies for safe IV practices (www.ashp.org/iv-summit). The strategies are outlined as follows:

- Standardizing product concentrations, patient care procedures, and equipment
- Developing toolkits and other resource materials to enhance the adoption of the recommendations
- Improving mechanisms for communicating in a timely manner specific information about medication errors that can reduce the likelihood of similar events occurring elsewhere

Common Pharmacy Technology

BAR CODING

To avoid dosing the wrong medication to the patient, bar coding systems at the bedside are being used in many institutions. When the nurse is about to administer a medication, he or she first scans the bar code of the patient's wristband against the bar code of the medication. If there is a discrepancy an alarm sounds, notifying the nurse of a problem. Although the electronic communication between physician, pharmacy, and nursing does reduce the number of errors, there are problems with the system. For example, if the nurse scans an alternative dose strength (e.g., two 5-mg tablets are substituted for one 10-mg tablet), the system reads this as an error. The nurse must then override the computer to administer the medication.

ROBOT RX MACHINES

Large robotic machines have been used for many years in some hospitals. Patient medication records are read by the machine through the use of bar

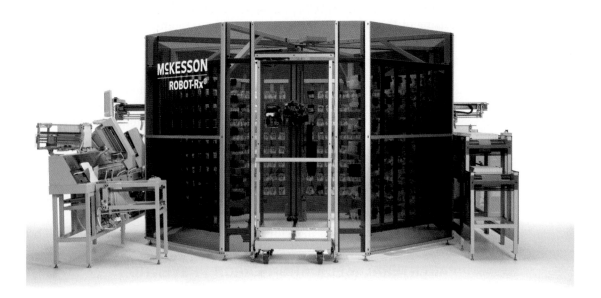

FIGURE 14-2 Robot Rx machine. (Courtesy of McKesson Corp., © 2011.)

coding; the appropriate medication's bar code is scanned from the package and then matched to the electronic medication administration record (E-MAR). Once verified, the machine will pull from a rack of prepacked unit dose medications that are stored within the unit. The medications are placed into a patient drawer, from which they can be delivered to the appropriate floor. These large fillers are expensive and require a large area to function. See Figure 14-2 for a robot Rx machine.

AUTOMATED DISPENSING SYSTEMS (ADS)

Automated Dispensing Systems (ADS) machines have been used for years in hospitals and institutions; ADS machines store unit-dosed medications and nursing supplies to be accessed by nurses on patient floors (see Figure 13-7). The pharmacy receives an order and enters it into the ADS computer, which then allows the nurse to access the medication via patient name. These systems work effectively if the medication in the drawer is correct; however, if the wrong medication is loaded into the drawer and the nurse fails to catch the mistake, then an error can occur. If, however, this system is coupled with bar coding, this greatly decreases the risk of errors. Each cubicle has an attached bar code that identifies the medication; when the technician attempts to fill the cubicle, he or she must match the bar code on the cubicle to the bar code on the medication. Then the nurse can use the bar code to match it to the patient.

COMMUNITY PHARMACY ADS MACHINES

For many years, automated dispensing systems have been used in community pharmacy. They are available in many different sizes to accommodate prescription load. Bar coding is used to verify the correct dosage is being dispensed to the correct patient. The following three main types of robotics are used in community pharmacy:

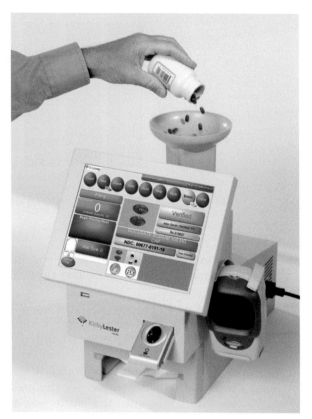

FIGURE 14-3 KL20. (Courtesy of Kirby Lester LLC, © 2011.)

- Tabletop automatic pill counters, such as model KL20 by Kirby Lester, are used for counting as well as verifying every order. The device instructs the technician to first scan the patient's prescription label and then scan the bottle of medication to ensure a match (of medication, dosage, and quantity to be dispensed). The device's touch-screen displays a picture of the medication as well as specific information about the drug. The tablets or capsules are then poured into a hopper and are counted electronically. The device estimates the correct vial size (in drams) to use. The medication is then dispensed into a tray, and the technician pours its contents into a vial. A technician can fill a typical prescription with a KL20 device in 3 to 6 seconds. (Figure 14-3).
- The second type of robotics in pharmacy are large wall units that use cassettes, such as Baker Cell systems. The number of cassettes is limited only by the wall space available, and each cassette holds an assortment of preloaded medications. Again, the bar code on the prescription label is scanned and the appropriate amount is then dispensed. The pharmacist then scans the bottle for a final check. A screen displays the correct appearance of the medication along with specific information on the drug.
- The third type uses robot technology, such as the SP 200 System by ScriptPro. This system is a fully automated robotic prescription dispensing system. It accepts prescription dispensing instructions from pharmacy computers and delivers filled and labeled vials at a rate of up to 100 prescriptions per hour (Figure 14-4).

There are many types of community pharmacy automated systems and software programs that are available, although they are very expensive and

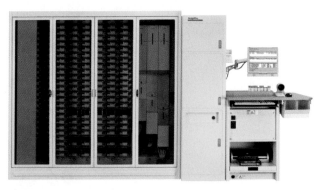

FIGURE 14-4 SP 200 robotic prescription dispensing system. (Courtesy of ScriptPro, © 2011.)

require training to use. More pharmacies are using these systems so they can fill more prescriptions in less time and concurrently reduce errors.

Patient Dose-Specific Orders

In the past, when patients required a large amount of liquids over a 24-hour period, a bulk bottle was placed in the patient's drawer. Also if the liquid was not available in unit dose form, it would be sent in bulk form. The nurse would pour the proper amount per the medication administration record (MAR) and use the liquid until the bottle was empty. The nurse would then send a refill request to the pharmacy. The bottles sometimes would be labeled with just the patient's name and room number. Because specific dosing instructions were not denoted on the bottle, there was an increased likelihood for the nurse to dose the liquid medication inappropriately. Also, opening and closing lids can increase the risk of contamination of a medication. The pharmacy must have control over each dose to ensure accuracy. The Joint Commission requires hospitals and institutions to prepack all liquid doses in oral syringes or containers. Each dose is prepared by the technician and is labeled with the patient's name, medical record number, and room number. In addition, the name of the drug, dose, strength, and time of administration are indicated on each dose. In this way, each dose is strictly controlled by the pharmacy. There are automated robots that can also fill and label doses, reducing the time needed by a technician to fill daily doses.

USP <797> Regulations

One of the regulations established by *USP <797>* addresses the problem of contamination of any type of sterile product. The adoption of *USP <797>* has been one of the most drastic changes made to any pharmacy that prepares sterile products, such as IVs and other parenterals. Because of the new regulations, many pharmacies are contracting their sterile preparations to companies that specialize and have met all guidelines of *USP <797>*. Chapter 12 lists specifics of *USP <797>* regulations.

Drug Labeling

Drug companies are urged to make several changes in their labeling of any type of medication that can be confusing or misinterpreted. Through the use of color coding and tall man and boldface lettering, drug selection errors are less likely to occur. For example, using tall man lettering for hydrOXYzine versus hydrALAzine helps differentiate the medications. Changes to drug stocking include placing "Name Alert" stickers on the bins holding problematic sound-alike or look-alike drugs or placing the bins in different areas of the pharmacy to reduce the possibility of pulling the wrong drug. Drug companies have been encouraged to name their new drugs differently from other medications to help reduce confusion.

BOXED WARNINGS

Certain medications that have been known to cause severe reactions have an additional warning to highlight the information on the package insert (official FDA-approved prescribing information). These warnings are often called Black Box Warnings because the warnings are inside an outlined black box on the package insert. The boxed warnings highlight any serious adverse effects of the drug being prescribed (Chapter 2).

Training and Education

One of the best ways to decrease errors is through training and education. Many states do not have standardized exams or use the national exam to pretest technicians. Some states do not even fingerprint or conduct a background check on pharmacy technicians. There are many schools that have pharmacy technician programs but do not have any accreditation or standards of learning. Many large pharmacies train their own employees to become technicians. The **Pharmacy Technician Certification Board (PTCB)** and ASHP have worked toward implementing training standards. In addition to certification it is important for the technician to consistently self-educate through staff meetings, continuing education, and journal reports.

Beyond certification and continuous training, technicians should always check each prescription three times throughout the filling process. If anything about the prescription seems unclear or confusing, the pharmacist should be notified immediately.

The **Pharmacy Technician Education Council** (PTEC) is an organization of instructors whose goals are to improve teaching techniques and competencies of students. Members include both Canadian and U.S. instructors. As technicians' initial training improves they are more able to address probable errors and to recognize questionable doses. More education is needed and must be continuously updated as technology and drug delivery methods change.

ASHP

This association has developed a model curriculum for pharmacy technician training. This model can be used in educational settings as well as in the pharmacy to ensure technicians are competent in all necessary areas. Several updates have been made to the model. The following four components are included in the guide:

* Goal statements, objectives, and instructional objectives
* A curriculum map with suggested sequencing of the modules of instruction
* Descriptors for each of the instruction modules
* A tracking document that identifies where teaching is offered for each objective and instructional objectives

ASHP also works with each individual state trying to institute programs and require national certification for all technicians.

Medication Reconciliation

The **Institute for Healthcare Improvement** (IHI) has defined medication reconciliation as the process of identifying the most up-to-date list of all the medications a patient is currently taking. The IHI reported that more than 50% of all errors in hospitals are due to poor communication of medication orders. The necessary information required to clearly analyze a patient's needs includes the following:

- Name of drug
- Dosage
- Frequency
- Route of administration

Reconciliation needs to be performed in all pharmacy settings, although each type of pharmacy must develop its own specific strategies. In institutional settings it is important to compare this current list of medications at the time of admission, at the time of any transfer within the facility, after surgeries, and at the time of discharge. The goal is to ensure the patient is being given the proper medications at all points as he or she moves through the health care system. In this way any errors can be identified promptly. The following three steps are involved in medication reconciliation:

- Verification—Attaining the patient's medication history and other medical information. This includes all medications and OTC drugs.
- Clarification—Making sure the medication and dosages are appropriate for the patient. The current physician's orders are compared to the patient's medication list.
- Reconciliation—Clinical decisions are made based on the comparison between the two drug lists. Resolving any observed discrepancies or errors through documentation and direct communication is the final step.

Reconciliation involves several parties—the patient, physician, nurse, and pharmacist. Orders must be rewritten each time the patient is transferred to or from the intensive care unit (ICU) or returns from surgery. In the past, physicians would sometimes write to "resume previous medications." This allowed misinterpretation of the medications being dosed. It was much easier to lose track of the medications the patient was taking. This resulted in adverse drug reactions and possible harm to the patient. The Joint Commission has since prohibited the use of these "blanket orders." At each point throughout the course of treatment the previous medications must be compared to the current orders. Normally, facilities use a reconciliation form (Figure 14-5) that can be viewed by the physician, nurse, and pharmacist. In addition, at the time of discharge, the community pharmacy must perform reconciliation. Finally, the patient must be informed about the current instructions as compared to any previous instructions.

Other Considerations

Other conditions that can help reduce errors when filling prescriptions include using good lighting to clearly read the label and checking the drug against the prescription. Also, filling protocol systems must be reviewed and altered if they can potentially cause an error. Decreasing the fear and anxiety of reporting errors should be implemented in all medical settings. Checking a prescription several times to ensure it is correct should also be implemented. Physicians should use the metric system when writing doses. In the future, all prescriptions

Patient Name
MRN

MEDICATION RECONCILIATION FORM

ADMISSION / POINT OF ENTRY RECONCILIATION

- The first nurse to interview the patient should initiate completion of this form. Additional nurses and clinicians may continue to use the same form for the same patient.
- Circle all sources of information: Patient   Caregiver   Rx bottle   EMS   Primary provider   Other:_____

ALLERGIES AND ADVERSE DRUG REACTIONS : _____

ACTIVE MEDICATION LIST				Date of Admission / Point of Entry:			RECONCILIATION
List below all medications patient was taking at time of admission. *(Dosing information REQUIRED, if available.)*							Continue on Admission?
Medication Name	Dose	Route	Frequency	Last Dose (Date/Time)	Date	Initials	Circle **Y** (yes) or **N** (no)*
1.							Y N
2.							Y N
3.							Y N
4.							Y N
5.							Y N
6.							Y N
7.							Y N
8.							Y N
9.							Y N
10.							Y N
11.							Y N
12.							Y N
13.							Y N
14.							Y N
15.							Y N
OTC Medications, Herbals, etc.							
							Y N
							Y N
							Y N
							Y N

*If order to be discontinued, see Admitting Note for comments.

Medication list recorded by RN/MD/PA/NP/LPN/RPh							
Initials	Print Name/Stamp	Signature	Date	Initials	Print Name/Stamp	Signature	Date

Reconciling Prescriber (MD/PA/NP/CNM)			
Print Name/Stamp	Signature	Title	Date

TRANSFER RECONCILIATION	DISCHARGE RECONCILIATION
<ul><li>See Physician Orders for active medication orders upon transfer.</li><li>See Medication Administration Record for last dose given.</li></ul>	<ul><li>See Patient Discharge Plan for list of medications patient should continue after discharge.</li><li>Discharge plan should include stopped medications.</li></ul>
Reconciling Prescriber (**Provide name, date, signature.**)	Reconciling Prescriber (**Provide name, date, signature.**)

☐   Check here if multiple pages needed. Please indicate: Page ____ of ____

FIGURE 14-5 Sample reconciliation form.

BOX 14-3 METHODS TO AVOID ERRORS IN THE PHARMACY

- Medication name alerts
- CPOE systems
- Bar coding
- ADS machines
- Software systems used for identification
- Pharmacy robots
- Tall man lettering
- Color coding
- Education
- Training
- Altering system factors such as clutter, lighting, workflow, distractions, interruptions, poorly designed procedures, stress, fear of reporting errors
- Patient dose-specific repackaging
- Medication reconciliation

should be electronic rather than written, because this will greatly improve clarity. Software systems must be improved to aid the pharmacy in identifying potential problems with dosing regimens.

There is no simple solution to prevent drug errors. It is true that many of the electronic software and hardware systems that are being implemented in pharmacy, institutions, physicians' offices, and clinics are helping to reduce errors, but these systems can malfunction. The ability to catch mistakes before they occur will always be the responsibility of the personnel involved in the prescribing, filling, and dosing of medications. For this reason it is imperative that every health care worker views drug error prevention as a priority. Only through continuous education and training can errors be controlled, now and in the future. A summary of practices that can be used to reduce the occurrence of medication errors is given in Box 14-3.

Through consistent monitoring and evaluation of drug errors, the number of errors can be greatly decreased. One must approach each action taken in the pharmacy and other medication settings as requiring 100% commitment to the goal of perfection. Manipulation and interpretation of drugs and drug orders can mean the difference between life and death to a patient. Reporting drug errors can help instigate a change in the current protocol of a pharmacy that can stop further errors of the same type from recurring. Technicians play an integral part in helping to identify errors.

DO YOU REMEMBER THESE KEY POINTS?

- The main causes of drug errors
- The increased risk of medication errors in pediatric and geriatric patients
- How medication reconciliation can reduce drug errors
- The three steps involved in medication reconciliation
- Look-alike, sound-alike drugs
- The types of automated systems used to decrease drug errors
- The areas where drug errors occur
- ISMP's guidelines on abbreviations that should be avoided
- Where to report an adverse drug event
- How *USP <797>* compliance can reduce drug errors
- The use of bar coding to verify medications
- How CPOE can reduce the number of confusing drug orders

Multiple choice questions

1. Of the reasons listed below, which one is NOT related to errors?
   A. Stress levels
   B. Orders arriving from different sources
   C. Multitasking
   D. Noise

2. Which of the following abbreviations should NOT be used according to ISMP?
   A. uD
   B. bid
   C. qod
   D. All of the above should not be used

3. ASHP strives to:
   A. Improve standards of learning for technicians
   B. Require the national certification of technicians
   C. Require the state registration of technicians
   D. All of the above are true

4. The Joint Commission's regulation concerning dosing patients includes:
   A. Preparing all oral medications in unit dose containers
   B. Using bar coding
   C. Using POS for ordering medications
   D. None of the above

5. A diabetic patient is ordered cefazolin in D_5W IV q8h. What possible problem may exist in this order?
   A. The dose is given too often.
   B. Cefazolin can only be given IM.
   C. D_5W may be the wrong solution because the patient has diabetes.
   D. A diabetic patient cannot be given cefazolin because of a possible allergic reaction.

6. Baker Cell systems can be used:
   A. In hospitals
   B. In community pharmacies
   C. In nursing homes
   D. Both A and C are correct

7. Which of the following contributes to drug errors?
   A. SR capsules versus regular capsules
   B. Look-alike drugs
   C. Lack of education
   D. All of the above

8. What changes have been made to pediatric OTC dosing?
   A. Pictograms
   B. New strengths in the medication
   C. New dosage forms
   D. All of the above

9. The most common IV medication(s) involved in overdosing is (are):
   A. Heparin
   B. Warfarin
   C. Insulin
   D. Both A and C

10. Drug errors can be reported to:
   A. The FDA's MedWatch
   B. ISMP MER Program
   C. IOM
   D. All of the above

11. Home health insurance coverage does NOT typically include:
   A. Medications
   B. Physicians' visits
   C. Consultation
   D. Home IV supplies

12. The organization that accredits pharmacy technician schools is:
   A. PTCB
   B. ASHP
   C. PTEC
   D. TJC

13. Education and training methods include:
   A. Continuing education
   B. Staff meetings
   C. Journal reports
   D. All of the above

14. Technicians need to be proficient in the following areas:
   A. Knowing normal medication doses
   B. Being aware of drugs that have similar looks and/or names
   C. Paying attention to detail
   D. All of the above

15. The most important factor in drug error prevention is:
   A. Automated systems
   B. Reporting drug errors
   C. Reporting and education of drug errors
   D. Medical intervention

True/False

If a statement is false, then change it to make it true.

_____   **1.** All errors can be solved through the use of automated machines.

_____   **2.** Seniors have more interactions with medications.

_____   **3.** Bar coding can decrease errors in giving the wrong medication.

_____   **4.** Black Box Warnings are printed on all medications.

_____   **5.** Medications wrongly taken at home are not counted as an error.

_____   **6.** Reported drug errors usually results in the person reporting the error being reprimanded.

_____   **7.** All errors can be avoided through education and training.

_____   **8.** Black Box Warnings are listed in the *PDR*.

_____   **9.** About one half of ER visits in urban areas are related to allergic reactions to antibiotics.

_____   **10.** Only pharmacists can load ADS machines with medications.

_____   **11.** Both physicians and nurses can use handheld devices for order entry or review.

_____   **12.** Humans will always commit errors.

_____   **13.** The FDA is the only reporting organization that tracks drug errors.

_____   **14.** Bar codes list the drug's expiration date, lot number, and amount of drug per container.

_____   **15.** Sound-alike and look-alike drugs should be kept in different areas of the pharmacy or labeled with Name Alert stickers.

TECHNICIAN'S CORNER

Read the order below: List drug(s) or sig(s) that may be mistaken in this order. Indicate what you would do if you were given this order. List at least three ways in which this order could have been safely transcribed.

BIBLIOGRAPHY

Am J Health-Syst Pharma-Vol 58 June 1, 2001. Developing and maintaining up-to-date training for pharmacy technicians.
www.ashp.org/s_ashp/docs/files/DevTechTraining.pdf

American Society of Hospital Pharmacies Guidelines on Preventing Medication Errors in Hospitals
www.ashp.org/s_ashp/docs/files/MedMis_Gdl_Hosp.pdf

Bates DW MD, MSC: Sustained-release Preparations and Medication Errors. *J General Internal Medicine* 2002 August; 17(8): 657-658
www.pubmedcentral.nih.gov/articlerender.fcgi?artid=1495086

Boyles S WebMD: Health News. Older Americans Take Risky Drug Combos. www.MedicineNet.com.

West D, R.Ph., Ph.D, Hastings J, Pharm. D, Earley A, Pharm. D, Candidate University of Arkansas for Medical Sciences, College of Pharmacy: An Economic Justification of the Use of Dispensing Technologies in Independent Community Pharmacies. www.ncpafoundation.org/downloads/asset_upload_file169_7723.pdf

FDA National Pharmacy: NCC MERP issues Guide to Help Non-hospital Settings Decrease Medication Errors. Referenced 9/09. www.nabp.net/ftpfiles/newsletters/nationalnews/NATL012004.pdf.

FDA Newsletter.

Human Longevity and Aging Research: Statement before the United States Senate, Special Committee on Aging. Richard J. Hodes, M.D. Director National Institute on Aging, June 3, 2003. www.nia.nih.gov/AboutNIA/BudgetRequests/HLAgingResearch.htm

International Essentials of Health Care Quality and Patient Safety. Joint Commission International. 2008. Referenced 8/09. www.jointcommissioninternational.org/common/pdfs/consulting/JCI-essentials-framework.pdf

J Gen Intern Med. 2002 August 17(8): 657-658 Sustained-release Preparations and Medication Errors Bates DW, MD, MSC. www.ashp.org/iv-summit

Medication Errors Injure 1.5 Million People and Cost Billions of Dollars Annually; Report Offers Comprehensive Strategies for Reducing Drug-Related Mistakes. www8.nationalacademies.org/onpinews/newsitem.aspx?RecordID=11623

Merck Manuals. Online Medical Library. Drug Errors. 2005. Referenced 9/09.

Drug Errors. www.merck.com/mmpe/sec20/ch302/ch302c.html

Merck Manuals. Online Medical Library. Drug Errors. 2005. Referenced 9/09.

Adverse Drug Effects in the Elderly. www.merck.com/mmpe/sec20/ch306/ch306d.html#CHDJHFCC

Modern Medicine. Drug Topics-Pharmacy mistake blamed for heparin overdoses at Texas hospital. July 11, 2008 by Mark R Lowery, Managing Editor. Source, DrugTopics.
www.modernmedicine.com/modernmedicine/Drug+Topics+Daily+News/Pharmacy-mistake-blamed-for-heparin-overdoses-at-T/ArticleStandard/Article/detail/529076

Recommendations to Reduce Medication Errors Associated with Verbal Medication Orders and Prescriptions. www.nccmerp.org/council/council2001-02-20.html

Siecker, Bruce Ph.D., R.Ph. Rx Errors, Mix-ups, and Near Misses.

To Err Is Human: Building a Safer Health System. November 11. Institute of Medicine.www.iom.edu/Object.File/Master/4/117/ToErr-8pager.pdf

Warfarin Interactions. www.mitamins.com/library/Drug/Warfarin.html

McCoy K: USA Today: http://www.usatoday.com/money/industries/health/2008-02-12-pharmacy-errors_N.htm)

Jones A, Como J: Assessment of medication errors that involved drug allergies at a university hospital, 2003. Accessed at www.medscape.com/viewarticle/458863).

Campaign to Prevent Antimicrobial Resistance in Healthcare Settings http://www.cdc.gov/drugresistance/healthcare/problem.htm

Hospitals & Health Networks. Hospital-acquired Infections: Leadership Challenges: http://www.hhnmag.com/hhnmag_app/jsp/articledisplay.jsp?dcrpath=HHNMAG/Article/data/10OCT2008/0810HHN_FEA_Dialogue&domain=HHNMAG

Prevention of medication errors in the pediatric inpatient setting, Pediatrics 112(2):431-436, Aug 2003. Available at http://aappolicy.aappublications.org/cgi/content/full/pediatrics;112/2/431).

Nursing error by Marc Green. Expanded version of Nursing error and human nature, J Nurs Law 9:37-44, 2004.

Smetzer JL, Cohen MR: (1998). Lessons from the Denver medication error/criminal negligence case: Look beyond blaming individuals. Hospital Pharmacy, 33, 640-657.

(Radwan C: Pharmacy technicians face states' scrutiny, regulation, Drug Topics, Aug 25, 2009. Available at http://drugtopics.modernmedicine.com/drugtopics/Associations/Pharmacy-technicians-face-states-scrutiny-regulati/ArticleStandard/Article/detail/621364).

Does computerized provider order entry reduce prescribing errors for hospital inpatients? A systematic review. Available at www.jamia.org/cgi/content/full/16/5/613.)

SECTION

two

Body Systems

Endocrine System

Objectives

UPON COMPLETING THIS CHAPTER, YOU SHOULD BE ABLE TO DO THE FOLLOWING:

- Write the generic and trade names for all drugs discussed in this chapter.

- List classifications and indications of each drug discussed.

- Name the major glands of the body.

- Describe the location and function of the glands discussed.

- Differentiate between the endocrine and exocrine glands.

- Explain the role of iodine in the metabolism of hormones of the thyroid gland.

- Explain the role of calcium in bones.

- Describe the causes and symptoms of osteoporosis.

- Describe the conditions caused by improper gland functioning.

- List the primary hormones that are produced in women and men.

- Explain the uses of androgen hormone replacement in men and women.

- List the causes of diabetes mellitus.

- Describe the differences between insulin-dependent diabetes mellitus and non–insulin-dependent diabetes mellitus.

- Explain the relationship between the central nervous system and the release of hormones from the adrenal gland.

- List the primary side effects of the medications discussed in the chapter.

- List the auxiliary labels required when filling prescriptions for hormones.

Addison's disease *Condition resulting in a decrease in levels of adrenocortical hormones such as mineralocorticoids and glucocorticoids, which causes symptoms including muscle weakness and weight loss*

Autocrine *Denoting a mode of hormone action in which a hormone binds to receptors on the cell and affects the function of the cell type that produced it*

Autoimmune disease *Condition in which a person's tissues are attacked by his or her immune system; abnormal antigen-antibody reaction*

Catecholamines *The hormones made in the brainstem, nervous system, and adrenal glands. They help the body respond to stress and prepare the body for the "fight or flight" response. They are important to heart rate, blood pressure, and nervous system functions*

Calcitonin *A thyroid hormone that helps regulate blood concentrations of calcium and phosphate and promotes the formation of bone*

Cretinism *Condition in which the development of the brain and body is inhibited by a congenital lack of thyroid hormone secretion*

Cushing's disease *Condition causing an increase in secretion of adrenocortical hormones; includes symptoms such as moon face (moon facies) and deposits of fat (buffalo hump)*

Cushing's syndrome *Although Cushing's disease is specifically caused by an adenoma of the pituitary gland that results in an increase in ACTH and cortisol levels, Cushing's syndrome is a complex set of symptoms that may have multiple causes (e.g., corticosteroid therapy)*

Diabetes mellitus *A complex disorder of carbohydrate, fat, and protein metabolism that is primarily a result of a deficiency or complete lack of insulin secretion from cells within the pancreas. Three primary types include the following: type 1 diabetes mellitus, an autoimmune process that is dependent on insulin to prevent ketosis; type 2 diabetes mellitus, adult-onset, ketosis-resistant diabetes that is non–insulin-dependent; gestational diabetes mellitus, occurs in women that become glucose intolerant during pregnancy*

Exophthalmos *Prominence (protrusion) of the eyeball out of the orbit; bilateral presentation commonly caused by increased thyroid hormone*

Glucose *Also known as a simple sugar; a very important carbohydrate in biology; it is the primary source of energy fuel for cells and its levels are measurable in the blood*

Goiter *Condition in which the thyroid gland is enlarged because of a lack of iodine; can be either a simple goiter or a toxic goiter (i.e., resulting from a tumor)*

Graves' disease *Condition caused by hypersecretion of thyroid hormones, symptoms include diffuse goiter, exophthalmos, and skin changes*

Homeostasis *The equilibrium pertaining to the balance of the body with respect to fluid levels, pH level, osmotic pressures, and concentrations of various substances*

Hormones *Chemical substances produced and secreted by an endocrine duct into the bloodstream that result in a physiological response at a specific target tissue*

Hypercalcemia *Elevated concentration of calcium in the blood*

Hyperglycemia *Elevated concentration of glucose in the blood*

Hypocalcemia *Low concentration of calcium in the blood*

Hypoglycemia *Low concentration of glucose in the blood*

461

Myxedema *Condition associated with a decrease in overall thyroid function in adults; also known as hypothyroidism*

Neuroblastomas *Tumors of the neural crest; neuroblastomas often originate in the adrenal glands*

Osteoporosis *Condition associated with a decrease of bone mass and softening of bones, resulting in the increased possibility of bone fractures*

Paget's disease of bone (osteitis deformans) *A focal disorder of bone remodeling resulting in weakened, deformed bones of increased mass and associated fractures*

Paracrine *Denoting a type of hormone function in which hormone synthesized in and released from one cell signals and binds to its receptor on other types of adjacent cells*

Pheochromocytoma *Tumors of the adrenal gland that produce excess adrenaline (epinephrine) and norepinephrine*

Simmonds' disease *A pituitary disorder that is a form of panhypopituitarism in which all pituitary secretions are deficient; usually caused by postpartum necrosis of the anterior pituitary*

Spermatogenesis *The process by which immature germ cells (spermatogonia) mature into spermatozoa (mature sperm); the process normally begins in male puberty*

Thyroxine (T$_4$) *A thyroid hormone derived from tyrosine (amino acid); influences metabolic rate*

Triiodothyronine (T$_3$) *A thyroid hormone that helps regulate growth and development and controls metabolism and body temperature; mainly produced through the metabolism of thyroxine*

COMMON DRUGS PRESCRIBED FOR HORMONAL CONDITIONS (NONINCLUSIVE LISTINGS)

Trade Name	Generic Name	Pronunciation	Trade Name	Generic Name	Pronunciation
Thyroid Hormones			Skelid	tiludronate disodium	(tye-**loo**-**droe**-nate **dy**-sow-dee-um)
Armour Thyroid	desiccated thyroid	(**des**-eh-kate-ed **thigh**-roid)			
Cytomel	liothyronine	(lie-oh-**thigh**-row-neen)	**Calcium Minerals**		
Synthroid, Levoxyl	levothyroxine	(lee-vo-**thigh**-rox-een)	Os-Cal, Tums	calcium carbonate	(**kal**-see-um **car**-bone-ate)
Thyrolar	liotrix	(lee-ow-**tricks**)		calcium gluconate	(**kal**-see-um **glue**-ko-nate)
Anti-Thyroid Agents			**Pituitary Hormones Affecting Adrenal Gland**		
PTU	propylthiouracil	(pro-pull-thigh-oh-**yoor**-ah-sill)	Acthar	corticotrophin or ACTH	(**kore**-tye-co-**troe**-pin)
Tapazole	methimazole	(meth-**em**-ah-zoll)	Cortrosyn	cosyntropin	(**koe**-sin-**troe**-pin)
Calcium Regulator			**Corticosteroids (Glucocorticoids)**		
Calcimar, Miacalcin	calcitonin-salmon	(cal-sit-**toe**-nen sa-men)	Aristocort	triamcinolone acetate	(trye-am-**sin**-oh-lone **as**-see-tate)
Bisphosphonates			Celestone	betamethasone	(beta-**meth**-i-sone)
Actonel	risendronate	(**rye**-sed-row-nate)	Cortef	hydrocortisone	(hye-droe-**kor**-ti-sone)
Aredia	pamidronate	(**pam**-i-**drow**-nate)	Decadron, Hexadrol	dexamethasone	(dex-ah-**meth**-ah-sone)
Boniva	ibandronate	(eye-**ban**-droe-nate)	Deltasone, Orasone	prednisone	(**pred**-ni-sown)
Didronel	etidronate disodium	(eh-tea-**droh**-nate **dy**-so-**dee**-um)	Depo-Medrol	methylprednisolone acetate	(**meth**-il-pred-**nis**-oh-lone **as**-see-tate)
Fosamax	alendronate	(a-**lend**-ron-ate)	Entocort EC	budesonide	(byoo-**dess**-oh-nide)
Reclast	zoledronic acid	(zole-**droe**-nick **as**-id)	Kenalog-10, Kenalog-40	triamcinolone	(trye-am-**sin**-oh-lone)

COMMON DRUGS PRESCRIBED FOR HORMONAL CONDITIONS (NONINCLUSIVE LISTINGS)—cont'd

Trade Name	Generic Name	Pronunciation
Medrol	methylprednisolone	(**meth**-il-pred-**nis**-oh-lone)
Prelone, Orapred, Pediapred	prednisolone	(pred-**nis**-oh-lone)
Solu-Cortef	hydrocortisone succinate	(hye-droe-**kor**-ti-sone suck-sin-ate)
Solu-Medrol	methylprednisolone sodium succinate	(**meth**-il-pred-**nis**-oh-lone **so**-de-um **suck**-sin-ate)
Mineralocorticoids		
Florinef	fludrocortisone acetate	(floo-**droe**-kor-ti-sone **as**-see-tate)
Estrogens		
Estrace, Climara	estradiol	(ess-tra-**dye**-ole)
Ogen	estropipate	(**ess**-trow-**pih**-pate)
Premarin, Cenestin	conjugated estrogens	(**kon**-juh-gat-ed **ess**-troe-jens)
Premphase, Prempro	conjugated estrogen/ medroxyprogesterone	(**kon**-ju-gated **ess**-troe-jen/ me-**drox**-ee-pro-**jes**-ter-own)
Progestins		
Aygestin	norethindrone acetate	(nor-**eth**-in-drone **as**-see-tate)
Megace	megestrol acetate	(me-**jes**-trall **as**-see-tate)
Prometrium	progesterone	(pro-**jes**-tur-own)
Provera	medroxyprogesterone	(me-**drox**-see-pro-**jess**-tur-own)
Insulin		
Rapid-acting		
Humalog	lispro	(**in**-su-lin **lis**-pro)
NovoLog	aspart	(**as**-part)
Apidra	glulisine	(**gloo**-lis-een)
Short-acting		
Humulin R, Novolin R	insulin human	(**in**-su-lin **reg**-yoo-lar)
Intermediate-acting		
Humulin N, Novolin N	isophane insulin human	(**eye**-soe-fane)
Lente	insulin zinc	(**in**-su-lin **zinc**)
Long-acting		
Levemir	detemir	(**de**-te-mir)
Lantus	glargine	(**glar**-jeen)
Premixed (combination intermediate- and short-acting insulin)		
Humulin 70/30, Humulin 50/50	isophane insulin/ insulin human	

Trade Name	Generic Name	Pronunciation
Novolin 70/30, Novolin 50/50	insulin isophane	
Humalog Mix 75/25	insulin lispro	
Oral Antidiabetic Drugs		
Biguanides		
Glucophage	metformin	(met-**four**-men)
Alpha-glucosidase inhibitors		
Precose	acarbose	(**ay**-car-bose)
Glyset	miglitol	(**mig**-li-tol)
Meglitinides		
Prandin	repaglinide	(re-**pag**-lih-nide)
Starlix	nateglinide	(na-**teg**-lin-ide)
Sulfonylureas—First Generation		
Diabinese	chlorpropamide	(klor-**pro**-pah-myde)
Tolinase	tolazamide	(toll-**laze**-ah-myde)
Orinase	tolbutamide	(toll-**butte**-ah-myde)
Sulfonylureas—Second Generation		
Amaryl	glimepiride	(gly-**mep**-ir-ide)
Glucotrol	glipizide	(**glip**-eh-zyed)
Micronase, DiaBeta	glyburide	(**glye**-burr-eyed)
Thiazolidinediones		
Actos	pioglitazone	(pye-oh-**glit**-ah-zone)
Avandia	rosiglitazone	(roes-i-**glit**-ah-zone)
Combination Agents		
Duetact	glimepiride/ pioglitazone	(gly-**mep**-ir-ide/ pye-oh-**glit**-ah-zone)
Metaglip	glipizide/metformin	(glip-eh-zyed/met-**for**-men)
ActoPlus Met	pioglitazone/metformin	(pye-oh-**glit**-ah-zone/ met-**for**-men)
Janumet	metformin/sitagliptin	(met-**for**-men/ **sye**-ta-**glip**-tin)
Miscellaneous Agents for Diabetes		
Januvia	sitagliptin	(**sye**-ta-**glip**-tin)
Byetta injection	exenatide	(ex-**en**-a-tide)

THE ENDOCRINE SYSTEM encompasses the production and secretion of **hormones** from glands. The Greek word *orme* means "to excite." This is exactly what hormones do. They activate specific target cells, causing a response. Many different types of hormones are produced in different glands. Endocrinologists are physicians who specialize in the study of glands and hormones. In this chapter we discuss the location and function of the major glands of the body. Major conditions affecting the endocrine system are discussed along with the types of agents used to treat them. All medication dosages listed are based on adult dosage unless otherwise indicated. Medical terminology related to the endocrine system is listed in Table 15-1. The following table lists common prefixes, suffixes, and root words used to define the endocrine system and the conditions that affect it.

MEDICAL TERMINOLOGY

Prefix	
Eu-	Good
Hyper-	Excessive, above
Hypo-	Deficient, below
Oxy-	Rapid, sharp
Pan-	All
Tetra-	Four
Tri-	Three
Suffix	
-agon	Assemble, gather
-emia	Blood condition
-in, -ine	A substance
-tropin	Stimulating the function of
-uria	Urine condition
Root words/combining forms	
Andr/o	Male
Calc/o, calci/o	Calcium
Cortic/o	Cortex, outer region
Dips/o	Thirst
Estr/o	Female
Gluc/o, glyc/o	Sugar
Home/o	Sameness
Hormon/o	Hormone
Kal/I	Potassium
Lact/o	Milk
Myx/o	Mucus
Natr/o	Sodium
Phys/o	Growing
Somat/o	Body
Ster/o	Solid structure
Toc/o	Childbirth
Toxic/o	Poison
Ur/o	Urine

Endocrine Anatomy

Three glands are located in the head: the pituitary gland, hypothalamus, and pineal gland. The pituitary gland produces hormones that affect other glands and specific organs of the body as shown in Figure 15-1. The hypothalamus, located above the pituitary gland, is a bridge between the nervous system and hormonal system. The hypothalamus secretes hormones that affect the pituitary

TABLE 15-1 Endocrine Structures, Medical Terms, and Functions

Term/Abbreviation	Definition	Primary Functions
adren/o	Adrenal glands	Influences metabolism and regulates electrolyte levels; also responds to stress
gonad/o	Gonads	Regulates maintenance of secondary sex characteristics
pancreat/o	Pancreatic islets	Controls blood sugar (glucose) levels
parathyroid/o	Parathyroid glands	Regulates calcium levels
pineal/o	Pineal glands	Influences both wake and sleep cycles
pituit/o, pituitar/o	Pituitary gland	Secretes hormones that affect activities of other endocrine glands
thym/o	Thymus	Affects immune system reaction
thyr/o, thyroid/o	Thyroid gland	Affects metabolism, growth, and activity of nervous system

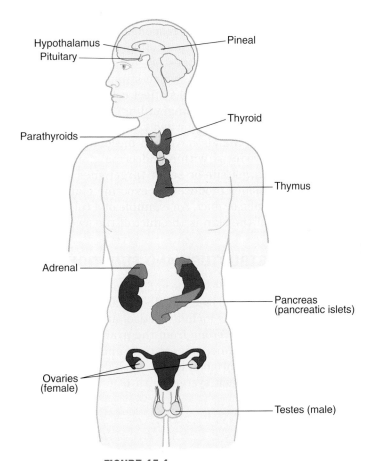

FIGURE 15-1 Endocrine anatomy.

gland. The pineal gland, located behind and below the hypothalamus, is involved in controlling circadian rhythms, sleep-wake patterns, and other body functions, primarily through the production of the hormone melatonin.

Located at the base of the neck, the thyroid gland is responsible for the following three hormones that affect metabolism: **thyroxine** (T_4), **triiodothyronine** (T_3), and **calcitonin**. The parathyroid glands, positioned slightly behind and above the thyroid gland, secrete a hormone called parathyroid hormone

(PTH), which helps maintain adequate calcium levels. Located lower in the chest is the thymus, which secretes hormones that play an important role in the immune system of the body. The two adrenal glands are located in the abdominal area, one gland positioned above each kidney; the adrenal glands secrete specific hormones (epinephrine and norepinephrine) linked to the stress responses of the body.

The largest gland is the pancreas, located behind the left kidney at the back of the abdominal wall. The pancreas is responsible for the production and secretion of hormones from cells called islets of Langerhans. The islets of Langerhans contain alpha cells that produce glucagon and beta cells that produce insulin. Glands that produce sex hormones are the ovaries in women and the testes in men. In women the ovaries secrete hormones such as estrogen and progesterone. In men the main hormone secreted is testosterone. Each of these hormones is also responsible for gender characteristics.

Description of Hormones

Hormones are responsible for many different human functions, including emotions. The actions of hormones are classified by the distance they travel. **Autocrine** hormones act on the same cell from which they are secreted, such as interleukin-2, which stimulates T cells (part of the immune system). The **paracrine** hormones affect cells that are in proximity or adjacent to the target cells (such as prostaglandins), and the endocrine hormones influence cells that are located farther away. The endocrine hormones are the focus of this chapter.

Glands have two mechanisms of action—endocrine or exocrine. Hormones produced within endocrine glands either enter the bloodstream to reach their target site or act at target sites near the site of hormone release, whereas hormones produced by exocrine glands are sent to the target organ or tissue via a tube or duct. An example of a tube or duct that secretes outwardly to the surface of the skin is the duct of the sweat glands.

STRUCTURE AND FUNCTION OF HORMONES

Hormones of the endocrine system are classified as proteins, steroids, and amines (Figure 15-2). Proteins include insulin, growth hormone (GH), and calcitonin. Steroids include cortisol and aldosterone from the adrenal cortex, estrogen and progesterone from the ovaries, and testosterone from the testes. The hormones thyroxine, epinephrine, and norepinephrine are examples of amines.

Hormone levels are balanced and maintained in a normal range through a feedback system with a mechanism similar to that of your home thermostat.

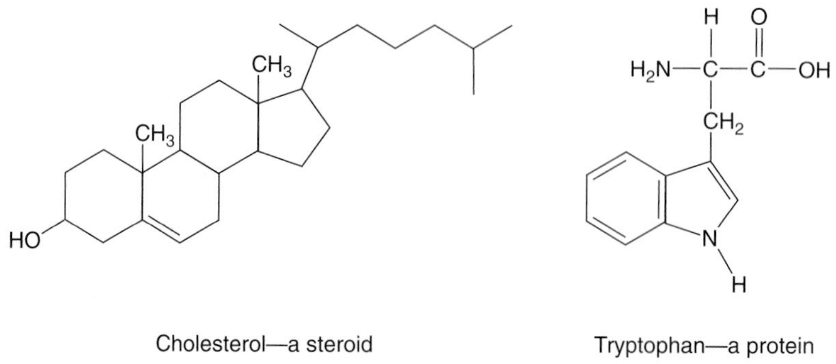

Cholesterol—a steroid   Tryptophan—a protein

FIGURE 15-2 Structures of a steroid and a protein molecule.

TABLE 15-2 Hormone Function

Hormone	Gland/Source	Functions
Adrenocorticotropic	Pituitary gland	Stimulates growth/secretions of adrenal cortex
Aldosterone	Adrenal cortex	Regulates salt/water balance
Androgen	Adrenal cortex/gonads	Influences sex-related characteristics
Antidiuretic	Pituitary gland	Helps control blood pressure
Calcitonin	Thyroid gland	Regulates calcium levels
Cortisol	Adrenal cortex	Regulates metabolism of proteins, fats, carbohydrates
Epinephrine	Adrenal medulla	Stimulates sympathetic nervous system
Estrogen	Ovaries	Regulates menstrual cycle; develops and maintains secondary sex characteristics
Follicle-stimulating	Pituitary gland	Secretes estrogen and promotes growth of ova in females; production of sperm in males
Glucagon	Pancreatic islets	Increases levels of glucose
Growth	Pituitary gland	Regulates growth of muscles, bones, and tissue
Human chorionic gonadotropin	Placenta	Secretes hormones throughout pregnancy
Insulin	Pancreatic islets	Transports glucose and converts excess glucose to glycogen storage
Lactogenic	Pituitary	Stimulates secretion of breast milk
Luteinizing	Pituitary	Stimulates ovulation in females; stimulates testosterone secretion in males
Melatonin	Pineal	Influences sleep-wake cycles
Norepinephrine	Adrenal medulla	Stimulates sympathetic nervous system
Oxytocin	Pituitary	Stimulates both uterine contractions and milk production during pregnancy
Parathyroid	Parathyroid	Regulates calcitonin levels, which in turn regulates calcium levels
Progesterone	Ovaries	Prepares uterus for pregnancy
Testosterone	Testicles	Influences sex-related characteristics in males
Thymosin	Thymus	Immune system
Thyroid	Thyroid	Affects metabolism
Thyroid stimulator	Pituitary	Promotes secretion of hormones by thyroid gland

However, hormones in general can be considered specialized keys that unlock specific doors. When the key enters the lock, a reaction takes place. As the hormone travels through the body, it does not react with any keyhole other than the ones it was made to fit. **Homeostasis** (balance) is disrupted if glands secrete too many or too few hormones; rather, a delicate balance must be maintained to produce the correct level of response. Table 15-2 provides a list of endocrine glands and their hormones as well as the functions of each hormone. If a gland ceases to produce hormone or secretes too much or too little hormone, various conditions of the endocrine system may result. Hormones perform many functions throughout the body, including the following:

- Maintain homeostasis—maintain normal physiological limits by increasing and decreasing blood glucose levels for energy use
- Prepare the body for an emergency situation—instigate the "fight or flight" reaction
- Participate in the development of the reproductive system—cause sexual maturity and reproductive functions, such as menstruation and pregnancy

MECHANISM OF ACTION

Receptor sites for hormones are located inside and outside of cells. Protein hormones fit into receptor sites outside cells, whereas steroid hormones enter into and attach to receptor sites inside the cell. Both mechanisms cause a reaction. The following are the three systems that influence the endocrine system:

- Negative feedback is the primary regulatory mechanism used to maintain homeostasis. In negative feedback a stimulus results in actions that reduce the stimulus. For example, insulin is secreted when blood **glucose** levels are high. The released insulin allows the cells to use glucose for energy, thus reducing glucose levels in the blood. As glucose levels drop, the stimulus for the secretion of insulin also decreases, and excess glucose is stored in the liver as glycogen.
- Positive feedback may also occur; however, in positive feedback a stimulus results in actions that further increase the stimulus. For example, during labor specific hormones are released that promote continued release of more hormones until a result is achieved: contractions result in the birth of a baby.
- The third response system is via the nervous system. Stressful situations can alter the production and secretion of specific hormones that, when released, prepare the body for the situation. For example, if a person is in an emergency, the body requires more energy; therefore chemicals such as epinephrine may be released, giving the body an extra boost of energy.

Functions of the Endocrine Glands

HYPOTHALAMUS

Located in the brain below the thalamus, the hypothalamus is a small organ that links the nervous system to the endocrine system. The hypothalamus stimulates the pituitary gland by neuronal impulses. The hypothalamus plays a key role in the regulation of several functions such as water balance, metabolism of fat and carbohydrates, body temperature, appetite, and emotions. This organ also produces releasing or inhibiting hormones that regulate the anterior pituitary gland. Hormones from the hypothalamus are also sent to the posterior pituitary gland where they are both stored and secreted.

PINEAL GLAND

The pineal gland is responsible for the production and secretion of melatonin. Melatonin is a chemical substance that helps to regulate the sleep-wake cycle. The target tissue of melatonin is the hypothalamus. Although this gland is small in adults, it is larger in small children. As a person ages, the pineal gland becomes smaller because of calcification and begins to function less effectively. The gland is affected by the retinal response to light; it secretes higher levels of melatonin at night and lower levels during the day. The effects of melatonin have been linked to the onset of puberty and the regulation of the menstrual cycle.

PITUITARY GLAND

The pituitary gland is analogous to the control tower of the endocrine system. The pituitary gland commonly is called the master gland of the endocrine system. The gland is composed of two portions—the anterior and posterior lobes. Although small, the anterior lobe synthesizes the hormones that stimulate many different organs (Table 15-3). Two hormones, oxytocin and antidiuretic hormone

TABLE 15-3 Hormonal Production of Anterior and Posterior Pituitary Gland

Abbreviation	Hormone	Target Tissue	Result
Anterior Pituitary Gland			
ACTH	Adrenocorticotropic hormone	Adrenal glands	Secretes glucocorticoids and adrenocortical hormones
FSH	Follicle-stimulating hormone	Ovaries in women; testes in men	Promotes estrogen secretion in women and sperm production in men
GH	Growth hormone	Tissues and bones throughout body	Promotes growth throughout childhood
LH	Luteinizing hormone	Ovaries in women; testes in men	Promotes progesterone production in women and testosterone production in men
	Prolactin	Mammary glands in women	Produces milk for lactation
TSH	Thyroid-stimulating hormone	Thyroid gland	Causes thyroid gland to produce thyroid hormones
Posterior Pituitary Gland			
ADH	Antidiuretic hormone	Kidneys	Causes resorption of water back into bloodstream
	Oxytocin	Uterus	Causes contraction of smooth muscle; also stimulates anterior pituitary lobe to produce prolactin

(ADH), are stored in the posterior portion of the pituitary gland. Oxytocin stimulates uterine contractions and cervical dilation during birth and lactation, and ADH (also known as vasopressin) affects the kidneys, cardiovascular system, and central nervous system. This entire pituitary system is regulated via negative feedback control from the nervous system (specifically the hypothalamus) and from the levels of other hormones.

THYROID GLAND

The thyroid gland is located at the base of the neck (Figure 15-3). This gland is responsible for producing and secreting three hormones: thyroxine (T_4), triiodothyronine (T_3), and calcitonin. Iodine is necessary within the thyroid gland to synthesize T_4 and T_3; each hormone is named to indicate the number of iodine atoms in its structure. T_4 and T_3 are transported via the bloodstream along with plasma proteins; the hormones pass through target cells into the interior of the cell, where they bind to a specific protein. This ultimate reaction helps trigger the rate of metabolism of proteins, fats (lipids), and sugars (carbohydrates) throughout the body; therefore T_3 and T_4 play an important role in the growth and homeostasis of the body. Calcitonin plays an active role in the regulation of calcium levels. Calcium is the major mineral found in bones. Calcium is also important for the proper functioning of muscle contractions, nerve impulses, and blood clotting. A constant level is maintained by three different hormones, including calcitonin. The function of calcitonin is to inhibit the resorption of calcium from the bone and kidney. Vitamin D (specifically 1,25-dihydroxycholecalciferol) and parathyroid hormone (PTH) are the two other hormones that help regulate calcium levels and are discussed in other sections of this chapter.

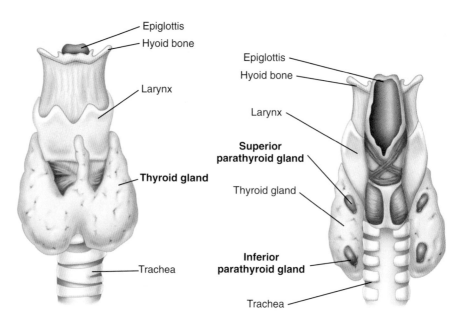

FIGURE 15-3 Thyroid and parathyroid glands. (From Thibodeau GA, Patton KT: *Anatomy and physiology,* ed 6, St Louis, 2007, Mosby.)

PARATHYROID GLANDS

Located behind the thyroid gland are the parathyroid glands (para meaning "across"). The parathyroid organ is composed of two sets of secreting glands. These glands are the primary regulators of calcium levels in the blood through the release of PTH. The glands can draw calcium out of the bone when needed, through a process called resorption, to increase the concentration of calcium in the blood. As PTH increases calcium levels in the blood by bone resorption, it also lowers phosphate levels in the blood, thus allowing more free calcium to be available.

ADRENAL GLANDS

The adrenal glands are located directly on top of each of the two kidneys. The adrenal glands secrete steroids (cortisol) and catecholamines. **Catecholamines** are hormones such as epinephrine, norepinephrine, and dopamine produced by the nerve tissue in the brain and the adrenal glands.

If the adrenal glands are dissected in a cross section, two layers of tissue can be seen: the medulla (located in the center) and the cortex (outer portion) of the gland. Each of the two layers within the adrenal gland is specific to its function.

The adrenal medulla synthesizes and secretes the catecholamines norepinephrine and epinephrine. These hormones are stored in the adrenal medulla until activated by the sympathetic nervous system. As mentioned previously, one of the functions of the endocrine system is to stimulate the "fight or flight" reaction. For instance, when the body encounters a stressful situation it prepares itself for fight or flight, depending on the situation. When the sympathetic nervous system is activated, the heart rate increases and the veins dilate to allow more blood to reach the skeletal muscles and to increase blood flow to the brain. Stored glucose is released into the bloodstream to fuel the body's increased metabolic rate. Epinephrine accounts for approximately 70% to 80% of the released catecholamines and norepinephrine 20% to 30%.

TABLE 15-4 Adrenal Hormones and Their Effects on the Body

Class of Hormones	Specific Hormone	Produced and Secreted	Effects
Glucocorticoids	Cortisol	Adrenal cortex	Increases blood glucose concentration; also has antiinflammatory and antiallergy effects
Mineralocorticoids	Aldosterone	Adrenal cortex	Increases urinary output, resulting in decreased potassium and hydrogen levels and increased sodium levels; keeps blood volume in balance
Sex hormones	Androgens in men	Adrenal cortex	Affects male and female characteristics such as hair growth and sex drive
	Estrogens in women	Adrenal cortex	Affects female sex drive, fat deposition, and bone formation

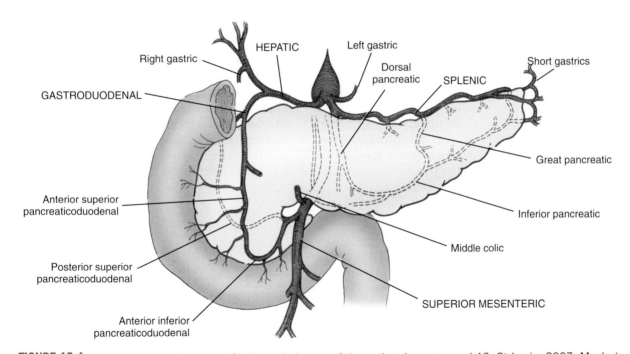

FIGURE 15-4 Pancreas. (From Rothrock JC: *Alexander's care of the patient in surgery,* ed 13, St Louis, 2007, Mosby.)

The cortex of the adrenal glands produces three types of hormones: glucocorticoids, mineralocorticoids, and sex hormones (i.e., androgens or estrogens) (Table 15-4). Glucocorticoids affect the metabolism of lipids, carbohydrates, and proteins. They increase glucose levels, reduce inflammation, and increase the capacity to cope with stressful situations. Mineralocorticoids are produced within the cortex but within a different layer than the glucocorticoids. Their function is to regulate the secretion of water and sodium by the kidney.

PANCREAS

The pancreas is the largest organ of the endocrine system (Figure 15-4). The exocrine function of the pancreas is the secretion of digestive enzymes into the small intestine. The endocrine function of the pancreas is to maintain energy homeostasis throughout the body. The gland accomplishes this by secreting glucagon and insulin, inhibiting the release of somatostatin. Glucagon is secreted in response to low blood glucose levels. This hormone triggers the liver to release stored glucose. Glucagon also triggers the release of fatty acids from adipose (fat) tissue for energy use. When blood glucose concentration is high, insulin is released into the bloodstream. This hormone targets tissues such as the liver, muscle, and adipose tissues to absorb excess glucose from the bloodstream, where it can be stored for later use. Somatostatin, secreted by the hypothalamus, inhibits the release of insulin and glucagon.

OVARIES

The two ovaries in women are responsible for the production (oogenesis) and secretion of one or, rarely, two eggs or more (ovulation) each month. Located on either side of the uterus, the ovaries sit above the uterus and are attached to the fallopian tubes, which connect the two organs. Although ovulation begins at puberty, it is not possible to become pregnant until the menstrual cycle begins. The ability to have children ends as the levels of the responsible hormones (such as estrogen) decline until the ovarian cycle stops. The ovaries secrete the hormones estrogen and progesterone; the ovaries are the primary source of estrogen in women. The function of estrogen is the development of breasts and genitals and the regulation of the menstrual cycle, which prepares the female for pregnancy. The anterior pituitary gland releases follicle-stimulating hormone (FSH) that triggers estrogen levels to increase, which causes luteinizing hormone (LH, another pituitary hormone) to be secreted. The combination of these two hormones triggers the cascade of events that causes ovulation. Figure 15-5 illustrates the anatomical location of the ovaries.

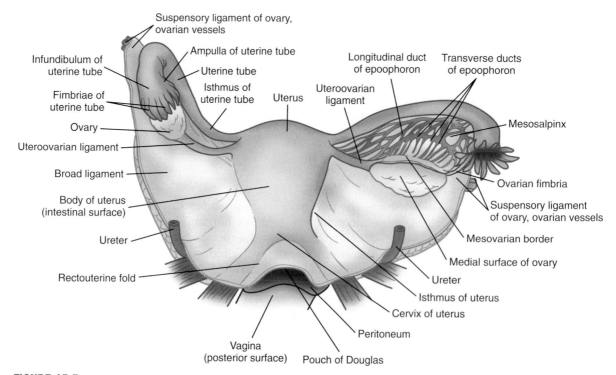

FIGURE 15-5 Ovaries. (From Rothrock JC: *Alexander's care of the patient in surgery,* ed 13, St Louis, 2007, Mosby.)

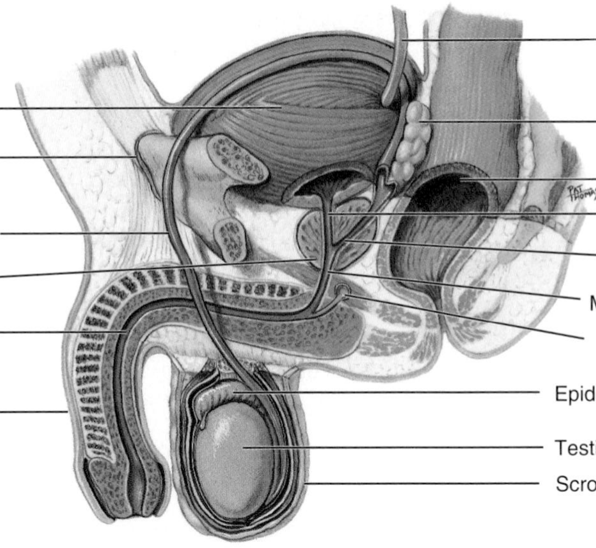

FIGURE 15-6 Testes. (From Applegate E: *The anatomy and physiology learning system,* ed 3, Philadelphia, 2006, WB Saunders.)

TESTES

The two testes in men are responsible for the production and secretion of sperm (**spermatogenesis**). The testes are located within the scrotum. Sperm production begins before the age of puberty and decreases with age, although most men produce sperm throughout their lifetime. Follicle-stimulating hormone (FSH) is released as puberty begins and causes the stored immature sperm cells to divide and mature. Each sperm contains one half of the genetic material that will be contributed to a new life during reproduction. The production of testosterone (also from the testes) is responsible for the growth of adjacent organs: prostate gland, seminal vesicles, vas deferens, and others. Testosterone is also responsible for secondary sex characteristics such as changes in voice pitch as a boy enters puberty and increased muscle development. This hormone also affects the differences in the physiques of men and women. Figure 15-6 shows the location of the testes.

Conditions of the Endocrine System and Their Treatments

Many different types of conditions and illnesses can affect the endocrine system. Causes can range from the effects of aging and genetic factors to conditions that affect another part of the body. The failure of the endocrine system to function correctly affects other areas of the body, such as heart, brain, and kidney function. Table 15-5 lists the common conditions and/or illnesses that affect the endocrine system.

TABLE 15-5 **Endocrine Conditions with Corresponding Glands and Hormones and Possible Treatments**

Condition/Disease	Gland	Due to	Effect	Possible Treatments
Acromegaly	Adrenal	Oversecretion of TSH	Excessive levels of TSH	Radiation, surgery
Adrenal hypofunction (Addison's disease)	Adrenal	Autoimmune process that destroys gland function, tuberculosis, removal of gland, hemorrhage, hypopituitarism, or tumor	Deficient levels of mineralocorticoids, glucocorticoids, and androgens	Hormone replacement
Cushing's syndrome	Adrenal	Excessive production of glucocorticoids stemming from pituitary gland or caused by tumor	Excessive levels of cortisol	Surgery or medication
Diabetes insipidus	Pituitary	Undersecretion of ADH	Low levels of vasopressin (antidiuretic hormone)	Medication: desmopressin (DDAVP)
Diabetes mellitus (type 1)	Adrenal/ pancreas	Underproduction or no production of insulin	A lack of insulin	Insulin replacement, education about condition
Diabetes mellitus (type 2)	Adrenal/ pancreas	Resistance to insulin	Insulin resistance	Oral antidiabetic agents or injectable insulin replacement if not controlled by oral agents; education about condition
Dwarfism	Adrenal	Undersecretion of growth hormone (GH)	Low levels of GH	GH replacement
Gestational diabetes	Adrenal/ pancreas	Underproduction of insulin during pregnancy	Temporary lack of insulin	Insulin replacement
Gigantism	Adrenal	Excessive production of GH	Excessive levels of GH	Radiation, surgery
Hyperaldosteronism (Conn's syndrome)	Adrenal	Benign tumor, malignant tumor, or unknown etiology	Excessive secretion of mineralocorticoids or aldosterone	Surgery, medication
Hyperparathyroidism (primary or secondary)	Thyroid	Tumor, genetic disorder, or multiple endocrine neoplasia	Oversecretion of PTH	Surgery, reduce calcium intake, diuresis
Hyperthyroidism (Graves' disease, Basedow's disease, thyrotoxicosis)	Thyroid	Genetic, immunologic factors	Increased secretion of T_3, T_4, calcitonin	Medication, surgery
Hypoparathyroidism	Thyroid	Idiopathic (autoimmune), acquired (from removal of gland)	Deficiency of PTH	Calcium and vitamin D replacement
Hypothyroidism (myxedema [adults], cretinism [children])	Thyroid or pituitary	Surgery, radiation therapy, autoimmune disease	Deficiency of thyroid hormones	Thyroid hormone replacement
Sexual dysfunction	Pituitary	Lack of hormone secretion	Decreased hormone levels: TSH < ACTH, FSH, LH	Hormone replacement
Sexual immaturity/ dysfunction	Female (ovaries) Male (testes)	Undersecretion	Deficiency of gonadocorticoids (androgens/estrogen/ progestins)	Hormone replacement
Simple goiter	Thyroid	Lack of dietary intake of iodine	Decreased levels of thyroid hormones	Medication
Thyroiditis (Graves' disease, myxedema)	Thyroid	Autoimmune condition or infection	Decreased levels of thyroid hormones	Medication

CONDITIONS OF THE PITUITARY GLAND AND HYPOTHALAMUS AND THEIR TREATMENTS

Gigantism and Acromegaly

Gigantism and acromegaly are two rare conditions that are progressive and involve an increase in levels of growth hormone. Hyperfunction of the pituitary gland can be caused by various tumor growths. If this condition is present in children, it is referred to as gigantism. The bones elongate, resulting in heights that have reached 8 feet. If this condition arises after normal bone growth has halted, it is called acromegaly and symptoms involve increased size of the head, tongue, nose, hands, feet, and toes; these conditions can lead to **hyperglycemia** (too much glucose in the blood) and **hypercalcemia** (too much calcium in the blood).

Prognosis. The outcome of gigantism if left untreated can be life-threatening, with death rates being 2 to 3 times higher than normal. These patients are susceptible to cardiovascular and respiratory complications. There are treatments available, and if they are successful the person may live a normal life.

Non–Drug Treatment. Treatment may involve removal of the tumor or growth, although any bone growth preceding removal cannot be reversed. Radiation therapy may be used as well. Most tumors of the pituitary gland tend to be benign.

Drug Treatment. The goal of treatment with medications may include shrinking the pituitary mass, restoring secretory patterns and serum levels to their normal state, and retaining normal pituitary secretion of other hormones to prevent recurrence of the condition. Agents such as bromocriptine, cabergoline (dopamine agonists), or octreotide (somatostatin analog) may be used to treat gigantism once its specific cause is diagnosed.

Hypopituitarism

Hypopituitarism (includes panhypopituitarism and dwarfism) is a condition that occurs secondary to destruction of all or part of the pituitary gland, resulting in the undersecretion of all anterior pituitary hormones. Panhypopituitarism is characterized by partial or total failure in the secretion of the anterior pituitary's vital hormones (corticotropin, thyroid-stimulating hormone [TSH], LH, FSH, human growth hormone [hGH], and prolactin) as well as the posterior pituitary hormone ADH. Partial and complete hypopituitarism occurs in both adults and children. A deficiency of hGH in children may result in hypoglycemia and short stature (growth failure), resulting in dwarfism. Gonadotropin deficiency (in older children) may lead to a delay in puberty. **Simmonds' disease** affects adults, causing a lack of menstruation in women and impotence in men. Corticotropin deficiency affects normal protein, carbohydrate, and lipid metabolism, resulting in **hypoglycemia**, fatigue, progressive emaciation (weight loss), and death. Most hypopituitarism conditions are caused by a tumor and involve the following disorders and treatments:

Disorders:
- Autoimmune disease
- Congenital defects
- Pituitary infarction (e.g., from hemorrhage)

Treatments:
- Partial or total hypophysectomy (surgery)
- Radiation treatments
- Treatment with chemical agents

Signs and symptoms develop slowly over time and vary depending on the severity of the condition. In adults, impotence, infertility, decreased libido, diabetes insipidus, hypothyroidism, and adrenocortical insufficiency may occur. An interruption in growth or the onset of puberty may occur in children. Dwarfism is not apparent at birth but appears during the first 3 to 6 months of age. Although the children are healthy, growth continues at about half the rate of normal growth with a final height of approximately 4 feet, which may not occur until the child reaches from 20 to 39 years of age.

Prognosis. Prognosis for hypopituitarism in children is good if treated early. If the condition is diagnosed and treated, the symptoms may be controlled or stopped. Left untreated, this disease can be fatal.

Non–Drug Treatment. Surgery may be necessary in the event of a tumor, although medication may still be needed throughout the patient's lifetime.

Drug Treatment. Treatment of pituitary hypofunction is directed at the underlying cause and replacement of needed hormones; also, the age of the child determines the hormones involved in replacement therapy. In the event of a deficiency of adrenocorticotropic hormone (ACTH), hydrocortisone or prednisone may be administered. In TSH deficiency, L-thyroxine may be prescribed. However, doses of these agents depend on the age of the patient. For gonadotropin deficiency, steroid replacement therapy would begin at puberty. A GH deficiency treatment may be prescribed in childhood through puberty.

Diabetes Insipidus

Diabetes insipidus is a rare disorder caused by a hormone deficiency of ADH (vasopressin), which prevents the kidney from producing too much urine. ADH is produced in the hypothalamus and stored in the posterior pituitary gland, and when needed it is released into the bloodstream. Causes of this condition include brain tumor or infection of the meninges (meningitis) or brain (encephalitis), and hemorrhage in or around the pituitary gland. A family history of diabetes insipidus may increase the risk of this condition. Kidneys that do not respond normally to the hormone cause the same type of condition and symptoms, and this condition is known as nephrogenic diabetes insipidus. Symptoms include excessive thirst, dehydration, rapid heart rate, low blood pressure, and constipation. It is important to note that diabetes insipidus is not diabetes mellitus, a more common condition that is treated with insulin or similar agents. Information and treatment for this type of diabetes are discussed under conditions of the pancreas.

Prognosis. Overall, the prognosis is good depending on the type and severity of the condition. Once controlled with treatment there are no limitations on activity or diet, including the intake of water.

Non–Drug Treatment. Treatment includes keeping a record of daily weight and prevention of dehydration. It is also suggested that the person wear a medical identification bracelet indicating his or her condition and prescribed medications.

Drug Treatment. Vasopressin or desmopressin acetate (synthetic forms of ADH) is typically prescribed to treat diabetes insipidus. Agents that can stimulate production of ADH such as chlorpropamide, carbamazepine, and clofibrate may also be used.

CONDITIONS OF THE THYROID GLAND AND THEIR TREATMENT

Hyperthyroidism

Hyperthyroidism is oversecretion of hormones from the thyroid gland and is primarily caused by three conditions: Graves' disease, goiter, or postpartum thyroiditis. **Graves' disease** is an autoimmune disorder; that is, the body's immune system attacks itself. The body manufactures antibodies to thyroid-stimulating hormone receptors (i.e., diffuse toxic goiter) that result in the production of more hormones that affect the thyroid gland, skin, and eyes. The reason for the attack on these areas is unknown. Inflammation and enlargement of the tissues in the orbit of the eye (causing the eyes to bulge, known as **exophthalmos**) only occurs in approximately 20% of persons affected by Graves' disease. Graves' disease affects more women than men, is more common between 30 and 50 years of age, and has a genetic component. There are three stages of Graves' disease:

1. Overactivity of the thyroid gland (may produce a goiter)
2. Inflammation of the tissues around the eyes, causing swelling
3. Thickening of the skin over the lower legs

A **goiter** gives the appearance of an enlarged neck and usually is caused by a nonmalignant tumor or nodules in or on the thyroid gland that are associated with excess production of thyroid hormone. Goiters are painless and range in size from barely discernible to the size of a grapefruit. If the goiter is small, it is not normally treated, since many goiters disappear on their own. If the goiter continues to grow then medications are used, reserving surgery only in those cases where medication is ineffective. Rare cases of goiter are associated with the lack of iodine in the diet; this is uncommon because most developed countries iodize salt.

Thyroiditis occurs in approximately 1 out of 20 women after childbirth. This type of thyroid problem causes little, if any, gland enlargement and is usually temporary and resolves within a few months of onset. Later, however, the thyroid gland may not produce enough hormones, resulting in chronic hypothyroidism. Viruses are another potential cause of hyperthyroidism, with the excessive amounts of T_3 and T_4 disappearing after the infection has been resolved. Although there are various causes of hyperthyroidism, the general symptoms are the same, including the following:

- Heat intolerance
- Nervousness
- Insomnia
- Fatigue
- Weight loss
- Muscle weakness
- Fast heart rate
- Hair loss
- Trembling hands

Prognosis. There are treatments available for all common types of hyperthyroidism; therefore the outlook for this condition is good.

Non–Drug Treatment. If a tumor exists, treatment could include surgery to remove the tumor. Radiation also may be used to destroy part of the thyroid gland.

Drug Treatment. For Graves' disease antithyroid agents can be used, such as methimazole and propylthiouracil (PTU), and both interfere with the thyroid gland's ability to make hormones. By far the most common treatment is the use of radioactive iodine, which destroys cells in the thyroid gland. This treatment is preferred because only thyroid cells absorb iodine and therefore the treatment does not harm any other cells in the body. In addition, the only side effect of iodine treatment is hypothyroidism resulting from the reduction in hormonal secretion.

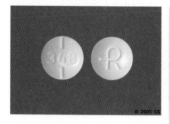

GENERIC NAME: propylthiouracil (PTU)
TRADE NAME: No trade named products available in United States; available in generic form.
INDICATION: Hyperthyroidism
COMMON ADULT DOSAGE: 300 to 450 mg daily in divided doses (initial dosage); 100 to 150 mg daily (maintenance)
SIDE EFFECTS: Nausea, headache, urticaria
AUXILIARY LABEL:
■ Take as directed.

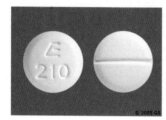

GENERIC NAME: methimazole
TRADE NAME: Tapazole
INDICATION: Hyperthyroidism
COMMON ADULT DOSAGE: 5 to 40 mg daily in divided doses (initial dosage); 5 to 15 mg daily (maintenance)
SIDE EFFECTS: Fever, rash, itching
AUXILIARY LABEL:
■ Take as directed.

Hypothyroidism

Hypothyroidism is a condition that occurs when the thyroid gland is unable to secrete sufficient levels of T_3 and T_4. This can be caused by a congenital deficiency referred to as thyroid aplasia (a lack of tissue or organ growth). Thyroid aplasia affects children who are born without a functional thyroid gland or any thyroid gland. The absence of the thyroid gland affects the growth of the child's body and the development of the nervous system. If the condition is not discovered early, the child's growth will be stunted (dwarfism), and the child will develop mental retardation (**cretinism**). Once hypothyroidism is diagnosed, thyroid medication must be administered for the lifetime of the patient, although any retardation that has already occurred is irreversible.

A lack of iodine in the diet can cause a deficiency in the production of thyroid hormones because iodine is necessary for the synthesis of T_3 and T_4. Hypothyroidism caused by iodine deficiency is not common in developed nations because of the addition of iodine to salt; patients with hypothyroidism rarely need iodine supplementation. Inflammation of the thyroid gland, known as thyroiditis, is an autoimmune condition. Tumors that affect the thyroid gland are usually benign (adenomas) and rarely are malignant (carcinoma).

Hypothyroidism is a common medical problem, and women older than 35 years are most commonly affected. Symptoms include increased sensitivity to cold, brittle fingernails, constipation, unexplained weight gain, and heavier menstrual periods. Hypothyroidism results in an overall decrease in energy and mental alertness. Before diagnosis and treatment with thyroid hormone replacement therapy, the patient with hypothyroidism often experiences cold intolerance, changes in appetite, weight gain, and hair loss. Hypothyroidism may cause the condition **myxedema**. Symptoms include skin that appears puffy and has a waxy appearance; the patient may also have dramatic changes in mental status if the condition is severe, such as myxedema coma.

Prognosis. If hypothyroidism is not treated, the symptoms may progress although it is not normally life-threatening. When treated appropriately through the use of medication, most patients do well.

Non–Drug Treatment. The main treatment for hypothyroidism caused by tumors is surgical removal of the tumor. In the case of thyroiditis, surgery may also be necessary to remove all or part of the thyroid gland.

Drug Treatment. Most patients with hypothyroidism do not have tumors and are managed with hormone replacement therapy. Thyroid hormone replacement agents need to be taken for life (one dose a day) because there are no other available treatments. Levothyroxine is most commonly preferred by many medical physicians because of its ease of dosing (i.e., uses one thyroid hormone, T_4) and the standardized manufacture of the products.

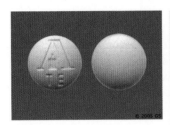

GENERIC NAME: thyroid (desiccated) (combined T_4-T_3 product)
TRADE NAME: Armour Thyroid, Westhroid
INDICATIONS: Hypothyroidism, thyroid cancer
COMMON ADULT DOSAGE: 60 to 120 mg once daily
SIDE EFFECTS: No major effects if correct dosage taken
AUXILIARY LABELS:

■ Take as directed.
■ Take with water on an empty stomach.

GENERIC NAME: levothyroxine sodium (T_4)
TRADE NAME: Synthroid, Levothroid, Levoxyl, Levo-T, Unithroid
INDICATION: Hypothyroidism
COMMON ADULT DOSAGE: 25 to 125 mcg once daily
SIDE EFFECTS: No major effects if correct dosage taken
AUXILIARY LABELS:

■ Take as directed.
■ Take with water on an empty stomach.

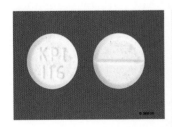

GENERIC NAME: liothyronine sodium
TRADE NAME: Cytomel, Triostat (T3)
INDICATION: Hypothyroidism
COMMON ADULT DOSAGE: 25 to 100 mcg once daily
SIDE EFFECTS: No major effects if correct dosage taken
AUXILIARY LABELS:

■ Take as directed.
■ Take with water on an empty stomach.

GENERIC NAME: liotrix (combined T_4-T_3 product)
TRADE NAME: Thyrolar, Euthroid
INDICATION: Hypothyroidism
COMMON ADULT DOSAGE: 60 to 120 mcg (based on T_4 content), taken once daily
SIDE EFFECTS: No major effects if correct dosage taken
AUXILIARY LABELS:

■ Take as directed.
■ Take with water on an empty stomach.

CONDITIONS OF THE PARATHYROID GLANDS AND THEIR TREATMENT

Hyperparathyroidism

Hyperparathyroidism is a condition in which there is an increased amount of parathyroid hormone (PTH) secreted into the bloodstream; it can arise from one or more of the four parathyroid glands. The most common cause of this condition is benign tumors. Another condition closely related is secondary parathyroid hyperplasia, in which all four glands are enlarged; this is linked to chronic renal disease. These two conditions are similar in that they both display increased calcium levels. This occurs because the increased levels of PTH promote the release of calcium into the bloodstream, which leads to bone weakening and an increased possibility of fractures (**Paget's disease**). In addition, the increased calcium level in the blood causes a buildup of calcium salts in the kidneys, which can cause kidney stones. Other side effects of hypercalcemia include muscle weakness, lethargy, and heart conduction changes.

Prognosis. The prognosis depends on the diagnosis of the condition. In some cases after removal of all or part of the affected gland, functioning may return to normal. Other patients may need to monitor their calcium intake for life. For those with renal failure, continuous dialysis may be necessary until a transplant is possible.

Non–Drug Treatment. Treatment depends on the underlying cause. Surgical removal of the entire or a section of the affected gland may be necessary. If the hyperparathyroidism is caused by improper kidney function, then transplantation or dialysis may be necessary to limit the disease process. Other treatments may include decreasing calcium levels by increasing fluid intake and/or limiting dietary intake of calcium.

Drug Treatment. The following drug monographs illustrate typical drugs used for hyperparathyroidism replacement therapy. Bisphosphonates may improve bone turnover. Medications termed "calcimimetics" are used to treat secondary hyperparathyroidism caused by kidney disease and are now also being used in the treatment of primary hyperparathyroidism; these agents (e.g., cinacalcet) reduce the amount of parathyroid hormone released by the parathyroid glands and are employed when surgery is not appropriate.

Bone Metabolism Regulators

GENERIC NAME: calcitonin-salmon injection
TRADE NAME: Miacalcin
ROUTE OF ADMINISTRATION: Injectable (refrigerate)
INDICATIONS: Paget's disease, hypercalcemia (used as short-term treatment); not common to use for postmenopausal osteoporosis since noninvasive intranasal form available
COMMON ADULT DOSAGE: Paget's disease, 50 units once daily IM or subcutaneously; hypercalcemia, 4 units/kg q12h; osteoporosis (injected intramuscularly or subcutaneously)
SIDE EFFECTS: Nausea, vomiting, diarrhea, facial flushing
AUXILIARY LABEL:
■ Refrigerate.

GENERIC NAME: calcitonin-salmon nasal spray
TRADE NAME: Fortical, Miacalcin
ROUTE OF ADMINISTRATION: Intranasal (refrigerate until opened)
INDICATION: Osteoporosis
COMMON ADULT DOSAGE: 200 units once daily intranasally for osteoporosis
SIDE EFFECTS: Runny nose or other sinus symptoms, nosebleed, nasal irritation, headache
AUXILIARY LABELS:
■ For nasal use only.
■ Discard after 30 days from first use.
■ Prime pump before first use.

Bisphosphonates

GENERIC NAME: etidronate sodium
TRADE NAME: Didronel
INDICATIONS: Paget's disease; also for bone growth after hip replacement surgery
COMMON ADULT DOSAGE: 5 to 10 mg/kg per day (may be given orally for up to 6 months or intravenously for 3 to 7 days; IV form is given in the institutional setting)
SIDE EFFECTS: Headache, gastrointestinal upset
AUXILIARY LABEL:
■ Take with full glass of water.
■ Take >30 minutes before first meal, other beverage, or medications; do not lie down for 30 minutes after dose.

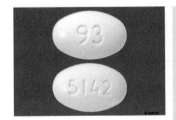

GENERIC NAME: alendronate
TRADE NAME: Fosamax
INDICATIONS: Paget's disease, postmenopausal osteoporosis
COMMON ADULT DOSAGE: Paget's disease, 40 mg orally once daily; osteoporosis, 10 mg once daily or 70 mg every week. Should be taken 30 minutes before breakfast
SIDE EFFECTS: Headache, gastrointestinal upset
AUXILIARY LABELS:
■ Take with full glass of water.
■ Take >30 min before first meal, other beverage, or medications; do not lie down for 30 minutes after dose.

GENERIC NAME: pamidronate
TRADE NAME: Aredia
INDICATIONS: Hypercalcemia caused by malignancy, Paget's disease, osteolytic metastases
COMMON ADULT DOSAGE: Hypercalcemia of malignancy, 60 to 90 mg IV over 2 to 24 hours; Paget's disease, 30 mg once daily IV × 3 days; osteolytic lesions, 90 mg IV over 2 hours every 3 to 4 weeks
ROUTE OF ADMINISTRATION: Intravenous infusion
SIDE EFFECTS: Headache, gastrointestinal upset

GENERIC NAME: zoledronic acid
TRADE NAME: Reclast
INDICATIONS: Paget's disease and osteoporosis
COMMON ADULT DOSAGE: Paget's disease, 5 mg IV at a constant infusion rate over no less than 15 minutes; given as 1 single dose; osteoporosis, 5 mg IV infusion given once yearly
ROUTE OF ADMINISTRATION: Intravenous infusion
SIDE EFFECTS: Headache, gastrointestinal upset
NOTE: This medication is administered by a health care provider in a health care setting.

Hypoparathyroidism

Malfunctioning of the parathyroid glands can cause hypoparathyroidism; decreased levels of PTH can result from removal of the parathyroid glands and, rarely, from a congenital or autoimmune disease. The result is **hypocalcemia**, which is the decrease in or lack of calcium; this calcium deficiency also reduces vitamin D levels in the body. Symptoms include muscle spasms, irregular heart contractions, and alteration of normal nerve conduction.

Prognosis. The prognosis is good, with replacement therapy administered for the patient's lifetime.

Non–Drug Treatment. The only treatment for hypoparathyroidism is the administration of the supplemental medications calcium and vitamin D.

Drug Treatment. Treatment is limited to replacement therapy with calcium and vitamin D supplements; examples are listed as follows:

Generic Name	Trade Name	Normal Adult Dosage for Hypoparathyroidism
Calcium Salts		
calcium carbonate	Tums	2-5 g PO daily given in divided doses
Vitamin D Preparations		
calcitriol	Rocaltrol, Calcijex	0.5-2 mcg PO once daily
dihydrotachysterol	DHT, Hytakerol	0.2-1.5 mg PO once daily
ergocalciferol	Calciferol, Drisdol	50,000-200,000 international units PO once daily

OSTEOPOROSIS MANAGEMENT AND TREATMENTS

Osteoporosis

Osteoporosis is the loss of calcium from the bones with insufficient replacement; this results in bones that become brittle and fracture easily. In nondiseased bone, as calcium is resorbed from the bone to maintain blood calcium levels, new calcium is formed at the same rate of loss. This maintains the strength of the bones. Estrogen plays an essential role in keeping bones strong and healthy in females. However, the decreasing levels of estrogen produced after menopause can make women susceptible to osteoporosis. Women who have had their ovaries removed, those who begin menopause at an early age, and those with irregular or infrequent periods are at higher risk of osteoporosis. Other factors that increase the risk of osteoporosis include long-term use of medications such as corticosteroids, medroxyprogesterone, and excessive thyroid hormones.

Prognosis. The prognosis of osteoporosis is good when treated early with dietary changes, exercise, and medication. If treated late there is usually some progression of the condition. Recent osteoporosis research has uncovered new treatments and prevention techniques that are helping Americans reduce their risk of acquiring this debilitating bone disease. According to the National Osteoporosis Foundation approximately 10 million people have osteoporosis and 34 million are estimated to have low bone mass which can lead to osteoporosis. The cost in 2005 was approximately $19 billion and is expected to rise to $25.3 billion by the year 2025 (http://www.nof.org/osteoporosis/diseasefacts.htm).

Non–Drug Treatments. It has been found that prevention against osteoporosis must be started early in life through lifestyle changes such as following an exercise program, eating a healthy diet, and refraining from smoking. Exercise helps to increase bone density, as does maintaining adequate intake of calcium and vitamin D. Calcium requirements can be met by drinking milk, eating cheese, or taking calcium supplements. New studies have shown that only 15 minutes of direct sunlight twice weekly (without the use of sunscreen) can supply enough vitamin D for the body.

Drug Treatments. Fosamax and Miacalcin are two examples of agents used to treat osteoporosis. Multivitamins that contain vitamin D may replace the sun's natural treatment. Several medications are being used to treat or prevent osteoporosis, including the following:

Trade Name	Generic Name	Normal Adult Dosage
Actonel	risedronate	5 mg PO once daily, or 35 mg once weekly, or 75 mg once daily × 2 days each month, or 150 mg once monthly
Boniva	ibandronate	2.5 mg PO once daily or 150 mg once monthly
Evista	raloxifene	60 mg PO once daily
Forteo	teriparatide (Subcut)	20 mcg subQ once daily
Fosamax	alendronate plus vitamin D	5-10 mg PO once daily, or 35 mg twice weekly, or 70 mg once weekly
Miacalcin	calcitonin-salmon (nasal spray)	1 spray, alternate nostril, once daily
	calcitonin-salmon (injectable)	100 units IM or Subcut every other day
Reclast	zoledronic acid	5 mg IV infusion once yearly

Osteoporosis Prevention

Bisphosphonates (see previous discussion) are often administered for osteoporosis prevention as well as for treatment. For prevention of osteoporosis in menopausal women, the following hormonal agents are representative of the many estrogen-containing products used (these should not be taken if pregnant or breast-feeding):

Trade Name	Generic Name	Common Adult Dosages
CombiPatch	estradiol/norethindrone acetate	Patch changed twice weekly
Alora, Estraderm, or Vivelle-Dot	estradiol patch	Patch changed twice weekly*
Climara or Menostar	estradiol patch	Patch changed every 7 days*
Estrace	estradiol	0.5 mg once daily*
Ogen	estropipate	0.75 mg once daily*
Premarin	conjugated estrogens	0.3 or 0.625 mg once daily*

*Continuous, daily unopposed estrogen is acceptable in women without a uterus. In women with an intact uterus, estrogen may be given cyclically or combined with a progestin for at least 10 to 14 days/month to minimize the risk of endometrial overgrowth and associated risks.

CONDITIONS OF THE ADRENAL GLANDS AND THEIR TREATMENT

Each adrenal gland consists of two portions—a cortex and a medulla. Diseases of the adrenal cortex range from overproduction to underproduction of steroids.

The cortex can be subdivided into three separate areas, each with its own specialized functions. Conditions affecting the cortex can be within one or more of the three areas. The three types of steroids produced include mineralocorticoids, glucocorticoids, and sex steroids. A decrease in secretion of these steroids can affect the levels of sodium, potassium, and chloride within the body; can alter carbohydrate metabolism; or can cause sexual problems.

Cushing's Syndrome

Cushing's syndrome is a rare condition affecting about 13 out of every 1 million people. It is caused by an oversecretion of the steroid cortisol into the bloodstream. Approximately 30% of Cushing's syndrome cases are caused by a tumor in the adrenal gland (normally noncancerous) that secretes cortisol. As cortisol is released from the adrenal glands symptoms develop that can include obesity, flushing of the face, hypertension, and thick, scaling skin. Other symptoms include overall weakness, fatigue, and slow-healing injuries. Osteoarthritis may also be experienced as bone deterioration is accelerated.

In approximately 70% of the cases of Cushing's syndrome, the cause is overproduction of corticotropin. The following three etiologies are associated with excess corticotropin production: hypersecretion of corticotropin from the pituitary glands, causing **Cushing's disease**; the presence of a corticotropin-releasing tumor located in another organ; or overmedication with corticosteroids (e.g., transplant recipients, persons with rheumatoid arthritis, or persons with severe asthma who must take corticosteroids as part of their treatment).

Prognosis. After a nonmalignant tumor is removed and treated, the prognosis is good. For those persons who are taking corticosteroids for severe conditions, the disadvantages must be weighed against the benefits of the medication.

Non–Drug Treatment. Adrenal gland tumors that cause Cushing's syndrome also require surgery. After excision of the tumor medication may be necessary. Chemotherapy may be indicated for a cancerous tumor. Persons suffering from Cushing's disease require either surgical excision of the tumor or radiation therapy.

Drug Treatment. Cushing's syndrome may require drug therapy such as mitotane, metyrapone, or aminoglutethimide, all of which decrease cortisol levels if the condition continues after surgery.

Addison's Disease

Addison's disease (that is, chronic adrenal insufficiency, hypoadrenocorticism, and hypocorticalism) is a rare hormonal disorder that is caused by a deficiency of cortisol in the bloodstream. In approximately 70% of persons suffering from Addison's disease, autoimmune disease causes dysfunction of the adrenal cortex. Less common causes include tuberculosis, fungal infection, or tumors that destroy the adrenal gland. Addison's disease results in the total necrosis of the adrenal cortex. Symptoms begin gradually and include fatigue, weight loss, nausea, and syncope.

Prognosis. Depending on the cause of this condition it is possible to correct the cortisol levels and return the adrenal gland to normal function, although the replacement therapy must be taken for the patient's life. If left untreated Addison's disease can be life-threatening.

Non–Drug Treatment. Surgery may be indicated for tumor removal. In addition, the patient may need to balance both potassium and sodium intake in the daily diet. Monitoring daily weight and recording daily intake and output of fluids may be necessary as well.

Drug Treatment. Treatment consists of replacement therapy with oral synthetic glucocorticoids and mineralocorticoids.

Mineralocorticoid

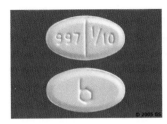

GENERIC NAME: fludrocortisone acetate
TRADE NAME: Florinef
INDICATION: Addison's disease
COMMON ADULT DOSAGE: 0.1 mg PO once daily
SIDE EFFECTS: Gastrointestinal upset
AUXILIARY LABEL:

■ Take as directed.

NOTE: *Under certain conditions, glucocorticoids can help the healing process of an inflamed or injured area. Following are glucocorticoid agents used for Addison's disease and for various inflammatory processes:*

Glucocorticoids

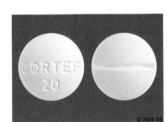

GENERIC NAME: hydrocortisone
TRADE NAME: Cortef
INDICATIONS: Adrenal deficiency, inflammation
COMMON ADULT DOSAGE: 20 to 240 mg PO once daily
SIDE EFFECTS: Gastrointestinal upset
AUXILIARY LABELS:

■ Take as directed.
■ Take with food.
NOTE: Additional dosage forms include the following injectables: hydrocortisone acetate, hydrocortisone sodium succinate (e.g., A-Hydrocort, Solu-Cortef). Dosages vary dependent on the condition treated and the individual response.

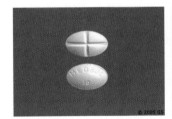

GENERIC NAME: methylprednisolone
TRADE NAME: Medrol
INDICATIONS: Inflammation, Addison's disease
COMMON ADULT DOSAGE: 4 to 48 mg PO once daily
SIDE EFFECTS: Gastrointestinal upset
AUXILIARY LABEL:

■ Take as directed.
NOTE: Methylprednisolone dose-packs are available in 21-tablet sets and are commonly dispensed to slowly taper the patient off the medication or to a maintenance level of continued medication.

GENERIC NAME: methylprednisolone acetate
TRADE NAME: Depo-Medrol
INDICATIONS: Addison's disease, inflammation
COMMON ADULT DOSAGE: 10 to 40 mg IM (for short-term use)
SIDE EFFECTS: Gastrointestinal upset
AUXILIARY LABEL:

■ None

GENERIC NAME: methylprednisolone sodium succinate
TRADE NAME: Solu-Medrol
INDICATIONS: Addison's disease, inflammation
COMMON ADULT DOSAGE: 10 to 40 mg IV or IM (for short-term use); common for doses to be higher for acute inflammation, such as 125 mg q6h
SIDE EFFECTS: Gastrointestinal upset
AUXILIARY LABEL:
■ None

GENERIC NAME: prednisolone; prednisolone sodium phosphate
TRADE NAME: Prelone Syrup; Pediapred, Orapred
INDICATION: Inflammation
COMMON ADULT DOSAGE: 5 to 60 mg once daily
SIDE EFFECTS: Gastrointestinal upset
AUXILIARY LABELS:
■ Take as directed.
■ Do not stop taking abruptly.
■ Take with food or milk.
■ Avoid alcohol.
NOTE: Syrup must be measured in calibrated dose-cup, oral syringe, or measuring spoon.

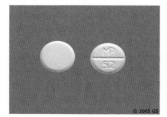

GENERIC NAME: prednisone
TRADE NAME: Deltasone, Predone
INDICATION: Inflammation
COMMON ADULT DOSAGE: 5 to 60 mg once daily
SIDE EFFECTS: Gastrointestinal upset
AUXILIARY LABELS:
■ Take as directed.
■ Do not stop taking abruptly.
■ Take with food or milk.
■ Avoid alcohol.
NOTE: Syrup must be measured in calibrated dose-cup, oral syringe, or measuring spoon.

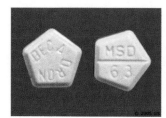

GENERIC NAME: dexamethasone
TRADE NAME: Decadron
INDICATIONS: Endocrine and allergic disorders, inflammation
COMMON ADULT DOSAGE: 0.75 to 9 mg PO once daily or divided into several doses daily (initial dose); maintenance dose varies
SIDE EFFECTS: Gastrointestinal upset
AUXILIARY LABELS:
■ Take as directed.
■ Take with food.

Adrenal Medulla

Most of the conditions that affect the adrenal medulla result from tumor growth. The two main types of tumors affecting the adrenal medulla are **neuroblastomas** and **pheochromocytomas**. Although neuroblastomas are known to grow rapidly and metastasize, they can be treated with chemotherapy, radiation, and surgical removal. Pheochromocytomas usually are benign and can cause hypertension. With surgical removal, the hypertension is relieved and the patient's prognosis is good.

Tech Note!

ENDOCRINE CONDITIONS OF THE PANCREAS GLAND AND THEIR TREATMENTS

The pancreas is responsible for the production and release of insulin. Insulin is important in the transportation of glucose into cells, where it is then either used for energy or stored as glycogen. Insulin also stimulates protein synthesis and releases fatty acids from fat deposits. A deficiency of insulin has a dramatic effect on the body's ability to access essential nutrients for fuel and storage. This condition is referred to as diabetes mellitus.

Diabetes Mellitus

One of the most well-known conditions that can affect the pancreas is **diabetes mellitus**. Diabetes mellitus (DM) is a chronic disease of either a deficiency in the production of insulin (type 1) or a resistance to insulin (type 2) because of disturbances in carbohydrate, protein, and fat metabolism. DM affects approximately 6% of the population of the United States with an estimated 50% of those afflicted not yet diagnosed. Diabetes is more common in women than men and the incidence rises with age. DM occurs in the following four forms that are classified by their cause.

Type 1. Type 1 diabetes is caused by destruction or defect in the beta cells of the pancreas. This results in undersecretion of insulin, thus making glucose transport ineffective. Type 1 is subdivided into two categories:

- Immune-mediated diabetes: The lack of insulin causes hyperglycemia and/ or ketoacidosis. Children and adolescents with immune-mediated diabetes can rapidly develop ketoacidosis. The effects of diabetic ketoacidosis (DKA) include dehydration that may ultimately cause shock and coma. The effects of hyperglycemia include the symptoms polyuria (frequent urination), polydipsia (excessive thirst), and polyphagia (excessive appetite); these are known as the three P's and are classic signs of type 1 diabetes. The loss of glucose via urination can cause dehydration, weight loss, and extreme hunger. Excessive urination is due to the absorption of fluids from tissues. Other symptoms include fatigue, which is caused by the lack of energy that is normally available from the metabolism of glucose. Type 1 immune-mediated diabetes beta cell destruction is more common in children than in adults. Most adults experience hyperglycemia unless they develop an infection or other stressor, which can cause ketoacidosis.
- Idiopathic diabetes: Persons diagnosed with idiopathic diabetes are prone to ketoacidosis.

Type 2. Most patients with type 2 diabetes are obese and have acquired insulin resistance. Most commonly adults are affected; however, the increasing prevalence of obesity in children has resulted in an increased incidence of children being diagnosed with type 2 diabetes.

Type 2 diabetes does allow insulin to be released from the beta cells; however, the receptors are insulin resistant and do not allow effective transport of glucose. Blood glucose levels are variable at best. The following co-morbidities are associated with a risk of type 2 diabetes:

- Obesity
- Lack of physical activity
- Hypertension
- History of gestational DM
- Older than age 45 years

- Strong family history of diabetes
- High levels of low-density lipoprotein cholesterol

Gestational Diabetes Mellitus (GDM). This type of diabetes occurs in women during pregnancy; blood glucose levels usually return to normal after childbirth. According to data from the American Diabetes Association gestational diabetes occurs in approximately 4% of women during pregnancy. GDM is only associated with pregnancy; weight gain and an increase in the concentrations of estrogen and placental hormones, which antagonize insulin, are its two precipitating factors. The effects may last only through the pregnancy period, although the condition must be treated through diet and possibly insulin injections. Some patients with gestational diabetes will have risk factors to develop type 2 diabetes mellitus later in life. For more information on gestational diabetes, visit www.diabetes.org/gestational-diabetes.jsp.

Other Specific Types. Some patients have diabetes as a result of a genetic defect or exposure to certain drugs or chemicals, and some patients may have combined features of both type 1 and type 2 DM.

Prognosis. With proper treatment and management of DM a person can lead a normal life, although it is necessary to be continuously monitored by a physician. Education in both diet and exercise is essential for a successful outcome.

Patients with diabetes are at risk for secondary complications if their condition is not well-controlled; these complications impact both quality and longevity of life. Macrovascular and microvascular complications of diabetes, and other conditions, include the following:

- Atherosclerosis (cardiac disease, including risk for heart attack)
- Erectile dysfunction (impotence)
- Gastroparesis
- Increased infections of the skin (feet), urinary tract (UTI's), and vagina (vaginitis)
- Nephropathy (kidney disease)
- Orthostatic hypotension
- Peripheral neuropathy

Non–Drug Treatment. The first line of treatment for patients with Type 2 DM is a change in lifestyle (i.e., following a strict diet and engaging in an exercise regimen) combined with meticulous hygiene. A diabetic diet must include the proper amount and combination of foods. Almost all foods are permissible in small amounts on an occasional basis. Both diet and exercise can regulate the amount of glucose in the bloodstream. Another important daily routine is to check the feet for swelling, redness, and warmth. Because of the lack of blood flow, the feet are numb and highly susceptible to infections, and the patient can be unaware of any damage.

For persons diagnosed with type 2 diabetes caused by obesity, weight loss is prescribed. With most persons, weight loss will help reverse the condition and some patients may not require any medication.

Drug Treatments. There are many medications available to treat DM and are prescribed based on the type of DM diagnosed.

For type 1 diabetes, insulin (given subcutaneously) is necessary. Two main types of insulin are used for type 1 DM: natural insulin, which is taken from animals such as pigs (porcine) or cows (bovine); and synthesized human insulin,

Tech Alert!

All insulin suspensions (e.g., NPH insulin) must be mixed before administration; they cannot be shaken but must be rolled between the hands several times in order to mix the solution before use. Insulin should never be shaken because this will break down the proteins and the insulin will become unusable. Also, when checking insulin stock, always check for proper consistency, clarity, and color. If there is any clumping or unusual coloration, alert the pharmacist before dispensing.

which is made in a laboratory and is chemically identical to human insulin. Persons who are newly diagnosed with type 1 DM are given the newer DNA recombinant human insulin. Some persons continue to take insulin derived from animals; however, most forms of animal-derived insulin are no longer marketed and patients in the United States have largely transitioned to human insulin. Injected insulin helps maintain the glucose levels of the blood. Short- and long-acting insulins are used to maintain metabolic homeostasis. Typical insulins prescribed are listed in Table 15-6.

Two types of dosage forms for injectable insulins are prefilled syringes or vials. Regular insulins are clear liquids, whereas mixtures of insulin combine two types of solutions that form a suspension. These latter include regular and isophane insulin combinations. A suspension is formed when solutions such as zinc are mixed with crystalline-type insulin, which precipitates and forms a milky mixture. Clear insulins do not need to be mixed before use, but suspensions need to be mixed to provide a uniform appearance and ensure proper dosing. Also, all insulins, while kept in the refrigerator in the pharmacy, should be at room temperature before being administered to the patient. Figure 15-7 shows a sample of the two types of insulin labels.

Patients with type 2 DM may require oral antidiabetic agents to limit insulin resistance and to control blood glucose levels; some patients with type 2 DM may require insulin as well. The drugs listed in Table 15-7 are examples of oral hypoglycemic agents used to treat type 2 DM. Many new drugs

TABLE 15-6 Commonly Prescribed Insulins for Insulin-Dependent Diabetes Mellitus (All Are Given Subcutaneously)

Type of Action	Generic/Brand Names	Onset of Action	Duration of Action
Rapid-acting	insulin lispro/Humalog, Humalog KwikPen, Humalog Pen, Humalog Cartridge	5-15 min	3-4 hr
Rapid-acting	insulin aspart/NovoLog, NovoLog FlexPen, NovoLog PenFill	5-15 min	3-4 hr
Short-acting	insulin regular/Humulin R, Humulin R (concentrated), Novolin R, ReliOn/Novolin R	30-60 min	6-8 hr
Intermediate-acting	isophane insulin/Humulin N, Humulin N Pen, Novolin N, ReliOn Novolin N	1-2 hr	14-20 hr
Intermediate-acting	insulin zinc/Humulin L	1-2 hr	14-20 hr
Long-acting	insulin glargine/Lantus	2 hr	Up to 24 hr
Long-acting	insulin detemir/Levemir (cartridges and prefilled syringes)	2 hr	Up to 24 hr
Mixed long- and short-acting insulins	isophane and regular insulin/Humulin 50/50, 70/30, Humulin 70/30 Pen, Novolin 70/30, ReliOn/Novolin 70/30	Biphasic	Up to 24 hr; has properties of both long-acting and short-acting insulins
Mixed long- and short-acting insulins	isophane and regular insulin/Humulin 50/50, 70/30, Humulin 70/30 Pen, Novolin 70/30, ReliOn Novolin 70/30 InnoLet, ReliOn/Novolin 70/30	Biphasic	Has properties of both long-acting and short-acting insulins
Mixed long- and short-acting insulins	lispro and lispro protamine/Humalog mix 50/50, Humalog mix 50/50 Pen, Humalog mix 50/50 KwikPen, Humalog mix 75/25, Humalog mix 75/25 Pen, Humalog mix 75/25 KwikPen	Biphasic	Has properties of both long-acting and short-acting insulins

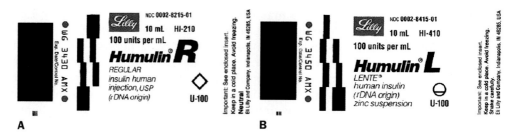

FIGURE 15-7 A, Humulin R (fast-acting). **B,** Humulin L (intermediate-acting).

TABLE 15-7 Antidiabetic Agents for Type 2 Diabetes Mellitus

Generic Name	Trade Name	Normal Maintenance Dosage Range for Adults
Oral Antidiabetic Agents That Control Glucose Levels in the Blood		
Meglitinides		
nateglinide	Starlix	120 mg tid with meals
repaglinide	Prandin	0.5-4 mg bid, tid, or qid with meals
Sulfonylureas		
chlorpropamide	Diabinese	100-250 mg bid
glimepiride	Amaryl	1-4 mg daily
glipizide	Glucotrol	5-10 mg daily
glyburide	Micronase, DiaBeta	1.5-20 mg daily
tolazamide	Tolinase	100-500 mg daily
tolbutamide	Orinase	500 mg daily
Oral Antidiabetic Agents That Decrease Insulin Resistance		
Alpha-glucosidase inhibitors		
acarbose	Precose	25-100 mg tid
miglitol	Glyset	50-100 mg tid
Biguanides		
metformin	Glucophage, Fortamet	Up to 2000 mg/day in divided doses
Thiazolidinediones		
pioglitazone	Actos	15-45 mg daily
rosiglitazone	Avandia	4-8 mg daily with or without food
Other Agents		
incretin mimetic		
exenatide	Byetta	10 mcg bid subcutaneously before meals
sitagliptin	Januvia	100 mg PO once daily
Agents Given for Type 1 and Type 2 DM		
Amylinomimetics		
pramlintide	Symlin	Taken subcutaneously just before each major meal
Antidote for Antidiabetic Agents or to Treat Severe Hypoglycemia		
glucagon	Glucagon	1 mg oral to 1 mg by injection

TABLE 15-8 Combination Oral Agents

Generic	Trade	Adult Maintenance Dose
glyburide/metformin	Glucovance	1.25/250 mg daily, may increase q 2 weeks
glipizide/metformin	Metaglip	Max 20 mg/2000 mg daily
rosiglitazone/metformin	Avandamet	Max 8 mg/2000 mg daily
pioglitazone/metformin	Actoplus Met	Max 45 mg/2550 mg daily
rosiglitazone/glimepiride	Avandaryl	Max 8 mg/4 mg daily
pioglitazone/glimepiride	Duetact	Max 30 mg/4 mg daily
repaglinide/metformin	PrandiMet	Max 10 mg/2500 mg daily
sitagliptin/metformin	Janumet	Max 100 mg/2000 mg daily
rosiglitazone/metformin	Avandamet	2 mg/500 mg to 8 mg/2000 mg daily

have been introduced to treat type 2 DM, because of the increasing incidence of this condition in the population. Because so many new agents are being marketed, it is important for technicians always to stay abreast of the various agents being used.

Combination Agents. A movement in the therapy for type 2 diabetes is toward multiple drug therapy. This therapy is considered advantageous to those persons suffering from type 2 DM who may not be able to control their condition by exercise and diet alone. There are several combination drugs that are prescribed to treat type 2 diabetes (Table 15-8).

Blood Glucose Meters. Patients with diabetes must monitor their blood glucose levels by taking a drop of blood using a small needle called a lancet. Although the finger is the most common location used for blood sampling, there are meters that allow blood to be taken from the forearm, thigh, or fleshy part of the hand. Blood sampling is done several times daily. The blood is then placed onto a strip that is inserted into a meter or directly on the meter. Meters will display a digital number on the screen that indicates blood glucose levels. There are a wide range of blood glucose meters available, including those that have memory so previous levels can be stored and those with large font size for persons with poor eyesight.

Regardless of the type of meter chosen it is important to keep the meter clean and the test strips in proper condition. Meters must be calibrated correctly for the current box of test strips and the strips must be at room temperature to work accurately. Technology has advanced the monitoring of glucose levels, and this has given consumers more choices for testing. Users must decide which type of meter best suits them. Considerations include those meters with varying blood sample size, data and computer compatibility, memory, alternative testing sites, and speakers for the visual impaired. Common diagnostic devices used for monitoring glucose levels via blood and urine are listed in Table 15-9.

Checking the glucose content of urine is another method for monitoring glucose levels in the diabetic patient, although it is not as accurate as blood glucose testing. Urine testing of glucose is not normally done unless it is not possible to obtain a blood sample. Urine testing can be helpful to test for ketones. If more fat is being burned instead of glucose, there will be an increase in the concentration of ketones in the urine, which indicates there is too little insulin available. When the strip contacts glucose in the urine, the strip changes color. The resulting color is compared with the chart provided, which indicates the amount of ketones in the urine. From the determination made, the patient can take the proper amount of insulin necessary to balance his or her system.

TABLE 15-9 Diagnostic Devices for Blood and Urine Analysis

Device	Manufacturer	Type of Meter	Tests for	Features
Chemstrip bG	Bio-Dynamics	Urine	Ketones	Strips: 100/bottle
Clinistix	Bayer Corp	Urine	Ketones	Strips: 50/bottle
Combistix	Bayer Corp	Urine	Ketones	Strips: 100/bottle
Diastix	Bayer Corp	Urine	Ketones	Strips: 50, 100/bottle
Clinitest	Bayer Corp	Urine	Ketones	Tablets: 36, 100/bottle
Glucostix	Bayer Corp	Blood	Glucose	Strips: 25, 50, 100/bottle
OneTouch	LifeScan	Blood	Glucose	Strips: 25, 50, 100/bottle; used with OneTouch brand meter
Contour Monitoring System	Ascensia	Blood	Glucose	240 memory with date and time; results in 15 sec; no coding required; PC downloading
DEX 2	Ascensia	Blood	Glucose	10-test strip disc; results in 30 sec; time-specific averages; PC downloading
FreeStyle Flash Kit	Abbott	Blood	Glucose	Multiple testing sites (forearm, upper arm, thigh, calf, fleshy part of hand); smallest sample size; backlit display and test light; results in 7 sec; 250-test memory with date and time; 14-day result average; 4 alarms for when to retest
Precision Xtra	Abbott	Blood	Glucose	Simple 2-step testing; simple icon-driven menu; result review with scroll option; no manual coding; tests both glucose (5 sec) and ketone levels
OneTouch Ultra	LifeScan	Blood	Glucose	Results in 5 sec; requires just speck of blood; may test on forearm
Elite	Ascensia	Blood	Glucose	Results in 30 sec; 10-action strip; 20 memories; small blood volume
OneTouch Select	LifeScan	Blood	Glucose	Results in 5 sec; 350-test memory; automatic 7-14 and 30 day averages; alternate testing sites (forearm/palm); English or Spanish
OneTouch UltraLink	LifeScan	Blood	Glucose	Wireless communication of test results; results in 5 sec; scrolling capabilities; monitors before and after meal averages
OneTouch UltraMini	LifeScan	Blood	Glucose	Results in 5 sec; available in pink, silver, and black

Hormones Secreted by the Ovaries and Their Uses

Many important hormones regulate the female reproductive system. Within the ovaries, many hormones are produced that are responsible for the secondary sex characteristics of the female body and for reproduction. The two main hormones produced are estrogen and progesterone. Estrogen is primarily responsible for the development of female organs, breasts, and female body contours caused by

TABLE 15-10 Examples of Alternate Routes of Administration of Estrogens

Trade Name	Generic Name	Common Usage	Dosage Form
Alora, Climara, Estraderm, Vivelle, Vivelle-Dot	estradiol	Reduces symptoms of menopause. Other uses include conditions that cause low levels of estrogen or after oophorectomy. This drug may be prescribed for teenagers who fail to mature at usual rate. In addition, Alora can be used for prevention of osteoporosis in conjunction with diet, exercise, and calcium supplements.	Patches
FemPatch, Esclim	estradiol	Reduces symptoms of menopause. Other uses include conditions that cause low levels of estrogen. This drug may be prescribed for teenagers who fail to mature at usual rate.	Patches
Elestrin, Divigel, Oestrogel	estradiol	Treats symptoms of menopause, specifically those associated with itching, burning, and dryness around vaginal area.	Topical gel in a metered-dose pump (Elestrin and Estrogel); gel packets (Divigel); pump-pack (Oestrogel)
Estrace	estradiol	Treats symptoms of menopause, specifically those associated with itching, burning, and dryness around vaginal area. Treats urgency or irritation of urination.	Vaginal cream with applicator
Estraderm, Esclim	estradiol	Reduces symptoms of menopause. May be used to prevent osteoporosis with diet, exercise, and calcium supplements. In addition, Estraderm may be used for estrogen replacement after oophorectomy.	Transdermal biweekly patches
Estrasorb	estradiol	Treats moderate to severe vasomotor symptoms of menopause.	Topical emulsion (foil-laminated pouches)
Estring, Femring	estradiol	Treats moderate to severe vasomotor symptoms of menopause and/or moderate to severe symptoms of vulvar and vaginal atrophy associated with menopause.	Ring (replace every 3 months)
Estrogel	estradiol	Treats moderate to severe vasomotor symptoms of menopause and/or moderate to severe symptoms of vulvar and vaginal atrophy associated with menopause.	Topical gel (metered-dose pump)
Evamist	estradiol	Treats symptoms of menopause.	Transdermal spray
Menostar	estradiol	Prevents osteoporosis in postmenopausal women.	Weekly patch
Premarin	conjugated estrogens	Treatment of dry, itchy external genitals and vaginal irritation due to vaginal degeneration due to menopause.	Vaginal cream with applicator

fat distribution. Estrogen also stimulates the growth of epithelial cells that line the uterus. Progesterone is secreted during the midpoint of the menstrual cycle and is responsible for changes in the uterus that prepare it for normal menstrual periods; progesterone is an important hormone during early pregnancy.

Treatment with an estrogen is indicated for the following:
- To correct estrogen deficiency; estrogen deficiency results in abnormal uterine bleeding, hypogonadism, decreased ovarian functioning, and post-menopausal osteoporosis
- For cancer therapy in the breast or advanced prostatic carcinomas

Treatment with a progestin is indicated for the following:
- To correct female hormonal imbalance that may cause amenorrhea, dysmenorrhea, or endometriosis
- To prevent pregnancy
- To maintain early pregnancy; certain dosage forms used during infertility protocols

See Chapter 24 for drugs used with these hormones.

There are many medications that are available in other routes of administration. These various drugs and dosage forms are listed in Table 15-10. Most topical sprays, gels, and transdermal patches are applied to the skin on the upper arm.

Conditions of the Testes and Their Treatment

The primary hormone secreted by males is androgen; testosterone is one of the main androgens. Testosterone regulates the development of secondary male sex characteristics. Testosterone also influences the growth and development of the musculoskeletal system and the production of sperm.

Treatment with testosterone or other androgens is indicated for the following:

- Testosterone deficiency resulting from cyst formation or removal of the testicles
- Treatment of delayed onset of puberty
- Certain types of breast carcinoma in women
- Certain types of anemia

See Chapter 24 for products that contain androgenic hormones.

DO YOU REMEMBER THESE KEY POINTS?

- The main glands of the endocrine system
- The main functions of the thyroid gland, pituitary gland, hypothalamus, adrenal glands, and pancreas
- The common diseases associated with the organs of the endocrine system
- The effect melatonin has on the body and the name of the gland that produces it
- How hormones regulate the reproductive system
- Which organs are linked to specific hormones
- Types of replacement therapies available to treat conditions of the reproductive system
- The locations of the primary calcium regulators and where secretion takes place
- The causes and types of diabetes
- The treatments of diabetes
- The differences between types of insulin
- The types of glucose meters available
- Routes of administration available for medicines containing estrogen

REVIEW QUESTIONS

Multiple choice questions

1. Three glands located in the head are the:
   A. Pineal, pituitary, and pancreas
   B. Hypothalamus, pituitary, and pineal
   C. Pituitary, exocrine, and endocrine
   D. None of the above

2. _____ hormones act on the same cell from which they are secreted, whereas _____ hormones must travel through the bloodstream to their target organ.
   A. Endocrine; autocrine
   B. Autocrine; paracrine
   C. Paracrine; endocrine
   D. Autocrine; endocrine

3. T_4 and T_3 are secreted from the:
   A. Thymus
   B. Adrenal gland
   C. Thyroid gland
   D. Pituitary gland

4. The endocrine system keeps the body in balance by a mechanism known as:
   A. Endocrine
   B. Exocrine
   C. Homeostasis
   D. Negative feedback

5. Thyroid-stimulating hormone, follicle-stimulating hormone, and adrenocorticotropic hormone are secreted from the:
   A. Hypothalamus
   B. Anterior pituitary gland
   C. Posterior pituitary gland
   D. Thyroid gland

6. The essential ions necessary for T_3 and T_4 production are:
   A. Proteins
   B. Carbohydrates
   C. Fatty acids
   D. Iodines

7. The endocrine gland(s) that help(s) regulate the kidneys and secrete(s) epinephrine and norepinephrine is (are) the:
   A. Parathyroid glands
   B. Pituitary gland
   C. Pancreas
   D. Adrenal glands

8. The most common causes of conditions affecting the endocrine system are:
   A. Tumors
   B. Cancer
   C. Congenital factors
   D. Smoking

9. The condition that affects children suffering from hypothyroidism is known as:
   A. Aphasia
   B. Cretinism
   C. Myxedema
   D. None of the above

10. The cause of diabetes is:
    A. The inability of the pancreas to secrete enough insulin to regulate glucose level
    B. A resistance to insulin that can affect the metabolism of glucose
    C. Other factors such as blindness or renal failure
    D. Both A and B

11. Glimepiride is used to treat:
A. Type 2 diabetes
B. Type 1 diabetes
C. Both type 1 and type 2 diabetes
D. None of the above

12. Which combination drug does NOT have metformin as a main ingredient?
A. Actoplus Met
B. Avandaryl
C. Glucovance
D. Metaglip

13. Which hormone is produced by the adrenal medulla and affects the parasympathetic nervous system?
A. Cortisol
B. Epinephrine
C. Melatonin
D. Oxytocin

14. Which of the following hormones is NOT produced by the pituitary gland?
A. Antidiuretic hormone
B. Calcitonin
C. Follicle-stimulating hormone
D. Growth hormone

15. Which of the following medications can be taken once a month?
A. Actonel
B. Boniva
C. Evista
D. Fosamax

True/False

If the statement is false, then change it to make it true.

_____ **1.** Acromegaly is a childhood disease caused by a deficiency of growth hormone.

_____ **2.** The hypothalamus links the central nervous system to the endocrine system.

_____ **3.** Hormones are produced in the primary gland and secreted from the target gland.

_____ **4.** Graves' disease is marked by the enlargement of the neck region.

_____ **5.** Types of insulin can be long-acting or short-acting.

_____ **6.** Aphasia is another term for hyperthyroidism.

_____ **7.** Persons with non–insulin-dependent diabetes mellitus usually need to make lifestyle changes, whereas those with insulin-dependent diabetes mellitus need insulin injections for life.

_____ **8.** Insulin helps maintain glucose levels in the pancreas.

_____ **9.** The two main hormones secreted by the ovaries are estrogen and progesterone.

_____ **10.** The hormone androgen is responsible for the development of male secondary sexual characteristics and also affects women's sex drives.

_____ **11.** The follicle stimulator is produced only in females.

_____ **12.** Excess glucose is converted into fat.

_____ **13.** The hormone aldosterone regulates the balance of salt and water.

_____ **14.** Estrogen is produced in the ovaries and regulates the menstrual cycle.

_____ **15.** Duetact is a combination drug composed of rosiglitazone and glimepiride.

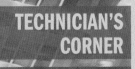

TECHNICIAN'S CORNER

Using a drug reference book or online drug source, determine whether there are any drug interactions between any of the following drugs:

Calcium carbonate (Os-Cal) 500 mg PO once daily
Levothyroxine (Synthroid) 0.1 mg PO once daily
Aspirin, enteric-coated, 325 mg PO once daily
Glipizide (Glucotrol) 5 mg PO once daily

BIBLIOGRAPHY

AMA (American Medical Association) Concise Medical Encyclopedia. 2006.

Chabner D-E: *The language of medicine*, ed 9, 2010, Saunders.

Damjanov I: *Pathology for the health professions*, ed 3, Philadelphia, 2005, Saunders.

Drug facts and comparisons, ed 63, St Louis, 2008, Lippincott Williams & Wilkins.

Gebhart F: Combination products offer alternative for type 2 diabetes patients, Drug Topics Oct 2005. Retrieved from www.drugtopics.com/drugtopics/article/articleDetail.jsp?id=184895

Hoffman R, M.D.: Panhypopituitarism, Updated: 9/25/08. Referenced: 9/09. http://organizedwisdom.com/helpbar/index.html?return=http://organizedwisdom.com/Simmonds'_Disease&url=www.emedicine.com/ped/topic1812.htm

National Osteoporosis Foundation: Osteoporosis: A debilitating disease that can be prevented and treated, 2008. Referenced 9/09. www.nof.org/osteoporosis/index.htm

Professional guide to diseases, ed 9, Ambler, PA, 2009, Lippincott Williams & Wilkins.

Rosenthal W: *New insights into osteoporosis management*, New York, 2004, Power$_X$-Pak CE/Jobson Publishing.

Rx Med: General illness information, Diabetes Insipidus. www.rxmed.com/b.main/b1.illness/b1.1.illnesses/DIABETES%20INSIPIDUS.htm

Salerno E: *Pharmacology for health professionals*, St Louis, 1999, Mosby.

Scanlon V, Sanders T: *Essentials of anatomy and physiology*, ed 5, Philadelphia, PA, 2007, FADavis.

Thibodeau G, Patton K: *Structure and function of the body*, ed 13, St Louis, 2007, Mosby.

Voet D: *Biochemistry*, ed 3, New York, 2004, Wiley.

16

Nervous System

Objectives

UPON COMPLETING THIS CHAPTER, YOU SHOULD BE ABLE TO DO THE FOLLOWING:

- Describe the major functions of the nervous system.

- Identify the main parts of a neuron.

- Describe how nerves function in transmitting impulses.

- List the primary neurotransmitters of the nervous system.

- Describe the differences between the central nervous system and the peripheral nervous system.

- Explain how the efferent system functions as opposed to the afferent system.

- Describe the major neurotransmitters of the peripheral nervous system and the central nervous system.

- Identify the types of drugs affecting the nervous system.

- Identify the differences between cholinergics and adrenergics, and their blocking agents.

- Give examples of conditions that affect the nervous system and describe how they are treated.

- List the drugs that affect the nervous system, explain their methods of action, and describe normal dosing.

- Identify the auxiliary labels for the drugs discussed.

TERMS AND DEFINITIONS

Afferent *The transmission of a neuronal impulse from the body toward the central nervous system*

Autonomic *Automatic or involuntary*

Autonomic nervous system *Division of the nervous system that controls the involuntary body functions; consists of sympathetic and parasympathetic divisions*

Axon *The part of a nerve cell that conducts impulses away from the cell body*

Blood-brain barrier *A barrier that exists in the brain as a result of special permeability characteristics of the capillaries that supply brain cells; these capillaries prevent certain solutes or chemicals from being transferred from the blood to the brain*

Brainstem *A section of the brain consisting of the medulla oblongata, pons, and midbrain; they connect the forebrain and cerebrum to the spinal cord*

Cell body *The main part of a neuron from which axons and dendrites extend*

Central nervous system *Consists of the brain and spinal cord; acts to coordinate sensory and motor control of body functions*

Cerebellum *Structure located posterior to the pons and medulla oblongata; responsible for posture, balance, and voluntary muscle movement*

Cerebrospinal fluid *A fluid that fills the ventricles of the brain and also occupies spaces of the brain or spinal cord and the arachnoid layer of the meninges*

Cervical *Pertaining to the neck region of the spinal cord; the region begins at the base of the skull and consists of the first seven vertebrae*

Coccyx *The small triangular bone located at the base of the spinal column; also known as the tailbone*

Dendrite *The part of a neuron that branches out to bring impulses to the cell body*

Efferent *The transmission of a neuronal impulse from the central nervous system toward the body*

Lumbar *The region of the spine that includes five vertebrae in the area between the ribs (thoracic spine) and the pelvis (sacral spine); also used to describe the area of the back around the waist*

Monoamine oxidases (MAOs) *Enzymes (includes MAO-A and MAO-B) found in nerve terminals, neurons, and liver cells; they inactivate chemicals such as tyramine, catecholamines, serotonin, and certain medications*

Nerve terminal *The end portion of the neuron where nerve impulses cause chemicals to be released; these chemicals (called neurotransmitters) cross a small space (called the synaptic cleft) to carry the impulse to another neuron*

Neuron *The functional unit of the nervous system, which includes the cell body, dendrites, axon, and terminals*

Neurotransmitters *Chemicals that are transmitted from one neuron to another as electrical nerve impulses*

Parasympathetic nervous system *Division of the autonomic nervous system that functions during restful situations; "breed or feed" part of the autonomic nervous system*

Peripheral nervous system *The division of the nervous system outside the brain and spinal cord*

Sacrum *The large triangular bone at the base of the spine; it connects superiorly with the last vertebra of the lumbar spine and inferiorly with the coccyx (tailbone). It is wedged between the two hip bones and helps form the pelvis.*

Somatic *The motor neurons of the peripheral nervous system that control voluntary actions of the skeletal muscles and provide sensory input (touch, hearing, sight)*

Sympathetic nervous system *Division of the autonomic nervous system that functions during stressful situations; "fight or flight" part of the autonomic nervous system*

Thoracic *Pertaining to the thorax area or the chest; essentially the region between the neck and abdomen; also describes the region of the spine that includes 12 vertebrae in the area between the neck (cervical spine) and lumbar (lumbar spine) regions*

COMMON DRUGS USED FOR CONDITIONS INVOLVING THE CENTRAL NERVOUS SYSTEM

Trade Name	Generic Name	Pronunciation	Trade Name	Generic Name	Pronunciation
Skeletal Muscle Relaxants			**Parkinson's Disease Agents**		
Dantrium	dantrolene	(**dan**-tro-lean)	Apokyn	apomorphine	(ah-poh-**mor**-feen)
Flexeril	cyclobenzaprine	(sigh-klo-**ben**-zah-preen)	Artane	trihexyphenidyl	(try-heks-ah-**fen**-a-dill)
			Cogentin	benztropine	(**benz**-tro-peen)
Lioresal	baclofen	(**back**-low-fen)	Comtan	entacapone	(en-**tak**-a-pone)
Norflex	orphenadrine	(or-**fen**-ah-dreen)	Eldepryl	selegiline	(se-**le**-ja-leen)
Parafon	chlorzoxazone	(klor-**zocks**-ah-zone)	Azilect	rasagiline	(ras-**aj**-il-een)
Robaxin	methocarbamol	(meth-o-**kar**-ba-mol)	Neupro	rotigotine	(row-**tig**-oh-teen)
Soma	carisoprodol	(kar-i-soe-**proe**-dole)	Mirapex	pramipexole	(**pram**-i-**pex**-ole)
			Parlodel	bromocriptine	(bro-mo-**krip**-teen)
Neuromuscular Blocking Agents			Requip	ropinirole	(row-**pin**-i-**role**)
Anectine	succinylcholine	(suck-si-nill-**koe**-leen)	Sinemet	carbidopa/levodopa	(**car**-bih-**doe**-pa/lee-vo-**doe**-pa)
Mivacron	mivacurium	(mih-vuh-**cure**-ee-um)			
Pavulon	pancuronium	(**pan**-kur-**row**-nee-um)	Symmetrel	amantadine	(ah-**man**-ta-deen)
None	vecuronium	(**vek**-you-**row**-nee-um)			
Zemuron	rocuronium	(row-kur-**oh**-nee-um)	**Migraine Agents**		
			Excedrin	acetaminophen (APAP)	(a-**seet**-a-**min**-oh-fen)
Dopamine Blockers					
Xenazine	tetrabenazine	(**tet**-rah-**ben**-a-zine)	Axert	almotriptan	(**al**-mow-**trip**-tan)
			Ergomar	ergotamine	(er-**got**-am-meen)
Anticonvulsants			Fiorinal	aspirin (asa)/butalbital/caffeine	(**as**-pir-in/byoo-**tal**-bi-tall/caf-**een**)
Cerebyx	fosphenytoin	(fos-**fen**-i-toyn)			
Depakene	valproic acid	(val-**pro**-ic **as**-id)	Frova	frovatriptan	(**froe**-va-**trip**-tan)
Depakote	divalproex sodium	(di-val-**pro**-ex so-de-um)	Imitrex	sumatriptan	(**soo**-mah-**trip**-tan)
Dilantin	phenytoin	(**fen**-i-toyn)	Maxalt	rizatriptan	(**rye**-za-**trip**-tan)
Felbatol	felbamate	(**fel**-ba-mate)	Midrin	acetaminophen/dichloralphenazone/isometheptene	(a-**seet**-a-**min**-oh-fen/dye-klor-al-**phen**-a-zone/eye-so-meh-**thep**-teen)
Keppra	levetiracetam	(**lee**-ve-ti-**ra**-se-tam)			
Klonopin	clonazepam (C-IV)	(kloe-**naz**-e-pam)			
Lamictal	lamotrigine	(la-**mow**-tri-jeen)			
Luminal	phenobarbital (C-IV)	(fee-no-**bar**-bi-tall)	Migranal	dihydroergotamine	(dye-hye-droe-er-**got**-a-meen)
Lyrica	pregabalin (C-V)	(pre-**ga**-bah-lin)			
Mebaral	mephobarbital (C-IV)	(mep-oh-**bar**-bi-tall)	Phrenilin	acetaminophen/butalbital	(ah-**seet**-ah-**min**-oh-fen/byoo-**tal**-bi-tal)
Mysoline	primidone	(**prim**-i-don)			
Neurontin	gabapentin	(**ga**-ba-**pen**-tin)	Relpax	eletriptan	(el-e-**trip**-tan)
Tegretol	carbamazepine	(kar-ba-**maz**-e-peen)	Treximet	sumatriptan/naproxen	(soo-ma-**trip**-tan/na-**prox**-en)
Topamax	topiramate	(toe-**pir**-ah-mate)			
Trileptal	oxcarbazepine	(**ox**-kar-**baz**-e-peen)	Zomig	zolmitriptan	(sol-mit-**trip**-tan)
Valium	diazepam (C-IV)	(dye-**az**-e-pam)			
Zarontin	ethosuximide	(**eth**-oh-**sux**-i-mide)	**Multiple Sclerosis Agents**		
Zonegran	zonisamide	(zoe-**nis**-a-mide)	Copaxone	glatiramer	(gla-**tir**-a-mer)
Vimpat	lacosamide	(la-**koe**-sa-mide)	Novantrone	mitoxantrone	(mye-toe-**zan**-trone)

COMMON DRUGS USED FOR CONDITIONS INVOLVING THE CENTRAL NERVOUS SYSTEM—cont'd

Trade Name	Generic Name	Pronunciation	Trade Name	Generic Name	Pronunciation
Tysabri	natalizumab	(nat-ta-**liz**-yoo-mab)	Mestinon	pyridostigmine	(pie-rid-o-**stig**-meen)
Zanaflex	tizanidine	(tye-**zan**-i-deen)	Prostigmin	neostigmine	(knee-oh-**stig**-meen)
Interferons for Multiple Sclerosis			**Alpha- and beta-Adrenergics (Sympathomimetics)**		
Avonex	interferon β-1a	(in-tur-**fear**-on **bay**-ta won ay)	Adrenalin	epinephrine	(ep-i-**nef**-rin)
			Levophed	norepinephrine	(nor-ep-i-**nef**-rin)
Betaseron	interferon β-1b	(in-tur-**fear**-on **bay**-ta won bee)	Intropin	dopamine	(doe-**pah**-meen)
			Alpha-Adrenergic Blocking Agents		
Agent to Treat Amyotrophic Lateral Sclerosis (ALS)			Cardura	doxazosin	(dok-sah-**zo**-sin)
Rilutek	riluzole	(ril-**you**-zole)	Hytrin	terazosin	(tur-ah-**zo**-sin)
			Minipress	prazosin	(pra-**zoe**-sin)
Alzheimer's Disease Agents			Regitine	phentolamine	(fen-**toll**-ah-meen)
Aricept	donepezil	(don-**nay**-pa-zil)			
Cognex	tacrine	(tac-**kreen**)	**Combined alpha- and beta-Adrenergic Blocking Agent**		
Exelon	rivastigmine	(ri-vas-**tig**-meen)	Normodyne	labetalol	(la-**bay**-ta-lol)
Namenda	memantine	(meh-**man**-teen)			
Razadyne	galantamine	(gal-**an**-ta-meen)	**Beta-Adrenergic Blocking Agents**		
			Brevibloc	esmolol	(es-**mo**-lol)
Myasthenia Gravis Agents			Lopressor	metoprolol	(me-**toe**-pro-lol)
	physostigmine	(phi-zo-**stig**-meen)	Tenormin	atenolol	(ah-**ten**-oh-lol)

T HE NERVOUS SYSTEM is a complex system controlling and coordinating the movements and many functions of the body. This includes both conscious and unconscious activities. Nerves also enable the body to perform internal functions involuntarily, such as the heart beating, the digestive system breaking down a meal, or the brain interpreting visual awareness. We take much for granted when it comes to the nervous system; however, if we lost a simple function, such as moving our eyes along a page of a book, it would be a devastating event in our lives. The nervous system is better understood when its divisions and the specific functions of each division are described. We begin with common medical terminology associated with the nervous system (NS) and a generalized overview of the NS and its main branches, describing some of the basic functions of each branch. An understanding of the NS and the way in which drugs affect the various levels is important. Some conditions that affect this system are discussed along with the medications that treat those conditions. Medical terms used for the nervous system are listed here.

NERVOUS SYSTEM MEDICAL TERMINOLOGY

Prefix	
a-	Without
intra-	Within
in-	Into or not

Suffix	
-al	Pertaining to
-algia	Pain
-cele	Hernia
-ia	Abnormal condition

NERVOUS SYSTEM MEDICAL TERMINOLOGY—cont'd

-ion	Condition or state of
-itis	Inflammation
-oma	Tumor
-pathy	Disease
-phasia	Speech disorder
-lepsy	Seizure

Root Words/Combining Forms

cephal/o	Head
cephalgia	Headache
crani/o	Cranium
encephal/o	Brain
hemat/o, hem/o	Blood
hydr/o	Water
mening/o	Meninges
meningocele	Congenital herniation of meninges through a defect in skull or spinal cord
my/o	Muscle
myel	Spinal cord
neur/o, neur/i	Nerves
lumbar	The part of the body located between the thorax and the pelvis
concuss	Shaken together
narc/o	Stupor

Conditions/Diseases

Alzheimer's disease	A progressive, degenerative disease of the brain that worsens over time resulting in death
Amyotrophic lateral sclerosis	A progressive neurological disease that results in degeneration of motor neurons resulting in death
Aphasia	Loss of speech
Bell's palsy	Paralysis of facial nerves; normally on one side; often temporary
Cerebrovascular accident	Sudden rupture or blockage of blood vessel in brain; also known as stroke
Concussion	Mild traumatic brain injury (MTBI); temporary loss of awareness and function may occur
Dystonia	Disorder that causes involuntary muscle spasms and contractions
Epilepsy	A recurring disorder of the nervous system resulting in seizures
Hematoma	Collection of blood trapped in tissue or body part as a result of ruptured or injured blood vessels
Hydrocephalus	Abnormally increased amount of CSF within ventricles of brain
Meningitis	Inflammation of meninges
Multiple sclerosis	An autoimmune disease of the CNS which destroys the myelin sheath causing muscle weakness, loss of speech and visual disturbances
Myasthenia gravis	A progressive disease of the skeletal muscles that impair nerve impulses following an autoimmune attack
Narcolepsy	Sleep disorder causing recurring episodes of falling asleep during day
Neuralgia	Nerve pain
Parkinsons disease	A degenerative disease characterized by tremors and muscular rigidity due to the loss of basal ganglia of the brain
Stroke	A sudden cerebrovascular accident; may be caused by embolism, hypertension, or hemorrhage that can cause impaired speech, coma, paralysis, convulsions, etc.
Tourette's syndrome	Inherited neuropsychiatric disorder characterized by multiple motor tics, lack of muscle coordination, and involuntary purposeless movements that are accompanied by grunts and barks

The Nervous System

The nervous system (NS) consists of sensory neurons positioned throughout the body. The following are the four main functions of the NS: transmission of impulses from sensory neurons to the **central nervous system** (CNS); interpretation of impulses sent to the CNS and transmission of a response to muscles or glands; coordination of the activities of all divisions of the nervous system; maintenance of homeostasis by responding to sensory changes in the body (e.g., temperature increase). The primary function of the nervous system is to keep the body in a balanced mode, which is referred to as homeostasis. The nervous system can be described as a complex, mainframe computer system with its network of nerves connected to the body much like the Internet is connected to millions of homes. The mainframe (CNS) is connected to computers (target sites) that interpret the signals; likewise, the computer extensions can send messages to the mainframe computer, where they can be interpreted and a response relayed (Figure 16-1).

The central nervous system (the mainframe) is divided between the brain and the spinal cord. An adult's brain weighs approximately 1.4 kg (3 pounds) and contains more than 100 billion neurons (i.e., nerve cells). The spinal cord weighs approximately 38 grams and is about half as long as the vertebral column (backbone).

The **peripheral nervous system (PNS),** located outside the CNS, consists of the afferent (sensory) and efferent (motor) branches. The **afferent division** transmits impulses from the body's organs to the CNS, where they are interpreted. The **efferent division** then relays the interpreted impulses to

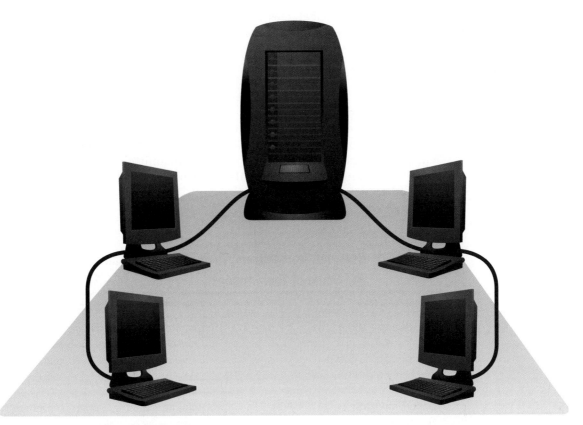

FIGURE 16-1 The nervous system is analogous to a mainframe computer (central nervous system) that communicates with other computers further away (peripheral nervous system).

the appropriate organ and triggers an effect. The efferent division is further divided into the **somatic** and **autonomic** divisions. The somatic system relays motor impulses to skeletal muscles throughout the body, and the **autonomic nervous system** transmits motor impulses to smooth muscle (e.g., blood vessels, stomach, liver), cardiac muscle (i.e., the heart), and glandular tissue. The autonomic nervous system consists of three branches: the sympathetic nervous system, the parasympathetic nervous system (PNS), and the enteric nervous system. Each is discussed later. The afferent branches carry impulses from the soft tissue areas and involuntary muscles of the body and other organs back to the CNS via visceral branches and the somatic branches. The various branches of the PNS allow the CNS to work at an optimal level because each area of the nervous system is in charge of a specific type of motor action or sensory response (Figure 16-2).

Remember, all the components of the nervous system are considered one organ system. We begin with the smallest functional part of the CNS—the neuron.

THE NEURON

The smallest unit of the nervous system is the **neuron**. Approximately 100 billion neurons, or nerve cells, make up the nervous system. Billions of nerves run throughout our bodies and carry messages (in the form of chemicals) back and forth from the nervous system.

The **cell body**, **dendrites**, **axon**, and the **nerve terminal** compose the four main sections of a neuron. As neurons branch out, forming a network of relay stations, they allow nerve impulses to travel from one neuron to another via small gaps called synapses. The dendrites are extensions that receive electrical impulses from the previous neuron's nerve terminal (or axon). The cell body processes the electrical message before it enters the axon. Many axons are covered by a special form of insulation called a myelin sheath; it consists of phospholipids and proteins and serves to accelerate impulse conduction (Figure 16-3).

Nerves are not separate from one another in the PNS but form bundles made of axons. In the PNS, bundles of cell bodies are called ganglions. However, within the CNS, the terminology differs—the axons are called tracts and the cell bodies are called nuclei or ganglia. The electrical impulses are transmitted from one neuron to another by various chemicals called **neurotransmitters**. When the impulse is activated by a neurotransmitter, a series of reactions take place to transmit the nerve impulse. Common neurotransmitters are listed in Table 16-1.

Tech Note!

The nervous system is composed of the CNS and the PNS. The CNS consists of the brain, brainstem, and spinal cord. The PNS carries messages from the body to the CNS, where they are interpreted. Then impulses are relayed from the brain and spinal cord outward to the rest of the body, where they trigger an effect. The PNS is divided into the somatic and autonomic divisions.

TABLE 16-1 Neuronal Transmitters, Their Most Important Clinical Locations, and Some of Their Actions

Neurotransmitter	Type of Response
Acetylcholine (PNS)*	Excitatory (skeletal muscles, gastrointestinal muscles); inhibitory (decreases heart rate)
Norepinephrine (PNS)	Excitatory (increases heart rate)
Epinephrine (PNS)	Excitatory (increases heart rate); inhibitory (bronchodilator)
Dopamine (CNS)	Helps to inhibit involuntary movement
Serotonin (CNS)	Helps to inhibit pain perception

CNS, Central nervous system; *PNS*, peripheral nervous system.

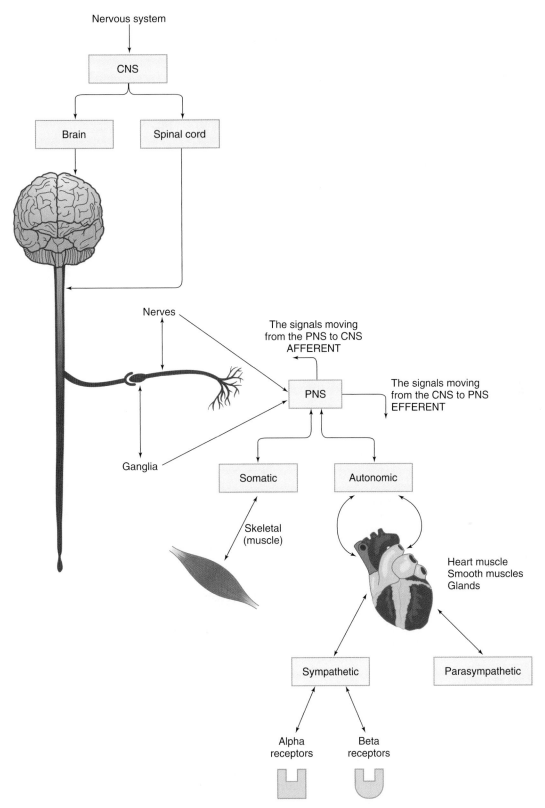

FIGURE 16-2 The nervous system: Divisions include the somatic and autonomic branches. The somatic division sends and receives impulses to and from the muscles whereas the autonomic system regulates both sympathetic and parasympathetic systems.

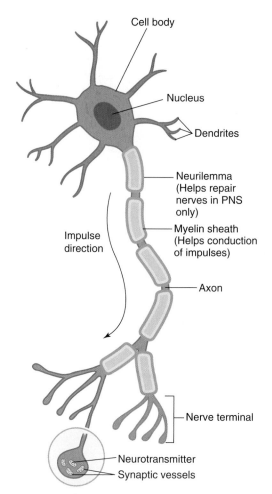

Cell body

Nucleus

Dendrites

Neurilemma
(Helps repair
nerves in PNS
only)

Myelin sheath
(Helps conduction
of impulses)

Impulse
direction

Axon

Nerve terminal

Neurotransmitter
Synaptic vessels

FIGURE 16-3 Neuron: Impulses travel down the axon into the nerve terminal, where they are released into the synaptic space between each neuron. Impulses then are transmitted to the following neuron via the dendrites, which extend out of the cell body. The spaces between segments of the myelin sheath are known as the nodes of Ranvier.

Tech Note!

Nerves are made of millions of axons. Each neuron consists of a cell body, dendrites, axon, and nerve endings. Electrical impulses travel along the nerves to and from the CNS via afferent and efferent branches. Impulses are generated by the change in polarity of the axon, which moves the impulse rapidly. This electrical conduction is aided by the myelin sheath. The impulse is started by neurotransmitters.

AFFERENT (SENSORY) NEURONS

The primary function of the afferent branch is to transfer information via electrical impulse from the peripheral area (outside the CNS) to the CNS. The afferent, or sensory, branch is composed of neurons that have long dendrites and short axons. The cell body is located within the PNS and the axon extends into the CNS.

EFFERENT (MOTOR) NEURONS

After the CNS receives a message, a response via nerve impulse travels through the efferent branch to a target muscle. The neurons in the efferent branch have short dendrites and long axons. The dendrites and cell body of the efferent neurons are located within the CNS, and the axons extend into the PNS (Figure 16-4).

NERVE TRANSMISSION

If we follow the conduction of a chemical message from one neuron to another, we would notice that three basic changes occur in the cell membrane:

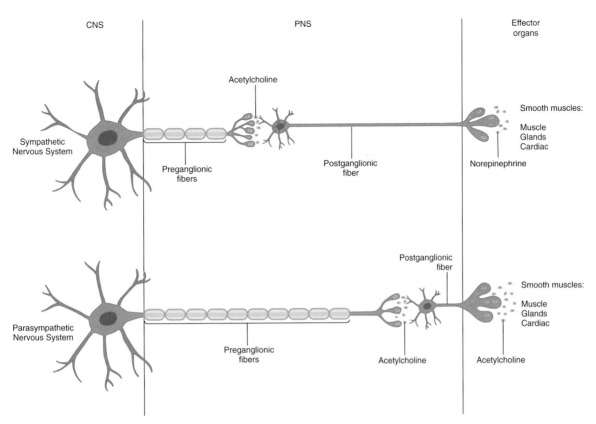

FIGURE 16-4 The afferent and efferent nerves and the areas innervated by the sympathetic and parasympathetic systems. Preganglionic and postganglionic nerves that make up the cell bodies and axon are shown.

polarization, depolarization, and repolarization. When the cell is in a resting state, there is an overall negative charge inside the neuron that consists of potassium (positive) and chloride ions (negative). The outside of the neuron is more positive, with sodium as the positive charge. At this point, the cell is polarized and waiting to be excited. When a neurotransmitter activates the cell membrane, an influx of sodium ions occurs, changing the negative charge inside the cell to a positive charge. This is called depolarization. The cell restores the resting state by allowing the inside positive charges (potassium ions) to escape. As the transition back to the resting state occurs, the cell actively transports the sodium back to the outside and allows the potassium to reenter the cell. The cell repolarizes, bringing the cell full circle and back to the resting stage (Figure 16-5). All of these steps occur in milliseconds!

Central Nervous System

Composed of the spinal cord and brain, the functions of the CNS are extensive. The following sections provide an overview of the primary functions of the CNS.

BRAIN

The brain is divided into several sections. The largest area of the brain is the cerebral cortex, which is composed of gray matter that lies over white matter. Gray matter consists of neuron cell bodies and dendrites and is where most of the neuronal activity takes place. These fibers are woven in a pattern, making up the contents of the brain. The gray area is where language, memory, and cognitive functions occur. The white matter consists of bundles of nerve fibers

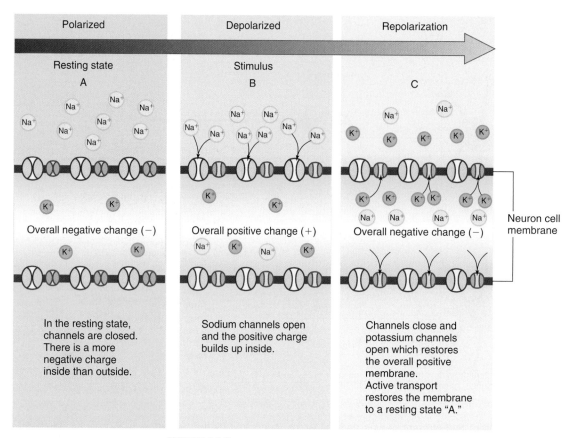

FIGURE 16-5 Neuronal impulse transfer cycle.

(myelinated axons). The white matter functions to communicate between other areas of the cerebral cortex and brain.

The folded mass that makes up the outer covering of the brain is what most people envision when they think of the human brain. This highly folded tissue is important because it increases the surface area of the brain, allowing for more activity. The cerebral cortex (referred to as the cerebrum) is composed of the left and right hemispheres (hemi meaning half). The two halves can communicate with each other by way of the corpus callosum (bundles of axons). Each of the two hemispheres is divided further into four different lobes, each having specific functions:

- Frontal lobe controls motor function, parts of speech, emotions, problem solving, reasoning, and planning.
- Parietal lobe is associated with orientation, recognition, sensation, and understanding language.
- Occipital lobe is in control of perception and interpretation related to vision.
- Temporal lobe is associated with auditory stimuli, long-term memory, and behavior.

The **brainstem** connects the brain to the spinal cord and consists of three main areas: the midbrain, pons, and medulla oblongata. These three areas are linked to many of the nerves within the brain (Figure 16-6). Specific functions of each part of the brainstem are listed below:

- Midbrain (i.e., mesencephalon): vision, hearing, eye movement, voluntary body movement

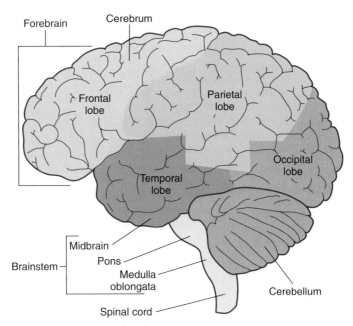

FIGURE 16-6 Lobes of the brain, cerebellum, and brainstem, which are all part of the central nervous system.

- Pons: motor control, sensory analysis
- Medulla oblongata: breathing or respiration, cardiac rate, force of contraction of the heart, and dilation of blood vessels

Located above the brainstem is the thalamus. The thalamus is a type of relay station that is involved in the transmission of messages between the brain and the spinal cord. The thalamus will send messages to the appropriate area within the cerebral cortex. Both the thalamus and the hypothalamus are part of a structure called the diencephalon.

The limbic system is composed of the hippocampus, amygdala, septal area, and the hypothalamus. All of these structures are linked to survival instincts. This includes hunger, thirst, defense, emotion, and reproduction. The limbic system also has a strong link to memory, which is necessary for the well-being and survival of the body. The specific functions are listed below and are all linked to the hypothalamus.

- Hippocampus: Plays a part in the transfer of short-term memory to long-term memory; responsible for memory navigation. New conditions that may be dangerous can be compared to past experiences to choose the best option.
- Amygdala: Responsible for memory, emotion, and fears. Essential in the flight-or-fight reaction associated with self-preservation.
- Septal area: Pleasure center related to pleasant sensations and those related to sexual experiences.

The hypothalamus is responsible for overall homeostasis; functions such as emotion, thirst, hunger, heart rate, control of the autonomic nervous system, and hormone production of the pituitary glands are under its control.

At the back of the brain near the brainstem is the **cerebellum;** this highly folded part of the brain is responsible for precise movements, such as maintaining balance and posture and coordinating movement.

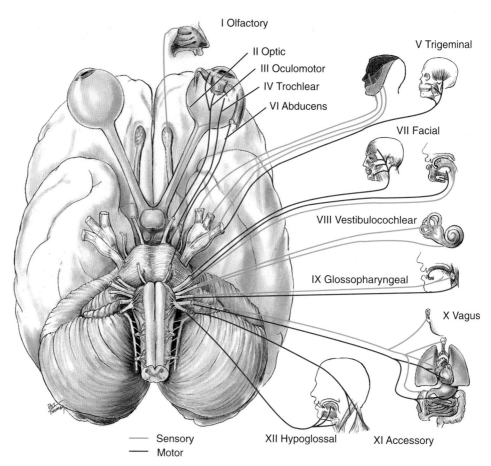

FIGURE 16-7 Cranial nerves. (From Applegate E: The anatomy and physiology learning system, ed 2, St Louis, 2006, Elsevier.)

CRANIAL NERVES

As shown in Figure 16-7, 12 pairs of cranial nerves originate within the brain matter. These nerves have specific functions and are designated by Roman numerals. The numbers represent the order in which the fibers are located within the brain from front to back. Most of these nerves have sensory and motor fibers, with three sets having sensory fibers only. Table 16-2 lists the primary functions for each set of cranial nerves I to XII.

SPINAL CORD

The spinal cord, located inside the vertebral column, serves as a pathway from the brain to the peripheral nervous system. The spinal nerves are protected by the vertebrae. Within the vertebrae an inner gray matter houses many nerve cells and an outer white matter contains nerve fibers. The meninges, a thin covering lining the inside of the bones, separate and protect the brain and spinal cord from the bony structures of the skull and spinal column, respectively. The brain and spinal cord also are cushioned by a watery liquid called the **cerebrospinal fluid** (CSF) and a double layer of cells known as the **blood-brain barrier** (BBB). The 31 bones of the vertebrae are compartmentalized between 8 **cervical**, 12 **thoracic**, 5 **lumbar**, 5 sacral (**sacrum**), and 1 coccygeal (**coccyx**) segment (Figure 16-8).

TABLE 16-2 Primary Functions of Cranial Nerves

Structure	Specific Nerve	Function	Specific Information about Structure	Type of Fiber
Brain ventricles		Filled with cerebrospinal fluid (CSF); CSF provides a type of shock absorption for brain. Ventricles connect to spinal cord. CSF produced at continuous rate, being replaced about 3 times daily.		
Cranial nerves		Composed of 12 pairs of nerves that are attached at base of brain and brainstem. Carry motor and sensory messages. Motor messages linked to muscles are involved in balance. Sensory messages, such as sight, hearing, taste, smell, and perception of balance, are all relayed to nerve impulses.		
I	Olfactory	Associated with smell. Mucous membranes of nose transmit information to region in cerebral cortex that processes and then sends a response to information.		Sensory
II	Optic	Associated with vision. Optic nerve receives an image that stimulates retina's rods and cones. These send messages via optic nerve, which ultimately travels through thalamus and then onto visual cortex, where they are processed.	Rods are responsible for black and white images and cones for color images	Sensory
III	Oculomotor	Oculomotor muscles are involved in movement of specific areas of eye and eyelid.		Motor
IV	Trochlear	Trochlear controls another area of eye involved in eye movement.		Motor
V	Trigeminal	Located in brainstem, trigeminal nerve provides sensation to face, scalp, mucous membranes in nose, mouth, and eyes. Also is responsible for nerves in the skin and muscles of jaw.		Sensory and motor
VI	Abducens	Abducens is third cranial nerve involved in eye movement.		Motor
VII	Facial	Involved in sensation of taste in front of tongue. Linked to face and head muscles; results in facial expressions.		Sensory and motor
VIII	Vestibulocochlear	Linked to inner ear (hearing) and responsible for sense of balance.	Small organs inside inner ear alert brain to changes in body position	Sensory
IX	Glossopharyngeal	Linked to sinus, back of tongue, soft palate, parotid gland, and reflex control of heart. Also plays a role in swallowing.		Sensory and motor
X	Vagus	Extends from brainstem through neck and then through chest and abdominal cavity. Involved in functions such as swallowing, breathing, speaking, heartbeat, and digestion. Linked to other nerves, receiving messages from ear, pharynx, esophagus, and chest and abdominal area.		Sensory and motor
XI	Spinal accessory	Composed of two divisions. Cranial branch controls muscles of pharynx, larynx, and palate, contributing to swallowing and movement through digestive tract. Spinal branch is involved in muscle movement of upper shoulders, head, and neck.		Motor
XII	Hypoglossal	Hypoglossal controls muscles of tongue.	Associated with autonomic nervous system	Motor

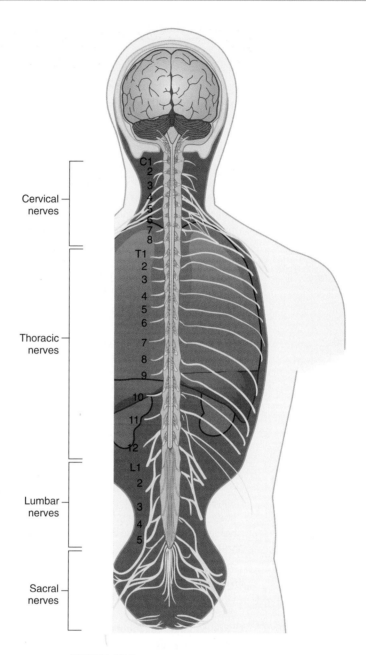

FIGURE 16-8 Segments of the spinal cord.

Tech Note!

The nerves of the brain crisscross so that the left side of the brain controls the right side of the body. Thus persons suffering from a stroke (blocked blood flow) on one side of the brain can lose the ability to move parts of the body located on the opposite side.

BLOOD-BRAIN BARRIER

Cerebrospinal fluid (CSF) protects the brain from being damaged by acting as a cushion if the outer skull is jolted. The blood-brain barrier (BBB) has the same protective function except it prevents molecules from entering and possibly damaging the brain via chemical reaction. Because it does allow certain chemicals to cross, it is considered a semipermeable membrane. However, the uniquely tight junctions and dense capillary network of these vessels are responsible for the limited transference of materials from the blood to the brain. In this way, the brain is independently protected from the rest of the body. Typical properties of the BBB include protection from bacteria that may be in the bloodstream. However, if an infection does occur in the brain, it is difficult to treat because defensive antibodies are too large to pass the BBB. Unfortunately, certain viruses

TABLE 16-3 Permeability of the Blood-Brain Barrier

	Type of Substance	Functions	Associated With
Substances That Cannot Pass BBB			
	Large molecules		
	Water-soluble molecules		
	Low-lipid molecules		
	Bacteria or viruses >500 Daltons 1 Dalton (Da) is a unit of mass about the size of a hydrogen atom		
Substances That Can Pass BBB			
	High-lipid molecules	Essential constituents of all cell membranes, such as endothelial cells	Brain function
	Oxygen	Nourishes brain	Brain function
	Glucose	Nourishes brain	Brain function
	Lipid-soluble molecules in drugs	Medication	
Substances That Are Weakened because of Protection from BBB			
	Melatonin	Regulates organism's environment (e.g., circadian rhythms)	Pineal gland
	Neuroactive peptides	Amino acids are building blocks of life and necessary for homeostasis	Pineal gland
Neuroactive peptides	Antidiuretic hormone	Conserves water for body	Pituitary gland
	Oxytocin	Involved in childbirth	Pituitary gland
	Area postrema	Allows toxic substances to be expelled	Vomit center
	Subfornical organ	Regulation of body fluids	Homeostasis
	Vascular organ	Chemosensory area that detects various molecules	Homeostasis
	Median eminence	Collects hormones produced by hypothalamus to be transferred to portal system	Pituitary gland

Tech Note!

The autonomic system is an involuntary branch of the PNS. The autonomic system is divided into sympathetic and parasympathetic divisions. The sympathetic system releases the neurotransmitter norepinephrine when we are stressed, and the parasympathetic system releases acetylcholine when we are at rest. Sympathetic ganglions synapse with many postganglionic fibers for a widespread effect, whereas parasympathetic preganglionic fibers synapse with fewer postganglionic fibers.

can easily pass the BBB because they are extremely small and often attach themselves to circulating immune cells that do cross into the brain. Certain regions of the brain have a weaker barrier from certain substances. This allows the brain to monitor the composition of the blood. In Table 16-3 specific substances that may or may not pass the BBB are listed.

Peripheral Nervous System (PNS)

The PNS is further divided into the autonomic and somatic systems, each having specific functions. Following is a description of these functions.

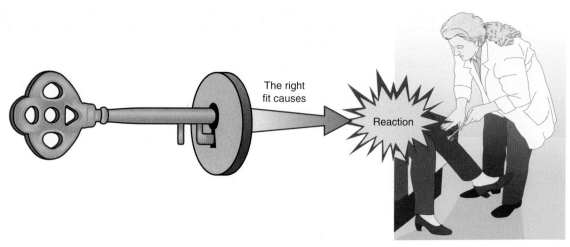

FIGURE 16-9 Lock-and-key mechanism: As the knee is tapped, impulses are sent to and from the brain. The neurotransmitters affect specific receptors that are interpreted. The reaction sent via neurotransmitters is to jerk the knee.

AUTONOMIC SYSTEM

The autonomic branch is called the autonomic nervous system (ANS) because it controls automatic functions. Automatic functions are unconscious body functions, such as heartbeat and breathing. The autonomic nervous system is called the involuntary nervous system and is subdivided further into three branches—sympathetic, parasympathetic, and enteric nervous systems. These systems serve to regulate organs, tissues, and blood vessels. They can perform this function in response to outside and inside stimuli with the use of specific neurotransmitters.

The autonomic system consists of two nerve fibers that carry impulses from the CNS to target tissue—preganglionic and postganglionic fibers. The ganglion is the area where the synapse (relay station) is located. The nerve fibers are either preganglionic or postganglionic, depending on whether they precede or follow the ganglia. Each neurotransmitter contacts its own specific receptor (the lock-and-key mechanism; Figure 16-9).

The nerve fibers of the enteric nervous system are configured in more of a meshwork to innervate the viscera (gastrointestinal [GI] tract, pancreas, gallbladder). When you get "butterflies in your stomach" before an exam, this is your enteric nervous system at work.

Sympathetic System

The areas of the CNS where the sympathetic nerves emerge are the thoracic and lumbar regions of the spinal cord. The function of the **sympathetic division** is to respond to stressful situations, such as the "fight or flight" response. During the fight-or-flight stress response, the sympathetic system shuts down the nonessential systems of the body. This redirects energy to other areas such as the muscular system. The nerves that are responsible for this type of behavior are composed of preganglionic neurons imbedded into the gray matter of the spinal cord. As the impulses travel through this gray matter, they synapse with long postganglionic neurons that innervate effector organs. The sympathetic preganglionic neurons synapse and affect many postganglionic neurons. This massive transfer of signals to many areas of the body allows human beings to respond quickly and powerfully to a situation. The sympathetic system also sends impulses to various organs and tissues for other emotional situations, such as anxiety, hate, and even stress. When you have an interview for a new job and

TABLE 16-4 Major Organ Response When Sympathetic System Is Activated

Organ/Tissue	Sympathetic Response
Heart	Increases force and rate of contraction; increases speed of conduction
Lung	Bronchi and bronchioles become dilated; secretions are suppressed
Blood vessels	Constricts all surface areas so person looks pale; increases circulation to areas where blood is most needed, such as gastrointestinal system, muscles, heart, and brain
Digestive system	Inhibition; decreases gastrointestinal motility and suppresses gastrointestinal secretions
Urinary system	Bladder wall relaxes; sphincter contracts
Liver	Increases release of glucose
Eyes	Pupils dilate for better vision; ciliary muscle relaxes for far vision
Adrenal medulla	Epinephrine is released into bloodstream
Sweat glands	Increases secretion

Tech Note!

In the CNS neurons are called nuclei whereas in the PNS they are called ganglia. Collections of axons in the CNS are called tracts; however, in the PNS they are called nerves.

your palms get sweaty, your heart rate increases, and your breathing becomes quick and shallow, you are experiencing a sympathetic reaction, but to a lesser degree than a person who is in fear for his or her life. Whether you are in a life-threatening situation or in minor stress, the sympathetic nervous system keeps the body in homeostasis through its fight-or-flight responses. Table 16-4 depicts the response of each major organ when affected by the sympathetic system. All of the nonessential energy-consuming functions, such as urination or digestion, are reduced while blood flow to large muscles, release of glucose from the liver, the heart rate, and other functions are increased. This sympathetic response is not mentally activated but rather is an instinctive or autonomic reaction.

Parasympathetic System

The sympathetic and parasympathetic systems have many differences. The **parasympathetic nervous system** can be thought of as the opposite or counterbalance to the sympathetic system; for this reason it has been called the "breed or feed" part of the autonomic system. In the parasympathetic system, nerves emerge from the brainstem and the sacral part of the cord. Another important difference is the location of the preganglionic nerves. In the parasympathetic system, these nerves are located in the gray matter of the brainstem or spinal cord. They exit the CNS and have a long preganglionic fiber. The impulse moves to the target organ, creating a response. One of the main functions of the parasympathetic system is activation of the digestive system. This function includes secreting acidic juices, increasing peristalsis, and inducing hormonal secretion of insulin. The parasympathetic system also slows the heart rate. The parasympathetic system functions while we rest and is inhibited only when the sympathetic system overrides it during periods of intense stress. Table 16-5 describes the organs and effects of the parasympathetic system.

SOMATIC SYSTEM

The somatic system is a network of nerves that relay messages to the CNS from the outside world and return messages back to the body. The spinal and cranial nerves are part of the somatic system. This system regulates the motor nerves

TABLE 16-5 Response of the Body Systems to Parasympathetic Stimulation

Organ/Tissue	Parasympathetic Response
Heart	Slows rate
Lungs	Dilates bronchi
Blood vessels	None
Digestive system	Increased motility; digestion takes place
Urinary system	Urinary bladder muscle contracts; sphincter relaxes
Liver	None
Eyes	Pupils constrict; ciliary muscle contraction for near vision
Adrenal medulla	None
Sweat glands	None

Tech Note!

Drugs that mimic the sympathetic system are called adrenergic drugs; those that block the actions of the sympathetic system are called adrenergic blockers. Drugs that mimic the parasympathetic system are called cholinergic drugs; those that block the actions of the parasympathetic system are called anticholinergics. **Monoamine oxidase** (MAO) enzymes are responsible for destroying excess neurotransmitters. Activators such as adrenergics and cholinergics increase the amount of neurotransmitters. MAO inhibitors (MAOIs) stop the monoamine oxidase enzymes from destroying the neurotransmitters. When various receptor blockers are used, they block the receptor sites of the neurotransmitters so that the impulse will not be transmitted, and the resultant action will not occur. When an agent blocks all receptors or all enzymes of a certain type, it is called nonselective. When an agent blocks a specific receptor or enzyme preferentially or exclusively, it is called selective.

that control voluntary actions of the skeletal muscles and impulses from sensory receptors. Receptor sites are sensitive to a stimulus and include smell, taste, touch, and hearing.

Neurotransmitters

Simply stated, neurotransmitters are chemicals that are located and released in the brain. They provide impulses that are emitted and sent from one nerve cell (neuron) to another. Neurotransmitters can either excite or inhibit (stop) nerve cells. Although there are more than 50 different types of neurotransmitters known, only a few of the primary neurotransmitters (NTs) will be discussed here. They influence our behavior depending on where they are activated in the brain. The impairment of NTs in the brain can cause various physical and mental disorders. Conditions such as multiple sclerosis, Alzheimer's disease, Parkinson's disease, and others are discussed later while mental disorders and medications employed in their treatment are discussed in Chapter 17.

MAIN NEUROTRANSMITTERS

The main neurotransmitters of the sympathetic system are norepinephrine and epinephrine. Dopamine is a precursor for norepinephrine and is found as a neurotransmitter within the CNS, specifically the basal ganglia.

Within the nerve ending are enzymes that either destroy excess norepinephrine or bind to it for future reuse. One set of enzymes responsible for this action are called **monoamine oxidases** (MAOs). Destruction of excessive amounts of norepinephrine is important because overexcitement can cause unwanted effects.

Four types of receptors are found opposite the sympathetic postganglionic fiber endings. α_1-Receptors are located in peripheral blood vessels, the heart, and the eyes. α_2-Receptors are located on smooth muscle. β_1-Receptors are located in heart muscle, and β_2-receptors are located in the respiratory system and elsewhere. Drugs that mimic natural sympathetic neurotransmitters are referred to as sympathomimetics or adrenergics, and the drugs used to block their actions are called sympatholytics or are named after the specific receptor they inhibit. The adrenergic agents that mimic the sympathetic nervous system are epinephrine and norepinephrine. Table 16-6 lists the uses for α- and β-sympathomimetics along with their effects.

Tech Note!

When a drug is designated as acting on an α-receptor or β-receptor, this indicates the location on the cell that is receptive to the substance. A physiological reaction then takes place.

TABLE 16-6 α- and β-Receptors and Their Effects on the Body Systems

Receptors	Effects
α₁	Heart contraction increases
	Eyes (pupils) dilate
	Peripheral vasoconstriction occurs
α₂	Smooth muscles contract
β₁	Heart rate increases
β₂	Bronchial muscles dilate
	Uterus relaxes

ADRENERGIC AGENTS AND ADRENERGIC BLOCKERS

Sympathomimetics or Adrenergic Agents

GENERIC NAME: epinephrine
TRADE NAME: Adrenalin, EpiPen
INDICATION: low blood pressure; used to treat heart attacks and shock
ROUTE OF ADMINISTRATION: injection
COMMON ADULT DOSAGE: 1 mg/mL
SIDE EFFECTS: headache, tachycardia, and high blood pressure
NOTE: Auxiliary label necessary for EpiPen.
AUXILIARY LABELS:

- For injection only.
- Use as directed.

Tech Note!

Although injectable drugs do not need an auxiliary label when administered by a physician or nurse, EpiPens (epinephrine auto injectors) do need auxiliary labels because these are carried by the patient for emergency use.

GENERIC NAME: dopamine
TRADE NAME: Intropin
INDICATION: In low doses, dopamine causes vasodilation and increased urine output; in moderate doses, it releases norepinephrine, which affects β₁-receptors, increasing heart rate; in high doses, it is used for patients suffering from circulatory shock.
ROUTE OF ADMINISTRATION: injection
COMMON ADULT DOSAGE: 1 to 5 mcg/kg per minute up to 50 mcg/kg per minute
SIDE EFFECTS: tachycardia, headache, vomiting

CHOLINERGIC AGENTS AND CHOLINERGIC BLOCKERS

The main neurotransmitter of the parasympathetic system is acetylcholine. Acetylcholine is important in the CNS and PNS. Acetylcholine works quickly and has a short duration of action. Two types of cholinergic agents are those that mimic acetylcholine and those that stop the destruction of acetylcholine by the enzyme acetylcholinesterase. Because these cholinergic drugs mimic the parasympathetic system, they are referred to as parasympathomimetics, whereas drugs that inhibit the cholinergic reaction by blocking the receptor are usually called anticholinergics. The main side effects of anticholinergics are dry mouth and a decreased urine output.

Parasympathetic receptors, which respond to the neurotransmitter acetylcholine, are located on smooth and cardiac muscle cells. Cholinergic blockers stop the response. They prevent acetylcholine from combining with the receptor, causing the nerve impulse to stop. This is useful when patients must be sedated or when their eyes have to be dilated by the optometrist.

Anticholinergic drugs have many uses, including for many of the conditions that are discussed later.

Conditions of the Nervous System and Their Treatments

Many disorders involve inappropriate or excessive muscle contractions. Some muscular disorders involve the wasting away (i.e., atrophy) of muscles from lack of use. Many of the following conditions are still without cures, and research continues to search for the cause and/or treatment. Some conditions are hereditary, whereas others may be random genetic mutations. Other disorders are being investigated to determine whether environmental conditions may increase the incidence of their occurrence. Because there are so many conditions, disorders, and diseases that can affect the brain and nervous system, only a sample of the major disorders is examined. For a list of websites that provide information on these and additional disorders, see Box 16-1.

BOX 16-1   CONDITIONS/DISEASES AFFECTING THE NERVOUS SYSTEM AND WEBSITES FOR ADDITIONAL INFORMATION

Alzheimer's disease: www.alz.org
American Chronic Pain Association: www.theacpa.org
Amyotrophic lateral sclerosis: www.alsa.org
Aphasia: www.aphasia.org
Ataxia: www.ataxia.org
Birth defects: www.birthdefects.org
Brain tumors: http://hope.abta.org/site/PageServer
Epilepsy: www.epilepsyfoundation.org
Lupus: www.lupusny.org
Multiple sclerosis: www.msaa.com
Muscular dystrophy: www.mdausa.org
Myasthenia gravis: www.myasthenia.org

Disorders and Stroke
Pain, chronic: www.theacpa.org
Parkinson's disease: www.pdf.org
Pediatric brain tumor: www.braintumorkids.org
Pediatric strokes: www.pediatricstrokenetwork.com
Polio: www.post-polio.org
Psychological disorders: www.apa.org
Restless legs syndrome: www.rls.org
Sleep disorders: www.sleepfoundation.org
Spinal cord injuries: www.spinalcord.org
Stroke: www.stroke.org
Stuttering: www.stutteringhelp.org
Vestibular disorders: www.vestibular.org

Government Institutes
National Institute of Neurological Disorders and Stroke: www.ninds.nih.gov/
National Institutes of Health, Office of Rare Diseases: *www.rarediseases.info.nih.gov*

GENERAL NERVOUS SYSTEM DISORDERS

Skeletal Muscle Pain

Pain in the muscles is a warning signal from the body. Although everyone experiences some pain at one time or another, severe injury or chronic pain may need additional care. Treatments include drug therapy and physical therapy, followed by surgery if these two treatment modalities are ineffective. Other causes of pain related to the nervous system include headaches, migraines, and various bone conditions affecting the skeletal system. Analgesics and nonsteroidal antiinflammatory drugs (including over-the-counter [OTC] medications) used to treat headache pain are discussed in Chapter 26. For chronic muscle pain that cannot be identified, the patient may be treated only with skeletal muscle relaxants. These medications can be central-acting or direct-acting.

Central-Acting Medications

Although the mechanisms of action of central-acting medications are not well known, the result of the medications is well documented. One of the most important effects of these agents is the depression of the CNS. These drugs affect the brainstem, thalamus, basal ganglia, and the spinal cord. Side effects include dizziness, drowsiness, blurred vision, and headaches. These agents are not intended for long-term use. These drugs are classified as smooth muscle relaxants. The main drugs used as smooth muscle relaxants follow, along with their primary indication, drug action, and necessary auxiliary labels. The normal dosage is based on an adult dose and/or range. In several instances the specific drug action currently is not known; therefore a general drug action is supplied. Auxiliary labels are placed on certain prescription bottles and contain brief information about the drug for the patient's reference. The information usually refers to side effects. For instance, if an auxiliary label states, "Take with food," the medication can cause stomach upset.

SMOOTH SKELETAL MUSCLE RELAXANTS

GENERIC NAME: baclofen
TRADE NAME: Lioresal
INDICATION: spasticity associated with multiple sclerosis or spinal cord injury
ROUTE OF ADMINISTRATION: oral, intrathecal
COMMON ADULT DOSAGE: usual oral dosage 5 mg tid; may increase by 5 mg every 3 days to a maximum of 20 mg qid if necessary
SIDE EFFECTS: dizziness, drowsiness, headache, insomnia, nausea, constipation
AUXILIARY LABELS:
- May take with food or milk.
- May cause dizziness or drowsiness.

NOTE: Intrathecal baclofen is used with an implantable pump for continuous infusion; it is never given by any other route.

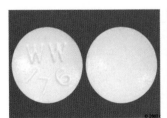

GENERIC NAME: carisoprodol
TRADE NAME: Soma
INDICATION: acute muscle pain
ROUTE OF ADMINISTRATION: oral
COMMON ADULT DOSAGE: 250 to 350 mg tid or qid
SIDE EFFECTS: dizziness, drowsiness, vertigo, upset stomach, headache
AUXILIARY LABELS:
- May cause dizziness or drowsiness.
- Take with food.
- Avoid alcohol.

GENERIC NAME: chlorzoxazone
TRADE NAME: Parafon Forte DSC
INDICATION: discomfort caused by muscle pain and spasms
ROUTE OF ADMINISTRATION: oral
COMMON ADULT DOSAGE: 250 to 750 mg tid to qid, tapering off dose as pain decreases
SIDE EFFECTS: dizziness, drowsiness, and stomach upset
AUXILIARY LABELS:

- May cause dizziness or drowsiness.
- Take with food.
- Avoid alcohol.

GENERIC NAME: cyclobenzaprine
TRADE NAME: Flexeril (immediate-release tablets [IR]), Amrix (extended-release capsules [ER])
INDICATION: acute muscle pain
ROUTE OF ADMINISTRATION: oral
COMMON ADULT DOSAGE: IR tablets, 5 mg tid (max 10 mg tid); ER capsules, 15 to 30 mg once daily; maximum use is 3 weeks for both IR/ER dosage forms
SIDE EFFECTS: dizziness, drowsiness, blurred vision, dry mouth
AUXILIARY LABELS:

- May cause dizziness or drowsiness.
- Avoid alcohol.
- Do not crush or chew capsules (Amrix ER).

GENERIC NAME: methocarbamol
TRADE NAME: Robaxin
INDICATION: acute muscle pain and muscle pain associated with tetanus
ROUTE OF ADMINISTRATION: oral, injection
COMMON ADULT DOSAGE: oral dosage, 1.5 g qid up to 8 g per day in severe cases
SIDE EFFECTS: drowsiness, dizziness; urine may change color to black, brown, or green
AUXILIARY LABELS:

- May cause dizziness or drowsiness.
- Avoid alcohol.
- Urine may change color.

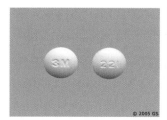

© 2005 GS

GENERIC NAME: orphenadrine
TRADE NAME: Norflex
INDICATION: acute muscle pain and bedtime leg cramps
ROUTE OF ADMINISTRATION: oral, injection
COMMON ADULT DOSAGE: oral dosage, 100 mg bid
SIDE EFFECTS: dizziness, drowsiness, blurred vision, fainting, dry mouth
AUXILIARY LABELS:

- May cause dizziness or drowsiness.
- Avoid alcohol.

GENERIC NAME: tizanidine
TRADE NAME: Zanaflex
INDICATION: disorders that produce muscle cramps, tightness, and spasms such as multiple sclerosis
ROUTE OF ADMINISTRATION: oral
COMMON ADULT DOSAGE: oral dosage, 4 mg q6-8h prn (max 36 mg/24 hr)
SIDE EFFECTS: dizziness, drowsiness, dry mouth
AUXILIARY LABELS:

- May cause dizziness or drowsiness.
- Avoid alcohol.
- Take with a full glass of water.

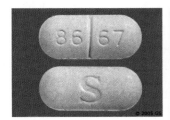

GENERIC NAME: metaxalone
TRADE NAME: Skelaxin
INDICATION: muscle spasms
ROUTE OF ADMINISTRATION: oral
COMMON ADULT DOSAGE: oral dosage, 800 mg tid to qid
SIDE EFFECTS: dizziness, drowsiness, headache, upset stomach
AUXILIARY LABELS:
■ May cause dizziness or drowsiness.
■ Avoid alcohol.

Direct-Acting Agents

Direct-acting agents work directly on the muscles by inhibiting calcium release, which results in decreased muscle response. Side effects include fatigue, dizziness, drowsiness, diarrhea, and respiratory depression (e.g., dantrolene, which is listed under Multiple Sclerosis). Commonly used oral agents are listed next. These are samples of combinations of agents that include a variety of popular analgesics and antiinflammatories.

MUSCLE RELAXANTS WITH ANALGESICS/ANTIINFLAMMATORIES

GENERIC NAME: carisoprodol/aspirin
TRADE NAME: Soma Compound
ROUTE OF ADMINISTRATION: oral
COMMON ADULT DOSAGE: 200 mg (based on carisoprodol component), one to two tablets 4 times daily
SIDE EFFECTS: dizziness, drowsiness
AUXILIARY LABELS:
■ May cause drowsiness.
■ Do not drink alcohol.

GENERIC NAME: carisoprodol/aspirin/codeine C-III
TRADE NAME: Soma Compound with Codeine
ROUTE OF ADMINISTRATION: oral
COMMON ADULT DOSAGE: one to two tablets 4 times daily
SIDE EFFECTS: dizziness, drowsiness
AUXILIARY LABELS:
■ May cause drowsiness.
■ Do not drink alcohol.

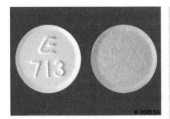

GENERIC NAME: orphenadrine/aspirin/caffeine
TRADE NAME: Norgesic
ROUTE OF ADMINISTRATION: oral
COMMON ADULT DOSAGE: 25 mg/385 mg/30 mg, one to two tablets every 6 to 8 hours
SIDE EFFECTS: dizziness, drowsiness
AUXILIARY LABELS:
■ May cause drowsiness.
■ Do not drink alcohol.

SPECIFIC CONDITIONS AFFECTING THE PERIPHERAL NERVOUS SYSTEM

Bell's Palsy

The condition **Bell's Palsy** causes the muscles in the face to become paralyzed as a result of trauma to cranial nerve VII. The paralysis can occur on one or both sides of the face. Bell's palsy affects approximately 40,000 people in the United States alone. Both women and men are equally affected by this condition; it is more prevalent in older adults than younger patients. Neither race nor genes play a role in acquiring this condition. However, having preexisting conditions such as diabetes or immunocompromised illnesses and being in the third trimester of pregnancy seem to increase the probability of acquiring Bell's palsy. Symptoms normally include rapid onset of facial paralysis (upon waking) although it may begin with dry eyes and tingling around the lips that progresses into Bell's palsy during the same day. Complete onset of the condition can take up to 2 weeks. It is common to feel very tired during the recovery period.

Prognosis. This condition is not contagious, or permanent. The prognosis is good for this condition if the symptoms are mild and many recover fully. Children who are affected have an even higher rate of recovery. Those who are immunocompromised tend to be predisposed to recurring Bell's palsy. About 50% of patients will recover within a relatively short time (days to weeks) and approximately 35% will recover in less than 1 year.

Non–Drug Treatment. Rest is the best treatment, allowing the immune system to effectively respond to this disease. Because of the numbness in the face, food particles can become lodged between the teeth and gums; therefore good oral hygiene is essential. Sunglasses should be worn to protect the eyes and OTC eyedrops can be used to treat dry eyes, resulting from decreased ability to blink. The ears can also be sensitive to noise; therefore it is common for patients with this condition to desire a quiet environment. Exercise is not recommended; pain can be treated with a hot, moist towel or gel packs.

Drug Treatment. Corticosteroid (e.g., prednisone) therapy is often recommended and should be given within 24 hours if possible and continued for 7 to 14 days for inflammation. If the condition is associated with the herpes virus for a particular patient, then oral acyclovir may also be prescribed.

Myasthenia Gravis (MG)

Myasthenia gravis is a rare autoimmune disorder that affects the transmission of electrical impulses from the CNS to muscles throughout the body. This results in muscle skeletal weakness, affecting areas such as the muscles of the throat, eye, and eyelid as well as muscles that voluntarily control facial movement. The immune system attacks and destroys the receptors that normally receive neuronal impulses from the neurotransmitter acetylcholine. A tumor within the thymus sometimes may be the cause of MG. If the cause is genetic, it is referred to as congenital myasthenia. Although the muscles in the face, eyes, and mouth are most commonly affected, the disease can affect other areas. Vocal and visual difficulties may occur, and drooping of the eyelids is a common side effect seen in persons suffering from this autoimmune disease. Muscles are easily fatigued and take a much longer time to recover from activity. This is a chronic disease that if not treated worsens over time. Myasthenia gravis affects more women than men; only 3 in 100,000 persons are affected in the United States. There are diagnostic tests to confirm the disease, including a blood test that detects the presence of acetylcholine receptor antibodies or immune molecules, which destroy the receptor sites.

Prognosis. Most patients with myasthenia gravis can lead normal lives. There are cases where the disease has a period of remission and medications can be stopped. Of persons with myasthenia gravis, 8 out of 10 can be helped; only rare cases result in respiratory failure. There is no cure for myasthenia gravis except in those cases caused by a tumor in the thymus (15% of cases).

Non–Drug Treatment. Surgery is performed to remove the thymus (thymectomy) if a thymic tumor is found. Another treatment is plasmapheresis: abnormal antibodies are removed from the patient's blood and a transfusion of normal antibodies (immune globulin) is used.

Drug Treatments. There are medications that can control myasthenia gravis. Certain drugs that block the destruction of acetylcholine, called anticholinesterase inhibitors, most often are used for treatment. Other drugs suppress the production of abnormal antibodies. Drug treatments are listed below.

Cholinergic medications are the main treatments for myasthenia gravis. The drug action is to block the destruction of the neurotransmitter acetylcholine by the enzyme acetylcholinesterase. They improve neuronal transmission and increase muscle strength. Side effects of the medications may occur because of overstimulation of the parasympathetic nervous system, resulting in nausea, vomiting, diarrhea, and severe abdominal pain. Other drugs such as azathioprine, cyclosporine, or cyclophosphamide may be administered to slow the progression of anti–acetylcholine receptor antibodies.

CHOLINERGIC AGENTS

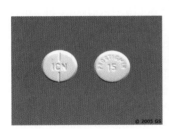

GENERIC NAME: neostigmine
TRADE NAME: Prostigmin
INDICATION: myasthenia gravis
ROUTE OF ADMINISTRATION: oral, injection
COMMON ADULT DOSAGE: oral dosage ranges from 15 to 375 mg daily, given in divided doses several times per day
SIDE EFFECTS: dizziness, headache, diarrhea, flatulence
AUXILIARY LABELS:
■ May take with food.
■ May cause dizziness or drowsiness.
■ Do not take if you are pregnant or plan on becoming pregnant.

GENERIC NAME: pyridostigmine
TRADE NAME: Mestinon
INDICATION: myasthenia gravis
ROUTE OF ADMINISTRATION: oral, injection
COMMON ADULT DOSAGE: oral dosage ranges from 70 mg to 1.5 g per day
SIDE EFFECTS: dizziness, headache, diarrhea, flatulence
AUXILIARY LABEL:
■ Do not take if you are pregnant or plan on becoming pregnant.

DISORDERS OF THE BRAIN AND/OR SPINAL CORD

Stroke

A **stroke** is the disruption of blood flow or the leakage of blood outside of vessel walls. Although there are several causes of stroke, most are attributable to ischemia. This is a decrease of blood flow to the brain when blood vessels are blocked by a clot or become too narrow. The brain is then deprived of oxygen and brain cells can die. Although the disruption is specific to the vascular system, it directly affects the nervous system and those functions that are associated with the NS. Four main blood vessels supply the brain with blood: two are in the anterior (front) area of the brain and two supply the posterior (back) of the brain. Strokes may also occur from a hemorrhage within the vessels of the brain when the vessels are either damaged or ruptured. The damage to the brain depends on the size of the blockage and how much brain tissue is harmed. The effects can range from weakness of a limb, to paralysis of one side of the body, to loss of the ability to speak. Several symptoms may occur when a person has a stroke. The most common effects include a severe headache, dizziness, visual difficulties, loss of balance or difficulty moving one side of the body, and weakness in the muscles of the facial area that can cause difficulty in speaking. A sudden weakness in half of the face or the entire body on one side occurs when the opposite side of the brain is damaged in certain areas. Those who experience involuntary emotional expression disorder (IEED) have episodes of emotional outbursts at inappropriate times. This neurological condition occurs when the brain is injured in the area that controls normal emotional response. Several factors may contribute to stroke and these include age, gender, race, and family history. More strokes occur in African Americans, Hispanics, and Asian/Pacific Islanders. Women are affected more often than men. Persons older than age 65 account for 75% of all stroke cases (www.strokecenter.org).

Prognosis. This is dependent on the severity of the damage to the brain, which can range from vascular dementia (memory loss) to depression. One of the most important factors affecting outcome is the time it takes to begin treatment. If a stroke is suspected, it is important to call 911 and to begin treatment as soon as possible. Quick treatment may reduce long-term symptoms. Depending on how quickly the stroke is treated and the severity of the blockage, some patients will never fully recover and may have muscle weakness, speech difficulties, sleep disorders, and sensations of numbness and tingling. For those who are bedridden, pain can occur from the lack of movement or may be a result of nerve damage. Most persons will require a strong support system; often family members become caregivers for the stroke patient. For those suffering from IEED there is no approved medication treatment at this time, although over time this condition may improve as the brain heals itself.

Non–Drug Treatment. Patients often must have extensive physical and/or speech therapy to regain their ability to function. This may take place in a rehabilitation hospital, an outpatient center, or the home. Many times support groups may help the survivor to cope with the emotional aspect of this condition.

Drug Treatment. Patients with ischemic strokes caused by blood clots who present to the emergency department quickly after the onset of symptoms may be treated with antithrombotic medications ("clot busters') to limit the potential damage to the brain. Hemorrhagic strokes may require neurosurgery. Most of the medical treatment for ischemic stroke is aimed at prevention of future strokes, and a range of medications that prevent blood from forming blockages and control cholesterol levels are used. Medications aimed at lowering cholesterol levels and high blood pressure are discussed in the cardiovascular system chapter (Chapter 23). Additional medications are often prescribed for depression and insomnia (see Antidepressants in Chapter 17). One of the most commonly prescribed over-the-counter medications for stroke prevention is aspirin (acetylsalicylic acid [ASA]) low dose (81 mg) taken daily. Warfarin may be prescribed to persons who are at high risk of stroke because of heart disease. Clopidogrel (Plavix) is an antiplatelet drug that works by a different mechanism than aspirin; it may or may not be administered with warfarin. The use of both aspirin and warfarin is discouraged because of the increased risk of bleeding.

ANTICOAGULANT

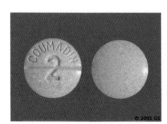

GENERIC NAME: warfarin

TRADE NAME: Coumadin

INDICATION: preventing blood clots

ROUTE OF ADMINISTRATION: oral, injection (in emergency only at hospital)

COMMON ADULT DOSAGE: based on prothrombin time (PT) or International Normalized Ratio (INR) results; most patients usually take from 1 to 10 mg per day, although rarely patients need higher dosage

SIDE EFFECTS: increased risk of bleeding

AUXILIARY LABELS:

- Take as directed.
- May take with or without food.
- Do not take with aspirin or NSAIDs.
- Avoid alcohol.
- Do not take if pregnant or plan on becoming pregnant.

ANTIPLATELET

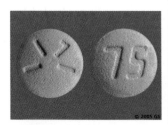

GENERIC NAME: clopidogrel

TRADE NAME: Plavix

INDICATION: preventing blood clots; used in persons who cannot take aspirin

ROUTE OF ADMINISTRATION: oral

COMMON ADULT DOSAGE: 75 mg daily

SIDE EFFECTS: increased risk of bleeding

AUXILIARY LABELS:

- Do not take with NSAIDs.
- Take with full glass of water.

Tech Note!

Stroke is the third leading cause of death in America and a leading cause of adult disability. Up to 80% of strokes are preventable.

Migraine Headache

Although scientists are still determining the triggers for a migraine, in some cases it seems to be linked to hormones. The triggers range from hormonal changes (e.g., before menstruation, during pregnancy, contraceptive use) to foods, stress, bright lights, and other changes in the environment. In some cases, there is no known etiology (cause). Drugs may also influence the frequency and severity of migraines. It is known that during a migraine headache serotonin levels drop; this causes the release of neuropeptides that travel to the meninges, where they result in dilation and inflammation of blood vessels. The result is a migraine headache. It consists of a set of symptoms that may include throbbing headaches, flashes of light, tingling in arms or legs, nausea, vomiting, and extreme sensitivity to light and sound. About 30 million people or 10% of the American population suffer from migraines and more women are affected than men. Types of migraines are listed in Table 16-7.

Prognosis. There is no cure at this time for migraine headaches. There is medication that can be taken once a migraine occurs and there are treatments to prevent migraines. Although it may be difficult to find the right drug or combination of drugs to control migraines, once the correct medication is determined migraines can be managed effectively and not interfere with the patient's lifestyle.

Non–Drug Treatment. Non–drug treatment includes using preventive measures (i.e., avoid triggers) and following an exercise regimen.

TABLE 16-7 Types of Migraines

Type	Description of Warning Signs	Note
Migraine with aura, classic migraine	Stars, bright lights, blind spots, distorted figures and shapes	Common for aura to precede attack by 60 min
Migraine without aura	Mood changes	Headaches may last up to 72 hr
Basilar artery migraine	Partial vision loss followed by vertigo, tinnitus, and sometimes tingling of fingers or toes lasting from minutes to 1 hr	Migraine headache is experienced before or during menstruation
Cluster headaches	Bouts of cluster periods can last from weeks to months; may go into remission for years	Occur in men more than women and occur at all ages, although more common in adolescence and middle-age people
Hemiplegic and ophthalmoplegic migraines	Severe, unilateral pain, with repeated headaches; neurological deficits in hemiplegic migraine may persist after headache is over	Rare type of migraine

Drug Treatments. For mild to moderate migraines the first line of treatment involves nonsteroidal antiinflammatory drugs (NSAIDs) or aspirin. For severe migraines triptans may be prescribed. Examples of triptans are listed below. Preventive medications include blood pressure medications (i.e., beta-blockers, calcium channel blockers), antidepressants (e.g., tricyclic antidepressants [TCAs], selective serotonin reuptake inhibitors [SSRIs]), some anticonvulsants (e.g., topiramate), and serotonin antagonists (e.g., methysergide). These may be prescribed as monotherapy or polytherapy depending on the person being treated. Pain-relieving medications range from NSAIDs to much stronger agents. Medications used to treat migraines and as prophylactic (preventive) therapy are listed in Table 16-8.

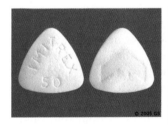

GENERIC NAME: sumatriptan
TRADE NAME: Imitrex
INDICATION: severe migraine
ROUTE OF ADMINISTRATION: oral, nasal
COMMON ADULT DOSAGE: oral, 50 to 100 mg upon onset of migraine, dose may be repeated if necessary (not to exceed 200 mg); nasal; 1 spray into nostril, may repeat in 2 hours (alternate nostrils) × 1 (max 40 mg/24 hr)
SIDE EFFECTS: dizziness, nausea, tiredness
AUXILIARY LABELS:
■ May cause dizziness or drowsiness.
■ For nasal use only (sumatriptan nasal dosage form).
NOTE: Should not be taken within 24 hours of an ergot preparation or another triptan. Use caution with other serotonergic agents (SNRIs, SSRIs).

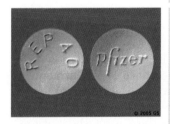

GENERIC NAME: eletriptan
TRADE NAME: Relpax
INDICATION: severe migraine
ROUTE OF ADMINISTRATION: oral
COMMON ADULT DOSAGE: 40 mg initial dose, may repeat 2 hr after initial dose (80 mg daily max)
SIDE EFFECTS: dizziness, nausea, tiredness
AUXILIARY LABEL:
■ May cause dizziness or drowsiness.
NOTE: Should not be taken within 24 hours of an ergot preparation or another triptan. Use caution with other serotonergic agents (SNRIs, SSRIs).

TABLE 16-8 Migraine Medications

Classification	Trade Name	Generic Name	Actions	Notes
To Be Given When Attack Occurs				
NSAIDs	Naprosyn, Anaprox	naproxen	Relieves pain and swelling	
	Motrin	ibuprofen	Relieves pain and swelling	
	Acular ophthalmic	ketorolac	Blocks substances to reduce pain and swelling	For use with ocular migraines
Ergotamines	Migranal nasal	dihydroergotamine	Narrows blood vessels in brain to relieve headache	Available in nasal solution;
	DHE 45	dihydroergotamine	Constricts blood vessels in brain	Used for prevention and treatment of cluster headaches; IV only
	Cafergot	ergotamine/ caffeine	Ergotamine narrows dilated blood vessels, reducing throbbing; caffeine increases effects of ergotamine	
Phenothiazine antiemetic agent	Compazine	prochlorperazine	Relieves nausea and vomiting symptoms; does not treat actual migraine	Available in oral dosage, injection, and suppositories
Triptans	Amerge	naratriptan	Relieves pain and swelling	
	Frova	frovatriptan	Relieves pain, light/sound sensitivity associated with migraines	
	Maxalt	rizatriptan	Relieves pain, sensitivity to light/ sound, nausea and vomiting associated with migraines	
	Relpax	eletriptan	Narrows blood vessels in brain to relieve headache	
	Zomig	zolmitriptan	Relieves headache pain and other symptoms of migraine	
	Imitrex	sumatriptan	Relieves pain, sensitivity to light/ sound, nausea and vomiting associated with migraines	Also available as injectable form
	Axert	almotriptan	Relieves headache pain and other symptoms of migraine	
Narcotics	Fioricet	acetaminophen (APAP), caffeine, butalbital	APAP reduces pain, caffeine increases effects of APAP, butalbital decreases anxiety and causes relaxation	
	Phrenilin with caffeine/ codeine	Codeine, APAP, caffeine	Codeine relieves pain, APAP helps to decrease pain, caffeine increases effects of APAP	
	Stadol NS	butorphanol	Helps to moderate severe pain	Controlled substance nasal spray, CI-V
To Be Taken as Prophylaxis				
Beta-blockers (BBs)	Tenormin	atenolol	Affects response to certain nerve impulses to prevent migraines	
	Lopressor	metoprolol		

Continued

TABLE 16-8 Migraine Medications—cont'd

Classification	Trade Name	Generic Name	Actions	Notes
Calcium channel blockers (CCBs)	Corgard	nadolol		
	Inderal	propranolol		
	Blocadren	timolol		
	Isoptin, Calan	verapamil	Reduces amount of narrowing of blood vessels in brain	
		diltiazem		
		nimodipine		
Antidepressants	Elavil	amitriptyline	Affects level of serotonin and other chemicals in brain to prevent migraines	
	Pamelor	nortriptyline		
	Vivactil	protriptyline		
SSRIs	Zoloft	sertraline	Affects level of serotonin and other chemicals in brain to prevent migraines	
Anticonvulsants	Depakote	divalproex sodium	Prevents migraines by restoring balance of NT in brain	
	Topamax	topiramate	Reduces frequency of migraines	

Pharmacist's Perspective
BY SUSAN WONG, Pharm D

What's New in Headache Management?

Many persons say, "I've got a migraine." What is a migraine headache? Migraines are a distinct type of headache with the following features: episodic, not continuous or daily, usually on one side of the head, may or may not be associated with aura, autonomic dysfunction (nausea, vomiting, photophobia), strong family history, and may be significantly disabling—not "just a headache." Daily throbbing headaches are more likely to be rebound headaches than migraines. Daily or near-daily throbbing headaches coupled with daily analgesic use are likely analgesic rebound headaches. Rebound headaches typically occur in migraine patients who get caught up in a cycle of frequent and excessive analgesic use. Management includes educating the patient about the cause of analgesic rebound, initiating preventive therapy, and tapering the patient off analgesics over several weeks.

The primary goal of management of migraine headaches is prevention. This involves identifying and eliminating risks or triggers for headaches such as fatigue, noise, bright lights, certain foods, and other lifestyle factors. Simple analgesics (aspirin, nonsteroidal antiinflammatory drugs) work well for acute attacks, especially in patients with mild to moderate pain in whom risks and trigger factors are under control. Antiemetics, such as metoclopramide or prochlorperazine, are useful additions if nausea is a prominent symptom. Analgesic combinations (e.g., Fiorinal or Midrin) and ergots (e.g., Cafergot, Ergostat) are usually effective for more severe migraines. Dihydroergotamine nasal spray (Migranal) has been a widely used migraine treatment; an injectable form has long been available for severe attacks requiring emergency treatment.

The "triptans"—e.g., sumatriptan (Imitrex), rizatriptan (Maxalt MLT), zolmitriptan (Zomig), naratriptan (Amerge), rizatriptan (Maxalt), frovatriptan (Frova), and eletriptan (Relpax)—are useful for patients whose migraines do not respond to other agents or for patients who are intolerant of other classes of agents. Compared with sumatriptan

(Imitrex), the new triptans are more selective 5-hydroxytryptamine (serotonin) agonists and offer greater oral bioavailability, a potentially improved risk-to-benefit ratio, and a potentially greater therapeutic benefit through a combination of peripheral and central effects.

Preventive drug therapy is indicated when a patient has frequent headaches (two or more per month) that create significant disability at home, school, or work (e.g., cancelled plans), causing significant emotional distress, or when a patient requires large quantities of medications to stop the pain quickly. Prevention should be part of a treatment plan that emphasizes behavioral changes and should be given an adequate trial to assess effectiveness (usually 2 to 3 months unless side effects are intolerable). Prescribing inadequate doses of preventive medications for brief periods is a major cause of therapeutic failure. Beta-blockers and tricyclic antidepressants remain the drugs of choice for migraine prevention. Propranolol is a very effective agent but may cause a decreased heart rate; it should be used with caution in patients with asthma. Failure of one beta-blocker does not preclude success with another.

Topiramate (Topamax) may be prescribed for prevention of migraines.

Your role as a technician is to pay attention to both the patient's complaints and the patient's requests for medication. If it seems as though the same patient is asking for over-the-counter pain or headache medicine in a large quantity or regularly, it should be a red flag, causing you to ask, "How often do you need to take this type of medicine? Are you using it for headaches or other pain? Does it help?" If any of the answers are more than just on an occasional basis, tell the pharmacist. Sometimes chronic use of over-the-counter medicines can be a problem because they can interfere with some prescription medicines, they can worsen or cause other problems, and, in the case of headaches, they actually can contribute to having more headaches (hence the description of analgesic rebound). A patient may ask you for recommendations regarding dietary supplements. Make sure the patient speaks with the pharmacist to obtain accurate information about the efficacy of the supplement; this may help prevent unnecessary use of the dietary supplement and the prevention of adverse drug interactions or side effects. ■

Epilepsy

Epilepsy is a seizure disorder in which there is hyperexcitability in some of the nerve cells in the brain. Diagnosis normally is based on an electroencephalogram (EEG). When an EEG is conducted, electrodes are attached to the head of the patient, and electrical impulses corresponding to brain waves are transferred onto paper strips that are interpreted by a physician. The two types of seizures are partial or generalized. Partial seizures affect only one hemisphere of the brain and may result in only a twitching of a limb without any loss of consciousness. Generalized seizures affect both hemispheres and have different levels of intensity, ranging from petit mal (the least violent) to grand mal seizures that are longer and more intense. Children often have petit mal seizures, causing them to stare into space for a time. In grand mal seizures, also known as tonic-clonic seizures, the person loses consciousness and falls to the ground; a period of widespread muscle spasms (tonic phase) is followed by a period of muscle relaxation (clonic phase). Injuries can occur depending on where and when the seizure takes place. The person having the seizure does not remember the episode. Other causes for seizure include head trauma or tumor, although often no cause is found. Box 16-2 outlines various seizure types.

Prognosis. Although there is still no known cure, most people live relatively normal lives with drug treatment or surgical intervention. There are social stigmas associated with this condition that can cause embarrassment and frustration. Certain states refuse to allow the issuance of drivers' licenses to patients with epilepsy, unless certain criteria are met, including a period in which the patient has been seizure-free. Women must consult with their physician about the risks of taking seizure medications while pregnant; however, it has been determined that there is more than a 90% chance that women with

BOX 16-2 TYPES OF SEIZURES

Partial Seizures

Simple partial motor type—Involves stiffening or jerking in one extremity followed by a tingling sensation in the same area. Consciousness is not normally lost although the seizure may progress into a generalized seizure.

Simple partial sensory type—Involves perceptual distortion including hallucinations.

Complex partial type—Effects vary and may include purposeless behavior. The patient experiences an aura immediately before the seizure begins that may include a pungent smell, nausea, a dreamy sensation, an unusual taste, or a visual disturbance. Behavior changes may include glassy stare, picking at one's clothing, aimless wandering, lip-smacking or lip-chewing motions, and unintelligible speech. May last from seconds to 20 minutes in duration. Mental confusion may continue after seizure.

Generalized Seizures

Absence (petit mal)—Brief change in level of consciousness, indicated by blinking or rolling the eyes, a blank stare, and slight mouth movements. Patient retains posture and seizures normally last no more than 10 seconds although seizures may repeat often throughout the day. Most often affects children.

Myoclonic (bilateral massive epileptic myoclonus)—Brief, involuntary muscular jerks of the body or extremities.

Tonic-clonic (grand mal)—Typically starts with a loud cry attributable to air rushing from lungs through vocal cords; patient falls to the ground, loses consciousness, and the body stiffens and then alternates between spasms and relaxation phases.

Akinetic seizure—General loss of postural tone and temporary loss of consciousness; also known as drop attack; often occurs in children.

Status epilepticus—Continuous seizure that can occur in all types of seizures and may be accompanied with a loss of consciousness and respiratory distress; is life-threatening. May occur as a result of abrupt withdrawal of anticonvulsant medications, head trauma, encephalopathy, or septicemia caused by meningitis.

epilepsy can have a healthy child (National Institute of Neurological Disorders and Stroke).

Non–Drug Treatment. If medication does not control seizures, surgery may be necessary to remove lesion(s) in the brain: however, surgery is not always effective.

Drug Treatments. Monotherapy (one drug) or polytherapy (more than one drug) may be prescribed. Anticonvulsants are normally prescribed to reduce the number of seizures. Anticonvulsants prevent abnormal impulses within the CNS by inhibiting one or more of the ions involved in nerve conduction, such as sodium, calcium, or potassium. Specific medications such as phenytoin (Dilantin) and carbamazepine (Tegretol) are commonly used to treat generalized tonic-clonic and partial seizures. Valproic acid and ethosuximide are prescribed for absence seizures. Often the dosage or type of medicine must be adjusted to help the patient become seizure-free. It is important for the patient to take the medication on time every day, as this will help avoid the possibility of seizures. Classes of agents used for treatment of seizures may include hydantoins, barbiturates, succinimides, carbonic anhydrase inhibitors (CAIs), and benzodiazepines. Both epilepsy classifications and agents used to treat them are listed in Table 16-9. Drug interactions are common with the anticonvulsants. In addition, it is extremely important not to alter or stop taking the prescribed medication

TABLE 16-9 Agents Used for Treatment of Epilepsy

Classification	Generic Name	Trade Name	Treats	Dosage Range (Adults, typical PO Doses)
Anticonvulsant	carbamazepine	Tegretol	Complex partial and generalized tonic-clonic seizures	Up to 1200 mg/day in 3-4 divided doses
Anticonvulsant	valproic acid	Depakene	All seizure types	Up to 1750 mg daily
Anticonvulsant	divalproex sodium	Depakote	All seizure types	15-60 mg/kg/day in divide doses 2-3 time per day
Anticonvulsant	divalproex sodium extended release	Depakote	All seizure types	
Anticonvulsant	acetazolamide	Diamox	All seizure types	250-1000 mg daily
Anticonvulsant	levetiracetam	Keppra	Partial seizures (all types)	1000-3000 mg daily
Anticonvulsant	pregabalin	Lyrica	Partial seizures (all types)	150-600 mg daily
Anticonvulsant	primidone	Mysoline	All seizure types	250-1000 mg daily
Anticonvulsant	gabapentin	Neurontin	Complex partial seizures	900-3600 mg daily
Anticonvulsant	vigabatrin	Sabril	Complex partial seizures	1000 mg/day or 500 mg bid
Anticonvulsant	carbamazepine extended release	Tegretol XR	Complex partial and generalized tonic-clonic seizures	600-1200 mg daily
Anticonvulsant	topiramate	Topamax	Partial seizures (all types)	25, 50, 100, 200 mg daily
Anticonvulsant	oxcarbazepine	Trileptal	Simple partial seizures	600-2400 mg daily
Anticonvulsant	lacosamide	Vimpat	Partial onset seizures	Oral: 50, 100, 150, 200 mg; injection: 200 mg
Anticonvulsant	ethosuximide	Zarontin	Absence seizures	500-1500 mg daily
Anticonvulsant	zonisamide	Zonegran	Simple partial seizures	100-600 mg daily
Anticonvulsant	felbamate	Felbatol	Partial seizures (all types)	120-3600 mg daily
Anticonvulsant	lamotrigine	Lamictal	All seizure types	100-500 mg daily
Antiepileptic agent	tiagabine	Gabitril	Partial seizures (all types)	32-56 mg daily
Antiepileptic agent	phenobarbital (C-IV)	Luminal	All seizure types	100 mg daily
Benzodiazepine	lorazepam	Ativan	All seizure types	1-10 mg daily
Benzodiazepine	clorazepate	Tranxene	Myoclonic, absence seizures, drop attacks	15-45 mg daily
Benzodiazepine	clonazepam	Klonopin	All seizure types	1.5-20 mg daily
Benzodiazepine	diazepam rectal gel	AcuDial	All seizure types	0.2-0.5 mg/kg
Hydantoin	phenytoin	Dilantin	Partial seizures (all types)	200-400 mg daily
Hydantoin	phenytoin extended release	Phenytek	Partial and generalized tonic-clonic	200-400 mg daily
			Emergency condition	**Injectables**
Benzodiazepine	diazepam	Valium	Status epilepticus	Injection: dosage varies
Benzodiazpine	lorazepam	Ativan	Status epilepticus	Injection: dosage varies
Hydantoin	phenytoin	Dilantin	Status epilepticus	Injection: dosage varies
Barbiturate	phenobarbital	Solfoton	Status epilepticus	Injection: dosage varies

unless instructed to do so by the physician. Examples of these types of interactions are listed below.

Phenytoin's effects may be increased, decreased, or altered if taken with these agents: alcohol, antacids, warfarin, diazepam, enteral feedings, estrogens, doxycycline, corticosteroids, sulfa drugs, ulcer medications such as cimetidine and ranitidine, and seizure medications such as valproate, carbamazepine, and ethosuximide.

Tegretol's concentration in blood may be raised to harmful levels with the following agents: cimetidine, clarithromycin, danazol, diltiazem, erythromycin, fluoxetine, isoniazid, itraconazole, niacinamide, propoxyphene, valproate, and calcium channel blockers.

EXAMPLES OF ANTICONVULSANTS

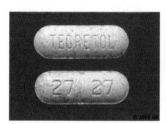

GENERIC NAME: carbamazepine
TRADE NAME: Tegretol; Tegretol-XR
INDICATION: all types of seizures
ROUTE OF ADMINISTRATION: oral
COMMON ADULT DOSAGE: 200 to 1200 mg/day in divided doses; dose divided bid for XR; dosage can vary widely
SIDE EFFECTS: dizziness, drowsiness, dry mouth, headache, diarrhea, constipation
AUXILIARY LABELS:
- May cause dizziness or drowsiness.
- Avoid alcohol.
- Take with food.
- Shake well (for oral suspension).
- Do not stop taking without consulting physician.

GENERIC NAME: gabapentin
TRADE NAME: Neurontin
INDICATION: all types of seizures
ROUTE OF ADMINISTRATION: oral
COMMON ADULT DOSAGE: 300 to 600 mg tid
SIDE EFFECTS: dizziness, drowsiness, blurred vision, nausea, vomiting, diarrhea, constipation, headache, insomnia, dry mouth
AUXILIARY LABELS:
- May take with or without food.
- Do not stop taking without consulting physician.
- May cause dizziness or drowsiness.

HYDANTOIN ANTICONVULSANTS

GENERIC NAME: phenytoin
TRADE NAME: Dilantin, Phenytek
INDICATION: most often for tonic-clonic seizures and partial seizures
ROUTE OF ADMINISTRATION: oral, injection
COMMON ADULT DOSAGE: 100 mg tid, although dosage can range widely
SIDE EFFECTS: dizziness, insomnia, nausea, vomiting, headache
AUXILIARY LABELS:
- May cause dizziness or drowsiness (for oral dosage form).
- Shake well before using (for suspension dosage form).
- Do not stop taking without consulting physician.

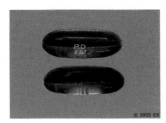

SUCCINIMIDE ANTICONVULSANT

GENERIC NAME: ethosuximide
TRADE NAME: Zarontin
INDICATION: absence (petit mal) seizures
ROUTE OF ADMINISTRATION: oral
COMMON ADULT DOSAGE: 250 mg twice daily initially. Up to 1.5 g given in two divided doses.
SIDE EFFECTS: drowsiness, nausea, vomiting, headache, loss of appetite
AUXILIARY LABELS:
- May cause dizziness or drowsiness.
- Do not stop taking without consulting physician.

Tech Note!

All controlled substances require an auxiliary label stating: "Federal law prohibits the transfer of this medication to anyone other than intended."

BARBITURATES (CONTROLLED SUBSTANCES)

GENERIC NAME: phenobarbital (C-IV)
TRADE NAME: Luminal
INDICATION: partial and generalized seizures; also used for sedation and other effects
ROUTE OF ADMINISTRATION: oral, injection
COMMON ADULT DOSAGE: oral dosage varies from 60 to 100 mg daily
SIDE EFFECTS: nausea and vomiting; also can cause respiratory depression if overdosed
AUXILIARY LABELS:
- Federal law prohibits the transfer of this medication to anyone other than intended.
- Do not drink alcohol.
- Do not stop taking medication without consulting physician.
- May cause drowsiness.

GENERIC NAME: mephobarbital (C-IV)
TRADE NAME: Mebaral
INDICATION: Epileptic convulsions; also used to treat anxiety
ROUTE OF ADMINISTRATION: oral
COMMON ADULT DOSAGE: 400 to 600 mg daily, usually at bedtime
SIDE EFFECTS: nausea and vomiting; also can cause respiratory depression if overdosed
AUXILIARY LABELS:
- Do not stop taking medication without consulting physician.
- Take with a full glass of water.
- Do not drink alcohol.

BENZODIAZEPINES (CONTROLLED SUBSTANCES)

GENERIC NAME: diazepam (C-IV)
TRADE NAME: Valium, Diastat rectal gel
INDICATION: status epilepticus, intermittent treatment of generalized tonic-clonic seizures
ROUTE OF ADMINISTRATION: oral, rectal gel, injection
COMMON DOSAGE: oral dosage, 2 to 10 mg bid to qid
SIDE EFFECTS: drowsiness
AUXILIARY LABELS:
- Federal law prohibits the transfer of this medication to anyone other than intended.
- Do not drink alcohol.
- Do not stop taking without consulting physician.
- For rectal use only (Diastat rectal gel device).

GENERIC NAME: clonazepam (C-IV)

TRADE NAME: Klonopin

INDICATION: seizures

ROUTE OF ADMINISTRATION: oral

COMMON ADULT DOSAGE: 0.5 mg tid up to maximum of 20 mg qid to control seizures

SIDE EFFECTS: drowsiness

AUXILIARY LABELS:

■ Federal law prohibits the transfer of this medication to anyone other than intended.

■ Do not drink alcohol.

■ Do not stop taking without consulting physician.

Alzheimer's Disease

Alzheimer's disease (AD) is a chronic progressive disease that causes memory loss, confusion, impaired judgment, personality changes, disorientation, and loss of language skills. AD is most common in the elderly although it can occasionally occur in younger adults. Alzheimer's disease affects approximately 7% of persons younger than 65 years; the incidence rises to 30% for persons older than 85. AD affects millions of elderly people, including some famous persons such as former President Ronald Reagan and actor Charlton Heston. According to the Alzheimer's Disease International 2009 report, there are 35 million people worldwide living with dementia and it is estimated this number will double every 20 years (www.alz.org). Although there are several other types of dementia (progressive conditions of deteriorating cognitive functions), AD is the most common and accounts for 50% to 70% of cases (www.alz.org). Because of the loss of neuronal synapses, the transfer of electrical stimuli is stifled; the memory banks cannot process information and memory loss occurs. Brain cells are replaced with deposits of protein often described as tangles and knots. The brain begins to shrink in size, and memory is affected.

Most persons lose some memory as they age; however, an abnormal loss of memory and basic mental function is called dementia. Other symptoms include inability to perform normally familiar tasks, difficulty talking, and disorientation in familiar surroundings. The sleep schedule in the patient often becomes reversed or altered as the disease progresses. Persons suffering from Alzheimer's disease lack the neurotransmitter acetylcholine, which is needed to transmit impulses properly. Many hypotheses have been proposed for the cause of Alzheimer's disease, including viruses, immunizations, and tainted water. The disease has been shown to have a genetic component as well.

Currently, there are three major categories in the progression of AD. Not all patients experience the onset and progression of AD in the same way, but a classification of disease progression helps the family and physician monitor the severity of the disease. These include early-stage, mid-stage, and late-stage categories (Box 16-3). Seven specific stages are used to classify the progression of AD. Researchers are making progress in determining the etiology of this disease but there is still no cure for AD.

Prognosis. Although medication may slow the progression of AD in some cases, the overall prognosis is grim. AD affects every individual differently as it progresses, but ultimately results in death. The deterioration of normal functions, such as swallowing, the inability to move, and the total absence of communicative or cognitive skills are seen in the final stage of the disease. Infections or other conditions attributable to the patient's physical and cognitive decline inevitably result in death.

Non–Drug Treatment. In addition to the use of drugs to help slow the advancing progression of this disease, patients usually need 24-hour care in skilled nursing

BOX 16-3 STAGES ASSOCIATED WITH ALZHEIMER'S DISEASE

Although this is a guide to the stages of AD, not all individuals show these signs in this order and the rate at which AD progresses varies from person to person.

Stage 1: No impairment or normal functioning
Normal function; does not show signs or symptoms of disease.

Stage 2: Very mild decline
Earliest signs of AD. Person is aware of memory loss; forgets familiar words and the location of common household items. No signs of AD seen upon physician's examination and within family unit or friends.

Stage 3: Mild cognitive decline
Signs appear as problems of memory loss continue. May not be able to remember names of people, reads less because of a decrease in memory retention, loses more items including those that are valuable, and exhibits a decline in planning or organization skills. Presence of disease becomes measurable in a clinical/medical interview.

Stage 4: Moderate cognitive decline
Mild or early-stage AD; deficiencies become evident as condition continues to progress. Decreased knowledge of recent occasions or current events in the world; cannot perform tasks related to more complex cognitive functions, such as managing finances, planning dinner functions, or performing mathematical calculations (such as counting backwards by 7). Person suffers reduced memory of personal history and may become withdrawn from individuals and group situations.

Stage 5: Moderately severe cognitive decline
Moderate or mild-stage AD; may include major gaps in memory and in daily activities. Person may not remember home address or phone number, may not remember day of week or month of year, and has trouble performing basic math manipulations (counting backwards by 2's). Still, person knows own name and names of immediate family members; does not require assistance with functions such as eating or using the toilet.

Stage 6: Severe cognitive decline
Moderately severe or mid-stage AD. Characterized by significant personality changes (e.g., becomes suspicious of caretakers, hallucinations), exhibits wandering behavior, occasionally forgets names of family members, cannot dress self or go to the toilet (increasing episodes of incontinence). May experience a disruption in sleep-wake cycle and may begin repetitive behaviors such as hand-wringing or shredding tissues.

Stage 7: Very severe cognitive decline
Severe or late-stage AD. Last stage of AD; person loses the ability to speak, control movements, or respond to environment. Eventually may lose ability to feed self, use the toilet, walk without assistance, or sit without support. May not be able to smile or hold head up, and as reflexes continue to decline muscles become rigid and swallowing is impaired.

facilities if their families cannot assume the responsibility. Education is important for the patient, family, and friends to help them understand the progression and effects of AD. In addition, changing the environment for the patient with AD can help resolve challenges and obstacles; for example, tasks should be divided into simple steps, noise should be kept to a minimum, and a daily routine should be followed for consistency.

Drug Treatment. Two classifications of drugs have been approved for use by the FDA to treat AD: cholinesterase inhibitors (which prevent the breakdown of acetylcholine) and memantine (lowers glutamate, a contributor to neuronal damage). Other medications such as nimodipine and physostigmine are sometimes used. Drug treatment may help delay the progression of the disease.

CHOLINESTERASE INHIBITORS

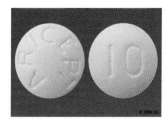

GENERIC NAME: donepezil

TRADE NAME: Aricept

DRUG ACTION: inhibits acetylcholinesterase, which is responsible for destroying acetylcholine; therefore it allows a higher concentration of acetylcholine to activate receptors

INDICATION: mild to moderate Alzheimer's disease

ROUTE OF ADMINISTRATION: oral

COMMON ADULT DOSAGE: 5 mg (first 4-6 weeks), then 10 mg daily if increase is needed. Maximum of 23 mg/day if advancing disease

SIDE EFFECTS: nausea, vomiting, and diarrhea; fatigue with initial dosing

AUXILIARY LABEL:

■ Take with or without food.

GENERIC NAME: tacrine

TRADE NAME: Cognex

DRUG ACTION: elevates acetylcholine concentrations in the cerebral cortex

INDICATION: mild to moderate Alzheimer's disease

ROUTE OF ADMINISTRATION: oral

COMMON ADULT DOSAGE: 10 mg qid (first 4 weeks); increase at 4-week intervals; 20 mg qid, 30 mg qid, 40 mg qid if tolerated

SIDE EFFECTS: upset stomach; most effects are caused by high dosage; nausea, vomiting, and diarrhea; can cause liver problems

AUXILIARY LABEL:

■ Take with food and water.

GENERIC NAME: rivastigmine

TRADE NAME: Exelon

DRUG ACTION: elevates acetylcholine concentrations in the cerebral cortex

INDICATION: mild to moderate Alzheimer's disease

ROUTE OF ADMINISTRATION: oral, transdermal (Exelon patch)

COMMON ADULT DOSAGE: oral, 1.5 mg bid × 2 weeks; at 2-week intervals may increase dose to 3 mg, 4.5 mg, and 6 mg bid

DOSAGE FOR THE PATCH: 4.6 mg daily initial dose to 9.5 mg daily maintenance

SIDE EFFECTS: loss of appetite, difficulty sleeping, dizziness, headache, diarrhea

AUXILIARY LABEL:

■ Take with food (oral).

GENERIC NAME: galantamine

TRADE NAME: Razadyne, Razadyne ER

DRUG ACTION: elevates acetylcholine concentrations in the cerebral cortex

INDICATION: mild to moderate Alzheimer's disease

ROUTE OF ADMINISTRATION: oral

COMMON ADULT DOSAGE: immediate release: 4 mg bid (first 4 weeks); 8 mg bid (second 4 weeks); then 12 mg bid. For extended-release capsules: 8 mg once daily (initially); up to 16-24 mg/day maintenance

SIDE EFFECTS: abdominal pain, anemia, blood in urine, diarrhea, dizziness

AUXILIARY LABELS:

■ Take with food and water.

■ May cause dizziness or drowsiness.

■ Do not crush or chew (extended-release capsules).

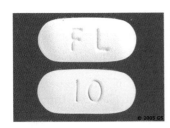

 Tech Note!

Tacrine is associated with liver damage and is dosed 4 times daily rather than once daily, as is donepezil. Therefore tacrine is not prescribed as often as donepezil in the AD population, because of issues with patient compliance, swallowing difficulties, and the risk of liver damage.

GENERIC NAME: memantine
TRADE NAME: Namenda
DRUG ACTION: Neuroprotective with mechanism different from other AD drugs; works in the cerebral cortex by targeting glutamate
INDICATION: mild to moderate Alzheimer's disease; may be taken concurrently with other cholinesterase inhibitors
ROUTE OF ADMINISTRATION: oral
COMMON ADULT DOSAGE: 5 mg daily × 7 days; then increase by 5 mg every week up to 10 mg twice daily max
SIDE EFFECTS: confusion, constipation, dizziness, headache, vomiting, sleepiness
AUXILIARY LABELS:
- Take with food and water.
- May cause dizziness or drowsiness.

Multiple Sclerosis (MS)

Multiple sclerosis is a chronic neurological condition that affects myelin and the cells that produce new myelin in the brain and spinal cord (CNS). Myelin sheaths cover the axon portion of neurons; they allow nerve transmission to proceed properly throughout the nervous system. MS involves deterioration of the myelin sheath, as shown in Figure 16-10. With multiple sclerosis the body begins to attack and destroy the myelin sheaths and the cells that produce myelin. The sheaths are replaced by plaques of sclerotic (hard) tissue. When this occurs, the electrical impulses cannot pass from one neuron to another, and the person fails to complete the movement he or she wishes to make. The cause is considered an autoimmune response to some unknown stimulus. The disease may be related to both hereditary and environmental factors.

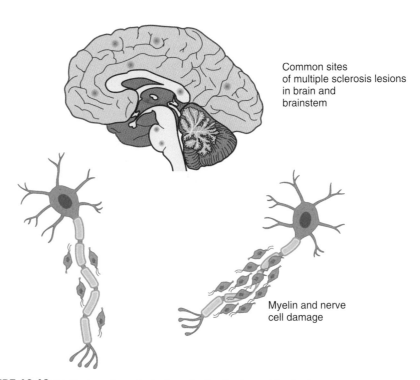

Common sites of multiple sclerosis lesions in brain and brainstem

Myelin and nerve cell damage

FIGURE 16-10 Multiple sclerosis lesions in the brain and brainstem.

Often diagnosis of the type of MS is difficult to determine because the symptoms vary widely. There are four disease courses, each having mild, moderate, or severe symptoms:

- Relapsing-remitting MS: Individuals with this type of MS experience attacks (i.e., flare-ups or relapses) of worsening neurological function. These can be followed by complete recovery periods (remission). This is the most common type of MS, affecting approximately 85% of MS patients.
- Primary-progressive MS: Individuals diagnosed with this type of MS have slowly worsening neurological functions from the onset of the disease. There are no distinct relapses or remissions. Approximately 10% of people suffer from this type of MS.
- Secondary-progressive MS: In this type of MS the disease worsens more steadily with or without occasional flare-ups, recovery periods, or plateaus. Many people develop this type of MS following an initial period of relapsing-remitting MS.
- Progressive-relapsing MS: With this type of MS people experience a steadily worsening disease from the onset of the condition and episodes of deteriorating neurological functions with each attack. A recovery period may or may not occur and there are no remission periods.

Symptoms range from mild to severe and may include muscle weakness, abnormal sensations such as numbness or tingling over any part of the body, vision change, and loss of coordination. There are three levels of symptoms of MS: the primary symptoms (first level) include weakness, numbness, tremor, paralysis, pain, loss of vision, loss of balance, and bowel and bladder dysfunction. Secondary symptoms (second level) occur from complications of the primary symptoms and include inactivity, poor posture, poor trunk control, and overall weakness resulting from muscle atrophy. The tertiary (third-level) symptoms must be managed by psychologists (for depression) and by physical and occupational therapists.

Prognosis. Because there is no clear disease course for MS, it is difficult to determine a prognosis. Most patients live a normal life, although there are persons who experience disease progression. Those who have frequent attacks initially or who are older than 40 years before symptoms occur tend to have a poor prognosis.

Non–Drug Treatment. Physical therapy may help the patient recover from attacks and may help with overall strength and balance.

Drug Treatment. The first treatment is disease-modifying immunotherapy to slow and minimize progression of the disease. These agents are referred to as the ABRC drugs (Avonex, Betaseron, Rebif, and Copaxone). In the second line of treatment, additional agents, such as steroids, are given to treat flare-ups that can last from 1 to 3 months. The third type of therapy involves treating the symptoms of MS using agents that manage fatigue, spasticity, tremors, pain, and depression.

ABRC AGENTS   INTERFERONS

GENERIC NAME: interferon β-1a
TRADE NAME: Avonex
INDICATION: multiple sclerosis
ROUTE OF ADMINISTRATION: injection
COMMON ADULT DOSAGE: 30 mcg intramuscularly every week
SIDE EFFECTS: dizziness, headache, stomach pain, runny/stuffy nose
AUXILIARY LABELS:
- Avoid alcohol.
- Keep medication away from heat and direct sunlight.
- Do not use if you are pregnant or plan on becoming pregnant.
- For intramuscular use only.
- May cause dizziness.
- Refrigerate.

GENERIC NAME: interferon β-1a
TRADE NAME: Rebif
INDICATION: multiple sclerosis
ROUTE OF ADMINISTRATION: injection
COMMON ADULT DOSAGE: (titration schedule) weeks 1 and 2, 4.4 mcg subcutaneously 3 times per week; weeks 3 and 4, 11 mcg subcutaneously 3 times per week; week 5 and beyond, 22 mcg subcutaneously 3 times per week
SIDE EFFECTS: headache, weakness or muscle pain, insomnia, swelling of hands and/or feet, skin rash, irregular menstrual periods, depression
AUXILIARY LABELS:
- Do not use if you are pregnant or plan on becoming pregnant.
- For subcutaneous use only.

GENERIC NAME: interferon β-1b
TRADE NAME: Betaseron
INDICATION: multiple sclerosis
ROUTE OF ADMINISTRATION: injection
COMMON ADULT DOSAGE: 0.25 mg subcutaneously every other day
SIDE EFFECTS: headache, weakness or muscle pain, insomnia, swelling of hands and/or feet, skin rash, irregular menstrual periods, depression
AUXILIARY LABELS:
- Do not use if you are pregnant or plan on becoming pregnant.
- For subcutaneous use only.

GENERIC NAME: glatiramer
TRADE NAME: Copaxone
INDICATION: multiple sclerosis
ROUTE OF ADMINISTRATION: injection
COMMON ADULT DOSAGE: 20 mg subcutaneously daily
SIDE EFFECTS: headache, weakness or muscle pain, insomnia, swelling of hands and/or feet, skin rash, irregular menstrual periods, depression
AUXILIARY LABELS:
- Do not use if you are pregnant or plan on becoming pregnant.
- For subcutaneous use only.
- Refrigerate.

ANTISPASMODIC MEDICATION

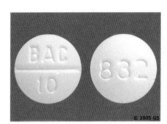

GENERIC NAME: baclofen
TRADE NAME: Lioresal
INDICATION: spasticity in multiple sclerosis and some spinal cord injuries
ROUTE OF ADMINISTRATION: oral
COMMON DOSAGE: increasing dosage over several weeks from 5 mg tid to 20 mg qid
SIDE EFFECTS: dizziness, drowsiness, headache, insomnia
AUXILIARY LABELS:

■ May cause dizziness or drowsiness.
■ Avoid alcohol.
■ Take with food.

CENTRAL-ACTING SMOOTH MUSCLE RELAXANT; ANTISPASMODIC

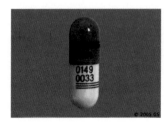

GENERIC NAME: dantrolene
TRADE NAME: Dantrium
INDICATION: spasticity from spinal cord injury, stroke, cerebral palsy, or multiple sclerosis
ROUTE OF ADMINISTRATION: oral
COMMON ADULT DOSAGE: 25 mg daily initially and slowly titrated up to 100 mg tid
SIDE EFFECTS: dizziness, drowsiness, diarrhea, constipation, headache, insomnia, difficulty swallowing, blurred vision, depression
AUXILIARY LABELS:

■ Take with a full glass of water.
■ May cause dizziness or drowsiness.
■ Avoid alcohol.

Parkinson's Disease

Parkinson's disease (PD) is a progressive disorder of the basal ganglia and is associated with the loss or deficiency of dopamine. The basal ganglia are a group of cells (gray matter) located in the medulla (white matter) of the cerebrum. The function of the basal ganglia is to regulate skeletal muscle tone and overall body movement. Dopamine is a natural chemical produced in the brain that inhibits movement. Acetylcholine activates the neurons, and dopamine inactivates them. If dopamine is lacking, then there is no cessation of movement. The overall degeneration of dopamine-producing neurons instigates the symptoms of Parkinson's disease (Figure 16-11).

The severity of symptoms increases over months to years. The most common symptoms include tremors, muscle rigidity, loss of balance, and hypokinesia and bradykinesia. Hypokinesia is a decrease in the range of motion, and bradykinesia involves an overall slowing of motion and performance of simple tasks, such as buttoning a shirt or eating. As this disease progresses, the patient's movement slows and eventually stops; the person becomes wheelchair-bound. Swallowing may become difficult, and speech may be slurred.

According to the Parkinson's Disease Foundation there are as many as 1 million Americans affected by PD, with 50,000 new cases being diagnosed annually. Signs of Parkinson's disease most commonly develop at approximately 60 years of age; however, it can occur between the ages of 21 and 40 years, and in this case is called young onset of Parkinson's disease (YOPD). This condition has affected millions of people, including famous persons such as Muhammad Ali, Janet Reno, and Michael J. Fox (Michael J. Fox Foundation). The cause is unknown; although researchers have found a genetic defect in some cases, whether the disease is genetic or environmental or a combination of both is still

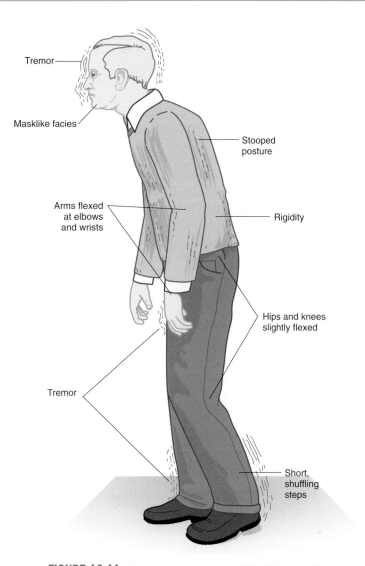

Tremor

Masklike facies

Stooped posture

Arms flexed at elbows and wrists

Rigidity

Hips and knees slightly flexed

Tremor

Short, shuffling steps

FIGURE 16-11 Symptoms and signs of Parkinson's disease.

unclear. Diagnosis is difficult because the disease can progress slowly. Doctors usually order computed tomography (CT) scans or magnetic resonance imaging (MRI) to rule out other possibilities. Often, administration of anti-parkinsonian agents is used to make the correct diagnosis of Parkinson's disease.

Prognosis. This disease varies from person to person, making a diagnosis difficult. Typically this is a slow progressive disorder that affects the person over decades rather than months or a few years. Many people can live somewhat normally with the help of medications, exercise, and maintenance of overall good health.

Non–Drug Treatment. Treatments include surgery and physical therapy. In certain cases surgery may be an alternative. Surgical interventions include insertion of a deep brain stimulator; that is, an electrode attached to a pulse generator (stored in the chest area) is implanted into the brain. The device can be wirelessly controlled and determines the pulse rate to the brain. This type of surgery is not a curative measure; instead, it may help treat the side effects of PD medications. Pallidotomy is another surgical procedure; it involves destroying certain brain cells that control movement and is fairly effective in reducing dyskinesias (involuntary movements) by 70% to 90%. There are risks with these types of surgeries, such as stroke.

Drug Treatment. Drug treatment began in the 1960s when it was discovered that the decrease in levels of dopamine was associated with PD. The normal course of treatment would have been to replace dopamine levels with the drug dopamine; however, dopamine cannot pass the blood-brain barrier (BBB). Therefore levodopa (L-dopa), a precursor to dopamine, was developed early in the treatment of PD; levodopa can cross the BBB and raise dopamine levels in the brain. Levodopa is still the primary agent used in treating PD, although newer agents that augment levodopa activity or the activity of dopamine are available. Agents used to treat PD, their method of action (MOA), and possible side effects are listed in Table 16-10.

TABLE 16-10 Medications Used to Treat Parkinson's Disease

Classification of Drug	Generic Name	Trade Name	MOA	Side Effects
L-Dopa	carbidopa/ levodopa	Sinemet	Levodopa is converted to dopamine after passing BBB; carbidopa stops destruction of levodopa outside BBB, allowing more L-dopa to cross into brain	Dyskinesias (involuntary movements)
Dopamine agonists	ropinirole	Requip	Bind to dopamine receptors, stimulating them to produce dopamine	Psychosis, edema, nausea and vomiting, fibrosis, and orthostatic hypotension
	bromocriptine	Parlodel		
	pergolide	Permax		
	apomorphine	Apokyn		
	pramipexole	Mirapex		
catechol-O-methyltransferase (COMT) inhibitors	entacapone	Comtan	Interfere with breakdown of L-dopa, allowing for more bioavailability of L-dopa in brain	Psychosis, diarrhea, abdominal pain, dry mouth, urine discoloration, orthostatic hypotension, and dyskinesias (caused by L-dopa buildup)
	tolcapone	Tasmar		
MAO-B inhibitors	selegiline	Eldepryl	Slows death of dopamine-producing neurons in brain, resulting in increased levels of dopamine	Insomnia, hallucinations, and orthostatic hypotension
	rasagiline	Azilect		
Anticholinergics	procyclidine	Kemadrin	Relax smooth muscle, which stops spasms	Blurred vision, constipation, dry mouth, nausea, vomiting, loss of appetite, light-headedness

EXAMPLES OF ANTI-PARKINSONISM DRUGS

GENERIC NAME: amantadine
TRADE NAME: Symmetrel
INDICATION: Parkinson's disease
ROUTE OF ADMINISTRATION: oral
COMMON DOSAGE: 100 bid to 100-200 mg once daily
SIDE EFFECTS: dizziness, drowsiness, dry mouth, headache, nausea, insomnia
AUXILIARY LABELS:

- ■ May cause dizziness or drowsiness.
- ■ Do not stop taking medication without consulting physician.

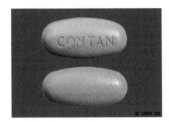

GENERIC NAME: entacapone
TRADE NAME: Comtan
INDICATION: to be used concurrently with carbidopa/levodopa to treat symptoms of PD
ROUTE OF ADMINISTRATION: oral
COMMON ADULT DOSAGE: 200 mg with each carbidopa/levodopa dose; max 8 times per day
SIDE EFFECTS: dizziness, drowsiness, constipation, diarrhea, nausea, change in color of urine
AUXILIARY LABELS:

- ■ Do not use with MAOIs.
- ■ May cause dizziness or drowsiness.
- ■ May cause urine to change to orange in color.

GENERIC NAME: levodopa/carbidopa
TRADE NAME: Sinemet
INDICATION: Parkinson's disease
ROUTE OF ADMINISTRATION: oral
COMMON ADULT DOSAGE: doses range from 25 mg/100 mg tid to 25 mg/250 mg tid
SIDE EFFECTS: confusion, nausea, vomiting, dry mouth, dizziness, drowsiness, headache, loss of appetite
AUXILIARY LABELS:

- ■ May cause dizziness or drowsiness.
- ■ Take on empty stomach 1 hr before meal or 2 hr after meal.
- ■ Do not use with nonselective MAOIs.

NOTE: Certain selective MAOIs can be used such as selegline (Eldepryl) and rasagiline (Azilect)

SELECTIVE MAO-B INHIBITOR

GENERIC NAME: selegiline
TRADE NAME: Eldepryl, Zelapar (disintegrating tabs)
INDICATION: Parkinson's disease
ROUTE OF ADMINISTRATION: oral
COMMON ADULT DOSAGE: dosing for Eldepryl: 5 mg bid along with other anti-Parkinson agents such as levodopa/carbidopa (Sinemet); dosing for Zelapar: 1.25 mg once daily × 6 weeks, may increase dose to 2.5 mg/day
SIDE EFFECTS: dizziness, dry mouth, light-headedness, nausea, vivid dreams, stomach pain
AUXILIARY LABELS:

- ■ May cause dizziness or drowsiness.
- ■ Take with food at breakfast and lunch (Eldepryl).

NOTE: Zelapar is taken before breakfast and without liquid; patient should not take food or liquid for 5 min before or after taking Zelapar.

ANTICHOLINERGICS PROLONG THE EFFECTS OF DOPAMINE BY INHIBITING THE REUPTAKE MECHANISM

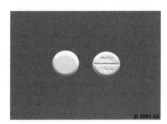

GENERIC NAME: benztropine
TRADE NAME: Cogentin
INDICATION: Parkinson's disease, normally used with other anti-Parkinson agents
ROUTE OF ADMINISTRATION: oral, injection
COMMON ADULT DOSAGE: oral dosages range from 0.5 to 6 mg per day, given once daily or bid, depending on dosage prescribed
AUXILIARY LABELS:
- May cause dizziness or drowsiness.
- Take with food.
- No alcohol.

GENERIC NAME: trihexyphenidyl
TRADE NAME: Artane
INDICATION: Parkinson's disease, normally used with other anti-Parkinson agents
ROUTE OF ADMINISTRATION: oral
COMMON ADULT DOSAGE: 2 to 5 mg bid to tid
AUXILIARY LABELS:
- May cause dizziness or drowsiness.
- Take with food.
- No alcohol.

DOPAMINE AGONISTS

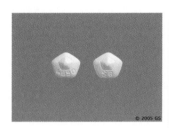

GENERIC NAME: pramipexole
TRADE NAME: Mirapex
INDICATION: Parkinson's disease; can be used with other anti-Parkinson agents; restless legs syndrome
ROUTE OF ADMINISTRATION: oral
COMMON ADULT DOSAGE: 2 to 5 mg bid to tid
SIDE EFFECTS: constipation, dizziness, drowsiness, abnormal dreams
AUXILIARY LABEL:
- May cause dizziness or drowsiness.

GENERIC NAME: ropinirole
TRADE NAME: Requip
DRUG ACTION: prolongs the effects of dopamine by inhibiting the reuptake mechanism
INDICATION: Parkinson's disease; can be used with other anti-Parkinson agents; restless legs syndrome
ROUTE OF ADMINISTRATION: oral
COMMON ADULT DOSAGE: start at 0.25 mg tid, raising each week by 0.25-mg increments to 1 mg tid
SIDE EFFECTS: constipation, dizziness, drowsiness, abnormal dreams
AUXILIARY LABEL:
- May cause dizziness or drowsiness.

Amyotrophic Lateral Sclerosis (ALS)

Amyotrophic lateral sclerosis (ALS) is a neurological condition resulting from degeneration *(trophic)* and hardening *(sclerosis)* of motor neurons in the spinal cord *(myo)*. Although this disease was first discovered in the mid-1800s, it is known in the United States as Lou Gehrig's disease, after the famous baseball player who contracted ALS. ALS is a progressive degeneration of the motor tract in the spinal cord. One theory is that it may be caused by the excitatory neurotransmitter glutamate at the synapse, leading to cell death. Although the motor functions of the body decrease, the mind is left unaffected. Those who suffer from this fatal disease describe it as being trapped inside a dying body. ALS occurs worldwide, affecting both men and women equally. The three classifications or types of ALS are as follows:

- Sporadic: This is the most common form in the United States, accounting for 90% to 95% of cases. The condition occurs randomly with no known etiology.
- Familial: This form of ALS may be associated with an inherited genetic mutation. It accounts for no more than 5% to 10% of cases in the United States.
- Guamanian: This form of ALS was named after an extremely high prevalence of ALS was observed in Guam and Trust Territories of the Pacific in the 1950s.

Symptoms vary widely and may include the following: twitching and cramping of the muscles (mostly in the hands and feet), loss of motor control in the hands and feet (resulting in tripping, falling, or dropping items), persistent fatigue, slurred speech, difficulty in projecting voice, and uncontrollable periods of laughing or crying. As the respiratory muscles become affected, dyspnea (shortness of breath) occurs followed by difficulty in swallowing and eventual paralysis and death.

Prognosis. There is no cure. The life expectancy is between 2 and 5 years from the time of diagnosis. Because the symptoms and their severity vary, there are many people who live beyond 5 years. Approximately 20% of people live longer than 5 years, and up to 10% live more than 10 years. Only 5% may live beyond 20 years. There are cases of persons with ALS where the symptoms have stopped progressing, and a small number of people experienced a reversal of the symptoms.

Non–Drug Treatment. In the early stages it is recommended to exercise (light aerobics) and stretch to maintain strength, reduce fatigue, and relieve depression. Changing dietary intake to foods that are softer and easier to swallow can help avoid choking. There are several products and devices to help persons with ALS, including neck collars to help support the head if/when the muscles become weak, braces, walkers or wheelchairs, shower seats, rails, ramps, and voice amplifiers.

Drug Treatment. Only riluzole has been developed specifically for treating ALS, and it only slows the progression of the disease by months. There are several agents being tested in clinical trials but at this time there are no other medications used to treat ALS. Other agents are used to treat various symptoms; these include muscle relaxants and antidepressants as well as medications to decrease excessive salivation.

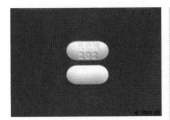

GENERIC NAME: riluzole
TRADE NAME: Rilutek
INDICATION: ALS
ROUTE OF ADMINISTRATION: oral
COMMON ADULT DOSAGE: 50 mg q12h
SIDE EFFECTS: nausea, dizziness, diarrhea, abdominal pain, cough, diarrhea, headache, loss of appetite; potential for liver damage.
AUXILIARY LABELS:
- Take on empty stomach 1 hr before meal or 2 hr after meal.
- Take medication at the same times daily.
- May cause dizziness or drowsiness.

Dystonia

This is a brain disorder that causes the nervous system to transmit improper signals to the muscles, resulting in involuntary muscle contractions and spasms. The movements can be very painful to the person and may involve a single muscle group or the entire body. Approximately 300,000 people in North America suffer from this neurological disorder. It affects all ages and both genders. Dystonias are believed to be related to an abnormality in the basal ganglia of the brain, where muscle contraction messages are processed. The neurotransmitters involved are gamma-aminobutyric acid (GABA), dopamine, acetylcholine, norepinephrine, and serotonin. Primary dystonia may be related to heredity with various patterns of gene expression. Secondary dystonia results from environmental or disease-related damage to the basal ganglia; this would include certain infections, reactions to certain drugs, trauma, stroke, exposure to heavy metals, or carbon monoxide poisoning. Approximately one half of all cases of dystonia are of unknown etiology and these cases are referred to as primary or idiopathic dystonia. Many people diagnosed with the primary type have inherited a genetic trait and a dominant gene may be passed onto offspring, who may show signs of the disease. However, the trigger is unknown and there is no cure at this time. The classifications or types of dystonia are based on the parts of the body they affect:

- Generalized dystonia: Affects most or all of the body
- Focal dystonia: Localized to a specific part of the body
- Multifocal dystonia: Two or more unrelated body parts are affected
- Segmental dystonia: Two or more adjacent body parts are affected
- Hemidystonia: Involves the arm and leg on the same side of the body

 Tech Note!

To date the best oral medication for treating generalized dystonia is tetrabenazine (TBZ), which is not available in the United States. TBZ can be obtained by prescription from Canada or the United Kingdom. TBZ is only approved for treating Huntington's disease in the United States.

Prognosis. Establishing a prognosis is very difficult because each person is different. However, if the disease presents during childhood, it seems to spread whereas in adulthood it may remain localized.

Non–Drug Treatment. Treatment ranges from surgery, to physical therapy, to deep brain stimulation. Relaxation and breathing techniques are also used as they may benefit the patient.

Drug Treatment. Agents used to treat dystonias include those that reduce the levels of acetylcholine, drugs that regulate GABA levels, and drugs that increase dopamine levels (dopamine agonists). There are some individuals who respond well to dopamine antagonists. Because of the varying effects of agents used, each person receives individualized medication treatment. Box 16-4 lists examples of these medications.

Tourette's Syndrome (TS)

Tourette's syndrome (TS) is a neurological disorder in the brain. Most often the disorder starts in children between the ages of 7 and 10 years. Symptoms include involuntary movements or vocal noises called tics. These tics may materialize as jerking motions that may involve the whole body and include kicking or stomping, blinking the eyes, or vocal sounds that range from clearing the throat to shouting and barking. Other symptoms include repetitive thoughts and compulsions. Sufferers can even cause self-inflicted damage by hitting or punching themselves. The vocalization of obscenities is referred to as coprolalia and obscene gestures are called copropraxia, both of which are not common with tic disorders. Symptoms vary widely and range from very mild to severe although most cases are mild. Effects may worsen with excite-

BOX 16-4 MEDICATIONS USED TO TREAT DYSTONIA

Agents That Reduce Levels of Acetylcholine
Artane (trihexyphenidyl)
Cogentin (benztropine)

Dopamine-Stimulating Agents
Sinemet (levodopa/carbidopa)
Parlodel (bromocriptine)
Mirapex (pramipexole)
Requip (ropinirole)
Permax (pergolide)
Mirapex (pramipexole)

Agents That Regulate GABA
Valium (diazepam)
Klonopin (clonazepam)
Ativan (lorazepam)
Lioresal (baclofen)

Miscellaneous Agents Used for the Following Symptoms:
Insomnia
Benadryl (diphenhydramine)
Lunesta (eszopiclone)
Ambien (zolpidem)

Spasms
Dilantin (phenytoin)
Depakote (divalproex sodium)
Myobloc (RimabotulinumtoxinB, formerly known as *Botulinum* toxin type B)
Flexeril (cyclobenzaprine)
Soma (carisoprodol)
Skelaxin (metaxalone)

Pain
Duragesic (fentanyl patches)

ment or anxiety. Specific causes of this syndrome are not known although it is believed to be a disorder in genes that control neurotransmitters in the brain. TS occurs in all ethnic groups and affects males 3 to 4 times more often than females.

Prognosis. There is no cure for TS although symptoms may decrease with aging. People do live a normal life span but may have to take medications for life.

Non–Drug Treatment. Currently there are no treatments available that can eliminate TS although relaxation techniques and/or biofeedback have been known to alleviate stress, which can trigger tics especially in mild cases. The only course of treatment is with medications. Education and tolerance of TS is also important for the person suffering from TS as well as for the public.

Drug Treatment. No medication will eliminate tics completely although there are a few agents that may lessen motor tics. Long-term use of certain neuroleptic agents may cause tardive dyskinesia. This causes involuntary movements,

TABLE 16-11 **Medications Used for Treatment of Tourette's Tics**

Generic Name	Brand Name	Most Common Adult Dosage	Side Effects
clonazepam	Klonopin	0.5-3 mg	Fatigue, irritability, dizziness, disinhibition
clonidine	Catapres patch or Catapres tablet	TTS-1 to TTS-3 (patch) or 0.1 mg (tablet)	Localized skin rash
fluphenazine	Prolixin	0.5-6 mg	Fatigue, weight gain, muscle rigidity, depression, photosensitivity, motor tardive dyskinesia
guanfacine	Tenex	0.5-3 mg	Fatigue, irritability, hypotension, sleep disturbance
haloperidol	Haldol	1-5 mg daily	Fatigue, weight gain, muscle rigidity, depression, photosensitivity, motor tardive dyskinesia
pimozide	Orap	1-10 mg	Fatigue, weight gain, muscle rigidity, depression, photosensitivity, motor tardive dyskinesia

drooling, tremor, and a flaccid face. If the medication is stopped, the symptoms disappear. Drugs that may be prescribed are listed in Table 16-11.

BUTYROPHENONE

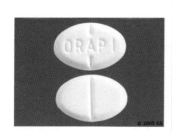

GENERIC NAME: pimozide
TRADE NAME: Orap
INDICATION: Tourette's syndrome; psychosis
ROUTE OF ADMINISTRATION: oral
COMMON ADULT DOSAGE: 1 to 2 mg once daily
SIDE EFFECTS: dizziness, drowsiness, insomnia, nausea, vomiting, diarrhea, constipation, dry mouth, blurred vision
AUXILIARY LABELS:
- Avoid grapefruit juice.
- May cause dizziness or drowsiness.
- Do not take with TCAs.
- Take with a full glass of water.

Miscellaneous Muscle Agents

When patients are taken into the OR (operating room) for surgery, these agents are used to cause relaxation of the muscles and to induce paralysis.

NEUROMUSCULAR BLOCKERS

Neuromuscular blocking agents are used with anesthetics when a patient is having surgery. Neuromuscular blockers relax skeletal muscles and induce paralysis. They are used to help place the patient on a ventilator and to suppress the patient's spontaneous breathing once a ventilator is in place. These agents can be divided into two major categories: depolarizing and nondepolarizing neuromuscular blockers. Depolarizing agents mimic the effects of the neurotransmitter acetylcholine (Ach); they block the membranes surrounding the neuromuscular junction, making it unresponsive to normal Ach-receptor interaction. Nondepolarizing agents bind to receptors and prevent transmission of impulses through the Ach neurotransmitters. Each type of neuromuscular blocker is used, depending on the length of anesthesia. Box 16-5 lists the names

BOX 16-5 CLASSIFICATION OF NEUROMUSCULAR BLOCKERS

Short-Acting (Effective 20-26 min)
mivacurium (Mivacron)
rocuronium (Zemuron)
succinylcholine (Anectine)

Intermediate-Acting
atracurium (Tracrium)
cisatracurium (Nimbex)
pancuronium (Pavulon)
vecuronium (Norcuron)

Long-Acting (Effective 75-100 min)
doxacurium (Neuro-Max)
pipecuronium (Arduan)

BOX 16-6 MEDICATIONS USED FOR CONSCIOUS SEDATION

Possible Combinations for Adults
- Ketamine, atropine (or glycopyrrolate), and benzodiazepine (e.g., midazolam). Ketamine works well for sedation in patients with asthma because it does not cause airway hyperreactivity
- Benzodiazepines (e.g., midazolam) and analgesic (common for short outpatient procedures, such as endoscopy)
- Systemic anesthetics (propofol or etomidate) and analgesic

Possible Combinations for Children
- Ketamine, atropine, and benzodiazepine (works best for children younger than 11 yr)
- Ketamine and benzodiazepine (may be used for children older than 11 yr)

of neuromuscular blockers and classifies them as short-acting, intermediate-acting, or long-acting. The action of the blocking agent can be prolonged with additional smaller dosages. Technicians may be responsible for filling floor stock orders for the OR with these medications.

CONSCIOUS SEDATION

Many hospitals prepare "conscious sedation packs" composed of various medications. Conscious sedation is a clinical technique that is used for various procedures such as colonoscopy and endoscopy that can cause anxiety and/or pain. The patient is put into a state of sedation, relaxation, and amnesia. There are three primary classes of drugs used: sedatives, analgesics, and miscellaneous anesthetics. The patient should be NPO (nothing by mouth) for at least 4 to 6 hours before the procedure if possible. Rarely is there a need to reverse the effects of the agents as they are titrated; however, if reversal is needed antidotes can be administered. For example, naloxone (Narcan) can be used to reverse the effects of narcotic analgesics. The pharmacy technician is responsible for preparing, delivering, and refilling these packs. Box 16-6 lists examples of the medications used for conscious sedation.

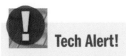

Tech Alert!

Remember the following sound-alike/look-alike drugs:

dopamine versus dobutamine
levodopa versus methyldopa
clonazepam, lorazepam, and clorazepate
esmolol versus Osmitrol
Trandate versus Tridrate

DO YOU REMEMBER THESE KEY POINTS?

- Generic and trade names of drugs discussed in this chapter
- The divisions of the nervous system and its branches
- The major divisions of the brain discussed in this chapter and their primary functions
- Conditions in which the sympathetic or parasympathetic systems are stimulated
- Medications that directly affect the sympathetic or parasympathetic system
- The composition of a neuron
- The anatomy of the ganglionic neuronal system with respect to the CNS
- The importance of the blood-brain barrier with respect to medications
- The major classifications of medications used on the sympathetic system and their side effects
- The major classifications of medications used on the parasympathetic system and their side effects
- Major conditions that affect the CNS
- Commonly used medications to treat conditions covered in this chapter
- Prognosis and non–drug treatments for the conditions covered
- Major functions of the blood-brain barrier
- Commonly used nervous system medical abbreviations

REVIEW QUESTIONS

Multiple choice questions

1. Cholinergic agents are stimulants of which system?
A. Nervous system
B. Sympathetic system
C. Parasympathetic system
D. None of the above

2. Afferent and efferent fibers have the function of:
A. Relaying messages to and from the central nervous system
B. Running the central nervous system
C. Stimulation
D. Inhibiting neuronal impulse transfers

3. Neurons are made of the following components EXCEPT:
A. Dendrites
B. Cell body
C. Nerve terminals
D. Amino acids

4. The area where a neurotransmitter crosses over to another neuron is called:
A. The nerve ending
B. The axon
C. The cell body
D. The synapse

5. All of the following are neurotransmitters EXCEPT:
A. Dopamine
B. Norepinephrine
C. Serotonin
D. Succinylcholine

6. Which of the following drugs is not used as a smooth muscle relaxant?
A. Baclofen
B. Cyclobenzaprine
C. Cerebyx
D. Soma

7. Which of the following system activities is NOT increased during a sympathetic response?
A. Digestive system
B. Heart
C. Lung
D. Liver

8. The part of the brain that controls memory, reason, and language skills is the:
A. Medulla oblongata
B. Cerebellum
C. Cerebrum
D. Brainstem

9. The area of the brain that controls breathing and cardiac functions is the:
A. Medulla oblongata
B. Right hemisphere
C. Left hemisphere
D. Thoracic spinal cord

10. The hypothalamus functions as the _____ of the body.
A. Thermostat
B. Appetite relay center
C. Memory
D. Both A and B

11. Which of the following medications used for Parkinson's disease can pass the blood-brain barrier?
A. Dopamine
B. Levodopa
C. Carbidopa
D. Both A and B

12. Which of the statements describing dopamine is inaccurate?
A. Dopamine is a naturally occurring substance within the body.
B. Dopamine allows for smooth movements of the muscle system.
C. Dopamine can be injected to replace low levels within the basal ganglia.
D. Dopamine is a precursor to norepinephrine.

13. Which of the following classes of drugs is used most often for epileptic seizures?
A. Barbiturates
B. Benzodiazepines
C. Hydantoins
D. All of the above may be used

14. Which of the types of seizures listed is typically caused by NOT taking medications?
A. Tonic-clonic
B. Absence seizures
C. Atonic type seizures
D. None of the above

15. The most common reason neuromuscular blocking agents are used is to:
A. Keep the patient asleep during an operation
B. Keep the patient from fighting a respirator (ventilator)
C. Stop all pain and movement while the patient is being intubated
D. Both B and C

16. _____ is converted into norepinephrine within the _____ system.
A. Acetylcholine, sympathetic
B. Epinephrine, sympathetic
C. Acetylcholine, parasympathetic
D. Dopamine, central nervous system

17. Which of the following statements is NOT true concerning the sympathetic system?
A. When activated, glucose is released from the liver.
B. All parasympathetic system functions stop.
C. It is responsible for the fight-or-flight reaction.
D. Drugs that activate this system are called cholinergics.

18. Of the components listed, which one is NOT housed in the brainstem?
A. Hypothalamus and thalamus
B. Pons
C. Midbrain
D. Medulla oblongata

19. The name of the enzyme that is responsible for destroying norepinephrine is:
A. Anticholinergic
B. Antiadrenergic
C. Acetylcholine
D. Acetylcholinesterase

20. _____ affect the sympathetic system, whereas _____ affect the parasympathetic system.
A. Cholinergics, anticholinergics
B. Cholinergics, adrenergics
C. Adrenergics, antiadrenergics
D. Adrenergics, cholinergics

True/False

If a statement is false, then change it to make it true.

_____ **1.** Gray matter makes up the brain, and white matter makes up the spinal cord.

_____ **2.** Homeostasis is when the body is in a sympathetic response mode.

_____ **3.** The peripheral nervous system can be divided into two divisions.

_____ **4.** The thalamus and hypothalamus link the nervous system to the endocrine system.

_____ **5.** The blood-brain barrier serves to prevent large molecules (such as toxins) from passing into the central nervous system.

_____ **6.** Carbidopa is an ingredient added to Sinemet to extend the life of the drug.

_____ **7.** Amyotrophic lateral sclerosis is a degenerative disease of the motor cells of the central nervous system that affects the myelin sheaths surrounding the neuronal axon.

_____ **8.** Tonic seizures involve stiffening of the muscles, whereas clonic is rapid jerking.

_____ **9.** Neuromuscular blocking agents block pain perception and muscle movement.

_____ **10.** Drugs that mimic the cholinergic neurotransmitters of the sympathetic system also are called sympathomimetics.

_____ **11.** Strokes occur equally in all racial and gender groups regardless of age.

_____ **12.** Various medications used as prophylactic treatment for migraine sufferers include calcium channel blockers and beta blockers.

_____ **13.** Mirapex and Parlodel are dopamine-stimulating agents used in dystonia.

_____ **14.** Conscious sedation medications include analgesics to decrease pain.

_____ **15.** The blood-brain barrier keeps all chemicals from entering the brain.

_____ **16.** The limbic system is composed of the hypothalamus, hippocampus, amygdala, and septal area.

_____ **17.** The nerve that controls hearing is the trochlear nerve.

_____ **18.** Medications used to treat migraines include triptans, NSAIDs, ergotamines, and pain relievers.

_____ **19.** Cholenergics have the side effect of causing dry mouth.

_____ **20.** If a person experiences a CVA this means the person had a stroke.

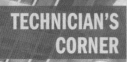

TECHNICIAN'S CORNER   Mr. Perkins was recently diagnosed with Parkinson's disease. He arrives at the pharmacy with a new prescription for Sinemat. What auxiliary labels are necessary?

BIBLIOGRAPHY

American Medical Association: *Concise medical encyclopedia*. 2006. Martin S, Lipsky MD, medical editor. Referenced 10/09

Applegate E: *The anatomy and physiology learning system*, ed 3, Philadelphia, 2006, Elsevier Health Services.

Drug facts and comparisons, ed 63, St Louis, 2008, Lippincott Williams & Wilkins.

McCuistion L, Gutierrez K: *Real-world nursing survival guide: pharmacology*, ed 1, Philadelphia, 2002, WB Saunders.

Potter P, Perry A: *Fundamentals of nursing*, ed 6, St Louis, 2004, Mosby.

Professional guide to diseases, ed 9, 2009, Lippincott. Referenced 10/09.

Thibodeau G, Patton K: *Structure and function of the body*, ed 13, St Louis, 2007, Mosby.

WEBSITES REFERENCED

Palsy B: www.bellspalsy.ws/. Referenced 09/10

Palsy B: www.ninds.nih.gov/disorders/disorder_index.htm. Referenced 09/10

Conscious Sedation. http://apps.med.buffalo.edu/procedures/conscioussedation.asp?p=8. Referenced 10/09

Dystonia. www.ninds.nih.gov/disorders/dystonias/detail_dystonias.htm Referenced 10/09

Migraines. www.migraineresearchfoundation.org/treatment.html. Referenced 10/09

Neuromuscular blocking agents. www.healthline.com/galecontent/neuromuscular-blockers

Stages of Alzheimer's. www.alz.org. Referenced 10/09

Stroke. www.stroke.org. Referenced 10/09

Tourette medications. www.tsa-usa.org/Medical/images/medications_and_tourettes_berlin.pdf. Referenced 10/09

Tourette Syndrome. www.tsa-usa.org/Medical/whatists.html. Referenced 10/09

Treatment of Dystonia. www.care4dystonia.org. Referenced 9/09

Psychopharmacology

Objectives

UPON COMPLETING THIS CHAPTER, YOU SHOULD BE ABLE TO DO THE FOLLOWING:

- List the major medications used for each of the conditions described in this chapter.

- List the most common side effects of each of the drugs discussed.

- Describe the main emotional conditions affecting the brain.

- Differentiate between clinical depression (major depressive disorder) and nonclinical depression (temporary sadness).

- List the types of insomnia that can occur and their possible causes.

- Differentiate between older and newer treatments for the mentally disabled.

- Distinguish the capabilities of a psychologist versus a psychiatrist.

- List the differences between the uses of monoamine oxidase inhibitors (MAOIs), tricyclic antidepressants (TCAs), and selective serotonin reuptake inhibitors (SSRIs).

- Describe attention deficit/hyperactivity disorder (ADHD) symptoms and treatments.

- Describe the types of non–drug therapy available for patients suffering from various mental disorders.

TERMS AND DEFINITIONS

Attention deficit/hyperactivity disorder (ADHD) *A physiological brain disorder that affects the ability to engage in quiet, passive activities or to focus one's attention; attributable to an imbalance of neurotransmitters in the brain*

Blood-brain barrier (BBB) *Special characteristics of capillaries that supply the brain cells act as a barrier to prevent certain solutes or chemicals from moving to the brain from the blood*

Cognition *Activities associated with thinking, learning, and memory*

Depression *A mental state characterized by sadness, feelings of loss and grief, and loss of appetite and that may include suicidal thoughts*

Electroconvulsive therapy *Also known as shock therapy; a carefully calibrated electrical current is administered to the anesthetized patient, causing a brief seizure that can relieve certain symptoms, such as depression*

Extrapyramidal symptoms *Often result from taking antipsychotic medications and include parkinsonism, dystonia, and tremors*

Insomnia *Difficulty falling or staying asleep*

Mania *A mood state characterized by excessive excitement, elevated mood, and exalted feelings; most often associated with bipolar disorder, where episodes of mania alternate (or cycle) with episodes of depression*

Neurosis *Mental disorder arising from stress or anxiety in the patient's environment without loss of contact with reality; phobias can be listed in this category; behavior usually does not fall out of social norms*

Neurotransmitter *Chemicals that are transmitted from one neuron to another as electrical nerve impulses that can also affect behavior*

Phobias *A continuous irrational fear of a thing, place, or situation that causes significant distress*

Psychosis *A mental illness characterized by loss of contact with reality; psychosis may be a true mental illness, or due to an underlying medical condition (e.g., dementia, drug withdrawal syndromes), or induced by substances such as medications, recreational drugs, or poisons*

Psychotherapy *Professional therapy that includes helping the patient work through personal problems that affect emotions and behaviors*

Schizophrenia *A group of mental disorders characterized by inappropriate emotions and unrealistic thinking*

Tardive dyskinesia *A type of dyskinesia (unwanted, involuntary rhythmic movements) attributed as potential side effects of taking dopamine antagonists such as phenothiazines or other medications (e.g., metoclopramide); the symptoms may continue even after discontinuation of the offending drug*

COMMON DRUGS USED FOR PSYCHOTHERAPEUTIC CONDITIONS

Trade Name	Generic Name	Pronunciation	Trade Name	Generic Name	Pronunciation
Agents for Psychosis and Bipolar Disorder			Seroquel	quetiapine	(kwe-**tye**-a-peen)
Atypical Antipsychotics			Zyprexa	olanzapine	(oh-lan-**zah**-peen)
Abilify	aripiprazole	(**ar**-i-**pip**-ra-zole)			
Clozaril, FazaClo	clozapine	(**kloe**-za-peen)	**Phenothiazine Antipsychotics**		
Fanapt	iloperidone	(**eye**-low-**per**-i-done)	Mellaril	thioridazine	(thy-oh-**rid**-ah-zeen)
Geodon	ziprasidone	(zi-**praz**-ih-dohn)	Prolixin	fluphenazine	(flew-**fen**-ah-zeen)
Invega	paliperidone	(**pal**-ee-**per**-i-done)	Serentil	mesoridazine	(meh-zoe-**rih**-da-zeen)
Risperdal	risperidone	(ris-**per**-ih-done)	Stelazine	trifluoperazine	(try-flew-**per**-ah-zeen)

Continued

COMMON DRUGS USED FOR PSYCHOTHERAPEUTIC CONDITIONS—cont'd

Trade Name	Generic Name	Pronunciation
Thorazine	chlorpromazine	(klor-**pro**-ma-zeen)
Trilafon	perphenazine	(per-**fen**-ah-zeen)

Tricyclic Antipsychotic

Loxitane	loxapine	(lock-**sah**-peen)

Antimanic

Eskalith	lithium	(**lith**-e-um)

Miscellaneous Antipsychotic Agents

Haldol	haloperidol	(**hal**-oh-**pear**-i-dol)
Navane	thiothixene	(**thye**-oh-**thick**-seen)
Orap	pimozide	(**pi**-moe-zyde)

Antidepressant Agents
Tricyclic Antidepressants (TCAs) and Related Agents

Anafranil	clomipramine	(klo-**mip**-ra-meen)
Asendin	amoxapine	(ah-**mox**-ah-peen)
Elavil	amitriptyline	(am-eh-**trip**-tah-leen)
Norpramin	desipramine	(des-**ip**-rah-meen)
Sinequan	doxepin	(**dox**-seh-pin)
Pamelor	nortriptyline	(nor-**trip**-tah-leen)
Tofranil	imipramine	(ih-**mip**-rah-meen)

Selective Serotonin Reuptake Inhibitors (SSRIs)

Celexa	citalopram	(si-**tal**-o-pram)
Lexapro	escitalopram	(**es**-sye-**tal**-oh-pram)
Luvox	fluvoxamine	(floo-**vox**-a-meen)
Paxil, Pexeva	paroxetine	(pa-**rox**-a-teen)
Prozac	fluoxetine	(flew-**ox**-eh-teen)
Zoloft	sertraline	(**sir**-tra-leen)

Selective Serotonin and Norepinephrine Reuptake Inhibitors (SSNRIs)

Cymbalta	duloxetine	(du-**lox**-uh-teen)
Effexor	venlafaxine	(**ven**-la-fax-een)
Pristiq	desvenlafaxine	(des-**ven**-la-**fax**-een)

Heterocyclic and Miscellaneous Antidepressants

Desyrel	trazodone	(trah-**zoe**-doan)
Remeron	mirtazapine	(mer-**taz**-ah-peen)
Wellbutrin	bupropion	(bew-**pro**-pe-on)

Monoamine Oxidase Inhibitors (MAOIs)

Trade Name	Generic Name	Pronunciation
Marplan	isocarboxazid	(eye-so-kar-**box**-a-zid)
Nardil	phenelizine	(fen-el-**zeen**)
Parnate	tranylcypromine	(tran-ill-**sip**-roe-meen)

Antianxiety Agents
Benzodiazepines for Anxiety

Ativan	lorazepam	(lor-**aze**-pam)
Serax	oxazepam	(ox-**aze**-pam)
Tranxene	clorazepate	(klor-**aze**-eh-pate)
Valium	diazepam	(dye-**aze**-eh-pam)
Xanax	alprazolam	(al-pra-**zoe**-lam)
Librium	chlordiazepoxide	(klor-**dye**-az-eh-**pox**-ide)

Miscellaneous Antianxiety Agents

BuSpar	buspirone	(byoo-**spye**-rone)
Equanil	meprobamate	(meh-pro-**bah**-mate)
Atarax	hydroxyzine HCl	(high-**drox**-ee-zeen)

Hypnotic Agents
Non-Benzodiazepine Hypnotics

Ambien	zolpidem	(zole-**pi**-dem)
Lunesta	eszopiclone	(e-zoe-**pik**-lone)
Rozerem	ramelteon	(ra-**mel**-tee-on)
Sonata	zaleplon	(**zal**-e-plon)

Benzodiazepine Hypnotics

Dalmane	flurazepam	(flure-**az**-e-pam)
Halcion	triazolam	(try-**az**-oh-lam)
Restoril	temazepam	(tem-**az**-e-pam)

ADD/ADHD Medications
Stimulants for ADD/ADHD

Adderall	amphetamine/ dextroamphetamine	(am-**fet**-a-meen/**dex**-troe-am-**fet**-a-meen)
Dexedrine	dextroamphentamine	(dex-troe-am-**fet**-a-meen)
Focalin	dexmethylphenidate	(dex-meth-il-**fen**-i-date)
Ritalin	methylphenidate	(meth-il-**fen**-i-date)
Vyvanse	lisdexamfetamine	(lis-**dex**-am-**fet**-a-meen)

SNRI for ADD/ADHD

Strattera	atomoxetine	(**a**-toe-**mox**-e-teen)

PSYCHOPHARMACOLOGY TERMINOLOGY

Word Combinations

Claustr/o	Barrier
Agor/a	Marketplace
Acr/o	Top
Pyr/o	Fire
Trichotill/o	Related to hair
Anxi/o	Anxiety
Somn	Sleep

PSYCHOPHARMACOLOGY TERMINOLOGY—cont'd

Suffixes

-mania	Madness
-lytic	To destroy
-ia	Abnormal condition
-lepsy	Seizure

Conditions

Anxiety	Feelings of apprehension, dread, and fear, with characteristics including tension, restlessness, tachycardia, dyspnea, and a sense of hopelessness
Attention deficit disorder (ADD)	Essentially a subtype of ADHD in which the patient is largely inattentive and has difficulty concentrating and completing tasks, without major components of motor restlessness or impulsivity found with hyperactive-impulsive subtype
Attention deficit/ hyperactivity disorder (ADHD)	A neurobehavioral disorder similar to ADD with the added symptom of motor hyperactivity and often impulsivity that is inappropriate to the level of the patient's age and development
Bipolar disorder	Characterized by alternating episodes of depression and mania or by episodes of depression alternating with mild excitement; formerly known as manic-depressive
Dementia	A slow progressive decrease in mental abilities marked by confusion and memory loss, beyond what is expected with the natural aging process
Depression	A mental state characterized by sadness, feelings of loss and grief, and loss of appetite and that may include suicidal thoughts
Insomnia	A symptom of a sleep disorder where there is difficulty falling or staying asleep
Psychosis	A mental illness characterized by loss of contact with reality; psychosis may be a true mental illness, or caused by an underlying medical condition (e.g., dementia, drug withdrawal syndromes), or induced by substances such as medications, recreational drugs, or poisons
Schizophrenia	A group of mental disorders characterized by inappropriate emotions and unrealistic thinking

OVER THE COURSE OF HISTORY, one of the most difficult studies of medicine has been the study of the brain because of its complexities—specifically, what makes individuals behave the way they do? Historically, a person suffering from mental illness who did not "fit" into "normal" society easily could have been institutionalized for life. Families would try to forget or hide their knowledge of a mentally ill relative. Electric shocks, straitjackets, isolation, and even physical punishment were traditional treatments. Few medications were available to help treat a mental disease. Most early medications treated the illness by sedating the patient so that he or she could not "act out." It was not until the 1950s that advancements were made in psychopharmacology.

Many different specialists are trained in the study of human emotions, feelings, and behavior, such as psychiatrists, psychologists, and counselors. Psychiatrists are medical doctors who have completed a residency in the field of psychiatry. A psychologist has a doctoral degree in psychology. Unlike psychiatrists, psychologists generally cannot write prescriptions (unless they meet specific state requirements), but they are trained extensively in the treatment of

TABLE 17-1 Types of Mental Disorders

Medical Term	Treatments	Medication Treatment if Applicable
Bipolar disorder	Medication and psychosocial treatments	Mood stabilizers
Depression	Psychotherapy, medications	Antidepressants
OCD	Psychotherapies and medications	Antidepressant (Clomipramine SSRI)
Phobias and panic attacks	Cognitive therapy, exposure therapy, and/or medication	Benzodiazepines, antidepressants
PTSD	Cognitive therapy, exposure therapy, and/or medication	Benzodiazepine antidepressant
Schizophrenia	Medication and psychosocial treatments	Antipsychotics

TABLE 17-2 Mental Health Websites

Website	Information	Other Attributes
www.mentalhelp.net	Free newsletter	Twitter interactive
www.nimh.nih.gov	Free newsletter	Really Simple Syndication for updates
http://mentalhealth.samhsa.gov	Free website information, e-mail updates	Free phone staff to answer questions, web chat, web cast
www.who.int/mental_health/en/	Free website information	RSS updates, information on statistics worldwide
http://learntobehealthy.org	Must be a member (membership is free); information and activities for kids and families	Concepts, lesson plans, web quests

mental illness through counseling. There are certain states that are considering allowing psychologists to prescribe certain medications under the approval of a physician. In addition to psychiatrists and psychologists, other professionals are available to counsel individuals with emotional problems, such as family counselors and clergy. For many persons, this type of therapy may be adequate for help through difficult times. A person suffering from a severe emotional, behavioral, or biological instability may need to be seen by a psychiatrist for proper diagnosis and treatment (Table 17-1). Depending on the diagnosis, a patient also may need to see a neurologist, a specialist of the nervous system. Many mental illnesses are caused by physiological disturbances within the nervous system (such as twitching) or by medical or physical conditions (such as emotional problems stemming from a brain tumor). According to the National Institute of Mental Health, approximately 57.7 million people, or more than 26% of the U.S. population, suffer from some type of mental disorder. Mental illness is the leading cause of disability in the United States and Canada. A list of mental health websites is found in Table 17-2.

Emotional Health

To evaluate a person's emotional health, a physician must evaluate the central nervous system (CNS) in addition to a person's social behaviors and the physical environment in which a person lives. The CNS can be divided into two main divisions—autonomic and somatic. The autonomic system works without conscious control, whereas the somatic system is under conscious control (see Chapter 16). The nervous system is an intricate network of chemical reactions that causes specific responses when activated. If any chemicals within the nervous system are imbalanced or cease to function normally, symptoms can appear as inappropriate behavior.

Psychiatric Disorders

Several different types of psychiatric disorders affect the brain. Most of these are due to a chemical imbalance of certain **neurotransmitters** (chemicals) such as serotonin and dopamine. It is not easy to diagnose or treat most psychiatric disorders because several conditions have similar or overlapping symptoms. Examples of psychological disorders will be discussed followed by the prognosis (future of the condition). Treatments (non–drug) and/or therapies are discussed first in this chapter followed by explanations of psychiatric conditions and the medications that are usually administered in their treatment.

NON–DRUG TREATMENTS

Because of the wide range of mental health conditions that exist, many alternative non–drug treatments are available. In the case of conditions that involve addictions or behavior disorders, many group therapies are available through nonprofit groups, such as Alcoholics Anonymous. Groups give patients a safe place to speak freely and without guilt. Another option is to participate in group therapy under the direction of a licensed professional (e.g., psychiatrist, psychologist, or counselor); in many cases, these forms of treatment are covered under medical insurance plans. For conditions that affect the whole family or a child, many family counselors specialize in group therapy within the family unit. Individualized counseling is an option available for more serious conditions or for patients who are uncomfortable speaking in the presence of a group. Cognitive therapy involves learning how to change present thinking, modify certain types of behavior, and improve communication skills. For persons who are suffering from severe crises, psychiatrists may prescribe medications or additional therapy. A once unconventional treatment, **electroconvulsive therapy** (i.e., shock therapy or ECT) has reemerged as a possible treatment for the relief of certain psychological conditions such as schizophrenia, mania, and severe depression. Through new medical advancements, this treatment is more precise and carefully monitored than in the past. ECT is only used when other options have been exhausted. Side effects can include memory loss, confusion, nausea/vomiting, and pain in the head, jaw, and muscles. Most side effects are temporary and symptoms such as nausea or headache can be treated with medications.

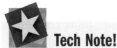

Tech Note!

Pharmacy technicians have knowledge of classifications of drugs as well as personal patient information. It is important to remember that all medical information should be kept private. If patient confidentiality is broken, the consequences possibly can be devastating to the patient. Patients' medications and conditions should never be discussed.

GENERAL PSYCHIATRIC DISORDERS

Depression

Everyone is depressed at one time or another during his or her lifetime. Most persons who experience **depression** do not seek medical help and recover within a short period. However, for those persons in whom the depression does not subside within a few weeks, professional attention may be necessary. This depressive state can range from prolonged feelings of extreme sadness to thoughts of suicide. Patients with manic-depressive disorder (also known as bipolar disorder) fluctuate between the two extremes of mania and depression. Other types of depression include postpartum depression (after pregnancy), seasonal affective disorder (SAD) (depression during winter months), and major depression. Major depression is the most common type of depression; the condition interferes with a person's ability to function normally; activities such as sleeping, eating, working, studying, and forms of enjoyment are disrupted. Many times this type of depression is associated with a serious illness or anxiety disorder. There is no known cause of depression. However, magnetic resonance imaging (MRI) has shown that certain areas in the brain of a depressed person appear different than those in a normal, nondepressed person's brain. These areas include those responsible for mood, thinking, sleeping, appetite, and behavior. Age, gender, and concurrent medical or psychological conditions all affect the way persons experience depression. For more information on depression visit www.nimh.nih.gov.

Medications used in the treatment of depression increase the levels of epinephrine and norepinephrine and serotonin in the bloodstream. Under normal circumstances, these neurotransmitters stimulate the brain as they are released and are then reabsorbed by the brain cells, where they are broken down by an enzyme called monoamine oxidase (MAO). When the levels of certain neurotransmitters are low, the brain is not stimulated. There are several agents used to treat depression that affect specific neurotransmitters.

Prognosis. Depression can be treated effectively in most cases using psychotherapy and/or antidepressant medications. Both short-term and long-term treatment options are available.

Non–Drug Treatment. Psychotherapy can help for short- or long-term depression. Interpersonal therapy (IPT) helps people learn how to deal with personal relationships that may be associated with their depression. Other forms of treatment include behavioral and **cognitive** therapy. Electroconvulsive therapy is an option for severe cases of ongoing depression that is not relieved by medications or traditional therapy sessions. For seasonal depression, light treatment may help to alleviate symptoms.

Drug Treatments. Agents that are commonly used to treat depression include selective serotonin reuptake inhibitors (SSRIs), serotonin norepinephrine reuptake inhibitors (SNRIs), tricyclic antidepressants (TCAs), and monoamine oxidase inhibitors (MAOIs). These agents help to increase the levels of two neurotransmitters: norepinephrine and serotonin. However, each type of agent accomplishes the relief of depression by a different drug action. Each method of action is discussed below under each agent.

Antidepressants

Selective Serotonin Reuptake Inhibitors. SSRIs specifically act to keep higher levels of serotonin in the brain. When serotonin level is increased, mood is elevated. Because SSRIs only block serotonin reuptake, these agents work differently than MAOIs and TCAs. Because SSRIs have a more selective mode of action, they are often preferable to treat depression and obsessive-compulsive disorders. The doses that follow are the maximum doses. Patients may be started at a lower dose initially, and the dose may be increased gradually to the maximum dosage. An important note is that patients cannot take MAOIs and SSRIs concurrently. There have been reports of death caused by this dangerous combination. Typically, these medications can take up to 6 weeks to achieve their full effectiveness.

SELECTIVE SEROTONIN REUPTAKE INHIBITORS (SSRIs)

GENERIC NAME: citalopram
TRADE NAME: Celexa
INDICATION: antidepressant
ROUTE OF ADMINISTRATION: oral
COMMON ADULT DOSAGE: oral, 20 mg, 40 mg, or 60 mg once daily
SIDE EFFECTS: insomnia, nausea, dizziness, drowsiness, sexual dysfunction, headache, constipation, dry mouth, and anorexia
AUXILIARY LABEL:
■ May cause dizziness and drowsiness.

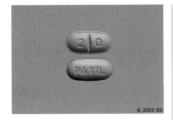

GENERIC NAME: paroxetine
TRADE NAME: Paxil, Paxil CR
INDICATION: depression, obsessive-compulsive disorder, panic disorder, PTSD
ROUTE OF ADMINISTRATION: oral
COMMON ADULT DOSAGE: depression, 20 mg once daily or Paxil CR 25 mg once daily; obsessive-compulsive disorder, 40 mg once daily
SIDE EFFECTS: insomnia, nausea, dizziness, drowsiness, sexual dysfunction, headache, constipation, dry mouth, and anorexia
AUXILIARY LABELS:
- Take with food.
- Do not drink alcohol.

GENERIC NAME: fluoxetine
TRADE NAME: Prozac, Prozac weekly, Sarafem
INDICATION: depression, obsessive-compulsive disorder, panic disorder, bulimia, premenstrual dysphoria (Sarafem)
ROUTE OF ADMINISTRATION: oral
COMMON ADULT DOSAGE: 60 mg once daily maximum; usually 10 to 20 mg daily; Prozac weekly contains 90 mg of medication to be taken once a week
SIDE EFFECTS: insomnia, nausea, dizziness, drowsiness, sexual dysfunction, headache, constipation, dry mouth, and anorexia
AUXILIARY LABELS:
- Take with food.
- Do not drink alcohol.

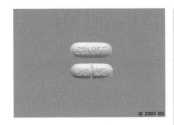

GENERIC NAME: sertraline
TRADE NAME: Zoloft
INDICATION: depression, obsessive-compulsive disorder, panic disorder, PTSD, social anxiety disorder
ROUTE OF ADMINISTRATION: oral
COMMON ADULT DOSAGE: 50 mg once daily up to 200 mg once daily
SIDE EFFECTS: insomnia, nausea, dizziness, drowsiness, sexual dysfunction, headache, constipation, dry mouth, and anorexia
AUXILIARY LABEL:
- Do not drink alcohol.

Serotonin Norepinephrine Reuptake Inhibitors. These antidepressants work on two neurotransmitters at the same time, serotonin and norepinephrine. They increase the levels of both neurotransmitters by inhibiting their reabsorption (reuptake) into the brain cells. The elevation of these chemicals affects the mood of the patient. SNRIs are also referred to as dual uptake inhibitors, and, along with psychotherapy, these agents may be the first treatment choice in treating moderate to severe depression.

SEROTONIN NOREPINEPHRINE REUPTAKE INHIBITORS (SNRIs)

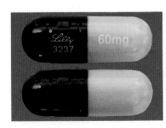

GENERIC NAME: duloxetine
TRADE NAME: Cymbalta
INDICATION: antidepressant, fibromyalgia
ROUTE OF ADMINISTRATION: oral
COMMON ADULT DOSAGE: 40 or 60 mg once daily
SIDE EFFECTS: nausea, vomiting, dizziness, insomnia, dry mouth, headache, diarrhea, loss of appetite
AUXILIARY LABEL:
- May cause dizziness and drowsiness.

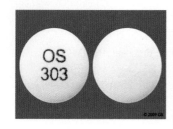

GENERIC NAME: venlafaxine
TRADE NAME: Effexor, Effexor XR
INDICATION: depression
COMMON ADULT DOSAGE: 75 to 225 mg/day in split dosages given twice daily or three times daily, Effexor XR given once daily
ROUTE OF ADMINISTRATION: oral
SIDE EFFECTS: dry mouth, elevated blood pressure, dizziness, drowsiness, sweating, sexual dysfunction
AUXILIARY LABELS:
- Do not drink alcohol.
- May cause dizziness and drowsiness.

Tricyclic Antidepressants. TCAs are used for depression, for obsessive-compulsive disorders, and in some cases for chronic pain. These agents inhibit (stop) the reuptake (the cells taking back excess amounts) of norepinephrine and serotonin. There are a wide range of concerns about TCAs in general. Worsening of symptoms in patients with heart disease, schizophrenia, seizure disorders, and renal or hepatic problems is a concern. Because of these adverse effects, TCAs are not the first line of treatment for depression. However, for some persons, they work well when all other medications fail. Side effects differ among the various types of TCAs and are described below.

TRICYCLIC ANTIDEPRESSANTS

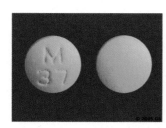

GENERIC NAME: amitriptyline
TRADE NAME: Elavil
INDICATION: depression
ROUTE OF ADMINISTRATION: oral
COMMON ADULT DOSAGE: 75 to 100 mg once daily (divided doses) up to 300 mg/day
SIDE EFFECTS: drowsiness, dry mouth, blurred vision, orthostatic hypotension, dizziness, and headache
AUXILIARY LABELS:
- May cause dizziness and drowsiness.
- Take with food.

GENERIC NAME: doxepin
TRADE NAME: Sinequan
INDICATION: depression, anxiety
ROUTE OF ADMINISTRATION: oral
COMMON ADULT DOSAGE: 50 to 150 mg once daily
SIDE EFFECTS: drowsiness, dry mouth, blurred vision, orthostatic hypotension, dizziness, and headache
AUXILIARY LABELS:
- May cause dizziness and drowsiness.
- May cause sensitivity to sunlight.

GENERIC NAME: imipramine
TRADE NAME: Tofranil
INDICATION: depression, enuresis (bed-wetting)
ROUTE OF ADMINISTRATION: oral (pamoate and hydrochloride)
COMMON ADULT DOSAGE: for depression, oral 75 to 150 mg once daily
SIDE EFFECTS: drowsiness, dry mouth, blurred vision, orthostatic hypotension, dizziness, and headache
AUXILIARY LABELS:
- May cause dizziness and drowsiness.
- Do not drink alcohol.

TABLE 17-3 Examples of Foods That Contain Tyramine

Foods	Additive
Cheese	Bacteria and fungi
Sour cream	Bacteria
Beer	Yeast
Wine	Yeast
Avocados	Bacteria
Soy sauce	Fungi
Yogurt	Bacteria
Chocolate	Caffeine
Tea	Caffeine
Coffee	Caffeine

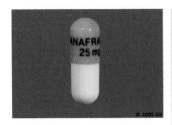

GENERIC NAME: clomipramine
TRADE NAME: Anafranil
INDICATION: obsessive-compulsive disorder, depression
ROUTE OF ADMINISTRATION: oral
COMMON ADULT DOSAGE: 25 mg once daily up to 100 mg/day given in divided doses
SIDE EFFECTS: drowsiness, dry mouth, blurred vision, orthostatic hypotension, dizziness, and headache
AUXILIARY LABELS:

- May cause dizziness and drowsiness.
- Do not drink alcohol.

Monoamine Oxidase Inhibitors (MAOIs). MAOIs mostly differ from TCAs and SSRIs by their side effects, which occur as the result of their nonselective inhibition of the MAO enzymes. Many food interactions occur with MAOIs that can lead to hypertension for the patient. Certain foods containing tyramine, such as red wine, aged cheeses, and cured meats, can be extremely dangerous to a patient taking MAOIs. In addition, foods that use bacteria or other microbes in their processing cause interactions. Produce such as raisins, bananas, avocados, and papaya can also cause adverse reactions with MAOIs. Many drugs must be avoided when a patient is taking an MAOI, including several over-the-counter drug products. Table 17-3 gives a sample list of foods with microbial ingredients that react with MAOI's. Because of the many food and drug interactions with MAOIs, they are reserved for use in patients who do not respond to TCAs or SSRIs or who have an adverse reaction to them. As mentioned previously, when dispensing MAOIs it is important to note that patients should avoid foods containing tyramine. Tyramine is a naturally occurring degradation product of the amino acid tyrosine, and is associated with blood pressure regulation. MAOIs inhibit the function of the enzyme monoamine oxidase, which breaks down tyramine in the body. Therefore when MAOIs are taken, tyramine can accumulate to very high levels, causing a dangerous increase in blood pressure. The following drugs are MAOIs.

MONOAMINE OXIDASE INHIBITORS (MAOIs)

GENERIC NAME: tranylcypromine
TRADE NAME: Parnate
INDICATION: depression
ROUTE OF ADMINISTRATION: oral
COMMON ADULT DOSAGE: 30 mg/day (divided doses) up to 60 mg/day
SIDE EFFECTS: gastrointestinal upset, insomnia, drowsiness, hypotension, dry mouth, and anorexia
AUXILIARY LABELS:
- Take with food.
- Do not drink alcohol.
- Avoid wine, cheese, chocolate while taking this medication.

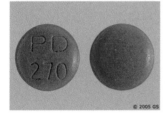

GENERIC NAME: phenelzine
TRADE NAME: Nardil
INDICATION: depression
ROUTE OF ADMINISTRATION: oral
COMMON ADULT DOSAGE: 15 mg three times daily up to 60 mg/day
SIDE EFFECTS: gastrointestinal upset, insomnia, drowsiness, hypotension, dry mouth, and anorexia
AUXILIARY LABELS:
- Do not drink alcohol.
- Avoid wine, cheese, chocolate while taking this medication.

GENERIC NAME: isocarboxazid
TRADE NAME: Marplan
INDICATION: depression
ROUTE OF ADMINISTRATION: oral
COMMON ADULT DOSAGE: 10 mg twice daily; may increase slowly up to 60 mg/day, if needed; rare to see doses >40 mg/day
SIDE EFFECTS: gastrointestinal upset, insomnia, drowsiness, hypotension, dry mouth, and anorexia
AUXILIARY LABELS:
- Do not drink alcohol.
- Avoid wine, cheese, chocolate while taking this medication.

Additional Antidepressants. The antidepressants discussed next do not fit into the previous categories because they do not have the same drug actions as the other antidepressants. In some cases the exact drug action is unknown; however, they are effective for some patients.

OTHER ANTIDEPRESSANTS

GENERIC NAME: trazodone
TRADE NAME: Desyrel
INDICATION: depression
ROUTE OF ADMINISTRATION: oral
COMMON ADULT DOSAGE: outpatient use: 150-400 mg/day split into divided doses
SIDE EFFECTS: dizziness, drowsiness, shortness of breath, chest pain, tachycardia, priapism
AUXILIARY LABELS:
- Take with food.
- May cause dizziness and drowsiness.
- Do not drink alcohol.

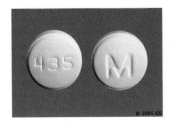

GENERIC NAME: bupropion

TRADE NAME: Wellbutrin, Wellbutrin SR, Wellbutrin XL

INDICATION: depression

ROUTE OF ADMINISTRATION: oral

COMMON ADULT DOSAGE: Wellbutrin, 100 to 150 mg three times daily; Wellbutrin SR, 150 to 200 mg once or twice daily; Wellbutrin XL, 150 to 450 mg/day given once daily

SIDE EFFECTS: dizziness, drowsiness, hallucinations, blurred vision; can cause seizures, especially with overdose; in addition priapism (prolonged erection of the penis) is linked to the use of bupropion

AUXILIARY LABELS:

■ Do not drink alcohol.

■ May cause dizziness and drowsiness.

NOTE: Another form of bupropion, Zyban, is used for smoking cessation; patients should not take Wellbutrin and Zyban together as this would result in overdose.

Anxiety Disorders

There are many different types of fears experienced by people. Anxiety can be expressed as a feeling of fear or dread, with symptoms ranging from rapid heart rate to trembling. Some of the most common disorders are outlined below along with their treatments. A **neurosis** is a mental or emotional disorder that is marked with a distorted view of reality (however, the distortion is not normally as severe as that seen with psychosis) that can lead to anxieties and phobias. Anxiety disorders can be divided into several different types; the diagnosis of each type is specific to the patient's symptoms. These range from panic disorders such as post-traumatic stress disorder (PTSD) and **phobias** to personality disorders such as obsessive-compulsive disorder (OCD) and obsessive-compulsive personality disorder (OCPD).

- Generalized anxiety disorder (GAD): This is a frequent condition in which a person experiences constant anxiety and worries about common problems in life (such as money or relationships) continuously over a period of 6 months or more.
- Social anxiety disorder: Also referred to as social phobia, the person experiences constant anxiety and extreme fear regarding being around others. The person with social anxiety disorder attempts to avoid situations in which he or she is exposed to groups of people or needs to speak or interact with people. The avoidance stems from overwhelming fears of being humiliated, being judged, and feeling uncomfortable; the condition disrupts the person's daily life and normal daily activities.
- Panic disorders are anxiety disorders in which the person experiences recurrent panic attacks. They can be triggered by a situational event from the person's past. During a panic attack, the person experiences severe apprehension, fear, and terror as well as physical complaints such as dizziness, heart palpitations, or shakiness. Severe panic disorders can lead to phobias and PTSD.
- PTSD follows any incident that has taken place that is either traumatic or terrifying to the person who experienced the event. Sights, sounds, and even smells can develop flashbacks, nightmares, and constant memories. Soldiers returning from war are a common group suffering from PTSD. Other persons who may suffer from PTSD include rape victims, those exposed to violence, and those diagnosed with a life-threatening medical illness. The symptoms of PTSD can occur at any time after the horrific event.
- Phobias: The term phobia is derived from the Greek word *phobos* (fear) and involves an irrational, persistent fear of situations, people, or things. The person suffering from a phobia experiences several symptoms including

TABLE 17-4 Examples of Types of Phobias

Phobia	Fear of
Acrophobia	Heights
Agoraphobia	Being in public places
Claustrophobia	Small enclosed spaces
Cynophobia	Dogs
Ophidiophobia	Snakes
Social phobia	Being in social situations where a person may be embarrassed or judged (i.e., social anxiety disorder)
Zoophobia	Animals

TABLE 17-5 Types of Obsessive-Compulsive Personality Disorders

OCD	
Kleptomania	The uncontrollable urge to steal that results in a thrill
Pyromania	The inability to stop the urge to set fires; derives pleasure from fire-setting
Trichotillomania	The overwhelming urge to pull one's own hair out; this includes hair from all parts of the body; results in bald spots
OCPD	
Hoarders	The need to collect insignificant items and cannot throw things away
Washers and cleaners	An irrational fear of disease and/or contamination; cleaning themselves and/or surroundings countless times daily
Checkers	The need to check and recheck objects such as door locks and switches; often believe something terrible will happen if they do not perform these rituals

rapid heart rate, shortness of breath, and trembling. Table 17-4 provides a list of several different types of phobias. Treatment ranges from psychotherapy to antianxiety medications.

- Personality disorders can often interfere with a person's daily activities. Examples of this type of condition are OCD and OCPD, which includes many different compulsions and obsessions. The difference between the two is that persons suffering from OCD feel sick and want to stop, whereas those with OCPD feel somewhat comfortable with their impulses. Table 17-5 lists examples of both types of disorders.

Prognosis. With proper diagnosis and treatment, including medication and ongoing therapy, persons can live relatively normal lives.

Non–Drug Treatments. Most persons require psychotherapy and behavioral therapy that can help the person learn to resist the urges, compulsions, or other triggers that cause the abnormal response. Cognitive behavioral therapy helps the person to change his or her negative styles of living, thinking, and behaving that lead to this type of behavior.

Drug Treatments. Primary medications used include antianxiety agents and selective serotonin reuptake inhibitors (SSRIs) (see Depression). SSRIs increase the levels of the neurotransmitter serotonin by decreasing (inhibiting) the reuptake mechanism of this neurotransmitter. Typically when serotonin is released into the synaptic cleft, it stimulates the next neuron and then returns to its original neuron. When this occurs, the production of more serotonin is stopped. It is believed that the low levels of serotonin are responsible for these types of conditions. Antianxiety medications can be used to help treat the patient's feelings of anxiety that can accompany the condition.

ANTIANXIETY MEDICATIONS

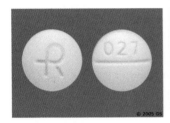

GENERIC NAME: alprazolam (C-IV)
TRADE NAME: Xanax
INDICATION: anxiety disorders
ROUTE OF ADMINISTRATION: oral
COMMON ADULT DOSAGE: 0.25 to 0.5 mg tid up to a maximum of 4 mg/day in divided doses
SIDE EFFECTS: drowsiness, dizziness, dry mouth
AUXILIARY LABELS:
■ May cause dizziness and drowsiness.
■ Do not drink alcohol.
NOTE: All benzodiazepine medications are schedule IV medications.

GENERIC NAME: buspirone
TRADE NAME: BuSpar
INDICATION: anxiety disorders, short-term relief of anxiety symptoms
ROUTE OF ADMINISTRATION: oral
COMMON ADULT DOSAGE: initial dose, 7.5 mg twice daily; max dose, 30 mg twice daily
SIDE EFFECTS: drowsiness, dizziness, nausea, insomnia
AUXILIARY LABELS:
■ May cause dizziness and drowsiness.
■ Do not drink alcohol.
■ Avoid grapefruit juice while taking this medication
NOTE: Should not be taken with MAO inhibitors.

Bipolar Disorder

The word **mania** is derived from the word *manic*. This disorder is characterized by excessive mood swings that range from manic (high) to depressive (low) states; it is also known as bipolar disorder, indicating the extreme mood swings. This disorder affects men and women equally. Specific symptoms of the mania include agitation, hyperactivity, inflated self-esteem, risky or reckless behavior, and decreased sleep requirements. The depression phase includes fatigue, loss of self-esteem, suicidal thoughts, social withdrawal from family and friends, and eating/sleeping disturbances.

Prognosis. With proper medications the symptoms can be controlled although many people stop taking their medications once they feel better. A strong support system is needed for continuing treatment.

Non–Drug Treatment. Psychotherapy can be used to help with the depressive phase. For those whose depressive state cannot be controlled by medications, electroconvulsive therapy may be an alternative form of treatment.

Drug Treatment. For the treatment of mania or bipolar illness with mixed features, mood-stabilizing drugs are used; lithium, some anticonvulsants (e.g., carbamazepine, divalproex, lamotrigine), and many atypical antipsychotic agents (e.g., aripiprazole, asenapine, olanzapine, quetiapine, risperidone, and ziprasidone) are useful and FDA-approved. Although the complete mechanism for lithium is not understood fully, it is believed to alter behavior by enhancing the uptake of serotonin and norepinephrine by nerve cells (see Chapter 16). This sets lithium apart from all the other psychiatric drugs, because it does not cause any major CNS changes such as sedation, feelings of euphoria, or depression.

ANTIMANICS

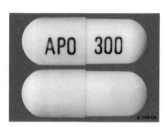

GENERIC NAME: lithium

TRADE NAME: Eskalith

INDICATION: treatment of manic episodes of bipolar disorder

ROUTE OF ADMINISTRATION: oral

COMMON ADULT DOSAGE: for acute mania, 600 mg three times daily or 900 mg twice daily; doses vary based on laboratory results of serum lithium levels

SIDE EFFECTS: dizziness, drowsiness, ataxia, hypotension, slurred speech, and weight gain; teratogenic

NOTE: All patients taking lithium must have their blood levels monitored regularly for toxicity. Because lithium toxicity levels are close to the necessary therapeutic levels, lithium therapy should be started only if the lithium levels can be monitored closely. It may take several weeks to see the desired effect of this agent.

AUXILIARY LABELS:

■ Do not drink alcohol.

■ May cause dizziness and drowsiness.

■ Take with food or milk.

■ Drink plenty of water.

NOTE: The effects of lithium are more powerful in older adults; therefore it is important that the elderly be monitored more closely.

Schizophrenia

Schizophrenia is a severe mental illness characterized by persistent, bizarre disturbances in thought processes for at least 6 months. These disturbances affect communication, perceptions, emotions, and behaviors. This condition is considered a **psychosis** because patients often become detached from reality. Patients are normally diagnosed with one of the following five different types of schizophrenia, depending on their symptoms:

• Paranoid schizophrenia: Primary symptoms include delusions or auditory hallucinations. Patients may have delusions in which they believe others are deliberately trying to poison them, harassing them, or spying or plotting against them. Auditory hallucinations include hearing voices that may comment on their behavior, order them to do something, or warn them of an impending threat. Not all symptoms may be present at one time; in severe cases there may be phases of worsening where other characteristics (present in other types of schizophrenia) may be observed, such as speaking incoherently or acting irrationally. This type of schizophrenia is the most common; however, patients are not necessarily considered as having a thought disorder or disorganized behavior. Some patients may be able to function normally at work and engage in relationships and not appear odd or unusual, and they may not feel compelled to discuss their symptoms.

• Disorganized schizophrenia: This type of schizophrenia affects the patient with unusual and disorganized thought processes. Patients may have difficulty organizing or connecting thoughts in a logical manner. Speech may be affected by being garbled or hard to understand. Another form of this type of schizophrenia is called "thought blocking," where the person loses their thought midsentence and later may make up unintelligible words instead.

Persons suffering from this type of schizophrenia may also appear to be emotionally unstable or their emotions seem inappropriate within the context of the situation, such as chuckling at a funeral service. Alternatively, they may exhibit a "flat affect," which is an immobile facial expression and/or a monotone voice.

- Catatonic schizophrenia: Patients with this type of schizophrenia may be clumsy and/or uncoordinated, exhibit involuntary movements and grimacing, or show unusual mannerisms. They may repeat certain motions and in certain cases become catatonic (immobile and unresponsive). This type of schizophrenia is rare.
- Residual schizophrenia: This type occurs in people experiencing long-term schizophrenia. The patient may no longer show any of the symptoms such as hallucinations, delusions, or disorganized speech, or symptoms may be mild. Instead, they do have symptoms including a flat affect and infrequent speech, even when forced to interact. These patients have a diminished ability to initiate and sustain planned activity, and a lack of pleasure throughout daily life. These individuals often neglect basic hygiene and require assistance with living activities. Others revolve between hospitalizations and periods of normalcy.
- Undifferentiated schizophrenia: This term is used to describe patients who meet the criteria for schizophrenia although their symptoms do not fall into the other forms described. Their symptoms can fluctuate at different points, resulting in uncertainty of diagnosis of a particular type of schizophrenia.

Although the cause is unknown some researchers believe schizophrenia may be linked by heredity or genetics. Children of schizophrenic parents have a greater chance of becoming schizophrenic, with the percentage as high as 40%. Even with this increased risk of schizophrenia, many people suffer from this condition and the disease is not linked to any one causation. Various psychosocial therapies are normally combined with medications in order to control the symptoms of schizophrenia.

Prognosis. Although there is no known cure for this condition there are effective treatments that can alleviate the symptoms, including therapy and medication. Patients who sustain a regimen of the appropriate medications and therapies throughout life have a better prognosis than patients who have periods of noncompliance. Relapses will occur if medication is stopped abruptly. Therefore compliance is the major limiting factor that will determine the outcome of this serious mental illness.

Non–Drug Treatments. Both professional counseling and a strong support system are key in the success of treatment; however, symptoms cannot be treated without the use of medications.

Drug Treatments. Drug treatments focus on eliminating the symptoms of the disease, improving the quality of life, and allowing the patient to live a productive life. Treatments are determined based on the phases of schizophrenia. These phases include acute, stabilizing, maintenance, or recovery. Often various medications and/or strengths of agents must be used before finding the most effective combination for the patient; this is because everyone responds differently to medications. Antipsychotic agents are used to treat schizophrenia and are available in two types: typical antipsychotics (first-generation agents) and atypical antipsychotics (second-generation agents), which are listed in Table 17-6. In addition to antipsychotics, the following agents may be used:

TABLE 17-6 Common Agents Used to Treat Schizophrenia

	Generic	Trade	Dosage Forms
Typical Antipsychotics			
	chlorpromazine	Thorazine	Tablets, injection
	fluphenazine	Prolixin	Tablets, elixir, injection, decanoate injection
	haloperidol	Haldol	Tablets, injection, solution decanoate injection
	loxapine	Loxitane	Capsules
	thioridazine	Mellaril	Tablets
	molindone	Moban	Tablets
	trifluoperazine	Stelazine	Tablets
	thiothixene	Navane	Capsules
Atypical Antipsychotics			
	aripiprazole	Abilify	Tablets, solution, injection, orally disintegrating tablets
	clozapine	Clozaril	Tablets
	iloperidone	Fanapt	Tablets
	olanzapine	Zyprexa	Tablets, orally disintegrating tablets, injection, long-acting depot injection
	paliperidone	Invega	Tablets extended release
	quetiapine	Seroquel	Tablets, tablets extended release
	risperidone	Risperdal	Film-coated tablets, solution, orally disintegrating tablets, long-acting depot injection
	ziprasidone	Geodon	Capsules, injection
	asenapine	Saphris	Sublingual tablets

- Antianxiety medications: Agents such as clonazepam (Klonopin) and diazepam (Valium) may be used to reduce anxiety and nervousness.
- Anticonvulsant medications: Agents such as carbamazepine (Tegretol) and valproate (Depakote) can help to stabilize and reduce the symptoms during a relapse.
- Antidepressants: Include various SSRIs (e.g., sertraline [Zoloft] or citalopram [Celexa]) or TCAs (e.g., nortriptyline ([Pamelor]). These agents can reduce the symptoms of depression that often occur with schizophrenia.

Typical Antipsychotics. These agents have a limited spectrum of therapeutic activity. One adverse reaction that can occur while taking these types of agents is **tardive dyskinesia** (TD). The symptoms include involuntary movement of the facial muscles, tongue, jaw, and head. If these symptoms appear, the medication must be stopped immediately because these effects can be irreversible. Another type of adverse effect that is related to overdosing is **extrapyramidal symptoms** (EPSs), which are side effects that mimic Parkinson's disease, causing the hands and head to shake. Drooling and a shuffling gait are present as well. These symptoms usually disappear if the medication strength is lowered or the medication is discontinued. It is believed typical antipsychotics completely block only one kind of dopamine receptor, which leaves other types of dopamine receptors unaffected.

PHENOTHIAZINES

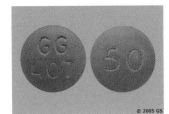

GENERIC NAME: chlorpromazine

TRADE NAME: Thorazine

INDICATION: manic-depressive reactions, schizophrenia, hyperactivity in children

ROUTE OF ADMINISTRATION: oral, injection, rectal

COMMON ADULT DOSAGE: 25 mg three times daily up to 400 mg once (every day)

SIDE EFFECTS: dizziness, drowsiness, ataxia, hypotension, slurred speech, and weight gain

AUXILIARY LABELS:

- May cause dizziness and drowsiness.
- Do not take if you become pregnant.
- Do not drink alcohol.

GENERIC NAME: trifluoperazine

TRADE NAME: Stelazine

INDICATION: psychotic disorders, anxiety

ROUTE OF ADMINISTRATION: oral, injection

COMMON ADULT DOSAGE: 1 to 5 mg once daily or twice daily

SIDE EFFECTS: drowsiness, dizziness, extrapyramidal symptoms, dry mouth, and tardive dyskinesia

AUXILIARY LABELS:

- May cause dizziness and drowsiness.
- Do not take if you become pregnant.
- Do not drink alcohol.

Atypical Antipsychotics. Atypical antipsychotic medications are effective at treating both positive and negative symptoms of schizophrenia. These agents also tend to have fewer side effects such as EPS and TD. Atypical antipsychotics tend to cause weight gain as a side effect, and use may lead to diabetes type 2 in some patients. Alternative antipsychotic agents are used to treat psychotic patients who do not respond well to other agents or who have adverse reactions to them. It is believed that compared to typical antipsychotics, atypical antipsychotics appear to block many kinds of dopamine receptors less completely.

ATYPICAL ANTIPSYCHOTICS

GENERIC NAME: clozapine

TRADE NAME: Clozaril

INDICATION: schizophrenia

ROUTE OF ADMINISTRATION: oral, injection, rectal

COMMON ADULT DOSAGE: 12.5 mg once or twice daily with increased increments of 25 mg/50 mg once daily; max 300 to 450 mg per day in divided doses by the end of 2 weeks

SIDE EFFECTS: dizziness, drowsiness, dry mouth, nausea, headache, weight gain

AUXILIARY LABELS:

- May cause dizziness and drowsiness.
- Do not drink alcohol.
- Take with or without food.

NOTE: There is a high risk of agranulocytosis with this medication. White blood cells are compromised, which can cause death. Blood tests must be done for the first 6 months of treatment. This medication should only be used for severe cases of schizophrenia that fail to be controlled by other agents or those patients who have recurrent suicidal behavior.

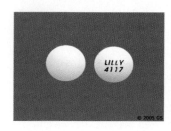

GENERIC NAME: olanzapine

TRADE NAME: Zyprexa

INDICATION: psychotic disorders

ROUTE OF ADMINISTRATION: oral, injectable

COMMON ADULT DOSAGE: (oral) 5 to 10 mg once daily; (intramuscularly) 10 mg daily

SIDE EFFECTS: headache, agitation, insomnia, constipation, weight gain

AUXILIARY LABEL:

■ Do not swallow; let dissolve in mouth (for ODT form).

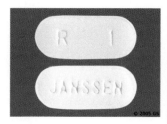

GENERIC NAME: risperidone

TRADE NAME: Risperdal

INDICATION: psychotic disorders and agitation in elderly persons

ROUTE OF ADMINISTRATION: oral, injectable

COMMON ADULT DOSAGE: 1 mg twice daily up to 8 mg once daily to twice daily

SIDE EFFECTS: headache, dizziness, agitation, insomnia, constipation, tardive dyskinesia, weight gain, dry mouth, drowsiness, decreased sex drive

AUXILIARY LABELS:

■ May cause dizziness or drowsiness.

■ Do not swallow; let dissolve in mouth for ODT form.

■ Store away from light or heat.

Long-acting antipsychotics (decanoates) are usually given once monthly (usually by a nurse or physician) for schizophrenia; Decanoates or depot agents tend to have a slower onset of action (24-72 hrs after injection), longer duration of action (average is 3 to 4 weeks) and may cause less drowsiness (http://www.mentalhealth.com/drug/p30-m03.html). The following are two of the most commonly used agents:

GENERIC NAME: haloperidol decanoate

TRADE NAME: Haldol

INDICATION: psychoses; Tourette's syndrome

ROUTE OF ADMINISTRATION: injection, oral

COMMON ADULT DOSAGE: 10 to 15 times the normal daily dose given once every month (maximum monthly dose should not exceed 100 mg)

SIDE EFFECTS: respiratory depression, tardive dyskinesia, drowsiness, orthostatic hypotension, and dry mouth

AUXILIARY LABELS:

■ Do not drink alcohol.

■ May cause dizziness and drowsiness.

GENERIC: fluphenazine decanoate

TRADE NAME: Prolixin

INDICATION: psychotic disorders

ROUTE OF ADMINISTRATION: oral, injection

COMMON ADULT DOSAGE: 10 to 15 times the normal daily dose, given once every month (maximum dose should not exceed 100 mg)

SIDE EFFECTS: respiratory depression, tardive dyskinesia, drowsiness, orthostatic hypotension, and dry mouth

AUXILIARY LABELS:

■ Do not drink alcohol.

■ May cause dizziness and drowsiness.

TABLE 17-7 Types and Description of Insomnia

Classification	Description
Transient insomnia	Lasting less than 1 week
Short term	Less than 3 weeks
Chronic	More than 3 weeks
Types of Insomnia (Based on Specific Times Insomnia Occurs)	
Initial	Difficulty falling asleep
Intermittent insomnia	Difficulty staying asleep
Terminal insomnia	Waking early and unable to fall back to sleep

OTHER CONDITIONS

Insomnia

Insomnia is not a disease but a symptom; the person cannot fall asleep, stay asleep, or both. Most people experience sleeping problems at certain times throughout life. Sleeping difficulties may need to be treated, depending on how often they occur. There are three general classifications of insomnia (Table 17-7). These are transient (lasting less than 1 week), short-term (less than 3 weeks), or chronic (more than 3 weeks). It is estimated that between 30% and 50% of the population have insomnia (www.emedicinehealth.com). It affects all age groups and women more than men. Causes for insomnia range from stressful situations, sleep interruptions, and pain to a side effect of withdrawal from certain substances such as addicting drugs and alcohol. Common foods that can contribute to insomnia include caffeine, coffee, tobacco, and alcohol. Various illnesses also can affect sleeplessness, such as sleep apnea, acid reflux disease, Parkinson's disease, and Alzheimer's disease. Insomnia can occur for many reasons, including side effects of drugs, whether they are over-the-counter (OTC) or prescription. Older persons commonly suffer from insomnia because of pain or physiological changes.

Prognosis. Depending on the cause of the insomnia, most persons can be treated effectively with medications.

Non–Drug Treatment. Good sleeping hygiene is a focus of behavioral therapy to treat insomnia. Behavioral therapy includes exercising regularly, maintaining a sleep schedule, avoiding alcohol and caffeine intake after certain times of the day, and keeping the bedroom quiet and at the right temperature. Relaxation therapy techniques include dimming lights, listening to soft music, or meditating before retiring.

Drug Treatment. For persons suffering from mild cases of insomnia there are many over-the-counter drugs available. Table 17-8 lists some of the most popular OTC agents. The main ingredient in OTC sedative and hypnotic agents is diphenhydramine. Diphenhydramine is classified as an antihistamine, and its most prevalent side effect is sleepiness, which in the case of insomnia is the desired effect. Diphenhydramine is often used in the hospital setting for this purpose. Acetaminophen and magnesium salicylate are analgesics added to sleep remedies, and are marketed for use to treat insomnia that is complicated by pain. OTC sedatives (see Table 17-8) are intended to treat short-term insomnia and work well. However, if the insomnia continues over a longer period, a prescription medication may be needed.

TABLE 17-8 Common (Adult Dosages) Over-the-Counter Medications Indicated For Insomnia

Active Ingredient(s)	Brand Name	Dosage Form	Strength(s)
Insomnia Agents			
doxylamine	Unisom Nighttime Sleep-Aid	Tablet	25 mg
	Medi-Sleep	Tablet	25 mg
diphenhydramine	Sominex	Tablet	25 mg
	Nytol	Tablet	25 mg
	Compoz Gel caps	Capsule	25 mg
	Simply Sleep	Tablet	25 mg
	Compoz Nighttime Sleep Aid	Tablet	50 mg
	40 Winks	Tablet	50 mg
	Unisom SleepMelts	Disintegrating tablet	25 mg
	Sominex	Tablet	50 mg
Insomnia and Pain Agent Combinations			
diphenhydramine/ acetaminophen	Extra Strength Tylenol PM	Tablet	25 mg/500 mg
	Excedrin PM Liquigels	Capsule	25 mg/500 mg
diphenhydramine/ acetaminophen	Nighttime Pamprin Powder packets	Powder	50 mg/650 mg
diphenhydramine/ ibuprofen	Advil PM	Capsule	25 mg/200 mg
acetaminophen/ diphenhydramine	Excedrin PM	Liquid	167 mg/8.3 mg
diphenhydramine/ magnesium salicylate	Extra Strength Doan's PM	Tablet	25 mg/500 mg

Tech Note!

Although non-benzodiazepine prescription medications were first marketed in the United States as not having the same side effects as benzodiazepines, some clinical studies found that they did produce the same adverse effects as benzodiazepines and hypnotics, including tolerance, dependence, and abuse; in addition, they were more expensive.

Several types of prescription medications can be used as sedatives, including benzodiazepines, non-benzodiazepines, and certain antidepressants. Although these medications can be effective they are best used when combined with non–drug treatments. Also, all sedatives can cause the person to become dependent upon them. Therefore they are not considered a permanent solution to insomnia. The elderly must be especially careful when combining OTC sleeping agents with their other prescription medications.

Benzodiazepines. Benzodiazepines have several effects on the body. They are known to affect parts of the brain, decreasing convulsions and affecting emotional stability. Effects within the spinal cord cause muscle relaxation, and benzodiazepines can cause sedation. Because these agents affect the CNS, they can decrease breathing rate. Their main uses are for anxiety and insomnia. Benzodiazepines are also used to control seizures and relax muscles.

The benzodiazepines are lipid (fat) soluble. This means that they can enter cells and tissues within the body that are made of lipids or are protected by a lipid barrier. The brain is a delicate and important area that must be protected from foreign bodies. The brain is protected by a **blood-brain barrier** that stops many chemicals from passing into the brain. Lipid-soluble drugs can pass through the blood-brain barrier, which is why mental function is changed after taking the medication. Excretion is through the urine. All the benzodiazepines are legend (prescription) drugs and are labeled controlled substances (schedule IV). A list of commonly prescribed benzodiazepines follows.

BENZODIAZEPINE HYPNOTICS

GENERIC NAME: temazepam (C-IV)
TRADE NAME: Restoril
INDICATION: insomnia
ROUTE OF ADMINISTRATION: oral
COMMON ADULT DOSAGE: 7.5 or 15 mg at bedtime
SIDE EFFECTS: drowsiness, dry mouth, amnesia, muscle weakness, nausea, vomiting
AUXILIARY LABELS:
- May cause dizziness and drowsiness.
- Do not drink alcohol.

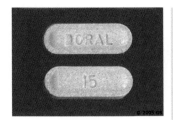

GENERIC NAME: quazepam (C-IV)
TRADE NAME: Doral
INDICATION: insomnia
ROUTE OF ADMINISTRATION: oral
COMMON ADULT DOSAGE: 15 mg 30 minutes to 1 hour before bedtime; may reduce to 7.5 mg once individual response is determined
SIDE EFFECTS: dizziness, drowsiness, amnesia, muscle weakness, headache, impotence, dry mouth
AUXILIARY LABELS:
- May cause dizziness and drowsiness.
- Do not drink alcohol.
- Take with a full glass of water.

Non-benzodiazepines. Zolpidem (Ambien), zaleplon (Sonata), and zopiclone (Imovane) and its active stereoisomer, eszopiclone (Lunesta), are effective medications to treat insomnia. Imovane is not available in the United States but is available in Canada. These agents appear less likely to cause excessive daytime sleepiness and amnesia. Ramelteon (Rozerem) is a unique agent that is a melatonin–receptor simulator, and it is not a controlled substance.

NON-BENZODIAZEPINE HYPNOTICS

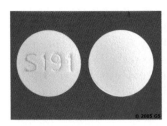

GENERIC NAME: eszopiclone (C-IV)
TRADE NAME: Lunesta
INDICATION: insomnia (falling and staying asleep)
ROUTE OF ADMINISTRATION: oral
COMMON ADULT DOSAGE: 2 mg at bedtime only
SIDE EFFECTS: daytime drowsiness, dizziness, headache, amnesia, dry mouth, nausea, loss of appetite
AUXILIARY LABELS:
- May cause dizziness and drowsiness.
- Do not drink alcohol.
- Take with a full glass of water.

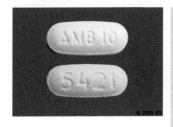

GENERIC NAME: zolpidem (C-IV)
TRADE NAME: Ambien, Ambien CR
INDICATION: insomnia (falling asleep)
ROUTE OF ADMINISTRATION: oral
COMMON ADULT DOSAGE: immediate release, 10 mg at bedtime; CR dosage form, 12.5 mg at bedtime
SIDE EFFECTS: daytime drowsiness, dizziness, headache, dry mouth, nausea, loss of appetite
AUXILIARY LABELS:
- May cause dizziness and drowsiness.
- Do not drink alcohol.
- Take with a full glass of water.

GENERIC NAME: zaleplon (C-IV)
TRADE NAME: Sonata
INDICATION: insomnia (falling asleep)
ROUTE OF ADMINISTRATION: oral
COMMON ADULT DOSAGE: 5 to 20 mg at bedtime
SIDE EFFECTS: daytime drowsiness, dizziness, headache, dry mouth, nausea, loss of appetite
AUXILIARY LABELS:
- May cause dizziness and drowsiness.
- Do not drink alcohol.

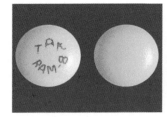

GENERIC NAME: ramelteon
TRADE NAME: Rozerem
INDICATION: insomnia (falling asleep)
ROUTE OF ADMINISTRATION: oral
COMMON ADULT DOSAGE: 8 mg within 30 minutes of bedtime
SIDE EFFECTS: dizziness, drowsiness, headache, nausea, diarrhea
AUXILIARY LABELS:
- May cause dizziness and drowsiness.
- Do not drink alcohol.
- Take on an empty stomach.

Barbiturates. Barbiturates are controlled substances. They were used for many years as sedatives for persons suffering from different conditions, such as seizures and insomnia, and as hypnotics before surgery. Barbiturates are differentiated by the time it takes them to become effective. They range from short- to long-acting and are listed in Table 17-9. Barbiturates act on the brainstem area, reducing nerve impulses to the cerebral cortex. Because barbiturates affect the respiratory system, nerves, and smooth muscles, their effects cause relaxation and sleep. If a low dose is given, barbiturates produce a mild sedative effect, whereas a high dose causes anesthesia. Examples of these agents include thiopental and methohexital, which are used in surgery to induce general anesthesia.

Side Effects. Several side effects are associated with the use of barbiturates, such as drowsiness, dizziness, nausea, vomiting, constipation, and a hangover effect after the drug dissipates. Because of the effect barbiturates have on the CNS and the respiratory system, barbiturates can cause death if the patient takes an overdose. Because of the many side effects produced by barbiturates, they are usually only of historical interest in the treatment of insomnia and

TABLE 17-9 Common Barbiturates

Schedule	Generic Name	Trade Name	Common Oral Adult Dosage	Length of Action	Route of Administration
C-IV	phenobarbital	Luminal	Sedative: 30-120 mg/day Seizures: 60-120 mg/day	Long acting	PO, IV, IM
C-IV	mephobarbital	Mebaral	Sedative: 32-100 mg tid/qid Seizures: 400-600 mg/day	Long acting	PO
C-III	butabarbital	Butisol	Sedation: 15-30 mg tid/qid Sleep: 50-100 mg Pre-op: 50-100 mg	Intermediate	PO
C-II	secobarbital	Seconal	Sleep: 100 mg Pre-op: 200-300 mg	Short acting	PO
C-II	pentobarbital	Nembutal	Pre-op: 1-3 mg/kg or 100-200 mg IM	Short acting	IV, IM

IM, Intramuscular; *IV,* intravenous; *PO,* oral; *pre-op,* preoperative; *qid,* 4 times a day; *tid,* 3 times a day.

have been replaced largely by non-benzodiazepine and benzodiazepine hypnotics. However, barbiturates are still used in many hospitals as anesthesia for surgery.

BARBITURATES

GENERIC NAME: phenobarbital (C-IV)
TRADE NAME: Luminal
INDICATION: insomnia (falling asleep), anxiety, certain types of seizures
ROUTE OF ADMINISTRATION: oral
COMMON ADULT DOSAGE: for insomnia, 100 to 200 mg at bedtime
SIDE EFFECTS: dizziness, drowsiness, headache, nausea, light-headedness, vomiting
AUXILIARY LABELS:
■ May cause dizziness and drowsiness.
■ Do not drink alcohol.

Attention Deficit/Hyperactivity Disorder (ADHD)
ADHD is a physiological brain disorder in which the person has difficulty focusing his/her attention or engaging in quiet, passive-type behavior, or both. Although this condition is present at birth it is not normally diagnosed until 4 or 5 years of age when the symptoms can be observed. It may be caused by a decrease in neurotransmitter levels attributable to reduced blood flow in specific areas of the brain. Boys are 3 times as likely as girls to be diagnosed with ADHD, which affects between 3% and 5% of school-age children. The symptoms and signs include impulsive, explosive, or irritable behavior. Although intelligence is not affected, work performance in school is sporadic because of the lack of the ability to focus on a task. Children that show signs of attention deficit without hyperactivity are normally diagnosed with attention deficit disorder or **ADD.** An older child or adult describes the symptoms as being easily distracted by irrelevant thoughts, sounds, or sights. Daydreaming is also a common symptom that can affect meeting deadlines, keeping track of school or work materials, and finishing assignments.

Prognosis. With proper treatment and understanding of this condition, the outlook for a normal productive life is very good.

Non–Drug Treatment. Education is extremely important in understanding this disorder. This normally involves the participation of several persons: parents, teachers, and therapists as well as the patient and physician. Treatment varies depending on the symptoms and the ability of the child to function at home and in school. Behavior modification, coaching, and supportive psychotherapy can help the patient cope with the disorder. To develop a treatment plan, parents are urged to understand the types of professionals available to treat the condition. The following list outlines the basic functions of each type of professional:

- Psychiatrists: Diagnose ADD and ADHD as well as prescribe medications.
- Psychologists: Diagnose ADD and ADHD, provide talk therapy, and explore feelings.
- Cognitive-behavioral therapists: Establish behavior modification programs at work, school, and/or at home. Create goals for behavior and achievement, and help families and teachers maintain rewards and consequences.
- Educational specialists: Teach techniques for succeeding in school; help children obtain accommodations from school (e.g., creating a quiet area to study, alternative testing). Advise families about assistive technologies (e.g., laptop computers, electronic planners).
- Behavioral coaches: Help adults find practical solutions to everyday problems. Teach organizational and time management techniques and methods to tackle procrastination and motivational problems

Drug Treatment. In certain cases the use of medications can help the patient. Stimulants are the most commonly used drugs followed by TCAs, antidepressants, mood stabilizers, and beta-adrenergic blockers that may help control the symptoms. Common CNS stimulants used include Ritalin (methylphenidate) and amphetamines such as Dexedrine (dextroamphetamine). For those who are prescribed these agents it is important to note that they are C-II drugs and patients can develop physical dependence (continued need to take). Persons who should not use methylphenidate or dextroamphetamine include those who have severe anxiety, glaucoma, overactive thyroid, Tourette's syndrome or a family history of Tourette's, heart defect, or irregular heartbeat; in addition, these drugs should be avoided if MAOIs have been taken within the previous 14 days. A list of agents used to treat ADD/ADHD is found in Table 17-10.

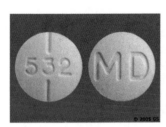

GENERIC NAME: methylphenidate C-II
TRADE NAME: Ritalin, Ritalin SR, Ritalin LA
INDICATION: ADD and ADHD
ROUTE OF ADMINISTRATION: oral
COMMON ADULT DOSAGE: immediate release formulas, 20 to 30 mg in divided doses (2 or 3 times) daily
COMMON CHILD DOSAGE: immediate release formulas, start with 5 mg twice daily with gradual increments of 5 mg to 10 mg weekly. Maximum: 60 mg/day
SIDE EFFECTS: dizziness, drowsiness, headache, loss of appetite, nausea, nervousness, stomach pain, trouble sleeping
AUXILIARY LABELS:
- May cause dizziness and drowsiness.
- Do not drink alcohol.
- Do not take MAOIs while using this medication.
- Take before meals (should be taken 30 to 45 minutes before meals).
- Do not stop medication abruptly.
NOTE: Not to be used in children under the age of 6 years.

TABLE 17-10 Agents Used to Treat ADD/ADHD. (Most products are for use in children >6 yr.; some extended-release products not acceptable for young children)

Trade Name	Generic Name	Dosage Forms	Notes
First-Line Treatment			
Ritalin and Ritalin LA or SR	methylphenidate, C-II	Tablets, LA: capsules, SR: tablets	LA: capsule form may be opened and sprinkled on food such as applesauce. SR: Tablet; do not crush, chew, or divide
Concerta		ER: Tablets	Do not crush, chew, or divide tablets.
Daytrana		Patch, transdermal	Apply topically once daily in AM; then remove after 9 hr.
Methylin		Chewable tablets: oral solution	
Metadate CD and ER		Tablets, CD: capsules, ER: tablets, ER	CD: Capsule form may be opened and sprinkled onto food such as applesauce. ER: Tablet; do not crush, chew, or divide.
Dexedrine and Dexedrine spansule SR	dextroamphetamine, C-II	Tablets, SR: spansules (capsules)	Do not crush, chew, or divide tablets or spansule.
Focalin, Focalin XR	dexmethylphenidate, C-II	Tablets, XR: capsules	XR: Capsule form may be opened and sprinkled onto food such as applesauce. Tablet; do not crush, chew, or divide.
Adderall, Adderall XR	amphetamine/ dextroamphetamine	Tablets, XR: capsules	XR: Capsule form may be opened and sprinkled onto food such as applesauce. Tablet; do not crush, chew, or divide.
Vyvanse	lisdexamfetamine	Capsules	Capsules may be opened and entire contents dissolved in a glass of water. Do not divide dose.
Strattera	atomoxetine	Capsules	May be taken with or without food. May be discontinued without tapering dose. Capsules should not be opened.

Medications and the Elderly

The elderly patient is likely to be more susceptible to the effects of psychotropic medications. Keep in mind that older persons are much more sensitive to certain medications because their bodies are not in the same condition as when they were younger. Because of the loss of muscle mass and changes in the functions of the organs, certain medications can become concentrated much easier than in a younger person. Organs such as the liver and kidneys take much longer to break down chemicals. According to the National Institute on Aging, older people over the age of 65 use more prescription and over-the-counter medications than any other age group. Because it is common for the elderly to take many medications at the same time, be sure to tell patients to inform the pharmacist of all the medications they are taking, including OTC drugs.

DO YOU REMEMBER THESE KEY POINTS?

- The main causes of insomnia
- The four types of depression discussed
- Various treatments for depression, including the types of agents used
- The differences between MAOIs, TCAs, and SSRIs
- The 5 types of schizophrenia discussed
- The circumstances under which a decanoate (long-acting) agent might be used
- The method of action of phenothiazines
- The major side effects of TCAs
- The foods that contain tyramine and why this knowledge is important if the person is taking MAOIs
- The reasons MAOIs are normally less popular than SSRIs and TCAs for treating depression
- The major OTC drugs that are available for treating insomnia
- The conditions that barbiturates are prescribed to treat and their schedules
- The conditions that benzodiazepines are prescribed to treat and their schedules

REVIEW QUESTIONS

Multiple choice questions

1. The blood-brain barrier protects the brain from:
   A. Toxins
   B. Drugs
   C. Large molecules
   D. All of the above

2. MAOIs should NOT be taken with which types of foods that are linked to high blood pressure?
   A. Meats, beer, and wine
   B. Meats, fruits, and wine
   C. Wine, meat, and dark green, leafy vegetables
   D. Wine, meat, and cheeses

3. A type of non–drug therapy for emotional problems may include:
   A. Family counseling
   B. Group therapy
   C. Visiting a psychologist
   D. All of the above

4. The illness that is marked by extremes in elevated and depressed moods is defined as:
   A. Schizophrenia
   B. Bipolar disorder
   C. Depression
   D. All of the above

5. Long-acting decanoate injections usually are given:
   A. Every other day
   B. Every week
   C. Every month
   D. In any of these combinations

6. The main neurotransmitters of the brain that are affected by benzodiazepines are:
   A. Dopamine
   B. Norepinephrine
   C. Epinephrine
   D. All of the above

7. Extrapyramidal effects that include shaky hands and head are caused mainly by:
   A. Overdosing MAOIs
   B. Overdosing TCAs
   C. Overdosing SSRIs
   D. All of the above

8. _____ is (are) the main drug(s) used for the treatment of manic phases of persons with bipolar disorder.
   A. TCAs
   B. SSRIs
   C. Lithium
   D. Diphenhydramine

9. The antidepressant class that has the most manageable side effects and is used for depression is:
   A. SSRIs
   B. MAOIs
   C. TCAs
   D. Benzodiazepines

10. SSRIs inhibit the reuptake inhibitors within the neuronal transmission, which increases the levels of:
    A. Norepinephrine
    B. Epinephrine
    C. Serotonin
    D. Dopamine

11. Which of the following terms are NOT used to describe types of this insomnia?
    A. Transient
    B. Severe
    C. Short-term
    D. Chronic

12. Which of the following conditions is NOT considered an anxiety disorder?
    A. PTSD
    B. Phobia
    C. OCD
    D. Schizophrenia

13. Cognitive therapy involves:
    A. Relearning how to think
    B. Electroconvulsive treatment
    C. Hypnosis treatment
    D. Antidepressant medications

14. The difference between OCD and OCPD is that persons with OCD _____, whereas those with OCPD _____.
    A. Feel they are sick, are okay with their behavior
    B. Take medications, do not take medications
    C. Have an early onset of the condition, have an onset that begins after adolescence
    D. None of the above

15. Lithium differs from other antipsychotic agents because it does not cause side effects such as:
    A. Sedation
    B. Depression
    C. Euphoria
    D. All of the above

True/False

If the statement is false, then change it to make it true.

_____ **1.** Tardive dyskinesia is a mental illness.

_____ **2.** Short-acting phenothiazines include oral fluphenazine (Prolixin), thioridazine (Mellaril), chlorpromazine (Thorazine), and trifluoperazine (Stelazine).

_____ **3.** Decanoate dosage forms include oral and parenteral.

_____ **4.** Persons taking SSRIs should avoid foods that contain tyramine.

_____ **5.** MAOIs are used less than SSRIs and TCAs because of their side effects.

_____ **6.** Insomnia can only be treated with prescription medications.

_____ **7.** Two of the most common auxiliary labels for benzodiazepines are "Take with plenty of water" and "Take with food."

_____ **8.** TCAs, MAOIs, and SSRIs can be used to treat bipolar behavior.

_____ **9.** Bipolar behavior also is referred to as a manic-depressive disorder.

_____ **10.** Hypnotic agents often are used to relax patients before procedures such as computed tomography scans.

_____ **11.** Non-benzodiazepine agents such as Z drugs do not have the same side effects as benzodiazepines and can be used long-term.

_____ **12.** All hypnotics and benzodiazepines are schedule IV drugs.

_____ **13.** Of the insomnia agents discussed, only eszopiclone is prescribed for both falling and staying asleep.

_____ **14.** Post-traumatic syndrome only affects soldiers returning from war.

_____ **15.** Extrapyramidal effects may cause drooling, shuffling gait, and the hands and head to shake.

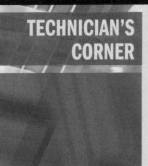

TECHNICIAN'S CORNER

The doctor has ordered Tofranil for a child who is 5 years old and weighs 45 lb. He orders 1.5 mg/kg per day to be given 3 times daily.

Is this dosage safe according to the *Drug Facts and Comparisons* recommendations?

How much drug per day would this child be given based on the dose ordered?

How much drug per dose would be given based on the dose ordered?

Is there a generic equivalent to Tofranil; if so, what other companies manufacture this drug?

BIBLIOGRAPHY

ADD & ADHD treatment, Referenced 10/09.www.helpguide.org/mental/adhd_add_treatments_coping.htm

AMA (American Medical Association) *Concise Medical Encyclopedia*. 2006.

Antipsychotics, Referenced 10/09 http://schizophrenia.emedtv.com/antipsychotics/antipsychotics-p2.html

Bipolar disorder, Referenced 10/09 www.nlm.nih.gov/MEDLINEPLUS/ency/article/000926.htm

Chabner D-E: *The language of medicine*, ed 9, 2010, Saunders.

Medications and Older People, FDA Consumer. Sept-Oct 1997 (Pub No FDA 03-1315C). Retrieved April 2006 from www.fda.gov/fdac/features/1997/697_old.html

Medicines: Use Them Safely. http://www.nyc.gov/html/dfta/downloads/pdf/health-meds.pdf

Non-benzodiazepines, Referenced 10/09. www.benzosupport.org/the_z_drugs.htm

Professional guide to diseases, ed 9, Ambler, PA, 2009, Lippincott Williams & Wilkins.
Types of OCD, Referenced 10/09. www.thehealthcenter.info/adult-ocd/types-of-obsessions-
and-compulsions.htm

WEBSITES

www.medterms.com
www.drugtopics.com/drugtopics
www.drugs.com

Respiratory System

Objectives

UPON COMPLETING THIS CHAPTER, YOU SHOULD BE ABLE TO DO
THE FOLLOWING:

- Define all terms used in this chapter and describe their role in the respiratory system.

- List the functions of the respiratory system.

- Describe the act of respiration—the exchange of oxygen and carbon dioxide between the air and cells in the body.

- Identify the components of the respiratory system outlined in this chapter.

- List the most common conditions that affect the lungs and the types of medications used to treat them.

- Differentiate between asthma and chronic obstructive pulmonary disease (COPD).

- Describe common respiratory tract infections such as colds, flu, pneumonia, sinusitis, and bronchitis.

- Describe other common respiratory conditions such as allergic rhinitis.

- List both generic and trade drug names covered in this chapter.

- List the classification and indication for each of the drugs described in this chapter.

- Choose the appropriate auxiliary labels when filling prescriptions for respiratory conditions.

- List the most common side effects for medications discussed in this chapter.

TERMS AND DEFINITIONS

Analgesic *A drug that reduces or eliminates pain*

Antipyretic *A drug that reduces or prevents fever*

Antitussive *A drug that can decrease the coughing reflex of the central nervous system*

Cough reflex *Response of the body to clear air passages of foreign substances and mucus by a forceful expiration*

Decongestant *An adrenergic drug that reduces swelling of the mucous membranes by constricting dilated blood vessels; decongestants reduce blood flow to nasal tissues, thus reducing nasal congestion*

Expectorant *A drug that helps remove mucous secretions from the respiratory system; it loosens and thins sputum and bronchial secretions for ease of expectoration*

Influenza *A respiratory tract infection caused by an influenza virus*

Metered dose inhaler *A device for supplying a predetermined dosage of medication(s) to the lungs through inhalation*

Nonproductive cough *A cough that does not produce mucous secretions from the respiratory tract*

Productive cough *A cough that expectorates mucous secretions from the respiratory tract*

Prophylaxis *Treatment given before an event or exposure to prevent the occurrence of a condition or symptom*

Sputum *Fluid (mucus) that is expectorated from the lungs and bronchial tissues*

Viscosity *The thickness of a solution or fluid*

COMMON DRUGS USED FOR RESPIRATORY CONDITIONS

Trade Name	Generic Name	Pronunciation	Trade Name	Generic Name	Pronunciation
Antihistamines			Claritin-D 12/24hr	loratadine/ pseudoephedrine	(lor-**at**-ah-**dean**/**soo**-doe-a-**fed**-rin)
Allegra	fexofenadine	(**fex**-oh-**fen**-a-deen)	Semprex-D	acrivastine/ pseudoephedrine	(**ak**-ri-vas-teen/ soo-doe-a-**fed**-rin)
Benadryl	diphenhydramine	(dye-fen-**high**-dra-meen)			
Chlor-Trimeton	chlorpheniramine	(klor-fen-**air**-ah-meen)	**Antitussives**		
Claritin	loratadine	(lor-**at**-ah-dean)	Delsym	dextromethorphan	(dex-troh-meht-**or**-fan)
Zyrtec	cetirizine	(se-**tir**-a-zeen)	Tessalon Perles	benzonatate	(ben-**zoe**-na-tate)
Antihistamine/Decongestant Combinations					
First Generation			**Antitussive/Antihistamine Combinations**		
Bromfed	brompheniramine/ pseudoephedrine	(brom-fen-**eer**-a-meen/ soo-doe-a-**fed**-rin)	Tussionex	hydrocodone/ chlorpheniramine	(**high**-droe-**koe**-doan/ **klor**-fen-**air**-ah-meen)
Deconamine	chlorpheniramine/ pseudoephedrine	(klor-fen-**eer**-a-meen/ soo-doe-a-**fed**-rin)	Phenergan/ codeine	promethazine/codeine	(pro-**meth**-a-zine/ **koe**-deen)
Rondec	carbinoxamine/ pseudoephedrine	(kar-bi-**nox**-ah-meen/ soo-doe-a-**fed**-rin)			
			Antitussive/Expectorant Combinations		
Second Generation			Hycotuss	hydrocodone/ guaifenesin	(**high**-droe-**koe**-doan/ gwi-**fen**-ah-sin)
Allegra-D	fexofenadine/ pseudoephedrine	(fex-oh-**fen**-a-deen/ soo-doe-a-**fed**-rin)			

COMMON DRUGS USED FOR RESPIRATORY CONDITIONS—cont'd

Trade Name	Generic Name	Pronunciation
Robitussin DM	guaifenesin/ dextromethorphan	(gwi-**fen**-ah-sin/ **dex**-troe- meth-**or**-fan)
Decongestants—Oral		
Sudafed	pseudoephedrine	(sue-doe-e-**fed**-dren)
Sudafed PE	phenylephrine	(**fen**-il-**ef**-rin)
Decongestants—Nasal		
Neo-Synephrine	phenylephrine	(**fen**-ill-**ef**-rin)
Afrin	oxymetazoline	(**ox**-e-**met**-azz-o-leen)
Expectorant		
Robitussin	guaifenesin	(gwi-**fen**-ah-sin)
Analgesic/Antihistamine/Decongestant Combinations		
Benadryl Allergy/ Cold	acetaminophen/ diphenhydramine/ phenylephrine	(a-**seet**-a-min-oh-fen/ dye-fen-**high**-dra-meen/ **fen**-il-**ef**-rin)
Analgesic/Cough Suppressant/Decongestant Combinations		
Comtrex Cold/ Cough Max Strength	acetaminophen/ dextromethorphan/ phenylephrine	(a-**seet**-a-min-oh-fen/ dex-troe-meth-**or**-fan/ **fen**-il-**ef**-rin)
Analgesic/Decongestant Combination		
Excedrin Sinus Headache	acetaminophen/ phenylephrine	(a-**seet**-a-min-oh-fen/ **fen**-il-**ef**-rin)
Cough Suppressant/Expectorant Combinations		
Certuss-D	dextromethorphan/ guaifenesin/ phenylephedrine	(dex-troe-meth-**or**-fan/ gwi-**fen**-ah-sin/ **fen**-il-e-**fed**-rin)
Cough Suppressant/Decongestant Combinations		
Respi-TANN	carbetapentane/ pseudoephedrine	(car-beta-**pen**-tane/ soo-doe-e-**fed**-rin)
P-V Tussin	hydrocodone/ pseudoephedrine	(high-droe-**koe**-dohn/ soo-doe-e-**fed**-rin)
Nucofed	codeine/ pseudoephedrine	(**koe**-deen/ soo-doe-eh-**fed**-rin)
Albatussin Pediatric	dextromethorphan/ phenylephrine	(dex-troe-meth-**or**-fan/ **fen**-il-**ef**-rin)
Decongestant/Antihistamine/Cough Suppressant Combinations		
Tussi-12D	carbetapentane/ phenylephrine/ pyrilamine	(car-beta-pen-tane/ **fen**-il-**ef**-rin/ peer-**il**-a-meen)
Decongestant/Antihistamine/Cough Suppressant/Analgesic		
NyQuil Muti-Symptom	acetaminophen/ dextromethorphan/ doxylamine/ pseudoephedrine	(a-**seet**-a-min-oh-fen/ dex-troe-meth-**or**-fan/ dox-il-a-**meen**/ **soo**-doe-e-**fed**-rin)

Trade Name	Generic Name	Pronunciation
Expectorant/Decongestant		
Prolex PD	guaifenesin/ phenylephrine	(gwi-**fen**-ah-sin/ **fen**-il-**ef**-rin)
Expectorant/Decongestant/Antihistamine Combinations		
Ryna-12X	guaifenesin/ phenylephrine/ pyrilamine	(gwi-**fen**-ah-sin/ **fen**-ill-**ef**-rin/ peer-**il**-a-meen)
Anticholinergics—Oral Inhalers		
Atrovent	ipratropium bromide	(**ip**-rah-**trow**-pea-um/ **bro**-mide)
Spiriva	tiotropium	(tye-oh-**troe**-pee-um)
Mucolytic		
Mucomyst	acetylcysteine	(a-**seet**-ill-**sis**-teen)
Bronchodilators		
Proventil HFA, Ventolin HFA	albuterol	(al-bu-**ter**-all)
Adrenalin	epinephrine	(ep-i-**nef**-rin)
Combivent	albuterol/ipratropium	(al-byoo-ter-ol/ **ip**-rah-**trow**-pee-um)
Isuprel	isoproterenol	(eye-so-pro-**tear**-in-all)
Alupent	metaproterenol	(met-a-pro-**tear**-in-all)
Foradil	formoterol	(for-**moe**-ter-ol)
Maxair	pirbuterol	(pur-**bu**-ter-all)
Serevent	salmeterol	(sal-**met**-er-ol)
Xopenex HFA	levalbuterol	(leh-val-**byoo**-ter-al)
Corticosteroids—Respiratory Inhalers		
Azmacort	triamcinolone	(try-am-**sin**-oh-lone)
AeroBid	flunisolide	(flew-**nis**-oh-lide)
Beclovent	beclomethasone	(beck-low-**meth**-ah-sone)
Flovent Diskus/ Flovent HFA	fluticasone	(floo-**tic**-ah-sone)
Pulmicort	budesonide	(byoo-**des**-oh-nide)
Mast Cell Stabilizers—Respiratory Inhalers		
Intal	cromolyn	(**krom**-oh-lin)
Corticosteroids—Nasal Inhalers		
Nasonex	mometasone	(moe-**met**-a-sone)
Rhinocort	budesonide	(byoo-**dess**-oh-nide)
Flonase	fluticasone	(floo-**tic**-ah-sone)
Mast Cell Stabilizers—Nasal		
Nasalcrom	cromolyn	(**krom**-oh-lin)
Immunomodulator		
Xolair	omalizumab	(**oh**-ma-**liz**-oo-mab)

COMMON DRUGS USED FOR RESPIRATORY CONDITIONS—cont'd

Trade Name	Generic Name	Pronunciation	Trade Name	Generic Name	Pronunciation
Leukotriene Inhibitors			Advair Diskus	fluticasone/salmeterol	(flu-**tick**-ah-sewn/ sal-**met**-er-ol)
Singulair	montelukast	(mon-tea-**loo**-cast)			
Accolate	zafirlukast	(zay-fur-**loo**-cast)	**Antitubercosis Agents**		
Zyflo	zileuton	(zi-**loo**-ton)	Generic only	isoniazid	(eye-**soe**-nye-a-**zid**)
			Myambutol	ethambutol	(e-tham-**byoo**-tole)
Xanthines			Generic only	pyrazinamide	(peer-ah-**zin**-a-mide)
Phyllocontin	aminophylline	(am-in-**off**-eh-lin)	Rifadin	rifampin	(rif-am-**pin**)
TheoDur	theophylline	(thee-**off**-ah-lin)	Streptomycin	streptomycin	(strep-**toe**-mye-sin)
Long-Acting Bronchodilator/Steroid Inhaler (Combination)					
Symbicort	budesonide/formoterol	(bue-**des**-oh-nide/ for-**moe**-ter-ol)			

Т HE LUNGS AND AIRWAYS play an important role in the body, working to keep us alive and well. We are acutely aware when the respiratory system is compromised. As seen in Figure 18-1, the respiratory system is composed of many structures, each having specific functions. For example, the lungs enable the body to extract oxygen from the atmosphere during inhalation and

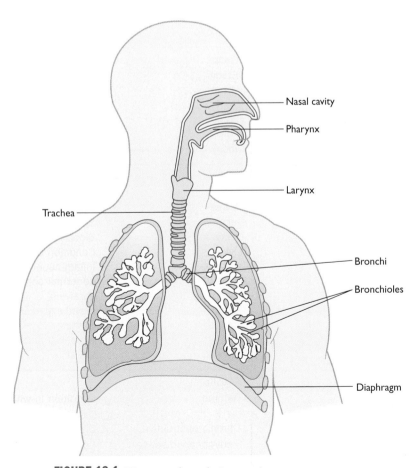

FIGURE 18-1 Diagram of respiratory system.

to remove carbon dioxide from the body during exhalation. The fine hairs of the nose and the mucosal lining of the bronchi act as filters to trap dust, microorganisms, and foreign particles. These unwanted particles are engulfed in mucus, propelled by cilia to the throat, and swallowed. In addition, the nose helps to heat and humidify cold, dry air so that it is more compatible with our body temperature. This chapter discusses the structures and functions of the components of the respiratory system, the events involved in the act of respiration, and the conditions that affect the respiratory system, including medications to treat them. The drug action, normal dosages, and any auxiliary labels that need to be affixed to prescriptions also are listed in this chapter.

RESPIRATORY TERMINOLOGY

Word Combinations	
Alveoli/o	Alveoli
Bronch/o, bronchi/o	Bronchi
Cyan/o	Blue
Epiglott/o	Epiglottis
Hem/o	Blood
Laryng/o	Larynx
Nas/o, rhin/o	Nose
Ox/i	Oxygen
Pharyng/o	Pharynx
Pleur/o	Pleura
Pneum/o, pulmon/o	Lungs, air
Sinus/o	Sinus
Thorac/o	Thorax, chest
Trache/o	Trachea

Prefixes	
Brady-	Slow
Hyper-	Excessive
Para-	Near
Phon-	Voice, sound
Poly-	Many
Tachy-	Rapid

Suffixes	
-al	Pertaining to
-dynia	Pain
-ectasis	Stretching
-emia	Blood
-isy	Condition of
-itis	Inflammation
-osis	Abnormal condition
-plegia	Paralysis
-pnea	Breathing
-ptysis	Spitting
-rrhea	Abnormal discharge
-thorax	Chest

Conditions	
Asthma	Condition in which narrowing and inflammation of airways impede breathing
Chronic obstructive pulmonary disease (COPD)	Disease that causes wheezing, tightness in chest, and coughing that produces large amount of mucus in airways and makes it difficult to breathe

RESPIRATORY TERMINOLOGY—cont'd

Croup	Childhood condition that causes obstruction of larynx, barking cough, and noisy breathing
Cystic fibrosis	Inherited disorder that causes production of very thick mucus in respiratory tract, causing difficulty in breathing and frequent respiratory tract infections
Influenza	Respiratory tract infection caused by an influenza virus
Laryngitis	Inflammation of larynx, causing loss of voice
Pleurisy	Inflammation of lining of lungs and lung cavities
Pneumothorax	Air in pleural spaces of lungs causes difficulty breathing
Pulmonary edema	Caused by fluid filling respiratory air sacs (alveoli) and bronchioles, impairing gas exchange in respiratory tract
Rhinitis	Irritation and inflammation of lining of nose, often accompanied by rhinorrhea (runny nose)
Sinusitis	Infection/inflammation of sinuses
Tuberculosis	Respiratory tract infection caused by bacterium *Mycobacterium tuberculosis*
Whooping cough	Also known as pertussis, a highly contagious respiratory disease caused by bacterium *Bordetella pertussis;* results in episodes of coughing ending in inspiration with a loud whooping sound

Tech Note!

Years ago, physicians quickly removed inflamed tonsils in children. Recently, it was discovered that the tonsils, which are part of the lymphatic system, help the body fight disease. Now physicians are less likely to perform a tonsillectomy as treatment for inflamed tonsils.

Structure and Function of the Respiratory System

The respiratory system resembles a large, multibranched tree that has been inverted. The large trunk is analogous to the trachea, and the two main branches represent the bronchi. The smaller branches are the bronchioles, and the leaves are the alveolar sacs where gas exchange takes place (Figure 18-2). Let us begin to take a more in-depth look at the respiratory tract, starting with the upper respiratory tract. The function of the respiratory system is to oxygenate the blood and remove carbon dioxide. The upper respiratory tract filters, warms, and moistens air before it enters the lower respiratory tract.

UPPER RESPIRATORY SYSTEM

The upper respiratory system is composed of the nose and nasal cavities, the pharynx (i.e., the throat), and the larynx (i.e., the voice box). A mucosal lining covers the inside of the respiratory tract. More than 125 mL (approximately ½ cup) of mucus is produced each day by the body. The mucus not only forms a protective blanket over much of the respiratory tract but also serves as an air purification mechanism by trapping inhaled irritants such as dust and pollens. The nasal septum separates the interior of the nose into two distinct cavities. The cavities also are lined by a mucous membrane with small microscopic hair-like structures called cilia. The function of the mucous membrane is to warm and moisten inhaled air. The cilia catch small dust particles in the air that we breathe. The nose also functions as the organ for the sense of smell and acts as a drainage system for tears from the eye. The pharynx is a tube approximately 5 inches long that is shared with the digestive system. Food passes into the esophagus and air flows through the trachea, also known as the windpipe. The tonsils, composed of lymphatic tissue, are located in the pharynx.

The larynx also is known as the voice box because it contains the vocal cords responsible for the sounds that we produce. Compared to men, the larynx of women is much smaller and does not protrude from the neck. This cartilage

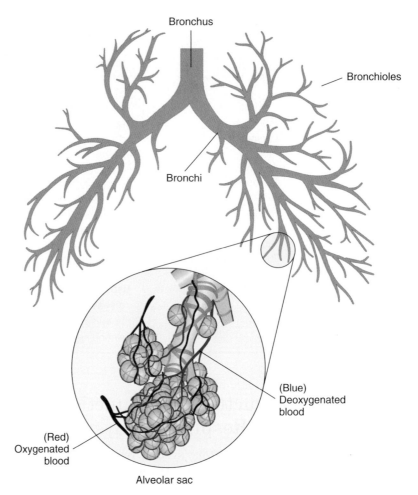

FIGURE 18-2 Bronchial tree.

(usually only visible in men) is referred to as the "Adam's apple." The vocal cords are in the larynx. They provide air distribution and voice production.

The epiglottis, a thin leaf-shaped structure, is located at the entrance of the larynx. Its function is to obstruct the trachea automatically when swallowing takes place to keep food, liquid, and saliva from entering the airway. If food enters the trachea rather than the esophagus, choking occurs. The epiglottis is formed by one piece of cartilage.

LOWER RESPIRATORY SYSTEM

The lower respiratory system is composed of the trachea, bronchial tree, and lungs. The trachea (windpipe) is approximately $4\frac{1}{2}$ inches long. It is lined with a mucous membrane that traps airborne particles; cilia (fine, microscopic, hair-like structures) then propel the particles upward, where they are swallowed. The trachea branches into two structures called the right bronchus and left bronchus, leading to the right and left lungs, respectively. The right bronchus is bigger than the left because the heart displaces some of the left side of the chest. The trachea has incomplete rings of cartilage reinforcing it so that it will not collapse when the neck is bent.

In turn, each bronchus branches into smaller bronchi and then into smaller bronchioles. The function of the bronchioles is to provide oxygen distribution and a passageway for air to reach the alveoli. The bronchioles end in millions of clusters of microscopic alveolar sacs deep in the lungs. It is in the alveolar sacs where respiration occurs—oxygen and carbon dioxide are exchanged in the tiny capillaries surrounding the alveoli. Oxygen diffuses from the alveoli into the bloodstream for use by the body and carbon dioxide passes from the blood into the alveoli for exhalation.

The lungs fill the chest cavity, except for the space occupied by the heart and large vessels. The lungs are divided into lobes: three in the right lung and two in the left. The right lung has a greater volume capacity, whereas the left lung is longer and has less capacity. The consistency of the lung is like that of a sponge because of the millions of alveolar sacs and their surrounding connective tissue. The lungs are separated from each other by the mediastinum, the region of the thoracic cavity in which the heart is located. The left lung has an indentation on its surface, called the cardiac notch, to accommodate the apex of the heart. The main function of the lungs is breathing, also known as pulmonary ventilation.

The pleural cavity is the area in which the lungs are located. The pleural membrane can be divided into the visceral pleura and the parietal pleura. The visceral pleura is attached directly to the surface of each lung while the parietal pleura lines the wall of the thorax. Within the parietal pleura, a small amount of fluid is produced that fills the gap between the visceral and parietal areas and surrounds the lungs. It serves to reduce friction between the lungs and the chest wall during breathing. At the base of the chest cavity is a major respiratory muscle called the diaphragm. This large dome-shaped muscle separates the chest cavity from the abdominal cavity. It contracts and flattens during inhalation, and it relaxes during exhalation.

RESPIRATION

The act of respiration can be divided into two distinct phases: inspiration, the movement of air into the lungs; and expiration, the movement of air out of the lungs. The thorax is another name for the chest cavity. The changes in the size and shape of the thorax during respiration cause a change in air pressure. This change in pressure, resulting from expansion and contraction of the chest wall caused by the raising and lowering of the diaphragm (breathing), causes air to move into and out of the lungs. As a person actively inhales (inspiration), the muscles of the diaphragm and intercostals contract. Specifically, the diaphragm flattens while the intercostal muscles expand the size of the chest cavity, resulting in an increase in the size of the thoracic cavity. This increased volume of the chest cavity causes the pressure inside the lungs to be lower than the atmospheric pressure, resulting in air flowing into the lungs. Expiration, however, is usually a passive response because, unlike inspiration, its mechanism of action does not require any energy. As the chest relaxes during expiration, the thorax returns to its resting size and shape. The reduction in the size of the thoracic cavity causes the pressure within the thorax to increase, and air flows from the lungs to outside the body.

EXCHANGE OF GASES

The air we breathe is composed of approximately 21% oxygen, 79% nitrogen, and less than 0.5% carbon dioxide. As we breathe, the lungs exchange inspired oxygen for carbon dioxide (waste) carried by the blood to the lungs. This waste then is expelled from our lungs. An average adult inhales approximately 250 mL of oxygen and produces approximately 200 mL of carbon dioxide per minute at rest.

After air travels through the bronchioles, it enters more narrow corridors (the alveolar sacs). In the alveolus, each oxygen molecule is able to move across

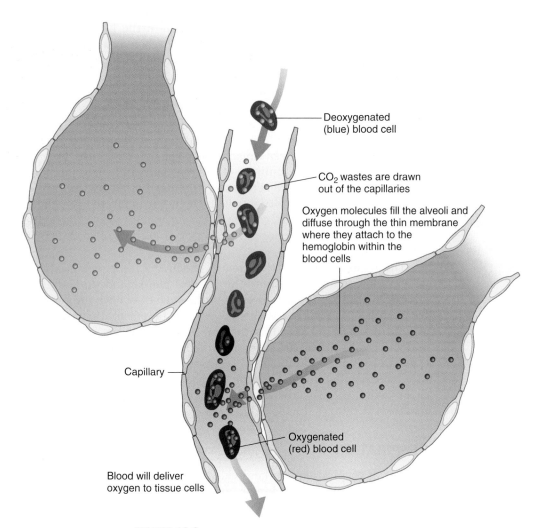

FIGURE 18-3 Exchange of oxygen and carbon dioxide.

the thin membrane into the waiting blood cells that are passing closely by on the other side of the membrane. The moving blood cells drop off carbon dioxide molecules before picking up oxygen molecules. The carbon dioxide molecules then move out of the lung capillary blood supply into the alveolar sacs and out of the body via expired air. The fully saturated blood moves into larger veins where it returns to the left atrium of the heart via four pulmonary veins. From the left atrium, blood flows into the left ventricle, where it is pumped through the aorta into the arteries, replenishing oxygen to all tissues and organs (Figure 18-3).

The regulation of respiration permits the body to adjust to varying demands for oxygen supply and carbon dioxide removal. This is done efficiently with help from the respiratory center within the medulla oblongata. The medulla is situated in the brainstem and is influenced by various receptors located in other areas of the body. The exchange of oxygen and carbon dioxide also helps keep the pH of our blood balanced. The body uses some of the carbon dioxide to make bicarbonate, which maintains the blood pH either by reducing the amount of hydrogen in the blood, causing the pH to become more alkaline, or by increasing the amount of hydrogen, making the blood more acidic. The blood pH must remain close to 7.4 to sustain life.

Tech Note!

Although we inhale 79% nitrogen with each breath, it is not used by the body. Instead, we exhale the nitrogen back into the atmosphere along with carbon dioxide and excess oxygen molecules.

TABLE 18-1 Types of Breathing Dysfunction

Condition	Description
Apnea	Respiration stops
Bradypnea	Slow breathing
Cyanosis	Lack of oxygen causes skin to turn blue-gray
Dyspnea	Labored or difficult breathing
Hyperventilation	Deep and rapid breathing
Hypopnea	Shallow, inadequate breathing
Orthopnea	Labored or difficult breathing while lying down
Tachypnea	Rapid breathing

BREATHING

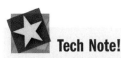

Tech Note!

The average respiratory rate for adults is 12 to 18 breaths per minute, whereas a child's rate is 40 breaths per minute.

Breathing is an involuntary mechanism. This means you do not have to think about it; the body automatically exhales and inhales when needed. The respiratory control center, located in the medulla in the brainstem, automatically controls the rate and depth of breathing. During inspiration, impulses in the inspiratory area of the respiratory center trigger the phrenic and intercostal nerves, causing the diaphragm and intercostal muscles, respectively, to contract, and inspiration occurs. As the lungs fill with air, nerve impulses originating in the expiratory area of the respiratory center trigger the muscles to relax, and expiration occurs.

Depending on the size of the person, breathing rates will vary: the smaller the size, the faster the rate of breathing. The breathing rates of small children can be twice as fast as the adult rate. The normal amount of air expelled from the lungs in a typical exhalation is approximately 500 mL, or 0.5 L, for an average adult, although the total lung capacity is more than 5 L of air. When a person is running, the body needs more oxygen than when sitting or sleeping. The elasticity of the lungs allows the capacity to vary widely depending on the need for oxygen. Table 18-1 lists common breathing problems.

SNEEZING

A common reflex action that occurs is sneezing. Breathing irritating materials, such as dust or dander, into the respiratory passageway causes the body to expel the foreign substance. The three mechanisms that cause someone to sneeze are (1) ciliary action, (2) peristaltic motion of the bronchioles, and (3) **cough reflex**. When foreign particles encounter the sensory receptors of the ciliary hairs, they trigger the reflex of deep inspiration, which then is followed by closure of the vocal cords. The vocal cords remain closed until the actual sneeze is underway, at which point the outward push of air expels the foreign material from the passageways, usually accompanied by a loud noise. Other examples of air movement include coughing, yawning, hiccupping, sighing, crying, and laughing.

Disorders/Conditions of the Respiratory System

UPPER RESPIRATORY SYSTEM

Many conditions affect the respiratory system. Some may be genetic, and others may be attributable to contagious infections, habits such as smoking, and other environmental factors. The symptoms of a respiratory illness are noticeable because of the abnormal breathing and coughing symptoms that typically accompany the various conditions. Although upper respiratory conditions are diverse,

TABLE 18-2 Conditions of the Upper Respiratory System

Upper Respiratory Conditions	Symptoms	Symptomatic Medication Treatment
Colds: viral	Stuffy nose, sore throat, sneezing, headache, muscle aches	Decongestants, antihistamines, analgesics
Influenza:* viral	Fever, chills, headache, muscle aches, fatigue, cough	Analgesics, antipyretics
Strep throat: bacterial	Fever, headache, vomiting, sore throat	Antibiotics, analgesics, antipyretics
Bronchitis:* bacterial, viral	Cough, shortness of breath (SOB), fatigue, chest pain	Bronchodilators, analgesics
Allergic rhinitis	Stuffy nose, congestion	Antihistamines/nasal corticosteroids
Sinusitis	Stuffy nose, headache, congestion	Antihistamines/nasal corticosteroids

*Bronchitis and influenza affect both upper and lower respiratory tracts.

similar types of medications are used to treat most of these conditions, which are often infectious. These include **antitussives**, **analgesics**, and **antipyretics**. For more severe conditions, which may involve bacterial infection or allergy, antibiotics and corticosteroids may be prescribed. Table 18-2 lists conditions, symptoms, and the types of medications used for their treatment. The following sections describe the causes and symptoms of typical respiratory disorders. Both nonmedical treatments and medications are listed with indication, side effects, route of administration, common dosages, and auxiliary labels if applicable. Many agents can be purchased over-the-counter (Chapter 8).

Common Cold

A cold is an infection of the nasal passages and upper respiratory tract normally caused by a rhinovirus. Because there are more than 140 cold viruses, the common cold has remained an untreatable illness; many medications are currently available that can alleviate the symptoms. Common symptoms include coughing, congestion, and sometimes wheezing within the upper respiratory tract. Other symptoms that accompany colds are rhinitis (inflammation and irritation of the lining of the nose), pharyngitis (sore throat), rhinorrhea (runny nose), and coughing. Efforts to reduce the transmission of the common cold usually focus on preventive measures to help limit spread of the viruses, such as good hygiene (e.g., hand washing, proper sneezing techniques) and use of sanitizers and occasionally face masks.

Prognosis. For most people colds are a part of life. With rest and time, a cold will run its course with no permanent damage. There are disorders, however, in which a cold can exacerbate a preexisting condition, such as persons with asthma, emphysema, and bronchitis or persons who are immunocompromised. For these patient populations care must be taken when using certain OTC medications because they may worsen an underlying condition. A physician or pharmacist can provide information on which agents to avoid. For a sample, see Box 18-1.

Non–Drug Treatment. Drinking plenty of water and getting enough rest are important when fighting a cold. To help relieve congestion that worsens at night, a vaporizer may be used. Gargling with warm salt water can help provide relief from a sore throat.

Drug Treatment. Common symptomatic treatments include decongestants, antihistamines, antitussives, and expectorants. These are available in a variety of dosage forms such as liquids, lozenges, nasal sprays, and oral tablets and

BOX 18-1 EXAMPLES OF CONDITIONS THAT MAY BE AFFECTED BY OTC MEDICATIONS

OTC medication side effects include elevated blood pressure and heart rate. Persons with liver or kidney disease should always check with a health care professional before product selection. Persons with the following conditions should also consult their physician before using the following OTC agents for colds or allergies:

Asthma: antihistamines, bronchodilators
Chronic bronchitis: antihistamines
Diabetes: decongestants
Emphysema: antihistamines
Glaucoma: decongestants, bronchodilators
Heart disease: decongestants, bronchodilators
High blood pressure: decongestants
Enlarged prostate: antihistamines, decongestants
Thyroid disease: decongestants

capsules (Table 18-3). In general, product selection should be aimed at the specific symptoms troublesome to the patient.

RELIEF OF SORE THROAT

GENERIC NAME: zinc combinations
TRADE NAME: Halls Zinc Defense
INDICATION: to decrease the duration of the common cold and for the relief of sore throat
ROUTE OF ADMINISTRATION: oral
COMMON ADULT DOSAGE: 5-mg lozenges as needed
SIDE EFFECTS: taste disturbance
AUXILIARY LABEL:
■ OTC agent; none needed

LOCAL ANESTHETICS FOR THROAT PAIN

GENERIC NAME: benzocaine/menthol
TRADE NAME: Chloraseptic relief strips
INDICATION: for the relief of sore throat
ROUTE OF ADMINISTRATION: oral
COMMON ADULT DOSAGE: 2 strips per dose (dissolved one at a time); may be repeated every 2 hours as needed, not to exceed recommended daily dose
SIDE EFFECTS: numbness of the throat and/or mouth
AUXILIARY LABEL:
■ OTC agent; none needed

GENERIC NAME: benzocaine, cetylpyridium chloride
TRADE NAME: Cepacol lozenges
INDICATION: for the relief of sore throat
ROUTE OF ADMINISTRATION: oral
COMMON ADULT DOSAGE: one lozenge every 2 hr as needed, not to exceed recommended daily dose
SIDE EFFECTS: numbness of the throat and/or mouth
AUXILIARY LABEL:
■ OTC; none needed

TABLE 18-3 Combination Agents Sold OTC for Symptoms of Colds, Hay Fever, Allergies, Flu, and Respiratory Tract Infections

Trade Name	Generic Combination	Indication	Dosage Forms
Albatussin Pediatric	dextromethorphan/ phenylephrine	Congestion and cough caused by colds, flu, or hay fever	Drops, syrup
Alka-Seltzer Plus Cold/Cough	acetaminophen/ chlorpheniramine/ dextromethorphan/ pseudoephedrine	Pain, sinus congestion, runny nose, sneezing, and cough caused by colds, upper respiratory tract infections, and allergies	Capsules, oral solution
Tylenol Cold	acetaminophen/ dextromethorphan/ phenylephrine	Pain, sinus congestion, runny nose, sneezing, and cough caused by colds, upper respiratory tract infections, and allergies	Capsules, oral solution
Benadryl Allergy plus Cold	acetaminophen/ diphenhydramine/ phenylephrine	Runny, stuffy nose, sinus congestion, sneezing, itchy nose, itchy or watery eyes, sore throat, cough, headache, and pain or fever caused by common cold or allergies	Tablets, syrup
Certuss-D	dextromethorphan/ guaifenesin/ phenylephrine	Stuffy nose, sinus congestion, cough, and chest congestion caused by common cold or flu	Extended release tablets
Comtrex Cold/ Cough Max Strength	acetaminophen/ dextromethorphan/ phenylephrine	Pain, congestion, and cough caused by colds, flu, or hay fever	Capsules, tablets
Excedrin Sinus Headache	acetaminophen/ phenylephrine	Pain and sinus congestion caused by colds, upper respiratory tract infections, and allergies	Tablets
Nucofed	codeine/ pseudoephedrine	Congestion and cough caused by colds, flu, or hay fever	Capsules
NyQuil Muti-Symptom	acetaminophen/ dextromethorphan/ doxylamine/ pseudoephedrine	Pain, sinus congestion, runny nose, sneezing, and cough caused by colds, upper respiratory tract infections, and allergies	Capsules
P-V Tussin	hydrocodone/ pseudoephedrine	Congestion and cough caused by colds, flu, or hay fever	Tablets
Respi-TANN	carbetapentane/ pseudoephedrine	Sinus congestion and cough caused by colds, upper respiratory tract infections, and allergies	Chewable tablets, liquid suspension
Ryna-12X, Decolate, Q-Tussin Pediatric	guaifenesin/ phenylephrine/ pyrilamine	Stuffy nose, sneezing, watery eyes, and cough caused by hay fever, colds, or flu	Tablets
Tussi-12D	carbetapentane/ phenylephrine/ pyrilamine	Sinus congestion, runny nose, sneezing, and cough caused by colds, upper respiratory tract infections, and allergies	Tablets
Zotex-GP	guaifenesin/ phenylephrine	Cough and stuffy nose caused by hay fever or common cold; also thins mucus to make cough more productive	Tablets

ANTITUSSIVES (REDUCE COUGHING)

GENERIC NAME: guaifenesin; dextromethorphan
TRADE NAME: Robitussin DM
INDICATION: nonproductive cough with chest congestion
ROUTE OF ADMINISTRATION: oral
COMMON ADULT DOSAGE: 10 mL every 4 hr up to a maximum of 6 doses/day
SIDE EFFECTS: nausea, dizziness, drowsiness
AUXILIARY LABEL:
- OTC; none needed

GENERIC NAME: dextromethorphan
TRADE NAME: Delsym
INDICATION: nonproductive coughs
ROUTE OF ADMINISTRATION: oral
COMMON ADULT DOSAGE: 10 mL every 12 hr; do not exceed 20 mL/day
SIDE EFFECTS: drowsiness, constipation; avoid alcohol may intensify drowsiness
AUXILIARY LABEL:
- none; OTC

Narcotic Antitussive/Expectorant. These agents may be prescribed for severe cases of uncontrollable coughing.

GENERIC NAME: hydrocodone and guaifenesin
TRADE NAME: Hycotuss Expectorant Syrup 100 mg/5 mL (C-III)
INDICATION: nonproductive cough (dry cough)
ROUTE OF ADMINISTRATION: oral
COMMON ADULT DOSAGE: 10 to 20 mg (2 to 4 mL) every 4 to 6 hours
SIDE EFFECTS: drowsiness, constipation, nausea, and vomiting
AUXILIARY LABELS:
- Do not drink alcohol.
- Alcohol intensifies the effects.
- Take with food.
- Take with plenty of water.

GENERIC NAME: promethazine/codeine
TRADE NAME: Phenergan/codeine (C-V)
INDICATION: severe cough
ROUTE OF ADMINISTRATION: oral
COMMON ADULT DOSAGE: 5 mL every 4 to 6 hours, not to exceed 30 mL in 24 hours
SIDE EFFECTS: nausea, vomiting, drowsiness, and constipation
AUXILIARY LABEL:
- May cause drowsiness
- May cause dizziness

GENERIC NAME: phenylpropanolamine/hydrocodone
TRADE NAME: Hycomine (C-III)
INDICATION: congestion and cough
ROUTE OF ADMINISTRATION: oral
COMMON ADULT DOSAGE: 5 mL every 4 hours as needed, not to exceed 30 mL in 24 hours
SIDE EFFECTS: drowsiness, constipation, nausea, and vomiting
AUXILIARY LABELS:
- Do not drink alcohol.
- Alcohol will intensify the effects.
- Take with food.
- Take with plenty of water.

Expectorants (Promote Coughing). **Expectorants** are agents that break up thick mucous secretions of the lungs or bronchi so that they can be expelled from the respiratory system through coughing. The main example of an expectorant is guaifenesin. Following administration of expectorants, the patient should be told to increase fluid intake to assist with thinning of mucous secretions.

EXPECTORANT (OTC)

GENERIC NAME: guaifenesin
TRADE NAME: Robitussin
INDICATION: chest congestion
ROUTE OF ADMINISTRATION: oral
COMMON ADULT DOSAGE: 200 to 400 mg (10 to 20 mL) every 4 hours, not to exceed 6 doses/day
SIDE EFFECTS: dizziness, headache, nausea, and vomiting

Nasal Decongestants (Sympathomimetics). **Decongestants** affect the adrenergic receptors of the vascular smooth muscle, causing vasoconstriction and a decrease in mucus production.

DECONGESTANTS (OTC)

GENERIC NAME: pseudoephedrine
TRADE NAME: Sudafed
INDICATION: nasal congestion
ROUTE OF ADMINISTRATION: oral, nasal
COMMON ADULT DOSAGE: 30 mg every 4 to 6 hours
SIDE EFFECTS: insomnia, restlessness; persons suffering from hypertension (high blood pressure) should use caution as pseudoephedrine may raise blood pressure
NOTE: Pseudoephedrine is now a regulated drug. Because of the misuse of a key component used in making the street drug methamphetamine, its OTC sales' quantity is now limited across the U.S. Refer to Chapter 2 for more information on this drug.

GENERIC NAME: phenylephrine
TRADE NAME: Sudafed PE (oral); Neo-Synephrine (nasal)
INDICATION: nasal congestion
ROUTE OF ADMINISTRATION: Sudafed PE (oral); Neo-Synephrine (nasal)
COMMON ADULT DOSAGE: Sudafed PE (oral), 1 to 2 tablets every 4 hours; Neo-Synephrine (nasal), 1 to 2 sprays every 4 hours
SIDE EFFECTS: nasal congestion; nasal decongestants may cause congestion if used longer than a few days; this is referred to as rebound congestion

GENERIC NAME: oxymetazoline
TRADE NAME: Afrin
INDICATION: nasal congestion; allergic rhinitis
ROUTE OF ADMINISTRATION: nasal spray
COMMON ADULT DOSAGE: 2 or 3 sprays every 10 to 12 hours
SIDE EFFECTS: nasal congestion; can cause rebound congestion if used longer than a few days

Laryngitis

Hoarseness is another problem affecting the vocal cords and may be caused by several conditions. Laryngitis is the temporary loss of speech resulting from an inflammation, irritation, or viral infection of the larynx. Both acute and chronic types of laryngitis occur and each must be treated differently. Acute cases are

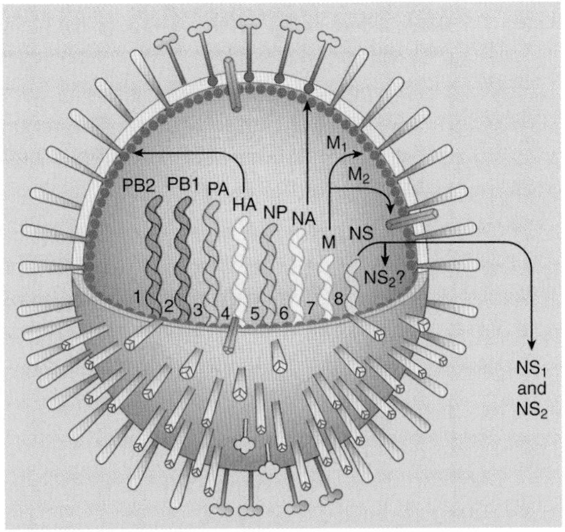

FIGURE 18-4 Influenza. (From Goldman M: *Procedures in cosmetic dermatology series: Photodynamic therapy*, ed 2, St Louis, 2008, Saunders/Courtesy Dr. Robert G. Webster.)

normally caused by viral infections or overuse of the vocal cords. Chronic laryngitis may result from other infections (such as sinusitis), gastroesophageal reflux disease (GERD), constant overuse of the voice (e.g., singers), or inhaled irritants.

Prognosis. Most cases will run their course and do not need to be treated. With proper lifestyle changes, laryngitis may be avoided. This involves not smoking, preventing or treating GERD, and avoiding irritants.

Non–Drug Treatment. Drinking plenty of water, using a hot humidifier, and resting the larynx are the best ways to treat laryngitis. Do not smoke.

Drug Treatment. There is no common medication to treat hoarseness; instead, resting the vocal cords should restore the voice within a couple of days. Lozenges soothe the throat. In extreme cases, corticosteroids can be used to reduce swelling.

Influenza

A more severe type of viral respiratory illness is known as the flu or **influenza** (Figure 18-4). Three types of viruses cause influenza: types A, B, and C. Type A can infect people, pigs, birds, seals, whales, horses, and other animals. Type B only affects humans, and type C viruses cause mild illness in humans. This infection attacks the respiratory system, including the nose, throat, bronchial tubes, and lungs. This illness strikes 50 million people each year (www.mayoclinic.com); each strain of virus usually is named after the region where it was first detected. Influenza is responsible for millions of dollars of lost wages and health care costs annually. Influenza can be deadly, especially to the very young, the elderly, or the immunocompromised.

Prognosis. With proper treatment most people recover from influenza; however, older persons or those with a weakened immune system can experience a slow recovery or even death. Obtaining a flu vaccine annually is the best way to avoid or lessen the risk of contracting influenza.

Non–Drug Treatment. Normally the best remedy is bed rest and drinking plenty of fluids.

BOX 18-2 VACCINATIONS (PREVENTION GUIDELINES)

All types of influenza vaccinations normally are given each influenza season (fall through spring in the United States). The recommendations of the Advisory Committee on Immunization Practices (ACIP) are listed below. For more information on vaccines and vaccinations, refer to Chapter 28.

- All persons 6 to 18 years of age
- Persons older than 50 years of age
- Women who will be pregnant during the influenza season
- Persons who have immunosuppression
- Persons who have chronic pulmonary, cardiovascular (except hypertension), renal, hepatic, cognitive, neurological, neuromuscular, hematological, or metabolic disorders
- Health care personnel
- Household caregivers of persons who are at high risk of contracting influenza

Drug Treatment. For severe influenza (types A, B) antivirals may be prescribed at the early onset of the symptoms (usually within 48 hours), to help shorten the course or lessen the severity of the illness. Some strains are resistant to antiviral medications. Vaccines are commonly given during the peak flu season. Guidelines for receiving vaccinations are listed in Box 18-2.

H1N1 (Swine Flu)

The H1N1 (swine flu) is a newer type of influenza that is being followed closely by the Centers for Disease Control and Prevention (CDC). Cases developed in the United States in April 2009. Originally it was referred to as the swine flu because of the similarities to the strains present in North American pigs. However, as the new virus was examined it was found to be more similar to infections noted in pigs from Europe and Asia. It was then given the name of H1N1 flu. The CDC has established that the illness is transferred from person to person in the same manner as the common flu (i.e., sneezing, coughing); however, the degree of contagion of the strain is unknown. The transfer of the virus is not through pork products; it is an airborne virus. Virtually all countries now have reported cases of the virus.

Prognosis. At this time, the CDC has no information on how widespread this influenza will become. Their primary goal is to compile the information gathered from all reported cases and to test the virus to determine whether it could evolve into a pandemic. Along with the CDC, the World Health Organization (WHO) and state and local health agencies are keeping track of the virus. Persons with weakened immune systems, children younger than 5 years, and pregnant women are at higher risk than the normal population. Normally, persons older than age 65 are also more susceptible to influenza; however, this does not appear to be the case with the H1N1 virus.

Non–Drug Treatment. Standard methods of prevention include adhering to meticulous hand hygiene, covering the mouth when sneezing or coughing, refraining from touching the eyes or mouth, and avoiding close contact with sick persons. A person who has H1N1 influenza may infect others 1 day before the manifestation of symptoms until 7 days after the onset of the illness. If infection occurs, the patient is advised to stay at home for 24 hours after symptoms are no longer present.

Drug Treatment. There is no active treatment for H1N1 influenza outside of typical supportive care. A vaccine to prevent the illness became available in the United States during late fall of 2009. In 2010, the annual influenza vaccine incorporated coverage of this new flu strain.

Rhinitis

Rhinitis is irritation and inflammation of the mucous membranes lining the nasal passage. It is caused by several different factors, including colds, influenza, allergens (see Allergies), air pollution, or strong odors (such as perfume, chemicals, or even certain medications). Rhinitis is either acute (e.g., colds or flu) or chronic (e.g., continuous or seasonal exposure to allergens). Common symptoms include runny and itchy nose, sneezing, congestion, and postnasal drip. Postnasal drip is due to the accumulation of mucus in the back of the nose and throat. Additional symptoms may include coughing, runny/watery eyes, and headache.

Prognosis. Rhinitis caused by colds or flu is normally short-lived, subsiding over several days, whereas chronic rhinitis is a continuing condition that may need treatment throughout life or every allergy season.

Non–Drug Treatments. Cold or flu viruses causing rhinitis can be treated with salt water; when used as an irrigating solution, salt water helps relieve postnasal drip symptoms. For allergens (see Allergies) causing rhinitis, symptoms can be lessened through several actions, including employing air purifiers or humidifiers within the home, using cotton bedding, keeping windows closed during pollen season, and avoiding live plants in the home. Animals that cause allergies should be bathed often to lessen dander.

Drug Treatments. The primary treatment for rhinitis regardless of the cause is nasal sprays, such as beclomethasone, flunisolide, budesonide, mometasone, and fluticasone, all of which are steroids that decrease inflammation within the nose. Additional medications include antihistamines and decongestants. Guaifenesin can be used to thin mucus, making it easier to expectorate. Allergy shots can also help those who suffer from seasonal or perennial allergies although this can only be done once the allergen is identified.

RX NASAL CORTICOSTEROIDS

GENERIC NAME: triamcinolone
TRADE NAME: Nasacort AQ
INDICATION: symptoms of hay fever and other nasal allergies
ROUTE OF ADMINISTRATION: nasal spray
COMMON ADULT DOSAGE: 2 sprays into each nostril once daily
SIDE EFFECTS: headache, minor nosebleed, sinus pain, cough, sore throat

GENERIC NAME: fluticasone
TRADE NAME: Flonase
INDICATION: symptoms of seasonal and perennial allergic rhinitis
ROUTE OF ADMINISTRATION: nasal spray
COMMON ADULT DOSAGE: 1 or 2 sprays into each nostril once daily.
SIDE EFFECTS: headache, minor nosebleed, sinus pain, cough, sore throat

Allergies

An allergy is the response of our immune system to an unrecognized substance. This response does not occur in all people and varies widely. In certain people, the allergic response can be severe to life-threatening. Types of allergens vary widely and include pollens, animal dander, foods, medications, chemicals, or environmental pollutants. Allergies are one of the most common types of respiratory problems, experienced by approximately 50 million people in the United States alone. Drinking plenty of fluids can thin the mucus associated with postnasal drip and aid in its expectoration. Symptoms and reactions include rash, hives, itching, and nasal congestion. Severe reactions can cause stomach pain, vomiting, wheezing, shortness of breath (SOB), low blood pressure, swelling of the throat, and anaphylactic (life-threatening) shock if left untreated.

Prognosis. If treated properly most allergic reactions can be controlled or the symptoms lessened. If the allergen is identified, allergy shots can be used to lessen the symptoms.

Non–Drug Treatment. Avoiding specific allergens is the best way to prevent an allergic reaction. If a reaction does occur, the type and severity of the allergic response determine whether treatment can be handled with or without medications. For allergic reactions caused by allergens in the home, removing and/or cleaning the irritant works best. Using a humidifier and/or air purifier may lessen the concentration of an airborne allergen. Foods and medications that need to be avoided should be documented in the patient's medical chart, and in certain cases wristbands should be worn that list allergies. Exposure to outdoor allergens can be lessened by wearing a face mask or by staying indoors on days in which environmental pollutants or pollen levels are high.

Drug Treatments. Many of the medications used for allergies mimic those used for colds. Allergy medications include oral, intranasal, ophthalmic, and topical antihistamines and/or decongestants. Many allergy medications can be obtained without a prescription as over-the-counter (OTC) drugs. Most OTC antihistamines cause drowsiness as a side effect; however, there are OTC medications now available that either have a mild sedative effect or cause no sedation at all. Other agents require a prescription, such as oral corticosteroids, intranasal or respiratory corticosteroids, leukotriene inhibitors, and epinephrine. In severe life-threatening cases, injectable epinephrine may be used to open airways. A list of both OTC and prescription medications available is found in Table 18-4.

OTC ANTIHISTAMINES

GENERIC NAME: diphenhydramine
TRADE NAME: Benadryl
INDICATION: coughs caused by colds or allergies
ROUTE OF ADMINISTRATION: oral, topical, injection
COMMON ADULT DOSAGE: 12.5 to 25 mg every 4 hours (not to exceed 150 mg every 24 hours)
SIDE EFFECTS: drowsiness, dry mouth, upset stomach, dizziness, headache

NONSEDATING RX ANTIHISTAMINES

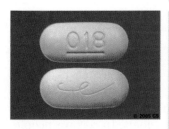

GENERIC NAME: fexofenadine
TRADE NAME: Allegra
INDICATION: seasonal allergies
ROUTE OF ADMINISTRATION: oral
COMMON ADULT DOSAGE: 60 mg twice daily or 180 mg once daily
SIDE EFFECTS: drowsiness, headache, upset stomach
AUXILIARY LABEL:
■ Take with water.

TABLE 18-4 Agents Used for the Treatment of Allergies

Examples of Trade Names	Generic Names	Indication	Dosage Forms
Over-the-Counter Allergy Agents			
Afrin, Nasacon, Duramist Plus, Nostrilla, Duration	oxymetazoline	Seasonal allergies	Nasal spray
Benadryl Allergy, Quenalin, Dytuss, Dytan	diphenhydramine	Hay fever, allergies, and cold symptoms	Tablets, chewable tablets, capsules, liquid
Chlor-Trimeton Allergy, Chlorphen, Aller-Chlor	chlorpheniramine	Symptoms of cold and/or allergies	Tablets, extended release tablets/ capsules, syrup
Claritin, Claritin RediTabs, Good Neighbor Loratadine, Alavert	loratadine	Seasonal allergies	Tablets, liquid, disintegrating tablets, chewable tablets
Dimetane, Dimetane Extentab, Dimetapp Allergy, Dimetapp Allergy Liquidgel	brompheniramine	Symptoms of cold and/or allergies	Tablets, extended release tablets, gelcaps, liquid
Neo-Synephrine, Vicks Sinex, Rhinall	phenylephrine	Seasonal allergies	Nasal spray
Sudafed PE-Quick-Dissolve Orally Disintegrating Strips	phenylephrine	Congestion caused by colds, flu, hay fever, and other allergies	Oral strips
Tavist Allergy, Good Sense Dayhist Allergy	clemastine fumarate	Symptoms caused by allergies	Tablets
Visine, Opti-Clear, Altazine, Geneye	tetrahydrozoline	Seasonal allergies	Ophthalmic eye drops
Behind-the-Counter Decongestants			
Sudafed, Sudanyl, Sudo-Tab, Ridafed, Genaphed, SudoGest	pseudoephedrine	Nasal congestion	Tablets, long-acting (LA) capsules, LA tablets, chewable tablets, liquid
Prescription Allergy Agents			
Allegra-D, Allegra-D 24	fexofenadine	Allergies	Tablets ER
Alrex, Lotemax	loteprednol	Allergic conjunctivitis	Ophthalmic eye drops
Beconase AQ, Vancenase AQ	beclomethasone	Nasal symptoms caused by seasonal or chronic allergies	Nasal inhaler
Claritin-D, Claritin RediTabs	loratadine	Allergies	Tablets, rapidly disintegrating tablets, and syrup
Dexacort	dexamethasone	Nasal symptoms caused by allergies and other seasonal reactions	Nasal inhaler
Flonase, Veramyst	fluticasone	Nasal symptoms caused by seasonal or chronic allergies	Nasal inhaler
Naphcon-A	naphazoline/pheniramine	Allergies	Ophthalmic solution
Naphcon, Vasocon	naphazoline	Allergic conjunctivitis	Ophthalmic solution
Nasacort AQ	triamcinolone	Nasal symptoms caused by seasonal or chronic allergies	Nasal inhaler
Nasonex	mometasone	Nasal symptoms caused by seasonal or chronic allergies	Nasal inhaler

TABLE 18-4 Agents Used for the Treatment of Allergies—cont'd

Examples of Trade Names	Generic Names	Indication	Dosage Forms
Optivar	azelastine	Allergic conjunctivitis	Ophthalmic solution
Patanol	olopatadine	Allergic conjunctivitis	Ophthalmic solution
Phenergan PE	promethazine/ phenylephrine	Congestion caused by colds, hay fever, or other allergic conditions	Syrup
Poly-Histine, Tri-Histine	pheniramine/pyrilamine/ phenyltoloxamine	Symptoms caused by colds, upper respiratory tract infections, and allergies	Syrup
Rhinocort	budesonide	Nasal symptoms caused by seasonal or chronic allergies	Nasal inhaler
Semprex-D	acrivastine/ pseudoephedrine	Nasal allergies	Tablets
Zaditor	ketotifen	Allergic conjunctivitis	Ophthalmic solution
Zyrtec, All Day Allergy	cetirizine	Symptoms of cold and/or allergies	Chewable tablets, liquid

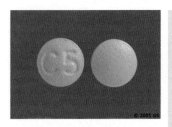

GENERIC NAME: desloratadine
TRADE NAME: Clarinex
INDICATION: allergic rhinitis
ROUTE OF ADMINISTRATION: oral
COMMON ADULT DOSAGE: 5 mg once daily
SIDE EFFECTS: dry mouth, headache
AUXILIARY LABEL:
■ Do not crush or chew tablet.

NONSEDATING OTC ANTIHISTAMINES

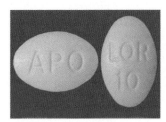

GENERIC NAME: loratadine
TRADE NAME: Claritin
INDICATION: symptoms caused by colds or allergies
ROUTE OF ADMINISTRATION: oral
COMMON ADULT DOSAGE: 10 mg once daily
SIDE EFFECTS: dry mouth

LOW-SEDATING OTC ANTIHISTAMINES

GENERIC NAME: cetirizine
TRADE NAME: Zyrtec
INDICATION: symptoms caused by colds or allergies
ROUTE OF ADMINISTRATION: oral
COMMON ADULT DOSAGE: 5 to 10 mg once daily
SIDE EFFECTS: dry mouth, sore throat, headache, tired feeling

LOWER RESPIRATORY SYSTEM

Conditions and disorders of the lower respiratory tract originate from the lungs although they affect the upper respiratory system as well (Table 18-5). The best way to avoid a respiratory tract infection of any kind is to wash your hands. Do

TABLE 18-5 Conditions of the Lower Respiratory System

Lower Respiratory Conditions	Symptoms	Medication Treatment
Asthma	Recurrent episodes of difficulty breathing, wheezing, cough, and production of thick mucus in airways caused by inflammation and bronchial spasms	Corticosteroids, leukotriene modifiers, bronchodilators, anticholinergics, and immunomodulators
Chronic bronchitis: bacterial, viral (contributes to COPD)	Coughing, wheezing, fatigue, excessive production of mucus	Cough suppressants, bronchodilators, expectorants
COPD: group of lung diseases including chronic bronchitis, emphysema, bronchiectasis	SOB, wheezing, tightness in chest, chronic cough, fatigue, loss of appetite/weight loss, frequent infections	Bronchodilators, steroids, supplemental oxygen
Croup: viral	Noisy breathing sounds, struggles to breath, high fever, agitation/irritability	Antipyretics, corticosteroids, antibiotics (if bacterial infection)
Emphysema: smoking, inherited deficiency of protein that protects elasticity of lungs (contributes to COPD)	SOB, wheezing, tightness in chest, fatigue, loss of appetite/weight loss	Bronchodilators, steroids, supplemental oxygen
Pleurisy: bacterial, viral	SOB, dry cough, fever, chills, chest pain	Antibiotics (if bacterial infection), NSAIDs
Pneumonia: bacterial, viral	Fever, cough, SOB, chills, chest pain, headache, muscle pain, fatigue, excessive sweating	Antibiotics, antipyretics, analgesics, cough suppressants, supplemental oxygen
Pulmonary edema: cardiogenic (e.g., heart failure), bacterial, viral, autoimmune conditions, clot, tuberculosis	Extreme SOB, wheezing, anxiety, excessive sweating, pale skin, chest pain	Diuretics, opioid analgesics, aspirin, hyper/hypotensive agents (depending on blood pressure)
Tuberculosis: bacterial (*Mycobacterium tuberculosis*)	Fever, chills, sweating, fatigue, weight loss	Antibiotics
Whooping cough: bacterial (*Bordetella pertussis*)	Dry coughing spasms, fever, nasal congestion, runny nose, watery eyes	Antibiotics

Tech Note!

Persons who are at higher risk should receive the flu vaccine annually. This includes health care workers. In addition, tuberculosis (TB) tests are normally required annually for health care workers employed in an institutional setting.

not sneeze or cough without covering your mouth. Most respiratory tract infections occur by this avenue.

Pneumonia

Pneumonia is an infection that causes acute inflammation in the airways of the lung, blocking them with thick mucus. One lobe (or many lobes) of one lung may be affected, or both lungs may be affected. The source for this infection can be bacterial, viral, fungal, chemical, or, in rare cases, parasitic. Once the organism enters the lung, it multiplies. As the body tries to fight the infection, fluid and pus fill the lungs, making breathing difficult. The most common bacterial organism causing community-acquired pneumonia is *Streptococcus pneumoniae* (Chapter 30); this organism causes a rapid onset of pneumonia. Hospital-acquired bacterial infections are commonly caused by gram-negative *Streptococcus aureus*. Older adults are at high risk, especially after an injury that requires them to remain in bed. Persons who have heart disease, alcoholics, drug users, and stroke victims are at higher risk of acquiring pneumonia. Persons with a weakened immune system are at a higher risk than most, but pneumonia can strike anyone.

Prognosis. Most people recover from pneumonia with rest and hydration, even those who acquire viral pneumonia. Of those who are admitted into a hospital, only a fraction die from this condition. Pneumonia may only occur once in a lifetime and will not permanently damage the lungs.

Non–Drug Treatment. Besides antibiotics, the best way to treat pneumonia is to get plenty of rest and to keep hydrated. Avoidance of irritants such as dust or pollution is helpful. The person should quit smoking because this will only worsen the condition.

Drug Treatment. Antibiotics can be used once the bacteria are identified, if the pneumonia is due to bacterial infection. Less often, fungal infections occur and they are treated with antifungals and other agents (Chapter 25). For all types of pneumonia, there are respiratory medications that may be used to treat the symptoms. These medications include bronchodilators and corticosteroids, which are used for other conditions such as asthma and chronic obstructive pulmonary disease (COPD). The following vaccines have been developed to prevent certain strains of bacterial and viral infections; for more information on vaccines, refer to Chapter 28.

Bacterial Vaccines
- Prevnar (used in children)
- Pneumovax (used in children, adolescents, and adults)

Viral Vaccines
- Influenza virus vaccine trivalent, types A and B (ages 18 years and older)
- FluMist Intranasal vaccine (2 to 49 years old)
- H5N1 influenza virus vaccine (18 to 64 years old)
- H1N1 virus vaccine (high-risk patients: children, adults 25 to 64 years old, pregnant women)

Asthma

Millions of persons suffer from asthma and it is a major childhood respiratory problem. Asthma is an inflammatory airway disease that can be caused by genetic defects or by a chronic allergic reaction to irritating substances in the environment. Asthma is classified as an inflammatory disease. The muscles around the bronchioles contract, narrowing the air passages so that air cannot be inhaled properly (Figure 18-5). In addition to this increase of resistance to airflow, the condition is worsened by edema and secretion of mucus into the airway. This causes the crackling sound heard during an asthma attack. In severe cases, the result is equivalent to suffocation as the brain is deprived of oxygen. Asthma is a chronic inflammatory condition of the lungs. Certain triggers can cause inflammation of the lining of the airways, production of mucus, and constriction of muscles within the airway. The symptoms include chest tightening, wheezing, and coughing that lead to airway obstruction. The most common triggers of asthma attacks are allergens caused by cats, smoke, exercise, stress, and environmental irritants. Approximately 34 million Americans have asthma. This is the leading cause of chronic illness and hospitalization in children (www.lungusa.org).

Prognosis. Using **prophylaxis** medications, most attacks can be avoided. With an acute attack the use of immediate relief agents can stop an asthmatic reaction. Patients with asthma will use medications for a lifetime. If left untreated, asthma can cause death.

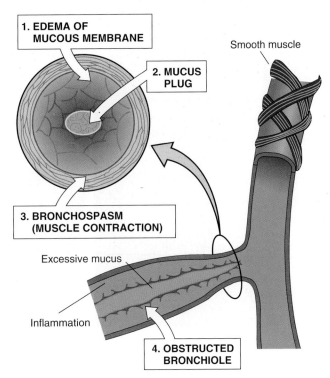

FIGURE 18-5 Asthma obstruction. (From Moscou, Snipe: *Pharmacology for Pharmacy Technicians*, ed 1, St Louis, 2009, Mosby.)

Non–Drug Treatments. Avoid triggers, such as excessive exercise and stress, to deter the onset of an attack. Breathing and relaxation techniques (yoga) can provide benefits to the person with asthma.

Drug Treatments. Although many medications can prevent or reverse asthma attacks, deaths are reported from asthma. Usually these deaths occur because many asthmatic persons do not have their medication available when an attack occurs or they delay going to an emergency room for treatment. There are two types of medications used in asthma patients: those used as a prophylaxis and those used when an attack occurs. Metered inhalers are often prescribed, and it is important for patients to learn how to use them properly so they obtain the correct dosage of medication (Figure 18-6, *A, B*).

Long-term control medications for asthma include corticosteroids, long-acting bronchodilators, leukotriene receptor antagonists, cromolyn, theophylline, and immunomodulators. Quick-relief (short-term) anticholinergic and short-acting beta-agonists are indicated for acute asthma attacks. Other uses of these classifications of medications may include conditions such as bronchitis and emphysema.

Corticosteroids. The drug action of corticosteroids includes acting as an antiinflammatory, thus lessening the constriction of the bronchial tubes. Corticosteroids also produce smooth muscle relaxation. Most can be given twice daily and may be effective as once daily doses in some patients. They are relatively non-toxic especially at low to moderate doses. Corticosteroids are recommended as the first line of treatment for long-term prophylaxis of asthma.

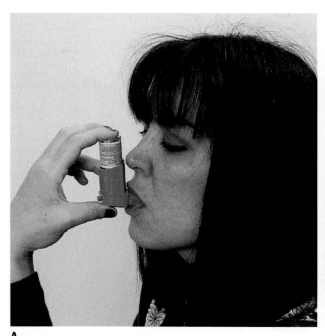
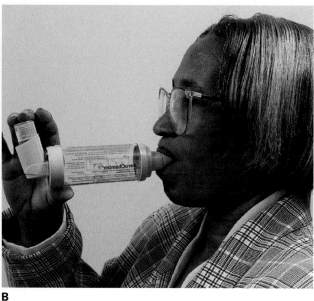

A

B

FIGURE 18-6 A, Proper use of an inhaler. **B,** Inhaler with spacer (e.g., AeroChamber). (From Elkin MK, Perry AG, Potter PA: *Nursing interventions and clinical skills*, ed 4, St Louis, 2007, Elsevier.)

GENERIC NAME: beclomethasone
TRADE NAME: oral, Beclovent, Vanceril; nasal, Beconase AQ, Vancenase AQ
INDICATION: prophylaxis of asthma attacks
ROUTE OF ADMINISTRATION: oral, nasal
COMMON ADULT DOSAGE: oral inhalant, 2 puffs 3 to 4 times daily; nasal inhalant, 1 spray into each nostril 3 to 4 times daily
SIDE EFFECTS: weight gain, bruising, and possible reduction in growth rate in adolescent children
AUXILIARY LABELS:
- Shake well.
- Take as directed.

GENERIC NAME: triamcinolone acetonide
TRADE NAME: Azmacort
INDICATION: prophylaxis of asthma attacks
ROUTE OF ADMINISTRATION: inhalation
COMMON ADULT DOSAGE: 2 puffs 3 to 4 times daily
SIDE EFFECTS: weight gain, bruising, and possible reduction in growth rate in children
AUXILIARY LABELS:
- Shake well.
- Take as directed.

GENERIC NAME: flunisolide
TRADE NAME: AeroBid, Nasalide
INDICATION: prophylaxis of asthma attacks (oral inhalation)
ROUTE OF ADMINISTRATION: inhalation, oral and nasal
COMMON ADULT DOSAGE: oral inhalant (AeroBid), 2 puffs twice daily
SIDE EFFECTS: weight gain, bruising, and possible reduction in growth rate in children
AUXILIARY LABELS:
- Shake well.
- Take as directed.

GENERIC NAME: fluticasone propionate
TRADE NAME: Flovent, Flonase
INDICATION: prophylaxis of asthma attacks
ROUTE OF ADMINISTRATION: oral and nasal inhalant and topical
COMMON ADULT DOSAGE: oral inhalation (Flovent), 2 to 4 puffs bid; nasal inhalation (Flonase), 2 sprays per nostril twice daily
SIDE EFFECTS: weight gain, bruising, and possible reduction in growth rate in children
AUXILIARY LABELS:
- Shake well.
- Take as directed.

Long-Acting Bronchodilators. These agents are recommended for chronic prophylaxis of asthma when used in conjunction with inhaled corticosteroids.

GENERIC NAME: salmeterol
TRADE NAME: Serevent
INDICATION: prophylactic use for asthma
ROUTE OF ADMINISTRATION: inhalant disk
SIDE EFFECTS: headache, nasal/sinus congestion, nervousness, stuffy nose, throat irritation
COMMON ADULT DOSAGE: 2 puffs bid (not meant for acute attacks; should not use more than once every 12 hours)
AUXILIARY LABEL:
- Use as directed.

Combination: Long-Acting Bronchodilator/Steroid Inhaler

GENERIC NAME: fluticasone propionate/salmeterol
TRADE NAME: Advair Diskus, Advair HFC
INDICATION: prophylactic use for asthma
ROUTE OF ADMINISTRATION: inhalant disk
COMMON ADULT DOSAGE: one blister dose as prescribed every 12 hours
SIDE EFFECTS: headache, dizziness, nausea, vomiting, diarrhea, dry mouth, stuffy nose, sore throat, hoarseness
AUXILIARY LABELS:
- Can cause dizziness.
- Use as directed.

Leukotriene Receptor Antagonists (Leukotriene Inhibitors). These agents are used for prophylaxis and chronic treatment of asthma or allergies.

GENERIC NAME: montelukast
TRADE NAME: Singulair
INDICATION: prophylaxis and chronic treatment of asthma, allergic rhinitis
ROUTE OF ADMINISTRATION: oral
COMMON ADULT DOSAGE: 10 mg once daily in the evening; 4- and 5-mg forms for pediatric use
SIDE EFFECTS: headache, heartburn, stomach pain, nausea, diarrhea, tooth pain, tiredness, stuffy nose, cough
AUXILIARY LABELS:
- Oral tablets: Take with full glass of water.
- Oral granules: Take with soft food. Do not take with water.

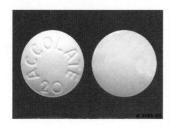

GENERIC NAME: zafirlukast
TRADE NAME: Accolate
INDICATION: prophylaxis and chronic treatment of asthma
ROUTE OF ADMINISTRATION: oral
COMMON ADULT DOSAGE: 20 mg 2 times daily
SIDE EFFECTS: headache, diarrhea
AUXILIARY LABEL:
■ Take 1 hr before meal or 2 hr after eating.

MAST CELL STABILIZERS

GENERIC NAME: cromolyn
TRADE NAME: Nasalcrom*
INDICATION: prevention of asthma attacks
ROUTE OF ADMINISTRATION: inhalant, nasal, and ophthalmic
COMMON ADULT DOSAGE: oral solution (Intal), 20 mg 4 times daily; nasal inhalant
    (Nasalcrom), 1 spray into each nostril 3 to 4 times daily
SIDE EFFECTS: bad taste in mouth, drowsiness, cough, throat irritation or dryness,
    wheezing
AUXILIARY LABEL:
■ none; OTC (nasal form)

_____

*Nasalcrom is nasal treatment

Medications for Acute Asthma Attacks

GENERIC NAME: albuterol
TRADE NAME: Proventil HFA, Ventolin HFA, AccuNeb
INDICATION: acute treatment of asthma; albuterol syrup and tablets are used as
    prophylaxis for asthma
ROUTE OF ADMINISTRATION: inhalant, liquid for nebulizer
COMMON ADULT DOSAGE: MDI, 2 puffs every 4 to 6 hours or as needed for rescue of
    acute attack; tablets or syrup, 2 to 4 mg 3 to 4 times daily
SIDE EFFECTS: headache, nervousness, stuffy nose, dizziness, insomnia, dry mouth,
    tremor, diarrhea, and cough
AUXILIARY LABELS:
■ For inhalers, shake well before using.
■ May cause dizziness.

Tech Note!

Spacers (generic term) may be used with certain inhalers; they are manufactured tubes that attach to the inhaler and have a one-way valve to allow the patient to inhale, not exhale, into the device, allowing more of the drug to reach the lungs. Examples are AeroChamber, OptiChamber, ProChamber, and Vortex. Some inhalers have incorporated spacers into their medication devices, such as triamcinolone and flunisolide HFA.

Chronic Obstructive Pulmonary Disease (COPD)

The three types of COPD are chronic bronchitis, emphysema, and bronchiectasis. Any long-term lung condition or exposure to lung irritants that damage the lungs can cause COPD. Emphysema is a condition that causes the destruction of the alveolar walls that eventually leads to a loss of elasticity of the lungs and heart failure. This can be caused by smoking, by exposure to environmental hazards (such as asbestos and fiberglass), or, in rare cases, by a genetic predisposition. Because normal exhalation requires elastic recoil of the lungs, the affected lungs allow air to be inhaled but cannot exhale all the air. The condition worsens as the surface area of the lungs becomes further reduced because of destruction of the alveolar walls (Box 18-3).

BOX 18-3 LUNG DISEASES THAT CAN LEAD TO COPD

- Bacterial infections in the lungs
- Interstitial lung disease (inflammation of the tissue surrounding the alveoli in the lungs)
- Lung cancer (malignant tumor in the lungs)
- Pneumonia (infection of one or both lungs)
- Pneumothorax (air accumulates in the chest but outside the lungs)
- Pulmonary edema (swelling from vessels to surrounding tissue caused by fluid)
- Pulmonary embolus (blood clot that enters into the lungs or airways, obstructing the vessel)
- Pulmonary fibrosis (scarring that occurs throughout the lungs)
- Pulmonary hypertension (abnormally elevated pulmonary arterial pressure)
- Sarcoidosis (inflammation that forms granulomas [small lumps] in tissues)
- Tuberculosis (infection of the lung caused by *Mycobacterium tuberculosis*)

Prognosis. COPD is a long-term condition although it can be managed with medication.

Non–Drug Treatment. Support groups can help COPD patients by the sharing of similar experiences. The person with COPD should stop smoking. In extreme cases, a lung transplant may be needed to remove parts of the affected lung.

Drug Treatment. Examples of the types of agents used are bronchodilators, corticosteroids, xanthines, and sympathomimetics. Examples are listed below.

CORTICOSTEROID/LONG-ACTING BRONCHODILATOR COMBINATIONS

GENERIC NAME: fluticasone/salmeterol
TRADE NAME: Advair HFA
INDICATIONS: COPD
ROUTE OF ADMINISTRATION: inhaler
COMMON ADULT DOSAGE: 2 inhalations two times daily
SIDE EFFECTS: tremors, headache, nausea, throat irritation, vomiting
AUXILIARY LABEL:
- Shake well before using.

GENERIC NAME: formoterol/budesonide
TRADE NAME: Symbicort
INDICATIONS: COPD
ROUTE OF ADMINISTRATION: inhalant
COMMON ADULT DOSAGE: 2 inhalations two times daily
SIDE EFFECTS: headache, back pain, nausea, vomiting, diarrhea, upset stomach, sore throat, stuffy nose
AUXILIARY LABEL:
- Shake well before using.

METHYLXANTHINE BRONCHODILATORS

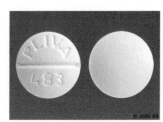

GENERIC NAME: theophylline, aminophylline
TRADE NAME: Theochron, Theo-24, Uniphyl
INDICATION: asthma and emphysema
ROUTE OF ADMINISTRATION: oral, inhalant, injection, rectal
COMMON ADULT DOSAGE: oral forms, 4-5 mg/kg or approximately 400 mg every 12 hours; dose varies depending on whether it is sustained release; for injection, infusion dose per hour varies based on weight and age of patient.
SIDE EFFECTS: shakiness, restlessness, and trembling
AUXILIARY LABEL:
■ Drink plenty of water.

Anticholinergics. Anticholinergics inhibit the action of acetylcholine, thus relaxing the smooth muscle of the bronchioles. These agents are used in the first-line treatment of COPD.

GENERIC NAME: ipratropium bromide
TRADE NAME: Atrovent
INDICATION: COPD, bronchospasms
ROUTE OF ADMINISTRATION: inhalant, oral and nasal
COMMON ADULT DOSAGE: oral inhalant, 2 puffs qid; nasal inhalant, 2 sprays into each nostril 2 to 3 times daily
SIDE EFFECTS: dry mouth
AUXILIARY LABEL:
■ Shake well.

GENERIC NAME: ipratropium/albuterol
TRADE NAME: Combivent, DuoNeb
INDICATION: COPD, bronchospasms
ROUTE OF ADMINISTRATION: inhalant, oral and nasal
COMMON ADULT DOSAGE: oral inhalant, 2 puffs qid; nasal inhalant, 2 sprays into each nostril 2 to 3 times daily
SIDE EFFECTS: dry mouth
AUXILIARY LABEL:
■ Shake well.

Tuberculosis

Worldwide, tuberculosis (TB) is the most common bacterial disease affecting the pulmonary system. This highly contagious disease is characterized by an infection within the lining of the lungs by a bacterium that needs oxygen to survive. The lungs provide an environment that is extremely oxygenated and where the causative bacteria, *Mycobacterium tuberculosis,* may reside for an extended time with few or no symptoms. When the immune system becomes weakened, the bacteria multiply and symptoms appear (Figure 18-7). There have been an increased number of tuberculosis cases over the last few years because of the emergence of drug-resistant strains. This occurs partly because many persons with tuberculosis do not complete their course of treatment once they feel better, allowing the bacterium not only to return but also to mutate, making it resistant to traditional drugs. Persons at high risk are those in a confined living space, such as a prison.

Prognosis. Tuberculosis can be cured if the prescribed medications are taken as directed. If left untreated, it can cause death.

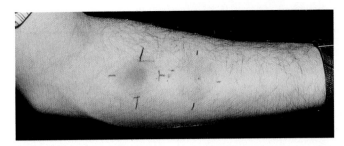

FIGURE 18-7 Positive result of a tuberculosis test. (From Zitelli BJ, Davis HW: *Atlas of pediatric physical diagnosis*, ed 5, St Louis, 2007, Mosby/Courtesy Dr. Kenneth Schuitt.)

Non–Drug Treatment. No non–drug treatments can be used to cure TB. Good hygiene should be used to prevent transmission of TB because it is extremely contagious. Keeping well hydrated and getting enough rest are important for recovery.

Drug Treatment. Most of the primary antituberculin agents are bactericidal. This means that they kill the bacterium that causes tuberculosis. These agents are used in combination for a course of treatment lasting many months. Although the medication used to treat tuberculosis is effective, many patients do not continue to take the medication once they are feeling better because they are unaware that the tuberculosis will return. In addition, one of the many side effects is nausea, which can complicate the lengthy treatment. For this reason, patients must be educated by their physicians about the importance of finishing their medication regimen to eradicate the bacteria completely from their system. The commonly used multiple medication treatment plans include isoniazid and rifampin given together as a daily dose. Another regimen includes isoniazid, streptomycin, and ethambutol. Another commonly used agent is pyrazinamide. Examples of the types of combination therapy are given in Table 18-6. These therapies can be given as a short or long course depending on the diagnosis. In the monographs that follow, specific side effects for each agent are listed along with the auxiliary labels and other drug information pertaining to that specific agent. To determine whether tuberculosis is cured entirely, **sputum** tests are required before treatment can stop.

ANTITUBERCULOSIS AGENTS

GENERIC NAME: isoniazid
TRADE NAME: Nydrazid
ROUTE OF ADMINISTRATION: oral, injection
SIDE EFFECTS: gastrointestinal upset
COMMON ADULT DOSAGE: 300 mg once daily 1 to 2 hours before or after meals (oral)
SIDE EFFECTS: tremors, shakiness, nausea, and vomiting; risk for liver dysfunction
AUXILIARY LABELS:
- Take on an empty stomach.
- Take as directed.
- Do not drink alcohol.
- Avoid certain foods such as fish or those containing tyramine, such as aged foods, due to some MAO inhibitor activity. Patient must not discontinue unless instructed to do so by physician.

TABLE 18-6 Examples of Tuberculosis Regimens

Trade Name	Generic Name	Adult Dosing	Comment
Regimen 1			
			Common regimens last 6 or 9 months
Rifadin	isoniazid rifampin	5 mg/kg/day 10 mg/kg/day	
Regimen 2			
			Streptomycin may be added to treatment if necessary (injection only)
Myambutol Streptomycin	isoniazid ethambutol streptomycin	5 mg/kg/day 15-25 mg/kg/day 500 mg to 1 g	Administered IM 3 times a week for first 3 months; given in severe cases of TB
Regimen 3			
			With four medications, alternate combination drugs may be used to replace 2 (long-term) to 3 (short-term) drugs
Myambutol Pyrazinamide	isoniazid ethambutol pyrazinamide	5 mg/kg/day 15-25 mg/kg/day 20-35 mg/kg/day	Doses of pyrazinamide may be taken 4 times daily if needed
Regimen 4			
			Rifapentine must be taken along with other TB agents such as ethambutol, isoniazid, pyrazinamide, or streptomycin
Priftin	rifapentine	150 mg twice weekly for 2 months followed by once a week dose for 4 months	Taken no less than 72 hr apart for first 2 months
Combination/Replacement Drugs			
			Combination drugs help with compliance for long-term therapy; each has its own specific time-frame of use as indicated
Mycobutin	rifabutin	300-mg capsule daily or 150-mg capsule twice daily	Alternative drug to replace rifampin; used for patients with HIV who are taking specific antiretroviral agents
Rifamate	isoniazid/ rifampin	2 capsules once daily	Not for initial therapy; may be taken for additional 4 months after initial 2 months of isoniazid, pyrazinamide, and rifampin
Rifater	isoniazid/ pyrazinamide/ rifampin	1 tablet daily	For first 2 months of initial therapy; must be followed by additional 4 months of treatment with isoniazid and rifampin

GENERIC NAME: rifampin
TRADE NAME: Rifadin
ROUTE OF ADMINISTRATION: oral
COMMON ADULT DOSAGE: 600 mg once daily 1 to 2 hours before or after meals
SIDE EFFECTS: orange to reddish urine and other excretions, tremors, shakiness, nausea, and vomiting
AUXILIARY LABELS:

- Take on an empty stomach.
- Take as directed.
- Special instructions: Patient must not discontinue unless instructed to do so by physician. Treatment normally lasts 6 to 9 months or 6 months if sputum culture is negative.

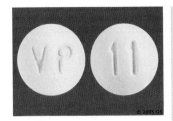

GENERIC NAME: ethambutol
TRADE NAME: Myambutol
ROUTE OF ADMINISTRATION: oral
COMMON ADULT DOSAGE: 800 mg to 1.2 g once daily
SIDE EFFECTS: gastrointestinal upset, nausea, vomiting, fever, or decrease in visual acuity
AUXILIARY LABEL:

- Take with food.

GENERIC NAME: pyrazinamide
TRADE NAME: (no trade name)
ROUTE OF ADMINISTRATION: oral
SIDE EFFECTS: nausea, vomiting, anorexia, myalgia, gout
NORMAL DOSAGE: 2000 mg once daily for 2 months
AUXILIARY LABEL:

- Take as directed.

EMERGENCY DISORDERS OF THE LUNGS

The following conditions affect the lungs and their lining, usually requiring hospitalization: pneumothorax, pulmonary embolism, and hemothorax. Pneumothorax (Figure 18-8) can be caused by COPD, tuberculosis, and chest wounds. Pneumothorax is characterized by a collapse of the alveoli resulting from air escaping into the pleural space. A pulmonary embolism occurs when an embolus

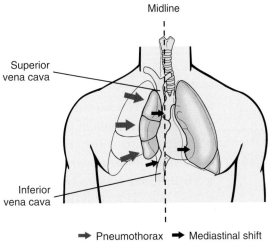

➡ Pneumothorax   ➡ Mediastinal shift

FIGURE 18-8 Pneumothorax.

(small blood clot that breaks away from its origin) blocks a branch of one of the pulmonary arteries, which extend from the right ventricle to the lungs. Hemothorax is the collapse of a lung resulting from blood leaking into the pleural space. All of these examples are serious conditions that need to be treated immediately, or death may result. Cancer of the respiratory tract can occur in any part of the respiratory system. Persistent hoarseness is one of the first signs of laryngeal cancer. Persons who smoke pipes, cigars, or cigarettes or those who have inhaled chemicals that contain hazardous particles are at higher risk than most. Treatments may include surgery, chemotherapy, radiation, or a combination of these treatment modalities.

If cardiopulmonary resuscitation (CPR) is started immediately when someone stops breathing, there is a good chance of reviving the person. Persons who collapse from cardiac arrest or respiratory arrest and children who have accidentally fallen into water and are not breathing are some of the types of victims who have been revived through the use of CPR. Most hospitals train pharmacy staff to learn CPR, free of charge. CPR training is in the best interest of all pharmacy technicians because they are in contact with the sick and with older adults daily.

Mucolytics

Mucolytics are agents that break up mucus that can obstruct the airway. Their mode of action is to act directly on the blockage, causing a breakdown of molecular bonds. This action decreases the **viscosity** of the mucus plug, thus allowing the mucus to be expectorated more easily or, if needed, to be suctioned out manually. Mucolytics are used in patients suffering from COPD and cystic fibrosis and for those patients with a tracheotomy. This type of medication is limited to acetylcysteine.

Tech Alert!

Remember the following sound-alike/look-alike drugs:

diphenhydramine versus dicyclomine or dimenhydrinate
hydrocodone versus hydrocortisone
epinephrine versus ephedrine
Alupent versus Atrovent
albuterol versus atenolol

MUCOLYTIC

GENERIC NAME: acetylcysteine
TRADE NAME: Mucomyst
DRUG ACTION: breaks the bonds between proteins responsible for mucus buildup; this decreases the viscosity of the mucus, allowing it to be expelled
INDICATION: COPD and cystic fibrosis; also used orally or parenterally (Acetadote) as an antidote to overdoses of acetaminophen
ROUTE OF ADMINISTRATION: inhalation
COMMON ADULT DOSAGE: inhalant, 10% (3 to 5 mL) to 20% (6 to 10 mL) 3 to 4 times daily
SIDE EFFECTS: nausea, vomiting, runny nose
AUXILIARY LABEL:
■ none (Most treatments are given in the hospital, although family members can be taught how to give respiratory treatments at home.)

DO YOU REMEMBER THESE KEY POINTS?

■ The main functions of the respiratory system
■ The major organs of the respiratory system
■ Common upper respiratory conditions
■ Common lower respiratory conditions
■ Medications used to treat respiratory conditions
■ Main side effects of the drugs discussed in this chapter
■ Major auxiliary labels that should be affixed to the container
■ Differences between emphysema, bronchitis, and asthma
■ Special instructions given for patients who are taking antituberculin agents
■ Types of contributing factors that can influence respiratory conditions

REVIEW QUESTIONS

Multiple choice questions

1. Which of the following statements is NOT true?
   A. Respiration is an involuntary response.
   B. Expiration is an active response.
   C. The diaphragm flattens while the intercostal muscles contract, increasing the size of the thoracic cavity and allowing for inspiration.
   D. Two phases describe respiration: expiration and inspiration.

2. The act of gas exchange within the lungs takes place specifically in the:
   A. Brainstem
   B. Brain
   C. Medulla
   D. Alveoli

3. The main function(s) of the cilia within the upper respiratory tract is (are):
   A. To smell
   B. To catch foreign material
   C. To warm and moisten air molecules
   D. Both A and C

4. The normal amount of air exhaled by an adult is:
   A. 0.25 L
   B. 0.5 L
   C. 1 L
   D. More than 5 L

5. Which of the following symptoms are not common in a typical cold?
   A. Laryngitis
   B. Congestion
   C. Wheezing
   D. Coughing

6. Pneumonia can be described as:
   A. Viral or bacterial in origin
   B. An upper respiratory tract infection
   C. Contagious
   D. Both A and C

7. A patient diagnosed with asthma might receive which of the following drugs as a prophylaxis?
   A. Narcotic antitussive
   B. Bronchodilator
   C. Xanthines
   D. Leukotriene receptor antagonist

8. Persons who smoke are more likely to suffer from:
   A. Bronchitis and emphysema
   B. Emphysema and asthma
   C. Bronchitis and asthma
   D. All of the above

9. Tuberculosis is on the rise mostly because of:
   A. Noncompliance with drug regimen
   B. Lack of money to buy medication
   C. Living in close quarters
   D. Both A and C

10. The function of gas exchange includes all of the following EXCEPT:
    A. Balancing the pH of the body
    B. Oxygenation of the bloodstream
    C. Discarding unused carbon dioxide
    D. Exchanging nitrogen for carbon dioxide

11. The specific site of exchange of oxygen across the membrane into the blood is:
- A. The pleural site
- B. The alveoli
- C. The lungs
- D. The bronchioles

12. All opioid antitussives should have the auxiliary label(s):
- A. Do not take with food.
- B. Do not drink alcohol.
- C. Take with plenty of water.
- D. Do not crush tablets.

13. COPD's symptoms include:
- A. Bronchitis and emphysema
- B. Emphysema and bronchiectasis
- C. Tuberculosis and emphysema
- D. Both A and B

14. Non–drug treatments for pneumonia include:
- A. Hydration
- B. Rest
- C. Quit smoking
- D. All of the above

15. Agents that break up thick mucous secretions of the lungs or bronchi so that they can be expelled from the system through coughing are called:
- A. Mucolytics
- B. Antitussives
- C. Expectorants
- D. Both A and C

True/False

If the statement is false, then change it to make it true.

_____ **1.** The highest percentage of gas in the air that we breathe is oxygen.

_____ **2.** The larynx also is known as the voice box.

_____ **3.** Viruses, bacteria, or both can cause colds.

_____ **4.** Influenza only strikes older adults.

_____ **5.** Allergies are caused by genetic traits.

_____ **6.** The main function of the epiglottis is to protect the vocal cords.

_____ **7.** Persons who smoke are not any more at risk of getting chronic obstructive pulmonary disease than nonsmokers.

_____ **8.** The overall effect of bronchodilators is vasodilation.

_____ **9.** Tuberculosis is caused by a bacterium and is not contagious.

_____ **10.** Asthma is caused by rupture of the alveolar sacs.

_____ **11.** Loss of the vocal cords is called laryngitis.

_____ **12.** Antitussives reduce pain.

_____ **13.** Annual influenzas are named after the region of origination.

_____ **14.** Opioid antitussives decrease the cough reflex by binding to opiate receptor sites located in the CNS.

_____ **15.** Only the symptoms of the common cold can be treated with medication.

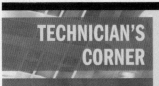

TECHNICIAN'S CORNER

List an over-the-counter medication for the relief of the following symptoms:

Cold (stuffy nose, cough, and fever)
Rhinitis (congestion, headache, and cough)
Allergies (itchy eyes; stuffy, runny nose; and congestion)

BIBLIOGRAPHY

AMA (American Medical Association) *Concise Medical Encyclopedia*. 2006.

Clayton B, Stock Y, Harroun R: *Basic pharmacology for nurses*, ed 14, Philadelphia, 2006, Elsevier Science.

Drug facts and comparisons, ed 63, St Louis, 2008, Lippincott Williams & Wilkins.

Favaro M: *Introduction to pharmacology*, ed 11, Philadelphia, 2008, Elsevier Health Services.

Grollman S: *The human body: its structure and physiology*, New York, 1965, Collier-Macmillan Limited.

Professional guide to diseases, ed 9, Ambler, PA, 2009, Lippincott Williams & Wilkins.

Seasonal Influenza Vaccination Resources for Health Professionals. 2009 Recommendations.

WEBSITES

Allergic rhinitis-immunotherapy. University of Maryland Medical Center. www.umm.edu/patiented/articles/how_decongestants_used_prevent_allergy_symptoms_000077_9.htm

Asthma: anatomy and function of the respiratory system. www.drgreene.com/21_1346.html

Drug interactions: What you should know. www.fda.gov/Drugs/ResourcesForYou/ucm163354.htm

Flu/Professionals/vaccinations. www.cdc.gov/

Visual and Auditory Systems

Objectives

UPON COMPLETING THIS CHAPTER, YOU SHOULD BE ABLE TO DO
THE FOLLOWING:

- List both trade and generic drug names covered in this chapter.

- Describe the functions of the eyes and ears.

- List the major components of the eyes and ears.

- Explain the drug action of the medications listed.

- Describe what causes glaucoma.

- Describe the different types of conjunctivitis and their treatments.

- List the various infections that affect the eyes and ears.

- Explain how medications work to relieve glaucoma.

TERMS AND DEFINITIONS: EYE

Accommodation *The change that occurs in the ocular lens when it focuses at various distances*

Aqueous humor *The fluid found in the anterior cavity of the eye, in front of the lens*

Cataract *Loss of transparency of the lens of the eye*

Cones *Photoreceptors in the retina of the eye responsible for color perception (daylight vision)*

Conjunctiva *Transparent protective mucous membrane that lines the underside of the eyelid*

Cornea *The transparent tissue covering the anterior portion of the eye*

Iris *Colored part of eye seen through cornea; consists of smooth muscles that regulate pupil size*

Lens *Flexible, clear covering of the retina that focuses on images*

Macula lutea *Yellow spot in the center of the retina responsible for central and high-acuity vision. The macula contains a pit in its center known as the fovea, which contains ganglion cells with a high concentration of cones. Any damage to the macula results in loss of central visual capacity*

Miosis *Contraction of the pupil*

Mydriasis *Dilation of the pupil*

Ophthalmic *Pertaining to the eye*

Orbit *Eye socket*

Pupil *Circular opening in the iris that allows light to enter*

Retina *Innermost layer of the eye; a complex structure that is considered part of the central nervous system (CNS); the retina contains photoreceptors (rods and cones) that transmit impulses to the optic nerve, as well as the macula lutea (a yellow spot in the center of the retina)*

Rods *Photoreceptors in the retina of the eye that respond to dim light and are responsible for black and white color perception (night vision)*

Sclera *White of the eyes*

Vitreous humor *Gel-like substance that fills the posterior cavity of the eye, between the lens and retina; helps to maintain shape of the eye*

TERMS AND DEFINITIONS: EAR

Acoustic nerve *The cranial nerve (CN VIII or vestibulocochlear nerve) that controls the senses of hearing and equilibrium and eventually leads to the cerebellum and medulla*

Auditory canal *A 1-inch segment of tube that extends from the external ear to the middle ear*

Auditory ossicles *The set of three small bony structures in the middle ear: the malleus, incus, and stapes*

Eustachian tube *A tubular structure in the middle ear that connects with the nasopharynx (throat); it functions to equalize pressure between the outside air and middle ear and to drain mucus*

Labyrinth *Inner ear consists of a bony labyrinth and a membranous labyrinth; bony labyrinth is composed of the vestibule, cochlea, and semicircular canals located in temporal bone; membranous labyrinth is series of membranous tubes found inside bony labyrinth*

Otic *Pertaining to the ear*

Tympanic membrane *A thin membrane that separates the external ear from the middle ear; also known as the eardrum*

COMMON DRUGS USED FOR CONDITIONS OF THE EYE

Trade Name	Generic Name	Pronunciation
Anticholinergics		
Cyclogyl	cyclopentolate	(sye-kloe-**pen**-toe-late)
Isopto Atropine	atropine	(**at**-roe-peen)
Isopto Homatropine	homatropine	(hoe-ma-**troe**-peen)
Isopto Hyoscine	scopolamine	(skoe-**poll**-a-meen)
Mydriacyl	tropicamide	(troe-**pik**-a-mide)
Adrenergic Agonists		
OcuClear	oxymetazoline	(**ox**-ee-**met**-tah-zoe-leen)
Propine	dipivefrin	(dye-**pie**-veh-frin)
Naphcon	naphazoline	(na-**faz**-oh-leen)
Visine	tetrahydrozoline	(tet-ra-hye-**droz**-oh-leen)
Alphagan P	brimonidine	(bri-**moe**-ni-**deen**)
Lopidine	apraclonidine	(app-rah-**kloe**-ni-deen)
Carbachol, Miostat	carbachol	(**kar**-ba-kall)
Antihistamine		
Emadine	emedastine	(**em**-e-**das**-teen)
Mast Cell Stabilizers		
Alomide	lodoxamide	(low-**dox**-a-mide)
Alocril	nedocromil	(ne-doe-**kroe**-mil)
Alamast	pemirolast	(pem-ir-**oh**-last)
Crolom	cromolyn	(**kroe**-moe-lin)
Antiinflammatories		
Acular	ketorolac	(**kee**-toe-**role**-ak)
Ocufen	flurbiprofen	(**flure**-bi-**pro**-fen)
Voltaren	diclofenac	(dye-**kloe**-fen-ak)
Combination Antihistamine/Mast Cell Stabilizer for Allergic Conjunctivitis		
Patanol	olopatadine	(oh-low-**pat**-a-deen)
Optivar	azelastine	(a-**zel**-as-teen)
Elestat	epinastine	(ep-**in**-nas-teen)
Zaditor	ketotifen	(**key**-toe-**tye**-fen)
Antiinfectives		
Aminoglycosides		
Genoptic	gentamicin	(**jen**-tah-**my**-sin)
Tobrex	tobramycin	(**toe**-bra-**my**-sin)
Antifungal		
Natacyn	natamycin	(**na**-ta-**my**-sin)
Antivirals		
Dendrid	idoxuridine	(eye-docks-**your**-eh-dean)
Vira-A	vidarabine	(vi-**dare**-ah-been)
Viroptic	trifluridine	(try-**floor**-eh-dean)
Fluoroquinolone Ophthalmics		
Besivance	besifloxacin	(be-se-**flox**-a-sin)
Chibroxin	norfloxacin	(nor-**flox**-a-sin)
Ciloxan	ciprofloxacin	(si-pro-**flox**-a-sin)
Ocuflox	ofloxacin	(oh-**flox**-a-sin)

Trade Name	Generic Name	Pronunciation
Vigamox	moxifloxacin	(mox-i-**flox**-a-sin)
Zymar	gatifloxacin	(gat-i-**flox**-a-sin)
Macrolides		
Ilotycin	erythromycin	(eh-**rith**-roh-**my**-sin)
AzaSite	azithromycin	(a-**zith**-row-**my**-sin)
Sulfonamide		
Bleph-10	sulfacetamide	(**sul**-fah-**set**-ah-mide)
Other Antibiotic Ophthalmics		
Polytrim	polymyxin B/ trimethoprim	(**pol**-ee-**mix**-in/ trye-**meth**-oh-prim)
Beta-Adrenergic Blocking Agents		
Betagan	levobunolol	(lee-voe-**byoo**-noe-lol)
Betaxon	levobetaxolol	(le-vo-be-**tax**-oh-lol)
Betoptic	betaxolol	(be-**tax**-oh-lol)
Ocupress	carteolol	(**car**-tee-oh-lol)
OptiPranolol	metipranolol	(me-ti-**pran**-oh-lol)
Timoptic	timolol	(**tim**-oh-lol)
Carbonic Anhydrase Inhibitors		
Azopt	brinzolamide	(brin-**zoh**-la-mide)
Diamox	acetazolamide	(a-**seet**-ah-**zole**-a-mide)
Neptazane	methazolamide	(**meth**-a-**zole**-a-mide)
Trusopt	dorzolamide	(dor-**zole**-a-mide)
Cholinergics		
Miochol-E	acetylcholine	(a-**seet**-ill-**koe**-leen)
Isopto-carbachol	carbachol	(**kar**-ba-kol)
Pilocar	pilocarpine	(pye-low-**kar**-peen)
Corticosteroids		
Decadron	dexamethasone	(**dex**-ah-**meth**-ah-sone)
FML	fluorometholone	(**floor**-oh-**meth**-oh-lone)
Maxidex	dexamethasone	(**dex**-ah-**meth**-ah-sone)
Pred Forte	prednisolone	(pred-**niss**-oh-lone)
Zylet	loteprednol	(low-te-**pred**-nol)
Immunologic Agent		
Restasis	cyclosporine	(sye-**klow**-spor-in)
Prostaglandin Agonists		
Lumigan	bimatoprost	(bye-**mat**-oh-prost)
Travatan	travoprost	(**trav**-oh-prost)
Xalatan	latanoprost	(la-**tan**-oh-prost)
Sympathomimetics		
Alphagan P	brimonidine	(brye-**moe**-ni-deen)
Osmotics		
Ophthalgan	glycerin anhydrous	(**glis**-er-in)
Osmitrol	mannitol	(**man**-ih-tole)

WE RELY ON OUR SENSES our entire lifetime. Although there are five major senses—sight, hearing, touch, smell, and taste—changes in vision and hearing can dramatically alter a person's life. Every day, from the moment we wake until the time we fall asleep, our senses are receiving and interpreting information; and our mind relies on the memories of sights and sounds. The ability to see enables us to navigate, whereas the ability to hear can prevent injuries (e.g., such as by walking into traffic). Both seeing and hearing are vital components in our ability to communicate with others. The conditions that can affect the eyes and ears may not seem as important as other conditions; however, the ramifications of neglecting these conditions can be earth-shattering. In this chapter, we discuss the major components of the eyes and ears, as well as major conditions that can affect these two senses and their common treatments. Although the five senses mentioned are commonly considered the only senses, equilibrium is another sense. It is closely associated with the sense of hearing and plays a role in our ability to maintain balance; it will be discussed later in this chapter.

The Eyes (Ophthalmic System)

As one of the five main sensors of the body, the eyes link the outside world and the mind. As images are perceived, they are translated into impulses that create lasting memories in the mind. The three different levels or categories of health care personnel who work in the field of eye care are opticians, optometrists, and ophthalmologists. Opticians are skilled in making lenses that compensate vision loss, but they cannot prescribe medication. Optometrists are trained to perform eye examinations and may prescribe certain medications for the eye. Ophthalmologists are physicians who treat major conditions affecting the eye, including performing eye surgery.

MEDICAL TERMS AND CONDITIONS OF THE EYE

Word Combinations	
Blephar/o	Eyelid
Irid/o	Iris
Kerat/o	Cornea (also means hard)
Ocul/o	Eye
Scler/o	White of the eye (also means hard)
Ophthalm/o	Eye
Macul/o	Spot
Presby	Old age

Prefixes	
Extra-	On the outside
Intra-	Within
Cor-	Pupil
Hyper-	Excessive, high above

Suffixes	
-ar/-ic	Pertaining to
-ologist	Specialist
-metrist	One who measures
-ptosis	Drooping/sagging
-ion	Condition
-it is	Inflammation
-ia	Abnormal condition
-edema	Swelling
-opia	Vision condition

MEDICAL TERMS AND CONDITIONS OF THE EYE—cont'd

Conditions	
Cataract	Film that grows on lens, causing loss of vision
Conjunctivitis	Inflammation of conjunctiva
Glaucoma	Increased pressure in eye, causing damage to retina and optic nerve
Hyperopia	Farsightedness
Macular degeneration	Gradual loss of central vision
Monochromatism	Color blindness
Myopia	Nearsightedness
Nyctalopia	Impaired vision at night; night blindness
Presbyopia	Lens becomes less flexible and muscles of ciliary body become weaker
Retinopathy	Disease of retina

ANATOMY OF THE EYE

The eye has several structures working in unison to help protect it, maintain its shape, and enhance vision. The eyebrows shade the eyes from light. More than 200 eyelashes work to catch debris, keep the eyes moist, and shade the eyes. The eye sits in a bony socket called the **orbit**. The position of the eyes allows for peripheral vision up to approximately 100 degrees. Covering the eyes are the eyelids, which are composed of four individual layers: the outer skin, the muscles, the connective tissue, and the **conjunctiva**. The muscles and fibers of connective tissues are under the skin within the lid. They allow the eyelid to open and close. The conjunctiva is a thin, transparent mucous membrane that covers the anterior eye, the eyelids, and the **sclera**. The natural reaction of blinking serves to protect the eye from foreign objects and allows lacrimal fluid (tears) to cleanse the eye. The lacrimal gland is located within the orbit; it secretes tears into the eye and has ducts that lead into the nasal cavity. Tears contain an enzyme called lysozyme that has antimicrobial properties. An overview of the anatomy of the eye is shown in Figure 19-1.

The **cornea** is a bulging transparent cover that allows light into the eye for visual acuity. The cornea is composed of connective tissue and is covered in a thin coating of epithelium. The cornea does not contain blood vessels to provide

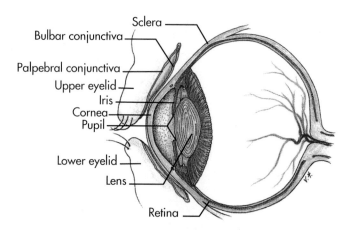

FIGURE 19-1 Anatomy of the eye. (From Potter PA, Perry AG: *Fundamentals of nursing*, ed 7, St Louis, 2009, Mosby.)

nourishment; instead, it is nourished by aqueous humor as well as oxygen from the atmosphere. The **aqueous humor** is found within the anterior portion of the eye, between the cornea and the lens. Many nerve fibers within the cornea are sensitive to pain. The sclera is attached to the cornea but wraps around to the back of the eyeball. Unlike the cornea, however, it is not transparent. The sclera is the protective white portion of the eye, and it contains many fibers and muscles. The optic nerve extends from the back of the eye through the sclera. The optic nerve sends images from the eye to the brain for interpretation. The fovea is a small pit located at the center of the **macula lutea;** the fovea is the area of highest visual acuity. From the front of the eye the sclera joins with the iris and the ciliary body. The **iris** is responsible for the color of the eye. The iris filters light. The largest space of the eye is an area called the posterior cavity, which is surrounded by the **lens,** ciliary body, and **retina.** The ciliary body forms a ring around the front of the eye. The ciliary body is responsible for holding the lens in place. When certain fibers in the eye contract, the choroid coat is pulled forward, shortening the ciliary body. This in turn thickens the lens, allowing for up-close focusing. The area between the lens and the retina is filled with a jelly-like substance called the **vitreous humor.** A function of the vitreous body is to hold the shape and form of the eye. The retina is a thin layer that contains layers of neurons, nerves, pigmented epithelium, and membranous tissues. Receptor cells (known as photoreceptors) of the retina are responsible for vision, and the neurons provide a path to the brain.

Six major muscles of the eye extend from the skeletal bones of the orbit. These muscles are responsible for the movement of the eye. The direction of movements is shown in Figure 19-2. Other important muscles include those that close and open the eyelid and dilate and constrict the pupil.

When focusing on a distant figure or in the dark, the **pupil** of the eye dilates (**mydriasis**), allowing more light to enter. When the eye is exposed to excessive light, the pupil constricts (**miosis**). Through complicated connections, visual information is transferred to the nerve endings located at the back of the eye, which then send information to the brain, causing the necessary change in the lens to adjust to the incoming image (i.e., **accommodation**). Aqueous humor is

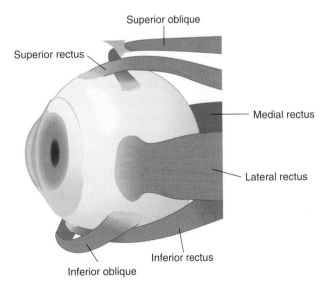

FIGURE 19-2 Eye muscles and direction of movement. Superior rectus rotates upward and inward; inferior rectus rotates downward and inward; medial rectus rotates inward; lateral rectus rotates outward; superior oblique rotates downward and outward; inferior oblique rotates upward and outward.

the watery fluid that functions both to maintain the shape of the anterior eye (i.e., between the cornea and the lens) and to nourish anterior compartment structures. Because aqueous humor is continuously synthesized, it must be released to maintain proper pressure within the anterior chamber. Excess aqueous humor drains through small ducts located near the sclera and cornea called the canals of Schlemm. The retina, located in the posterior eye, contains the nerve endings that transmit electrical impulses to the brain. The retina also contains the rods and cones, photoreceptors that are responsible for vision in dim light (i.e., rods) and for color vision (i.e., cones).

VISION

Each area of the eye has a specific function. As an image passes through the lens, it reaches the back of the eye, the retina. The rods and cones are located in the retina. **Rods** are responsible for sight in dim light and produce only an image in black and white. **Cones** detect color and can produce an image in bright light. As the rods and cones synapse (connect) with nerve endings, the signals are sent through the optic nerve to the brain. The occipital lobe of the brain is responsible for visual interpretation.

Conditions That Affect the Eye

A variety of conditions can affect the eye. Depending on the cause, treatment can range from medication to surgery. Over the past decade there have been many new developments in corrective lens treatment. For conditions such as myopia (nearsightedness), laser surgery is becoming an alternative to wearing glasses. For certain persons who are blind, a new surgical technique implants new lenses, restoring vision to some individuals. As new techniques become available, potentially many more eye conditions will be treated and even cured.

Many combinations of **ophthalmic** medications are available by prescription. Combination drugs treat the eye with several medications at once. Keeping eye solutions sterile is imperative because foreign objects instilled into the eyes can cause damage or infection. Patients are counseled by the pharmacist to avoid touching the medication and contaminating it. In addition, most medications should not be instilled into the eyes while one is wearing contact lenses. In this section, commonly used medications for examinations and conditions of the eye are discussed. Because dosages vary depending on age and severity of the condition, only adult dosages will be listed unless otherwise noted. In Box 19-1 pharmacy abbreviations and terms are listed that will be used throughout this chapter for dosing, side effects, and descriptions.

COMMON CONDITIONS

Allergies

When the body comes into contact with an irritant or foreign object, mast cells are produced; they release histamine, which causes inflammation of the blood vessels in an effort to fight the allergen. When the eyes are exposed to allergens, they become itchy, red, and watery. This condition can occur at any time; however, seasonal allergies are the most common. Seasonal allergies are the allergic reactions caused by the release of pollen from trees, grasses, and flowers. Other causes of allergies include pet dander, molds, dust mites, cigarette smoke, and other exhaust fumes that can either cause or exacerbate (worsen) the condition.

BOX 19-1 ABBREVIATIONS

Q or q	Every
N/V	Nausea/vomiting
bid	Twice daily
tid	Three times daily
qid	Four times daily
gtt	Drop(s)
soln	Solution
susp	Suspension
oint, ung	Ointment
H/A	Headache

Terms

Analgesics	Agents that lessen pain
Antipyretics	Agents that lower temperature/fever
NSAIDs	Nonsteroidal antiinflammatory drugs, agents that reduce inflammation

Abbreviations That Should NOT Be Used*

OD	Right eye
OS	Left eye
OU	Both eyes
AD	Right ear
AS	Left ear
AU	Both ears
QOD	Every other day
QD	Daily
HS	Bedtime
Q hs	At bedtime

*Do not use these abbreviations; see Chapter 14.

Prognosis. There is no cure for allergies. However, persons with allergies should adhere to the medication regimen prescribed by their physicians, avoid irritants, and limit outdoor activities if possible.

Non–Drug Treatment. Avoiding irritants will diminish allergic reactions. Also, staying indoors during the daytime (i.e., when pollen levels are highest) in an environment cooled by air conditioning may also be beneficial. Monthly allergy shots can be given for allergic rhinoconjunctivitis (i.e., affecting the nose and eyes) to relieve all symptoms of eye allergies.

Drug Treatments. A wide variety of conditions can affect the eyes, ranging from allergies to bacterial, viral, or fungal infections. If the eye is infected, the type of antiinfective prescribed will depend on the causative organism. There are several agents that can be used to treat allergies, such as mast cell stabilizers, antihistamines, and decongestants. Mast cell stabilizers function by preventing mast cells from releasing chemicals that cause inflammation. These are available as ophthalmic solutions and suspensions as well as systemic agents. Antihistamines inhibit the release of histamine from nerve endings, which results in common symptoms of itching and inflammation. By inhibition of the histamine receptors, the effects of seasonal allergies and other allergens can be lessened. Decongestants are used to dry mucous secretions caused by allergies and hay fever. Decongestants act on the specific receptors that cause constriction of the mucous membrane, thus lessening congestion. Table 19-1 lists

TABLE 19-1 Ophthalmic Decongestants, Antihistamines, and Mast Cell Stabilizers*

Generic Name	Trade Name	Availability
Decongestants		
naphazoline	VasoClear-A	OTC
naphazoline	AK-Con, NaphaForte	Prescription
oxymetazoline	Visine L.R., OcuClear	OTC
phenylephrine	Neofrin, AK-Dilate	Prescription
tetrahydrozoline	Visine	OTC
Antihistamines		
olopatadine	Patanol, Pataday	Prescription
emedastine	Emadine	Prescription
azelastine	Optivar	Prescription
epinastine	Elestat	Prescription
ketotifen	Claritin Eye, Zaditor	OTC
Antihistamine/Decongestant Combinations		
pheniramine/naphazoline	Visine-A	OTC
Mast Cell Stablizers		
lodoxamide	Alomide	Prescription
nedocromil	Alocril	Prescription
pemirolast	Alamast	Prescription
cromolyn	Crolom	Prescription

*Patients must read the package insert and follow manufacturer's recommended dosage. Dangerous side effects may occur if ophthalmic over-the-counter agents are used by patients with glaucoma and certain conditions.

decongestants, antihistamines, and mast cell stabilizers. These agents are indicated for allergies resulting from pollen or other allergens.

ANTIALLERGY AGENTS

GENERIC NAME: emedastine
TRADE NAME: Emadine
INDICATION: allergic conjunctivitis
ROUTE OF ADMINISTRATION: ophthalmic
COMMON ADULT DOSAGE: 1 to 2 drops twice daily to four times daily into affected eye
SIDE EFFECTS: eye irritation, blurred vision
AUXILIARY LABEL:
■ For the eye.

GENERIC NAME: lodoxamide
TRADE NAME: Alomide
INDICATION: allergic conjunctivitis
ROUTE OF ADMINISTRATION: ophthalmic
COMMON ADULT DOSAGE: 1 to 2 drops twice daily to four times daily into affected eye
SIDE EFFECTS: eye irritation, blurred vision
AUXILIARY LABEL:
■ For the eye.

BOX 19-2 MAIN TREATMENTS FOR INFLAMMATION AND INFECTION

Antibiotics
Antifungals
Antihistamines
Antivirals
Corticosteroids
Decongestants
Nonsteroidal antiinflammatory drugs

GENERIC NAME: nedocromil
TRADE NAME: Alocril
INDICATION: allergic conjunctivitis
ROUTE OF ADMINISTRATION: ophthalmic
COMMON ADULT DOSAGE: 1 to 2 drops twice daily into affected eye
SIDE EFFECTS: eye irritation, blurred vision, unusual watering of the eyes
AUXILIARY LABEL:
■ For the eye.

Inflammation Caused by Infection or Injury

Corticosteroids. Corticosteroids are potent agents used to relieve inflammation resulting from infection or injury. They commonly are used postoperatively to decrease swelling. These agents should not be used any longer than necessary because they compromise the effectiveness of the immune system, resulting in a slower rate of healing. Corticosteroid ophthalmic dosage forms include solutions, suspensions, and ointments. Side effects may include a temporary burning sensation, blurred vision, eye pain, or headaches. Most of the agents used to decrease inflammation are solutions or suspensions. Suspensions need to be shaken well before use. Steroids reduce the inflammatory response by decreasing macrophage movement and the release of compounds associated with swelling and pain. If they are used over a long period, they can decrease antibody production. Treatments used for inflammation and/or infection are listed in Box 19-2.

ANTIINFLAMMATORY, CORTICOSTEROIDS

GENERIC NAME: prednisolone
TRADE NAME: Pred Forte (suspension)
INDICATION: inflammation
ROUTE OF ADMINISTRATION: ophthalmic
COMMON ADULT DOSAGE: 1 to 2 drops four times daily into affected eye
SIDE EFFECTS: eye irritation, blurred vision, unusual watering of the eyes
AUXILIARY LABELS:
■ For the eye.
■ Shake well before using.

GENERIC NAME: dexamethasone

TRADE NAME: Decadron phosphate (solution and ointment), Maxidex* (suspension)

INDICATION: inflammation

ROUTE OF ADMINISTRATION: ophthalmic

COMMON ADULT DOSAGE: 1 to 2 drops into affected eye(s) hourly during the daytime and every 2 hours at night until inflammation decreases; then decrease as directed (usually to every 4 hours)

SIDE EFFECTS: eye irritation, blurred vision, itching, sensitivity to light

AUXILIARY LABELS:

- For the eye.
- Use as directed.
- Shake well before using.

---

*If suspension is used, apply the label "Shake well before using."

Nonsteroidal Antiinflammatory Drugs (NSAIDs). NSAIDs inhibit the enzyme cyclooxygenase, which is responsible for the synthesis (creation) of prostaglandins. Prostaglandins are related directly to the mechanisms that are responsible for inflammation and the pain associated with it. Ophthalmic NSAIDs are available in solution only. Flurbiprofen and suprofen are indicated for intraoperative miosis. Diclofenac and ketorolac also relieve pruritus (itching) caused by allergies.

GENERIC NAME: flurbiprofen

TRADE NAME: Ocufen

INDICATION: Allergies; may be used to treat postoperative inflammation after cataract surgery

ROUTE OF ADMINISTRATION: ophthalmic

COMMON ADULT DOSAGE: 1 drop into affected eye every 30 minutes beginning 2 hours before surgery for a total of 4 drops

SIDE EFFECTS: eye irritation, blurred vision, itching

AUXILIARY LABELS:

- For the eye.
- Use as directed.

GENERIC NAME: ketoprofen ophthalmic

TRADE NAME: Acular

INDICATION: allergies

ROUTE OF ADMINISTRATION: ophthalmic

COMMON ADULT DOSAGE: 1 drop into affected eye(s) 4 times daily

SIDE EFFECTS: eye irritation, itching, headache

AUXILIARY LABELS:

- For the eye.
- Use as directed.

GENERIC NAME: diclofenac 1% soln

TRADE NAME: Voltaren

INDICATION: reduce pain, swelling, and light sensitivity (also used before and after surgery)

ROUTE OF ADMINISTRATION: ophthalmic

COMMON ADULT DOSAGE: 1 drop to affected eye(s) 4 times daily

SIDE EFFECTS: mild stinging or itching of the eyes, swollen eyelids

AUXILIARY LABEL:

- For the eye.

Conjunctivitis

This contagious condition, also known as "pink eye," is common in day care centers. Conjunctivitis is an acute inflammation of the conjunctiva that is caused by viruses, bacteria, fungus or allergies. Each type of conjunctivitis is treated differently although the symptoms of this condition are the same. The eye becomes red and a yellow discharge crusts over the eyelashes (occurs mostly after sleep); in addition, the eyes may burn and itch and cause blurred vision. Newborns can acquire a neonatal form of conjunctivitis (ophthalmia neonatorum) as they pass through the birth canal. Immediate prophylaxis must take place or the infant may lose his or her eyesight. Conjunctivitis attributable to allergies is discussed under Allergies.

Prognosis. With proper care and treatment this condition can be treated without any lasting effects. If left untreated, scarring may occur or even loss of eyesight in newborns. In children and adults viral infections normally last no more than 1 week without any medical treatment.

Non–Drug Treatment. Placing a warm compress onto the eyelids can relieve pain. The patient should wash hands frequently and avoid touching the eyes to prevent reintroduction of bacteria and proliferation of the infection. Towels and other personal care items should not be shared. Many forms of conjunctivitis are easily disseminated. If the patient wears contact lenses, the use of the lenses should be discontinued until the infection is resolved.

Drug Treatment. The treatment for conjunctivitis depends on its origin. When a virus causes conjunctivitis, there is no treatment because this form is similar to a "cold" of the eye and will run its course. For allergies, antihistamine eye drops are used. In the case of ophthalmia neonatorum, newborns are treated with erythromycin ointment at birth to deter infection.

Antiinfective Agents. Antiinfective agents are commonly used for conjunctivitis. The severe inflammation and discomfort of conjunctivitis can be treated with many different antibiotics. The physician determines the medication according to the cause of the infection. If the infection is viral, an agent such as vidarabine may be used. If the infection is fungal, natamycin may be prescribed. If the infection is bacterial, a wide variety of antibiotics can be used depending on the specific microbe. For many bacterial infections a wide-spectrum antibiotic, such as gentamicin or ciprofloxacin, may be used. Other popular ophthalmic drugs used to treat conjunctivitis and other infections of the eye are combinations that can treat both infection and inflammation at the same time. A list of combination agents is found in Table 19-2. Types of conjunctivitis are listed in Table 19-3.

OPHTHALMIC SULFONAMIDES

The actions of sulfonamides are bacteriostatic. Sulfonamides are effective against both gram-negative and gram-positive organisms. Sulfonamides block the formation of folic acid required by microbes.

TABLE 19-2 Antiinfective Combination Ophthalmics

Trade Name	Ingredients	Class of Drug	Indication
FML-S Suspension	fluorometholone 0.1%, sulfacetamide 10%	Steroid, antibiotic	Inflammatory/bacterial infection conditions of eye
Blephamide	prednisolone acetate 0.2%, sodium sulfacetamide 10%	Steroid, antibiotic	Inflammatory/bacterial infection conditions of eye
TobraDex Suspension	dexamethasone 0.1%, tobramycin 0.3%	Steroid, antibiotic	Inflammatory/bacterial infection conditions of eye
Zylet	loteprednol/tobramycin	Antihistamine, antibiotic	Inflammatory/bacterial infection conditions of eye
Pred-G	gentamicin/prednisolone	Steroid, antibiotic	Inflammatory/bacterial infection conditions of eye
Tobraflex	tobramycin/fluorometholone	Antibiotic, steroid	Inflammatory/bacterial infection conditions of eye
Neosporin	neomycin 3.5 mg/mL, polymyxin B sulfate 10,000 units/mL, bacitracin zinc 400 units/g	Antibiotics	Infection
Neocidin	gramicidin 0.025 mg, neomycin 1.75 mg/mL, polymyxin B sulfate 10,000 units/mL	Antibiotics	Infection

---

GENERIC NAME: sulfacetamide sodium

TRADE NAME: Bleph-10 (solution, ointment)

INDICATION: bacterial infections

ROUTE OF ADMINISTRATION: ophthalmic

COMMON ADULT DOSAGE: 1 to 2 drops into lower eyelid every 1 to 4 hr initially; for ointment, apply a thin ribbon four times daily and at bedtime

SIDE EFFECTS: eye irritation, itching, sensitivity to light

AUXILIARY LABELS:

■ For the eye.

■ Use as directed.

WARNING: This medication should not be used if the solution darkens. Avoid contamination.

Aminoglycosides. Aminoglycosides are a potent group of medications. Because of their wide spectrum of activity, they also can be used for some microbial-resistant strains. Side effects and adverse effects include burning, stinging, and photosensitivity. Their mechanism of action is the inhibition of bacterial protein synthesis. Aminoglycosides are bactericidal and are used to treat gram-negative and gram-positive microbes.

GENERIC NAME: gentamicin

TRADE NAME: Genoptic (solution), Garamycin (ophthalmic ointment)

INDICATIONS: bacterial infections

ROUTE OF ADMINISTRATION: ophthalmic

COMMON ADULT DOSAGE: solution, instill 1 to 2 drops every 2 to 4 hr; ointment, apply ½ inch q3-4h, twice daily to three times daily

SIDE EFFECTS: eye irritation, itching, sensitivity to light

AUXILIARY LABELS:

■ For the eye.

■ Use as directed.

TABLE 19-3 Viral/Nonviral Conjunctivitis

Types of Conjunctivitis (Nonviral)	Condition	Causes	Notes
Environmental			
	Allergic conjunctivitis	Pollen, dander, or other allergen	
	Vernal conjunctivitis	Recurrent hypersensitivity that may be genetic	Occurs mostly in summertime or hot climates
Bacterial (staphylococcal, streptococcal forms)	Neonatal conjunctivitis	Any bacteria that may enter eye area This includes normal flora present in women's vaginal area that passes onto infant at birth Infection, irritation, or blocked tear duct	Most hospitals treat newborns with erythromycin or azithromycin to prevent infection of eye
	Ophthalmia neonatorum	*Neisseria gonorrhoeae* (STD),* where child contracts infection while passing through birth canal	Most hospitals treat newborns with erythromycin or azithromycin to prevent infection of eye
	Chlamydial neonatal conjunctivitis	Bacterium *Chlamydia trachomatis* (STD), where child contracts infection while passing through birth canal; rare in U.S.	Because infection is not limited to eyes this must be treated with systemic antibiotics such as erythromycin
	Trachoma	Chronic form of *Chlamydia trachomatis* (STD) bacterial infection	High risk of blindness
Diseases	Keratoconjunctivitis sicca	Lack of tears as one ages	
	Systemic lupus	Autoimmune disease	
	Crohn's disease	Abnormal immune response	Causes eye inflammation as an extraintestinal symptom in some patients
	Rheumatoid arthritis	Abnormal immune response	
Contact lenses		Rubbing eyes or touching contacts after touching infected surfaces	
Chemical exposures		Chlorine chemicals in a swimming pool, other chemical exposures	
Viral conjunctivitis			
Pink eye		Viral or bacterial infection of conjunctiva	

*STD, Sexually transmitted disease.

> **GENERIC NAME:** tobramycin
> **TRADE NAME:** Tobrex (solution and ointment)
> **INDICATION:** bacterial infections
> **ROUTE OF ADMINISTRATION:** ophthalmic
> **COMMON ADULT DOSAGE:** solution, instill 1 to 2 drops every 4 hours; ointment, apply twice daily to three times daily
> **SIDE EFFECTS:** eye irritation, itching, sensitivity to light
> **AUXILIARY LABELS:**
> ■ For the eye.
> ■ Use as directed.

Macrolides. The antiinfective erythromycin is available only in ointment form for ophthalmic use. Side effects may include stinging, burning, itching, and inflammation.

This agent is bacteriostatic but can be bactericidal if used in high doses. Erythromycin is used to treat mostly gram-positive and some gram-negative microbes. Erythromycin ophthalmic ointment is most commonly used as a prophylactic treatment for newborns to prevent ophthalmia neonatorum (gonorrhea infection of the eye).

> **GENERIC NAME:** erythromycin
> **TRADE NAME:** Ilotycin
> **INDICATION:** bacterial infections
> **ROUTE OF ADMINISTRATION:** ophthalmic
> **COMMON ADULT DOSAGE:** instill ½ inch 2 to 8 times daily, depending on the type and severity of the eye infection; in neonates, the ointment is applied once within 1 hour of birth for prevention
> **SIDE EFFECTS:** eye irritation, itching, sensitivity to light
> **AUXILIARY LABEL:**
> ■ For the eye.

Antifungals. Fungal conjunctivitis is relatively rare. Specific fungal infections must be treated with agents that can attack the specific metabolism of the invading fungus. The primary ophthalmic agent for superficial eye infections is natamycin, a fungicidal agent. The only noted adverse effect is a possible sensitivity to the formulation. The specific method of action involves the antifungal drug binding to the cell membrane of the fungus. When this occurs, the stability of the membrane is jeopardized, and the cell membrane deteriorates, killing the fungus. Safety has not been established in children and pregnant or lactating women.

Tech Note!

The best way to avoid conjunctivitis is to wash your hands before touching the eyes. Other possible ways to come into contact with this infection include sharing towels, pillows, and even computer keyboards.

> **GENERIC NAME:** natamycin
> **TRADE NAME:** Natacyn (suspension)
> **INDICATION:** fungal infections (blepharitis, conjunctivitis, or keratitis only)
> **ROUTE OF ADMINISTRATION:** ophthalmic
> **COMMON ADULT DOSAGE:** to treat fungal conjunctivitis, 1 drop four to six times per day over a minimum of 14 days
> **SIDE EFFECTS:** eye irritation, itching, sensitivity to light
> **AUXILIARY LABELS:**
> ■ For the eye.
> ■ Shake well before using.

Antivirals. The three most common viral infections of the eye are herpes simplex, keratitis, and conjunctivitis. The aim of antiviral therapy is to interrupt or alter the synthesis of new virions at a specific step during replication, thus rendering the virion inactive. Many of the viruses that affect the eyes are more common in persons who are immunocompromised, such as those diagnosed with acquired immunodeficiency syndrome (AIDS). Side effects may be sensitivity to light, stinging, or mild burning sensation. The general method of action for these antiviral agents is at the point where the attacking virus is using the host's deoxyribonucleic acid (DNA) to replicate. This results in a malformation of various components necessary for properly working virions.

GENERIC NAME: idoxuridine
TRADE NAME: Dendrid
ROUTE OF ADMINISTRATION: ophthalmic
INDICATION: viral infection, infections caused by herpes simplex virus
COMMON ADULT DOSAGE: initially, 1 drop into eye(s) every hour during the day and every 2 hours at night; may decrease over time as determined by physician
SIDE EFFECTS: eye irritation, itching, sensitivity to light
AUXILIARY LABELS:
- For the eye.
- Take as directed.

GENERIC NAME: vidarabine
TRADE NAME: Vira-A (ointment)
ROUTE OF ADMINISTRATION: ophthalmic
INDICATION: viral infections and those caused by herpes virus
COMMON ADULT DOSAGE: apply thin ribbon of ointment to lower eyelid 5 times daily at 3-hour intervals
SIDE EFFECTS: eye irritation, itching, sensitivity to light
AUXILIARY LABELS:
- For the eye.
- Use as directed.

GENERIC NAME: trifluridine
TRADE NAME: Viroptic (solution)
ROUTE OF ADMINISTRATION: ophthalmic
INDICATION: viral infection
COMMON ADULT DOSAGE: 1 drop into affected eye every 2 hours while awake for a maximum of 9 drops; then treatment may decrease to 1 drop every 4 hours while awake (for 7 days) for a maximum of 7 drops per day
SIDE EFFECTS: eye irritation, itching, sensitivity to light
AUXILIARY LABELS:
- For the eye.
- Use as directed.
- Must be refrigerated.

Cataracts

Cataracts are a condition caused by the formation of protein deposits on the lens. Vision is impaired because light cannot fully penetrate the cloudy lens to reach the retina and the optic nerve. Eventually a person's vision becomes blurred, and if the cataract is left untreated, it can cause blindness. Symptoms that occur with cataracts include double vision, cloudy or blurry vision, and nighttime vision difficulties.

In fact, cataracts are the leading cause of blindness worldwide, followed by glaucoma. In the United States, more than 22 million people have cataracts; by the age of 80 years more than half of all people in the United States will either

TABLE 19-4 Types of Cataracts

Types of Cataracts	Due to	Description/Notes
Congenital (family history)	Cataracts developed in fetal stage (in womb); are present at birth	Reasons include genetic mutations before birth, infections (viral/bacterial), or drug reactions attributable to mother taking certain antibiotics
Age-related	Aging process; cataracts more prevalent with age; cataracts in persons >60 yr can cause blindness	Clumps of protein, often in older adults, cloud lens; lens begins to change to a brownish color, which can lead to inability to detect colors
Pediatric	Overlooking congenital form or trauma to eyes	Surgery can be done just days after birth
Secondary	Another disease condition	Marfan syndrome is a mutation of the gene responsible for making filbrillin 1 (connective tissue producer); among its symptoms are early cataracts and glaucoma
Trauma	Injury to eye at any age	Either blunt or penetrating trauma directly to ocular lens
Environmental	Exposure to certain types of radiation	Sunlight and ultraviolet radiation over many years can cause damage to lens
Toxic/drug induced	Side effects of certain drugs (corticosteroids)	Other drugs associated with drug-induced cataracts include TCAs,* Phenothiazines, miotics

*TCAs, Tricyclic antidepressants.

have a cataract or have undergone cataract surgery (National Institutes of Health, 2008). There are various types/causes of cataracts (Table 19-4), which determines the subsequent treatment. The mechanism of action that results in cataract formation is still unknown. Factors that exacerbate the problem include irritants to the eye such as cigarette smoke and environmental factors.

Prognosis. It is not possible to deter a person's likelihood to develop cataracts; however, cataracts do not grow back if surgery is performed successfully.

Non–Drug Treatment. Often eyewear is prescribed—eyeglasses or contacts that can restore vision problems. Surgery is another option; in this procedure the cloudy lens of the eye is replaced with an artificial lens cover. Following surgery, the eyes should be protected by wearing sunglasses and avoiding cigarette smoke and other irritants.

Drug Treatment. There are no current medications that can be used for long-term treatment of cataracts. Mydriatic-cycloplegic drugs are used in the diagnosis of cataracts (dilated eye examinations) and to treat inflammation after surgery has been performed. Mydriatic eye drops can be used to help dilate the pupil and increase the amount of light that passes through the cloudy lens. A cycloplegic paralyzes the ciliary muscle (making it impossible to focus on near objects). Examples of these agents include atropine, cyclopentolate, homatropine, and tropicamide. The purpose of most ophthalmic medications is to control glaucoma, treat infection or inflammation, or manipulate pupil dilation. For an overview of some of the mydriatic agents used before eye surgery, refer to Table 19-5.

TABLE 19-5 **Commonly Used Agents for the Treatment of Glaucoma**

Classification of Drug	Generic Name	Trade Name	Indication	Side Effects
Beta-adrenergic blocking agents	betaxolol	Betoptic	Open-angle glaucoma	Burning, stinging, eye irritation
	carteolol	Ocupress		
	levobunolol	Betagan		
	metipranolol	OptiPranolol		
	timolol	Timoptic		
Carbonic anhydrase inhibitors	dorzolamide	Trusopt	Lower IOP* in open-angle or angle-closure glaucoma	
	methazolamide	Neptazane		
	brinzolamide	Azopt		
Miotics, intraocular	carbachol	Miostat	Open-angle or angle-closure glaucoma	Blurred vision, irritation, myopia, headache
Miotics, ophthalmic	pilocarpine	Isopto-Carpine	Glaucoma	
	dipivefrin	Propine	Elevated IOP	Burning, stinging, eye irritation
Sympathomimetics	brimonidine	Alphagan P	Open-angle glaucoma	
Prostaglandin	bimatoprost	Lumigan	Elevated IOP agonist	
	latanoprost	Xalatan		
	travoprost	Travatan		

*IOP, Intraocular pressure.

ANTICHOLINERGICS

GENERIC NAME: cyclopentolate
TRADE NAME: Cyclogyl, Cyclate, AK-Pentolate
INDICATION: for dilation and relaxation of the pupil
ROUTE OF ADMINISTRATION: ophthalmic
COMMON ADULT DOSAGE: 1-2 drops into each eye as prescribed
SIDE EFFECTS: blurred vision, sensitivity to sunlight, mild stinging of the eye or swelling of the eyelids
AUXILIARY LABEL:
■ For the eye.

CHOLINERGICS—MIOTICS

GENERIC NAME: acetylcholine
TRADE NAME: Miochol-E
INDICATION: used for eye surgery
ROUTE OF ADMINISTRATION: ophthalmic
COMMON ADULT DOSAGE: 5- to 20-mg injection before or after suture is in place
SIDE EFFECTS: headaches and decreased night vision
AUXILIARY LABEL:
■ For the eye.

BOX 19-3 TYPES OF GLAUCOMA*

Primary (Includes Angle-Closure or Open-Angle Conditions)
Acute congestive: Also called angle-closure glaucoma; this refers to the closure of the anterior chamber, possibly resulting from genetic defects.
Chronic simple: Also called open-angle glaucoma; this refers to the increase in intraocular pressure rather than a closed duct. About 90% of persons suffering from glaucoma have this type of condition.
Treatment: Correction by medication or surgery (laser).

Secondary
This condition may result from an existing eye condition or may occur following cataract extraction.
Treatment: Correction or control by medication.

Congenital
This condition exists because of genetic predisposition.
Treatment: Correction by surgery.

*See Table 19-5 for agents used to treat glaucoma.

GENERIC NAME: diclofenac 1% soln
TRADE NAME: Voltaren
INDICATION: postoperative ophthalmic inflammation and pain; also used for allergies
ROUTE OF ADMINISTRATION: ophthalmic
COMMON ADULT DOSAGE: 1 to 2 drops into affected eye within 1 hour before surgery; after surgery, 1 drop into affected eye four times daily for 2 weeks
SIDE EFFECTS: eye pain, redness, watering, sensitivity to light, white patches on eyes
AUXILIARY LABELS:
- For the eye.
- Use as directed.

Glaucoma

Glaucoma is a group of ophthalmic disorders characterized by high intraocular pressure (IOP) that can damage the optic nerve. If untreated, it can lead to peripheral vision loss and ultimately blindness. Two main causes for this condition are overproduction of aqueous humor and blockage of the ducts that drain excess aqueous humor. The three types or levels of glaucoma are listed in Box 19-3. Depending on the degree of severity, a wide range of medications and treatments are available. The treatments for glaucoma are aimed at controlling intraocular pressure.

Prognosis. Although glaucoma is the second leading cause of blindness worldwide (Glaucoma Research Foundation), it can be treated before it leads to this irreversible condition. With the use of glaucoma medications this condition can be successfully managed for many years.

Non–Drug Treatment. Surgery can be used to implant drainage valves for the outflow of aqueous humor. Alternatively, in some cases corrective lenses can be used for glaucoma treatment.

Drug Treatment. Treatment of glaucoma focuses on decreasing IOP by increasing drainage of, or reducing the production of, aqueous humor. Ophthalmic dosage forms include drops, suspensions, and ointments; in some cases, medicated inserts may be prescribed. Five classifications of drugs can be used topically to treat glaucoma: beta-adrenergic blockers, carbonic anhydrase inhibitors, miotics, sympathomimetics, and prostaglandin agonists. Because these drugs are specific in their actions, the right diagnosis is important in order to prescribe the correct medication. In many cases, more than one medication is used.

Beta-Adrenergic Blockers. The beta-adrenergic blockers are referred to as beta-blockers. These medications lower the intraocular pressure in open-angle glaucoma. These agents affect a specific site within the adrenergic system (also known as the sympathetic system). By binding to a beta site, the blockers prevent the activation of the beta-adrenergic response (i.e., the sympathetic or "fight or flight" response), which affects many body systems (see Chapter 16). Specifically, in the eye beta-adrenergic blockers prevent constriction of blood vessels in the eye, and therefore aid in the drainage of aqueous humor, reducing intraocular pressure. Most ophthalmic agents are nonspecific and can bind to both beta-receptor sites; however, betaxolol is beta-1 selective.

GENERIC NAME: betaxolol
TRADE NAME: Betoptic (solution), Betoptic-S (suspension)
ROUTE OF ADMINISTRATION: ophthalmic
INDICATION: open-angle glaucoma
COMMON ADULT DOSAGE: 1 drop into eye(s) twice daily
SIDE EFFECTS: mild stinging, itching of the eyes, dry eyes, swollen eyelids, headache, dizziness, insomnia
AUXILIARY LABEL:
■ For the eye.
■ Shake well before using (suspension).

GENERIC NAME: carteolol
TRADE NAME: Ocupress
ROUTE OF ADMINISTRATION: ophthalmic
INDICATION: open-angle glaucoma or ocular hypertension
COMMON ADULT DOSAGE: 1 drop twice daily
SIDE EFFECTS: burning, stinging, headache, fatigue, nausea
AUXILIARY LABEL:
■ For the eye.

GENERIC NAME: levobunolol
TRADE NAME: Betagan
INDICATION: chronic open-angle glaucoma or ocular hypertension
ROUTE OF ADMINISTRATION: ophthalmic
COMMON ADULT DOSAGE: 1-2 drops once (0.5% soln) or twice daily (0.25% soln) into affected eye(s)
SIDE EFFECTS: burning, stinging, headache, fatigue, nausea
AUXILIARY LABEL:
■ For the eye.

GENERIC NAME: metipranolol
TRADE NAME: OptiPranolol
INDICATION: glaucoma or intraocular hypertension
ROUTE OF ADMINISTRATION: ophthalmic
COMMON ADULT DOSAGE: 1 drop twice daily into affected eye(s)
SIDE EFFECTS: burning, stinging, headache, fatigue, nausea
AUXILIARY LABEL:
■ For the eye.

> **GENERIC NAME:** timolol
> **TRADE NAME:** Timoptic, Timoptic-XE (gel-forming solution)
> **INDICATION:** open-angle glaucoma
> **ROUTE OF ADMINISTRATION:** ophthalmic
> **COMMON ADULT DOSAGE:** 1 drop twice daily into affected eye(s); Timoptic-XE dosage, 1 drop twice daily into affected eye(s)
> **SIDE EFFECTS:** stinging of the eye, blurred vision, drooping eyelid, headache, dizziness
> **AUXILIARY LABEL:**
> ■ For the eye.
> **SPECIAL NOTE:** Patient must be instructed to invert and shake Timoptic-XE container once before each application. A pharmacist shows the patient this process at the time of consultation.

Carbonic Anhydrase Inhibitors. Carbonic anhydrase inhibitors are medications used to treat glaucoma. These medications sometimes are prescribed with other miotic and osmotic ophthalmic agents. These agents inhibit the enzyme carbonic anhydrase, and thereby decrease the formation of aqueous humor. By directly applying these medications to the eye, the intraocular pressure is reduced in persons suffering from chronic simple open-angle glaucoma. In persons suffering from secondary (angle-closure) glaucoma, carbonic anhydrase inhibitors can be used only for a short duration to lower the intraocular pressure in order to perform surgery. Carbonic anhydrase inhibitors can be applied locally to the eye, or may be given systemically (orally, e.g., methazolamide).

> **GENERIC NAME:** dorzolamide
> **TRADE NAME:** Trusopt
> **INDICATION:** open-angle glaucoma or preoperatively for procedures to treat angle-closure glaucoma
> **ROUTE OF ADMINISTRATION:** ophthalmic
> **COMMON ADULT DOSAGE:** 1 drop three times daily into affected eye
> **SIDE EFFECTS:** eye irritation, such as blurring, and stinging sensation
> **AUXILIARY LABEL:**
> ■ For the eye.

> **GENERIC NAME:** brinzolamide
> **TRADE NAME:** Azopt
> **INDICATION:** open-angle glaucoma or preoperatively for procedures to treat angle-closure glaucoma
> **ROUTE OF ADMINISTRATION:** ophthalmic
> **COMMON ADULT DOSAGE:** 1 drop three times daily into affected eye
> **SIDE EFFECTS:** eye irritation, such as blurring, and stinging sensation
> **AUXILIARY LABELS:**
> ■ For the eye.
> ■ Shake well before using.

CARBONIC ANHYDRASE INHIBITOR—ORAL

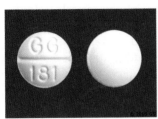

GENERIC NAME: methazolamide

TRADE NAME: Neptazane

INDICATION: open-angle glaucoma or preoperatively for procedures to treat angle-closure glaucoma

ROUTE OF ADMINISTRATION: oral

COMMON ADULT DOSAGE: 50 to 100 mg twice daily or three times daily

SIDE EFFECTS: increased urination, pain in lower back, pain or burning while urinating, dizziness, constipation, headache

AUXILIARY LABEL:

■ May cause drowsiness.

Miotics. Miotics are similar to carbonic anhydrase inhibitors regarding the types of glaucoma that they treat. These medications reduce the intraocular pressure by increasing the outflow of aqueous humor from the eye. Within the classification of miotics are direct-acting agents and indirect-acting agents. Direct-acting agents lower the intraocular pressure by contracting the ciliary muscle around the eye, increasing the outflow of aqueous humor. Certain ophthalmic drugs are injectable and are used in eye surgery. Indirect agents inhibit an enzyme (cholinesterase) that causes ciliary muscle contraction, reducing the resistance of the aqueous humor outflow. The result is the same in either case.

CHOLINERGICS—MIOTICS

GENERIC NAME: carbachol, Isopto-carbacho

TRADE NAME: Miostat, Isopto-carbachol

INDICATION: long-term treatment for open-angle glaucoma

ROUTE OF ADMINISTRATION: ophthalmic (Isopto-carbachol), intraocular (Miostat)

COMMON ADULT DOSAGE: 1 to 2 drops, max 3 times a day into affected eye, (Isopto-carbachol)

SIDE EFFECTS: headaches and decreased night vision

AUXILIARY LABEL:

■ For the eye.

GENERIC NAME: pilocarpine

TRADE NAME: Pilocar, Isopto-Carpine

INDICATION: long-term treatment for open-angle glaucoma

ROUTE OF ADMINISTRATION: ophthalmic

COMMON ADULT DOSAGE: 1 drop three to four times daily into affected eye

SIDE EFFECTS: headaches and decreased night vision

AUXILIARY LABEL:

■ For the eye.

Sympathomimetics. The name *sympathomimetics* refers to mimicking or "acting like" the sympathetic system. The primary agent, phenylephrine, helps to constrict blood vessels in the nasal and sinus passages. Most of the agents in this class are intended specifically for persons suffering from allergies and congestion in the eyes. When the sympathetic system is activated (see Chapter 16), the vessels in the eyes contract, the pupils dilate, and the ciliary muscle relaxes. The result is an increase in drainage and, with certain agents, a decrease in aqueous humor production. These medications are used to treat open-angle glaucoma and are often used in conjunction with other antiglaucoma agents to reduce intraocular pressure.

GENERIC NAME: brimonidine
TRADE NAME: Alphagan P
INDICATION: used commonly along with miotics to treat glaucoma
ROUTE OF ADMINISTRATION: ophthalmic
COMMON ADULT DOSAGE: 1 drop three times daily into affected eye
SIDE EFFECTS: blurriness and, if overused, redness of the eyes.
AUXILIARY LABEL:
■ For the eye.
■ Do not take MAOIs while using this medication.

Prostaglandin Agonists. Several agents are indicated to treat glaucoma under this classification: latanoprost, bimatoprost, travoprost, and unoprostone. These medications reduce the intraocular pressure by increasing the outflow of aqueous humor.

GENERIC NAME: latanoprost
TRADE NAME: Xalatan
INDICATION: open-angle glaucoma and to decrease intraocular pressure
ROUTE OF ADMINISTRATION: ophthalmic
COMMON ADULT DOSAGE: 1 drop once in the evening into affected eye
SIDE EFFECTS: possible change in iris color (becomes darker)
AUXILIARY LABELS:
■ For the eye.
■ Protect from light.
■ Possible permanent change in eye color, thickening and darkening of eyelashes, darkening of eyelids.

GENERIC NAME: bimatoprost
TRADE NAME: Lumigan
INDICATION: to decrease intraocular pressure
ROUTE OF ADMINISTRATION: ophthalmic
COMMON ADULT DOSAGE: 1 drop once in the evening into affected eye
SIDE EFFECTS: mild eye irritation, stinging after use, dry or watery eyes
AUXILIARY LABELS:
■ For the eye.
■ Possible permanent change in eye color, thickening and darkening of eyelashes, darkening of eyelids.

Blindness

Blindness is a lack of vision that can be partial or complete. Complete blurriness of vision can be due to diabetic retinopathy. Macular degeneration results in

Tech Note!

A new bimatoprost formulation (Latisse) is indicated for the thickening of eyelashes. It is used to treat hypotrichosis (i.e., less than normal amount of hair) of the eyelashes.

blindness of central vision and the presence of only peripheral vision. If the field of vision is limited to a small circular opening in the middle, this condition is called retinitis pigmentosa, and blurriness of the center of vision with darkened perimeters is indicative of glaucoma. Depending on the cause, new treatments are available that possibly can reverse the effects. For example, if glaucoma is left untreated, it can cause total blindness; however, if diagnosed in the early stages it can be successfully managed with a variety of ophthalmic medications (see Glaucoma).

Prognosis. The outcome of blindness varies depending on the cause. For many conditions such as cataracts, glaucoma, and infections there are medications and surgical treatments that can prevent blindness. For other conditions such as macular degeneration the disease process can be slowed, while certain genetic conditions such as anophthalmia result in permanent blindness (Table 19-6). Those conditions that cause partial blindness can be treated with visual aids.

Non–Drug Treatment. The most common treatments for visual impairment include glasses, magnifying glasses, sunglasses, or surgery (e.g., lens implants, removal of causative effect).

TABLE 19-6 Causes of Blindness

Causes of Blindness		Websites for More Information
Cataracts	Cloudiness of eye lens	www.nei.nih.gov
Glaucoma	Intraocular fluid cannot drain from eye ducts, increasing intraocular pressure	www.globalaigs.org
Diabetic retinopathy	Blood vessels that supply retina grow abnormally and rupture; retina may detach	www.diabetes.org
Age-related macular degeneration (ARMD)	Macula (center of visual acuity; responsible for clear, straight-ahead vision) degenerates, causing loss of sight	www.aoa.org
Retinitis pigmentosa	Degeneration of retina and choroid; inherited progressive condition	www.genome.gov
Examples of Less Common Eye Conditions		
Achromatopsia	Genetic/inherited: Little or no cone cell functions, causing color blindness, extreme light sensitivity, nystagmus	www.blindness.org
Aniridia	Genetic eye condition in which iris is absent or underdeveloped	
Anophthalmia	Eyes did not grow in utero; if 1 eye develops, may have some vision; no known cause	
Choroideremia	Inherited condition causing progressive loss of vision attributable to lack of a specific protein; results in degeneration of choroid and retina and eventual blindness	
Stargardt's disease	Juvenile degeneration/progressive inherited condition; lipid deposits in retinal pigment lining under macula, leading to blindness	
Usher's syndrome	Condition of both eyes and ears In eyes disorder is called retinitis pigmentosa, causing night blindness; balance problems also present	
Monochromastism	Abnormal or missing rods/cones	

BOX 19-4 PROPER USE OF EYE DROPS

Basic steps for the use of eye drops are as follows:

1. Wash hands.
2. Tilt head backward or lie down and gaze upward.
3. Gently pull lower eyelid down and away from the eye to form a pouch.
4. Place dropper directly over the eye. Avoid contact of the dropper with the eye or any other surface such as fingers.
5. Look upward just before applying a drop.
6. After instilling the drop, look downward for several seconds.
7. Release the lid slowly and close eyes gently.
8. With eyes closed, use fingertips to apply gentle pressure to the inside corner of the eye for 3 to 5 minutes (this prevents the solution from becoming part of the naso-lacrimal drainage, where the drug could enter the systemic circulation; temporary occlusion helps prevent systemic side effects and may improve drug efficacy).
9. Do not rub the eye or squeeze the eyelid, and try not to blink.
10. Do not rinse the dropper.
11. If more than one type of eye drop is being used, wait at least 5 minutes before administering the second agent.
12. For ointments, follow steps 1 to 3. Then apply $\frac{1}{4}$ to $\frac{1}{2}$ inch of ointment with a sweeping motion inside the lower eyelid by squeezing the tube gently and slowly releasing the eyelid. Close the eye for 1 to 2 minutes and roll the eyeball in all directions. Remove any excess ointment from around the eye with a tissue. If using more than one kind of ointment, wait 10 minutes before applying the second ointment.

Drug Treatment. Depending on the type of visual impairment, there are many ophthalmic treatments, such as antibiotics, IOP reducers, and other agents. For many persons, a corneal transplant may correct blindness. Another type of treatment for certain damaged corneal linings is stem cell transplant. This may reverse blindness through regeneration of a new membrane lining.

Miscellaneous Ophthalmic Agents

Agents such as artificial tears commonly are purchased over-the-counter. They are used for the relief of dry eyes and irritation that may occur. Their ingredients include sodium chloride, buffers to adjust for pH, and other additives to prolong their effects. The only dosage form is a solution, but they are available in various strengths and in combination with various ingredients. Although each tear product has somewhat different ingredients, all contain sodium chloride and all are used for the same reasons. Box 19-4 lists application techniques used for instillation of ophthalmic solutions.

Artificial tear inserts are also available by prescription for dry eye syndrome or severe keratoconjunctivitis. Another agent that can be used is Restasis (cyclosporine) eye drops; Restasis helps alleviate chronic dry eyes caused by inflammation. Table 19-7 lists examples of the most common types of artificial tears.

The Ears (Auditory System)

The human ear is not only responsible for hearing but also for balance, equilibrium, and many communication skills. The ear is composed of three major sections: the external, middle, and inner ear (Figure 19-3).

TABLE 19-7 Artificial Tear Products

Trade Name	Manufacturer	Ingredients
Tear Drop	Parmed	polyvinyl alcohol, NaCl, EDTA,* benzalkonium chloride
Artifical Tears	Various manufacturers	polyvinyl alcohol, povidone, NaCl, chlorobutanol
Cellufresh	Allergan	carboxymethylcellulose, NaCl, KCl, sodium lactate
Refresh	Allergan	polyvinyl alcohol, povidone, NaCl
Just Tears	Blairex	benzalkonium chloride, EDTA, polyvinyl alcohol, NaCl
Murine	Ross	polyvinyl alcohol, povidone, benzalkonium chloride, dextrose, EDTA, NaCl, sodium bicarbonate, sodium phosphate

*EDTA, Ethylenediaminetetraacetic acid.

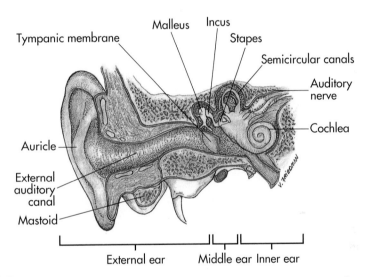

FIGURE 19-3 Anatomy of the ear. (From Potter PA, Perry AG: *Fundamentals of nursing,* ed 7, St Louis, 2009, Mosby.)

COMMON DRUGS USED FOR CONDITIONS OF THE EAR

Trade Name	Generic Name	Pronunciation	Trade Name	Generic Name	Pronunciation
Anesthetic			**Swimmer's Ear**		
Auralgan	antipyrine/ benzocaine	(an-tee-**pie**-reen/ **ben**-zoe-kane)	Swim-EAR	isopropyl alcohol/ anhydrous glycerin	(**eye**-so-pro-pal **al**-ko-hall/ an-**high**-dros glis-**sir**-in)
			Acetasol HC	acetic acid/ hydrocortisone	(as-**seet**-ik as-id/ hydro-**kor**-ti-sone)
Otitis Externa					
Earwax Removal			**Otic Broad-Spectrum Antibiotic**		
Cerumenex	triethanolamine polypeptide oleate-condensate	(tri-eth-an-**oh**-la-meen pol-e-**pep**-tide **oh**-lee-ate **kon**-den-sate)	Chloromycetin	chloramphenicol	(klor-am-**fen**-eye-kol)

COMMON DRUGS USED FOR CONDITIONS OF THE EAR—cont'd

Trade Name	Generic Name	Pronunciation	Trade Name	Generic Name	Pronunciation
Fluoroquinolones			**Penicillins**		
Cetraxal	ciprofloxacin	(**sip**-row-**flock**-a-sin)	Amoxil	amoxicillin	(am-**ox**-i-**sil**-in)
Floxin	ofloxacin	(oh-**floks**-ah-sin)	Augmentin	amoxicillin/	(am-**ox**-i-**sil**-in/
				clavulanate	**clav**-ue-la-nate)
Otic Antibiotic Combination					
Cortisporin Otic	hydrocortisone/	(**hi**-drow-**core**-tah-zone/	**Cephalosporins**		
	neomycin/	**knee**-oh-**my**-sin/	Omnicef	cefdinir	(**sef**-dih-near)
	polymyxin B	**pol**-ee-**mix**-in B)	Ceftin	cefuroxime	(**sef**-you-**rox**-eem)
			Vantin	cefpodoxime	(**sef**-poe-**dox**-eem)
Fluoroquinolone/Corticosteroid Combinations			Cedax	ceftibuten	(**sef**-tie-**bue**-ten)
Ciprodex	ciprofloxacin/	(sih-pro-**flock**-sah-sin/			
	dexamethasone	dex-ah-**meth**-ah-sone)	**Beta-Lactam (Carbacephem)**		
Cipro HC	ciprofloxacin/	(sih-pro-**flock**-sah-sin/	Lorabid	loracarbef	(lor-a-**kar**-bef)
	hydrocortisone	**hi**-drow-**core**-tah-zone)			
			Macrolide/Sulfa Combination		
Oral Antibiotics			E.S.P.	erythromycin/	e-RITH-row-MY-sin/
Macrolides				sulfisoxazole	SUL-fi-SOX-a-zole
Zithromax	azithromycin	(a-**zith**-row-**my**-sin)			
Biaxin	clarithromycin	(kla-**rith**-row-**my**-sin)			

MEDICAL TERMS AND CONDITIONS OF THE EAR

Word Combinations	
Tympan/o	Tympanic membrane
Audi/o	Hearing
Ot/o	Ear
Py/o	Pus
Myring/o	Eardrum

Prefixes	
Mon-	One
Bi-	Two

Suffixes	
-ologist	Specialist
-rrhea	Flow or discharge
-rrhagia	Bleeding, excessive flow
-algia	Pain
-it is	Inflammation

Conditions of the Ear	
Deafness	Partial or complete loss of hearing
Noise-induced hearing loss	Repeated exposure to loud noises causes nerve damage and hearing loss
Otalgia	Earache
Otitis externa	Inflammation of outer ear canal; also known as swimmer's ear
Otitis media	Inflammation of middle ear caused by infection
Otomycosis	Otitis externa caused by fungal infection
Ototoxicity	Hearing loss resulting from medications
Presbycusis	Gradual loss of hearing that occurs as one ages
Sensorineural hearing loss	Damage of auditory nerve or hair cells in inner ear
Tinnitus	Ringing or buzzing in one or both ears
Vertigo	Loss of balance, dizziness

ANATOMY OF THE EAR

External Ear

The most exterior part of the ear is called the auricle. This area is composed of cartilage and skin and serves as an entrance for sound waves. The auricle transmits sound waves through the external **auditory canal**. This canal, measuring approximately 1 inch long, leads to the **tympanic membrane** (eardrum) inside the ear. This membrane has two major functions:

- Protection of the middle ear from foreign objects
- Transmission of sound waves to the middle ear

The transmission is possible because of the vibration caused when sound hits the membrane, much the same way a drum skin vibrates and carries sound when struck with a drumstick. Cerumen (a waxy substance) is produced by glands inside the ear.

Middle Ear

Vibrations from the tympanic membrane are carried into the middle ear. This cavity (space) contains three small bony structures called **auditory ossicles**. These are as follows:

- Malleus (hammer)
- Incus (anvil)
- Stapes (stirrup)

These three small bones are connected to each other and transmit the sound waves that enter the cavity. Another area in the middle ear is the **eustachian tube**. This tube leads to the nasopharynx. When swallowing, yawning, or movement of the jaw occurs, the eustachian tube opens and relieves the change in pressure between the outside and inside atmosphere.

Inner Ear

After the transmission of sounds through the ossicles, the stapes (last ossicle) then continues the transfer of sound into the third section of the ear called the inner ear. This fluid-filled area is called the **labyrinth** and is composed of many components that process and transmit the audible sounds via nerve impulses (via **acoustic nerve**) to the brain, where the sound then is interpreted. The two important areas or divisions of the labyrinth are the following:

Perilymph (bony labyrinth)	Composed of three main structures: cochlea, vestibule, and semicircular canal
Membrane division	Lines the bony division; areas include sacs and tubes that run throughout the inner ear and aid in sound wave transference

The three main structures within the bony division are in proximity to one another and have separate but important functions as described in Box 19-5 (Figure 19-4).

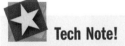

Tech Note!

When climbing altitudes in a car or plane, the eustachian tube relieves the decreased pressure from the outside by causing a "pop" of the ear. This causes equalization between the two pressure levels.

CONDITIONS AFFECTING THE EAR

Various conditions can affect the quality of hearing, including infections, earwax accumulation, damage to the eardrum, and genetic defects (Table 19-8). Most infections of the ear are viral in nature; however, bacterial infections may follow. Depending on the strain of bacterial infection, certain preparations are

BOX 19-5 THREE MAIN AREAS OF THE INNER EAR AND THEIR FUNCTIONS

Cochlea

This area is coiled and consists of three fluid-filled canals. The small, hair-like structures found here are connected to the acoustic nerve (i.e., the vestibulocochlear nerve [CN VIII]) that transmits impulses to the brain. As the sound waves enter, the hairs bend and create impulses that are transmitted to the acoustic nerve.

Vestibule

The vestibule is located between the cochlea and the semicircular canals and is responsible for equilibrium and balance. Small, hair-like cells are affected by gravity and when they move nerve impulses are transmitted to the brain, specifically to the cerebellum and midbrain areas. Thus equilibrium is maintained. This gives human beings a sense of direction and orientation.

Semicircular Canals

Three semicircular canals are filled with a fluid that helps with the transfer of messages via the acoustic nerve. Small, hair-like fibers behave as sensors, moving back and forth as the person moves forward, backward, or stops. The signals sent from two of these canals provide information to the brain about the orientation of the body when at rest, whereas the third canal sends information pertaining to the body when in motion.

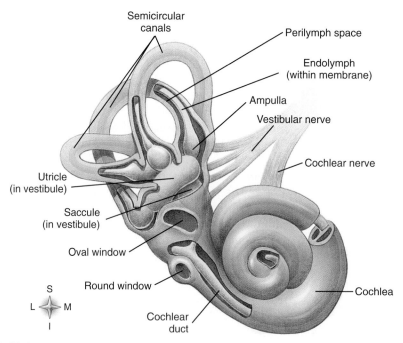

FIGURE 19-4 Anatomy of the inner ear. (From Thibodeau GA, Patton KT: *Anatomy and physiology,* ed 6, St Louis, 2007, Mosby.)

available—bactericidal or bacteriostatic. Bactericidal agents kill the bacteria, whereas bacteriostatic agents limit bacterial growth (see Chapter 30). Drugs that are bacteriostatic are used to assist the body's immune system in the battle against bacteria. Table 19-9 lists otic agents along with their indication for use. Almost all ear preparations contain several major ingredients such as antibiotic combinations or antibiotics and steroids. Table 19-10 lists additives and their active ingredient in some of the otic preparations. Combination drugs are listed in Table 19-11.

TABLE 19-8 Hearing Conditions

Hearing Condition	Due to	Symptom(s)	Treatment
Auditory neuropathy	After sounds enter ear, signals are disrupted between inner ear and brain	Mild to severely hearing-impaired	Hearing implants or aids
Autoimmune inner ear disease (AIED)	Body's immune system attacks its own cells in ear	Slow to rapid loss of hearing in the first ear and then quickly in the other	Corticosteroids, methotrexate, cochlear implant, or hearing aid
Noise induced	A single exposure to loud noise (such as an explosion) or continuous loud noise from workplace or music; damage to inner ear hair cells and nerves	Hearing loss can be immediate with single exposure or gradual over time with continuous exposure	Hearing aid may help
Otosclerosis	Abnormal growth of bone (most often stapes) in middle ear, causing hearing loss	Gradual loss of hearing, starting with low-pitched sounds	Surgery followed by hearing aid in certain instances
Ototoxicity	Chemicals and/or drugs that damage inner ear, affecting both balance and hearing	Temporary to permanent hearing loss, loss of balance, or both	No treatment once hearing loss occurs Rapid removal of causative agent(s) may stop or reduce effects

TABLE 19-9 Ear Preparations*

Generic Name	Trade Name	Availability	Indication
acetic acid	Domeboro	Over-the-counter (OTC)	Used for external ear infections and prophylaxis of swimmer's ear
benzocaine, benzethonium chloride, glycerin, PEG† 300	Americaine	Prescription	Used for pain within ear caused by swimmer's ear and infections
carbamide peroxide, glycerin, propylene glycol, sodium stannate	Debrox	OTC	Used to remove earwax
triethanolamine polypeptide oleate-condensate	Cerumenex	OTC	Used to remove earwax
isopropyl alcohol, anhydrous glycerin	Swim-EAR	OTC	Used for swimmer's ear

*Many of the otic preparations are combination drugs.
†*PEG,* Polyethylene glycol.

TABLE 19-10 Major Ingredients in Otic Preparations

Agents	Classification	Indication
acetic acid	Antibacterial, antifungal	Infection
dexamethasone	Steroid	Antiinflammatory
hydrocortisone	Steroid	Antiinflammatory

TABLE 19-11 Combination Otics

Trade Name	Active Generic Ingredients	Drug Classes	Indications
Acetasol HC	hydrocortisone 1%, acetic acid 2%	Steroid/antimicrobial	Inflammation, itching
Auralgan	benzocaine 1.4%, antipyrine 5.4%	Anesthetic/analgesic	Otitis media
Domboro	acetic acid 2% in aluminum acetate solution	Antibacterial/antifungal	Otitis externa
Mediotic-HC	chloroxylenol 0.1%, pramoxine 1%, hydrocortisone 0.01%	Antibiotic/topical anesthetic/steroid	Infection/pain
Cipro HC	ciprofloxacin 0.2%, hydrocortisone 1%	Antibiotic/steroid	External infection/ inflammation
Cortisporin-TC	neomycin 3.3 mg, hydrocortisone 1%, 3 mg colistin, 0.5% thonzonium bromide/mL	Antibiotic/steroid/steroid facilitator	External ear infection

Deafness

Deafness is the loss of hearing caused by damage to the auditory nerve. A normal loss of hearing occurs as one ages, resulting from the cumulative effects of loud noises. The small, hair-like structures in the middle ear can break with loud noise and the hairs become less able to bend. Unfortunately, once the hairs break they do not regenerate, and over time a loss of hearing can occur. Another cause is the buildup of earwax, which can lessen hearing although complete deafness is rare. There are several causes of hearing impairment or complete loss, including the following:

- Aging (normal process)
- Heredity (genetic)
- Infections (bacterial or viral)
- Loud noises (music or machinery)
- Medications (aminoglycosides)
- Trauma (blunt trauma)

Prognosis. Depending on the cause of deafness and treatment, hearing can either be restored or be improved. Because of the technological advancements of hearing aids and implants, many people who would have suffered from severe or total hearing loss in the past can now hear.

Non–Drug Treatment. Hearing aids and implants (cochlear) are the primary treatments that do not involve drugs.

Drug Treatment. Depending on the cause of this condition there are several medications that can be used to treat the symptoms. These are listed below under each condition covered.

Otitis Media

Otitis media is an infection in the middle ear (earache) and often is associated with inflammation of the eustachian tube, which courses from the middle ear to the nasopharynx. The lining of the middle ear and nasopharynx is a single continuous membranous structure. This is why a sore throat can lead to a middle ear infection, as often is seen in children. Antiinfectives can treat the infection. However, many times because of recurring infections in children, pediatricians insert small tubes that allow drainage from the middle ear and eustachian tube, which lessens the occurrence of infections. Common symptoms of otitis media include fever, nausea and vomiting, earache, hearing problems, and a feeling of pressure in the ear.

Prognosis. The recovery from otitis media is good with proper treatment. If left untreated, this can cause damage to the ear and hearing.

Non–Drug Treatment. Most earaches are caused by viruses and will resolve on their own in several days. Placing a warm compress onto the ear can help relieve pain.

Drug Treatment. Antiinfectives are used to treat ear infections; antihistamines, decongestants, and analgesics are used to treat symptoms of otitis media. If the infection is severe, a systemic antibiotic may be prescribed, such as amoxicillin or sulfamethoxazole/trimethoprim. There are many otic antiinfectives available as well.

Oral Antibiotics (Systemic)

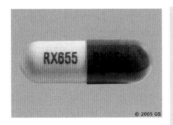

GENERIC NAME: amoxicillin
TRADE NAME: Amoxil, Amoxil Pediatric suspension, chewable tablets
INDICATION: bacterial infection of ear, nose, throat
ROUTE OF ADMINISTRATION: oral
COMMON ADULT DOSAGE: adult dose, 500 mg every 12 hours; pediatric, >3 months, 90 mg/kg/day in divided doses every 12 hours
SIDE EFFECTS: diarrhea, tooth discoloration in children
AUXILIARY LABELS:
- Shake well.
- Refrigerate.
- "Use by" label.

TRADE NAME: Bactrim, Septra
GENERIC NAME: sulfamethoxazole/trimethoprim suspension
INDICATION: acute otitis media
ROUTE OF ADMINISTRATION: oral
COMMON ADULT DOSAGE: adult dose, 20 mL every 12 hours for 10 to 14 days; pediatric, 2 months and older, dosage is based on weight ranges
SIDE EFFECTS: dizziness, ringing in the ears, painful or swollen tongue, insomnia, joint pain
AUXILIARY LABELS:
- Shake well before using.
- Refrigerate.
- "Use by" label.

Otic Antibiotics. Antibiotics may be prescribed in the following situations: following ear tube insertion, in the presence of an inner ear infection with eardrum perforation, or for outer ear infections.

TRADE NAME: Ciprodex
GENERIC NAME: ciprofloxacin/dexamethasone otic suspension
INDICATION: acute otitis externa, otitis media when ear tubes are present
ROUTE OF ADMINISTRATION: otic
COMMON ADULT DOSAGE: 4 drops placed into affected ear 2 times daily for 7 days
SIDE EFFECTS: ear discomfort such as pain or itching
AUXILIARY LABELS:
- Shake well.
- For the ear only.

> **TRADE NAME:** Cipro HC
> **GENERIC NAME:** ciprofloxacin/hydrocortisone otic suspension
> **INDICATION:** acute otitis externa, otitis media when ear tubes are present
> **ROUTE OF ADMINISTRATION:** otic
> **COMMON ADULT DOSAGE:** 3 drops placed into affected ear two times daily for 7 days
> **SIDE EFFECTS:** Headache, itching of the ear
> **AUXILIARY LABELS:**
> - Shake well.
> - For the ear only.

Cerumen Buildup

As mentioned previously, the glands near the tympanic membrane naturally produce a waxy substance referred to as cerumen. This is a normal process; the cerumen acts as a barrier to infection (that is, acts as an antibacterial agent). As the amount of wax increases, it will migrate out of the ear. If excessive wax accumulates, is not removed, or dries, it can impede hearing quality. It may be necessary for a physician to remove this waxy buildup to perform an examination or to improve hearing quality.

Prognosis. If treated appropriately hearing will improve, although if left untreated symptoms may include partial hearing loss, tinnitus (ringing of the ears), earache, itching, or discharge.

Non–Drug Treatment. Earwax removal is performed using an irrigation kit that includes a saline solution and an ear syringe. Using warm water and the solution, the ears are purged of excessive wax. Other treatments include using a few drops of mineral oil, glycerin, or hydrogen peroxide in the ear to soften the wax for a few days; warm water is then used to irrigate the wax out of the ear. Avoid using cotton swabs to clean earwax because they will push the wax further into the ear.

Drug Treatment

> **TRADE NAME:** Cerumenex
> **GENERIC NAME:** triethanolamine polypeptide oleate
> **INDICATION:** earwax removal
> **ROUTE OF ADMINISTRATION:** otic
> **COMMON DOSAGE:** fill ear canal with solution; allow it to sit for 15-30 minutes covered by cotton ball; remove cotton, place tip of syringe into ear, and gently squeeze to allow wax and liquid to drain
> **SIDE EFFECTS:** may cause some irritation
> **NOTE:** OTC, for the ear only

> **TRADE NAME:** Debrox
> **GENERIC NAME:** carbamide peroxide
> **INDICATION:** earwax removal
> **ROUTE OF ADMINISTRATION:** otic
> **COMMON DOSAGE:** apply proper amount of eardrops into ear canal; leave for at least 5 minutes; may use cotton to plug ear
> **SIDE EFFECTS:** temporary decrease in hearing after use, mild feeling of fullness in ear or itching
> **NOTE:** OTC, for the ear only

Ototoxicity

Certain medications can cause toxic levels of chemicals to accumulate in the cochlear hair cells, which may cause hearing damage known as ototoxicity. This

TABLE 19-12 **Medications That Cause Ototoxicity or Tinnitus**

Class	Specific Drugs
Aminoglycosides	gentamicin, tobramycin, amikacin
Macrolides	clarithromycin, erythromycin
Analgesics	aspirin, salicylates, nonsteroidal antiinflammatory drugs (NSAIDs)
Loop diuretics	furosemide, ethacrynic acid
Antineoplastics	cisplatin and platinum-containing agents
Antimalarials	quinine
Antiarrhythmics	quinidine
Glycopeptide antibiotics	vancomycin

injury to the auditory nerve may include a ringing or buzzing within the ears (tinnitus). This can progress to permanent ear damage if left untreated. Balance also may be affected. Specifically, aminoglycosides have been known to cause ear damage if given in high enough doses over a long period. Drugs listed in Table 19-12 have been noted to have ototoxic side effects. Daily patient assessment is necessary when these drugs are prescribed; dosages should be sufficient to avoid permanent damage yet effective enough to fight bacterial infections.

Prognosis. The prognosis can be difficult to assess. Although many cases of ototoxicity reverse themselves after drug treatment is discontinued, others may cause permanent damage. Also, hearing loss may not occur until after several weeks of drug treatment.

Non–Drug Treatment. In most cases there is no treatment once permanent hearing loss occurs. In rare cases amplification may be used depending on the cause of hearing loss and if the drug is withdrawn soon enough.

Drug Treatment. There is no drug treatment to restore hearing.

Steroid and Antibiotic Combination

TRADE NAME: Cortisporin
GENERIC NAME: neomycin/polymyxin B sulfate/hydrocortisone soln, susp*
INDICATION: steroid and antibiotic
ROUTE OF ADMINISTRATION: otic
COMMON ADULT DOSAGE: 3 drops instilled three or four times daily
AUXILIARY LABELS:
■ For the ear.
■ Shake well before using.

*If suspension is used, apply the label "Shake well before using."

MISCELLANEOUS OTIC PREPARATION

TRADE NAME: Auralgan Otic
GENERIC NAME: antipyrine and benzocaine otic
INDICATION: anesthetic, analgesic, and cerumen removal adjunct
ROUTE OF ADMINISTRATION: otic
COMMON ADULT DOSAGE: fill ear canal with 2-4 drops; insert saturated cotton pledget; repeat three or four times daily, use limited to 2-3 days
SIDE EFFECTS: minimal to none
AUXILIARY LABEL:
■ For the ear.

Tech Note!

There are many ophthalmic agents, particularly antibiotics and corticosteroids, that commonly are prescribed for ear treatment. This is acceptable because the ophthalmic preparations are sterile and can be used in the ear. However, otic preparations cannot be used in the eye because they are not sterile; in addition, the pH and other qualities of otic formulations may injure the eye.

Miscellaneous Otic Preparations

TRADE NAME: EarSol-HC
GENERIC NAME: 1% hydrocortisone, alcohol, propylene glycol, dermoprotective factor yerba santa, benzyl benzoate
INDICATION: itching of the ear
ROUTE OF ADMINISTRATION: otic
COMMON ADULT DOSAGE: insert 4-6 drops into ear three to four times daily
SIDE EFFECTS: minimal to none
AUXILIARY LABEL:
■ none; available OTC

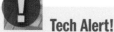

Tech Alert!

Remember the following sound-alike/look-alike drugs:

Timoptic versus Viroptic
Tobrex versus TobraDex
prednisone versus
    prednisolone
carteolol versus
    carvedilol

TRADE NAME: Domeboro Otic
GENERIC NAME: acetic acid 2% in aqueous aluminum acetate solution
INDICATION: superficial infections of external ear canal and their prevention—astringent and antimicrobial agent
ROUTE OF ADMINISTRATION: otic
COMMON ADULT DOSAGE: 4 to 6 drops every 2-3 hours
SIDE EFFECTS: minimal to none
AUXILIARY LABEL:
■ For the ear.

DO YOU REMEMBER THESE KEY POINTS?

■ The main structures of the eye
■ The functions of rods and cones
■ Conditions that can affect the eye
■ The definition of glaucoma and the medications used to treat it
■ Agents used to treat infections of the eye
■ The main structures of the ear
■ The three bony structures that make up the labyrinth of the inner ear
■ Conditions that affect the ear
■ The reason children suffering from colds and flu often have ear infections
■ The names and functions of various ear preparations
■ The eye and ear medications that are available over-the-counter or by prescription
■ The auxiliary labels necessary for eye and ear medications
■ The reasons eardrops cannot be used in the eye

REVIEW QUESTIONS

Multiple choice questions

1. The cornea is responsible for:
   A. The color of the eye
   B. Lubrication of the eye
   C. Protection of the eyeball
   D. Visual acuity

2. The substance that bathes the eye with nutrition is the:
   A. Conjunctiva
   B. Aqueous humor
   C. Vitreous humor
   D. Blood

3. Glaucoma is a condition of the eye that results from:
   A. Narrowing of eye blood vessels
   B. A lack of aqueous humor
   C. Intraocular pressure
   D. Age

4. Glaucoma can be divided into three types; these are:
   A. Acute congestive, chronic simple, and congenital
   B. Primary, secondary, and congenital
   C. Angle-closure, open-angle, and chronic
   D. None of the above

5. Which of the following medications is NOT a beta-adrenergic blocker?
   A. Timoptic
   B. Betoptic
   C. Betagan
   D. Trusopt

6. Miotics act by:
   A. Contraction of ciliary muscles, increasing outflow of aqueous humor
   B. Inhibition of beta sites that then relax vessels, allowing proper drainage of aqueous humor
   C. Inhibition of anhydrase, thus lessening the formation of aqueous humor
   D. The drug action is not clear

7. Of the various antiinfectives used to treat eye conditions, which works as a bacteriostatic at low doses and as a bactericidal at high doses?
   A. Aminoglycosides
   B. Sulfacetamide sodium
   C. Erythromycin
   D. Natacyn

8. The cavity of the middle ear contains all the following structures EXCEPT:
   A. Cochlea
   B. Malleus
   C. Incus
   D. Stapes

9. The structure within the inner ear responsible for balance is the:
   A. Semicircular canal
   B. Vestibule
   C. Cochlea
   D. Answers A and B

10. Which of the following ingredients is used to treat inflammation of the ear?
    A. Dexamethasone
    B. Benzethonium chloride
    C. Acetic acid
    D. Boric acid

11. The types of agents used to treat otitis media include all of the following EXCEPT:
    A. Antiinfectives
    B. Steroids
    C. Antivirals
    D. Antiemetics

12. Treatments for blindness include:
    A. Medications
    B. Implants
    C. Glasses
    D. Both B and C

13. If the hair-like structures inside the inner ear are damaged:
   A. They can be repaired by surgery
   B. They can be treated with medication
   C. They will regenerate themselves
   D. The effects are irreversible

14. Which of the following ophthalmic agents are commonly used before eye surgeries?
   A. Miotics
   B. Corticosteroids
   C. Aminoglycosides
   D. Mydriatics

15. Ototoxicity can be caused by:
   A. Analgesics
   B. Aminoglycosides
   C. Antineoplastics
   D. All of the above

True/False

If the statement is false, then change it to make it true.

_____ **1.** The eye is located in an area called the socket.
_____ **2.** The back of the eye is oxygen-rich through blood vessels.
_____ **3.** The occipital lobe in the brain is responsible for interpretation of images.
_____ **4.** Conjunctivitis is inflammation of the cornea.
_____ **5.** Otic drugs may be prescribed to be used in the eye or ear.
_____ **6.** The ossicles of the ear are located in the middle ear and are composed of four bones.
_____ **7.** The eustachian tube connects the middle ear to the throat.
_____ **8.** Debrox is an agent available over-the-counter for earwax removal.
_____ **9.** Otitis media is an infection and inflammation of the inner ear.
_____ **10.** The tympanic membrane is a covering at the entrance of the middle ear.
_____ **11.** Oral antibiotics are often used to treat ear infections.
_____ **12.** Cataracts can develop at any time, including in the womb.
_____ **13.** Pink eye is caused by a virus.
_____ **14.** Retinitis pigmentosa causes night blindness.
_____ **15.** Ototoxicity is an irreversible ear condition.

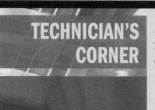

TECHNICIAN'S CORNER

Look up the following agents in *Drug Facts and Comparisons,* and list the following information on each drug: both generic and trade names, normal dosage, strength(s), indication, and auxiliary labels.

Auralgan otic
Blephamide
Timolol

BIBLIOGRAPHY

AMA (American Medical Association) *Concise Medical Encyclopedia.* 2006.

Drug facts and comparisons, ed 63, St Louis, 2008, Lippincott Williams & Wilkins.

Edmunds M: *Introduction to clinical pharmacology,* ed 6, Philadelphia, 2009, Elsevier Health Services.

Glaucoma Research Foundation: www.glaucoma.org/learn/glaucoma_facts.php.

Hitner N: *Basic pharmacology*, ed 4, New York, 1999, Glenco.

McCuistion L, Kathleen G: *Real-world nursing survival guide: pharmacology*, ed 1, Philadelphia, 2002, WB Saunders.

Professional guide to diseases, ed 9, Ambler, PA, 2009, Lippincott Williams & Wilkins.

Salerno E: *Pharmacology for health professionals*, St Louis, 1999, Mosby.

Thibodeau G, Kevin P: *Structure and function of the body*, ed 13, St Louis, 2007, Mosby.

WEBSITES

Conjunctivitis: http://emedicine.medscape.com/article/797874-overview

National Institutes of Health: www.nei.nih.gov

National Institutes of Health, 2008: www.nlm.nih.gov/medlineplus/magazine/issues/summer08/articles/summer08pg14-15.html

National Marfan Foundation: www.marfan.org

World Health Organization: Glaucoma is the second leading cause of blindness globally: Article: In focus 2004;82:887-888. www.who.int/bulletin/bulletin_board/83/infocus11041/en/-15.html

Integumentary System

Objectives

UPON COMPLETING THIS CHAPTER, YOU SHOULD BE ABLE TO DO THE FOLLOWING:

- List the major components of skin anatomy.
- List eight types of noninfectious skin conditions and their treatments.
- List four types of infectious skin conditions and their treatments.
- Determine the proper strength of sunscreen necessary to protect skin from ultraviolet rays.
- Define the various forms of acne.
- Describe psoriasis and the types of medications used to treat this skin condition.
- List the degrees of burn injury and describe the depth and severity of damage of each classification of burn.
- Define the functions of the sebaceous and sweat glands, nails, and hair.
- Identify the conditions that affect the nails and hair and their treatments.
- Describe the use of immunosuppressants to treat psoriasis.

TERMS AND DEFINITIONS

Acne vulgaris *Commonly known as pimples, acne occurs when the pores of the skin are clogged with oil or bacteria*

Analgesic *A drug that relieves pain by reducing the perception of pain*

Antiinflammatory *A drug that reduces swelling, redness, and pain and promotes healing*

Antiseptic *A substance that slows or stops growth of microorganisms on surfaces such as skin*

Comedone *A blackhead; a plug of keratin and sebum within a hair follicle that is blackened at the surface*

Dermis *A thick layer of connective tissue that contains collagen*

Desquamation *A process of shedding the top layer of the skin, also known as exfoliation; this process may be a normal process or may be associated with disease*

Epidermis *The outermost layer of the skin composed of the stratum corneum or horny layer, the keratinocytes (squamous cells), and the basal layer; also contains melanin, a pigment that contributes to the color of skin and hair*

Keratolytic *A drug that causes shedding of the outer layer of the skin*

Prophylaxis *Treatment given before an event or exposure to prevent the occurrence of a condition or symptom*

Pruritus *Itching*

Sebaceous glands *Skin glands responsible for the secretion of oil called sebum*

Sebum *An oily/waxy substance that lubricates the skin and retains water to provide moisture*

Skin protectant *A substance that acts as a barrier between the skin and an irritant*

Subcutaneous layer *The deepest layer of the skin that consists of fat cells and collagen; serves to protect the body and conserve heat*

Sweat glands *Found in the dermis; activated in response to increased body temperature to cool the body*

Urticaria *Also known as hives; red welts that arise on the surface of the skin; often attributable to an allergic reaction but may have nonallergic causes*

COMMON DRUGS USED FOR SKIN CONDITIONS

Trade Name	Generic Name	Pronunciation	Trade Name	Generic Name	Pronunciation
Antibacterials			Lamisil	terbinafine	(**ter**-bin-a-feen)
Achromycin	tetracycline	(**tet**-ra-**sye**-kleen)	Lotrimin	clotrimazole	(kloe-**trim**-a-zole)
Bacitracin	bacitracin	(bass-ih-**tray**-sin)	Nizoral	ketoconazole	(**kee**-toe-**kon**-a-zole)
Bactroban	mupirocin	(myoo-**peer**-oh-sin)	Tinactin	tolnaftate	(tol-**naf**-tate)
Cleocin T Gel	clindamycin	(klin-da-**mye**-sin)			
Dynapen	dicloxacillin	(dye-**klox**-a-sil-in)	**Antivirals**		
Eryderm	erythromycin	(er-**ith**-ro-**mye**-sin)	Zovirax	acyclovir	(a-**sye**-klo-veer)
Neomycin	neomycin	(ne-oh-**mye**-sin)	Famvir	famciclovir	(fam-**sye**-kloe-vir)
Neosporin	neomycin/bacitracin polymyxin b sulfate	(**nee**-oh-**mye**-sin/ **bas**-i-**tray**-sin/ **pol**-ee-**mix**-in)	Valtrex	valacyclovir	(val-ay-**sye**-kloe-vir)
			Biologics		
			Amevive	alefacept	(ah-**leh**-fa-cept)
Antifungals			Enbrel	etanercept	(ee-**tan**-er-sept)
Desenex	miconazole	(mi-**kon**-a-zole)	Humira	adalimumab	(ay-da-**lim**-yoo-mab)
Diflucan	fluconazole	(flue-**kon**-a-zole)	Remicade	infliximab	(in-**flix**-i-mab)
			Stelara	Ustekinumab	(**yoo**-sti-**kin**-ue-mab)

Continued

COMMON DRUGS USED FOR SKIN CONDITIONS—cont'd

Trade Name	Generic Name	Pronunciation	Trade Name	Generic Name	Pronunciation
Corticosteroids			**Miscellaneous Psoriasis Agents**		
Triderm	triamcinolone acetonide	(trye-am-**sin**-oh-lone)	Drithrocreme, Micanol	anthralin	(**an**-thrah-lin)
Cortaid	hydrocortisone	(hi-**droe**-cor-te-sone)	Denorex, DHS Tar, Doak Tar,	coal tar	(kohl tar)
Cordran	flurandrenolide	(flur-an-**dren**-oh-lide)	Theraplex T		
Cutivate	fluticasone propionate	(floo-**tik**-a-sone)			
			Retinoids		
Decadron (oral)	dexamethasone	(dek-se-**meth**-a-sone)	Differin	adapalene	(a-**dap**-a-leen)
Diprolene	betamethasone	(bay-ta-**meth**-a-sone)	Retin-A, Retin-A Micro, Avita	tretinoin	(tret-**in**-oin)
Lidex	fluocinonide	(floo-oh-**sin**-oh-nide)			
Temovate	clobetasol propionate	(kloe-**bay**-ta-sol)	Tazorac	tazarotene	(ta-**zar**-oh-teen)
			Soriatane	acitretin	(**a**-si-**tre**-tin)
Topicort	desoximetasone	(des-**ox**-ih-**met**-ah-sone)	**Topical Vitamin D**		
			Dovonex	calcipotriene	(cal-sih-poh-**try**-een)
Beta-val	betamethasone valerate	(bay-ta-**meth**-a-sone)			
			Miscellaneous Agents		
Westcort	hydrocortisone valerate	(hi-**droe**-cor-te-sone)	Caladryl Clear	pramoxine/zinc acetate	(pram-**ox**-een/ **zink** as-ee-**tate**)
Immunosuppressants			Clearasil Max Strength	benzoyl peroxide	(ben-**zoyl** per-**ox**-ide)
Imuran	azathioprine	(ay-za-**thye**-oh-preen)	Wart Off, Compound W	salicylic acid	(**sal**-i-**sil**-ik **as**-id)
Rheumatrex Dose Pak	methotrexate	(meth-oh-**trex**-ate)			
Sandimmune, Neoral	cyclosporine	(sye-**kloe**-spor-een)			
Immune Response Modifier					
Aldara	imiquimod	(im-**i**-kwi-mod)			

T HE TERM *INTEGUMENTARY* means covering. The integumentary system is composed of the skin, hair, and nails. The skin is one of the most abused organs of the body system. Skin withstands damage from weather, detergents, scratches, cuts, and bruises, and it repairs itself repeatedly. Like other organs, it must be nourished, oxygenated, and maintained. In return, it functions to protect the body, regulate temperature, and act as a sensor to stimuli. This chapter will cover the anatomy of the skin, hair, and nails to reveal their functions; then we will explore the conditions that can affect the integumentary system as well as common treatments.

MEDICAL TERMS AND CONDITIONS OF THE SKIN

Word Combinations and Prefixes	
Alopec	Baldness
Contus	Bruise
Crypt	Hidden
Cutane/o, dermat/o, derm/o	Skin
Cyst/o	Cyst
Dia-	Through or complete
Epi-	Above

MEDICAL TERMS AND CONDITIONS OF THE SKIN—cont'd

Follicul	Hair follicle
Hemat/o	Blood
Hidr/o	Sweat glands
Hirsut	Hair
Hyper-	Excessive
Integument	Covering
Melan/o	Black
Myc	Fungus
Onych/o	Nails
Par-	Near
Pil/i, pil/o	Hair
Phor-	Movement
Purpur	Purple
Seb/o	Sebaceous glands

Suffixes

-ia, -ic, -ism	Condition
-it is	Inflammation
-ologist	Specialist
-oma	Tumor
-osis, -esis, -ism	Abnormal condition
-ous	Pertaining to
-phagia	Swallowing or eating
-plasty	Surgical repair
-rrhea	Flow or discharge

Conditions

Albinism	An inherited condition in which little or no melanin is made
Alopecia	Partial or complete loss of hair from head or body; may result in baldness; skin appears white
Clubbing	Abnormal condition of fingers and nails, leading to abnormal curving of nails and drumstick-like appearance of fingers
Folliculitis	Inflammation of hair follicles
Hematoma	A trapped blood clot that swells under tissues or nails
Hirsutism	Presence of excessive hair in females in areas where it would normally be minimal or absent
Koilonychia	Spoon-shaped appearance of nails (concave)
Lesions	Any change in tissues of skin caused by injury or disease
Miliaria	Heat rash
Onychocryptosis	Ingrown nail
Onychomycosis	Fungal infection of nails
Onychophagia	Biting of nails
Seborrhea	Overproduction of sebum
Urticaria	Skin eruption characterized by well-defined, red-margined wheals that are usually result of allergic reaction to foods, drugs, or insect bites; in some cases cause is nonallergenic

Skin Anatomy

The skin is the largest organ of the body. It is made of various layers that contain nerves, glands, hair, and blood vessels. The function of the skin is to protect the body against heat, cold, light, dehydration, and infection. It does this by regulating the temperature of the body as well as by storing fat and water for replenishment. The nerves allow the skin to detect pain, heat, and cold. The thicker layer of skin found on the soles of the feet and palms of the hands acts as a

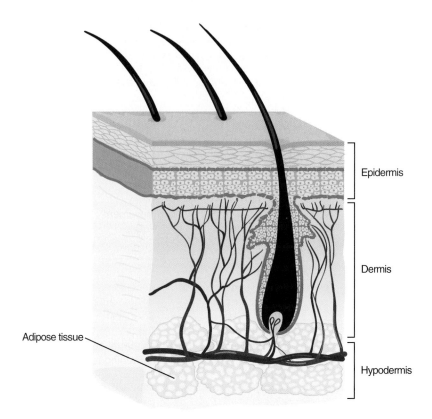

FIGURE 20-1 Skin anatomy.

protective layer. Most of the body surface area is covered with hair, the follicles of which are embedded in the dermis.

The top portion of the skin—the **epidermis**—can be divided into three main layers: the horny outer layer, squamous cells, and the basal layer (Figure 20-1). The epidermis is the outermost layer and protects the layers below it. The epidermis also contains melanocytes, which produce skin pigment (i.e., melanin). The epidermis does not have a blood supply of its own; instead, it receives nutrition from the tissues surrounding it. A thin layer of skin cells flakes off (i.e., exfoliates) and the cells are replaced as they die. The basal layer is responsible for the production of new cells. As new skin cells are made, they push the older cells upward and this becomes the outer layer of the epidermis. Beneath the epidermis are the dermis and the subcutaneous layer.

The **dermis** is a thick layer of connective tissue that contains collagen; it is located under the epidermis. Collagen is made of interwoven flexible fibers and helps support other structures such as the blood vessels, glands, and nerves. Below the dermis lies the **subcutaneous layer or hypodermis.** This is the deepest layer and contains fat cells (i.e., lipocytes) that store fat, which in turn insulates the body. Fat in the skin helps cushion the body against injury and serves as a food reserve in case of emergency. All areas of the skin receive nourishment, except for the epidermis.

HAIR AND NAILS

Hair is made of proteins called keratin, and is similar to the top layer of the skin. The hair has roots that are embedded in the skin's dermis, and the base contains melanocytes (cells that produce melanin) that are responsible for the color of hair. As one gets older, the melanocytes stop producing the chemical melanin and the hair begins to turn gray.

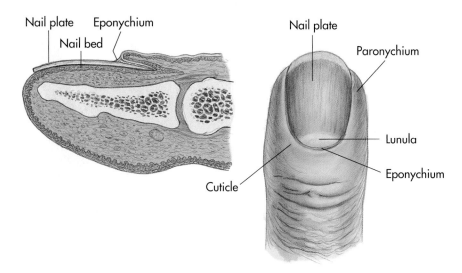

FIGURE 20-2 Nail anatomy. (Redrawn from Thompson JM et al: *Mosby's clinical nursing,* ed 5, St Louis, 2001, Mosby.)

Nails are composed of keratin as well, although they are more dense than hair. Nails cover the top surface at the end of the toes and fingers. The nail root is embedded into the epidermis and provides protection to the surface of the toes and fingers. The lunula is the small white portion located at the base of the nail. The cuticle is composed of keratin at the base and the sides of the nail. The paronychium surrounds the nail and consists of a softer tissue (Figure 20-2).

GLANDS

The two types of glands that are within the layers of the skin are the sebaceous and sweat glands. The **sebaceous glands** are located within the dermal layer of the skin and secrete an oily substance called sebum. **Sebum** lubricates the skin and retains water to keep the skin and hair soft and supple. Sebum is transported by ducts to hair follicles, where this oily substance resides. Sebaceous glands can be found everywhere on the skin except the palms of the hands and soles of the feet.

Sweat glands are much smaller than sebaceous glands and are very prevalent in the soles of the feet and palms of the hands (Figure 20-3). The composition of sweat is mainly water with a very low concentration of salt. When these glands are activated, sweat escapes through pores on the skin. As the temperature rises, the nervous system signals the glands to perspire, allowing sweat to flow onto the surface of the skin, where it evaporates; as it does this, the body is cooled.

Conditions Affecting the Skin, Hair, and Glands

Many different types of agents can be used to treat conditions of the integumentary system. Injuries, genetic conditions, and diseases of the skin will be covered. Many childhood diseases cause outbreaks on the surface of the skin and are discussed in Chapter 28. Allergies are discussed in Chapter 26. We begin with a short overview of common conditions and treatment with medications and/or non–drug treatments. In addition, the prognosis or outcome of these conditions will be explored. The skin will be covered first, divided into noninfectious and infectious conditions, followed by conditions of the nails and hair.

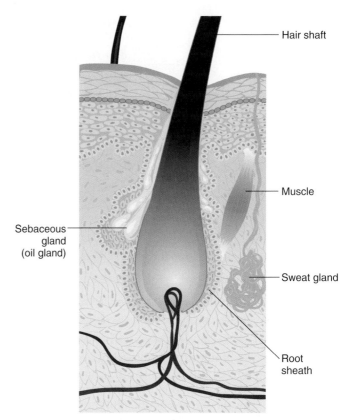

FIGURE 20-3 Glands of the skin.

NONINFECTIOUS SKIN CONDITIONS

Most skin conditions can be divided into the following two categories:

1.   Noninfectious inflammatory conditions
2.   Infectious inflammatory conditions

Many products are available that work well in treating noninfectious skin conditions, although if the symptoms continue it is recommended that the patient consult a physician. Infectious inflammatory conditions are much more serious because they can be transferred from person to person; therefore the patient should see a physician immediately for the proper treatment. Many of these conditions must be treated with prescription drugs. It is usually recommended that the patient consult a physician for the proper diagnosis.

Acne, sunburns, and hives are common skin conditions that are often treated at home. These are examples of noninfectious inflammatory conditions. Growths on the surface of the skin are common and not all are cancerous. Noncancerous-type growths are referred to as benign growths, while cancerous types are called malignant. These are discussed further under Skin Cancer and in oncology in Chapter 29.

Acne Vulgaris

Acne vulgaris (aka:acne) is a common condition in which inflammation of the sebaceous glands produces pustules, papules, comedones, and scars. The popular belief that eating too much candy or greasy foods causes acne is incorrect. These foods do not cause acne, although they can worsen existing acne. Although

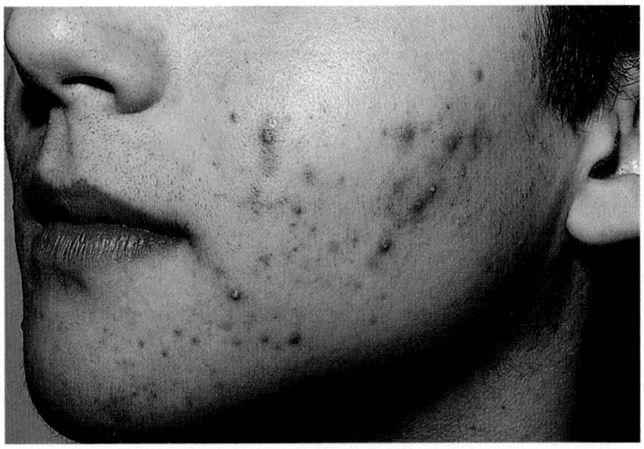

FIGURE 20-4 Acne. (From Callen JP et al: *Color atlas of dermatology,* ed 2, Philadelphia, 2000, Saunders.)

inflammation occurs, it is not caused by infection but rather by hormonal changes.

Hormones have an ability to enlarge the glands of the skin. Two of the most productive glands are the **sweat glands,** which can become clogged, and the **sebaceous glands,** which produce sebum. When sebum production increases, it traps bacteria at the base of the hair follicle, and the likelihood of acne increases. The increased production of androgens (hormones) during puberty leads to increased sebum production. At the same time, the obstructed outflow of sebum and bacteria in hair follicles dilates a lipid (fat) sac called the **comedone.** When this occurs, the bacteria *Propionibacterium acnes* multiply, leak from pores, and release oily chemicals onto the dermis, which causes inflammation. *P. acnes* is a bacterium that normally increases around adolescence and may add to the inflammatory process (Figure 20-4).

Symptoms include a greasy residue on the surface of the skin. Lesions may be located on the face, back of the neck, the chest, shoulders, back, and upper arms. Lesions are classified into five different categories:

1. Whiteheads are small papules without inflammation.
2. Blackheads are open comedones that can have either single or multiple heads.
3. Papules are small, red, inflamed follicular spots.
4. Pustules are various sizes of pus-filled sites that are inflamed.
5. Scars (caused by popping and scratching pimples) may occur in some instances after the healing process has finished and are normally permanent.

Prognosis. Depending on the type of acne present, the length of time varies before the symptoms will disappear. Typically, as adolescents reach maturity the outbreak of acne decreases, though scarring can occur in more severe cases of acne.

Non–Drug Treatment. The most effective non–drug treatment for acne is to keep the skin clean and free from bacteria by using cleansing agents that will decrease sebum production and exfoliate (i.e., remove) dead skin cells. Although cleaning is clearly important, excessive cleansing can irritate the skin, worsening the condition. A new FDA-approved treatment called blue light therapy is used to treat inflammatory acne vulgaris (caused by *P. acnes*) that has not

TABLE 20-1 Topical Acne Treatments

Treatment	Action	Examples	Dosage Form
Benzoyl peroxide	Kills *P. acnes;* removes excess oils from skin and removes skin cells that clog pores	Clearasil 10% Desquam 5%, 10% Oxy 10% Neutrogena 3.5%	Cream Gel Liquid Mask
Salicylic acid	Slows shedding of cells inside hair follicles, which prevents pores from clogging Breaks down both blackheads and whiteheads	Noxzema Anti-Acne Stridex Dermalogica	Gel Pads Gel
Sulfur and resorcinol	Remove dead skin cells that clog pores and removes excess oils	Clearasil Acne Control Liquimat light/medium	Topical Lotion
Alcohol and acetone	Remove dirt and oils from skin	Seba-Nil liquid cleanser Tyrosum	Liquid Liquid, packets
Retinoids	Increase dryness and reduce acne formation	Retin-A, Altinac, Avita, or Retin-A Micro (tretinoin) Differin (adapalene) Tazorac (tazarotene)	Cream or gel Cream or gel Cream or gel

responded to other treatments. The blue light does not contain UV light, which can damage skin.

Drug Treatments. Mild acne is treated with topical agents such as benzoyl peroxide, which helps dry the skin, and salicylic acid, which increases skin turnover. More severe inflammatory acne may require the use of topical or systemic antibiotics or topical retinoids in addition to **keratolytics**. Prescription antibiotics such as tetracycline (orally), erythromycin (orally or topically), and clindamycin (topically) may be prescribed. Topical retinoid agents such as tretinoin (Retin-A Micro, Avita) increase the growth of skin around the acne areas, which causes **desquamation** (exfoliation) of the skin and removes dead skin cells, decreasing the formation of comedones (Table 20-1). With retinoid treatment, the acne may seem to worsen initially but usually improves over several weeks. Oral retinoids such as isotretinoin (Claravis, Sotret) are reserved for the treatment of severe, recalcitrant nodular acne (aka: cystic acne); these agents require that the prescriber, the pharmacy, and the patient be enrolled in a special program called i-PLEDGE. The program is intended to reduce the risk of fetal exposure to the medication, because systemic retinoids are known teratogens (cause fetal harm).

GENERIC NAME: tetracycline
TRADE NAME: Sumycin
INDICATION: moderate to severe cases of acne
ROUTE OF ADMINISTRATION: oral
COMMON ADULT DOSAGE: 125 to 250 mg four times daily for 1-2 weeks, then decrease to 125 to 500 mg daily
SIDE EFFECTS: mild nausea, vomiting, loss of appetite, diarrhea
AUXILIARY LABELS:
■ Do not take with dairy products.
■ Take on an empty stomach.
■ Take with a full glass of water.

GENERIC NAME: tretinoin
TRADE NAME: Retin-A, Renova (cream only)
INDICATION: acne vulgaris
ROUTE OF ADMINISTRATION: topical
COMMON ADULT DOSAGE: applied once daily before bedtime to affected area(s)
SIDE EFFECTS: dry skin, itching, peeling, redness, and stinging
AUXILIARY LABEL:
■ For external use only.

GENERIC NAME: isotretinoin
TRADE NAME: Claravis, Sotret
INDICATION: severe acne
ROUTE OF ADMINISTRATION: oral
COMMON ADULT DOSAGE: 1 mg/kg/day divided into 2 doses for 15 to 20 weeks; may be decreased if nodule count decreases more than 70% before completing treatment
SIDE EFFECTS: abnormal skin sensations, bleeding and redness or swelling of the gums, changes in menstrual flow, chapped lips, dizziness, headache, itching, nervousness, sweating, voice changes, mood changes, and dry eyes, nose, and mouth
AUXILIARY LABELS:
■ Do not use if you are pregnant or planning on becoming pregnant.
■ Take with food.

Sunburn

Sunburn is due to constant overexposure to the sun; excessive exposure may cause the skin to blister. Symptoms of a sunburn include painful, reddening skin. Severe sunburn may result in swelling and blistering of the skin as well as fever, chills, and/or weakness. Several days following the exposure the skin may begin to peel in the burned areas (normally occurs in fair-skinned people) with itching of the affected area(s). These areas are more sensitive to further sunburn for several weeks. Each episode of sunburn raises the likelihood of deoxyribonucleic acid (DNA) mutations from ultraviolet A (UVA) and ultraviolet B (UVB) rays, with the potential for precancerous changes to the skin and a risk of skin cancer later. UVA radiation is UV light with the longest wavelength and makes up 95% of UV light. It is carcinogenic because the longer waves can penetrate deep into the epidermis and dermis of the skin. Cancer can occur from this deep penetration, as well as discoloration of the prematurely aged skin. UVB radiation is medium wavelength and comprises only 5% of UV light. It is responsible for producing the sunburn as it penetrates into the epidermis or outer layer of the skin, and can cause cancer. To protect oneself from both of these harmful ultraviolet rays, one must wear the proper amount of skin protection factor (SPF).

The two types of **skin protectants** are sunscreens and sunblocks. Sunscreens protect the skin from UVA and UVB rays by allowing the skin protectant to absorb the ultraviolet rays, rendering them harmless. Sunblocks are essentially physical sunscreens; they function by reflecting the ultraviolet rays away from the skin. Ultimately, the best protection one can provide the skin is a sunblock/sunscreen combination. To judge how much protection a sunscreen or sunblock will provide, multiply the amount of time it takes you to burn (with no protection) times the SPF number. For example, if it takes you only 10 minutes to burn and you wear an SPF 20 sunblock, your coverage would last about 200 minutes (i.e., 20 × 10), or about 3.2 hours. Reapplication is necessary based on the type of activity in which you are participating. For swimmers, there are water-resistant and waterproof agents that increase longevity of the product from 40 to 80 minutes, respectively, before it must be reapplied. Because

TABLE 20-2 Skin Protection Factor Guide Coverage of Sunscreen*

Skin Type	Skin Characteristics after 10 Min of Sun Exposure	Coverage	Consideration of Agents
I Very Fair Skin	Burns easily/rarely tans	20 to 50 SPF[†]	Lotion gives better coverage than oil agents
II Fair Skin	Burns easily/tans minimally	12 to 50 SPF	15 SPF is minimum level that should be used
			Lotions give better coverage than oil agents
III Light Skin	Burns moderately/tans gradually	8 to 30 SPF	Below 15 SPF is considered too low*[†]
IV Medium Skin	Burns minimally/tans well	4 to 15 SPF	Below 15 SPF is considered too low[†]
V Dark Skin	Rarely burns/always tans	2 to 8 SPF	Below 15 SPF is considered too low[†]
VI Very Dark Skin	Does not burn	2 to 4 SPF	Below 15 SPF is considered too low[†]

*It is recommended that a minimum SPF 15 should be used for all skin types.
[†]*SPF,* Skin protection factor.
[‡]According to American Melanoma Foundation/Skin Cancer Foundation.

ultraviolet rays are always present, even on cloudy days, it is suggested that sunscreen (no less than 15 SPF) be worn daily. See Table 20-2 for sunscreen absorption and reflecting abilities.

Certain people may burn particularly easily or develop exaggerated skin reactions to sunlight. This condition is called *photosensitivity*. The signs of photosensitivity may include development of a rash when exposed to the sunlight outside or even indoor lighting from fluorescent lights (less common). The amount of sensitivity varies from person to person. Symptoms may include red skin rash with blisters, scaly patches, or raised spots on areas exposed to the sun. Both itching and burning may occur and last for several days afterward. Normally the reaction to sunlight gradually lessens with subsequent exposures. The causes of photosensitivity may include contact with chemicals (e.g., perfumes, plants), systemic medications (e.g., sulfonamides, tetracycline, fluoroquinolones, thiazide diuretics), or herbs (e.g., St. John's wort) or the presence of a disease process, such as the autoimmune disease systemic lupus erythematosus (SLE) or porphyria (a metabolic disorder that is normally hereditary).

Prognosis. Sunburns usually take several days to disappear; the damaged skin begins to peel off with the new skin underneath replacing the damaged skin. Several years of this type of damage can lead to skin cancer.

Non–Drug Treatments. The best way to deter sunburn is to prevent overexposure. Wear protective clothing and a cap with a broad rim to keep the sun off the face and skin. Taking shelter in the shade is another way of avoiding sunburn; other preventive measures that are recommended by the Skin Cancer Foundation and American Melanoma Foundation are the following:

- Stay in the shade between 10 AM and 4 PM, when the sun's rays are most intense.
- Avoid tanning salons.
- Avoid deliberate sunbathing.
- Apply 1 ounce of sunscreen to the entire body 30 minutes before going outside and repeat every 2 hours; this should be done even on cloudy days and during the winter months.
- Apply lip balm containing sunscreen.

- Choose a wide-spectrum sunscreen (UVA/UVB) and apply when going outside for more than 20 minutes.
- Wear sunglasses to protect the eyes; a wide-brim hat is also recommended.
- Keep newborns out of the sun.
- Use sunscreens on children over the age of 6.
- To help ease the pain associated with a sunburn, a cold compress to the affected area(s) can be used along with cooling agents such as aloe vera. These agents are available in both gel and ointment forms.
- See your physician every year for a professional skin exam.

Choosing a Sunscreen. There are dozens of sunscreens available; however, choosing one with an SPF of 15 or more will provide the best protection. Dosage forms vary from sprays to gels. The best products are those that are PABA-free. PABA (i.e., *para*-aminobenzoic acid) absorbs UV rays similarly to oxybenzone; however, PABA is believed to cause damage to DNA, thus increasing the risk of skin cancer. Table 20-3 lists a few of the many available brands of sunscreens.

Drug Treatments. Severe sunburns caused by sun overexposure or those burns enhanced by photosensitivity agents (such as oral beta-carotene, steroids, or other medications) may be treated with topical OTC agents such as aloe vera gel or Cortaid (hydrocortisone/aloe). If the sunburn is extremely severe, topical agents such as Silvadene cream may be prescribed to prevent infection (see Burns).

TABLE 20-3 Choosing a Sunscreen*

SPF	Dosage Form	Product	Ingredients	Notes
SPF 15	Gel	Hawaiian Tropic 15 Plus	octyl methoxycinnamate, octocrylene, enzophenone-3, menthyl anthranilate	PABA-free; waterproof
SPF 15	Lip balm	ChapStick Sunblock 15	padimate, oxybenzone, cetyl alcohol, petrolatum, lanolin, isopropyl myristate, parabens, mineral oil, titanium dioxide	
SPF 15	Spray	Coppertone Sport Sunblock Spray	ethylhexyl *p*-methoxycinnamate, 2-ethylhexyl salicylate, homosalate, oxybenzone, alcohol	PABA-free; waterproof
SPF 15	Lotion	Nivea Sun	Also contains octyl methoxycinnamate, octyl salicylate, benzophenone-3, 2-phenylbenzimidazole-5-sulfonic acid	PABA-free; waterproof
SPF 18	Lotion	Bullfrog Sport	benzophenone-3, octocrylene, octyl methoxycinnamate, octyl salicylate, titanium dioxide, diazolidinyl urea, EDTA, parabens, vitamin E	Waterproof
SPF 30	Cream	Neutrogena No-Stick Sunscreen	octyl methoxycinnamate, homosalate, benzophenone-3, octyl salicylate	EDTA, parabens, dizolidinyl urea
SPF 30	Lip balm	Blistex Ultraprotection	Also contains homosalate, menthyl anthranilate, octyl methoxycinnamate, octyl salicylate, oxybenzone, dimethicone	PABA-free; waterproof
SPF 30	Lotion	Australian Gold Face Zinc Oxide	octocrylene, octyl methoxycinnamate, zinc oxide	

*These are just a few of the many sunscreens available over-the-counter. NOTE: Formulations may change widely from year to year; always check current product labels.

GENERIC NAME: hydrocortisone/(OTC)
TRADE NAME: Cortaid, Caldecort, Hycort, Westcort
INDICATION: inflammation of the skin
ROUTE OF ADMINISTRATION: topical
COMMON ADULT DOSAGE: apply a small amount to the affected area(s) as directed on label
SIDE EFFECTS: skin redness, burning, itching or peeling, thinning of the skin, blistering of skin
AUXILIARY LABEL:
■ none

Urticaria

Urticaria is also called hives. These superficial bumps range in size and are extremely itchy. They are commonly caused by a hypersensitivity to food, environment, or drugs and can occur anywhere on the body; they also can be spread easily within hours of onset. Topical agents can be used for hives and other noninfectious inflammatory skin rashes. Some cases of urticaria are idiopathic, or of unknown cause. They can disappear as rapidly as they appear.

Prognosis. Hives may dissipate within several hours even without treatment. However, those resulting from an allergic reaction may require treatment to dissipate or to improve patient comfort. Removal of the allergen or root cause will help them disappear.

Non–Drug Treatment. Applying a cold, wet compress can help to alleviate the **pruritus** (i.e., itching) that accompanies hives.

Drug Treatment. Antihistamines are used to treat the symptoms of urticaria. Topical medications also include local anesthetics, which numb the pruritus (Table 20-4). Diphenhydramine lotion (Caladryl Pink, Benadryl) is a commonly sold topical treatment; however, topical use may cause sensitization of the skin and therefore these products are often not recommended. If an antihistamine is needed, an oral one, such as oral diphenhydramine, can dramatically reduce the appearance of hives and itching; a side effect of this agent is sleepiness.

GENERIC NAME: pramoxine/zinc acetate (OTC)
TRADE NAME: Caladryl Clear, Clear Calamine
INDICATION: skin irritation and itching
ROUTE OF ADMINISTRATION: topical
COMMON ADULT DOSAGE: apply to affected area(s) 3 to 4 times daily following the directions on label
SIDE EFFECTS: dryness, itching
AUXILIARY LABEL:
■ OTC, shake well before use

TABLE 20-4 Examples of Topical Antiinflammatory Products

Product	Trade Names	Dosage Forms
Corticosteroids		
hydrocortisone (OTC, Rx)	Hytone, Hycort	Cream, ointment
triamcinolone in Orabase (Rx)	Kenalog in Orabase	Dental paste
desoximetasone (Rx)	Topicort 0.05%, 0.25%	Gel
fluocinonide (Rx)	Lidex	Solution
	Lidex-E	Extended cream

GENERIC NAME: diphenhydramine (OTC)
TRADE NAME: Benadryl
INDICATION: allergies, hives, itching, and rashes
ROUTE OF ADMINISTRATION: oral
COMMON ADULT DOSAGE: 25 mg PO q6h as needed; follow directions on label or as directed by prescriber
SIDE EFFECTS: dizziness, drowsiness, headache, dry mouth
AUXILIARY LABEL:
■ none

Skin Cancer

Any abnormal growth of new skin tissue that results in a malignancy is known as skin cancer. Melanomas are cancerous skin growths emanating from moles and areas of the skin that may have been sunburned. There are three main types of skin cancer: melanoma, squamous cell, and basal cell cancer (non-melanomas). The most aggressive and severe type of cancer is melanoma; in 2009 more than 68,720 people in the United States were diagnosed with this type of cancer, of which 8650 died (American Cancer Society). Typically the appearance of melanomas on the skin is marked by an irregular shape, elevation off the skin, discoloring, and changes in size, and can occur anywhere on the body. Melanomas start in the lower part of the epidermis within the melanocytes (cells that color the skin). Risk factors for skin cancer include previous sun damage, genetics, and exposure to radiation from tanning booths. Those individuals with light-colored or freckled skin, red- or blond-haired people, and Caucasians ages 20 years and older are at higher risk. The normal course of treatment is dependent on the stage or severity of the cancer. Basal cell cancer grows very slowly, occurs on the surface of the skin, and is usually due to sun damage. This type of cancer usually first appears on the face and it rarely spreads to other areas. Squamous cell skin cancer normally occurs on other parts of the body (besides the face) that have been overexposed to the sun, but this type of cancer can spread to the lymph nodes and other organs within the body. Figure 20-5 shows several types of skin cancer.

Prognosis. The prognosis of any cancerous cells depends on several factors such as early detection (Box 20-1), effective treatment, and a strong support system. With skin cancers the outcome is very good if detected early, although constant awareness is necessary to catch any new areas of the skin that are changing in a suspicious way. Regularly scheduled visits with the physician play an important role in early detection.

Non–Drug Treatment. Prevention is the best treatment of many skin cancers, including protection from harmful sunrays. Once cancer is suspected, the stage or severity of the cancer must be diagnosed. The first line of treatment is surgery to remove the area of concern. Treatments include photodynamic therapy or radiation therapy. Both squamous and basal cell carcinomas are less severe and can be treated with various therapies (Box 20-2).

Drug Treatment. If the cancer is deep in the skin tissue, topical chemotherapy can be used. This type of treatment is used when there are large areas of cancer that cannot be removed. An example is topical fluorouracil (5-FU), which is an antimetabolite that inhibits cancer cells from synthesizing DNA. 5-FU is used to treat basal cell and squamous cell cancers on the surface of the skin. For more information on chemotherapeutic agents see Chapter 29.

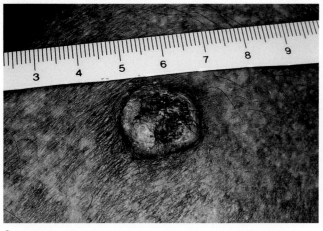

A

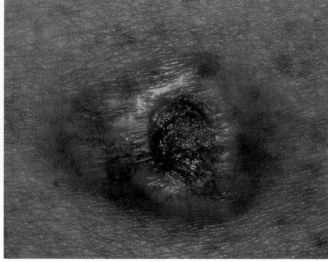

B

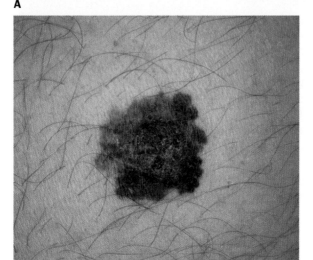

C

FIGURE 20-5 Types of skin cancer: **A,** Squamous cell; **B,** Basal cell; **C,** Malignant melanoma. (**A** From Noble J: *Textbook of primary care medicine*, ed 3, Philadelphia, 2001. Mosby.) (**B** From Goldman L, Ausiello D: *Cecil textbook of medicine*, ed 23, Philadelphia, 2003, Saunders.) (**C** From Townsend C, Beauchamp RD, Evers BM, Mattox K: *Sabison textbook of surgery*, ed 18, Philadelphia, 2008, Saunders.)

BOX 20-1 DETECTION OF POSSIBLE SKIN CANCER

Check yourself on a regular basis for skin cancer using the ABCD method. This will take only a few minutes and may allow you to catch skin cancer in the early stages. Stand in front of a mirror and examine your entire body for any moles that may be present. Remember, not all moles look the same on every person; they can be different colors (red, black, brown), flat, raised, round, oval, or even irregularly shaped from the beginning. By examining yourself you can determine if any suspicious changes have taken place; if this occurs, see your dermatologist.

A—Asymmetry
Moles should appear symmetrical. This means both halves of the mole should look alike or be a mirror image of one another.

B—Border
The border of moles should be well defined and clear. The border should not be fuzzy, blotchy, or irregular in any way.

C—Color
The color of moles needs to be monitored to note if there are any changes, such as the mole changing from light to dark in color.

D—Difference
Check your skin on a regular basis (such as every month) to see if any moles have changed or appear different from the other moles on your body.

BOX 20-2 CANCER TREATMENTS

Radiation therapy—Uses high-energy radiation focused on the abnormal growth to kill cancerous cells. Radiation therapy can be given one to several times, depending on the severity of the cancer. Used when surgery or other options are not possible.

Photodynamic therapy—A photosensitizing agent is either applied to the cancer cells or injected into the skin. After a few days, a laser is focused on the area; the laser activates the photosensitizing agent and destroys the cancer cells. This type of treatment is used on superficial cancers.

Surgery

Excisional skin surgery—Removal of the growth and margin (area surrounding growth) with a scalpel. The skin is examined under a microscope to determine if all cancer cells have been removed.

Electrodesiccation and curettage—Removal of the cancer with the use of a curette (a sharp excisional instrument) followed by application of an electric current to control bleeding and kill any remaining cancer cells. This type of treatment is used to remove small basal cell skin cancers.

Cryosurgery—Liquid nitrogen is applied directly to the skin growth; the extreme cold burns the skin. Used when other surgeries are not possible or when cancers are in an early stage or affect the upper layer of the skin.

Laser surgery—A narrow beam of light is used to remove the cancer cells. Used for growths that are on the outside surface of the skin.

Grafts—The cancerous area is removed and new skin is grafted onto the area. The new skin comes from another area of the body, and both areas must receive care until healed.

Medication

Chemotherapy—Fluorouracil (5-FU) in cream form is used topically on skin containing cancer cells.

Imiquimod—Used to treat basal cell cancer; it is applied to the top layer of the skin on cancer cells.

Biological therapy—Monoclonal antibodies, growth factors, and vaccines are used to boost the immune system.

GENERIC NAME: fluorouracil

TRADE NAME: Efudex, Fluoroplex, Carac

INDICATION: superficial basal cell carcinoma, scaly overgrowth of skin

ROUTE OF ADMINISTRATION: topical

COMMON ADULT DOSAGE: applied once a day to the skin where lesions appear, using enough to cover the entire area with a thin film

SIDE EFFECTS: skin irritation, dryness, severe scaling or peeling, rash, redness, pain or sores

AUXILIARY LABELS:

■ For topical use only.

■ Avoid contact with eyes, nose, and mouth.

■ Do not use if pregnant or breastfeeding.

■ Sunlight precautions.

NOTE: must be applied using gloves or with a nonmetal applicator; thoroughly wash hands after application

---

Stasis Dermatitis and Ulcers

Stasis dermatitis (varicose eczema) is a condition attributable to the buildup of fluids under the skin that can cause ulcers. The open sores that are left in the

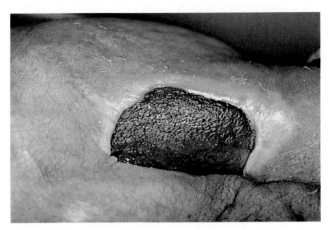

FIGURE 20-6 Ulceration.

TABLE 20-5 Examples of Topical Antibacterial Products

Product	Trade Names	Dosage Forms
bacitracin (OTC)	Bacitracin	Ointment
neomycin (OTC)	Neomycin	Ointment
polymyxin B sulfate, neomycin, bacitracin (OTC)	Neosporin	Ointment, cream
mupirocin 2% (Rx)	Bactroban, Centany	Ointment, cream
retapamulin 1% (Rx)	Altabax	Ointment

skin are called ulcers. Ulcers are common in the ankles and feet because of the lack of circulation in those areas. Poor circulation can cause stasis dermatitis resulting in ulcerative sores. Many external ulcers are caused by bedsores from lying in bed too long without activity, and these often affect the elderly. These sores are slow to heal and may harbor methicillin-resistant *Staphylococcus aureus* (MRSA). This highly contagious and resistant infection must be treated with a strong antibiotic, and cases must be reported to the county health department. In the case of ulcers, the wound must be kept moist and sterile. In addition, antibiotics are prescribed. The patient usually has a lab sample taken after treatment to ensure there is no evidence of methicillin-resistant *Staphylococcus aureus*. Symptoms include pruritus, pain, skin lesions, and swelling of legs, ankles, or other areas that have an ulcer or dermatitis. (Figure 20-6).

Prognosis. Stasis dermatitis can be a chronic condition and may need to be consistently treated by wearing special stockings, elevating the legs and feet, and taking medication.

Non–Drug Treatment. Circulation in the lower extremities can be increased and edema can be decreased by wearing elastic compression stockings. Also, elevating the feet above the level of the heart can reduce swelling. Activity can also improve circulation. The areas of ulceration should be free of external pressure as well.

Drug Treatment. Topical antibiotics such as mupirocin (Bactroban, Centany) may be applied to control some infections. See Table 20-5 for a list of topical and oral antibiotics.

GENERIC NAME: mupirocin (Rx)
TRADE NAME: Bactroban, Centany
INDICATION: prevent infection
ROUTE OF ADMINISTRATION: topical, cream or ointment
COMMON ADULT DOSAGE: apply to affected area(s) three times daily for 10 days or as directed by physician
SIDE EFFECTS: burning, headache, nausea, stinging
AUXILIARY LABEL:
■ For topical use only.
NOTE: If condition does not improve in 3 to 5 days, patient should be reevaluated.

GENERIC NAME: metronidazole (Rx)
TRADE NAME: MetroGel
INDICATION: inflammatory pustules of rosacea; off-label for select malodorous wounds
ROUTE OF ADMINISTRATION: topical
COMMON ADULT DOSAGE: apply to affected area(s) once daily as directed by physician
SIDE EFFECTS: mild burning or stinging when medication is applied, numbness in hands and feet, cough, stuffy nose, sore throat (cold symptoms), headache, and dry, scaly itchy skin
AUXILIARY LABEL:
■ For topical use only.

Psoriasis

Psoriasis is a common, noninfectious inflammatory skin disorder. It has been related to genetics, especially those cases with an early onset (ages 40 years and younger), and may last a lifetime. The onset of this painful disorder is usually during the teen years but can occur later in life. Persons can suffer from mild to severe cases of this disease. This condition is not contagious, although the lesions appear inflamed. Most affected areas are around the joints, limbs, neck, and even scalp and often appear as plaques of silvery scales that vary in size (Figure 20-7).

Prognosis. There is no cure for psoriasis. Constant treatment must be given to keep the outbreaks to a minimum. Treatment with various medications can help in some instances. Approximately 5% to 10% of people in the United States who have psoriasis develop arthritis and joint pain. For these persons, additional

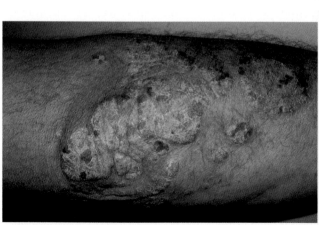
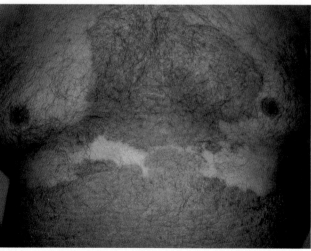

A   B

FIGURE 20-7 Psoriasis. (From Lookingbill D, Marks J: *Principles of dermatology*, ed 4, Philadelphia, 2006, Saunders.)

medications are often prescribed such as nonsteroidal **antiinflammatory** drugs (NSAIDs), sulfasalazine and methotrexate, and biological modifiers; these are normally prescribed by a rheumatologist.

Non–Drug Treatment. For mild psoriasis (covering 3% to 10% of the body), using a high-quality moisturizer will both keep the skin moist and help to control flare-ups. After softening the affected area(s), gently remove the psoriatic crusts; however, this must be done carefully so the skin does not become irritated. By removing these crusted areas, the moisturizer is able to be better absorbed into the skin. The greasier lotions (emollients) that trap moisture work better than nongreasy lotions or moisturizers. However, it may take time to determine which products are most effective.

Phototherapy (or UV exposure treatments) may be used to cause mild sunburn of the skin and subsequent peeling in patients with more serious disease. This is done in a gradual manner over many months using UV light. Another form of light therapy involves use of the excimer laser, which is used for mild to moderate psoriasis. These treatments require fewer sessions because only UVB wavelengths are used. Both types of light treatments cause the skin cells to decrease in replication, which also decreases overall scaling and inflammation.

Drug Treatment. Treatment depends on the type of psoriasis, the extent of the disease, and the patient's response. Although there is no cure, measures can be taken for palliative care (i.e., care focused on pain, symptoms, and the stress of a condition). Three types of agents are used to treat psoriasis: topical agents, phototherapy, and systemic agents. Application of topical agents over the affected area(s) is usually the first line of treatment. Occlusion therapy uses moisturizers or topical medication applied to the skin, and then wrapped with tape, fabric, or plastic. This keeps the area moist, allowing the medication to penetrate more deeply and work more effectively. This treatment should be done under the supervision of a dermatologist because it can lead to problems such as thinning of the skin. Bath soaks using agents such as Aveeno (colloidal oatmeal) can be purchased OTC and may reduce pruritus and discomfort of the skin in mild cases of psoriasis. Tar-based shampoos or preparations may be prescribed for treatment of the scalp. Some tar-based preparations can be used in whirlpools if large areas of the patient's body are affected. After treatment to soften the scales of psoriasis, they can be removed with a soft brush while bathing. Calcipotriene (Dovonex) is a common prescription topical agent applied to plaques to control skin turnover.

Immunosuppressants may help refractory psoriasis. More potent topical drugs such as corticosteroids may be used to manage psoriasis. Creams may be applied after bathing to facilitate absorption and overnight use of occlusive dressings. Small stubborn plaques may require steroidal injection. The mechanism of action of potent corticosteroids is the suppression of T cells and other constituents that cause inflammation and an increase in cell growth. Thus these agents must be used carefully because they impede the immune system. Biological agents such as Amevive (alefacept) may be used in patients who require systemic therapy to control skin plaques and improve skin appearance. Enbrel (etanercept), Remicade (infliximab), and Rheumatrex (methotrexate) are used in treating psoriatic arthritis to prevent progression of joint damage. For a list of agents used to treat psoriasis, see Table 20-6.

Another method to reduce the rapid cell growth seen in psoriasis includes exposure to ultraviolet B (UVB) light or natural sunlight. Tar preparations or coal tar itself may be applied to affected areas for about 15 minutes before light exposure or may be left on overnight and wiped off the following morning. A thin layer of Vaseline (petroleum jelly) may be applied before UVB exposure.

TABLE 20-6 Agents Used to Treat Psoriasis (Most Are Rx)

Classification of Agents	Generic Name	Brand Name	Dosage Form	Indication/Type of Action
Corticosteroids	betamethasone	Diprolene	Gel, cream, ointment, topical aerosol, lotion	Corticosteroids decrease skin inflammation and itching These agents have medium to very high potency depending on type and strength of each agent
	clobetasol propionate	Temovate	Ointment and cream	
	fluocinolone	Synalar	Ointment	
	fluocinonide	Lidex	Cream and ointment	
	flurandrenolide	Cordran	Ointment	
	fluticasone propionate	Cutivate	Ointment	
	hydrocortisone	Aveeno Anti Itch Cream, Cortaid	Cream	OTC forms available
	hydrocortisone valerate	Westcort	Cream	
	triamcinolone acetonide	Triderm	Ointment and cream	
	betamethasone valerate	Valisone	Cream and ointment	
	desoximetasone	Topicort	Cream, gel, and ointment	
Antipsoriatic agent	methotrexate	Rheumatrex	Tablet	Rheumatrex is used to treat plaque psoriasis or psoriatic arthritis It interferes with growth of rapidly growing cells
Coal tar preparations	coal tar	DHS Tar, Doak Tar, Theraplex T	Shampoo, bath oil, ointment, cream, gel, lotion, paste	Tar reduces itching and slows production of excess skin cells OTC forms available
Immunomodulator	alefacept	Amevive	Solution for injection (intramuscular or intravenous)	Fusion protein that suppresses immune system to slow production of skin cells
Immunosuppressive	cyclosporine	Sandimmune, Neoral	Capsules, oral solution	Cyclosporine is used to treat severe psoriasis
Monoclonal antibody	adalimumab	Humira	Solution for injection (subcutaneous)	TNF* blocker indicated for treatment of psoriatic arthritis
Immunomodulator	etanercept	Enbrel	Solution for injection (subcutaneous)	TNF blocker indicated for treatment of plaque psoriasis and psoriatic arthritis
Monoclonal antibody	infliximab	Remicade	Solution for injection (intravenous infusion)	TNF blocker indicated for treatment of plaque psoriasis and psoriatic arthritis

Continued

TABLE 20-6 Agents Used to Treat Psoriasis (Most Are Rx)—cont'd

Classification of Agents	Generic Name	Brand Name	Dosage Form	Indication/Type of Action
Monoclonal antibody	ustekinumab	Stelara	Solution for injection (subcutaneous)	Stelara mimics body's own antibodies (part of immune system) and blocks proteins that contribute to overproduction of skin cells and inflammation
Psoralens	methoxsalen	Oxsoralen-Ultra	Oxsoralen: lotion; 8-MOP* and Oxsoralen-Ultra: capsules; Uvadex: 8-MOP solution	Psoralens make skin more sensitive to light and sun They are used with UVA light to treat psoriasis
Topical retinoid	tazarotene	Tazorac	Gel, cream	Retinoids control psoriasis and reduce redness of skin They can also be used with phototherapy
Oral retinoid	acitretin	Soriatane	Capsule	
Tree bark extract	anthralin	Dithranol, Anthra-Derm, Drithocreme	Cream, ointment, paste	Anthralin slows production of excess skin cells
Vitamin D analog	calcipotriene	Dovonex	Scalp solution, cream, ointment	Dovonex is used to treat moderate psoriasis It slows production of excess skin cells

*8-MOP, 8-Methoxypsoralen; *TNF,* tumor necrosis factor.

UVB treatments can extend for up to 6 months with each session lasting longer than the previous session; they can be done on an outpatient basis. This type of treatment may result in remission of the condition for a longer period and prevents the need for hospitalization.

In the patient with severe chronic psoriasis a combination of tar baths and UVB treatment may be necessary. An alternate therapy uses anthralin instead of tar or the combination of psoralens with exposure to high-intensity UVA.

CORTICOSTEROIDS

GENERIC NAME: betamethasone
TRADE NAME: Diprolene
INDICATION: psoriasis
ROUTE OF ADMINISTRATION: topical
COMMON ADULT DOSAGE: apply to affected area as a thin film from 1 to 2 times daily
SIDE EFFECTS: skin redness, burning, itching or peeling, thinning of skin, blistering of skin
AUXILIARY LABEL:
■ For topical use only.

GENERIC NAME: fluocinonide
TRADE NAME: Lidex
INDICATION: psoriasis
ROUTE OF ADMINISTRATION: topical
COMMON ADULT DOSAGE: apply to affected area as a thin film from 2 to 4 times daily
SIDE EFFECTS: skin redness, burning, itching or peeling, thinning of skin, blistering of skin, swollen hair follicles, blisters, pimples, or crusting of treated skin
AUXILIARY LABEL:
■ For topical use only.

IMMUNOMODULATORS

GENERIC NAME: cyclosporine
TRADE NAME: Sandimmune, Neoral, Gengraft
INDICATION: refractory plaque-type psoriasis
ROUTE OF ADMINISTRATION: oral
COMMON ADULT DOSAGE: initially, 2.5 mg/kg/day, given in 2 divided doses; max 4 mg/kg/day in divided doses
SIDE EFFECTS: increased blood pressure, tremors, increased hair growth, headache, diarrhea, constipation, vomiting, numbness, gingivitis
AUXILIARY LABEL:
■ Take as directed.

VITAMIN D ANALOG

GENERIC NAME: calcipotriene
TRADE NAME: Dovonex
INDICATION: psoriasis
ROUTE OF ADMINISTRATION: topical
COMMON ADULT DOSAGE: apply a thin layer to affected area(s) once or twice daily and rub in gently and completely
SIDE EFFECTS: burning, itching, redness, swelling, dryness or peeling of the skin
AUXILIARY LABEL:
■ For topical use only.

Burns

Burns range in severity from first-degree to fourth-degree, with the fourth-degree burn being the most severe. If the degree of the burn or the size of the burn is substantial (second, third, or fourth degree), the patient may undergo surgery to replace the damaged layers of skin. This is done by removing healthy skin from another part of the body. The new skin then is thinned through a rolling process and then adhered by staples to the damaged skin area. This is a painful process. Burn hospitals require specialized solutions and medications from the pharmacy in order to treat patients who stay in the burn unit. First-degree burns can normally be treated at home (Box 20-3).

Prognosis. Many times both first-degree and second-degree burns heal by themselves with simple care if they are small in size. Scarring is a common outcome of third-degree (Figure 20-8) and fourth-degree burns, or even loss of limb(s) depending on the severity and body surface area involved. The healing process can take a long time and may involve rehabilitation if tissues, muscles, and tendons are damaged. The patient with severe burns over a large surface area can be at high risk for infection, sepsis, and death.

BOX 20-3 BURN DEGREES

First—Only the outer layer (epidermis) of the skin is burned. The skin becomes red and swells, and pain is often present. This is a minor burn unless it involves portions of the hands, feet, face, groin, buttocks, or a major joint. Holding the burned area under cold water and using first aid creams such as bacitracin and over-the-counter (OTC) analgesic agents are the common course of treatment.

Second—When the first layer of the skin (epidermis) burns through to the second layer (the dermis), blisters form and the skin becomes very red and sometimes splotchy. Severe pain, swelling, and sometimes blisters can occur. If the area is no larger than 3 inches (7.5 cm) the same treatments as those used for first-degree burns can be employed. Otherwise, antibiotic ointments may be applied. If severe, hospitalization for the administration of IV antibiotics may be necessary.

Third—When all the layers of the skin are burned, tissue damage occurs. These injuries are painless but can cause severe damage to the fatty tissue, muscles, and even the bones. These burns do not heal without treatment. Damaged tissue may be removed surgically and replaced with skin grafts. Analgesics are used to treat pain.

Fourth—The worst burns are those that penetrate the deepest layers of the skin including muscles, tendons, and bones. Shock can occur in the person with fourth-degree burns because of fluid changes in the body. Replacement IV fluids may be given. Surgery is performed to remove all the burned skin and tissue. Additional surgeries may be necessary to repair and replace lost skin. Strong analgesics are normally required to control pain.

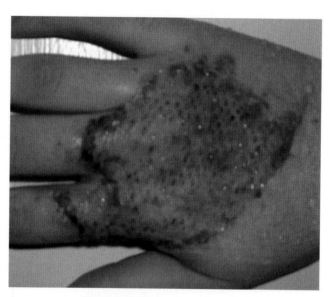

FIGURE 20-8 Third-degree burn.

Non–Drug Treatment. If the burn is minor (first- or second-degree and an area no larger than 3 inches in diameter), then first cool the burn by rinsing it in cool water for about 5 minutes. This conducts heat away from the burn. Do not use ice, which can damage the tissues. Remove any jewelry (e.g., rings) close to the affected area, because jewelry may become constrictive if there is swelling. Cover the affected area with a loose sterile gauze. For severe burns, seek medical help immediately (call 911). Elevating the part of the body burned is advised; also covering the burn with a cool, moist, sterile bandage or clean, moist cloth is suggested. Do not remove burnt clothes if they are present, but make sure nothing is smoldering. Do not place the burned areas under cold water, as this may cause shock. Seek medical help immediately.

Drug Treatment. Treatment may vary depending on the type of burn. For example, there are chemical and electrical burns as well as burns from fire. Topical medications used may include silver cream (Silvadene [sulfadiazine]) and bacitracin ointment.

> **GENERIC NAME:** sulfadiazine
> **TRADE NAME:** Silvadene
> **INDICATION:** prevent infection of second- or third-degree burns
> **ROUTE OF ADMINISTRATION:** topical
> **COMMON ADULT DOSAGE:** apply a thin layer to the affected area twice per day as directed by physician
> **SIDE EFFECTS:** areas of dead skin, burning sensation, red and raised rash on the body, skin discoloration
> **AUXILIARY LABEL:**
> ■ For topical use only.
> **NOTE:** Apply with sterile gloves.

Canker Sores

Canker sores are small topical ulcers that tend to disappear within 2 weeks; they are located in the soft tissue of the mouth—inside the cheeks, lips, base of the gums, or under the tongue. Canker sores are not contagious and there is no known cause although it is believed they appear related to an immune system response. They can be related to stress, poor nutrition, food allergies, immunosuppression, and menstrual periods.

Prognosis. Many canker sores will heal within a couple of weeks.

Non–Drug Treatment. Avoid chewing gum, hard foods, and irritating foods to reduce mouth irritation.

Drug Treatment. Treatments vary from mouth rinses and topical pastes to oral medications and nutritional supplements if necessary. See Table 20-7 for a list of treatments.

> **GENERIC NAME:** Orabase with benzocaine (OTC)
> **TRADE NAME:** Anbesol, Orajel
> **INDICATION:** canker sores, teething pain, or other sources of minor pain
> **ROUTE OF ADMINISTRATION:** topical
> **COMMON ADULT DOSAGE:** use the smallest amount necessary to numb the affected area; up to 4 times per day
> **SIDE EFFECTS:** mild stinging, burning, or itching where medication is applied
> **AUXILIARY LABEL:**
> ■ none

> **GENERIC NAME:** dexamethasone oral solution
> **TRADE NAME:** generically available (0.5 mg/5 mL)
> **INDICATION:** inflammation
> **ROUTE OF ADMINISTRATION:** oral
> **COMMON ADULT DOSAGE:** 0.5 mg swish and spit up to 3 times daily (off-label use)
> **SIDE EFFECTS:** acne, dry skin, thinning skin, bruising or discoloration, dizziness, headache, nausea
> **AUXILIARY LABEL:**
> ■ Take as directed.

TABLE 20-7 **Canker Sore Treatments**

Generic Name	Trade Name	Indication
Mouth Rinses (Rx) (Suspensions Containing)		
dexamethasone	Decadron	To reduce pain and inflammation
tetracycline	Sumycin	To speed healing time and reduce pain; used only for secondary bacterial infections
Topical Pastes/Gels (OTC and Rx)		
triamcinolone acetonide	Kenalog in Orabase Rx	Reduces inflammation and pain
fluocinonide	Lidex Gel Rx	Reduces inflammation
Miscellaneous Medications*		
cimetidine	Tagamet Rx	Normally used for heartburn and ulcers
colchicine	Colchicine Rx	Normally used for gout
oral steroids	Various Rx	Used to reduce inflammation and pain
Nutritional Supplements (OTC)		
folic acid	Folate	Prophylaxis and/or speeds healing
pyridoxine	Vitamin B_6	Prophylaxis and/or speeds healing
cyanocobalamin	Vitamin B_{12}	Prophylaxis and/or speeds healing
zinc		Prophylaxis and/or speeds healing
Anesthetics (OTC)		
benzocaine 20%	Orajel, Anbesol	Helps to reduce pain by numbing area
Orabase/benzocaine	Orabase B	Reduces pain

*Medications not intended for canker sore treatments or when other treatments have failed to work; these medications have shown success in the treatment of canker sores and must be prescribed by a physician.

INFECTIOUS INFLAMMATORY SKIN CONDITIONS

Although infectious skin conditions treated with prescription drugs are common, certain conditions such as warts, tinea infections (such as athlete's foot), cold sores, and lice can be treated with OTC medications. Recurrent or resistant cold sore, lice, or fungal infections will require physician consultation and treatment. Other infections of the skin such as herpes or impetigo must be treated with prescription medications.

Warts
A common wart is caused by a virus that results in growths on the skin. Verruca plana are commonly seen in children and may appear on areas such as the hands, face, and neck. Plantar warts are found on the bottom of the foot, and may be tender. Common warts are caused by human papillomavirus (HPV) (Figure 20-9, *A*). A physician should be seen for appropriate treatment, which may include drug treatment, liquid nitrogen (freezing) application, or surgical removal. Genital warts are different than common warts; they are caused by specific strains of the human papillomavirus (HPV); genital warts are a sexually transmitted disease. Genital warts can be linked to cervical cancer and must receive adequate medical treatment (Figure 20-9, *B, C*).

Prognosis. Warts are contagious, although most disappear on their own within 6 months.

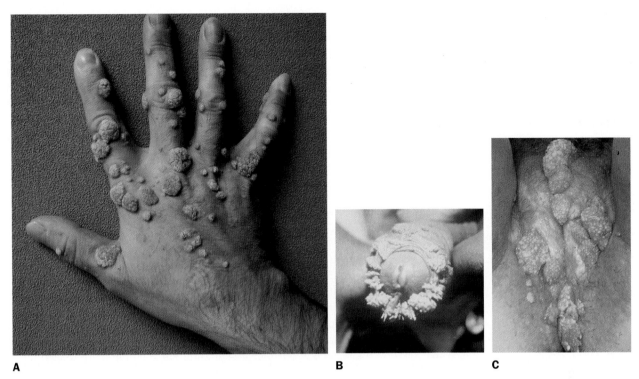

FIGURE 20-9 A, HPV (common warts). **B,** Genital warts, male. **C,** Genital warts, female. (**A** From Lookingbill D, Marks J: *Principles of dermatology*, ed 4, Philadelphia, 2006, Saunders.) (**B, C** From Monahan and Neighbors, 1998/Courtesy New York City Health Department)

TABLE 20-8 Over-the-Counter (OTC) Products to Treat Common Warts

Product	Trade Names	Dosage Forms
Salicylic acid	Wart Off	Liquid
	Compound W	Liquid, gel, medicated strips
	Dr. Scholls Freeze Away wart remover	Liquid
	Compound W Freeze	Liquid

Non–Drug Treatment. If no actions are taken, common warts will normally disappear over time. A non–drug treatment that is effective for common warts or for genital warts does not exist. The best strategy for genital warts is prevention of sexual transmission. Gardasil (human papillomavirus vaccine) is used in young women and female adolescents to prevent genital warts and cervical/vaginal cancer.

Drug Treatment. For common warts OTC agents that contain salicylic acid or that freeze the wart can be used. When applied, the wart becomes dislodged from the skin. Fluorouracil topical (Carac, Efudex, Fluoroplex) works by interfering with skin cell growth; it is usually reserved for resistant plantar warts. Fluorouracil must be applied topically while wearing gloves or nonmetal applicators. Other treatments are listed in Table 20-8. For genital warts, Aldara (imiquimod) or podofilox (topical gel or solution) may be prescribed.

Tech Note!

Dermatophytosis, commonly called tinea, can affect the scalp, body, nails, hands, feet, groin, and bearded skin. Infections are caused by dermatophytes (fungus) of the genera *Trichophyton, Microsporum,* and *Epidermophyton.* Transmission of the fungus can occur through direct contact with infected lesions, with infections present on the skin of cats and dogs, and with soiled or contaminated clothing or articles such as shoes, towels, or shower stalls. Tinea pedis (athlete's foot) is a common condition affecting the toes and soles of the feet.

GENERIC NAME: salicylic acid (OTC)
TRADE NAME: Compound W Wart Removal Gel
INDICATION: common warts, including plantar warts
ROUTE OF ADMINISTRATION: topical
COMMON ADULT DOSAGE: follow skin preparation instructions on product label; this product is applied once or twice daily as needed (until wart is removed) for up to 12 weeks
SIDE EFFECTS: skin irritation
AUXILIARY LABEL:
■ none
NOTE: Wash hands after application.

GENITAL WARTS

GENERIC NAME: imiquimod
TRADE NAME: Aldara
INDICATION: external genital warts around the genital and rectal areas
ROUTE OF ADMINISTRATION: topical
COMMON ADULT DOSAGE: apply as directed by physician once daily or 3 times per week at bedtime; allow medication to stay on skin for 6 to 10 hours and then wash the area thoroughly with soap and water; repeat until warts are gone (up to 16 weeks)
SIDE EFFECTS: skin site reactions such as itching, burning, redness, skin rash, scabbing, crusting
AUXILIARY LABELS:
■ For topical use only.
■ Not for mouth, eye, or vaginal use.
NOTE: Wash hands after application.

Athlete's Foot

Athlete's foot is caused by a fungus of the species *Trichophyton rubrum.* The name of a tinea infection depends on where it is located. Tinea pedis (athlete's foot) causes scaling and blisters between the toes. Severe infection can cause inflammation of the skin on the entire sole and may include relentless pruritus and pain when walking. The infection can be spread by contact from shower floor surfaces or clothing, and by sharing socks. Direct contact must be made to transfer the fungal infection (Figure 20-10).

Other types of tinea include the following:

- Tinea barbae (bearded skin)
- Tinea capitis (hair of the head)
- Tinea corpus (ringworm of the skin)
- Tinea cruris (groin, also known as "jock itch")
- Tinea manuum (hands)
- Tinea unguium (nails)

Prognosis. In most cases the prognosis is excellent if antifungals are used and the feet are kept clean and dry. Through education on proper care of the feet, this condition can be completely avoided.

Non–Drug Treatment. The infection can be prevented with good hygienic practices. Keeping the feet dry and in clean, comfortable socks and shoes helps prevent athlete's foot. Exposing the feet to air whenever possible is also helpful. Avoid walking barefoot in community showers or other places where transmission may be possible.

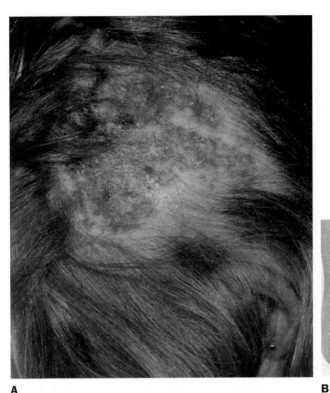

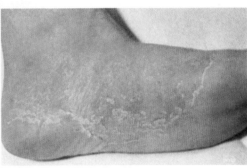

FIGURE 20-10 A, Tina capitis (head). **B,** Tina pedis (athlete's foot).

TABLE 20-9 Antifungal Products to Treat Athlete's Foot

Product	Trade Names	Dosage Forms
tolnaftate	Tinactin	Cream, solution, spray, ointment, powder
miconazole	Desenex or Croex Powder	Powder, spray powder
clotrimazole	Desenex AF, Lotrimin AF	Solution, lotion, cream
terbinafine	Lamisil	Solution
ketoconazole	Nizoral	Cream, gel

Drug Treatment. Most treatments involve topical agents available over-the-counter or by prescription in stronger strengths. Antifungals are used to kill fungus and treat athlete's foot; they are usually in powder or spray form. Skin infections causing chronic thickening of the skin and other unresolved infections normally require oral antifungals. If the infection affects the nails, systemic therapy may be needed to clear the nail infection completely (see Acute Paronychia Onycomycosis). Common agents used to treat athlete's foot are listed in Table 20-9.

GENERIC NAME: clotrimazole (OTC)
TRADE NAME: Desenex AF, Lotrimin AF
INDICATION: athlete's foot and other fungal infections of the skin
ROUTE OF ADMINISTRATION: topical
COMMON ADULT DOSAGE: apply a small amount of the cream twice daily for 2 to 4 weeks
SIDE EFFECTS: none
AUXILIARY LABEL:
■ none

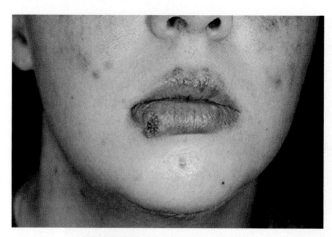

FIGURE 20-11 Herpes simplex.

> **GENERIC NAME:** tolnaftate (OTC)
> **TRADE NAME:** Tinactin
> **INDICATION:** athlete's foot
> **ROUTE OF ADMINISTRATION:** topical
> **COMMON ADULT DOSAGE:** apply agent (gel, cream, lotion, powder, or spray) twice daily for 2 to 6 weeks
> **SIDE EFFECTS:** none
> **AUXILIARY LABEL:**
> ■ none

Herpes

Herpes is a viral outbreak of the skin that causes painful blister-like eruptions. The two different types of herpes are herpes simplex (HSV-1 and HSV-2 viruses) and herpes zoster (varicella-zoster virus), and both can be painful. Herpes simplex is a form of virus that usually causes welts and sores around the mouth (cold sores) or vaginal area (herpes genitalis). This type of herpes is a sexually transmitted disease and commonly is treated with a prescription antiviral. Both types of herpes affect the nervous system, and persons are prone to repeated outbreaks (Figure 20-11) when the immune system becomes weakened. The pain can be intense as the sores form around nerve endings.

Herpes zoster is a painful blistering of the skin causing lesions on the head, neck, arms, and legs. This condition is caused by varicella-zoster virus, the same virus that causes chickenpox. After a person contracts chickenpox, the virus can lay dormant in the nerves of the body for many years. When the virus becomes active once again, it causes shingles. Outbreaks occur along nerve tracks on one side of the body. Symptoms include pain, burning, or tingling, and symptoms may occur before the rash appears.

Prognosis. Although there is no cure for herpes, there are medications that can lessen the amount and length of outbreaks. For shingles, the virus will disappear on its own, although later outbreaks can occur especially if the immune system is weakened. In rare cases, either temporary or permanent weakness or paralysis may occur if the motor nerves have been affected. A chickenpox vaccine (Varivax) is available to prevent chickenpox in children and a vaccine (Zostavax) is available for the prevention of shingles in adults. Zostavax can also prevent

TABLE 20-10 Herpes Medications

Generic Name	Trade Name	Dosage Forms	Available
Genital Herpes Treatments			
valacyclovir	Valtrex	Tablets	Rx only
famciclovir	Famvir	Tablets	Rx only
acyclovir	Zovirax	Tablets, ointment	Rx only
Oral Herpes			
acyclovir	Zovirax	Cream, tablets	Rx only
famciclovir	Famvir	Tablets	Rx only
penciclovir	Denavir	Cream	Rx only
valacyclovir	Valtrex	Tablets	Rx only
docosanol	Abreva	Cream	OTC
Anesthetics for External Pain Relief			
tetracaine	Viractin	Cream, ointment, solution	OTC
lidocaine	Zilactin-L	Cream, lotion, solution, spray, film	OTC

further attacks of shingles; however, the adult vaccine is given only to those persons over the age of 60.

Non–Drug Treatment. Keeping the affected area clean and dry helps the healing process for both types of herpes. For genital herpes, wearing loose-fitting undergarments may help prevent chafing. Proper nutrition, exercise, and rest help strengthen the immune system. Rest is recommended for shingles. Avoid direct contact with others to avoid transmission of infection.

Drug Treatment. Antiviral medications may be used to alleviate the side effects along with analgesics for pain. Drugs such as acyclovir (Zovirax) topical ointment may be prescribed for cold sores attributable to herpes simplex. Depending on the site of the outbreak and the frequency of outbreaks, systemic therapy may be needed. Some patients follow **prophylactic** medication regimens to reduce the incidence of outbreaks. Acyclovir may be given orally, as can valacyclovir (Valtrex) and famciclovir (Famvir) (Table 20-10).

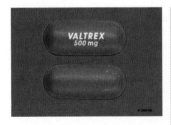

GENERIC NAME: valacyclovir
TRADE NAME: Valtrex
INDICATION: genital herpes, shingles
ROUTE OF ADMINISTRATION: oral
COMMON ADULT DOSAGE: recurrent episodes of genital herpes: 500 mg twice daily for 3 days; shingles: 1 g three times daily for 7 days
SIDE EFFECTS: nausea, stomach pain, headache, dizziness, joint pain, mild skin rash, stuffy nose, sore throat
AUXILIARY LABEL:
■ Take with a full glass of water.

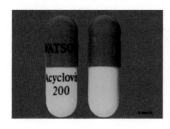

GENERIC NAME: acyclovir
TRADE NAME: Zovirax
INDICATION: genital herpes, shingles
ROUTE OF ADMINISTRATION: oral, topical, injection
COMMON ADULT DOSAGE: oral (genital herpes): 200 mg every 4 hours 5 times daily for 10 days; oral (herpes zoster, shingles): 800 mg every 4 hours, 5 times daily for 10 days
SIDE EFFECTS: diarrhea, nausea, vomiting, general feeling of bodily discomfort; if dehydrated can cause kidney problems
AUXILIARY LABEL:
■ Take with a full glass of water.

Impetigo

Impetigo is a highly contagious condition caused by streptococcal organisms or *Staphylococcus aureus* (see Chapter 30). The bacteria can enter the body through broken skin caused by animal bites, injury or trauma, or insect bites, although impetigo may appear where there is no break in the skin. Areas affected include the face, limbs, and abdomen. A thick yellow crust is formed, sores are itchy and oozing, and blistering is common. The infection is contagious because of the lesions' discharge.

Prognosis. The sores of impetigo heal slowly although they rarely cause scarring. Children may have recurrences of the condition.

Non–Drug Treatment. Keeping the skin clean by washing several times daily with an antibacterial soap is recommended to remove crusted skin and oozing discharge. The condition is very contagious. Sheets, towels, and clothing should be washed frequently to help prevent the spread of infection. Isolation may be advised to decrease transfer of the bacteria to others.

Drug Treatment. Treatment includes topical antibiotics such as mupirocin 2% ointment (Bactroban, Centany) or retapamulin 1% ointment (Altabax); these are effective for limited areas and have the advantage of no systemic side effects. Oral antibiotics are used for more extensive cases of impetigo or for those patients who have concurrent systemic symptoms. Antibiotics used include penicillins (e.g., dicloxacillin or Augmentin) or cephalosporins (e.g., Keflex or Ceftin) as first choices; erythromycin may be used but is typically a second-line antibiotic.

GENERIC NAME: retapamulin
TRADE NAME: Altabax
INDICATION: impetigo
ROUTE OF ADMINISTRATION: topical
COMMON ADULT DOSAGE: apply a thin layer to affected area(s) twice daily for 5 days or as directed by prescriber
SIDE EFFECTS: mild pain, redness, itching, headache, diarrhea
AUXILIARY LABEL:
■ For topical use only.
NOTE: Wash hands after application.

CONDITIONS OF THE HAIR

Lice

Head lice are caused by the parasite *Pediculus humanus capitis*. Many children come home from school with head lice. Lice can be transferred easily

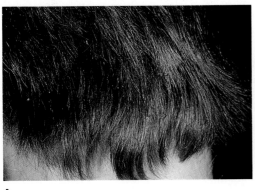
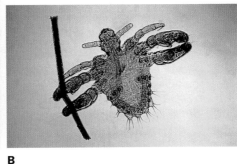

A **B**

FIGURE 20-12 A, Head louse. **B,** Crab lice. (**A** From Callen JP et al: *Color atlas of dermatology,* ed 2, Philadelphia, 2000, Saunders; Courtesy Dr. Robert Zax. **B** from Auerbach PS: *Wilderness medicine,* ed 5, St Louis, 2007, Mosby.)

when children use the same hair brush. Other ways to transmit lice include sleeping next to someone with lice and sharing clothes with someone who has lice. Symptoms include itching, sores on the head, and a tickling feeling of something moving in the hair. Several products on the market treat this infestation. Treatment of the whole family is important even though the infestation affects only one child (Figure 20-12A).

Another type of lice affects the pubic area (commonly called crabs) and is spread through sexual contact. Other areas that the lice can be found include hair on the legs, armpits, mustache, beard, eyebrows, and eyelashes of adults (if lice are found on the eyelashes or eyebrows of children, it is considered head lice). Symptoms include pruritus and visible nits (lice eggs) or crawling lice in the genital area (Figure 20-12B).

Prognosis. If treated correctly by following the directions given on the treatment package, lice can be easily eliminated.

Non–Drug Treatment. All brushes, combs, and hats must be cleaned in hot, soapy water or alcohol and should not be shared. Wash all bed linens in hot water and dry for at least 20 minutes on the hottest setting. Dry clean those items that are not washable. Place all stuffed animals and blankets for at least 2 weeks in a sealed plastic bag to ensure the lice (if any are present) die. Vacuum the floor and furniture. For genital lice in adults that also are present in the eyebrows or eyelashes, removing lice with your fingers is recommended. Never use medicated treatments on or around the eyes. For genital lice, sexual contact should be avoided until the lice are adequately treated. Physical removal of all nits is essential to adequately treat lice of any type.

Drug Treatment. OTC agents are available, such as Nix (permethrin) topical cream rinse, Medi-Lice, Pronto, and Tegrin LF (pyrethrins and piperonyl butoxide) as shampoos. Prescription treatments include Ovide (malathion) topical and Kwell (lindane) shampoos and lotions; these are reserved for resistant cases. Lindane may cause neurotoxicity and seizures if improperly used; patient counseling on proper use is essential to safety. A new prescription treatment is Denzyl alcohol (Ulesfia).

For treatment of pubic lice a pediculicide such as permethrin or pyrethrin is used; prescription therapies are reserved for resistant cases.

GENERIC NAME: permethrin (OTC)
TRADE NAME: Nix
INDICATION: lice
ROUTE OF ADMINISTRATION: topical
COMMON ADULT DOSAGE: use enough solution to saturate hair and scalp; leave on for 10 minutes and then rinse with water; remove eggs (nits) with comb provided; apply second treatment in 7-10 days if needed
SIDE EFFECTS: itching, mild burning or stinging, redness, swelling
AUXILIARY LABEL:
■ none

CONDITIONS OF THE NAIL

Acute Paronychia and Onychomycosis

Nails on both hands and feet endure daily abuse and can become damaged. Bacterial and fungal infections or trauma can occur that may discolor, deform, or cause detachment of the nail. Acute paronychia is normally due to a staphylococcal infection. Onychomycosis is an infection of the nails; if caused by tinea fungi it is referred to as tinea unguium. Infection normally starts at the tip of one or more toenails. It produces thickening, discoloration, and crumbling of the nail, possibly destroying the entire nail. Infections attributable to the genus *Candida* are referred to as onychomycosis. The nails become red and swollen with a darkened nail bed. Occasionally pus will be discharged and the nail may become separated from the nail bed. Most infections of the nails are superficial and rarely become systemic; therefore they are typically treated with topical agents. If, however, a fungal infection is systemic, agents such as ketoconazole or fluconazole may be prescribed. The nail conditions listed in Box 20-4 are those that may require treatment with medication.

Prognosis. With proper treatment the prognosis is good. Although nails may have to be removed, they do grow back and their absence does not alter normal activities.

Non–Drug Treatment. Patients should be educated about avoiding direct contact with high-risk areas in public places to avoid further infections. Good hand hygiene is paramount in keeping the nails in good condition. In certain cases a combination of oral and topical agents along with surgical removal of the affected nails may be necessary.

Drug Treatment. The type of treatment used for onychomycosis depends on the type of infection and the number of affected nails. The severity of the condition will also determine the dosage form and length of treatment needed. Certain infections can be treated with topical antifungals such as ciclopirox olamine 8%

⭐ Tech Note!

Soap and water have always been a good way to remove bacteria from our skin; however, they do not necessarily kill all bacteria. **Antiseptics** are necessary for the health care worker because they do kill and/or inhibit the growth of germs. Unfortunately, both good and bad germs are killed when these agents are used. It is wise not to overuse antiseptics because bacteria have the capability to mutate into strains that are not necessarily inhibited or destroyed. Using gloves can reduce the necessity of constant hand hygiene, and therefore help skin stay more hydrated. See proper techniques for washing hands and gloving in Chapter 12. Learn more about microbial growth in Chapter 30.

BOX 20-4 NAIL CONDITIONS

Condition	Due to:
Koilonychia	Iron deficiency
Onycholysis	Psoriasis or fungal infection
Onychomycosis	Fungal infections caused by tinea or candidiasis
Blue-green nails	*Pseudomonas* infection
Black nails	Subungual melanoma
Yellow nail syndrome	Lymphedema pleural effusions, bronchiectasis, AIDS patients

lacquer solution. Oral therapy may be prescribed either alone or in addition to topical treatments. Oral antifungals such as terbinafine provide higher cure rates than previously used agents (itraconazole, griseofulvin); treatment durations allow for outgrowth of healthy nail(s).

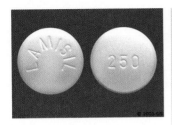

GENERIC NAME: terbinafine
TRADE NAME: Lamisil
INDICATION: onychomycosis
ROUTE OF ADMINISTRATION: oral
COMMON ADULT DOSAGE: 250 mg once daily for 6 weeks (fingernails) or for 12 weeks (toenails)
SIDE EFFECTS: diarrhea, abdominal pain, hives, itching, and altered taste
AUXILIARY LABEL:
■ Take as directed.

DO YOU REMEMBER THESE KEY POINTS?

■ The importance of skin protection against UVA and UVB rays
■ The differences between infectious inflammatory and noninfectious inflammatory conditions
■ The degrees of a burn and their treatments
■ Treatments used for psoriasis
■ Treatments used for canker sores
■ Types of acne and their treatments
■ How skin protectants are rated for protection
■ Common topical antiinflammatories

REVIEW QUESTIONS

Multiple choice questions

1. The skin has many functions. Which of the following is NOT one of its main functions?
  A. Regulates temperature of the body
  B. Acts as a sensor to a stimulus
  C. Protects the internal organs from the elements
  D. All of the above

2. The terms *UVA* and *UVB* relate to the:
  A. Amount of sun that a person can withstand
  B. Ultraviolet rays of the sun
  C. Wavelength of rays emitted from the sun
  D. Both B and C

3. If you burn easily and rarely tan and you decide to use an SPF 10 product, how long can you be exposed to the sun before you will need to reapply the lotion?
  A. 10 minutes
  B. 100 minutes
  C. 1 hour
  D. 10 hours

4. Common warts are caused by:
  A. Viruses
  B. Bacteria
  C. Fungi
  D. Unclean skin

5. To treat lice, all of the following items and/or people should be treated EXCEPT:
   A. The entire family of the person infected with lice
   B. The person infected with lice
   C. Bedding and stuffed animals
   D. Anyone who has shared a comb or clothing

6. Herpes zoster is a condition that:
   A. Affects mostly children who have not contracted chickenpox
   B. Is highly contagious at all stages
   C. Is caused by the same virus that is responsible for HPV
   D. Is caused by the dormant virus that causes chickenpox

7. The medication fluocinonide is used to treat:
   A. Warts
   B. Psoriasis
   C. HPV
   D. Athlete's foot

8. Which of the medications below could be used to treat pruritis of the skin?
   A. Tolnaftate
   B. Salicylic acid
   C. Bacitracin
   D. Caladryl

9. Impetigo can be treated with all of the following methods EXCEPT:
   A. Keep the skin clean and dry
   B. Use both oral and topical bacterial antibiotics
   C. Use a topical antiviral
   D. Wash with antibacterial soap

10. All of the following statements are true concerning stasis dermatitis EXCEPT:
   A. Those persons most affected by stasis dermatitis are those who are bedridden
   B. Stasis dermatitis must be treated with oral antibiotics such as metronidazole to heal the infection
   C. MRSA can occur in open ulcers caused by stasis dermatitis
   D. Symptoms of stasis dermatitis include swelling of legs, ankles, and other areas that may be affected

True/False

If the statement is false, then change it to make it true.

_____ **1.** Betamethasone (Diprolene) is a high-level corticosteroid that can be used for skin conditions such as psoriasis.

_____ **2.** The skin is the largest organ of the body.

_____ **3.** Herpes simplex and herpes zoster are caused by the same bacterial infection.

_____ **4.** Athlete's foot is caused by bacteria.

_____ **5.** Acne is caused by hormone levels, not eating habits.

_____ **6.** The epidermis contains the blood vessels and nerves that nourish the skin.

_____ **7.** Waterproof sun lotion increases the longevity of effectiveness by 40 minutes.

_____ **8.** Psoriasis is an infectious, inflammatory condition of the skin.

_____ **9.** Tetracycline is available as an over-the-counter antibacterial product used for acne.

_____ **10.** Many cases of urticaria are idiopathic.

BIBLIOGRAPHY

AMA (American Medical Association) *Concise Medical Encyclopedia.* 2006.
American Cancer Society: *Cancer facts and figures 2009,* Atlanta, GA, 2009, American Cancer Society.

Graham-Brown R, Bourke J: *Mosby's color atlas and text of dermatology*, ed 2, Philadelphia, 2007, Elsevier.

Professional guide to diseases, ed 9, Lippincott, 2009. Reference 10/09.

WEBSITES

American Cancer Society: www.cancer.org/downloads/STT/500809web.pdf

Carey M, MD: Burns: From Treatment to Prevention. InterMDnet 2008. www.thedoctorwillseeyounow.com/articles/other/burns_23/

Pubic Lice (Crabs): Source cdc.gov. 4/26/2006.

www.medicinenet.com/pubic_lice_crabs/article.htm

Skin cancer treatments: http://cancertrials.nci.nih.gov/cancertopics/wyntk/skin/page9

Statistic on melanoma: www.cancer.gov/cancertopics/types/melanoma/

Levy S, MD. Sunscreens and Photoprotection. January 13, 2009 http://emedicine.medscape.com/article/1119992-overview

Skin Cancer Guidelines: http://www.skincancer.org/skin-types-and-at-risk-groups.html

21

Gastrointestinal System

Objectives

UPON COMPLETING THIS CHAPTER, YOU SHOULD BE ABLE TO DO THE FOLLOWING:

- Identify the anatomy of the digestive system that is covered in this chapter.

- List the most common conditions affecting the digestive system.

- List both trade and generic names of drugs covered in this chapter.

- Explain the differences between stool softeners, laxatives, and bulk-forming laxatives.

- Describe the drug action of the medications covered in this chapter.

- Explain the types of treatments used for ulcers, including lifestyle modifications.

- Distinguish between common ulcers and those caused by *Helicobacter pylori,* and explain why the treatments are different.

- Explain causes of diarrhea, constipation, flatulence, and emesis.

- List the different types of treatments for each of the conditions discussed.

TERMS AND DEFINITIONS

Absorption (gastrointestinal) *The processes describing the movement of nutrients, fluids, and medications from the gastrointestinal tract into the bloodstream*

Amino acids *Molecules that make up proteins*

Carbohydrates *Chemical compounds that contain carbon, hydrogen, and oxygen; examples include sugars, glycogen, starches, and cellulose*

Chyme *The soupy consistency (semifluid consistency) of food after mixing with stomach acids and digestive enzymes as it passes into the duodenum (first part of small intestine)*

Digestion *The mechanical, chemical, and enzymatic action of breaking food into molecules that can be used in metabolism*

Excretion *Elimination of waste products and other remnants of metabolism, primarily through stools and urine*

Ingestion *The act of taking in food, liquid, or other substances (e.g., medications)*

Peristalsis *The contraction and relaxation of the tubular muscles of the esophagus, stomach, and intestines that moves substances from the mouth to the anus*

COMMON DRUGS FOR THE GASTROINTESTINAL SYSTEM

Trade Name	Generic Name	Pronunciation	Trade Name	Generic Name	Pronunciation
H₂-Antagonists			Metamucil	psyllium	(**sill**-ee-um)
Axid	nizatidine	(nye-**zah**-tih-deen)	MiraLAX	polyethylene glycol 3350	(pol-ee-**eth**-il-een **glye**-kol)
Pepcid	famotidine	(fa-**mo**-ta-deen)	Phillips' MOM	magnesium hydroxide	(mag-**nee**-see-um/ hye-**drock**-side)
Tagamet	cimetidine	(sy-**met**-ta-deen)			
Zantac	ranitidine	(ra-**nit**-ta-deen)	Senokot, Ex-Lax	senna	(**sen**-ah)
Proton Pump Inhibitors			**Antidiarrheals**		
AcipHex	rabeprazole	(rah-**bep**-rah-zole)	Imodium AD	loperamide	(low-**pear**-ah-myde)
Dexilant	dexlansoprazole	(dex-**lan**-soe-pra-zole)	Lomotil	diphenoxylate/ atropine	(die-fen-**ox**-i-late/ **at**-row-peen)
Nexium	esomeprazole	(es-o-**mep**-rah-zole)	Pepto-Bismol	bismuth subsalicylate	(**biz**-muth sub-suh-**li**-suh-late)
Prevacid	lansoprazole	(lan-**sew**-prah-zole)			
Prilosec	omeprazole	(oh-**mep**-rah-zole)			
Protonix	pantoprazole	(pan-**tow**-prah-zole)	**Constipation-Predominant Irritable Bowel Syndrome and Chronic Idiopathic Constipation**		
Zegerid	omeprazole/ sodium bicarbonate	(oh-**mep**-rah-zole/ **so**-dee-um by-**kar**-bon-ate)	Amitiza	lubiprostone	(loo-**bee**-pros-tone)
			Severe Diarrhea-Predominant Irritable Bowel Syndrome		
Anticonstipation Agents (Laxatives and Stool Softeners)			Lotronex	alosetron	(a-**low**-se-tron)
Citrucel	methycellulose	(meth-ill-**cell**-you-lows)			
Chronulac	lactulose	(**lak**-tyoo-lose)	**Antinausea/Antiemetics**		
Colace	docusate sodium	(**dok**-yoo-sate **sow**-dee-um)	**Antivertigo/Anticholinergic Antiemetics**		
Dulcolax	bisacodyl	(by-saw-**co**-dill)	Antivert	meclizine	(**meck**-la-zeen)
FiberCon	calcium polycarbophil	(**kal**-ce-uhm pol-ee-**kar**-bow-phyl)	Dramamine	dimenhydrinate	(die-men-**hi**-dra-nate)
			Transderm Scōp	scopolamine	(sko-**pole**-la-meen)
Fleet	mineral oil	(min-**uh**-ral oy-il)			
Glycerin, Babylax, Colace Glycerin	glycerin anhydrous	(**glis**-ir-in)	**Phenothiazine and Related Antiemetics**		
			Compazine	prochlorperazine	(pro-klor-**pear**-ah-zeen)

Continued

695

COMMON DRUGS FOR THE GASTROINTESTINAL SYSTEM—cont'd

Trade Name	Generic Name	Pronunciation	Trade Name	Generic Name	Pronunciation
Phenergan	promethazine	(pro-**meth**-a-zeen)	Zofran	ondansetron	(on-**dan**-see-tron)
Tigan	trimethobenzamide	(try-meth-oh-**ben**-za-mide)	Reglan	metoclopramide	(mea-toe-**clow**-prah-myde)
Torecan	thiethylperazine	(thye-eth-ill-**per**-a-zeen)			
			Antispasmodics/Anticholinergics		
Antinauseants and Antiemetics			Cystospaz	hyoscyamine	(hye-oh-**sigh**-a-meen)
Aloxi	palonosetron	(**pal**-oh-**noe**-se-tron)	Levsin	hycoscyamine	(hye-oh-**sky**-a-meen)
Anzemet	dolasetron	(doe-**las**-eh-tron)	**Antiflatulence Agent**		
Kytril, Granisol, Sancuso	granisetron	(gra-**ni**-se-tron)	Mylicon	simethicone	(sye-**meth**-i-cone)
			Antiulcer Agent/Gastric Mucosa Protectant		
			Carafate	sucralfate	(soo-**kral**-fate)

T HE DIGESTIVE TRACT EXTENDS from the mouth to the anus. It processes ingested substances, such as food and fluids, so they can be absorbed and used by the body. Foods are broken down from large substances into small molecules that can be absorbed readily into the bloodstream and used for energy production, in protein synthesis, and as enzymes for essential metabolic reactions. As food is broken down, nutrients are absorbed, and all nonessential food elements are excreted through the feces or urine. The common analogy used to describe the entire gastrointestinal system is one long tube that runs through the body. This description is adequate for most of the functions that are covered in this chapter. However, a pharmacy technician should be aware of various important functions. These areas are covered more thoroughly as they pertain to medications. Many medications are available over-the-counter (OTC) to treat the symptoms of the digestive tract and the intestines. Because of the ease of self-treatment by purchasing OTC medications, many patients believe it is unnecessary to consult their physician or pharmacist about possible interactions of OTC drugs with legend (prescription) drugs or the effect of OTC medications on underlying health conditions. Many interactions need to be considered when filling new prescriptions for patients.

GASTROINTESTINAL MEDICAL TERMINOLOGY

Word Combinations

An/o	Rectum/anus
Cholecyst/o	Gallbladder
Col/o, colon/o	Large intestine
Diverticul/o	Diverticulum
Duoden/o	Duodenum
Enter/o	Intestine
Esophag/o	Esophagus
Gastr/o	Stomach
Gingiv	Gums
Halit	Breath
Hemat/o	Blood
Hepat/o	Liver
Hiat/i	Opening
Ile/i	Ileum
Jejun/o	Jejunum
Lith/o	Stone (calcification)
Metabol/o	Change
Odont/i	Tooth

GASTROINTESTINAL MEDICAL TERMINOLOGY—cont'd

Or/o	Mouth
Orth/o	Straight or normal
Pancreat/o	Pancreas
Pharyng/o	Pharynx
Pept/o	Digest
Proct/o	Rectum, anus
Pyr/o	Fever
Rect/o	Rectum
Sial/o	Saliva
Splen/o	Spleen
Stom/o, stomat/o	Mouth

Prefixes

Dys-	Difficult
Hyper-	Excessive
Peri-	Around

Suffixes

-eal, ic, al	Pertaining to
-emesis	Vomiting
-ism	Condition
-ologist, -ist	Specialist
-osis	Abnormal condition
-pepsia	Digestion
-phagia	To swallow or eat
-rrhea	Flow or discharge
-um	Latin ending for noun

Conditions

Appendicitis	Inflammation of appendix
Botulism	Bacterial infection caused by *Clostridium botulinum*
Cholera	Bacterial infection caused by *Vibrio cholerae*
Constipation	Difficult or infrequent defecation; often accompanied by dry, hard stools and/or sluggish bowel activity
Crohn's disease	Form of inflammatory bowel disease, a systemic autoimmune disorder that primarily involves GI tract; may occur in any part of GI tract from mouth to anus
Diarrhea	Frequent, watery, loose stools
Diverticulitis	Inflammation of diverticulum located in colon
Dyspepsia	Pain or discomfort while digesting food
Dysphagia	Difficulty in swallowing
Enteritis	Inflammation of small intestine
Gastritis	Inflammation of stomach lining
GERD	Gastroesophageal reflux disease; acid backflow into esophagus
Hematemesis	Blood present in vomit
Hemorrhoids	Veins, muscles, and/or tissues push through anal opening
Hiatal hernia	Defect in diaphragm that allows a portion of stomach to pass through diaphragm opening into chest cavity
Peptic ulcer	Disease where one or more raw areas develop in membrane lining of stomach, esophagus, and duodenum; affected areas are damaged by digestive enzymes and acid secreted by stomach
Pyrosis	Heartburn, burning sensation in upper abdomen
Typhoid fever	Bacterial infection caused by *Salmonella typhi*
Ulcer	Lesion on mucosal surface of gastrointestinal tract
Ulcerative colitis	Form of inflammatory bowel disease, a systemic illness characterized by chronic inflammation and ulceration of large intestine (colon)

Form and Function of the Gastrointestinal System

The four main functions of the gastrointestinal system are digestion, absorption, metabolism, and excretion. Within the gastrointestinal tract, the various organs perform these functions 24 hours a day. The gastrointestinal system is controlled by the parasympathetic nervous system. The parasympathetic nervous system is the part of the nervous system that balances with the sympathetic system in controlling many of the functions of the body (see Chapter 16). When we are at rest, the parasympathetic nervous system is at work in body systems such as the gastrointestinal system. Each organ within the gastrointestinal tract completes specific tasks. This chapter examines the gastrointestinal system from the time food is ingested until it is expelled. This chapter also discusses additional organs, including the liver, pancreas, and gallbladder, that assist the gastrointestinal tract in **digestion**.

Anatomy of the Gastrointestinal System

When thinking about the gastrointestinal system, most people consider the stomach as the primary organ. However, by the time food has arrived to the stomach, it has already begun its transformation from a solid food. Let us begin by looking at the overall system of the gastrointestinal tract (Figure 21-1). The organs discussed in this chapter, in sequence, are the mouth, salivary glands,

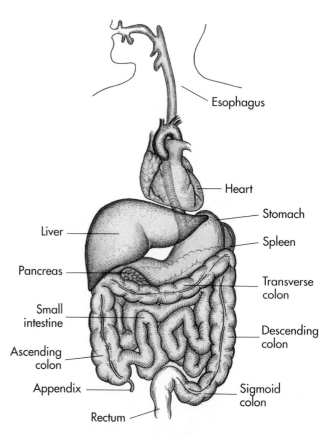

FIGURE 21-1 Anatomy of the gastrointestinal system (including mouth, pharynx, esophagus, stomach, and intestines). (From Potter PA, Perry AG: *Fundamentals of nursing,* ed 7, St Louis, 2009, Mosby.)

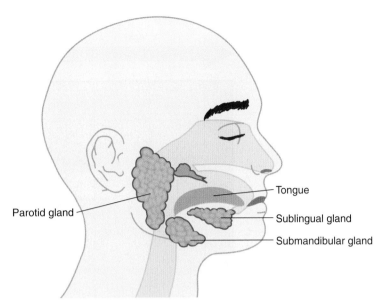

FIGURE 21-2 Major glands of the mouth.

pharynx, and esophagus (ingestion); followed by the stomach and small intestine (absorption); the large intestine (excretion); and finally the rectal area (elimination).

INGESTION

The mouth begins the process of digestion by physically breaking down food into smaller pieces through the act of chewing. In addition to the action of the teeth chewing food into smaller pieces (i.e., mastication), salivary glands begin to secrete an enzyme called amylase that initiates the chemical breakdown of food. The mouth has three pairs of salivary glands that are responsible for the beginning of food digestion: sublingual, submandibular, and parotid. The sublingual and submandibular glands are located below the tongue and jaw, respectively. Each parotid gland is located immediately in front of the ear (Figure 21-2).

Another function of the saliva besides enzymatic breakdown of food is to moisten the esophagus so that food can be swallowed easily. With help from the tongue, the food is swallowed and makes its way into the pharynx (i.e., the throat). The pharynx connects the mouth to the esophagus and contains the epiglottis. The function of the epiglottis is to obstruct the trachea so that food does not enter the respiratory tract, causing choking. **Peristalsis** action in the esophagus propels food downward into the stomach. As the food arrives in the stomach, it enters into an acidic environment in which further chemical breakdown will occur (Figure 21-3).

When activated by food, gastric juices are secreted in the stomach. The gastric juices are composed of intrinsic factor, enzymes, and hydrochloric acid; the gastric juices have a pH of 2 in the stomach lumen. The enzymatic function of the stomach is important because it allows the intestines to absorb the nutrients and chemicals and use them for metabolic processes. However, this acidic environment also destroys many medications that enter into the stomach, which is why several medications need special coating for protection. Alternatively, some medications (e.g., parenteral medications) need to be administered in a totally different form to bypass the stomach and its acidic environment. To help balance this extremely acidic pH, the inner mucosal lining of the stomach is alkaline for protection. An additional protective mucosal lining prevents the acid from eating through the stomach wall. The function of the stomach muscles is

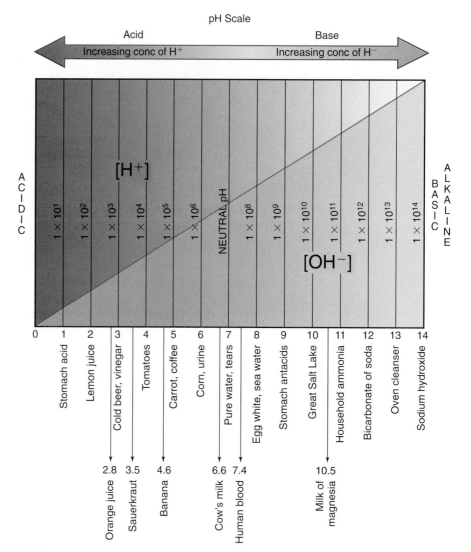

FIGURE 21-3 pH scale ranges from 1 (the most acidic) to 14 (the most basic). Normal human blood is pH 7.4, approximately the midpoint of the range.

to help with digestion by a churning action that mixes the food. The acid helps to eliminate bacteria that have been ingested and activates the enzymes that break down food. An important chemical produced, pepsinogen, becomes an active enzyme in the stomach called pepsin. When the churning and chemicals have converted the solid substances into small pieces, the acidic, semifluid mixture that remains is referred to as **chyme**. The chyme then leaves the stomach and passes through the pyloric sphincter, the muscle that forms the division and opening into the small intestine. The pyloric sphincter must relax in order for the chyme to pass. This is a reflex action.

ABSORPTION

Absorption of nutrients takes place within the small intestine. The vitamins and minerals move through the lining of the gut. Molecules of glucose, **amino acids**, and fatty acids begin to circulate into the body fluids. The blood becomes another avenue that nutrients must travel to reach their ultimate destination—the cells. Without the process of absorption, our cells would not be nourished and would die. Nutrients are used for energy and as building blocks for larger

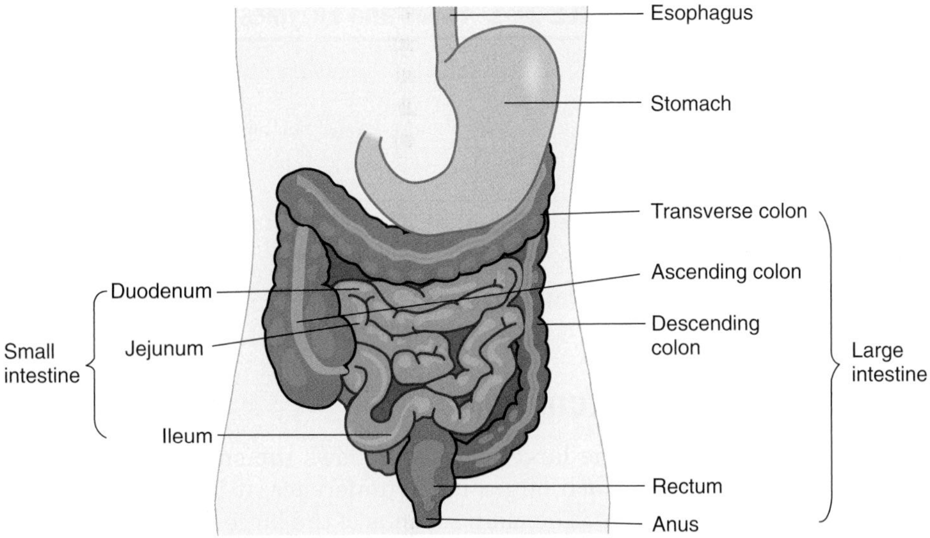

FIGURE 21-4 Intestinal tract (including duodenum, jejunum, and ileum).

complex chemicals. The act of building molecules is known as anabolism, whereas breaking down molecules to release energy is known as catabolism. The overall process is called metabolism (see Chapter 30).

The small intestine is about 6 meters (m) long and is responsible for the final steps in the digestion of food. The materials that are not digested or absorbed from the small intestine pass into the large intestine. The structure of the small intestine is congruent with its function—to absorb nutrients from the foods we eat. To do this, it must be able to make contact with as much of the broken-down food as possible and for as long as possible. The small intestine accomplishes this by being extremely long. Because there is limited space in a human body, the small intestine must fold upon itself to conserve space. In addition, the inside of the lining of the small intestine is formed in such a way that it folds back and forth, which also increases the overall surface area to provide maximum exposure to ingested substances (Figure 21-4).

The small intestine can be divided further into three sections: the duodenum, jejunum, and ileum. Each has a specific function and contribution to the breakdown and absorption of food. The duodenum is at the beginning of the small intestine and is about 25 cm long. The duodenum also is connected to the liver and pancreas, from which it receives secretions that mix with the chyme from the stomach. In addition to the liver and pancreas, the gallbladder also helps in the digestion of food. The gallbladder releases the stored bile to help in the dispersion of fats. The next section of the small intestine is the jejunum, which is much longer (about 2.5 m). The ileum is the most distal section, measuring about 3.5 m in length.

Within these three sections of the small intestine most of the food and oral drug absorption takes place. Intestinal secretions have a more alkaline pH, allowing for good absorption of nutrients. Various enzymes continue to break down specific foods such as sugar, protein, and fat (Table 21-1). The amount of secretions produced depends on how much food or chyme is present. Nutrients and drugs absorb into the bloodstream from the small intestine through several processes, including diffusion and active transport. Various transport processes available in the walls of the small intestine help carry important nutrients and drugs to the bloodstream. Each villus (fingerlike projection) on the surface of the small intestine has a network of capillaries and fine lymphatic vessels. The epithelial cells of these villi transport nutrients and drugs from the lumen into

TABLE 21-1 Foods and Enzymes That Digest Them

Food	Enzyme*
Proteins	Peptidase
Sugars	Maltase, sucrase, lactase
Fats	Lipase

*Words ending in -ase indicate that the substance is an enzyme.

the capillaries. Any substances that are not absorbed or remain undigested pass to the large intestine.

EXCRETION

The large intestine follows the small intestine. Although the large intestine is much larger in circumference, it is not as long as the small intestine (only 1.5 m). The main sections of the large intestine used in excretion include the cecum, colon, rectum, and anus. The colon comprises most of the length of the large intestine. Although some absorption continues in the large intestine, it is limited to water and electrolytes. The substances moving through this portion of the intestine are not chyme but are transformed into solid fecal matter as water and electrolytes are absorbed into the bloodstream.

The rectum is the shortest section of the intestinal tract and connects to the anal canal. The rectum is usually empty except during defecation. The amount of time for normal passage of fecal material can range from 3 to 5 days. Within the anal canal, the internal anal sphincter is under involuntary control and is responsible for the urge to defecate. The external anal sphincter is voluntary, giving the person control of the bowels.

AUXILIARY ORGAN FUNCTIONS

The chemical contribution of the auxiliary organs (pancreas, liver, and gallbladder) to digestion is only one of their many functions. All three organs have ducts that lead to the duodenum. In the duodenum, the enzymes from the pancreas meet the contents from the stomach and actively metabolize various foods. Foods such as proteins, **carbohydrates**, and fats must be converted from complex molecules to simple molecules. Proteins are large molecules that are broken down into peptides—first by pepsin in the stomach and then by trypsin and chymotrypsin (from the pancreas) in the duodenum. Carbohydrates arrive in the stomach as large sugar molecules and are converted into disaccharides; in the duodenum, they are further broken down into monosaccharides and are absorbed and used for energy. Fats begin their process of digestion in the duodenum, where they encounter bile produced by the liver and stored in the gallbladder. These long carbon chains of fat are more difficult to metabolize. They are first made water-soluble by a process called emulsification and then are broken down further by enzymes called lipases.

The appendix, attached to the cecum of the large intestine, is a small worm-shaped lymphatic structure that has no apparent function within the digestive system. If the lining of the appendix becomes inflamed, appendicitis results, which requires removal of the appendix (appendectomy).

Conditions Affecting the Gastrointestinal System

Numerous conditions can affect the gastrointestinal system. These conditions affect different sections of the gastrointestinal (GI) tract and may include any of the structures from the mouth to the anus (Table 21-2). Those conditions that

TABLE 21-2 **Conditions of the Upper/Lower GI System**

Condition	Symptoms	Cause	Treatments
Upper GI System			
Canker sores	Mouth ulcers: not contagious	Not known: may be due to certain drugs, allergies, hormonal disorder, infection, trauma, stress	½ tsp salt in 8 oz water (rinse mouth); numbing agents: Orabase, Orajel; antibiotics for infections
Cold sores	Mouth ulcers/blisters: contagious	Viral infection (herpes simplex type 1)	Antivirals, OTC agents for relief of symptoms only; Lipactin gel, Zilactin, lip balm, ibuprofen or acetaminophen for pain
Bacterial infections	Infections of mouth, throat, pancreas, liver, and gallbladder	Bacterial and viral Bacterial and fungal in mouth or throat	Antibiotics or antivirals prescribed once specific causes are identified
Stomatitis	Inflammation of mucous lining in mouth; may involve cheeks, gums, tongue, lips, and roof/ floor of mouth; painful, oral bleeding, bad breath	Infection (viral/bacterial), poor dental hygiene, cheek biting, allergic reaction, post chemotherapy treatment	Good oral hygiene; antibiotics for infection; analgesics for pain
Achalasia	Food, saliva accumulate in esophagus; chest pain, heartburn, difficulty belching	Rare disease of muscles in esophagus, making it difficult to swallow; caused by tightened esophageal sphincter (valve)	No known cure; treated with Botox injections, oral medications to relax sphincter (Isordil, verapamil), pneumatic dilation (balloon inserted), surgery to cut sphincter muscle
GERD	Dysphagia, chest/back pain	Backflow of gastric juices that enter esophagus	OTC or Rx medications (antacids, H_2-antagonists, proton pump inhibitors)
Lower GI System			
Crohn's disease	Abdominal pain, weight loss, diarrhea	Congenital or acquired chronic inflammation of colon and terminal ileum	Corticosteroids, immunosuppressants, antidiarrheals; surgery is last resort
Ulcerative colitis	Rectal bleeding, pain	Congenital or acquired chronic inflammation of large intestine	Corticosteroids, immunosuppressants, antidiarrheals; surgery is last resort
Hemorrhoids	Rectal bleeding, pain	Lesions caused by enlargement/inflammation of veins in rectum	Topical corticosteroids (hydrocortisone), topical anesthetics (Americaine)
Diverticulitis	Rectal bleeding, inflammation, bowel obstruction	Protrusions of colon wall resulting from weakened intestinal wall	Surgery, corticosteroids, antibiotics
Irritable bowel syndrome (IBS)	Diarrhea, constipation, abdominal cramping, bloating, and gas	Syndrome of large intestine; no known cause	Amitiza for pain and constipation; antispasmodics (Bentyl) for spasms

Continued

TABLE 21-2 Conditions of the Upper/Lower GI System—cont'd

Condition	Symptoms	Cause	Treatments
Gastroenteritis	Diarrhea, abdominal pain, vomiting, headache, fever, chills, loss of appetite	Inflammation of lining of intestines caused by virus, bacteria, or parasites	Hydration; in severe cases, antiemetics; analgesics for pain (non-NSAIDs); antibiotics if linked to specific microbe
Ancillary Organs			
Pancreatitis	Digestive enzymes back up and cause inflammation of pancreas	Cystic fibrosis, alcoholism, severe hypertriglyceridemia, some medications; heredity; other underlying condition	Pancreatic enzyme replacement to improve GI function; removal or treatment of underlying cause; analgesics for pain; in most serious cases, surgery to remove pancreas or open ducts to relieve blockage
Hepatitis, cirrhosis	May lead to loss of function; liver cannot produce enzymes that aid in dissolving fats and loses capacity to perform detoxification	Hepatitis (primarily caused by virus); cirrhosis (scarring); alcoholic or nonalcoholic steatosis (fatty liver); alcoholism; cancer; drug toxicity	Hepatitis B (Epivir, Hepsera); hepatitis C (ribavirin, interferon); chemotherapy for cancer; liver transplant
Cholecystitis	Diarrhea, nausea/ vomiting, severe pain	Cholecystitis caused by gallstones; inflammation or blockage of digestive enzymes	Analgesics for pain, surgery to remove gallbladder

affect digestion include commonly occurring and recurring conditions, such as heartburn, upset stomach, and gastroesophageal reflux disease (GERD). In the upper and lower bowels, constipation or diarrhea may occur in both acute and chronic forms. More severe illnesses—such as Crohn's disease, ulcers, and others—can be exacerbated by consistent stress. Other gastric conditions can be caused by bacterial infections, food allergies, and tumors. Genetic defects, such as the lack of specific chemicals that are necessary for the proper function of this system, may also be a cause of a condition or disease state. This section begins with a discussion of conditions of the mouth and then the gastrointestinal tract. Examples of drugs used to treat each specific condition will be covered.

MOUTH AND THROAT CONDITIONS

The mouth is subject to daily bacterial exposure. The lack of good oral hygiene is the most common reason for acquiring a mouth condition. Ulcers or inflammation of the gums can occur within the mouth cavity, causing pain and discomfort. In addition, the condition of the teeth plays an important role in the initial breakdown of food. The throat may become inflamed because of colds or the flu or through straining of the vocal cords. Symptoms of throat inflammation include sore throat and fever. Treatments for the mouth and throat include mouthwashes, sprays, lozenges, or troches. Many agents contain alcohol or phenol bases. These agents are antiseptics and are effective at destruction of bacteria. Benzocaines, phenols, and menthol have anesthetic effects.

Tech Note!

The abbreviated term *s/s* means "swish and swallow" or can mean "swish and spit." This is a common order for a nystatin oral suspension used for yeast infections (thrush) of the mouth or throat.

Tech Note!

Antacids may interact with many medications by preventing proper drug absorption. For example, patients taking certain antibiotics such as tetracycline and ciprofloxacin should not take antacids containing calcium, magnesium, or aluminum at the same time because the antacid can bind to and decrease the absorption of the antibiotic. Administration times of drugs should be spaced at proper intervals to help avoid interactions.

STOMACH CONDITIONS

The high acid content of stomach fluids causes a number of commonly experienced gastrointestinal conditions (Table 21-3). These conditions are known more commonly as upset stomach, indigestion, or heartburn. Antacids are the types of drugs normally used for occasional dyspepsia (upset stomach) or heartburn. They decrease the acid content of the stomach. Most remedies for relief of these occasional symptoms may be purchased OTC. Single-ingredient antacids are listed in Table 21-4. Other conditions of the stomach include GERD and peptic ulcers. Stomach disorders may require prescribed medications if OTC agents do not relieve the symptoms. The following sections cover the specifics of various stomach conditions and the medications used to treat them.

GERD

GERD can occur when the upper sphincter (opening) at the top of the stomach relaxes. This allows acidic contents from the stomach to back up into the esophagus. This causes the burning sensation that most persons feel in their chest or throat. Many OTC antacid medications contain simethicone because of the

TABLE 21-3 Gastrointestinal Conditions

GI Conditions	Cause	Symptoms	Treatments May Include
Hyperacidity or dyspepsia	Overproduction of acidic secretions or decrease of chemicals that help deactivate excessive acidic secretions between meals Small areas within stomach lining are eroded away, causing painful sore Normally caused by poor eating habits Linked to stomach ulceration, acid reflux disease, and cancer	Pain in stomach, nausea, sour belching, indigestion	Avoid trigger foods that cause upset such as those high in fat or spicy meals. Increase fiber and exercise; decrease red meat and alcohol. Stop smoking.
Gastric ulcer	Open sores in lining of stomach can be caused by *H. pylori* infection, NSAIDs, or hypersecretory diseases (e.g., Zollinger-Ellison syndrome)	Abdominal pain, nausea/vomiting, dark blood in stools	Antibiotics if cause is due to infection, antacids, H_2-blockers (e.g., famotidine, ranitidine), PPIs (e.g., rabeprazole, esomeprazole). Avoid trigger, NSAIDs.
Duodenal ulcer	Normally caused by *H. pylori* infection, peptic ulcer, NSAIDs	Abdominal pain, nausea/vomiting, dark blood in stools	Treatments are same as for gastric ulcers.
Barrett's esophagus	Long-term exposure to acid/bile that causes changes in lower esophagus, caused by GERD; increases risk for dysplasia/cancer	Heartburn, difficulty swallowing	Nonsurgical treatments include thermal therapy, balloon catheter and focal radiofrequency ablation, photodynamic therapy, liquid nitrogen and carbon dioxide cryotherapy, and endoscopic mucosal resection. Surgery is used as last resort.
Gastritis	Stomach mucosal irritation and inflammation; can be linked to stress, medications, infection, autoimmune disease, alcohol, bile reflux, *H. pylori* infection, NSAID use	Belching, nausea/vomiting, bloating/fullness in abdomen, burning sensation	Use agents that coat stomach lining (sucralfate), H_2-blockers, PPIs, antiemetics, and antibiotics if caused by infection.

TABLE 21-4 Over-the-Counter Antacid Agents (Single Ingredient)

Active Ingredient	Trade Name	Dosage Forms	Strengths
aluminum hydroxide (AlOH)	Amphojel	Tablets	600 mg
	AlternaGEL	Liquid	600 mg/5 mL
magnesium hydroxide	Milk of Magnesia	Liquid	400 mg/5 mL
	Phillips' Chewable	Chewable tablets	311 mg
	Concentrated Phillips' Milk of Magnesia	Liquid	800 mg/5 mL
sodium citrate	Citra pH	Solution	450 mg/5 mL

common occurrence of flatulence (gas) that accompanies gastric upsets. Gas also can be a side effect of carbonates, which are major ingredients in antacids.

Prognosis. With medications and a change in diet, the outlook for GERD is extremely good. Most people recover fully.

Non–Drug Treatments. A change in eating habits can help decrease the event of GERD. If medication and diet are not effective, then surgery is the final option; however, surgery is rarely needed because of the effectiveness of medical management.

Drug Treatments. In addition to antacids, histamine$_2$-antagonists (H$_2$-antagonists) are used to treat GERD and ulcers. Agents such as cimetidine and ranitidine block H$_2$-receptors located within the lining of the stomach. Proton pump inhibitors (PPIs) are a third type of agent used for the treatment of GERD. PPIs inhibit gastric acid secretion within the stomach lining by blocking the final enzymatic reaction before acid secretion. This makes proton pump inhibitors effective; thus they usually are prescribed for more severe cases of GERD. Depending on the strength of these agents will determine whether they are available OTC or require a prescription.

Antacids. Antacids include a variety of additives such as aluminum carbonate, sodium bicarbonate, calcium carbonate, magnesium hydroxide, and aluminum hydroxide. These ingredients each act in their own way to change the pH level in the stomach. Compounds containing cations (positively charged ions, such as aluminum, magnesium, calcium) act as buffers, decreasing acidity within the stomach. Table 21-5 lists examples of key products used in combination to alter pH.

Histamine$_2$-Antagonists. H$_2$-Antagonists bind to H$_2$-receptor sites, reducing acid secretion. They are well-tolerated agents, and rare side effects of histamine antagonists include drowsiness, headache, and rash. The prescription (Rx) strength typically is stronger than the OTC brand and must be filled in the pharmacy. Although most of the prescription agents have normal dosages approved by the FDA for specific medical conditions, many physicians allow patients to take an H$_2$-antagonist on an as-needed basis for occasional indigestion.

Tech Note!

Histamine$_1$-receptors are found throughout the body—in smooth muscles, vascular endothelial cells, the heart, and the central nervous system. Agents that block H$_1$-receptors, which are used to treat the effects caused by histamine (released in an allergic reaction), are called antihistamines. Histamine$_2$-receptors are found primarily in the stomach's parietal cells, and agents designed to target these receptors preferentially are called H$_2$-antagonists.

TABLE 21-5 Over-the-Counter Combination Antacids

Active Ingredients	Trade Name(s)	Dosage Forms OTC	Strengths of Active Ingredients
aluminum hydroxide and magnesium trisilicate	Gaviscon	Chewable tablets	AlOH 80 mg, magnesium trisilicate 20 mg
aluminum hydroxide and magnesium hydroxide	Alamag	Suspension	AlOH 225 mg, MgOH 200 mg
aluminum hydroxide, magnesium hydroxide, and simethicone	Gelusil	Chewable tablets	AlOH 200 mg, MgOH 200 mg, simethicone 20 mg
	Maalox Regular Strength Antacid/Mylanta	Suspension	AlOH 200 mg, MgOH 200 mg, simethicone 20 mg
	Extra-Strength Mintox Plus	Liquid	AlOH 500 mg, MgOH 450 mg, simethicone 40 mg
calcium carbonate and magnesium carbonate	Marblen	Liquid	Calcium carbonate 520 mg, magnesium carbonate 400 mg
calcium carbonate and simethicone	Maalox Max Strength	Chewable tablets	Calcium carbonate 1000 mg, simethicone 60 mg
sodium bicarbonate, acetaminophen (APAP), and citric acid	Bromo Seltzer	Effervescent granules	Sodium bicarbonate 2781 mg, APAP 325 mg, citric acid 2224 mg
sodium bicarbonate, aspirin, and citric acid	Original Alka-Seltzer	Effervescent tablets	Sodium bicarbonate 1916 mg, aspirin 325 mg, citric acid 1000 mg
sodium bicarbonate, citric acid, and potassium bicarbonate	Gold Alka-Seltzer	Effervescent tablets	Sodium bicarbonate 958 mg, citric acid 832 mg, potassium bicarbonate 312 mg

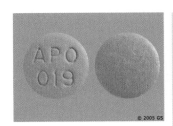

© 2005 GS

GENERIC NAME: cimetidine

TRADE NAME: Tagamet (Rx: 300, 400, 800 mg), Tagamet HB (OTC: 100, 200 mg)

INDICATION: GERD, erosive esophagitis, gastric ulcer, duodenal ulcer treatment and prophylaxis (OTC for heartburn and indigestion)

ROUTE OF ADMINISTRATION: oral, intravenous

COMMON ADULT DOSAGE: oral dosage Rx, GERD, 400 mg four times daily or 800 mg bid

AUXILIARY LABELS:

■ Take with food.
■ May cause drowsiness.

GENERIC NAME: ranitidine

TRADE NAME: Zantac (Rx: 150, 300 mg), Zantac 75, Zantac 150 (OTC: 75, 150 mg)

INDICATION: GERD, erosive esophagitis, gastric ulcer, duodenal ulcer treatment and prophylaxis (OTC for heartburn and indigestion)

ROUTE OF ADMINISTRATION: oral, intravenous

COMMON ADULT DOSAGE: oral dosage Rx, GERD, 150 mg twice daily

AUXILIARY LABELS (Rx):

■ Take with food.
■ May cause drowsiness.

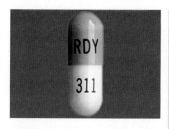

GENERIC NAME: nizatidine
TRADE NAME: Axid Pulvules (Rx: 150, 300 mg), Axid AR (OTC: 75 mg)
INDICATION: GERD, erosive esophagitis, gastric ulcer, duodenal ulcer treatment and prophylaxis (OTC for heartburn and indigestion)
ROUTE OF ADMINISTRATION: oral
COMMON ADULT DOSAGE: oral dosage Rx, GERD, 150 mg twice daily
AUXILIARY LABEL (Rx):
■ May cause dizziness and drowsiness.

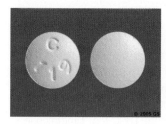

GENERIC NAME: famotidine
TRADE NAME: Pepcid (Rx: 20, 40 mg), Pepcid AC (OTC: 10, 20 mg)
INDICATION: GERD, erosive esophagitis, gastric ulcer, duodenal ulcer treatment and prophylaxis (OTC for heartburn and indigestion)
ROUTE OF ADMINISTRATION: oral, intravenous
COMMON ADULT DOSAGE: oral dosage Rx, GERD, 20 mg twice daily
AUXILIARY LABEL (Rx):
■ May cause dizziness and drowsiness.
SPECIAL NOTE: Suspension needs a "shake well" auxiliary label.

Proton Pump Inhibitors (PPIs). Proton pump inhibitors are used primarily in the treatment of GERD and peptic ulcers. Most of these agents are available as a delayed-release form or buffered (such as Zegerid) and can be taken once daily. The mechanism of action for all proton pump inhibitors is to block gastric acid secretion in the stomach. At this time, the only PPI available over-the-counter is Prilosec OTC and Prevacid 24 hour.

GENERIC NAME: omeprazole
TRADE NAME: Prilosec (Rx: 10, 20, 40 mg) (OTC: 20 mg tablets)
INDICATION: gastric ulcer, duodenal ulcer, GERD, erosive esophagitis; OTC for frequent heartburn occurring 2 or more days per week for up to 2 weeks
ROUTE OF ADMINISTRATION: oral
COMMON ADULT DOSAGE: dosage varies depending on the severity of the condition; a common dose is 20 mg once daily; OTC dosage 20 mg daily for up to 14 days
SIDE EFFECTS: diarrhea, nausea, vomiting, headache, stomach pain, gas
AUXILIARY LABELS (Rx):
■ Take before meals.
■ Do not crush or chew.
NOTE: Capsule granules may be sprinkled on 1 tablespoon of applesauce and taken immediately.

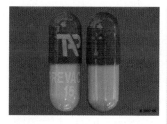

GENERIC NAME: lansoprazole
TRADE NAME: Prevacid (Rx only: 15, 30 mg; OTC: 15 mg)
INDICATION: GERD, duodenal ulcer, gastric ulcer, NSAID-induced ulcer prophylaxis, erosive esophagitis
ROUTE OF ADMINISTRATION: oral, intravenous form available
COMMON ADULT DOSAGE: dosage varies depending on the severity of the condition; common dose is 15 to 30 mg once daily
SIDE EFFECTS: diarrhea, nausea, vomiting, headache, stomach pain, gas
AUXILIARY LABELS:
■ Take before meals.
■ Do not crush or chew.
NOTE: Capsule granules may be sprinkled on 1 tablespoon of applesauce and taken immediately.

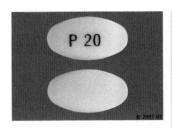

GENERIC NAME: pantoprazole
TRADE NAME: Protonix (Rx only: 20, 40 mg)
INDICATION: GERD, erosive esophagitis
ROUTE OF ADMINISTRATION: oral, intravenous form available
COMMON ADULT DOSAGE: dosage varies depending on the severity of the condition; a common dose is 40 mg once daily
SIDE EFFECTS: diarrhea, nausea, vomiting, headache, stomach pain, gas
AUXILIARY LABEL:
- Do not crush or chew.

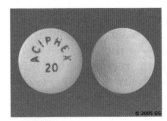

GENERIC NAME: esomeprazole magnesium
TRADE NAME: Nexium (Rx only: 10, 20, 40 mg)
INDICATION: GERD, duodenal ulcer, erosive esophagitis, and prophylaxis for NSAID-induced ulcer
ROUTE OF ADMINISTRATION: oral
COMMON ADULT DOSAGE: dosage varies depending on the severity of the condition; a common dose is 20 mg once daily
SIDE EFFECTS: diarrhea, nausea, vomiting, headache, stomach pain, gas
AUXILIARY LABELS:
- Take 1 hour before meals.
- Do not crush or chew.

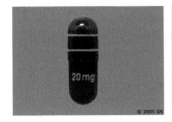

GENERIC NAME: rabeprazole sodium
TRADE NAME: AcipHex (Rx only: 10, 20 mg)
INDICATION: GERD, duodenal ulcer, erosive esophagus
ROUTE OF ADMINISTRATION: oral
COMMON ADULT DOSAGE: dosage varies depending on the severity of the condition; a common dose is 20 mg once daily
SIDE EFFECTS: diarrhea, nausea, vomiting, headache, stomach pain, gas
AUXILIARY LABEL:
- Do not crush, chew, or split tablet.

GENERIC NAME: dexlansoprazole
TRADE NAME: Dexilant (Rx only: 30, 60 mg)
INDICATION: erosive esophagitis, GERD
ROUTE OF ADMINISTRATION: oral
COMMON ADULT DOSAGE: dosage varies depending on the severity of the condition; common dosage is 60 mg once daily for initial treatment
SIDE EFFECTS: diarrhea, nausea, vomiting, headache, stomach pain, gas
AUXILIARY LABEL:
- Do not crush, chew, or split tablet.

Tech Note!

Patients often need assistance in determining how to treat upset stomach and/or heartburn. Pharmacists should be consulted because they can differentiate between common problems versus possible conditions that may be the underlying cause of the patient's symptoms. A pharmacist either can suggest the proper treatment or can refer the patient to his or her physician for an evaluation. In addition, since many OTC stomach agents can interact with prescription medications, it is important that most patients avoid self-treatment, which could cause more harm than good.

Peptic Ulcer Disease (PUD)

Peptic ulcer disease is a chronic condition that causes sores (ulcers) in the lining of the stomach and/or duodenum (small intestine); occasionally ulcers may also appear in the esophagus. The main symptom of PUD is abdominal pain; the pain is often relieved by ingesting food or taking antacids. Hyperacidity attributable to drugs (such as nonsteroidal antiinflammatory drugs [NSAIDs]) and infection with bacteria (*Helicobacter pylori*) are the leading causes of PUD, damaging the lining of the stomach, duodenum, or esophagus and causing ulcerations. The bacterium *Helicobacter pylori* is a contributor in up to 80% of all peptic ulcers and may be acquired through infected water or food and by person-to-person contact. *H. pylori* is treated with a combination of antibiotics and acid-blocking medications. Ulcers are often diagnosed either with barium-enhanced x-rays or with endoscopy.

Prognosis. With proper treatment of antibiotics and acid-reducing medications along with good hygiene, the outcome is excellent.

Non–Drug Treatment. One of the most important ways to reduce the possibility of contracting *H. pylori* is to wash your hands. This reduces the spread of the bacteria. Avoid long-term use of NSAIDs when possible; NSAIDs can cause ulcers by interfering with the protective prostaglandins in the stomach. If NSAID therapy is needed, some agents may be taken to prevent ulcers (for example, PPIs). Do not smoke. Cigarette smoking not only contributes to ulcer formation but also increases the risk of ulcer complications such as ulcer bleeding and perforation. Contrary to popular belief, foods such as alcohol, coffee, colas, and spicy foods have no proven role in ulcer formation. Similarly, there is no conclusive evidence to suggest that life stresses contribute to ulcer disease. However, many conditions can co-exist and the prescriber may recommend ingestion of a bland diet, avoidance of aggravating foods, or use of stress reduction techniques.

Drug Treatments. PUD caused by *Helicobacter pylori* will require antibiotics as a course of treatment. *H. pylori* is a gram-negative bacillus. The bacterium can embed itself into the mucosal lining of the stomach, duodenum, and rectum. *H. pylori* is the cause of gastritis and peptic ulcers and is linked to cancer of the stomach. Six laboratory tests can be performed to confirm the presence of *H. pylori* (Table 21-6). Table 21-7 lists the current treatment regimens that have been approved by the FDA for eradication of *H. pylori*. Treatments may consist of two, three, or four agents to be given simultaneously. PPIs are added to promote ulcer healing. For relief of abdominal pain a variety of antacids can be used.

INTESTINAL CONDITIONS

Two of the most common symptoms affecting the intestinal tract are diarrhea and constipation. These can be caused by various infections of the gastrointestinal system. Infections by bacteria, viruses, and parasites typically result in symptoms of diarrhea. Tumors and other obstructions can cause constipation; however, most cases of diarrhea or constipation are isolated symptoms that can be treated with OTC medications. In addition, medications are among one of the most common causes of diarrhea or constipation; therefore to alleviate potential problems, many physicians prescribe stool softeners along with routine medications that are likely to cause constipation.

Patients who require a bowel resection, such as for the removal of a tumor, may be required to wear an ileostomy or colostomy bag. Ostomy bags are

TABLE 21-6 Diagnostic Tests to Confirm *Helicobacter pylori*

Diagnostic Test	Use
Blood test	Confirms bacteria by elevated levels of antibody to *H. pylori*
Urea breath test	Carbon-labeled urea is given to patient; on exhaling, a change in urea to ammonia detects presence of bacteria
Tissue biopsy	After obtaining biopsy, four different laboratory tests can be performed to confirm *H. pylori*

TABLE 21-7 *Helicobacter pylori* Regimens

Regimen Options	Initial Treatment	Followed by	Additional Agents/Notes
1	Omeprazole 40 mg daily and clarithromycin 500 mg three times a day for 2 weeks	Omeprazole 20 mg once daily for 2 weeks	NOTE: This regimen is indicated for patients who are allergic or intolerant to amoxicillin
2	Bismuth subsalicylate 525 mg four times daily and metronidazole 250 mg four times daily and tetracycline 500 mg four times daily for 2 weeks		H$_2$-Receptor antagonist therapy as directed for a total of 4 weeks. Started at beginning of treatment
3	Lansoprazole 30 mg two times daily and amoxicillin 1 g two times daily and clarithromycin 500 mg three times daily for 10 days		
4	Lansoprazole 30 mg three times daily and amoxicillin 1 g three times daily for 2 weeks		NOTE: This regimen is indicated for patients who are allergic or intolerant to clarithromycin or for resistance to clarithromycin
5	Omeprazole 20 mg two times daily and clarithromycin 500 mg two times daily and amoxicillin 1 g two times daily for 10 days		NOTE: A common alternative regimen is metronidazole (50 mg) with clarithromycin (500 mg) both given twice daily, with a PPI such as omeprazole 20 mg bid or lansoprazole 30 mg bid.

attached to the abdominal wall with adhesive strips; wearing an ostomy bag allows the patient to empty the intestinal contents into the bag through the stoma (ostomy opening). The site of the ostomy varies depending on the location of the resection. Because the intestinal tract is responsible for most nutrient absorption, if the ostomy site is close to the stomach, fewer nutrients can be absorbed through the intestine and must be provided to the patient. Other than having to empty the ostomy bag a few times during the day and changing the tubing twice weekly, a person can live a normal life with an ostomy. The following list provides brief descriptions of the types of ostomies:

- Colostomy: Surgical creation of an opening (stoma) in the abdominal wall to allow feces to pass from the bowel through the opening, rather than through the anus. A colostomy may be temporary or permanent (e.g., cancer of colon or rectum).
- Ileostomy: A surgical opening made in the ileum onto the abdominal wall to allow for the passage of feces. Performed in cases of cancer of the colon, severe or recurrent Crohn's disease, or ulcerative colitis.

Another common condition is excess gas in the intestines that can cause pain and distention of the stomach or intestines, which can be uncomfortable as well as embarrassing. When this is expelled, it is referred to as flatulence (passing gas from the anus). The source of this gas is from intestinal bacteria that normally coat our intestines. As the bacteria digest the foods we eat (sugars, starch, cellulose), they produce hydrogen and/or methane as a by-product. OTC agents are available to treat this condition.

Diarrhea

An abnormal increase in the frequency, fluidity, or volume of bowel movements (more than three soft, loose, or watery bowel movements per day) is considered diarrhea. Abdominal cramping, gas, and general discomfort may accompany diarrhea. Diarrhea is not a condition but is a symptom of another underlying disorder. There are two types of diarrhea: acute and chronic. Acute is short-term (often caused by viral and bacterial infections), whereas chronic symptoms continue several weeks. Other causes include disorders of the colon (colitis), gastrointestinal tumors, or a metabolic disorder. Although treatment depends on the cause, the symptoms of diarrhea can be treated with antidiarrheal agents.

As diarrhea continues, vital fluids and electrolytes are lost through the intestines. Death can occur if fluids and electrolytes are not replaced and the diarrhea is not managed. Persons who are most susceptible to this danger are older adults and young children. There are several types of bowel problems one may experience (Box 21-1). Many conditions have symptoms including diarrhea; therefore if symptoms are not controlled (using OTC agents) within a few days, diagnosis may be necessary in order for proper treatment. However, children younger than 3 years, patients who have a fever, and anyone with diarrhea for more than 2 days should be evaluated by a physician. Treatment for diarrhea often consists of agents that have an absorbent and/or protectant quality.

Prognosis. In many cases diarrhea is short-lived and resolves without treatment. Other patients will need treatment with medication, and in rare cases surgery may need to be performed. With proper eating/drinking habits and treatment, this condition does not interfere with most people's daily activities.

Non–Drug Treatments. Resting and drinking clear fluids (for example, oral rehydrating solutions such as Pedialyte) until the diarrhea subsides are commonly suggested by physicians to avoid dehydration and electrolyte loss.

Drug Treatments. Several agents, OTC and prescription, can treat this condition. OTC drugs include medications such as Kaopectate, FiberCon, and Pepto-Bismol. More potent drugs or controlled substances require a prescription. Agents such as Lomotil (diphenoxylate/atropine) or paregoric are meant for short-term use because they can become less effective with continued use.

BOX 21-1 BOWEL PROBLEMS

Constant bowel movements: Having a BM immediately after eating a meal
Incomplete evacuation: Feeling of another BM soon after the first; having a BM is difficult
Rectal urgency: Sudden urge to have a BM; toilet must be close by
Fecal incontinence: Inability to control BMs

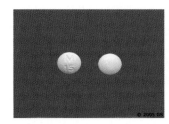

GENERIC NAME: diphenoxylate/atropine, schedule C-V
TRADE NAME: Lomotil
ROUTE OF ADMINISTRATION: oral
INDICATION: acute or chronic noninfectious diarrhea
DRUG ACTION: slows intestinal motility; reduces spasms in stomach, intestines, bladder
COMMON ADULT DOSAGE: 2.5 to 5 mg four times daily, then 2-3 times per day prn; maximum 20 mg/day
SIDE EFFECTS: dry mouth, dizziness, drowsiness
AUXILIARY LABELS:
■ May cause dizziness and drowsiness.
■ Do not drink alcohol.
■ Drink plenty of water.

GENERIC NAME: loperamide
TRADE NAME: Imodium (Rx), Imodium AD (OTC)
ROUTE OF ADMINISTRATION: oral
INDICATION: acute or chronic noninfectious diarrhea
DRUG ACTION: slows gastrointestinal motility and increases viscosity of fecal matter
COMMON ADULT DOSAGE: 2 mg following each loose stool (maximum 16 mg/day × 2 days)
SIDE EFFECTS: dizziness, drowsiness, dry mouth

GENERIC NAME: bismuth subsalicylate
TRADE NAME: Pepto-Bismol (OTC)
ROUTE OF ADMINISTRATION: oral
INDICATION: heartburn, indigestion, stomach upset, nausea, diarrhea
DRUG ACTION: antisecretory and antibacterial effects in gastrointestinal tract
COMMON ADULT DOSAGE: 2 tablets or 30 mL (liquid) prn, not to exceed 8 doses in 24 hours
SIDE EFFECTS: stools may appear grayish black
AUXILIARY LABEL:
■ None for OTC items; advise patient to shake suspension well before each use.
NOTE: Remember this is a salicylate and should not be used in those with aspirin allergy.
NOTE: Children's Pepto contains calcium carbonate, an antacid; it is not used for diarrhea, Children <12 years should not take bismuth subsalicylate products.

Constipation

Constipation is a condition in which the feces are hard and dry. Bowel movements are infrequent or irregular. Many people have a bowel movement once a day to several times daily, while others may normally have as few as three bowel movements a week. The ease of the bowel movement is more important than the frequency when defining constipation. Most people can treat temporary constipation themselves through diet changes or OTC agents; however, if other symptoms are present (weight loss, abdominal pain, or rectal bleeding), a more serious condition may be the cause. Certain medications can cause constipation such as narcotic pain medications (e.g., codeine, oxycodone), antidepressants (e.g., amitriptyline, imipramine), anticonvulsants (e.g., phenytoin, carbamazepine), calcium channel blockers (e.g., diltiazem, nifedipine, verapamil), and aluminum-containing antacids (such as Amphojel or Basaljel).

Prognosis. Constipation can be managed in most cases by either dietary modifications or medications. Lifestyle need not be altered. When constipation is a symptom of a more serious disease, such as a tumor, surgery or chemotherapy may be necessary to treat the underlying bowel condition.

Non–Drug Treatments. Non–drug treatments suggested to avoid constipation include the ingestion of adequate dietary fibers, found in fruits and vegetables, in the daily diet. Roughage also aids in good digestion and elimination. In addition to a well-balanced meal plan, drinking plenty of water also helps prevent constipation. For the prevention of constipation, the following guidelines are usually recommended:

- Increase fluids: Drink at least 8 to 10 glasses of water daily because fluids help keep the intestinal contents in a semisolid state, making it easier to pass stools. Stimulate bowel movements by drinking hot coffee, warm lemonade, iced liquids, or prune juice before breakfast or in the evening.
- Add fiber: Increased dietary intake of fiber (such as from whole-grain cereals) contributes to intestinal bulk and induces peristalsis (movements). Because too much fiber irritates the intestines, fiber content should be monitored. In addition, fresh fruits (with skins) as well as raw and unrefined vegetables should be added to the diet for additional bulk.
- Exercise: Including moderate exercise (such as walking) into the daily routine can help as well.

What to avoid:

- Fats should be limited. Although they can help soften intestinal contents, they can cause diarrhea.
- Laxatives and enemas should be limited. Frequent use of sodium biphosphate should be avoided because it is hypertonic and can absorb as much as 10% of the colon's sodium content or draw intestinal fluids into the colon, causing dehydration.

Drug Treatments. Stool softeners pull water and fatty compounds into the intestine to aid in elimination. Hyperosmotic agents work by osmosis, increasing pressure within the bowels by absorbing water, similar to bulk-forming agents. For stubborn bouts of constipation, a stimulant may be used. These agents increase the peristalsis within the intestines (specifically the colon), which forces the contents to be expelled. Abdominal cramping is also a common occurrence from using laxatives that are more powerful. Persons who constantly take stimulant laxatives eventually may become dependent on them; therefore it is recommended that laxatives be used only as a short-term treatment (not more than 1 week) before seeking medical attention. Other evacuants consist of enemas to attain the same results. Table 21-8 lists examples of laxatives available. Dosage forms include oral and rectal agents.

NOTE: Bowel evacuants are also used to empty the intestines before a procedure or surgery. The solutions contain polyethylene glycol and replacement electrolytes because the intestines are not able to absorb the necessary ions from the expelled fecal material. Typically, the patient must drink approximately 2 to 4 liters (2000 to 4000 mL) of solution within a relatively short time. Staying at home is recommended after administration of bowel evacuants because of the rapid onset of action and the need for frequent elimination.

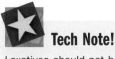

Tech Note!

Laxatives should not be used in children younger than 6 years unless instructed to do so by a pediatrician.

Bulk-Forming Laxatives. Bulk-forming agents (e.g., psyllium) function by absorbing water from the body to increase the moisture and overall bulk of the stools, allowing for easier elimination. A positive aspect of these agents is that they can be taken over long periods and can be used for both constipation and diarrhea. Examples of bulk-forming agents include FiberCon (polycarbophil) and Citrucel (methylcellulose).

TABLE 21-8 Laxatives

Anticonstipation Agents	Ingredients	Normal Adult Dosage	Route of Administration
Over-the-Counter Laxative			
Phillips' Milk of Magnesia	magnesium hydroxide	30-60 mL prn	PO (orally)
Fleet Sodium Phosphates	sodium phosphate, sodium biphosphate	20-30 mL prn	PO
Stimulants			
Ex-Lax	senna	1 tablet at bedtime	PO
MiraLAX	polyethylene glycol	17 g/day	PO
Bulk-Producing Laxatives			
FiberCon	500 mg calcium polycarbophil	2 caplets once to twice daily (max 4 g/day)	PO
Rectal			
Fleet Laxative	bisacodyl	1 suppository once daily	PR (per rectum)
Fleet Mineral Oil	mineral oil	1 enema once daily	PR
Prescription Osmotic Laxative			
Cephulac	lactulose	15-30 mL once daily	PO
Bowel Evacuant (OTC)			
HalfLytely, GoLYTELY	polyethylene glycol, sodium sulfate, sodium bicarbonate, sodium chloride, potassium chloride	2-4 L	PO
Magnesium Citrate	magnesium citrate	240 mL once daily	PO

GENERIC NAME: psyllium (OTC)
TRADE NAME: Metamucil
INDICATION: constipation
ROUTE OF ADMINISTRATION: oral
DRUG ACTION: holds water within the intestine, allowing stools to pass
COMMON ADULT DOSAGE: 1 tablespoonful daily in 8 ounces of water or juice
SIDE EFFECTS: bloating, gas, cramping
NOTE: Should be taken with at least 8 oz of fluid to avoid choking. Psyllium also is used to reduce cholesterol levels in persons with hyperlipidemia.

Emollient Laxatives (Stool Softeners). Docusate improves the ability of water within the colon to penetrate and mix with stool. The increased water content softens the stool. Often stool softeners are used as a preventive measure rather than to treat constipation. These agents work gently and are very effective.

GENERIC NAME: docusate sodium (DSS) or docusate calcium (OTC)
TRADE NAME: Colace, Kaopectate Stool Softener (formerly Surfak)
INDICATION: constipation
ROUTE OF ADMINISTRATION: oral, rectal (enema)
DRUG ACTION: retains fat and water in bowels, allowing stools to pass
COMMON ADULT DOSAGE: orally, 50 to 240 mg once daily
SIDE EFFECTS: well tolerated; if stools become too soft, may reduce dosage; liquid forms must be diluted before administration to reduce risk of throat irritation

Stimulant Laxatives. Stimulant laxatives cause the muscles of the small intestine and colon to propel their contents rapidly. They also increase the content of water in the stool, either by reducing the absorption of water in the colon or by causing additional secretion of water in the small intestines. Examples of stimulants include senna compounds and castor oil.

> **GENERIC NAME:** bisacodyl (OTC)
> **TRADE NAME:** Dulcolax
> **INDICATION:** constipation
> **ROUTE OF ADMINISTRATION:** oral, rectal (suppository or enema)
> **DRUG ACTION:** acts by increasing absorption of water by intestine's mucosal lining, softening stool
> **COMMON ADULT DOSAGE:** 10 mg orally or rectally once daily as needed
> **SIDE EFFECTS:** may cause crampy abdominal pain, dizziness, nausea; rectal use may cause perianal irritation

> **GENERIC NAME:** senna (OTC)
> **TRADE NAME:** Senokot
> **INDICATION:** constipation (also used for constipation from opioid agents)
> **ROUTE OF ADMINISTRATION:** oral
> **DRUG ACTION:** irritates intestinal wall and causes osmotic gradient, softening stools
> **COMMON ADULT DOSAGE:** 30 mg once to twice daily
> **SIDE EFFECTS:** GI irritation, nausea, abdominal cramping

Hyperosmolar Laxatives. These agents are indigestible, unabsorbable compounds that remain within the colon and retain water that is already in the colon. The result is softening of the stool. Examples include Colace Glycerin (glycerin), MiraLAX (polyethylene glycol), and Kristalose (lactulose).

> **GENERIC NAME:** glycerin (OTC)
> **TRADE NAME:** Colace Glycerin, Fleet Babylax
> **INDICATION:** constipation
> **ROUTE OF ADMINISTRATION:** rectal
> **DRUG ACTION:** irritates intestinal wall and causes osmotic gradient, softening stools; rectal lubricant
> **COMMON ADULT DOSAGE:** one suppository rectally once daily as needed
> **SIDE EFFECTS:** fecal urgency because of fast onset of action, perianal irritation
> **AUXILIARY LABEL:**
> ■ For rectal use only.

Selective Chloride Channel Activators. These agents increase the secretion of chloride ions from the cells of the intestinal lining into the lumen. Water follows the sodium ions to the lumen and the water softens the stool, making it easier to expel.

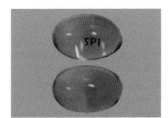

> **GENERIC NAME:** lubiprostone (Rx)
> **TRADE NAME:** Amitiza
> **INDICATION:** chronic idiopathic constipation, irritable bowel syndrome
> **ROUTE OF ADMINISTRATION:** oral
> **COMMON ADULT DOSAGE:** chronic idiopathic constipation dosage: 24 mcg two times daily; irritable bowel syndrome: 8 mcg two times daily
> **SIDE EFFECTS:** stomach pain, nausea, bloating, gas
> **AUXILIARY LABEL:**
> ■ Take with food and water.

Flatulence

Flatulence is normally caused by the by-products (nitrogen, carbon dioxide, methane) of the microbial breakdown of certain food(s) (see Chapter 30); flatulence is also known as passing gas, or flatus. This gas originates in the intestines and the anus expels it. Sugars (lactose, sorbitol, fructose) and starches (rice, wheat, certain vegetables) may pose a problem because they may be difficult to digest. Persons who are lactose-intolerant lack the enzyme lactase; this enzyme is located in the lining of the intestines, and without it the person cannot metabolize the carbohydrate lactose; this results in poor digestion of milk products.

Another cause of flatulence may result from poor absorption of foods in the small intestine, allowing more undigested food to reach the bacteria in the colon. Sometimes the bacteria are present in the small intestine, where the food has not had a chance to be digested, and bacteria will begin producing gas; this is called bacterial overgrowth of the small intestine. Although excessive gas is normally accompanied by flatulence, it may not be evident; there are other ways gas can escape. Gas may be eliminated by absorption into the body or used by other bacteria, or eliminated at night while the person is sleeping. Other causes of gas include overeating and pancreatic insufficiency. Symptoms are discomfort (bloating feeling) and pain within the abdominal cavity.

Prognosis. With proper treatment, flatulence can be greatly reduced. However, the patient should be educated that flatulence is a normal digestive process that everyone experiences, although levels of gas production may vary.

Non–Drug Treatment. For those suffering from lactose intolerance, using soy products is an option. Alternatively, persons who are lactose-intolerant can ingest replacement enzymes (lactase supplements) similar to those found in the lining of the intestines. Eliminating trigger foods that cause gas, such as cabbage or onions, can lessen symptoms. For pancreatic insufficiency, specific enzyme replacements can be taken with meals. Beano, an OTC product, contains an enzyme (alpha-D-galactosidase) that helps to break down sugars in vegetables so they can be absorbed, thus eliminating gas in the intestines.

Drug Treatment. OTC medications used for the treatment of gas contain simethicone as the primary ingredient. This medication is available in tablets, chewable tablets, and liquid for children (Table 21-9).

Antiflatulence Medications. These agents relieve pain attributable to excess gas by allowing the gas bubbles to combine for easier passage of gas. These agents are often used on babies, children and adults.

TABLE 21-9 Over-the-Counter Combination Antacid-Antiflatulence Agents

Trade Name	Generic Name	Common Dosage
Maalox Extra-Strength Tablets	aluminum hydroxide, magnesium hydroxide, simethicone	Usually taken after meals or as needed
Tempo Tablets	aluminum hydroxide, magnesium hydroxide, calcium carbonate, simethicone	Usually taken after meals or as needed
Mylanta Liquid	aluminum hydroxide, magnesium hydroxide, simethicone	Usually taken after meals or as needed

> **GENERIC NAME:** simethicone
> **TRADE NAME:** Gas-X, Mylicon, Phazyme
> **INDICATION:** for the relief of gas and abdominal distention caused by gas
> **DRUG ACTION:** decreases the surface tension of gas bubbles, preventing gas pockets
> **ROUTE OF ADMINISTRATION** oral
> **COMMON ADULT DOSAGE** 40 to 80 mg up to four times daily after meals and at bedtime as needed
> **SIDE EFFECTS:** none

Irritable Bowel Syndrome (IBS)

Irritable bowel syndrome is a common condition that is marked by chronic or periodic diarrhea alternating with constipation. This disorder is generally associated with psychological stress; however, it can result from physical factors such as changing hormonal levels during the menstrual cycle, ingesting irritants (coffee, raw fruits/vegetables), or being lactose-intolerant.

Prognosis. Although there is no cure for IBS, the prognosis is good with supportive treatment or avoidance of a known irritant.

Non–Drug Treatment. Avoiding specific irritants is one of the leading non–drug treatments; irritants can include foods or stress factors. A warm compress applied to the abdomen along with rest is usually suggested for relief. A high-fiber diet can help to control constipation. Foods that may cause symptoms of IBS include gas-producing foods, sugarless chewing gum and candy, coffee, and alcohol. Stress management techniques along with regular exercise (to reduce tension) can help in many cases.

Drug Treatment. Often antispasmodics (dicyclomine) are prescribed to manage IBS; however, if this agent is used over a long period of time the patient may become dependent on it. Other agents used to treat various symptoms of IBS include antidiarrheals (e.g., Lomotil, Imodium), which slow intestinal movements; bile acid sequestrants (e.g., cholestyramine), which prevent bile acids from stimulating the colon and thereby relieve diarrhea; and alosetron (Lotronex) for those patients with diarrhea-type IBS who have not responded to other treatments. Antidepressants or antianxiety agents may also be prescribed to treat symptoms of depression or anxiety that often accompany this condition. Patients with constipation-type IBS may respond to lubiprostone (Amitiza).

Antispasmodics. Antispasmodics relieve or prevent spasms of the muscles in the stomach through anticholinergic effects and direct action on the gastrointestinal smooth muscles.

> **GENERIC NAME:** dicyclomine
> **TRADE NAME:** Bentyl
> **INDICATION:** irritable bowel syndrome
> **ROUTE OF ADMINISTRATION:** oral
> **COMMON ADULT DOSAGE:** 20 mg four times daily
> **SIDE EFFECTS:** drowsiness, dizziness, headache, blurred vision, nausea, vomiting, constipation, bloating, stomach pain
> **AUXILIARY LABEL:**
> ■ Take with a full glass of water.

Serotonin. Serotonin inhibits serotonin receptors in the gastrointestinal tract, reducing cramping, pain, and discomfort within the stomach and the diarrhea caused by IBS.

GENERIC NAME: alosetron
TRADE NAME: Lotronex
INDICATION: irritable bowel syndrome, diarrhea prominent
ROUTE OF ADMINISTRATION: oral
COMMON ADULT DOSAGE: 0.5 mg twice daily
SIDE EFFECTS: mild stomach discomfort, nausea, bloating, or gas
AUXILIARY LABEL:

■ Take with a full glass of water.

NOTE: This agent is to be used in women suffering from IBS who have had diarrhea for at least 6 months. It has not shown to be effective in men with IBS.

NOTE: Infrequent but serious adverse effects have occurred with the use of Lotronex, including ischemic colitis and severe constipation that may result in hospitalization and, in rare cases, blood transfusion, surgery, and death.

NOTE: Patient must read and sign a patient-physician agreement form before getting a prescription.

Crohn's Disease

Crohn's disease is a chronic inflammatory disease of the intestines that can cause ulcerations in the small and large intestinal lining; however, it can affect the digestive tract anywhere from the mouth to the anus. Crohn's disease is closely related to ulcerative colitis and together they constitute inflammatory bowel disease (IBD). In Crohn's disease, there is a blockage in the intestinal wall that leads to edema and eventually inflammation, ulceration, and stenosis (narrowing). Over time this narrowing and stiffness of the intestine stops all bowel movements. In addition, ulcers may puncture holes in the wall of the bowel and bacteria from within the bowel can spill into the abdominal cavity, causing infection. Although the exact cause of Crohn's disease is unknown, both autoimmune and genetic factors are thought to play a role. Symptoms include cramping, tenderness, flatulence, nausea, fever, and diarrhea. Symptoms may mimic appendicitis with a steady, colicky pain of the right lower quadrant.

Prognosis. The prognosis depends on the severity of the condition. With proper lifestyle changes and medication to control Crohn's disease, the outcome can be good.

Non–Drug Treatment. Effective treatment requires lifestyle changes, which include physical rest and a restricted diet. Trigger foods must be identified and avoided. In debilitated patients, parenteral nutrition may be necessary to maintain nutritional status while resting the bowels. Vitamin B$_{12}$ injections along with the administration of various supplements as well as the elimination of dairy products may be prescribed. Surgery (colectomy with ileostomy) may be necessary to correct bowel perforation, massive hemorrhage, fistulas, or acute intestinal obstruction.

Drug Treatment. To control inflammation, agents such as 5-aminosalicylates (5-ASA); Azulfidine (sulfasalazine) or Asacol (mesalamine) are normally prescribed first. Corticosteroids (prednisone) and immunomodulators such as Imuran (azathioprine) or Prograf (tacrolimus) may be prescribed if 5-ASA drugs are not effective or if the condition is severe. Biological agents such as Remicade (infliximab) or Humira (adalimumab) may also be prescribed. If infection occurs because of the overgrowth of bacteria in the small intestine, antibiotics such as ampicillin, sulfonamide, tetracycline, metronidazole, or cephalosporins may be prescribed. Antidiarrheals are used to control diarrhea, and fluid/electrolyte replacement is necessary to counteract dehydration.

Biological Agents. Biological agents are proteins that recognize, attach to, and block a substance called tumor necrosis factor (TNF). TNF is a cytokine and is made by macrophages in the body. Although TNF plays an important role in fighting off tumor cells it is linked to the inflammatory response mechanism; agents such as infliximab lower the levels of TNF, thus reducing inflammation caused by Crohn's disease.

GENERIC NAME: infliximab
TRADE NAME: Remicade
INDICATION: Crohn's disease, ulcerative colitis
ROUTE OF ADMINISTRATION: IV infusion
COMMON ADULT DOSAGE: 5 mg/kg infused IV and then 2 and 6 weeks later; followed by maintenance regimen of 5 mg/kg every 8 weeks thereafter
SIDE EFFECTS: headache, mild stomach pain, back pain, runny or stuffy nose, tiredness
AUXILIARY LABELS:
- For infusion only.
- Keep vials refrigerated before use.

NOTE: Usually administered by physician or nurse in a medical setting.
NOTE: Each prescription of Remicade comes with an extra patient information sheet called a Medication Guide.
NOTE: Serious, life-threatening infections leading to hospitalization have occurred; in rare cases, death may occur.

Ulcerative Colitis

Ulcerative colitis is a disease that causes inflammation and sores in the lining of the large intestine or colon. Ulcerative colitis only affects the colon and rectum while Crohn's disease can affect the entire gastrointestinal system. Although ulcerative colitis can affect any person of any age, it is most likely to occur in those 30 years of age and younger. There is no definitive cause for ulcerative colitis although it is believed to be an immune condition in which the immune system is overreacting to normal bacteria in the digestive tract; it is also possible that other types of bacteria or viruses may cause this disease. Symptoms include stomach pain, cramps, bloody diarrhea, or bleeding from the rectum. Some people may experience fever, loss of appetite, and weight loss. In severe cases, people may have diarrhea up to 20 times daily.

Prognosis. Because there is no cure for ulcerative colitis, living with the symptoms can be quite difficult. There are many lifestyle changes that must be made, including adjusting dietary intake, employing stress reduction techniques, and being part of a strong support system. In severe cases, surgery may be necessary although it should not limit normal activities.

Non–Drug Treatment. Eating a healthy diet and participating in therapeutic counseling may help the patient cope with the difficulties of this condition.

Drug Treatment. Depending on the severity of the symptoms, various agents can be prescribed. For mild symptoms antidiarrheals, corticosteroids, or 5-ASA may be used for a short time. For moderate to severe symptoms both corticosteroids and aminosalicylates may need to be prescribed for a time. Many of the medications used for ulcerative colitis are the same as those used for Crohn's disease.

Antiinflammatory. Mesalamine's method of action is not entirely known; however, it is believed to reduce the levels of prostaglandins, which are responsible for inflammation of the colon.

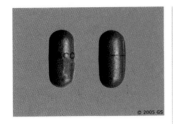

GENERIC NAME: mesalamine
TRADE NAME: Asacol
INDICATION: mild to moderate ulcerative colitis, Crohn's disease
ROUTE OF ADMINISTRATION: oral, rectal
COMMON ADULT DOSAGE: ulcerative colitis: oral tablet (Asacol): 2 tablets three times a day for 6 weeks; rectal suppository (Asacol): 1 suppository two times daily; rectal enema (mesalamine): 60 mL (rectal instillation) once a day
SIDE EFFECTS: diarrhea, dizziness, flulike symptoms, gas, headache, nausea, stomach pain
AUXILIARY LABELS:

■ May cause dizziness; take with a full glass of water.
■ Suspension enema: Shake well before using. For rectal use only.
■ Suppository: For rectal use only.

Emesis

Emesis is another term for vomiting. This violent reaction of the body is controlled by the medulla oblongata located within the brain. Known as the chemoreceptor trigger zone (CTZ) or nausea zone, this small area of the brainstem can be activated by smell, pain, medication, motion sickness (originating in the inner ear), and even emotions. When the chemoreceptor trigger zone is activated, chemical signals are sent via the nervous system to the vomit center, which then relays the message to the stomach, where muscles of the diaphragm, stomach, esophagus, and salivary glands work together to cause the vomiting reflex.

Although most persons have experienced nausea and vomiting, it is usually an isolated event. Other causes of emesis include food/drug poisoning, overconsumption of alcohol, or a postsurgical reaction to anesthesia. Persons who are subjected to certain chemotherapeutic agents as a part of cancer treatment must deal with extreme nausea and vomiting. The chemotherapy agents activate the chemoreceptor trigger zone, causing emesis as a common side effect. Variations of emesis are listed in Box 21-2.

Prognosis. If left untreated, severe dehydration and a decrease in electrolyte levels (potassium, sodium) as well as alkalosis may occur, requiring a longer recovery period. Treating the underlying cause or condition normally will alleviate emesis.

Non–Drug Treatments. Depending on the reason for vomiting, certain non–drug treatments can be extremely effective. Do not overeat or eat too quickly. To prevent transfer of infectious causes of vomiting, avoid undercooked foods and wash hands before eating. If nausea occurs, eating a soda cracker or toast can sometimes help. One of the most important considerations is that dehydration

BOX 21-2 **VARIATIONS OF EMESIS**

Projectile vomiting: Sudden/forceful vomiting
Retching: Making an effort to vomit; some are unproductive (dry heaves)
Delayed vomiting: May occur days after chemotherapy treatment
Anticipatory vomiting: Vomiting caused by anticipation of unpleasantness; often occurs with patients who have previously received medications, like chemotherapy, that caused vomiting
Cyclical vomiting: Occurs on a cycle, often associated with migraine headaches

can occur with continued vomiting; replacing the lost liquids and electrolytes is a vital aspect of treatment.

Drug Treatments. Drugs used to treat this condition are referred to as antiemetics. Most antiemetics require a prescription because of their side effects and possible misuse. Agents that do not affect the chemoreceptor trigger zone can be purchased OTC and usually are used for motion sickness. Depending on the underlying cause(s) of emesis, it may be treated with or without medications. Medications include anticholinergics, antidopaminergics, H₁-antihistamines, cannabinoids (dronabinol), corticosteroids (dexamethasone, methylprednisolone), and benzodiazepines (lorazepam). Agents such as corticosteroids, serotonin antagonists, and benzodiazepines are often used before emetic chemotherapies to prevent emesis.

Antidopaminergics. These have an antimuscarinic effect, lessening vomiting. Muscarinic pertains to the effects of the neurotransmitters acetylcholine (ACh) and dopamine on the nerves of the parasympathetic nervous system. Agents that have an antimuscarinic effect bind to muscarinic receptors, blocking the binding of ACh and dopamine. Metoclopramide passes the blood-brain barrier and reduces the effects of dopamine on the chemoreceptor trigger zone. Its prokinetic effect also improves GI motility and the emptying of stomach contents.

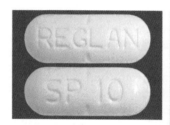

GENERIC NAME: metoclopramide
TRADE NAME: Reglan
INDICATION: for the relief of nausea and vomiting, also used for gastroparesis
ROUTE OF ADMINISTRATION: oral, intravenous
COMMON ADULT DOSAGE: nonchemotherapeutic dose: 5-10 mg before meals and at bedtime as needed; chemotherapeutic adult dosage: 10 mg in 50 mL of normal saline over 30 minutes; given once before chemotherapy treatment, may repeat every 2 hours × 2 doses or every 3 hours for 3 doses
SIDE EFFECTS: diarrhea, drowsiness, restlessness
AUXILIARY LABELS:

- May cause dizziness and drowsiness.
- Alcohol may intensify this effect.

Phenothiazines. These agents block dopamine receptors in the brain, decreasing the effects of specific neurotransmitters on the chemoreceptor trigger zone, which is responsible for nausea.

GENERIC NAME: prochlorperazine
TRADE NAME: Compro, Compazine
INDICATION: for the relief of nausea and vomiting
ROUTE OF ADMINISTRATION: oral, intravenous
COMMON ADULT DOSAGE: oral: 5 mg three to four times daily as needed; injection: 5 to 10 mg intramuscularly every 3 or 4 hours (not to exceed 40 mg per day) (may also be given IV)
SIDE EFFECTS: dizziness, drowsiness, dry mouth, rash, fever, headache
AUXILIARY LABELS:

- May cause dizziness and drowsiness.
- Alcohol may intensify this effect.
- Drink plenty of water.

Miscellaneous Antiemetics. The mechanism of action of miscellaneous antimetics is not entirely known but is believed to be associated with the CTZ.

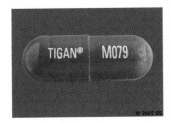

GENERIC NAME: trimethobenzamide
TRADE NAME: Tigan
INDICATION: for the relief of nausea and vomiting
ROUTE OF ADMINISTRATION: oral, intramuscular
COMMON ADULT DOSAGE: oral: 300 mg PO three to four times daily
SIDE EFFECTS: dizziness, drowsiness, diarrhea, headache, blurred vision
AUXILIARY LABELS:

■ May cause dizziness and drowsiness.
■ Alcohol may intensify this effect.
■ Drink plenty of water.

Serotonin Receptor Antagonists (5-HT$_3$-Antagonists). The mechanism of action of these agents is not fully understood. It is known that they block a specific receptor (5-HT$_3$) that is present in the chemoreceptor trigger zone as well as other areas. Examples of these types of agents include the following:

- granisetron (Granisol, Kytril, Sancuso)
- dolasetron (Anzemet)
- alosetron (Lotronex)
- palonosetron (Aloxi)

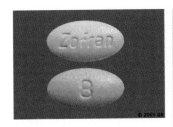

GENERIC NAME: ondansetron
TRADE NAME: Zofran
INDICATION: for the relief of nausea and vomiting; used with chemotherapy
ROUTE OF ADMINISTRATION: oral, injectable
DRUG ACTION: affects chemoreceptor trigger zone directly by blocking serotonin in brainstem and gastrointestinal tract
COMMON ADULT DOSAGE: Oral: 8 mg 30 minutes before chemotherapy treatment; then 8 mg 8 hours after dose followed by 8 mg every 12 hours for several days
SIDE EFFECTS: fever, headache, constipation, diarrhea
AUXILIARY LABELS:

■ Take as directed.
■ Do not drink alcohol.

Antihistamines/Anticholinergics. Used for motion sickness and allergies, these drugs have an anticholinergic effect that decreases vomiting. They inhibit the action of acetylcholine at muscarinic receptors (see Antidopaminergics).

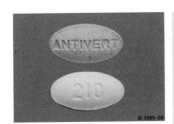

GENERIC NAME: meclizine
TRADE NAME: Antivert (Rx: 12.5, 25, 50 mg), Bonine (OTC: 25 mg)
INDICATION: to relieve nausea and vomiting resulting from motion sickness
ROUTE OF ADMINISTRATION: oral
COMMON ADULT DOSAGE: oral: 12.5 to 25 mg 1 hour before exposure to stimulus
SIDE EFFECTS: dizziness, drowsiness, dry mouth
SPECIAL NOTE: Meclizine is also available in 25- and 50-mg tablets but requires a prescription.

GENERIC NAME: dimenhydrinate
TRADE NAME: Dramamine (OTC: 50 mg)
INDICATION: to relieve nausea and vomiting resulting from motion sickness
ROUTE OF ADMINISTRATION: oral, intramuscular, intravenous
COMMON ADULT DOSAGE: oral: 50 to 100 mg every 4-6 hours
SIDE EFFECTS: dizziness, drowsiness, dry mouth

GENERIC NAME: scopolamine
TRADE NAME: Transderm Scōp (transdermal form)
INDICATION: for the relief of nausea and vomiting associated with motion sickness or following recovery from anesthesia
ROUTE OF ADMINISTRATION: transdermal skin patch
COMMON ADULT DOSAGE: apply one patch behind ear 4 hours before event; change patch every 3 days, alternating side of application
SIDE EFFECTS: dizziness, drowsiness, headache
AUXILIARY LABELS:

- May cause dizziness and drowsiness.
- Alcohol may intensify this effect.

MISCELLANEOUS CONDITIONS

Poisoning

A poison includes anything that can injure or kill via its chemical actions. Although most substances are ingested orally, there are several ways poisoning or overdose can occur. These include inhalation, absorption through the skin, biting or stinging from a venomous animal, IV injection, and exposure to radiation.

The type of chemical ingested determines the corresponding treatment. Symptoms of poisoning may include excessive salivation, nausea/vomiting (N/V), trouble breathing, seizures, or confusion. If poisoning should occur, the proper steps should be taken quickly. Options include calling the poison prevention line or Emergency Medical Services (911). The poison prevention call center is staffed with pharmacists and nurses who can help you determine how to proceed. If you must take a person who has been poisoned to the hospital, it is important to bring the container of the ingested substance so the appropriate course of action can be taken.

A common antidote used in emergency rooms for oral ingestions is activated charcoal. This odorless and tasteless agent has the consistency of tar and can absorb toxins in the stomach and intestines to prevent or limit absorption. Antidotes may be given in the emergency room and effectively work on overdoses of acetaminophen (Tylenol), aspirin, barbiturates, digitalis, tricyclic antidepressants, and others (Table 21-10). Other types of antidotes include those that reverse the effects of various snake and spider bites.

TABLE 21-10 Antidotes

Poisoning Antidotes	Causative Agents
atropine	Mushrooms, phosphates
N-acetylcysteine (Acetadote)	Acetaminophen
Kayexalate	Potassium/electrolytes
naloxone	Opioids
Digibind	Digoxin
flumazenil	Benzodiazepines
glucagon	Beta-blockers
deferoxamine	Iron
sodium bicarbonate	Tricyclic antidepressants (TCAs), salicylates (e.g., aspirin)

BOX 21-3 POISONOUS SNAKES AND SPIDERS

Most snake and spider bites are not from poisonous species and may only require first aid. Those listed below are poisonous (lethal). Antivenins, if available, are made from the venom of the same species it treats.

Types of Snakes
Rattlesnakes: diamondback, Mojave, Pacific
Copperheads: broad-banded, Northern, Southern
Cottonmouths: Eastern, Florida, Western
Coral snakes: Arizona, Texas, Eastern, Western

Types of Spiders
Funnelweb spiders
Brown recluse
Redback jumping spider
Black widow spider

Prognosis. The prognosis varies depending on how quickly treatment is initiated as well as the poison involved. In most cases, the person recovers with no long-term effects.

Non–Drug Treatment. Vomiting can relieve or eliminate poisons such as those caused by food ingestion.

Drug Treatment. The main agents used for poisonings are emetics (to induce vomiting), absorbents, or antidotes. Emetics (e.g., ipecac syrup) trigger the CTZ to cause the patient to vomit, eliminating the causative agent. Absorbents such as activated charcoal are used to deter absorption of the toxin(s). Antidotes either reverse the effects of the poison ingested or prevent the poison from working (Box 21-3). Depending on the area where venomous types of species are found, pharmacies stock antivenins to be used by the emergency department.

Lavage. Emergency treatment can consist of gastric decontamination or lavage. The protocols for this type of response are specific depending on the agent ingested and are not without possible adverse effects of their own. For gastric lavage a 36- to 40-gauge tube (hose) with multiple holes is placed down the throat of the patient. The patient normally will be left in a seated position while the contents empty from the stomach. Care must be taken because aspiration may occur with lavage.

Ipecac Syrup. The use of ipecac is no longer routinely recommended by poison experts.

Activated Charcoal. The absorption capabilities of activated charcoal are great, with only 1 g of charcoal needed to absorb 100 to 500 mg of poisonous agent. However, there are risks with charcoal as well; it is not effective with ethanol or certain metals (lithium or iron). Charcoal may cause emesis (risking aspiration) that can cause tissue damage if the substances ingested are caustic. Also, any additional use of medications may be impeded because of the absorption properties of charcoal.

Tech Alert!

Remember these sound-alike/look-alike drugs:

simethicone versus
   cimetidine
Mylanta versus Mynatal
Phazyme versus
   Phenerzine
hydroxyzine versus
   hydralazine
Prevacid versus
   Pravachol or Prinivil
metoclopramide versus
   metolazone
ranitidine versus
   amantadine
Zantac versus Zofran

General Information

Because the gastrointestinal system can be affected by outside forces—such as bacteria, viruses, parasites, medications, and emotions—this system is a complicated one. Numerous OTC remedies are available to consumers to treat a variety of symptoms. As the median age increases across America and around the world, the amount of routine medication that is taken to help deter illness is increasing. Imbalances that affect the gastrointestinal system can alter the amount of nutrients the body can absorb and the chain reaction that allows for the chemical breakdown of food. If this chain reaction is affected, side effects may occur. By reducing stress, eating a well-balanced diet, and exercising, the gastrointestinal tract is better able to remain in good working condition. However, those who are diagnosed with a more severe condition have many medications and sometimes surgery available to treat their illness. If at all possible, it is important to take care of the gastrointestinal system before problems occur.

DO YOU REMEMBER THESE KEY POINTS?

- The major parts of the digestive system
- The pH of the stomach and its importance
- The functions of the stomach and intestines
- The major conditions covered in this chapter that affect the gastrointestinal system
- The agents used to treat common conditions such as indigestion
- The ingredients used in antacids
- The generic names of the medications covered in this chapter
- The difference between GERD and *H. pylori* infection
- The treatment for *H. pylori* infection
- The difference between laxatives such as cathartics and stool softeners

REVIEW QUESTIONS

Multiple choice questions

1. The primary functions of the gastrointestinal system include all of the following EXCEPT:
   A. Digestion
   B. Absorption
   C. Secretion
   D. Metabolism
   E. All of the above are GI functions

2. Auxiliary organs to the gastrointestinal system include all those listed EXCEPT:
   A. Pancreas
   B. Liver
   C. Gallbladder
   D. Appendix

3. The function of the epiglottis is to:
   A. Break down food particles
   B. Digest food
   C. Block off the tracheal tube
   D. Aid in peristalsis

4. The pH of the stomach is acidic, and its function is to:
A. Help in digestion by breaking down food into chyme
B. Help move food through the intestines
C. Help the absorption of food in the stomach
D. Help in metabolism

5. The pyloric sphincter is located _____ and allows chyme to pass when _____.
A. At the top of the stomach; relaxed
B. At the base of the stomach; tense
C. At the opening of the small intestine; tense
D. At the opening of the small intestine; relaxed

6. The type of medication that can be used for prevention and treatment of chemo-induced emesis is:
A. Meclizine
B. Ondansetron
C. Dramamine
D. All of the above

7. Bile is made by the _____ and stored by the _____.
A. Gallbladder; liver
B. Liver; gallbladder
C. Pancreas; gallbladder
D. Liver; pancreas

8. Excretion takes place mainly in the:
A. Stomach
B. Small intestine
C. Large intestine
D. Rectum

9. A person diagnosed with gastroesophageal reflux disease may receive which of the following medications?
A. Calcium carbonate
B. Ranitidine
C. Omeprazole
D. All of the above

10. Which medication listed below would not be used to prevent emesis?
A. Pepto-Bismol
B. Meclizine
C. Docusate sodium
D. Both A and C

11. Antidopaminergic agents have the effect of:
A. Causing dizziness/drowsiness as a side effect
B. Inhibiting the CTZ
C. Both A and B
D. None of the above

12. PUD is associated with:
A. *H. pylori*
B. GERD
C. Nonsteroidal antiinflammatory drugs
D. Both A and C

13. Agents used to treat Crohn's disease and ulcerative colitis include all of the following EXCEPT:
A. Antispasmodics
B. Anticholinergics
C. Corticosteroids
D. Aminosalicylates

14. Medications used to treat *H. pylori* include:
- A. Antibiotics, PPIs, and antifungals
- B. Antivirals, PPIs, and antibiotics
- C. PPIs, H$_2$-antagonists, and analgesics
- D. H$_2$-Antagonists, analgesics, and antibiotics

15. Ulcers that can be attributed to hyperacidity include all those listed EXCEPT:
- A. Peptic
- B. Duodenal
- C. Gastroesophageal reflux disease
- D. *Helicobacter pylori*

True/False

If the statement is false, then change it to make it true.

_____ **1.** Chyme is an acidic mixture of small food particles.

_____ **2.** Anabolism is the breaking down of molecules, whereas catabolism is the building of molecules; each represents a part of metabolism.

_____ **3.** Proteins are broken down into simple sugars by enzymatic actions.

_____ **4.** Most antacids should be given twice daily, once in the morning and at bedtime.

_____ **5.** Simethicone is an antacid that is added to many stomach medications.

_____ **6.** H$_2$-Receptors are located in the lungs.

_____ **7.** Carbonates are used to balance pH concentrations.

_____ **8.** The drug action for proton pump inhibitors is that they inhibit gastric secretions and block enzymes.

_____ **9.** Aluminum and magnesium can cause diarrhea as a side effect.

_____ **10.** *H. pylori* is a gram-positive microbe that infects the esophagus.

_____ **11.** Antivenin is made from the venom of the species that produces the poison.

_____ **12.** Antiemetic routes of administration include oral, rectal, and topical medications.

_____ **13.** The same virus causes canker and cold sores.

_____ **14.** The treatment for *H. pylori* is normally given over several weeks to months.

_____ **15.** Treatments for poisonings include emetics, absorbents, and antidotes.

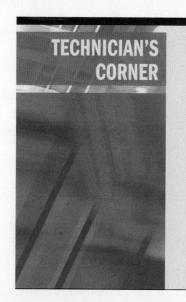

TECHNICIAN'S CORNER

A. A patient arrives in your pharmacy to fill a prescription. The prescription reads: codeine 30 mg; take one to two tablets every 4 to 6 hours as needed for pain. The quantity indicates #100.

What over-the-counter medication probably was prescribed by the physician or will be suggested by the pharmacist at the time of consultation and why?

B. A patient who tested positive for *Helicobacter pylori* arrives at the pharmacy and gives you a prescription for the following agents:

Clarithromycin

Omeprazole

Metronidazole

Question: What would be the recommended strengths and the dosing of these medications? Also, give the length of time the medications should be taken. How is it determined when the medications should be stopped?

BIBLIOGRAPHY

AMA (American Medical Association) *Concise Medical Encyclopedia*. 2006.

Brunton L, John L, Keith P: *Goodman and Gillman's the pharmacological basis of therapeutics*, ed 11, Elmsford, 2005, McGraw-Hill.

Drug facts and comparisons, ed 63, St Louis, 2008, Lippincott Williams & Wilkins.

Koda-Kimble M, Joseph G: *Applied therapeutics: the clinical use of drugs*, ed 9, Philadelphia, 2008, Lippincott Williams & Wilkins.

McKenry LM, Salerno E: *Mosby's pharmacology in nursing*, ed 21, St Louis, 2001, Mosby.

WEBSITES

Cincinnati Children's Hospital Medical Center: Drug and Poison Information Center/DPIC: syrup of ipecac no longer recommended. Retrieved 10-05 from www.cincinnatichildrens.org/svc/alpha/d/dpic/ipecac

Dopamine receptor antagonists: www.pharmacorama.com/en/Sections/Catecholamines_7_4.php

General Principles of Poisoning: www.merck.com/mmpe/print/sec21/ch326/ch326b.html www.aafp.org/afp/20020401/1367.html

Helicobacter pylori and Peptic Ulcer Disease. www.cdc.gov/ulcer/keytocure.htm#fda

Juckett G, M.D., M.P.H, John H, M.D. 2002. American Family Physician. Venomous Snakebites in the United States: Management Review and Update.

Poisoning. www.emedicinehealth.com/poisoning/article_em.htm

Stomatitis. Healthline. www.healthline.com/galecontent/stomatitis-3#definition

22

Urinary System

Objectives

UPON COMPLETING THIS CHAPTER, YOU SHOULD BE ABLE TO DO THE FOLLOWING:

- List both trade and generic names covered in this chapter.
- Describe the location and functions of the kidneys.
- Explain the functions of the nephrons.
- Describe the location and functions of the bladder.
- Differentiate between kidney tubular secretion and reabsorption.
- List the most common conditions that affect the urinary system.
- Describe the drug action of various diuretics discussed in this chapter.
- List the most commonly used diuretics.
- Describe dialysis treatments and the medications that are prescribed to persons requiring dialysis.
- List the auxiliary labels necessary when filling diuretic prescriptions.
- Describe the two common types of incontinence and explain their causes.
- List medications prescribed to treat incontinence and explain the exercises that can be used to manage incontinence.

Absorption (renal) *Within the kidneys: the intake of liquids, solutes, and gases*

Acidification *The conversion to an acidic environment*

Acidosis *The increase in the blood's acidity resulting from the accumulation of acid or loss of bicarbonate; the pH of blood is decreased*

Alkalosis *The increase in the blood's alkalinity resulting from the accumulation of alkali or reduction of acid content; the pH of blood is increased*

Blood urea nitrogen (BUN) *A test that measures the nitrogen in the blood in the form of urea*

Dialysis *The passage of a solute through a semipermeable membrane to remove toxic materials and to maintain fluid, electrolyte, and pH levels of the body system when the kidneys are malfunctioning*

Distribution *Within the kidneys: the mechanism by which elements are sent throughout the body system*

Diuretic *An agent that increases urine output and excretion of water from the body*

Electrolyte *Charged elements called cations (which have positive charges) and anions (which have negative charges); in the human body, some key electrolytes are sodium, chloride, potassium, calcium, and magnesium*

Excretion *Elimination of waste products through stools and urine*

Kidney stones *Solid mineral deposits that form in the urinary tract*

Metabolism (renal) *Within the kidneys: the mechanism by which chemical transformation takes place*

Micturition *Urination*

Nephron *The filtering unit of the kidneys*

Nosocomial infection *An infection that originates in the hospital or institutional setting*

Osmosis *The diffusion of water from low solute concentrations to higher solute concentrations, across a semipermeable membrane*

Renal artery *One of the pair of arteries that branch from the abdominal aorta; each kidney has one renal artery*

Renal failure *The inability of the kidneys to function properly*

Renal fascia *The membranous tissue that surrounds and supports the kidneys*

Renal vein *The vein in which filtered blood from the kidneys is sent back into the body's circulatory system; each kidney has one renal vein*

Tubular reabsorption *The conservation of protein, glucose, bicarbonate, and water from the glomerular filtrate by the tubules*

Tubular secretion *A function of the nephron where ions, toxins, and water are secreted into the collecting duct to be excreted*

Urea *The main nitrogenous constituent of urine and final product of protein metabolism; formed in the liver*

Ureter *The tube that carries urine from the kidneys to the bladder; each kidney has one ureter*

Urethra *The tube that carries urine from the bladder to the urethral sphincter for elimination from the body*

COMMON DRUGS FOR THE URINARY SYSTEM

Trade Name	Generic Name	Pronunciation	Trade Name	Generic Name	Pronunciation
Diuretics			**Alkalinizing Agents**		
Carbonic Anhydrase Inhibitor			Urocit-K	potassium citrate	(poe-**tass**-ee-um sih-trate)
Diamox	acetazolamide	(ah-see-ta-**zoe**-la-myde)			
			Hematopoietic Agents (for Anemia in Chronic Renal Failure)		
Loop Diuretics			Epogen,	epoetin alfa	(eh-**poh**-ee-tin al-fah)
Bumex	bumetanide	(byew-**met**-ah-nide)	Procrit		
Demadex	torsemide	(**tore**-sea-myde)	Aranesp	darbepoetin alfa	(dar-be-**poe**-e-tin **al**-fa)
Edecrin	ethacrynic acid	(eth-a-**krin**-ik **as**-id)	**Iron Supplements**		
Lasix	furosemide	(feur-**oh**-sah-myde)	Feosol	ferrous sulfate	(fair-**us** sul-**fate**)
Osmotic Diuretics			**Vitamin D Analogs to Prevent Renal Osteodystrophy**		
Osmitrol	mannitol	(**man**-ah-tol)	Rocaltrol	calcitriol	(**kal**-si-**trye**-ol)
Potassium-Sparing Diuretics and Diuretic Combinations			**Urinary Tract Infection Agents**		
Aldactone	spironolactone	(spir-own-oh-**lak**-tone)	**Urinary Analgesic Agents**		
Aldactazide	hydrochlorothiazide/ spironolactone	hye-droe-klor-oh -**thy**-a-zide/ spir-own-oh-**lak**-tone)	Pyridium	phenazopyridine	(fen-**ay**-zoe-**pir**-i-deen)
Dyrenium	triamterene	(try-**am**-tur-een)	**Antimicrobials Used for UTIs and Other Infections of the Urinary System**		
Dyazide, Maxzide	hydrochlorothiazide/ triamterene	(hye-droe-klor-oh-**thy**-a-zide/ try-**am**-ter-een)	Amoxil, Trimox	amoxicillin	(am-**oks**-i-sil-in)
			Cipro	ciprofloxacin	(sip-roe-**flox**-a-sin)
Midamor	amiloride	(ah-**mill**-or-ide)	Declomycin	demeclocycline	(**dem**-e-kloe-**sye**-kleen)
Moduretic	hydrochlorothiazide/ amiloride	(hye-droe-klor- oh-**thy**-a-zide/ ah-**mill**-oh-ride)	Duricef	cefadroxil	(**sef**-a-**drox**-il)
			Floxin	ofloxacin	(oh-**flox**-a-sin)
			Keflex	cephalexin	(cef-a-**lex**-in)
Potassium Replacement Supplements			Macrobid, Macrodantin	nitrofurantoin	(**nye**-troe-fue-**ran**-toin)
Micro-K, Klor-Con, K-Tab, K-Dur, Slow-K, K-Lor	potassium chloride	(po-**tass**-ee-um **klor**-ide)	Monurol	fosfomycin	(fos-fo-**my**-sin)
			Principen, Omnipen	ampicillin	(**am**-pi-**sil**-in)
			Septra, Bactrim	sulfamethaxazole/ trimethoprim	(sul-fa-meth-**ox**-a-zole/ trye-**meth**-oh-prim)
Klor-Con Ef	potassium bicarbonate	(po-**tass**-ee-um bi-**kar**-bow-nate)	Vibramycin	doxycycline	(**dox**-i-**sye**-kleen)
Thiazide and Similar Drugs			**Urinary Incontinence Agents**		
Diuril	chlorothiazide	(klor-oh-**thigh**-ah-zide)	Ditropan, Oxytrol, Gelnique	oxybutynin	(**ox**-i-**bue**-ti-nin)
Ezride, Microzide	hydrochlorothiazide	(hye-droe-klor- oh-**thy**-a-zide)			
Thalitone	chlorthalidone	(klor-**thal**-ah-doan)	Toviaz	fesoterodine	(**fes**-oh-**ter**-oh-deen)
Lozol	indapamide	(in-**dap**-ah-myde)	Detrol	tolterodine	(tol-**ter**-oh-deen)
Zaroxolyn	metolazone	(me-**toe**-lah-zone)	VESIcare	solifenacine succinate	(sol-ee-**fen**-a-sin)
Chronic Kidney Disease Agents			Enablex	darifenacin	(dar-e-**fen**-a-sin)
Common Phosphorus Binding Agents			Sanctura	trospium chloride	(trose-**pee**-um)
PhosLo	calcium acetate	(**kal**-see-uhm **ass**-eh-tate)	**Antispasmotic**		
Renagel, Renvela	sevelamer	(se-**vel**-a-mer)	Urispas	flavoxate	(fla-**vox**-ate)

WHEN THE BODY IS IN BALANCE (EQUILIBRIUM), this is known as homeostasis. The urinary system is one of two systems that help create and maintain homeostasis. The other system is the respiratory system (Chapter 18). The kidneys are the major organs of the urinary system; they are responsible for performing urinary system functions, such as the following: maintenance of the chemical compositions of the electrolytes, fluids, and tissues within the body, including acid-base balance; preservation of normal blood pressure; production of certain hormones, including the active form of vitamin D, renin, and erythropoietin. This chapter discusses the location and function of the various parts of the kidneys. This chapter also provides an overview of the conditions that can affect the urinary system along with some of the medications used to treat these conditions.

URINARY MEDICAL TERMINOLOGY

Word Parts	
Cyst/o	Urinary bladder
Glomerul/o	Glomeruli
Home/o	Sameness
Nephr/o, ren/o	Kidneys
Olig/o	Scant
Pyel/o	Renal pelvis
Ur/o, urin/o	Urine
Ureter/o	Ureters
Urethr/o	Urethra

Prefixes	
An-	Without
Diur-	Output of urine
Dys-	Painful
Hydro-	Water
Hyper-	Excessive or increased
Hypo-	Deficient or decreased
Lith-	Stone
Noct-	Night
Poly-	Many
Pyo-	Pus

Suffixes	
-algia	Pain
-cele	Hernia
-chrome	Color
-ectasis	Enlargement or stretching
-emia	Blood condition
-itis	Inflammation
-lithiasis	Presence of stones
-osis	Abnormal condition
-ostomy	Create an opening
-pathy	Disease
-ptosis	Drooping
-rrhagia	Abnormal or excessive flow
-stasis	Maintenance of constant level
-stenosis	Abnormal narrowing
-tic	Pertaining to
-uresis	Urination
-uria, -ur	Urine

Continued

URINARY MEDICAL TERMINOLOGY—cont'd

Conditions	
Congestive heart failure	Inability of heart to pump blood efficiently and meet body demands; often causes edema, including pulmonary edema; may cause kidney dysfunction because of decreased circulation to organs, or may be a complication of end-stage kidney failure
Cystitis	Inflammation of bladder
Edema	Local or generalized condition in which body tissues retain an excessive amount of fluid
Incontinence	Loss of control over excretion of urine or feces
Nocturia	Having to urinate excessively at night
Prostatitis	Inflammation of prostate; condition may present with urinary tract infection
Pyelonephritis	Urinary tract infection that has ascended to renal pelvis, with inflammation of kidney
Urethritis	Inflammation of urethra
Urinary tract infection	Infection of kidney, bladder, or urethra
Urolithiasis or nephrolithiasis	Kidney stones

Anatomy

The kidneys are located inside the upper abdominal cavity, between the third thoracic and twelfth lumbar vertebrae. One kidney is positioned on each side of the vertebral column (Figure 22-1). The right kidney is located a little lower than the left kidney because the liver is positioned directly above the right kidney and displaces it. A fibrous connective tissue called the **renal fascia** holds the kidneys stationary. The shape of the kidneys is similar to the shape of a kidney bean with a small indentation called the hilus. Blood enters the kidneys at the hilus via the **renal artery**. Blood is then filtered within the kidney as it passes through a series of structures. Important ions such as sodium and chloride are reabsorbed into the body and circulatory system. The **renal vein** and ureter leave the kidney at the hilus. The renal vein returns the blood to the body after it has undergone the filtration process. The **ureter** carries wastes removed from the blood to the bladder, where the waste is stored for excretion (Figure 22-2).

The bladder is similar to a holding tank that can expand. When the bladder becomes full, we feel the urge to urinate. The urine is eliminated through the **urethra,** which is a short tube leading from the bladder to the outside of the body.

FUNCTION OF THE KIDNEYS

The kidneys play an important role in our daily lives. Wastes develop from the normal metabolism of active tissues, such as muscles, as well as from the digestion of food. After the body absorbs the necessary nutrients, the wastes are sent to the bloodstream. Ultimately, the blood is filtered as it passes through the kidneys and the cleansed blood (and other vital components such as proteins) is returned to the body system. The filtered wastes enter the urinary system and are ultimately excreted through the urine. Excretion is one of the four major important functions of the body:

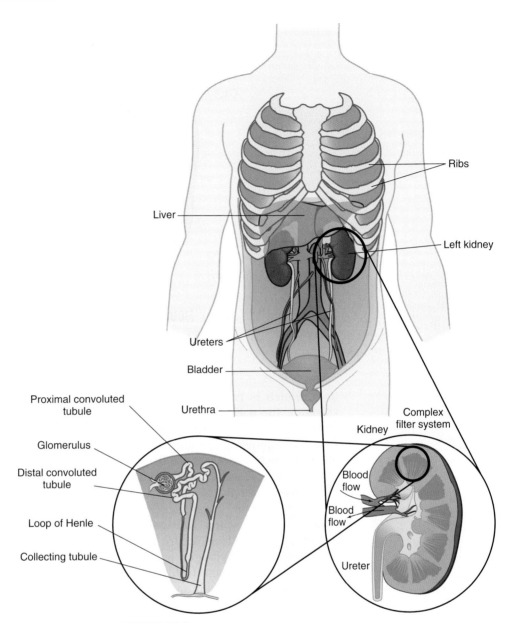

FIGURE 22-1 Anatomy of urinary tract and nephrons.

1. **Absorption:** The intake of liquids, solids, and gases into the body fluids and tissues
2. **Distribution:** The way in which chemicals or drug agents are separated and sent throughout the body
3. **Metabolism:** The chemical changes and reactions occurring within the body system; metabolism includes anabolism (building up processes) and catabolism (breaking down processes)
4. **Excretion:** The elimination of chemicals and substances from the body system

The bladder has walls that can expand to hold approximately 1000 mL (1 L) of urine if necessary; however, the usual volume of urine contained in the bladder at any one time is about 250 to 300 mL under normal conditions. The adult human body excretes about 960 mL of urine per day. Urine contains

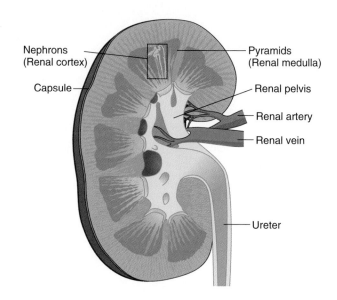

FIGURE 22-2 Anatomy of the kidney.

urea, which is produced by the liver. **Urea** is a form of nitrogen that, upon standing for a time in the presence of oxygen, changes to ammonia, which causes the characteristic smell of urine. The kidneys also have an important function: balancing the fluid content of the body. Most of the body is composed of fluids such as water, blood, and plasma and various ions such as chloride, potassium, and sodium. The kidneys balance ions within the blood and eliminate excess ions in the blood. If excessive ions are not eliminated and either an abundance or a deficit occurs, conditions such as metabolic acidosis or **alkalosis** can develop. **Acidosis** occurs when too many free hydrogen ions are present, and alkalosis occurs when there is either retention of bicarbonate or excessive loss of hydrogen ions. Although the kidneys are only about the size of a fist, they manage to filter about 50 gallons of blood products every day. Plasma travels through an amazing 140 miles of tubules contained inside the kidneys.

NEPHRON FUNCTION

The functional units of the kidneys are termed **nephrons**; they are responsible for the regulation of fluids, solutes, and wastes. Each kidney contains millions of microscopic nephrons (Figure 22-3). Each nephron is shaped like an inverted pyramid with many twists and turns of its tubules; the nephrons are active 24 hours a day. The following is a systematic look into the filtering process by following the flow of blood as it enters the kidney:

1. The renal artery enters the kidney and divides into progressively smaller vessels until it becomes afferent arterioles. Blood then passes from the afferent arterioles into a cluster of capillaries called the glomerulus. Each glomerulus is surrounded by a double-layered epithelial cup that resembles a baseball glove; this structure is called Bowman's capsule.
2. Blood cells, platelets, and large proteins cannot pass through the capillaries of the glomerulus into Bowman's capsule. Only plasma can pass through the

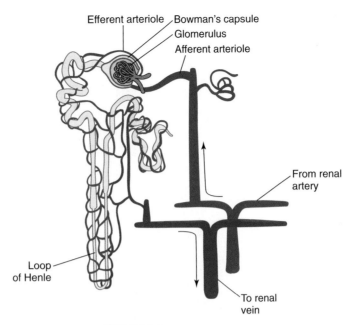

FIGURE 22-3 Nephron anatomy.

glomerulus. Plasma is the liquid component of blood, which is mostly water. However, some of the components of plasma are still too large to leave the capillaries, such as albumins and globulins. Other components of plasma include toxins that may accumulate in the blood. These are very small; they can leave the capillaries easily and enter Bowman's capsule.

3. The filtrate from Bowman's capsule then travels down the descending tubule (also called the proximal convoluted tubule) and up the ascending tubule (called the distal convoluted tubule). The U-turn part of the nephron is called the loop of Henle.

4. As the filtrate passes through the nephron tubules, various nutrients, water, and important chemical ions such as sodium, chloride, and potassium are pulled out of the filtrate (i.e., reabsorbed) and returned to the plasma to be used for cellular nourishment. At the same time, other ions in the tubules (such as those in excess) are excreted.

5. The filtrate, now called urine, travels from the nephrons to the collecting ducts.

6. The collecting ducts empty directly into the ureter.

7. The ureter extends from the hilus of each kidney directly to the bladder.

8. The bladder empties the urine into the urethra and the urine travels out of the body.

Tech Note!

Sodium is an important electrolyte that helps conduct nerve impulses and balance fluid in the body; sodium content is regulated through reabsorption in the kidneys.

Tubular Reabsorption

The first function of the nephrons is **tubular reabsorption**. Important molecules are separated from the filtrate into their individual components in this process. Some of these molecules eventually are excreted in urine, whereas others—such as glucose (sugar), water, sodium, chloride, and amino acids (proteins)—reenter the plasma. This takes place at various points in the proximal convoluted tubule, distal convoluted tubule, and loop of Henle (Figure 22-4).

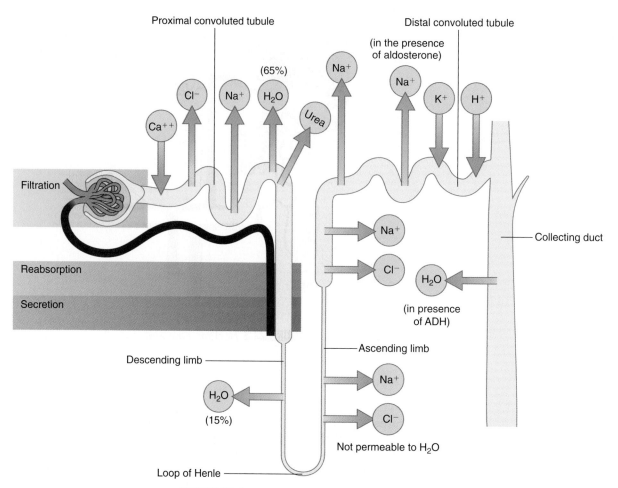

FIGURE 22-4 Tubular reabsorption and secretion.

The kidneys balance the acid-base content of the body. Two mechanisms affect the balance of ions. The first is ion exchange. Sodium ions are pulled out of the tubules and are exchanged for hydrogen ions. As sodium accumulates on the outside of the proximal convoluted tubules, it creates an osmotic gradient, and water molecules are drawn toward the higher concentration of sodium; this is called **osmosis** (Figure 22-5). The overall effect is a decrease in excreted water. Ion exchange also can take place in the distal convoluted tubule. As sodium ions exit the distal convoluted tubule, they are exchanged for potassium ions. The loop of Henle has a different transport mechanism called active transport. Instead of an exchange of ions, there is a one-way uptake of sodium and chloride from the loop of Henle. These ions return to the circulatory system. Most of the sodium that enters the renal system is returned to the circulatory system.

Tubular Secretion

Tubular secretion is another major function of the nephrons. This function takes place throughout the nephron. Various ions, toxins, and water are secreted into the collecting duct. First, molecules such as toxins, water-soluble molecules, and excess or unnecessary chemicals are excreted. Weak acids, such as aspirin and penicillin; weak bases, such as narcotic analgesics; metformin; and antihis-

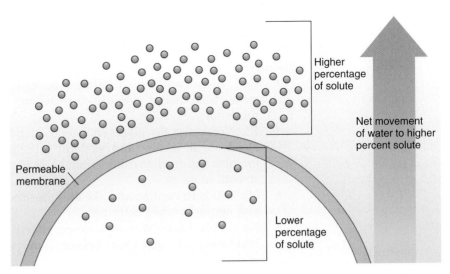

FIGURE 22-5 Also known as an osmotic gradient, the smaller water molecules gravitate toward the highly concentrated sodium ions.

tamines are some of the types of chemicals that are secreted and eliminated. The second function of secretion is to allow the kidneys to regulate the pH of the blood through urine acidification. **Acidification** is the process of eliminating extra hydrogen ions through the urine. This is why urine has an acid content between a pH of 4 and 5, whereas the pH of blood is maintained at approximately 7.4.

As hydrogen ions are taken into the nephron tubules, they combine with other molecules to produce bicarbonate. This then is released into the bloodstream where it regulates the overall pH of the body, helping to maintain homeostasis. Bicarbonate is a buffer. A buffer has the ability to bind hydrogen (which creates a basic environment) or release hydrogen (which creates an acidic environment), balancing the blood pH. To put it another way, an acid can release hydrogen ions, whereas a base can remove hydrogen ions by binding to them. The extra hydrogen ions are taken into the tubules and eventually are excreted.

The kidneys are also responsible for the production of renin, an enzyme that plays a role in maintaining water balance in the body. When the body is under stress (causing a loss of fluids), the kidneys secrete renin. The renin is released into the bloodstream where it transforms angiotensinogen to angiotensin I, which circulates throughout the system. Angiotensin I is transformed in the liver into angiotension II. The formation of angiotensin II activates the adrenal cortex, which begins to excrete aldosterone (hormone); the aldosterone circulates back to the kidneys, where it activates the kidneys to increase the reabsorption of fluids. This overall effect increases the volume of fluids throughout the body, which increases blood pressure.

THE IMPORTANCE OF ELECTROLYTES

An important function of the kidneys is to maintain homeostasis by balancing the levels of **electrolytes** (free ions) within the body. To understand the importance of electrolytes not only in the urinary system but also for the entire body system, we must look at specific cations and anions (see Chapter 31)—the cations Na^+ (sodium), K^+ (potassium), Ca^{2+} (calcium), and Mg^{2+} (magnesium); the anions Cl^- (chloride), PO_4^{3-} (phosphate), and HCO_3^- (bicarbonate).

The following is a list of functions of each electrolyte:

Cations:

- Ca^{2+}: Bone and teeth formation, cell membrane integrity, cardiac conduction, nerve impulse conduction, muscle contraction, hormone secretion
- K^+: Necessary for glycogen (sugar) deposits in the liver (to maintain blood sugar levels) and skeletal muscles (for energy); aids in nerve impulse and cardiac conduction; helps in contraction within skeletal and smooth muscles
- Mg^{2+}: Aids in cardiac and skeletal muscle excitability, enzyme activities, and neurochemical activities
- Na^+: Maintains water balance, nerve impulse transmission, and regulation of acid-base balance; participates in cellular chemical reactions

Anions:

- Cl^-: The main anion in the transport of sodium, hydrogen, and potassium; essential to acid-base balance
- HCO_3^-: The most important chemical that acts as a buffer; it is essential for the proper acid-base balance for the body system
- PO_4^{3-}: Aids as a buffer to balance acid-base regulation within cells; promotes normal neuromuscular action and participates in carbohydrate metabolism; essential for formation and strength of bones and teeth; also necessary for many biochemical pathways (such as production of energy, cell division)

Conditions Affecting the Urinary System

It seems as though it would be impossible for individuals to survive without the constant functioning of both kidneys; however, many persons live with just one kidney. The kidneys are so efficient that as little as 20% of a kidney needs to function in order for a person to survive. In spite of the kidney's resiliency and efficiency, it is still very important for people to closely monitor their diet, medications, and activities to maintain kidney health. It is reassuring to know, however, that many persons can live normal lives with only one kidney or partial kidney function. In some cases, however, dialysis or even kidney transplants may be necessary.

Other conditions that can affect the kidneys and urinary system in general include blockages or infections of the kidney, ureter, bladder, or urethra. If there is residual urine that does not leave the bladder, infection can result. Drinking plenty of water is one of the most effective ways of taking care of the urinary system because it helps to cleanse the body of toxins and other unwanted chemicals. Table 22-1 lists other common conditions affecting the urinary system.

COMMON CONDITIONS

Renal Failure

Renal failure is the loss of kidney function. Many possible causes can lead to either acute or chronic renal failure, such as accidents, toxic agents, genetic diseases, or certain illnesses. Older persons suffer from renal impairment more

TABLE 22-1 Conditions Affecting the Urinary System

Condition	Effect
Anuria	Lack of urine: less than 100 mL over 24 hours
Cystitis	Inflammation of bladder
Edema	Increased fluid in cells, tissues, and/or cavities
Glomerulonephritis	Inflammation of glomeruli
Hyperkalemia	Excessive increase in potassium in blood
Hypokalemia	Excessive decrease in potassium in blood
Incontinence	Lack of control of urination or defecation
Kidney stones	Concretions in kidneys that may cause obstruction of urine output
Oliguria	Scant urine output: between 100 and 400 mL over 24 hours
Polyuria	Excessive or large volume of urine within a certain time
Pyelonephritis	Inflammation of kidney, often associated with infection
Renal failure	Kidney no longer functions
Sepsis	A serious medical condition characterized by a whole-body inflammatory state and presence of known or suspected serious infection
Uremia	Excess urea in blood
Urethritis	Inflammation of urethra
Urolithiasis	Kidney stones made of calcium or salts
Urinary tract infection	Infection of urinary tract caused by microorganisms

TABLE 22-2 End-Stage Renal Disease Symptoms*

System	Effect
Cardiovascular	Hypertension, congestive heart failure
Respiratory	Pulmonary edema, dyspnea
Gastrointestinal	Nausea, vomiting, gastrointestinal bleeding
Endocrine	Hyperparathyroidism
Ocular	Hypertensive retinopathy
Nervous	Fatigue, confusion, seizures

*Other symptoms include problems with the skin, nerves, blood, and metabolism as well as psychological problems.

often than younger adults. As a kidney ages, it is less able to compensate for fluid imbalances of the body. Diabetes mellitus and uncontrolled hypertension are the most common causes of chronic renal failure in adults in the United States. Other persons who are at risk of renal failure include those with human immunodeficiency virus, leukemia, or Hodgkin's disease or those with genetic predispositions (Table 22-2). Congestive heart failure (CHF) may cause renal failure by reduction of necessary blood flow to the kidneys. A common genetic disease that can cause renal failure is polycystic renal disease. This disease can affect a person in childhood or in adulthood. The kidney becomes enlarged and filled with cysts, and if progression of the disease process is fast, the kidney eventually fails. In many cases, the deterioration of the kidneys can be slowed using medications.

As renal failure progresses, every part of the body is affected because of the buildup of waste products and an imbalance of fluids. Early symptoms include fatigue, headache, shortness of breath (SOB), sudden weight changes, and edema. Symptoms progress to include a loss of appetite and anemia. As waste products continually accumulate in the blood, the organs cannot function properly and begin to shut down, causing bone weakness, decreased mental alertness, and coma. CHF may occur as a result of the buildup of fluids in the entire body, especially the lungs, which causes difficulty breathing.

Prognosis. Keeping both sugar intake and blood pressure under control is extremely important to facilitate a more normal lifestyle. However, lifestyle quality depends on the amount of damage the kidneys have sustained. Diet and medications can help but cannot reverse the damage, and the course of chronic renal failure slowly progresses to end-stage renal disease (ESRD). When a person has lost too much kidney function or has end-stage renal disease, renal replacement therapies (i.e., dialysis or transplant) are the only alternatives. Although transplants are relatively common and have a high rate of success, unfortunately there are not enough donors to supply kidneys. Many patients whose names are on transplant waiting lists must wait for years. While they wait, dialysis is the patient's only option. Sometimes a transplant may not be an option because the donor's kidneys are not compatible with the recipient's tissue type. In addition, many times individuals do not want to have surgery to replace their kidneys.

Non–Drug Treatment. Patients with chronic renal failure must learn to manage their dietary intake, limiting foods that are high in phosphates (e.g., colas) and dairy products (e.g., milk, cheese). Other considerations should be given to sodium intake to manage hypertension, which negatively impacts the kidneys.

Dialysis is the procedure used to remove waste products from the blood of patients with end-stage renal disease. This treatment replaces the normal kidney function of removing wastes and balancing fluids. Two major methods are in use today: hemodialysis and peritoneal dialysis. A third type—nocturnal dialysis—may be yet another choice. Although each of these types of dialysis has drawbacks, they are life-sustaining treatments. Negative aspects of dialysis include the additional medications that patients must take to further balance pH and fluids, the inconvenience of having to be stationary for a length of time, and the fact that even sophisticated machinery cannot perform as efficiently as one's own kidneys.

Hemodialysis requires the patient to visit a clinic or hospital for treatment. A vein shunt (needle puncture with a reinforced opening) is used to connect the patient's bloodstream to the dialysis machine. The dialysis machine uses a mechanical filtration system to clean a small but steady stream of blood from the patient's body. Patients undergoing this treatment feel good afterward; however, over time, toxins accumulate and patients begin to feel ill. Although the length of treatment varies, traditional hemodialysis normally takes 3 or more hours 2 to 3 times weekly.

Peritoneal dialysis is an alternative to hemodialysis. The patient's bloodstream is connected to a bag of osmotic solution. A catheter plug is implanted into the abdominal cavity for administration and removal of the solution. The osmotic solution flows into the peritoneal cavity. The peritoneal membrane is a thin lining that encases the organs of the abdomen, including the stomach, liver, spleen, and kidneys. The osmotic solution works in the same fashion as the sodium gradient works in the kidneys. As the solution is allowed to fill the cavity, wastes are pulled into the solution, where they can be drained from the cavity into an empty bag attached to the outside of the abdominal wall. This treatment usually is done several times daily to keep toxin levels to a minimum. Treatment can be done at home (continuous ambulatory

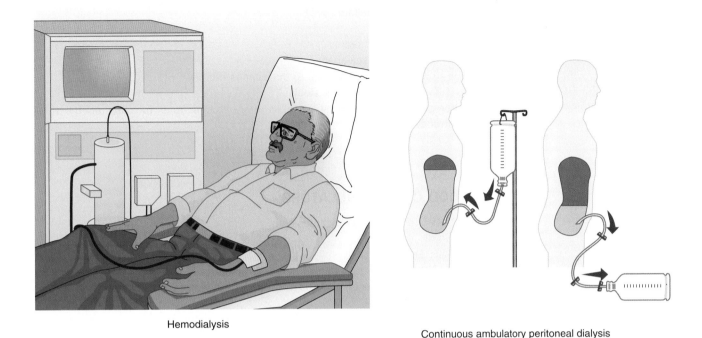

Hemodialysis

Continuous ambulatory peritoneal dialysis

FIGURE 22-6 Two types of dialysis.

peritoneal dialysis [CAPD]); however, peritoneal dialysis can be performed in clinics if the patient cannot afford a home health nurse for assistance (Figure 22-6). It is important that aseptic technique be used when performing this type of dialysis in order to avoid peritonitis, an infection within the abdominal cavity.

Nocturnal continuous cycle peritoneal dialysis or nocturnal hemodialysis is another form of dialysis that allows the patient to receive treatment while sleeping. Dialysis treatment is done using the help of a portable peritoneal or hemodialysis machine, 8 to 12 hours per night. Because the process can be performed slowly over the course of the night (most nights of the week), patients often feel better and have a reduced risk of complications. Patients do not have to wait between treatments, which is when they begin to feel the effects of toxic buildup; in addition, patients do not have to spend several hours immobilized at a dialysis clinic. If dialysis is done in a home setting, the patient must be able to troubleshoot problems with the machinery if there is a malfunction. Finally, the patient usually must have a home health nurse to help with the treatment.

Drug Treatment. Persons receiving dialysis have to be careful of their fluid and salt intake. With any of these treatments, a loss of ions and nutrients must be replaced with supplements each time dialysis is performed. One of the most common side effects of end-stage renal disease is anemia. For this condition, iron and erythropoietin are given to the patient. Iron supplements can increase the oxygen-carrying capacity of the hemoglobin. Hemoglobin is a protein within the red blood cells that carries oxygen with the help of iron. Other medications may include vitamin replacement, blood pressure agents, and phosphorus-lowering medications such as calcium carbonate, calcium acetate, and sevelamer.

IRON SUPPLEMENT

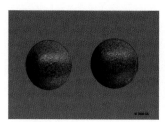

GENERIC NAME: ferrous sulfate (OTC)

TRADE NAME: Feosol

ROUTE OF ADMINISTRATION: oral

INDICATIONS: iron deficiency anemia

COMMON ADULT DOSAGE: 325 mg one to three times per day

SIDE EFFECTS: constipation, black stools

NOTE: Iron supplements normally are taken with a stool softener to counteract the side effect of constipation

RED BLOOD CELL STIMULATORS

GENERIC NAME: epoetin alfa (erythropoietin)

GENERIC NAME: epoetin alfa

TRADE NAME: Epogen, Procrit

ROUTE OF ADMINISTRATION: subcutaneous or intravenous

INDICATION: anemia secondary to end-stage renal disease or resulting from chemotherapy

COMMON ADULT DOSAGE: for dialysis patients: 75 units/kg three times weekly; doses adjusted for hemoglobin levels; once maintained, a larger dose may be administered just once per week.

SIDE EFFECTS: hypertension, headache, nausea/vomiting (N/V); may cause thrombosis

AUXILIARY LABELS:

- Refrigerate.
- Do not shake.
- Protect from light.

GENERIC NAME: darbepoetin alfa

TRADE NAME: Aranesp

ROUTE OF ADMINISTRATION: subcutaneous or intravenous

INDICATION: anemia secondary to end-stage renal disease or resulting from chemotherapy

COMMON ADULT DOSAGE: for dialysis patients: 0.45 mcg/kg once weekly; doses adjusted for hemoglobin levels

SIDE EFFECTS: hypertension, headache, N/V; may cause thrombosis

AUXILIARY LABELS:

- Refrigerate.
- Do not shake.
- Protect from light.

PHOSPHORUS BINDING AGENTS

GENERIC NAME: calcium carbonate (OTC)

TRADE NAME: TUMS

ROUTE OF ADMINISTRATION: oral

INDICATION: reduce phosphate absorption from diet (phosphate binder)

COMMON ADULT DOSAGE: 500-2000 mg three times daily with meals; adjusted based on calcium and phosphate levels

SIDE EFFECTS: constipation

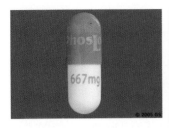

GENERIC NAME: calcium acetate (Rx only)
TRADE NAME: PhosLo
ROUTE OF ADMINISTRATION: oral
INDICATION: reduce phosphate absorption from diet (phosphate binder)
COMMON ADULT DOSAGE: 1334 mg (2 tablets or gel caps) three times daily with meals; adjusted based on calcium and phosphate levels
SIDE EFFECTS: constipation
AUXILIARY LABELS:
- Protect from moisture.
- Take with meals.

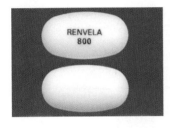

GENERIC NAME: sevelamer (Rx only)
TRADE NAME: Renagel, Renvela
ROUTE OF ADMINISTRATION: oral
INDICATION: reduce phosphate absorption from diet (phosphate binder)
COMMON ADULT DOSAGE: 800-1600 mg three times daily with meals; dose based on phosphate levels
SIDE EFFECTS: headache, heartburn, N/V, constipation
AUXILIARY LABELS:
- Protect from moisture.
- Take with meals.

AGENT TO REDUCE RISK OF RENAL OSTEODYSTROPHY (WEAK BONES)

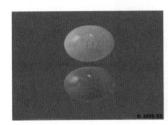

GENERIC NAME: calcitriol
TRADE NAME: Rocaltrol
ROUTE OF ADMINISTRATION: oral
INDICATION: prevention of weak bones secondary to renal failure
COMMON ADULT DOSAGE: for dialysis patients: 0.25 to 1 mcg/day for most patients; based on serum calcium levels and other parameters
SIDE EFFECTS: minimal to no common side effects; hypocalcemia and associated symptoms if dose is too high
AUXILIARY LABEL:
- Do not crush or chew.

Edema

Edema is a condition of excess fluids in the tissues, often occurring in the extremities. Fluids are normally stored in the blood and interstitial spaces (spaces around cells). As a result of various conditions, fluids can accumulate in the blood and in the interstitial spaces of tissues (Box 22-1). There are two types of edema: pitting and nonpitting. Pitting is observed when an indentation on the surface of the skin can be made by applying pressure, often caused by high-salt diets or congestive heart failure (CHF) (Figure 22-7). Nonpitting edema does not leave a skin indentation and is more difficult to treat because the causes may be due to an underlying condition, such as myxedema or a lymphatic system disorder.

In CHF the heart cannot handle the normal volume of blood and begins to pump less; thus the kidneys receive less blood. The kidneys' response signals indicate that there is a lack of blood content in the body, and the kidneys respond by retaining salt and fluid. As fluid volume increases, the heart muscle weakens further, putting more stress on the heart and creating the vicious cycle of CHF (see Chapter 23).

BOX 22-1 SOME CAUSES OF EDEMA

Chronic venous insufficiency: Attributable to poor blood flow caused by a weakness in the veins; often seen in older and obese people

Cirrhosis: Chronic hepatic disease characterized by destruction and fibrotic regeneration of hepatic cells.

Heart failure: Decreased ability to function properly because of overload. Can occur after myocardial infarction or be due to CHF, cardiomyopathy, or coronary artery disease (CAD)

High salt intake: Can cause fluids to be retained in cells if kidneys cannot eliminate excess sodium and fluids

Kidney disease: Inability of the kidneys to function properly in regulation of fluids. Due to hypertension, diabetes, or any condition affecting any part of the renal system

Thrombophlebitis: Inflammation of the vein due to clot formation. Can be caused by trauma, inactivity, and varicose veins

Underlying conditions (e.g., heart failure, kidney disease) can also cause the kidneys to retain sodium

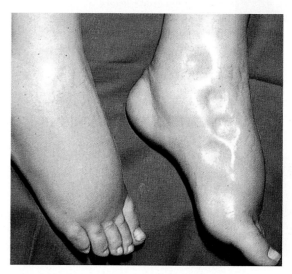

FIGURE 22-7 Pitting edema. (From Bloom A, Ireland J, Watkins P: *A colour atlas of diabetes,* ed 2, St Louis, 1992, Mosby.)

Prognosis. In many cases edema may be a temporary condition that corrects itself within a couple of days. Causes of temporary edema include high altitude, exercise, or medication. For those persons who suffer from chronic forms of edema, medication and dietary intake can control this condition. Those with CHF must take medication for their entire life.

Non–Drug Treatment. Avoid salt and/or restrict the intake of foods processed with salt; refrain from high volumes of fluid intake. Once swelling has occurred, elevating the legs above chest level will help move the fluid toward the heart and reduce edema for some patients. Do not sit for long periods as this increases the pooling of fluids in feet and legs. Support stockings can also be worn to help deter the buildup of fluids.

Drug Treatment. The choice to treat edema with medications will be determined by its underlying cause. For example, medication-induced edema is not likely to respond to diuretic treatment. For most causes of edema, the main drugs prescribed are diuretics. Classes of **diuretics** include the thiazides, thiazide-like agents, loop diuretics, potassium-sparing diuretics, carbonic anhydrase inhibitors, and osmotic diuretics. Each classification is discussed along with its drug action and a listing of an example of each medication. The normal dosage given is for an adult maintenance dose for edema. Certain diuretics (e.g., loop diuretics, thiazides, and potassium-sparing agents) are effective for the treatment of chronic hypertension; they lower blood pressure by reducing blood volume, cardiac output, and systemic vascular resistance.

Thiazides and Thiazide-like Agents. Thiazides and thiazide-like agents act by inducing an equal increase in the urinary excretion of the ions sodium and chloride. These agents accomplish this by inhibiting the normal process of reabsorption of sodium and chloride within the distal convoluted tubule. They also lower the urinary excretion of calcium and increase the loss of potassium. Their onset of action is rapid. Because of the loss of potassium, a potassium supplement may be taken concurrently with this type of medication if it is prescribed chronically, unless other drugs that preserve potassium are used at the same time. Thiazides can also be used for hypertension and to prevent formation of kidney stones.

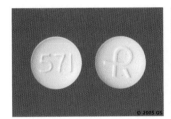

GENERIC NAME: indapamide
TRADE NAME: Lozol
INDICATION: edema
ROUTE OF ADMINISTRATION: oral
COMMON ADULT DOSAGE: 2.5 mg PO once daily
SIDE EFFECTS: headache, dizziness, upset stomach
AUXILIARY LABELS:

- Take with food or milk.
- Do not crush tablet.

GENERIC NAME: hydrochlorothiazide
TRADE NAME: Ezride, Microzide
INDICATION: edema
ROUTE OF ADMINISTRATION: oral
COMMON ADULT DOSAGE: 12.5 to 50 mg daily or intermittently
SIDE EFFECTS: may cause gastrointestinal upset and photosensitivity
AUXILIARY LABELS:

- Take with food or milk.
- May cause photosensitivity.

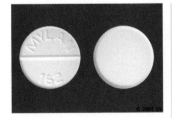

GENERIC NAME: chlorothiazide
TRADE NAME: Diuril
INDICATION: edema
ROUTE OF ADMINISTRATION: oral, intravenous
COMMON ADULT DOSAGE: oral: 0.5 to 1 g per day, in 1-2 divided doses
SIDE EFFECTS: may cause photosensitivity
AUXILIARY LABELS:

- Take with food or milk.
- May cause photosensitivity.

Tech Alert!

Common side effects for all thiazides include frequent urination. For this reason, they normally are to be taken early in the day to avoid nocturia.

GENERIC NAME: metolazone
TRADE NAME: Zaroxolyn
INDICATION: edema
ROUTE OF ADMINISTRATION: oral
COMMON ADULT DOSAGE: 5 to 20 mg once daily
SIDE EFFECTS: may cause photosensitivity
AUXILIARY LABELS:

- Take with food or milk.
- May cause photosensitivity.

Loop Diuretics. Loop diuretics inhibit reabsorption of sodium and chloride in the proximal convoluted tubule, distal convoluted tubule, and loop of Henle. Because of the strong action of these agents, a great deal of potassium is lost with urination; potassium supplementation is often needed to maintain homeostasis. Loop diuretics normally are prescribed to be taken early in the day to avoid excessive urination at night (nocturia).

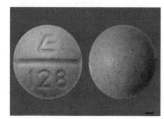

GENERIC NAME: bumetanide
TRADE NAME: Bumex
INDICATION: edema
ROUTE OF ADMINISTRATION: oral, intravenous
COMMON ADULT DOSAGE: 0.5 to 2 mg once or twice daily
SIDE EFFECTS: may cause gastrointestinal upset, dizziness, light-headedness
AUXILIARY LABELS:

- Take with food or milk.
- May cause dizziness.

GENERIC NAME: torsemide
TRADE NAME: Demadex
INDICATION: edema
ROUTE OF ADMINISTRATION: oral, intravenous
COMMON ADULT DOSAGE: 10 to 20 mg once daily
SIDE EFFECTS: may cause dizziness, light-headedness
AUXILIARY LABELS:

- May cause dizziness.
- May cause photosensitivity.

SPECIAL NOTE: Torsemide does not need to be taken with food or milk.

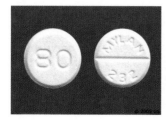

GENERIC NAME: furosemide
TRADE NAME: Lasix
INDICATION: edema
ROUTE OF ADMINISTRATION: oral, intravenous
COMMON ADULT DOSAGE: 20 to 80 mg once daily
SIDE EFFECTS: may cause gastrointestinal upset
AUXILIARY LABEL:

- Take with food or milk.
- May cause dizziness.
- May cause photosensitivity.

Potassium-Sparing Agents. Because potassium-sparing agents function primarily in the distal convoluted tubule and inhibit sodium reabsorption, which decreases potassium loss, they do not cause large amounts of potassium to be excreted in the urine. With these types of agents, it is recommended that patients avoid consuming large quantities of potassium-rich foods.

Table 22-3 lists combination drugs composed of potassium-sparing and thiazide or loop diuretics, along with their indication, dosage form, and auxiliary labels.

TABLE 22-3 **Combination Diuretics (Potassium-Sparing)**

Generic Name	Trade Name	Dosage Form	Strength	Normal Dosage	Auxiliary Label
amiloride/hydrochlorothiazide (HCTZ)	Moduretic	Tablet	5 mg/50 mg	1-2 tablets daily	Take with food Photosensitivity
spironolactone/HCTZ	Aldactazide	Tablet	25 mg/25 mg	1-2 tablets daily	Take with food Photosensitivity
	Aldactazide	Tablet	50 mg/50 mg	1-2 tablets daily	Take with food Photosensitivity
triamterene/HCTZ	Dyazide	Capsule	37.5 mg/25 mg	1-2 capsules daily	Take with food Photosensitivity
	Maxzide-25	Tablet	37.5 mg/25 mg	1-2 tablets daily	Take with food Photosensitivity
	Maxzide	Tablet	75 mg/50 mg	1 tablet daily	Take with food Photosensitivity

POTASSIUM-SPARING DIURETICS

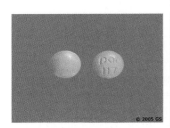

GENERIC NAME: amiloride
TRADE NAME: Midamor
INDICATION: edema
ROUTE OF ADMINISTRATION: oral
COMMON ADULT DOSAGE: 5 to 10 mg per day with food
SIDE EFFECTS: may cause gastrointestinal upset, dizziness, headache, visual disturbances
AUXILIARY LABELS:
- Take with food.
- May cause dizziness.

GENERIC NAME: spironolactone
TRADE NAME: Aldactone
INDICATION: edema
ROUTE OF ADMINISTRATION: oral
COMMON ADULT DOSAGE: for edema: 25 to 200 mg per day
SIDE EFFECTS: may cause drowsiness, mental confusion, breast enlargement in males (long-term use)
AUXILIARY LABEL:
- May cause dizziness and drowsiness.
- Take with food.

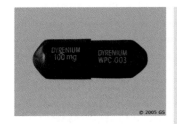

GENERIC NAME: triamterene
TRADE NAME: Dyrenium
INDICATION: edema
ROUTE OF ADMINISTRATION: oral
COMMON ADULT DOSAGE: 100 mg twice daily after meals
SIDE EFFECTS: may cause gastrointestinal upset, headache
AUXILIARY LABEL:
- Take after meals.

Carbonic Anhydrase Inhibitors. Carbonic anhydrase inhibitors inhibit the enzyme carbonic anhydrase. Carbonic anhydrase inhibitors include acetazolamide, dichlorphenamide, and methazolamide. They inhibit the transport of bicarbonate from the proximal tubule, causing less reabsorption of sodium and an increased excretion of sodium, potassium bicarbonate, and water. These diuretics are relatively weak, and they are not commonly used in the treatment of edema. Most of these agents more commonly are used to treat glaucoma (see Chapter 19) or for the treatment of altitude sickness. Side effects include possible gastrointestinal upset, photosensitivity, dizziness, tingling, and drowsiness.

CARBONIC ANHYDRASE INHIBITOR

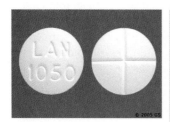

GENERIC NAME: acetazolamide
TRADE NAME: Diamox
INDICATION: edema caused by CHF or medications
ROUTE OF ADMINISTRATION: oral, intravenous
COMMON ADULT DOSAGE: 250 to 375 mg every other day in the morning or for 2 days followed by 1 day of rest; 1 day of rest in the regimen allows kidney recovery to maintain effectiveness
AUXILIARY LABELS:
■ Take with meals.
■ May cause dizziness.

Osmotic Diuretics. Osmotic diuretics inhibit tubular reabsorption of water by increasing the osmolarity of the glomerular filtrate. They are used for prophylaxis of acute renal failure when the glomerular filtration rate (GFR) is reduced. The only agent used for the treatment of edema is mannitol (Osmitrol), which forces urine production in people with acute kidney failure. The increased urine production helps to prevent kidney failure and also contributes to elimination of toxic substances from the body. Dosage is based on the patient's weight and is given intravenously. Other uses include reduction of intraocular pressure from glaucoma (Chapter 19).

Kidney Stones

Kidney stones are small clumps of material (usually calcium, magnesium, or uric acid salts) that form in the kidney from substances that pass through the renal system. Hundreds of thousands of Americans experience a condition known as urolithiasis (kidney stones) every year. Although stones most commonly are found in persons between the ages of 20 and 55, they can affect anyone. They occur at a somewhat higher percentage in Caucasians than African Americans, and they tend to have a genetic component. One of the first signs of a kidney stone is pain while urinating. Often stones will pass without treatment; for stones that cannot be excreted, a physician is needed. Additional symptoms that may occur with a blocked kidney include fever, vomiting, blood in urine, and extreme pain in the lower side or back.

Different types of stones can form at different locations within the urinary tract (Figure 22-8). Many substances pass daily through the urinary system; some people are more prone to the formation of kidney stones. Table 22-4 lists the different types of stones along with their characteristics and treatments.

Prognosis. Patients have several options for stone removal and prevention. Through dietary changes and medication, one can limit the possible development of more stones. Most kidney stones should not limit daily activities. Most medications used to prevent formation of stones may need to be prescribed for the patient's lifetime.

Non–Drug Treatment. If the stone is small enough, there may be no need for treatment outside of pain management and fluids; the stone will usually pass on its own. For larger stones, there are a variety of procedures that can be used, based on the composition of the stone. Lithotripsy is the use of shock waves to

Tech Alert!

Mannitol is available only in injectable solution. Mannitol must be stored at a temperature from 15° to 30° C (59° to 86° F) because it has a tendency to crystallize at lower temperatures because of its high sugar content (e.g., the solution is supersaturated at room temperature). If mannitol does crystallize, it can be placed for short periods in 80° C water with periodic vigorous shaking or can be autoclaved at 121° C for 20 minutes at 15 psi (pounds per square inch). The vials cannot be placed in a microwave or they may explode. Mannitol should not be administered until it is at room temperature or slightly below, and the drug requires a filter for infusion. This is a common question on the Pharmacy Technician Certification Board exam.

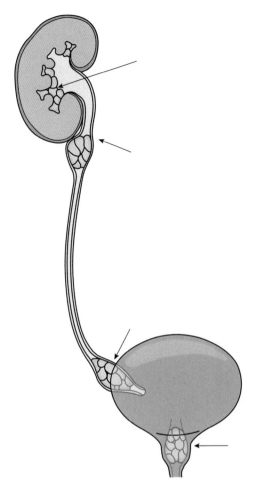

FIGURE 22-8 Common locations of kidney stones. (From Monahan F et al: *Phipps' medical-surgical nursing: health and illness perspectives*, ed 8, St. Louis, 2007, Mosby.)

TABLE 22-4 Kidney Stones: Characteristics and Treatments

Type	Possible Cause	Characteristic	Treatment
Cystine	Genetic	Defect in transport of cystine across kidney and gastrointestinal tract that causes buildup of cystine	Penicillamine; alkalinize urine
Uric acid	Gout, genetic	Seen more in men, especially Jewish men	Allopurinol, potassium citrate, diet change (reduce purines)
Struvite	Urinary tract infection	Seen more in women	Antimicrobials, surgery
Calcium phosphate	Hyperparathyroidism or oxalate stones	Appearance of struvite or oxalate stones	Treat hyperparathyroidism; alkalinize urine; reduce soda intake
Calcium oxalate	Genetic, idiopathic hypercalciuria	Small stones, seen more in men	Increase water intake; decrease oxalate in diet

break up kidney stones; it can be performed while the patient sits in water or the surgeon can direct an ultrasonic device toward the stones while the patient is in the operating room. Ureteroscopes are lighted instruments that are inserted through the urethra; the stone is then retrieved by the physician with the help of an attached camera and endoscopic instruments. A more invasive procedure would require surgery to remove the stone(s). Drinking plenty of water is important because this helps to flush out any small stones and may help prevent the formation of future stones. Another measure to reduce the incidence of kidney stones is to limit caffeinated fluids such as coffee, tea, and sodas. Depending on the types of stones affecting the kidneys, certain foods should be avoided to deter further formation.

Drug Treatments. Analgesics can be used for relieving pain; common OTC drugs include a variety of nonsteroidal antiinflammatory drugs (NSAIDs). Calcium channel blockers (CCBs; e.g., nifedipine) and alpha-blockers (e.g., tamsulosin, Flomax) can acclerate the passage of stones and thereby reduce pain. The mechanism of action of CCBs is unclear; however, it is known that they act on the ureter. Agents used to prevent calcium stones include thiazides and potassium citrate. Agents to prevent formation of uric acid stones are allopurinol and potassium citrate. Captopril, tiopronin, and potassium citrate can help deter the formation of cystine stones. Antibiotics are also used if infection occurs.

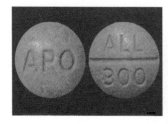

GENERIC NAME: allopurinol
TRADE NAME: Zyloprim
INDICATION: uric acid kidney stones
ROUTE OF ADMINISTRATION: oral
COMMON ADULT DOSAGE: 200-300 mg once daily OR in divided doses
SIDE EFFECTS: N/V, diarrhea, dizziness or drowsiness; serious hypersensitivity and rashes
AUXILIARY LABELS:
■ May cause dizziness/drowsiness.
■ Take with a full glass of water.

GENERIC NAME: potassium citrate
TRADE NAME: Urocrit-K
INDICATION: calcium kidney stones, uric acid kidney stones
ROUTE OF ADMINISTRATION: oral
COMMON ADULT DOSAGE: 10-20 mEq three times daily with meals; maximum dosage of 100 mEq/day depending on lab values of urinary citrate
SIDE EFFECTS: N/V, diarrhea, gas
AUXILIARY LABEL:
■ Take with food.

Urinary Tract Infection (UTI)

A urinary tract infection is an infection (either bacterial or fungal) of any part of the urinary tract (kidneys, bladder, ureters, and/or urethra). Each year, approximately 8 million people consult their physician for a UTI, with the majority of patients being women. The most common UTI is caused by the bacterium *Escherichia coli* (*E. coli*) from the colon. If it reaches the urethra, it can travel upward and multiply, infecting various parts of the renal system. If the infection is focused in the urethra, it is called urethritis. Cystitis indicates infection/inflammation of the bladder, and pyelonephritis is infection/inflammation of the kidney. Sexually transmitted diseases (STDs) are another cause of UTIs. Persons with various preexisting conditions may be more likely to have infections. Immunocompromised people and patients with diabetes are at risk because of a weakened immune system. Symptoms vary with each type of infection but can include painful, burning sensation when urinating, fever, lack of urine output, cloudy or bloody urine, nausea, and vomiting.

Prognosis. The prognosis for UTIs is good if proper treatment is taken.

Non–Drug Treatment. There are several precautions that can be taken to ensure that bacteria do not enter the urethra. These include the following: wipe from front to back after urination or defecation; take showers instead of baths; make sure the genital area is cleaned both before and after sexual intercourse; urinate following intercourse to flush the urethra of introduced bacteria.

Drug Treatment. Antimicrobial agents are the main course of treatment for most UTIs, although it depends on proper identification of pathogens that are responsible. For bacterial infections, medication such as Septra, or a cephalosporin or fluoroquinolone type agent may be prescribed. For symptomatic fungal urinary tract infections, fluconazole (Diflucan) or other antifungal agents may be prescribed. If the infection is caused by *Chlamydia* or is an uncomplicated gonorrheal infection, a tetracycline drug may be indicated although it is not effective for treatment of all types of STDs. Specific drug action for these antibiotics is given in Chapter 25. The following are three examples of medications used specifically for uncomplicated UTIs caused by strains of *E. coli* and *Enterococcus faecalis*. Table 22-5 lists the most common agents used to treat the various causes of UTIs. Even though most symptoms will disappear in a few days, it is important that the entire course of medication be finished.

Tech Note!

An infection that is acquired by the patient while in the hospital or an institutional setting is a **nosocomial infection.** Many nosocomial urinary tract infections are caused by catheterization or cystoscopic examinations. Regardless of the cause, it is important to determine the specific organism in order to prescribe the proper medication.

ANTIINFECTIVE ANTIBIOTIC

GENERIC NAME: fosfomycin
TRADE NAME: Monurol
INDICATION: acute cystitis/uncomplicated UTI in women
ROUTE OF ADMINISTRATION: oral granules
COMMON ADULT DOSAGE: 3-g packet in 90 to 120 mL (3-4 ounces) of cold water, given as a single dose
SIDE EFFECTS: nausea, diarrhea, abdominal cramps, flatulence
AUXILIARY LABELS:

■ Mix in water.
■ May cause diarrhea.
■ May cause nausea.
■ Important: Finish all of this medication unless otherwise directed by prescriber.

UTI ANTIBIOTIC

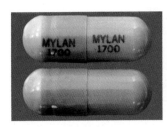

GENERIC NAME: nitrofurantoin
TRADE NAME: Macrobid, Macrodantin
INDICATION: acute cystitis/uncomplicated UTI
ROUTE OF ADMINISTRATION: oral
COMMON ADULT DOSAGE: Macrobid: 100 mg twice daily; Macrodantin: 50 to 100 mg four times daily
SIDE EFFECTS: nausea
AUXILIARY LABELS:

■ May cause brownish urine.
■ Important: Finish all of this medication unless otherwise directed by prescriber.

NOTE: Female patients should avoid taking if breast-feeding an infant <1 month of age.

TABLE 22-5 Treatments for Urinary Tract Infections* (Based on Oral Adult Dosages Unless Otherwise Indicated)

Generic Name	Trade Name	Type of Infection†	Normal Adult Dosage
Antibiotics			
Sulfonamides with Trimethoprim			
sulfamethoxazole/ trimethoprim	Septra DS, Bactrim	Uncomplicated UTIs	Septra DS: 1 DS tablet q12h
Penicillins			
amoxicillin	Amoxil	Uncomplicated UTIs	500 mg q12h
Penicillin and Beta-Lactamase Inhibitor Combination			
amoxicillin/ clavulanate	Augmentin	Drug-resistant UTIs caused by *Enterococcus* or *S. saprophyticus*†	500 mg q12h
Fluoroquinolones			
norfloxacin	Noroxin	UTIs or cystitis caused by *E. coli, E. faecalis, Klebsiella, P. mirabilis, Staphylococcus* strains, *P. vulgaris, S. aureus, E. cloacae, S. marcescens*	400 mg q12h
ofloxacin	Floxin	UTIs or cystitis caused by *E. coli, E. faecalis, Klebsiella, P. mirabilis, Staphylococcus* strains, *P. vulgaris, S. aureus, E. cloacae, S. marcescens*	200 mg q12h
Nitrofurantoins			
nitrofurantoin	Macrodantin	UTIs caused by *E. coli, Klebsiella,* enterococci, *S. aureus*	50-100 mg q6h
nitrofurantoin	Macrobid	Acute cystitis caused by strains of monohydrate/macrocrystals of *E. coli* or *S. saprophyticus*	100 mg q12h
Tetracyclines			
tetracycline	Sumycin	Uncomplicated gonorrhea caused by *C. trachomatis*	500 mg q6h 500 mg qid
doxycycline	Vibramycin	Uncomplicated gonorrhea Chronic UTIs	100 mg q12h × 1 day, then 100 mg/day 100 mg q12h
minocycline	Minocin	Nongonococcal urethritis caused by *C. trachomatis*	100 mg q12h
demeclocycline	Declomycin	Gram-positive and gram- negative bacteria	150 mg qid or 300 mg bid
First-Generation Cephalosporins			
cephalexin	Keflex	UTIs or acute prostatitis caused by *E. coli, P. mirabilis, K. pneumoniae*	250 mg q6h or 500 mg q12h
cefadroxil	Duricef	UTIs caused by *E. coli, P. mirabilis, Klebsiella*	For cystitis: 1-2 g/day For all other UTIs: 1 g bid
Second-Generation Cephalosporins			
cefaclor	Ceclor	UTIs, cystitis, and pyelonephritis caused by *E. coli, P. mirabilis, Klebsiella,* and coagulase-negative staphylococci	250-500 mg q8h

TABLE 22-5 Treatments for Urinary Tract Infections* (Based on Oral Adult Dosages Unless Otherwise Indicated)—cont'd

Generic Name	Trade Name	Type of Infection†	Normal Adult Dosage
cefuroxime	Ceftin	Uncomplicated UTIs caused by *E. coli* or *K. pneumoniae*	250 mg bid
loracarbef	Lorabid	UTIs caused by *E. coli* or *S. saphrophyticus* Pyelonephritis caused by *E. coli*	200 mg/day 400 mg q12h
Third-Generation Cephalosporins			
cefpodoxime	Vantin	Uncomplicated UTIs Acute, uncomplicated urethritis caused by *N. gonorrhoeae,* including penicillinase-producing strains	100 mg q12h 200 mg × 1 dose
ceftriaxone	Rocephin	Complicated and uncomplicated UTIs caused by *E. coli, P. mirabilis, P. vulgaris, M. morganii,* or *K. pneumoniae*	500 mg to 1 g bid (IV or IM only)
Miscellaneous Antibiotics			
trimethoprim	Trimpex	UTIs caused by *E. coli, P. mirabilis, Klebsiella, Enterobacter* spp., coagulase-negative *Staphylococcus* (used for drug-resistant stains)	100 mg q12h
fosfomycin	Monurol	Acute cystitis in women due to *E. coli, E. faecalis*	3 g (dissolve 1 sachet) × 1 dose
Urinary Analgesics			
phenazopyridine	Pyridium	Relieves pain, urgency, discomfort caused by UTIs	200 mg tid
methenamine	Urised	Relieves bladder spasms	2 tabs qid
flavoxate	Uripas	Relieves dysuria, nocturia, pain, frequency, bladder spasms	100 mg tid to qid

*Duration of treatment is dependent on agent used, severity of the infection (complicated versus uncomplicated), and other factors. Please see individual prescribing information for more detail.
†*C. trachomatis,* Chlamydia trachomatis; *E. cloacae,* Enterobacter cloacae; *E. faecalis,* Enterococcus faecalis; *K. pneumoniae,* Klebsiella pneumoniae; *M. morganii,* Morganella morganii; *N. gonorrhoeae,* Neisseria gonorrhoeae; *P. mirabilis,* Proteus mirabilis; *P. vulgaris,* Proteus vulgaris; *S. aureus,* Staphylococcus aureus; *S. marcescens,* Serratia marcescens, *S. saprophyticus,* Staphylococcus saprophyticus.

CEPHALOSPORIN ANTIBIOTIC

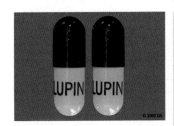

GENERIC NAME: cephalexin
TRADE NAME: Keflex
INDICATION: acute cystitis/uncomplicated UTI or acute bacterial prostatitis
ROUTE OF ADMINISTRATION: oral
COMMON ADULT DOSAGE: UTI: 500 mg q12h; prostatitis: 500 mg q6h
SIDE EFFECTS: mild N/V, diarrhea, dizziness
AUXILIARY LABELS:

- Important: Finish all of this medication unless otherwise directed by prescriber.
- May cause dizziness.
- Take with food or milk.

TABLE 22-6 Drugs Commonly Used to Treat Bacterial Prostatitis

Generic Name (Brand Name)	Usual Oral Adult Dosage for Prostatitis
sulfamethoxazole/trimethoprim (Septra DS)*	1 DS tablet twice daily
ciprofloxaxin (Cipro)	500 mg twice daily
levofloxacin (Levaquin)	500 mg once daily
ofloxacin (Floxin)	400 mg twice daily
norfloxacin (Noroxin)	400 mg twice daily
cephalexin (Keflex)	500 mg q6h
doxycycline (Vibramycin)	100 mg twice daily

*Septra DS is usually the drug of choice; if allergy or treatment failure, then a fluoroquinolone is often used. A tetracycline is added if *Chlamydia* is a potential cause.

Prostatitis

Inflammation of the prostate gland, which surrounds the urethra, is referred to as prostatitis. This condition can interfere with the ability to urinate. Symptoms include painful urination and difficulty urinating. The patient often has a concurrent urinary tract infection; the organism typically responsible is *E. coli*. This condition affects mostly young and middle-aged men. Risk factors include trauma and infection of the urethra or a urinary catheter. Treatment includes alpha-blockers to relax the affected area and improve urinary flow and analgesics for pain. Selection of an antibiotic must include the choice of a drug that penetrates the prostate gland tissue. For a list of antibiotics used to treat prostatitis, see Table 22-6. For information on the prostate gland, see Chapter 15.

Prognosis. Medications that treat prostatitis are usually prescribed for a longer duration than those used to treat UTIs. In fact, it may take 1 month or longer to eradicate a chronic infection.

Non–Drug Treatment. Bed rest and adequate hydration (at least 8 oz of water daily) are important while recovering from prostatitis. Other supportive treatments include sitz baths to relieve pain.

Drug Treatment. Antibiotics are chosen based on the specific organism identified and may first be given intravenously for up to 1 week, followed by oral administration. For infections caused by a sexually transmitted disease, an injection of ceftriaxone followed by a 10-day course of doxycycline or floxacin may be administered.

Incontinence

A common condition that affects millions of Americans is incontinence, which is the loss of control over urination and/or defecation. This chapter will discuss the issue of urinary incontinence. Older adults, especially females, are more prone to this condition; women who have multiple pregnancies tend to develop this condition later in life because of the stretching of pelvic muscles during childbirth. The weakening of these muscles can worsen over time. Micturition is the term commonly used to describe urination. Although the bladder can store almost 1 L of fluid, receptors are triggered when the bladder fills about halfway. Even after urinating, there is always a small amount (approximately 100 mL) of urine left in the bladder. When coughing or sneezing occurs, there may be enough force placed on the bladder to release a small amount of urine. This is called stress incontinence. Weight gain also can intensify this type of condition. Urge incontinence is involuntary urination resulting from a sudden, uncontrollable impulse to urinate. Urge incontinence has several causes, such as decreased

TABLE 22-7 Types of Urinary Incontinence

Type	Possible Causes	Possible Treatment
Stress	Relaxed pelvic muscles because of lower estrogen levels, multiple pregnancies	Kegel exercises; weight loss; vaginal estrogen creams or rings
Urge	In most cases specific cause not identified; neurological dysfunction may contribute in some patients (e.g., underlying central nervous system disorders such as Alzheimer's disease, Parkinson's disease, spinal cord injury, stroke, tumors, and bladder disorders)	Anticholinergic agents; treat underlying cause or condition; vaginal estrogen creams
Reflex	Central nervous system disorder	Treat underlying cause or condition; surgery; alpha-adrenergic blockers
Functional	Age: older adults lose mobility and balance	Change in environment; timed voiding; implement care plan for person
Overflow	Hyperplasia, bladder neck obstruction following surgery	Catheterization; bethanechol to increase bladder contractions; surgery

bladder capacity, infection, or irritation. In addition, increased fluid intake, including alcohol or caffeine ingestion, can increase the risk.

Types of urinary incontinence are listed in Table 22-7.

Prognosis. Often incontinence can be overcome if the patient seeks help from his or her physician. If incontinence cannot be corrected by exercise or medication, certain medical procedures or surgery (in some cases) can alleviate the problem.

Non–Drug Treatment. The most common non–drug therapy for most types of incontinence is the Kegel exercise. This is an exercise that involves strengthening of the pelvic floor muscles. The exercise requires that the patient tighten the muscles around the pelvis in the same fashion as he or she would to hold urine; Kegel exercises can be performed standing or sitting. The exercise regimen typically prescribed is sets of 10 exercises performed 10 times daily over several weeks.

Drug Treatment. The following are samples of the types of medications commonly used to treat incontinence.

ANTICHOLINERGIC

GENERIC NAME: trospium chloride
TRADE NAME: Sanctura, Sanctura XR
INDICATION: overactive bladder (OAB) with symptoms of urge urinary incontinence, urgency, and frequency
ROUTE OF ADMINISTRATION: oral
COMMON ADULT DOSAGE: Sanctura: 20 mg twice daily; Sanctura XR: 60 mg every AM
SIDE EFFECTS: dry mouth, constipation
AUXILIARY LABELS:

- Do not crush, break, or chew.
- Take on an empty stomach.
- Avoid taking with alcohol (Sanctura XR).

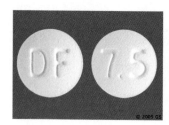

GENERIC NAME: darifenacin hydrobromide
TRADE NAME: Enablex EX
INDICATION: overactive bladder (OAB) with symptoms of urge urinary incontinence, urgency, and frequency
ROUTE OF ADMINISTRATION: oral
COMMON ADULT DOSAGE: 7.5 to 15 mg once daily
SIDE EFFECTS: dry mouth, diarrhea, nausea, dizziness, headache
AUXILIARY LABELS:
- May cause dizziness.
- May take with or without food
- Do not crush, break, or chew.

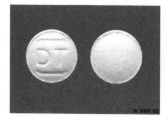

GENERIC NAME: tolterodine tartrate
TRADE NAME: Detrol, Detrol LA
INDICATION: overactive bladder (OAB) with symptoms of urge urinary incontinence, urgency, and frequency
ROUTE OF ADMINISTRATION: oral
COMMON ADULT DOSAGE: Detrol: 1 to 2 mg twice daily; Detrol LA: 2 to 4 mg once daily
SIDE EFFECTS: dizziness, drowsiness, blurred vision
AUXILIARY LABELS:
- Do not take if breast-feeding.
- May cause dizziness.
- Do not crush, break, or chew.

 Tech Alert!

Remember the following sound-alike/look-alike drugs:

Urised versus Urispas
chlorthalidone versus
    chlorothiazide
Bumex versus Buprenex
furosemide versus
    torsemide
metolazone versus
    metoclopramide
Ditropan versus
    diazepam

GENERIC NAME: oxybutinin
TRADE NAME: Ditropan, Ditropan XL, Oxytrol (Patch), Gelnique (topical gel)
INDICATION: overactive bladder (OAB), muscle spasms of the bladder and urinary tract
ROUTE OF ADMINISTRATION: oral, transdermal
COMMON ADULT DOSAGE: 5 mg 2 to 3 times daily; transdermal patch: apply patch every 3 to 4 days; transdermal gel: apply 1 packet topically once daily
SIDE EFFECTS: dizziness, drowsiness, blurred vision, dry mouth, headache, nausea, mild constipation
AUXILIARY LABELS:
- Take with a full glass of water.
- May cause dizziness/drowsiness.
- Do not crush, break, or chew (Ditropan XL).
- Transdermal patch or gel: For topical use only.

DO YOU REMEMBER THESE KEY POINTS?
- The location of the kidneys
- The functions of the kidneys
- The major components of the kidneys and urinary tract
- The functions of the glomerulus
- The conditions that require dialysis and the types of dialysis available
- The various types of medications that dialysis patients must receive
- The drug action of diuretics
- The major conditions affecting the urinary system and their treatments

REVIEW QUESTIONS

Multiple choice questions

1. Blood enters the kidneys through the:
   A. Renal fascia
   B. Renal artery
   C. Renal vein
   D. Hilus

2. All of the following are components of the nephron EXCEPT the:
   A. Glomerulus
   B. Urethra
   C. Bowman's capsule
   D. Loop of Henle

3. When taking loop diuretics, it should be necessary to take which of the following supplements?
   A. Potassium
   B. Calcium
   C. Multivitamins
   D. All of the above

4. The _____ is where sodium is transported actively along with chloride.
   A. Proximal convoluted tubule
   B. Distal convoluted tubule
   C. Loop of Henle
   D. Glomerulus

5. Edema commonly is associated with all of the following conditions EXCEPT:
   A. Hypertension
   B. Congestive heart failure
   C. Glaucoma
   D. Nephritis

6. Buffers have the ability to prevent:
   A. Large changes in pH
   B. Edema
   C. Renal failure
   D. Blood loss

7. Plasma is a component of:
   A. Buffers
   B. Water
   C. Blood
   D. Dialysis

8. Which of the following classifications of medications include diuretics?
   A. Blood formers
   B. Thiazides
   C. Carbonic anhydrase inhibitors
   D. Both B and C

9. An example of active transport is when:
   A. Sodium is exchanged for hydrogen
   B. Potassium is exchanged for sodium
   C. Sodium and chloride leave the nephron
   D. Bicarbonate leaves the nephron

10. Loop diuretics and thiazides:
    A. Have a slow mechanism of action
    B. Cause a loss of potassium
    C. Cause a loss of sodium
    D. Must be taken with a potassium-sparing agent

11. The heart's inability to pump sufficient blood volume to and from the body system, causing a host of conditions, is best described as:
A. CAD
B. CHF
C. MI
D. None of the above

12. Kidney stones can be caused by:
A. Calcium phosphate or struvite
B. Uric acid or cystine
C. Struvite or calcium oxalate
D. All of the above

13. Which class(es) of drugs listed below may be used to treat UTIs caused by *Chlamydia*?
A. Tetracyclines
B. Fluoroquinolones
C. Cephalosporins
D. Both A and B

14. Which of the procedures can be used to treat certain kidney stones?
A. Lithotripsy
B. Ureteroscopes
C. Surgery
D. All of the above

15. Which of the medications below is NOT a potassium-sparing agent?
A. Midamor
B. Lasix
C. Demadex
D. Both B and C

True/False

If the statement is false, then change it to make it true.

_____ **1.** The connective tissue that holds the kidneys in place is called the peritoneal membrane.

_____ **2.** All food is metabolized and excreted by the kidneys.

_____ **3.** When giving thiazide diuretics, a potassium replacement is not necessary.

_____ **4.** A blood urea nitrogen test measures the uric nitrogen content within the liver.

_____ **5.** Tetracyclines are often used to treat gonorrhea.

_____ **6.** Weak acids and bases are reabsorbed via the nephron.

_____ **7.** Waste products from the kidneys are called urine.

_____ **8.** Urine pH is between 4 and 6, which is acidic.

_____ **9.** The two mechanisms of reabsorption include ion exchange and active transport.

_____ **10.** Epoetin is given to dialysis patients to counteract iron deficiency.

_____ **11.** Kidney stones can be treated with medication alone.

_____ **12.** UTIs are most often caused by bacterial, viral, and fungal infections.

_____ **13.** Keflex can be used to treat both UTIs and prostatitis caused by *E. coli*.

_____ **14.** Incontinence is the lack of control over urination and/or defecation.

_____ **15.** Pyridium can be given to patients with UTIs to relieve pain and discomfort.

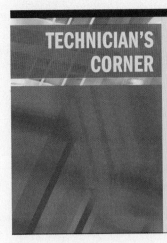

TECHNICIAN'S CORNER

Ms. Lewis went to the physician because of swelling in her legs and shortness of breath. After blood tests and a physical examination, she was diagnosed with congestive heart failure. The physician prescribed the following medications to be filled in the pharmacy:

Spironolactone 25 mg 1 tablet every AM
Furosemide 20 mg 1 tablet every AM

Question

What are the classifications of these medications, and what auxiliary labels will you place on the vial? Also, what medication, if any, did the physician omit that you would bring to the attention of the pharmacist?

BIBLIOGRAPHY

Campbell N, Jane R: *Biology*, ed 8, Redwood City, 2007, Benjamin/Cummings.

Clayton B, Yvonne S, Renae H: *Basic pharmacology for nurses*, ed 14, Philadelphia, 2006, Elsevier Science.

Drug facts and comparisons, ed 63, St Louis, 2008, Lippincott Williams & Wilkins.

Heitkemper M, et al: *Medical-surgical nursing: assessment and management of clinical problems*, ed 7, St Louis, 2007, Mosby.

Lacy C, et al: *Lexi Comp's drug information handbook*, ed 18, Hudson, 2009, Lexi-Comp.

Potter P, Anne P: *Fundamentals of nursing*, ed 6, St Louis, 2004, Mosby.

Salerno E: *Pharmacology for health professionals*, St Louis, 1999, Mosby.

Stedman's concise medical dictionary for health professionals, ed 3, Baltimore, 1997, Williams & Wilkins.

Wilson B, Margaret S, Kelly S: *Prentice Hall nurse's drug guide 2009*, Upper Saddle River, 2008, Prentice Hall.

WEBSITES

National Kidney and Urologic Diseases Information Clearinghouse: http://kidney.niddk.nih.gov/Kudiseases/pubs/stones_ez/

23

Cardiovascular System

Objectives

UPON COMPLETING THIS CHAPTER, YOU SHOULD BE ABLE TO DO THE FOLLOWING:

- List both trade and generic names covered in this chapter.
- Describe the location and function of the heart.
- Name the four chambers of the heart.
- Explain how the heart receives nourishment.
- List the major disease states of the heart.
- Explain the possible causes of coronary artery disease, congestive heart failure, and hypertension.
- List the three types of angina.
- Describe how hypertension and hyperlipidemia can contribute to heart conditions.
- Compare the differences between arteriosclerosis and atherosclerosis.
- List the drugs used to treat heart conditions.
- List the drugs used to treat hypertension.
- Apply the correct auxiliary labels to the drugs covered.
- Describe the indications for and mechanisms of the following classifications of drugs:

  Angiotensin-converting enzyme inhibitors
  Anticoagulants
  Beta-blockers
  Calcium channel blockers
  Diuretics
  Nitrates
  Thrombolytics

Artery *A vessel that carries oxygenated blood from the heart to the tissues of the body*

Capillary *Extremely small vessel that connects the ends of the smallest arteries (arterioles) to the smallest veins (venules), where exchange of nutrients, waste products, O_2, and CO_2 occurs; blood vessels at cellular level*

Coagulation *To solidify or change from a fluid state to a solid state, as in forming a blood clot*

Diuretic *An agent that increases urine output and excretion of water from the body*

Embolism *The formation of a clot from any foreign substance that obstructs a vessel*

Endocardium *The thin membrane that lines the interior of the heart; inner layer of the heart wall*

Enzyme *A protein that accelerates a reaction by reducing the amount of energy required to initiate a reaction; also called a biological catalyst*

Epicardium *The outer layer of the heart wall; the inner layer of the pericardium*

Myocardium *The middle muscular layer of the heart wall; consists of cardiac muscle tissue*

Pericardium *Fluid-filled membrane that surrounds the heart; also called pericardial sac*

Syndrome *A set of conditions that occur together*

Thrombin *An enzyme that is formed in coagulating blood from prothrombin; thrombin reacts with fibrinogen and converts it to fibrin, which is essential in the formation of blood clots; thrombin levels tested by performing a prothrombin time or partial thromboplastin time blood test*

Thrombolytic *Medication used to break up a thrombus or blood clot*

Vein *A vessel that carries deoxygenated blood to or toward the heart*

Venae cavae *The large veins that carry deoxygenated blood from the upper (superior vena cava) and lower (inferior vena cava) parts of the body to the right atrium of the heart*

EXAMPLES OF CARDIOVASCULAR AGENTS

Trade Name	Generic Name	Pronunciation	Trade Name	Generic Name	Pronunciation
Alpha-Blocker Antihypertensives			Norpace	disopyramide	(dye-so-**peer**-a-mide)
Cardura	doxazosin	(dok-**sah**-zo-sin)	Pronestyl, Procanbid	procainamide	(pro-**cane**-ah-mide)
Hytrin	terazosin	(tur-**ah**-zoh-sin)			
Minipress	prazosin	(**pra**-zoe-sin)	Quinidex	quinidine	(**kwin**-ah-deen)
			Rythmol	propafenone	(proe-pa-**feen**-none)
Centrally Acting Antihypertensives			Tikosyn	dofetilide	(doe-**fet**-ah-lide)
Aldomet	methyldopa	(meth-ill-**doe**-pah)			
Catapres	clonidine	(**klon**-ih-deen)	**Angiotensin-Converting Enzyme Inhibitors (ACE Inhibitors or ACEIs)**		
	reserpine	(re-**sir**-peen)	Accupril	quinapril	(**kwin**-a-pril)
			Altace	ramipril	(ray-**mi**-pril)
Antiarrhythmics			Capoten	captopril	(**cap**-tow-pril)
Betapace, Betapace AF	sotalol	(soe-**ta**-lol)	Lotensin	benazepril	(ben-**ayz**-ah-pril)
			Mavik	trandolapril	(tran-**dole**-a-pril)
Cordarone, Pacerone	amiodarone	(a-mi-**oh**-da-rone)	Monopril	fosinopril	(foe-**sin**-oh-pril)
Lanoxin	digoxin	(di-**jox**-in)	Prinivil, Zestril	lisinopril	(lih-**sin**-oh-pril)

Continued

EXAMPLES OF CARDIOVASCULAR AGENTS—cont'd

Trade Name	Generic Name	Pronunciation
Univasc	moexipril	(moe-**ex**-a-pril)
Vasotec	enalapril	(eh-**nal**-ah-pril)

Angiotensin Receptor Blockers (ARBs)

Trade Name	Generic Name	Pronunciation
Atacand	candesartan	(kan-de-**sar**-tan)
Avapro	irbesartan	(erb-ba-**sar**-tan)
Cozaar	losartan	(low-**sar**-tan)
Diovan	valsartan	(val-**sar**-tan)
Micardis	telmisartan	(tel-meh-**sar**-tan)
Teveten	eprosartan	(eh-pro-**sar**-tan)

Beta-Blockers (BBs)

Trade Name	Generic Name	Pronunciation
Brevibloc	esmolol	(**es**-mo-lol)
Inderal	propranolol	(pro-**pran**-oh-lol)
Kerlone	betaxolol	(be-**tax**-oh-lol)
Lopressor	metoprolol	(meh-toe-**pro**-lol)
Sectral	acebutolol	(a-se-**byoo**-toe-lol)
Tenormin	atenolol	(ay-**ten**-oh-lol)
Trandate	labetalol	(lah-**bet**-ah-lol)
Visken	pindolol	(**pin**-doe-lol)

Calcium Channel Blockers (CCBs)

Trade Name	Generic Name	Pronunciation
Calan, Isoptin	verapamil	(ver-**ap**-ah-mill)
Cardene	nicardipine	(nye-**kar**-de-peen)
Cardizem	diltiazem	(dill-**tie**-ah-zem)
DynaCirc	isradipine	(iz-**ra**-di-peen)
Norvasc	amlodipine	(am-**low**-di-peen)
Plendil	felodipine	(fe-**low**-de-peen)
Procardia	nifedipine	(nye-**fed**-ih-peen)
Sular	nisoldipine	(nye-**sol**-di-peen)

Anticoagulant

Trade Name	Generic Name	Pronunciation
Coumadin	warfarin	(**war**-far-in)
Heparin	heparin	(heh-par-in)

Low-Molecular-Weight Heparins (LMWHs)

Trade Name	Generic Name	Pronunciation
Fragmin	dalteparin	(**dal**-te-**par**-in)
Lovenox	enoxaparin	(ee-nox-**ap**-a-rin)

Antiplatelet Agents

Trade Name	Generic Name	Pronunciation
Aggrenox	aspirin/dipyridamole	(**as**-pir-rin/ dye-peer-**id**-a-mole)
Bayer	aspirin	(**as**-pir-rin)
Plavix	clopidogrel	(kloh-**pid**-oh-grel)
Pletal	cilostazol	(sil-oh-**sta**-zol)
Ticlid	ticlopidine	(tye-**kloe**-pi-deen)

Nitrate Antianginals

Trade Name	Generic Name	Pronunciation
Imdur, Monoket	isosorbide mononitrate	(**eye**-soe-**sor**-bide **mon**-oh-**nye**-trate)
Isordil	isosorbide dinitrate	(**eye**-soe-**sor**-bide dye-**nye**-trate)
Nitrostat, Tridil	nitroglycerin	(**nye**-troe-**glis**-sir-rin)
Minitran, Nitro-Dur	nitroglycerin patches	(**nye**-troe-**glis**-sir-rin)

Piperazine Antianginal

Trade Name	Generic Name	Pronunciation
Ranexa	ranolazine	(ra-**noe**-la-zeen)

Antihyperlidemic Agents

Trade Name	Generic Name	Pronunciation
Lovaza	omega-3-acid ethyl esters	(oh-**may**-ga 3 **as**-id **eth**-il **es**-ters)
Niacor	niacin	(**nye**-a-sin)
Zetia	ezetimibe	(eh-**zet**-eh-mi-be)

Fibrates

Trade Name	Generic Name	Pronunciation
Lopid	gemfibrozil	(gem-**fib**-row-**zil**)
Antara, Lipofen, Tricor	fenofibrate	(**fen**-no-**fye**-brate)
TriLipix, Fibricor	fenofibric acid	(**fen**-oh-fye-**brik as**-id)

HMG-CoA Reductase Inhibitors ("Statins")

Trade Name	Generic Name	Pronunciation
Zocor	simvastatin	(sym-vah-**stat**-in)
Livalo	pitavastatin	(pit-**av**-a-**stat**-in)
Lipitor	atorvastatin	(a-**tor**-va-stat-in)
Altoprev, Mevacor	lovastatin	(low-**vah**-stat-in)
Pravachol	pravastatin	(**prav**-ah-stat-in)
Crestor	rosuvastatin	(row-**soo**-va-stat-in)
Lescol	fluvastatin	(**floo**-va-stat-in)

Bile Acid Sequestrant Agents

Trade Name	Generic Name	Pronunciation
Colestid	colestipol	(koe-**les**-ti-pole)
Questran	cholestyramine	(koe-**les**-teer-a-meen)
WelChol	colesevelam	(**koe**-le-**sev**-e-lam)

Diuretics

Trade Name	Generic Name	Pronunciation
Aldactone	spironolactone	(spear-**on**-oh-**lak**-tone)
Ezride, Microzide	hydrochlorothiazide	(hye-dro-klor-o-**thy**-zide)
Bumex	bumetanide	(byew-**met**-ah-nide)
Demadex	torsemide	(**tore**-se-mide)
Diamox	acetazolamide	(ah-see-ta-**zole**-a-mide)
Diuril	chlorothiazide	(klor-oh-**thye**-a-zide)
Dyrenium	triamterene	(try-**am**-tur-reen)
Lasix	furosemide	(feur-**oh**-sah-myde)
Lozol	indapamide	(in-**dap**-ah-mide)
Zaroxolyn	metolazone	(meh-**tole**-uh-zone)

Vasodilators

Trade Name	Generic Name	Pronunciation
Apresoline	hydralazine	(high-**dral**-ah-zeen)
Loniten	minoxidil	(min-**ox**-i-dill)
NTG	nitroglycerin	(nye-troe-**glih**-sur-rin)

Agents to Reverse Anticoagulation

Trade Name	Generic Name	Pronunciation
Mephyton	phytonadione, vitamin K_1	(fy-toe-na-**dye**-own)
Protamine	protamine sulfate	(pro-**toe**-mean)

Thrombolytics

Trade Name	Generic Name	Pronunciation
Kinlytic	urokinase	(**your**-oh-**kye**-nase)
Activase	alteplase (t-PA)	(**al**-teh-**place**)
Retavase	reteplase	(reh-**teh**-place)
TNKase	tenecteplase	(ten-**ek**-te-place)

MEDICAL TERMINOLOGY OF THE CARDIOVASCULAR SYSTEM

Word Parts

angi/o, vas/o	Vessel
arteri/o	Artery
ather/o	Plaque
capill/o	Capillary
card/o, cardi/o	Heart
hem/o, hemat/o	Blood
my/o	Muscle
phleb/o, ven/o	Vein
thromb/o	Clot

Prefixes

brady-	Slow
end-	Within
endo-	Within
epi-	Upon, on, by, or near
isch-	To hold back, suppress
lipid-	Fat
peri-	Surrounding
tachy-	Rapid
valvul-	Valve

Suffixes

-ar, -ial	Pertaining to
-cytes	Cells
-emia	Blood condition
-ia, -ism	Condition
-itis	Inflammation
-lytic	Destroy
-stenosis	Abnormal narrowing
-um, -us	Singular noun ending

Conditions

Angina	Severe, often constricting pain affecting pectoral, or chest, region caused by lack of oxygen to heart cells
Arrhythmia	Irregular rhythm of heart
Arteriosclerosis	Thickening and loss of elasticity (hardening) of arterial walls caused by multiple conditions; atherosclerosis is most common form
Atherosclerosis	Buildup of fatty materials or plaque, usually of cholesterol, in arterial blood vessels
Bradycardia	Abnormally slow heart rate
Carditis	Inflammation of heart
Congestive heart failure (CHF)	Inability of heart to pump efficiently and meet body's demands
Coronary artery disease (CAD)	Abnormal condition affecting heart's arteries that results in narrowing of lumen of coronary arteries and lowering of oxygen and nutrient delivery to heart muscle
Essential hypertension	High blood pressure in which no known cause can be found
Hyperlipidemia	Abnormally high concentration of lipids in blood
Hypertension	High blood pressure
Hypotension	Low blood pressure
Myocardial infarction	Death of a portion of heart muscle
Stroke	Impaired cerebral blood flow caused by thrombosis, hemorrhage, or embolism
Tachycardia	Abnormally rapid heartbeat
Transient ischemic attack (TIA)	Temporary reduction of oxygen and blood in a portion of brain

THE CARDIOVASCULAR SYSTEM is a network of many complex interactions. These interactions involve the blood, lungs, arteries, and veins of the body and the heart muscle itself. We begin with an overview of the anatomy of the heart, followed by the most common conditions that affect the heart. The last section of this chapter discusses the treatments available for heart conditions, with particular emphasis on the medications used. Technicians fill many prescriptions for heart medications over their careers, and it is important to learn basic information about the classifications to assist the pharmacist.

Anatomy of the Heart

The heart is located in the chest cavity between the lungs. The heart is a large muscle that initiates systemic arterial pulse waves, causing blood to circulate throughout the body and supply it with nutrition and oxygen (Figure 23-1). Extending from the heart are large blood vessels called arteries. These arteries flow into smaller vessels called arterioles and then ultimately into very small blood vessels called **capillaries**. From the capillaries, oxygen and nutrients are exchanged throughout the tissues.

A normal heart beats from 60 to 100 times per minute and is about the size of a person's fist. The heart is surrounded by connective tissue called the **pericardium,** which in turn is anchored by ligaments to the chest wall and diaphragm. The heart wall is composed of three main layers:

1. *Endocardium* (inner layer): The endocardium has a smooth accordion pleat–like surface, which allows the heart wall to collapse when it contracts.
2. *Myocardium* (middle muscular layer): The myocardium is the heart muscle that contracts.
3. *Epicardium* (outer layer): The epicardium is the outer layer of the heart wall. This is also the inner layer of the pericardium. The coronary arteries that supply the heart with oxygenated blood and the coronary veins that return deoxygenated blood to the heart are located in the epicardium.

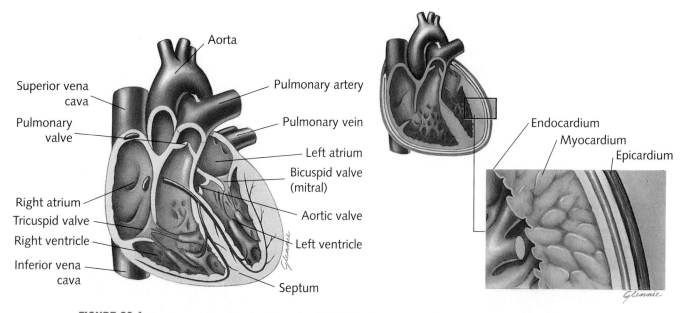

FIGURE 23-1   Anatomy of the heart. (From Gerdin J: *Health careers today*, ed 4, St Louis, 2007, Mosby.)

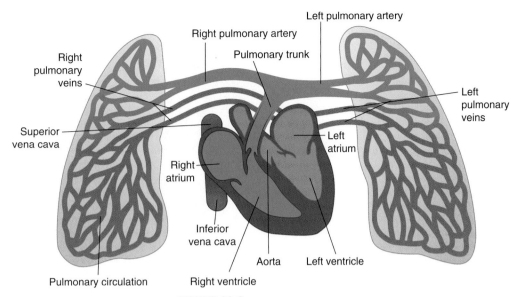

FIGURE 23-2 Blood oxygenation.

OXYGENATION

The heart has two pumps, each of which is composed of two chambers (Figure 23-2). The first two chambers are the right atrium and the right ventricle. Blood circulates through the body, exchanging oxygen, nutrients, and other substances to tissues and organs. The blood returns to the heart via two large **veins** called the superior and inferior **venae cavae**. The superior vena cava transports blood from the upper portion of the body, and the inferior vena cava carries blood from the lower portion of the body. The blood travels through the right atrium into the right ventricle. The right ventricle contracts, expelling blood into the pulmonary **arteries**; the pulmonary arteries carry blood to the lungs, where blood is fully oxygenated by the air that we breathe (see Chapter 18). The left atrium of the heart then receives the fully oxygenated blood from the lungs via the pulmonary veins. Blood then is passed into the left ventricle through the mitral valve. The left ventricle then contracts, expelling the blood into the aorta. In the aorta the blood initiates a pulse wave that carries it to all parts of the body (Figure 23-3). Although the heart is an efficient organ, it still must be oxygenated just like other organs. The main arteries that supply blood to the heart are called the coronary arteries.

CARDIAC CONDUCTION SYSTEM

The cardiac conduction system provides the electrical charge that makes the heart pump. This system is a lifetime battery that keeps our heartbeats in rhythm. This cardiac conduction system is operated by two nodes: the sinoatrial and atrioventricular nodes. The sinoatrial node is located in the upper right atrium wall (this is where the impulse begins). The signal then is sent down to the atrioventricular node, located in the septum between the right atrium and the right ventricle. As the cardiac impulse is sent from the sinoatrial to the atrioventricular node, it also is transmitted to the muscle fibers that run throughout the atria. From the atrioventricular node the impulse is conducted to the ventricles to initiate a ventricular beat by stimulation of the bundle branches and Purkinje fibers.

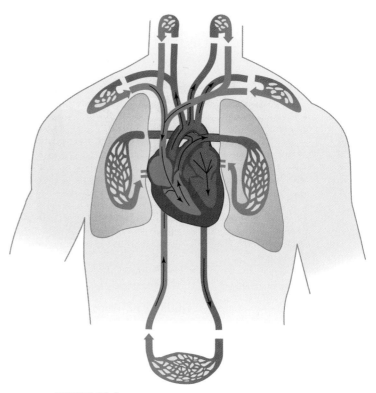

FIGURE 23-3 Circulation of blood through the body.

The Cardiac Cycle

The series of events that occur for one complete heartbeat is called the cardiac cycle. This cycle is composed of two sequences:

1. Systole: The myocardium squeezes blood from the heart chamber into the pulmonary artery or aorta.
2. Diastole: Blood is allowed to refill the chambers (relaxation). During diastole, the atria contract to pack 20% more blood into the ventricles. Most of the body's blood supply is cycled every minute through the heart.

Conditions Affecting the Heart

Cardiovascular diseases are responsible for 1 death every 37 seconds (american-heart.org). Diseases and conditions affecting the health of the heart include heart failure, heart attack, high blood pressure (BP), diabetes, obesity, high cholesterol level, stroke, arrhythmias, and congenital heart disease. Despite the widespread incidence of heart disease, available advancements in health care, new medications, and surgical techniques are helping individuals live longer. In addition, lifestyle changes—such as refraining from smoking, following an exercise regimen, and eating fewer high-fat foods—have helped lessen the incidence of cardiovascular diseases. Box 23-1 describes common cardiovascular conditions.

Both non–drug and drug treatments are covered for each condition as well as the prognosis (outcome). The common dosages for medications are based on recommendations for adults. In addition to the indications listed, many of the medications can be used for other conditions per the physician's recommendation. Table 23-1 lists the classifications of drugs used in the cardiovascular system. Combination drugs are listed in Table 23-2.

BOX 23-1 COMMON CONDITIONS AND DEFINITIONS

Angina pectoris: Pain and pressure in the chest caused by a lack of proper blood flow and oxygenation to the heart muscle

Arrhythmia: Irregular heartbeats resulting from a malfunction in the conduction system

Arteriosclerosis: A disease of the arterial vessels resulting from thickening, hardening, and loss of elasticity in the arterial walls

Atherosclerosis: A form of arteriosclerosis resulting from the buildup of fatty plaques in the walls of the arteries

Congestive heart failure (CHF): A condition in which the heart is unable to pump the amount of blood needed to meet the requirements of the body

Coronary artery disease (CAD): A term used to describe blood vessel disorders that affect the coronary arteries

Hyperlipidemia: High or excessive amounts of lipid (fat) in the blood that lead to arteriosclerosis and atherosclerosis

Hypertension: High blood pressure, which is considered a series of measurements with systolic pressure greater than 140 mm Hg and diastolic pressure greater than 90 mm Hg

Myocardial infarction (MI): Death of an area of heart muscle attributable to interruption of its blood supply through occlusion of the coronary arteries; also known as a heart attack.

Prehypertensive state: Blood pressure in the range of 120/80 to 139/89 mm Hg

Thrombosis: The formation of a blood clot within the vascular system

COMMON CONDITIONS

Hypertension

Hypertension is defined as intermittent or persistent elevation in diastolic or systolic blood pressure. High blood pressure is a prevalent problem in the United States, affecting millions of Americans. This disease also is known as the "silent killer" because there are usually no obvious signs of its presence. When a cause for hypertension cannot be established, the person is considered to have essential hypertension; of those with hypertension, essential hypertension is present in 19 out of 20 persons. One out of 20 persons has an identifiable cause for hypertension, such as medications, certain kidney diseases (such as glomerular nephritis), and diseases of the adrenal glands (such as Cushing's syndrome). Hypertension with a known cause is called secondary hypertension. When blood pressure suddenly rises to extremely high levels, it is known as malignant hypertension. This condition may occur in people who already have hypertension and may cause a life-threatening condition (called hypertensive crisis) that requires hospitalization and treatment to prevent or lessen the damage to the heart, kidneys, brain, and blood vessels. Some people who have advanced hypertension may have symptoms such as nosebleeds and/or headaches; however, most people do not have any symptoms, which is why it is important to monitor blood pressure, which can allow early detection and treatment. Whatever the cause of hypertension, the result is that the heart must work much harder to pump blood through the chambers and out into the body. Hypertension also can result from various conditions and risk factors such as those listed in Box 23-2.

The continuous overload on the coronary system also contributes to the development of atherosclerosis (hardening of the arteries) and can cause small ruptures of vessels within the heart. Common signs of high blood pressure can be confused with other symptoms not associated with hypertension, such as blurred vision, headache (H/A), and shortness of breath (SOB). Patients with hypertension should be informed by their physicians and pharmacists that many over-the-counter agents can affect their blood pressure. This includes

TABLE 23-1 **Drug Classifications**

Drug Classification	Use	Generic Name	Trade Name	Effect
ACE inhibitors	Hypertension	benazepril	Lotensin	Prevent blood vessel constriction
		lisinopril	Prinivil	
		captopril	Capoten	
		ramipril	Altace	
		fosinopril	Monopril	
		moexipril	Univasc	
Beta-blockers	Hypertension	nadolol	Corgard	Reduce workload of heart
		metoprolol	Lopressor	
		pindolol	Visken	
		bisoprolol	Zebeta	
		acebutolol	Sectral	
Calcium channel blockers	Hypertension	verapamil	Calan, Isoptin	Increase blood flow and decrease vessel constriction in heart
		diltiazem	Cardizem	
		nifedipine	Adalat, Procardia	
Bile acid sequestrants	Hypercholesterolemia	cholestyramine	Prevalite, Questran	Lower cholesterol
		colestipol	Colestid	
Statins	Hypercholesterolemia	atorvastatin	Lipitor	Lower cholesterol
		lovastatin	Mevacor	
		pravastatin	Pravachol	
		simvastatin	Zocor	
Diuretics	Edema	hydrochlorothiazide	Ezride, Microzide	Reduce body fluids
		chlorothiazide	Diuril	
		furosemide	Lasix	
		bumetadine	Bumex	
		spironolactone	Aldactone	
		triamterene	Dyrenium	
		metolazone	Zaroxolyn	
Nitrates	Angina	nitroglycerin	Nitrostat, Nitro-Dur	Relax blood vessels, allowing more blood to reach heart
		isosorbide dinitrate	Dilatrate-SR, Isordil	
Antiplatelet agents	Thrombosis	aspirin	Bayer, Ecotrin	Prevent blood clot formation
	Thrombosis	clopidogrel	Plavix	

antihistamines, decongestants, and ingredients in many different cold and allergy remedies.

Prognosis. With proper diet (and medications, if necessary) hypertension can normally be controlled.

Non–Drug Treatment. Individuals should have their blood pressure measured regularly throughout their lifetime to evaluate blood pressure for elevations or to seek medical attention if necessary. Three categories of hypertension are based on diastolic readings and two categories are based on systolic readings, as explained in Box 23-3. Even a mild case of hypertension can lead to problems later in life because of the extra work placed on the heart.

There are many risk factors that cannot be changed, such as family history. However, the following lifestyle changes can help reduce high blood pressure:

TABLE 23-2 **Classifications of Combination Drugs**

Drug Combinations	Use	Generic Name	Trade Name
ACE inhibitor/diuretic	Hypertension	captopril/HCTZ	Capozide
		fosinopril/HCTZ	Monopril HCT
		losartan/HCTZ	Hyzaar
		valsartan/HCTZ	Diovan HCT
		candesartan/HCTZ	Atacand HCT
		enalapril/HCTZ	Vaseretic
BB/diuretic	Hypertension	atenolol/HCTZ	Tenoretic
		propranolol/HCTZ	Inderide, Inderide LA
	HTN, angina, prevent MI	metoprolol/HCTZ	Lopressor HCT
Aldosterone Antagonist/diuretic	CHF, edema	spironolactone/HCTZ	Aldactazide
Angiotensin II antagonists/CCB	Hypertension and treat heart failure	amlodipine/valsartan	Exforge
	Hypertension	amlodipine/olmesartan	Azor
ACE inhibitor/CCB		diltiazem/enalapril	Teczem
		trandolapril/verapamil	Tarka
		enalapril/felodpine	Lexxel
Angiotensin II antagonist/CCB/ diuretic		amlodipine/valsartan/HCTZ	Exforge HCT
CCB/statin	Hypertension/ hypercholesterolemia	amlodipine/atorvastatin	Caduet
Statin/nicotinic acid	Lowers cholesterol, prevents heart disease	lovastatin/niacin	Advicor
		simvastatin/niacin	Simcor
Statin/Lipid absorption blocker	Lowers cholesterol	ezetimibe/simvastatin	Vytorin
Statin/Platelet inhibitor	Lowers cholesterol	pravastatin/aspirin	Pravigard PAC

ACE = Angiotensin Converting Enzyme; BB = Beta Blocker; CCB = Calcium Channel Blocker.

BOX 23-2 **EXAMPLES OF CONDITIONS THAT CAN LEAD TO HYPERTENSION**

Common Conditions or Factors That May Increase Risk for Hypertension
Adrenal gland conditions such as hyperthyroidism
Diabetes mellitus
Heart conditions such as coronary artery disease, atherosclerosis, angina, cardiomyopathy, congestive heart failure
Kidney conditions such as glomerular nephritis
Medications such as oral contraceptives, nasal decongestants
Pregnancy

Risk Factors for Essential Hypertension
1. Genetic
   Age
   Gender
   Race
2. Lifestyle
   Diet
   Anxiety
   Alcohol consumption
   Sodium intake
   Obesity
   Sedentary habits

BOX 23-3 CLASSIFICATION OF BLOOD PRESSURE MEASUREMENTS

First or top measurement (systolic blood pressure [SBP]): this represents the pressure in the arteries during contraction of the ventricles.

  Normal SBP: ≤120 mm Hg
  Prehypertensive state: between 120 and 139 mm Hg
  HTN (stage 1): 140 to 159 mm Hg
  Severe HTN (stage 2 HTN): ≥160 mm Hg

Second or bottom measurement (diastolic pressure [DBP]): this represents the pressure in the arteries during relaxation of the ventricles (the heart is at rest).

  Optimal DBP: <80 mm Hg
  Prehypertensive state: between 80 and 89 mm Hg
  HTN (stage 1): 90 to 99 mm Hg
  Severe HTN (stage 2 HTN): ≥100 mm Hg

- Maintain a healthy weight.
- Exercise regularly (moderate to vigorous exercise for 30 to 60 minutes per day on most or all days of the week).
- Avoid high-sodium foods such as potato chips, pickles, canned soups, and cold cut meats as well as table salt (reduce to about 1.5 g per day).
- Increase intake of fruits and vegetables daily to increase potassium intake. Potassium lowers blood pressure.
- Limit alcohol intake (no more than 2 drinks per day).
- Avoid high-sodium antacids and over-the-counter cold and sinus medications.
- Reduce stress through daily relaxation techniques.
- Stop smoking because this leads to atherosclerosis, which increases blood pressure.
- Follow the DASH diet (Dietary Approaches to Stop Hypertension), which encourages:
  - Vegetables
  - Fruits
  - Whole grains
  - Fish
  - Poultry
  - Nuts
  - Low fat
- Discourage the following foods:
  - Fats
  - Red meat
  - Sweets
  - Sugar-containing beverages

Persons with reduced kidney function should consult their physician before starting the DASH diet, because it is rich in potassium, which is not recommended for persons with kidney disorders.

Drug Treatment. If patients fail to achieve the desired blood pressure by making substantial changes in their lifestyle habits, medications may be prescribed. Treatment of hypertension (HTN) is given by a step-care approach as described in Box 23-4. Diuretics are commonly used to treat HTN although there are many medications available that are effective in controlling hypertension, including angiotensin-converting enzyme inhibitors (ACE inhibitors), beta-blockers (BBs), and calcium channel blockers (CCBs) (see ABCDs for the heart; see Types of

BOX 23-4 APPROACHES TO CONTROLLING HIGH BLOOD PRESSURE

Therapy   **Example of Medication**
Separate or in combination with medication
Lifestyle changes   None
DASH diet   None

Stage 1 hypertension: SBP 140-159 mm Hg or DBP 90-99 mm Hg in patients without other conditions (such as heart, kidney disease, recurrent stroke prevention, or diabetes). The following may be used alone or in combination:

Drug Class	Example(s)
Diuretics (thiazide type)	hydrochlorothiazide (HCTZ)
Angiotensin-converting enzyme inhibitors (ACEIs)	enalapril, lisinopril
Beta-blockers (BBs)	atenolol, metoprolol
Calcium channel blockers (CCBs)	verapamil
Angiotensin receptor blockers (ARBs)	losartan

Stage 2 hypertension: SBP 160 mm Hg or DBP 100 mm Hg or greater in patients without concurrent conditions (such as those listed previously). Patients should receive two-drug combination:

Thiazide diuretic with ACEI, ARB, CCB, or beta-adrenergic blocker
Centrally acting adrenergic blocker: clonidine
For patients with one or more disease states present (heart failure, post-MI, high coronary disease risk, diabetes, chronic kidney disease, or recurrent stroke prevention), treatment may include the following depending on the indication:
    Heart failure: diuretic, beta-adrenergic blocker, ACE inhibitor, ARB, or aldosterone antagonist
    High coronary disease risk: diuretic, beta-adrenergic blocker, ACE inhibitor, or CCB
    Diabetes: diuretic, beta-adrenergic blockers, ACE inhibitor, or CCB
    Chronic kidney disease: ACE inhibitor, or ARB
    Post-MI: ACE inhibitor, beta-adrenergic blocker, or aldosterone antagonist
    Recurrent stroke prevention: diuretic, or ACE inhibitor

Medications Used for Heart Conditions later in this chapter). These medications are covered separately; information includes drug action, side effects, and commonly used auxiliary labels on prescription vials.

An important note is that hypertension and edema can affect patients concurrently. Edema results from the excessive amount of fluid that is retained in the body tissues (see Chapter 22). This extra fluid must be pumped throughout the body system, which causes activation of the renin-angiotensin-aldosterone system (RAS), which in turn raises blood pressure. Drugs such as ACE inhibitors can reduce edema by blocking certain hormones and peptides (proteins) in the RAS cascade that trigger vasoconstriction. This reduces the production of excess fluid and decreases vasoconstriction. Diuretics can lower hypertension by reducing the reabsorption of sodium and water by the kidneys. This results in lowered circulating fluid volume.

Risk factors for cardiovascular disease and stroke, such as hypertension and hyperlipidemia, occur simultaneously (i.e., are co-morbid conditions) in many cases. Combination drugs are constantly being added to the list of antihypertensive and antilipidemic drugs to treat both conditions at the same time. Combination drugs, in general, allow for better compliance by the patient. If the patient has fewer medications to take, the patient is more likely to take them. Table 23-3 lists a small sample of the various combination drugs.

TABLE 23-3 Examples of Combination Drugs

Trade Name	Dosage Form	Strength
Antihypertensives		
ACE Inhibitor/Diuretic Combinations		
Capozide	captopril/HCTZ	25 mg/15 mg; 25 mg/25 mg; 50 mg/15 mg; 50 mg/25 mg
Lotensin HCT	benazepril/HCTZ	5 mg/6.25 mg; 10 mg/12.5 mg; 20 mg/12.5 mg; 20 mg/25 mg
Micardis HCT	telmisartan/HCTZ	40 mg/12.5 mg; 80 mg/12.5 mg; 80 mg/25 mg
Prinzide	lisinopril/HCTZ	10 mg/12.5 mg; 20 mg/12.5 mg; 20 mg/25 mg
Uniretic	moexipril/HCTZ	7.5 mg/12.5 mg; 15 mg/12.5 mg; 15 mg/25 mg
Vaseretic	enalapril maleate/HCTZ	10 mg/25 mg
Zestoretic	lisinopril/HCTZ	10 mg/12.5 mg; 20 mg/12.5 mg; 20 mg/25 mg
Beta-Blocker/Diuretic Combinations		
Inderide	propranolol/HCTZ	40 mg/25 mg; 80 mg/25 mg
Tenoretic	atenolol/chlorothalidone	50 mg/25 mg; 100 mg/25 mg
Ziac	bisoprolol fumarate/HCTZ	2.5 mg/6.25 mg; 5 mg/6.25 mg; 10 mg/6.25 mg
CCB/ACE Inhibitor Combinations		
Lotrel	amlodipine/benazepril HCl	2.5 mg/10 mg; 5 mg/10 mg; 5 mg/20 mg; 5 mg/40 mg; 10 mg/20 mg; 10 mg/40 mg
Tarka	trandolapril/verapamil	1 mg/240 mg; 2 mg/180 mg; 2 mg/240 mg; 4 mg/240 mg
Diuretic Combinations		
Dyazide	triamterene/HCTZ	37.5 mg/25 mg
Maxzide	triamterene/HCTZ	37.5 mg/25 mg; 75 mg/50 mg
Moduretic	amiloride/HCTZ	5 mg/50 mg
Lipid-Lowering and Antiplatelet Agent		
Pravigard	pravastatin/buffered aspirin	20 mg/81 mg
Lipid-Lowering and CCB Agent		
Caduet	amlodipine/atorvastatin	2.5 mg/10 mg; 2.5 mg/20 mg; 2.5 mg/40 mg; 5 mg/10 mg; 5 mg/20 mg; 5 mg/40 mg; 5 mg/80 mg; 10 mg/10 mg; 10 mg/20 mg; 10 mg/40 mg; 10 mg/80 mg

Hypotension

A person suffering from hypotension has low blood pressure. There are several types of hypotension (Box 23-5). A common problem that persons can experience is orthostatic hypotension. This occurs because a large amount of blood remains in the lower extremities (ankles and feet). When one stands quickly, the blood returning to the heart is decreased considerably, and the body responds by increasing the heartbeat, compensating for the lack of blood flow. This results in a feeling of light-headedness. Side effects of hypotension include syncope (fainting) and/or vertigo (dizziness). For persons who have chronic hypotension, physicians may recommend midodrine, which causes vasoconstriction, raising the blood pressure. Causes of low blood pressure are listed in Box 23-6.

Prognosis. With proper medical treatment and lifestyle changes, hypotension can be greatly, if not totally, controlled.

Non–Drug Treatment. If a person is not symptomatic, mild hypotension usually requires no treatment. Adjustments in medications may alleviate orthostatic

BOX 23-5 TYPES OF HYPOTENSION

Orthostatic
This is caused by standing up quickly from a sitting or lying position. Onset can be due to prolonged bed rest, pregnancy, dehydration, diabetes, or heart problems

Neurally mediated hypotension
A drop in blood pressure (BP) after standing for long periods of time. Affects mostly young people; the left ventricle signals the brain the BP is too high. Heart rate is lowered, causing low blood pressure (LBP)

Postprandial hypotension
Sudden drop in BP after eating. Affects older adults, persons with high blood pressure, and persons with Parkinson's disease

Multiple system atrophy with orthostatic hypotension
Rare disorder (Shy-Drager syndrome) causes damage to the nervous system, causing LBP

BOX 23-6 CAUSES OF HYPOTENSION

Pregnancy
Due to increased volume of blood circulation, BP may drop; this is normally temporary and BP returns to normal levels after giving birth

Blood loss
Due to trauma

Dehydration
Due to loss of water; fluid content decreases, causing hypotension; this can occur with mild dehydration as well

Deficiency of certain nutrients in diet (e.g., vitamin B_{12} or folate)
Due to a lack of vitamins that play a role in forming new red blood cells, causing anemia and leading to hypotension

Severe infection or septicemia
Due to an infection of the whole body system that can cause septic shock and hypotension

Severe allergic reaction: anaphylaxis
Due to a severe life-threatening reaction (foods, insect bites, venom), leading to hypotension and death

Heart problems: bradycardia, MI, heart failure, heart valve problems
Due to decreased blood pressure, leading to decreased circulation

Endocrine problems: hypothyroidism, hyperthyroidism, hypoglycemia, diabetes
Due to low or high hormone dispersion, or low blood glucose levels that can trigger hypotension

Medications (not limited to examples: diuretics, BBs, alpha-blockers, Parkinson's drugs, antidepressants)
Due to the side effects of agents taken for other conditions

hypotension or hypotension resulting from medication. Increasing salt intake raises blood pressure. This can only be done if an increase in salt does not affect any other ongoing condition. Drinking more water helps to increase fluid volume in the bloodstream and relieves dehydration. To prevent blood from pooling in the lower extremities, support stockings can be worn. Avoid alcohol because it causes dehydration, which can worsen hypotension. Moving or standing up slowly can lessen the onset of dizziness. To avoid postprandial hypotension (BP drops after eating), eating smaller meals more often and limiting high-carbohydrate foods may help. Caffeinated drinks may help to raise blood pressure although this should only be done if approved by the patient's physician.

Drug Treatment. The agents used to treat neurally-mediated postural hypotension include fludrocortisone (increases blood volume) and midodrine (raises blood pressure).

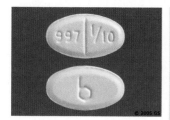

GENERIC NAME: fludrocortisone
TRADE NAME: Florinef
INDICATION: conditions that lose sodium; postural neurally mediated hypotension; Addison's disease; adrenogenital syndrome
ROUTE OF ADMINISTRATION: oral
COMMON ADULT DOSAGE: 0.1 to 0.2 mg once daily
SIDE EFFECTS: decreased appetite, dizziness, headache, weakness, muscle cramps
AUXILIARY LABEL:
■ Take with food or milk.

GENERIC NAME: midodrine
TRADE NAME: ProAmatine
INDICATION: postural hypotension
ROUTE OF ADMINISTRATION: oral
COMMON ADULT DOSAGE: 10 mg three times per day given at 4-hour intervals during daytime hours; usual maximum is 30 mg/day
SIDE EFFECTS: headache, nervousness, dry mouth, blurred vision

Hyperlipidemia

Hyperlipidemia (also known as hypercholesterolemia) is the increase of lipids (specifically cholesterol) in the bloodstream that leads to hardening of the arteries (atherosclerosis). This increases the incidence of angina, heart attack, and stroke. When discussing fats (lipids) in the body, it is important to recognize that cholesterol is only one type of lipid and performs many vital functions, including the synthesis of steroid hormones and cell membranes. When persons eat foods that are high in fat, they are ingesting too much cholesterol and other fatty acids, which our bodies cannot eliminate. Instead, these fatty substances float throughout the bloodstream where they can latch onto large arteries and middle-sized arteries of the heart and brain. Hypercholesterolemia can also result from certain inherited conditions. The most widespread genetically associated disorder is familial hypercholesterolemia. Because hyperlipidemia is known to lead to atherosclerosis, it is important to obtain an accurate cholesterol level measurement. Factors such as family history and lifestyle are important parts of the assessment as well. These may indicate the likelihood of experiencing further problems. The guidelines for specific cholesterol readings are listed in Box 23-7. Blood tests are used to measure serum levels of cholesterol, fat, and protein—or lipoproteins. Lipoproteins transport cholesterol throughout the body systems and can be classified as either low-density lipoproteins (LDLs) or high-density lipoproteins (HDLs). A third type of lipoprotein, very low density lipoprotein (VLDL), is a precursor to LDL. Large lipoproteins with low density (i.e., LDLs or "bad" cholesterol) carry cholesterol to the tissues, where it becomes lodged in blood vessel walls and contributes to atherosclerosis. On the other

BOX 23-7 U.S. GUIDELINES FOR CHOLESTEROL MEASUREMENTS

These levels do not necessarily include thresholds for those patients with an added risk of MI; desirable lipid levels for individuals with diabetes and other risk factors may vary from this list.

Overall cholesterol: Overall cholesterol level present in the blood. Necessary for production of hormones in proper levels.
  Good: <200 mg/dl
  Borderline high: 200-239 mg/dl
  High: ≥240 mg/dl

LDL: Low-density lipoprotein cholesterol (also known as bad cholesterol). Both saturated and trans–fatty acids increase LDL level.
  Good: 100-129 mg/dl
  Borderline high: 130-159 mg/dl
  High: 160-189 mg/dl
  Very high: ≥190 mg/dl

HDL: High-density lipoprotein cholesterol (also known as good cholesterol). Diets composed of fiber, vegetables, and fruits increase HDL level. Helps to remove cholesterol from bloodstream.
  Best: ≥60 mg/dl
  Okay: 50-59 mg/dl
  Poor: <50 mg/dl (women), <50 mg/dl (men)

Triglycerides (three molecules of fatty acids): A type of fat derived from animal proteins, vegetables, and certain carbohydrates. Increased amounts lower HDL level and increase LDL level.
  Good: <150 mg/dl
  Borderline high: 150-190 mg/dl
  High: 200-499 mg/dl
  Very high: ≥500 mg/dl

hand, high-density lipoproteins (i.e., HDLs or "good" cholesterol) remove cholesterol from the arteries and transport it to the liver. Besides cholesterol measurements, other factors that determine the treatment approach include family history, lifestyle habits, and the patient's personal medical history.

Prognosis. In severe cases, bypass surgery or cardiac stenting may be indicated for persons who are already suffering from atherosclerosis and may not respond to medications and lifestyle changes, as well as for post–myocardial infarction (post-MI) patients.

Non–Drug Treatment. By eating a healthy diet and engaging in regular exercise, many persons can lower their lipid content. Diet and lifestyle changes (exercise, weight control, and cessation of smoking) can be a good initial approach for patients without other major risk factors for heart disease; such changes are usually implemented for 6 months before remeasurement of cholesterol levels. Patients with significant risk factors for heart disease and stroke or those with familial hyperlipidemia may incorporate drug treatments immediately, along with diet and lifestyle changes, to reduce their risk of serious events.

Drug Treatment. For persons at high risk because of family history or those who have high levels that do not decrease through diet and exercise, medication treatments are available (referred to as antihyperlipidemics). Niacin is available in some products over-the-counter (OTC); however, due to the high doses needed and the possibility of side effects, the drug is usually only used under a physician's prescription. It is more commonly added to other drug therapies for cholesterol rather than used as a single agent.

Antihyperlipidemics. The classes of drugs that make up the antihyperlipidemics include bile acid sequestrants, fibrates, and hydroxymethylglutaryl-coenzyme A (HMG-CoA) reductase inhibitors (also known as "statins"). The "statins" specifically inhibit an enzyme responsible for one of the first steps in the overall conversion of fats into cholesterol. They raise the high-density lipoprotein (HDL) level and decrease the LDL and VLDL cholesterol levels. They effectively reduce LDL by greater than 30%. Statins are considered first-line drug treatments because of their proven efficacy in helping patients reach LDL goals and reducing the incidence of cardiac endpoints such as heart attack and stroke. Bile acid sequestrants, such as cholestyramine, increase the loss of cholesterol, specifically LDLs, through *increased* defecation. Many agents effectively help reduce cholesterol in this manner. The fibrates, such as gemfibrozil and fenofibrate, work specifically to lower VLDL cholesterol levels by inhibiting the extraction of free fatty acids, which reduces the ability of the liver to produce triglycerides. Fibrates also increase HDL levels; however, the specific mechanism of action is not well-known. Nicotinic acid (a form of niacin) reduces cholesterol, triglyceride, and VLDL levels, which leads to an overall decrease in LDL levels and an increase in HDL levels; the exact mechanism is not well known. The recommended maintenance doses for adults are listed in the following drug monographs.

BILE ACID SEQUESTRANTS

GENERIC NAME: cholestyramine
TRADE NAME: Questran, Questran Light, Prevalite
INDICATION: high cholesterol, especially LDL; also for pruritus associated with biliary stasis
ROUTE OF ADMINISTRATION: oral (powder)
COMMON ADULT DOSAGE: initially, 4 g once or twice daily before meals; maximum 24 g/day in divided doses
SIDE EFFECTS: constipation, flatulence
AUXILIARY LABELS:

■ Take before meals.
■ Take with plenty of fluids.

SPECIAL NOTE: Powder form should be mixed into 60 to 180 mL of liquid. Other medications should be taken 4 to 6 hours apart from cholestyramine to avoid interference with absorption.

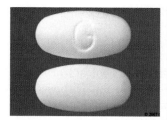

GENERIC NAME: colestipol
TRADE NAME: Colestid
INDICATION: high cholesterol, especially LDL
ROUTE OF ADMINISTRATION: oral (tablet, granules for suspension)
COMMON ADULT DOSAGE: initially, 5 g once or twice daily; maximum 30 g/day in divided doses
SIDE EFFECTS: constipation, flatulence
AUXILIARY LABELS:

■ Do not chew or crush (tablets).
■ Take with plenty of fluids.

SPECIAL NOTE: Granule form should be mixed into at least 90 mL of liquid, or with a highly fluid soup or applesauce. Other medications should be taken at least 1 hour before or at least 4 hours after colestipol to avoid interference with absorption.

HMG-COA REDUCTASE INHIBITORS ("STATINS")

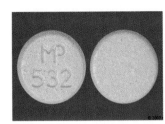

GENERIC NAME: lovastatin
TRADE NAME: Mevacor, Altoprev
INDICATION: high cholesterol, especially LDL
ROUTE OF ADMINISTRATION: oral
COMMON ADULT DOSAGE: 10 to 80 mg once daily or in 1-2 divided doses; Altoprev:
  10-60 mg once daily at bedtime
SIDE EFFECTS: nausea, constipation, diarrhea, stomach upset, gas
AUXILIARY LABELS:
- Take with meals.
- Do not drink grapefruit juice.
- Altoprev: Do not crush, cut, or chew.

GENERIC NAME: simvastatin
TRADE NAME: Zocor
INDICATION: high cholesterol
ROUTE OF ADMINISTRATION: oral
COMMON ADULT DOSAGE: 5 to 80 mg once daily, usually in the evening
SIDE EFFECTS: H/A, abdominal pain
AUXILIARY LABEL:
- Do not drink grapefruit juice.

GENERIC NAME: pravastatin
TRADE NAME: Pravachol
INDICATION: high cholesterol, also increases HDL
ROUTE OF ADMINISTRATION: oral
COMMON ADULT DOSAGE: 10 to 80 mg once daily
SIDE EFFECTS: dizziness, H/A, heartburn
AUXILIARY LABEL:
- May cause dizziness.

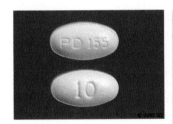

GENERIC NAME: atorvastatin
TRADE NAME: Lipitor
INDICATION: high cholesterol; lowers the risk of heart attack, coronary heart disease,
  stroke
ROUTE OF ADMINISTRATION: oral
COMMON ADULT DOSAGE: 10 to 80 mg once daily
SIDE EFFECTS: H/A, nausea, constipation, bloating, gas
AUXILIARY LABELS:
- Do not drink grapefruit juice.
- Take with or without food.
- Avoid alcohol.

FIBRIC ACID ANTIHYPERLIPIDEMIC

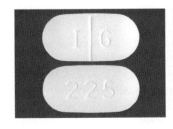

GENERIC NAME: gemfibrozil
TRADE NAME: Lopid
INDICATION: very high cholesterol, triglycerides; lowers risk of MI or other heart
  complications
ROUTE OF ADMINISTRATION: oral
COMMON ADULT DOSAGE: 600 mg twice daily, before morning and evening meals
SIDE EFFECTS: dizziness, drowsiness, N/V, diarrhea, constipation, upset stomach
AUXILIARY LABEL:
- May cause dizziness/drowsiness.

CHOLESTEROL ABSORPTION INHIBITOR

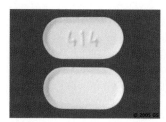

GENERIC NAME: ezetimibe
TRADE NAME: Zetia
INDICATION: hypercholesterolemia
ROUTE OF ADMINISTRATION: oral
COMMON ADULT DOSAGE: 10 mg once daily
SIDE EFFECTS: diarrhea, joint pain, fatigue

MISCELLANEOUS ANTIHYPERLIPIDEMIC

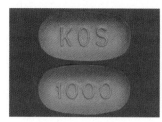

GENERIC NAME: nicotinic acid
TRADE NAME: Niaspan, Niacor (both Rx only) (NOTE: For any forms of niacin over-the-counter, read drug facts for dosage.)
INDICATION: hyperlipidemia and hypertriglyceridemia
ROUTE OF ADMINISTRATION: oral
COMMON ADULT DOSAGE: Niacor: 1-2 g three times daily with or following meals; Niaspan: 500 mg at bedtime initially, then 1-2 g/day at bedtime after titration
SIDE EFFECTS: flushing, may cause photosensitivity
AUXILIARY LABELS:

- May cause photosensitivity.
- Niaspan extended release: Do not crush, cut, or chew.

Transient Ischemic Attacks (TIAs) and Strokes

Transient ischemic attacks are caused by a short duration of reduced oxygenation of the brain that can be due to atherosclerotic cerebrovascular disease. TIAs are almost the same as ischemic attacks, except the duration is much shorter for TIAs and also there is no permanent loss of function. Transient attacks may last only a few minutes or may occur many times over the span of a day. The plaque causes narrowing of the blood vessels, which leads to a reduction of blood flow. If this plaque accumulates to form a blood clot, a thrombosis is created. This eventually may obstruct the vessel, causing a stroke. TIAs sometimes are referred to as mini-strokes and are considered a possible precursor to a stroke.

Two types of strokes are an ischemic (clot) stroke or a hemorrhagic (bleeding) stroke. Hemorrhagic strokes are caused by weakened vessels or aneurysms in the brain that cause a vessel to rupture. When a vessel is ruptured, blood flows into areas of the brain, causing damage; additional injury is caused by the lack of oxygenated blood flow to areas of the brain where it is needed. Most of the symptoms of TIAs and strokes may appear rapidly and include vision or hearing problems, weakness on one or both sides of the body, dizziness, slurred speech, and sudden severe headache. One of the main chronic causes of TIAs and strokes is high blood pressure (hypertension). Besides hypertension, other contributing factors may lead to the likelihood of a stroke. Persons with diabetes, high cholesterol levels, heart problems, and obesity are at higher risk. Also certain lifestyle habits such as smoking, lack of exercise, and excessive alcohol intake can add to the damage of the vessels in the body system.

Prognosis. The incidence of having more than one episode of TIA is increased based on preexisting conditions. TIAs may be a precursor to a stroke. About one third of those who experience a TIA will have an acute stroke in the future. Only through management of the underlying conditions can the likelihood of further TIAs or a stroke be lessened.

If a patient shows TIA symptoms, certain diagnostic tests can be conducted to determine the likelihood of more TIAs or even an impending stroke. Common diagnostic tests include computed tomography and magnetic resonance imaging scans (MRI). A computed tomography scan shows whether a clot is present and whether it is ischemic or hemorrhagic. Magnetic resonance imaging is used to diagnose brain vessel abnormalities that may be involved in a hemorrhagic stroke.

Non–Drug Treatment. Reducing the factors that contribute to the underlying causes is one of the necessary changes that should be made. This includes stopping smoking, reducing fat and alcohol consumption, losing weight if necessary, exercising, and eating a balanced diet.

Nonfatal strokes are one of the most common causes of disability, resulting in possible brain damage and lengthy physical therapy. Through lengthy rehabilitation, sometimes the unaffected portion of the brain can learn to assume the functions that were lost because of the stroke.

Drug Treatment. TIAs are treated by improving arterial blood flow to the brain so that a stroke can be avoided. In the case of a TIA, patients may be treated with antiplatelet medication such as aspirin to decrease the risk of platelets clumping and forming a clot, or with anticoagulants such as warfarin. Usually the last resort is carotid artery surgery to remove arterial plaque.

The main agents used to treat an acute ischemic stroke in progress would be thrombolytics such as tissue plasminogen activator (t-PA, Activase) if indicated. Therapy must be given within 3 hours of the onset of the symptoms of the event, after the patient has received evaluation to rule out intracranial bleeding. More information on thrombolytics is given later in this chapter under the section titled Thrombosis.

Although many medications are used to prevent the onset of a TIA or stroke, there are few medications available to reduce the effects of a stroke once it has occurred. Nimodipine is one agent used specifically to reduce vascular spasms in the cerebral arteries following a form of stroke called a subarachnoid hemorrhage (SAH); it is not used for other types of ischemic or hemorrhagic stroke.

CALCIUM CHANNEL BLOCKER

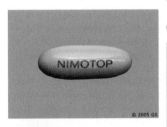

GENERIC NAME: nimodipine
TRADE NAME: Nimotop
INDICATION: reduce spasms following subarachnoid hemorrhage
ROUTE OF ADMINISTRATION: oral
COMMON ADULT DOSAGE: oral, 60 mg (2 × 30-mg capsules) q4h × 21 days; or if the patient cannot take it orally, extract the contents from the capsule* and give ORALLY, flushing it with 30 mL of normal saline afterward
SIDE EFFECTS: dizziness
AUXILIARY LABELS:

■ Give on an empty stomach.
■ Do not give with grapefruit juice.
■ Protect from light.

*NOTE: If the capsule cannot be swallowed, a hole should be made in both ends of the capsule with an 18-gauge needle, and the contents of the capsule extracted into a syringe. A parenteral syringe can be used to extract the liquid inside the capsule, but the liquid should ALWAYS be transferred to an oral syringe that cannot accept a needle and that is designed for oral or NG tube or PEG administration only. Label the oral syringe "Not for IV Use." The contents should then be administered and washed down a tube with 30 mL of normal saline (0.9%).

Tech Alert!

Proper preparation of Nimotop doses is essential. **DO NOT** administer Nimotop intravenously or by other parenteral routes. Death and serious life-threatening adverse events have occurred when the contents of Nimotop capsules have been injected parenterally.

Angina Pectoris

Angina pectoris results from a decrease in blood flow to the heart, which causes chest pain. Pain can vary from minor to severe. Decreased blood flow can be caused by factors such as hardening of the arteries (atherosclerosis), hypertension, cigarette smoking, and diabetes. Environmental and genetic influences also can play a role in acquiring angina (chest pain). Three types of angina are the following:

1. Stable angina
2. Variant angina
3. Unstable angina

In classic stable angina the patient can experience short ischemic episodes of pain, in which a mild deficiency of oxygen has occurred. Patients may feel as though there is a weight on the chest accompanied with a sharp pain. This pain can occur in the chest, neck, arms, teeth, and jaw. Many times this type of an angina attack occurs after exercise, excessive activity or emotional stress; therefore the episodes are usually predictable.

Another type of angina is variant angina (AKA: Prinzmetal's angina). This type may not be related to atherosclerosis; instead the patient experiences very painful spasms of the coronary artery that can occur spontaneously. Variant angina does not occur after physical exercise or stress, instead it usually occurs when the patient is at rest, often between the hours of midnight and 8 a.m.

The third type is unstable angina, which may worsen in a person with a known history of angina attacks, and usually occurs at rest or is more severe in pattern than the patient's usual symptoms. Unstable angina is caused mainly by obstruction of the arteries from atherosclerosis, and may include rupture of an atherosclerotic plaque. Because unstable angina may be a sign of an impending heart attack, it requires immediate medical attention.

All three types of angina pain are treated with medications such as nitrates. In addition to medications, the patient may be required to make certain lifestyle changes that may decrease the likelihood of these attacks. In addition, surgery may be performed to bypass the blockage.

Prognosis. The prognosis of angina depends on the type of angina and the severity of the condition. A history of heart conditions such as arrhythmias or heart attacks also influences the outcome.

Non–Drug Treatment. Modifying behaviors to lessen angina attacks include stopping smoking, reducing stress, losing weight, lowering blood pressure and cholesterol levels, and controlling any underlying conditions such as hypertension or abnormal cholesterol levels. Surgical procedures may be used to relieve occlusion in some patients. Procedures include coronary artery bypass graft (CABG) or stent implantation. Percutaneous transluminal coronary angioplasty (PTCA) is an alternative for patients who cannot undergo surgery although it may be used along with coronary artery stenting. A stent is a small, cylindrical wire tube device that is inserted into the affected artery, providing a framework to hold the artery open. The stent is placed by inserting a catheter through a vein and guiding the stent to the site. Stents can be uncoated or coated with a slow-release medication that keeps the artery from clotting and ultimately closing. Medication (clopidogrel, aspirin, etc.) must be taken after such a procedure regardless of which type of stent is used.

Drug Treatment. Nitrates, calcium channel blockers, and beta-blockers are commonly used to treat and prevent angina. A newer agent for angina is ranolazine (Ranexa). Probably one of the most prescribed antianginal agents is nitroglycerin. Millions of individuals carry nitroglycerin sublingual tablets in their

Doctor David Gall
1000 Archway
St. Louis, MO
ph: 816-555-5555

Patient name: _B. Jones-Lewis_

Address: _106 Nutree Way_ Date: _1-30-03_

℞: NTG 0.4mg sl #100

Take 1 sl q 5 mm x3

y no relief call 911

D. Gall

Dr. Signature

Refills: 6 DEA # _____

FIGURE 23-4 Nitroglycerin sublingual tablet prescription.

pockets or purses in the event of an acute angina attack. Nitroglycerin has many dosage forms, including capsules, topical patches, paste, and sublingual spray. The sublingual tablets and injectable forms are used for emergencies.

Nitrates. Nitrates are vasodilators; that is, they dilate the arteries to permit an increase of blood flow through the heart muscle. They also reduce the workload of the heart. Because more oxygenated blood is allowed to enter the arteries, less blood is returned to the heart, thereby decreasing the workload. Isosorbide dinitrate or mononitrate and nitroglycerin are the common nitrate agents used for the treatment of angina. Both isosorbide dinitrate and nitroglycerin are available as sublingual tablets, which are effective because of their rapid absorption; the medication bypasses the gastrointestinal system and enters directly into the bloodstream for a more rapid onset of action. Figure 23-4 shows a common nitroglycerin prescription order.

Nitroglycerin sublingual is functional for only 6 months after opening the container. In addition, it must be kept in a dry area and in the original light-protected glass container to prevent the active agent from deteriorating. Table 23-4 provides a list of the nitrate agents and their dosage forms. Another form for acute relief is translingual nitroglycerin spray. The patient sprays one or two metered doses under the tongue with a maximum of three sprays in a 15-minute period. Sublingual dosages are kept at the patient's bedside in an institution, or constantly with the ambulatory individual, for emergency relief of angina attacks. In the hospital, nitroglycerin is often given by IV infusion for a variety of circumstances, including the treatment of unstable angina.

For chronic treatment of angina to prevent attacks, longer-acting nitrate dosage forms are available. Transdermal dosage forms (nitroglycerin) or oral dosage forms (e.g., isosorbide dinitrate or mononitrate) are available. The nitroglycerin transdermal patches normally are applied once daily in the morning and are removed at bedtime to decrease the possibility of tolerance to the medication. Ointment tubes are available in 60-g, 30-g, and 1-g unit dose sizes. The ointment dosage form also includes papers premarked in $\frac{1}{2}$-inch increments for delivering the proper amount of ointment. The ointment is squeezed onto the paper in increments of $\frac{1}{2}$ inch to 2 inches (similar to toothpaste placed on a toothbrush), then placed on the chest.

Tech Note!

Patients taking nitrates CANNOT receive or use certain drug treatments for erectile dysfunction such as sildenafil (Viagra), vardenafil (Levitra), or tadalafil (Cialis). Taking these drugs together may result in serious, life-threatening low blood pressure.

TABLE 23-4 Common Nitrate Agents

Trade Name	Generic Name	Dosage Form	Normal Usage
Tridil	nitroglycerin	Injectable for dilution for infusion	Emergency
NTG in D_5W	nitroglycerin	Injection pre-mixed infusion	Emergency
Nitrostat	nitroglycerin	Sublingual tablets	Emergency
Nitro-Time	nitroglycerin	Sustained-release capsules	Routine medication
Nitro-Dur	nitroglycerin	Nitroglycerin patches	Routine medication
Nitro-Bid	nitroglycerin	Ointment 2% with papers	Routine medication
Monoket, Imdur	isosorbide mononitrate	Tablets, extended-release tablets	Routine medication
Isordil	isosorbide dinitrate	Sublingual tablets	Emergency
Dilatratese-SR, Isochron, Isoditrate, Isordil	isosorbide dinitrate	Tablets, capsules, sustained-release tablets	Routine medication

Tech Note!

When filling a prescription for nitroglycerin sublingual tablets (e.g., Nitrostat), never take the tablets out of the glass container in which they are packaged. Instead, place the glass container within a larger plastic vial on which the label is attached. Other containers include the box type, which holds four small glass vials each containing 25 tablets and which has a space on the box for the drug label.

Other agents commonly used for the chronic treatment of angina include beta-blockers, calcium channel blockers, and the novel agent ranolazine (Ranexa), which also reduces heart ischemia through a different mechanism than other available agents. Ranolazine can often be added to existing standard angina therapies, because the drug does not lower heart rate or blood pressure. Compared to nitrates, it also does not interact with medications for erectile dysfunction.

Myocardial Infarction (MI)

If coronary blood flow to an area of the heart becomes entirely blocked because of a thrombus or **embolism**, that area of heart muscle cannot receive the necessary oxygen. This results in the death of that part of the heart muscle, a condition known as myocardial infarction. The onset of an MI is experienced differently from person to person and may not be treated quickly if the patient is unaware that his or her symptoms indicate a heart attack. Depending on the severity of the blockage, the patient may have an MI from which he or she can recover over time or a massive MI that weakens the heart permanently or may even result in death.

Prognosis. Many people survive an MI because of prompt medical treatment. There are several classes of drugs that can manage various conditions and lifestyle changes that can reduce the recurrence of another MI. If necessary, a bypass can be performed to reroute blood flow. Some patients are at high risk for either heart arrhythmia, heart failure, or other complications following an MI.

Non–Drug Treatment. The many medications that are available for post-MI patients have been discussed previously in this chapter. With the continued use of a variety of agents and a change in lifestyle, many patients live a normal life span. Cardiac rehabilitation, dietary changes, and reduction of risk factors (e.g., smoking) are all important actions to implement after a heart attack. However, if the patient's MI was severe or if the condition of the coronary arteries is such that blockages present place the patient at high risk, an intervention such as bypass surgery may be necessary. Bypass surgery creates new routes for blood flow to the heart muscle. Veins are transplanted from the legs and are used to reroute blood flow around the damaged vessel(s) within the heart. Newer techniques allow surgeons to conduct bypass surgery without opening the chest wall. This less invasive technique enables the patient to recover more quickly. For more information on innovative treatments in cardiac surgery, visit the American Heart Association online (www.heartassociation.org).

Drug Treatment. Because of the severity of an MI the longer the area within the heart is blocked from blood flow, the more damage is done. The death of the tissue can be severe enough to cause death. Most people are admitted to the hospital via the emergency room, where they may require a variety of medications, all given parenterally. Following an MI, drug treatment goals are to reduce the mortality (risk of death) of the patient and to prevent reinfarction. After an MI, the heart undergoes structural changes, and another major goal of drug therapy is to maximize and preserve the remaining function of the left ventricle, and to avoid heart arrhythmia and heart failure. Many medications are used, including beta-blockers, ACE inhibitors, statins, and aspirin and other antiplatelet medications (e.g., clopidogrel [Plavix]). The treatments chosen are dependent on the individual patient's history, type of infarction, and types of procedures that may have been performed.

Arrhythmia

A person with coronary artery disease can develop arrhythmias (irregular heartbeats), also known as dysrhythmias. As previously discussed earlier in this chapter under Cardiac Conduction System, the heart beats in a regular rhythm. This is accomplished via special fibers that run throughout the heart. The pacemaker is located in the sinoatrial node. Many factors influence the efficient operation of the pacemaker, including chemical balance. If an imbalance results from chemicals (e.g., electrolytes) or oxygen, then irregular heartbeats can occur. Most patients receive short-term treatment in the emergency room. Once stabilized, the patient may be discharged home. If so, long-term medications can be prescribed to help maintain the heart's normal rhythm.

Prognosis. The outcome of an arrhythmia depends on its location and severity. Arrhythmias originating in the atrium may ultimately be controlled with medications or other treatment. Ventricular tachycardia or fibrillation is more deadly. All arrhythmias have the potential to be fatal; the risk varies from person to person.

Non–Drug Treatment. In severe cases in which medications cannot correct the continuing problem of arrhythmias, a pacemaker implant may be the only alternative.

Drug Treatment. The medications used in treating arrhythmias are called antiarrhythmic agents. Quinidine sulfate, procainamide, amiodarone, sotalol, and verapamil are common agents that may be prescribed. The following drug monographs list common antiarrhythmics and their indications.

Drug Action. Antiarrhythmic agents affect the conduction system and induce regular heartbeats. Lidocaine is used in an emergency situation to treat arrhythmias resulting from MIs and other conditions. Quinidine sulfate and procainamide reduce the speed of the conduction system and treat tachycardia (rapid heartbeat) and other arrhythmias. The injectable form of procainamide normally is used in life-threatening tachycardia episodes in an emergency. Disopyramide slows the heart rate. Again, the injectable form is used in life-threatening tachycardia similar to procainamide. Verapamil slows the conduction system at the atrioventricular node and stabilizes cardiac rhythm.

Antiarrhythmics. Antiarrhythmics are agents that correct an irregular heartbeat by restoring normal rhythm; they can also help the heart work more efficiently by slowing the heart rate when it beats too fast or by helping it beat more regularly. Commonly used antiarrhythmics include sotalol, propafenone, and amiodarone.

Tech Note!

Serious medication errors can occur because of the similar names of quinidine and quinine. Quinine is an antimalarial agent; quinidine is a cardiac agent. These two medications are often close to one another on a pharmacy shelf and have been mistaken for one another. This can result in a dangerous error.

GENERIC NAME: quinidine sulfate, quinidine gluconate

TRADE NAME: Quinidex (oral), Quinalan (intravenous)

INDICATION: irregular heartbeat

ROUTE OF ADMINISTRATION: sulfate (immediate release), gluconate (extended-release tablets); gluconate injection (intramuscular, intravenous)

COMMON ADULT DOSAGE: quinidine gluconate ER oral: initially, 324 mg two or three times daily; then adjusted to patient response and drug levels

SIDE EFFECTS: gastrointestinal upset

AUXILIARY LABELS:

- Do not crush or chew extended-release tablet.
- Take with food.
- Take as directed.

GENERIC NAME: procainamide

TRADE NAME: Procanbid extended-release; Pronestyl, Pronestyl SR

INDICATION: life-threatening irregular heartbeat

ROUTE OF ADMINISTRATION: oral, injection (intramuscular, intravenous)

COMMON ADULT DOSAGE: Procanbid oral: usually 50 mg/kg/day, given in divided doses q12h; dosage of procainamide in general is determined based on weight and age of patient and therapeutic monitoring

SIDE EFFECTS: bitter taste, anorexia, GI upset, or diarrhea; hypotension with parenteral use

AUXILIARY LABELS:

- Take as directed.
- Take with or without food.
- Do not break, crush, or chew extended-release form.

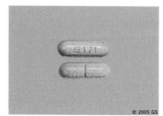

GENERIC NAME: sotalol

TRADE NAME: Betapace and Betapace AF

INDICATION: irregular heartbeat; Betapace is for ventricular arrhythmias, Betapace AF for atrial fibrillation

ROUTE OF ADMINISTRATION: oral

COMMON ADULT DOSAGE: ventricular arrhythmias: initially 80 mg bid, then 120-160 mg bid; for a-fib: initially 80 mg twice daily, up to 160 mg twice daily

SIDE EFFECTS: gastrointestinal upset, slow heart rate, fatigue, dizziness, shortness of breath

AUXILIARY LABELS:

- Do not take at same time as antacids.
- Take as directed.

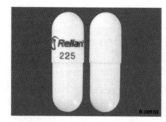

GENERIC NAME: propafenone

TRADE NAME: Rythmol, Rythmol SR

INDICATION: irregular heartbeat

ROUTE OF ADMINISTRATION: oral

COMMON ADULT DOSAGE: Rythmol: 150-225 mg q8h; Rythmol SR: 225-425 mg q12h

SIDE EFFECTS: gastrointestinal upset; dizziness, nausea and/or vomiting, unusual taste, constipation, and blurred vision

AUXILIARY LABELS:

- Take as directed.
- Do not crush, cut, or chew (extended-release capsules).

GENERIC NAME: amiodarone
TRADE NAME: Cordarone, Pacerone
INDICATION: irregular heartbeat
ROUTE OF ADMINISTRATION: oral, injectable (in hospital only)
COMMON ADULT DOSAGE: dependent on type of arrhythmia; usual maintenance doses range from 200 to 600 mg once daily
SIDE EFFECTS: fatigue, tremor, neuropathy, photosensitivity, skin discoloration, nausea and/or vomiting, constipation, visual changes; may cause thyroid disorders or lung or liver problems
AUXILIARY LABELS:

- Take as directed.
- May cause photosensitivity.
- Avoid grapefruit juice.

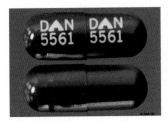

GENERIC NAME: disopyramide
TRADE NAME: Norpace, Norpace CR (controlled-release)
INDICATION: serious ventricular arrhythmias
ROUTE OF ADMINISTRATION: oral
COMMON ADULT DOSAGE: 150 mg q6h; controlled release: 300 mg q12h
SIDE EFFECTS: dry mouth, dizziness, drowsiness, difficulty urinating, constipation, blurred vision
AUXILIARY LABELS:

- Take as directed.
- May cause dizziness/drowsiness.
- Do not break, crush, or chew extended-release form.

GENERIC NAME: lidocaine PFS (prefilled syringes, IV)
TRADE NAME: Xylocaine
INDICATION: acute management of ventricular arrhythmias
ROUTE OF ADMINISTRATION: injection or intravenous drip
COMMON ADULT DOSAGE: 50 to 100 mg IV bolus, then followed by IV infusion at a rate of 1-4 mg/min (or approximately 20-50 mcg/kg/min); adjustments guided by patient response and drug levels; convert to other antiarrhythmic therapy as soon as possible to avoid drug toxicity with prolonged use
SPECIAL NOTE: This medication is often kept in emergency rooms and other areas where crash carts are located. These carts are used in code blue situations. In the emergency department and intensive care units, a code blue* occurs when a patient is having a heart attack or stops breathing.

---

*Color codes may differ between hospitals

Congestive Heart Failure (CHF)

Congestive heart failure is usually a progressive disease in which the heart cannot pump enough blood to the body. Effective treatments are available to help patients with CHF, but there is no cure. Edema complicates CHF because the kidneys compensate for the lack of blood flow by retaining more fluid in the body. This fluid increases the heart's workload, further weakening it. Eventually the heart can no longer pump adequately to meet body demands. The best way to avoid CHF is to prevent the main conditions that lead to it, such as myocardial infarction, hypertension, and coronary artery disease. Other conditions that may cause CHF include valvular heart disease, congenital heart defects, cardiomyopathy, and endocarditis. Symptoms of CHF include fatigue, shortness of breath (SOB) during activities of daily living or when lying down, edema in the legs and ankles, increased heart rate, coughing, and a decreased ability to concentrate.

Prognosis. CHF can be treated in several ways although certain conditions that are associated with the onset of CHF cannot be reversed. Through the use of medications and lifestyle changes the life span of a person suffering from CHF is greatly improved; it is a lifelong condition that needs to be controlled.

Non–Drug Treatment. There are a number of changes that can influence the severity of CHF. These include reduction of salt intake, cessation of smoking, loss of weight, rest and modification of daily activities, and reduction of stress. When lifestyle changes and/or medications are ineffective, the alternative may be surgery. If valvular or congenital heart disease is the source of a patient's congestive heart failure, surgery may correct the defects and improve heart function.

Drug Treatment. The goal of all drug treatments is to improve the ease and efficiency of heart function. The most common treatment for CHF is cardiac glycosides. The only cardiac glycoside available in the United States is digoxin. Additional agents include ACE inhibitors, angiotensin II receptor blockers (ARBs), select beta-blockers, and diuretics (see ABCDs for the heart; see Types of Medications Used for Heart Conditions later in this chapter). Cardiac glycosides increase the forcefulness of the pumping of the heart but not the oxygen requirements. Specifically, they inhibit the sodium-potassium pump, which works within the heart to increase contractility. In arrhythmias, a suppression of the atrioventricular node increases the regularity of the heartbeat and decreases the conduction speed and force (velocity); thus (in both cases) the heart works smarter, not harder. Patients must take their medications exactly as directed. **Diuretics** often are prescribed concurrently. They increase urine output, thus decreasing the overall fluid retention (see Chapter 22) and allowing the heart to function more efficiently.

CARDIAC GLYCOSIDE

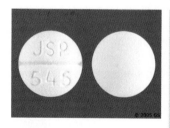

GENERIC NAME: digoxin
TRADE NAME: Lanoxin
INDICATIONS: treatment of CHF and certain atrial arrhythmias
ROUTE OF ADMINISTRATION: oral, injection (intravenous [preferred], intramuscular)
COMMON ADULT DOSAGE: 0.125 to 0.25 mg once daily (the dosage and frequency of dosing must be adjusted for body weight and renal function of the patient)
SIDE EFFECTS: nausea and vomiting, diarrhea, dizziness; visual changes may occur as a symptom of toxicity
AUXILIARY LABELS:
- Take as prescribed.
- Do not stop taking medication without consulting physician.

SPECIAL NOTE: The antidote for an overdose of digoxin or symptomatic toxicity is digoxin immune Fab (e.g., Digibind). This agent binds to the digoxin molecule, and it then is excreted from the body. This treatment must be done in the emergency department and the antidote is available in injectable form only.

Tech Note!

The pharmacy technician should be aware that the pulse rate should be measured each day before taking digoxin. If the pulse rate is less than 60 beats/min, the patient should consult a physician before taking the medicine.

Diuretics Used for Congestive Heart Failure–Related Edema. Different diuretic agents can be used to help reduce edema. With thiazides and loop diuretics, an important consideration is the large amount of potassium lost in the urine. For this reason, both classes of drugs may be supplemented with potassium. Diuretics also are given along with one or more of the listed agents to decrease the effects of sodium retention. Frequent urination leading to a decrease in edema is the main outcome with the use of diuretics. An example is the agent hydrochlorothiazide (HCTZ). However, some agents are known as *potassium sparing*.

BOX 23-8 CLASSIFICATION OF DIURETIC AGENTS

Thiazides
Loop diuretics
Potassium-sparing diuretics
Carbonic anhydrase inhibitors
Osmotic diuretics

These include agents such as triamterene (and combinations of this drug with HCTZ) and spironolactone; others are listed in Box 23-8. A maximum of two examples of each type of diuretic is given because a more extensive list is provided in Chapter 22.

THIAZIDE AND THIAZIDE-LIKE DIURETICS

GENERIC NAME: hydrochlorothiazide
TRADE NAME: Microzide, Ezide
INDICATION: edema, CHF, hypertension
ROUTE OF ADMINISTRATION: oral
COMMON ADULT DOSAGE: 25 to 50 mg daily as a single dose or 2 divided doses
SIDE EFFECTS: diarrhea, constipation, blurred vision, mild stomach pain
AUXILIARY LABEL:

■ Avoid alcohol.

GENERIC NAME: metolazone
TRADE NAME: Zaroxolyn
INDICATION: edema, CHF, hypertension
ROUTE OF ADMINISTRATION: oral
COMMON ADULT DOSAGE: 2.5 to 20 mg once daily
SIDE EFFECTS: dizziness, H/A, blurred vision
AUXILIARY LABELS:

■ Take with food or milk.
■ May cause dizziness.
■ Avoid alcohol.

Loop Diuretics. Loop diuretics work specifically in the loop of Henle within the renal tubules (see Chapter 22). They have a rapid onset of action and cause large amounts of urine to be excreted. They often are prescribed for patients who have edema caused by CHF and hypertension. Their side effects include increased urination, possible gastrointestinal upset, orthostatic hypotension, and photosensitivity. Because these agents work rapidly and may cause greatly increased urine output, it is advised that the patient take them in the morning or early in the day to limit nocturia.

LOOP DIURETICS

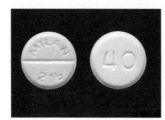

GENERIC NAME: furosemide
TRADE NAME: Lasix
INDICATION: edema associated with CHF and other conditions, hypertension
ROUTE OF ADMINISTRATION: oral, injection (intravenous, intramuscular)
COMMON ADULT DOSAGE: 20 to 80 mg once daily or in divided doses
SIDE EFFECTS: dizziness, H/A, diarrhea, constipation, blurred vision
AUXILIARY LABELS:
- May cause dizziness.
- May cause photosensitivity.

GENERIC NAME: bumetanide
TRADE NAME: Bumex
INDICATION: edema, CHF
ROUTE OF ADMINISTRATION: oral, injection (intramuscular, intravenous)
COMMON ADULT DOSAGE: 0.5 to 2 mg once daily
SIDE EFFECTS: dizziness, H/A, mild nausea or stomach pain
AUXILIARY LABELS:
- Take with food or milk.
- May cause photosensitivity.

Potassium-Sparing Diuretics. Potassium-sparing agents reduce potassium loss in the urine by interrupting sodium reabsorption within the distal tubules of the kidney. Because of their location of action, they prevent a large amount of potassium from being excreted in the urine. Their side effects are similar to those of other diuretics (such as possible gastrointestinal upset), but they also may cause dizziness, drowsiness, headache, and diarrhea. The following is a commonly used agent.

POTASSIUM-SPARING DIURETIC

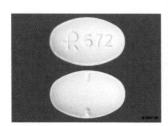

GENERIC NAME: spironolactone
TRADE NAME: Aldactone
INDICATION: CHF, edema due to various conditions, primary hyperaldosteronism, hypertension
ROUTE OF ADMINISTRATION: oral
COMMON ADULT DOSAGE: range: 50 to 200 mg/day in single or divided doses; usual dose for CHF initially is 50 mg twice daily
SIDE EFFECTS: dizziness, H/A, mild nausea, vomiting, stomach pain, gas, gynecomastia
AUXILIARY LABELS:
- Take with food or milk.
- May cause dizziness and drowsiness.
- Avoid alcohol.

Carbonic Anhydrase Inhibitors. Carbonic anhydrase inhibitors (CAIs) specifically inhibit the enzyme carbonic anhydrase. These agents work to reduce edema by inhibiting hydrogen ion secretion by the renal tubule, which causes the loss of ions such as sodium and potassium. Acetazolamide also is used to reduce intraocular pressure, which is the cause of glaucoma (see Chapter 19).

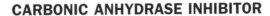

CARBONIC ANHYDRASE INHIBITOR

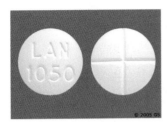

GENERIC NAME: acetazolamide
TRADE NAME: Diamox
INDICATION: edema due to CHF or medications
ROUTE OF ADMINISTRATION: oral, intravenous
COMMON ADULT DOSAGE: 250 to 375 mg every other day in the morning or for 2 days followed by 1 day of rest; 1 day of rest in the regimen allows kidney recovery to maintain effectiveness against edema
AUXILIARY LABELS:
- Take with meals.
- May cause dizziness.

Coronary Artery Disease (CAD)

Coronary artery disease is a condition in which the arteries of the heart do not receive proper oxygenation because of conditions such as atherosclerosis and arteriosclerosis. Symptoms include hypertension, angina pectoris, hyperlipidemia, and myocardial infarction.

Atherosclerosis is a **syndrome** (more than one condition) that affects arterial blood vessels. Inflammation occurs as a result of the lifelong buildup of small plaques, mainly composed of lipids (i.e., fats such as cholesterol), and the clumping of platelets. Although these plaques and platelets can occur anywhere in the large arteries of the body, they tend to accumulate in the arteries throughout the heart, restricting blood flow. Over time small injuries can occur in the vessel wall. When damage occurs to the arterial wall the body responds by sending macrophages and T-lymphocytes to fight the plaques; however, instead of eliminating plaques, these lymphocytes increase the blockage. This cycle continues, eventually causing total blockage or bleeding into the plaque, and this can result in a heart attack or stroke. Although atherosclerosis is a common effect of the aging process, lipid deposits have been observed in young children as well. Many risk factors can be linked to the development of atherosclerosis and eventual coronary artery disease.

Arteriosclerosis is a condition that is due to the thickening, loss of elasticity (hardening), and calcification of the arterial walls. This condition can be caused by hypertension, hyperlipidemia, diabetes, and normal aging.

Prognosis. CAD is one of the leading causes of death in both men and women. This may be due partially to the fact that following their first heart attack (MI), many people do not make the necessary changes in their lifestyle or adhere to their medication regimen to avoid further complications or MIs. Another factor is the difficulty of determining when a complication will occur. With proper medication in addition to lifestyle changes, many people can live with CAD and reduce their risk factors for MI and stroke.

Many available surgical treatments provide relief of symptoms although lifestyle changes are still necessary. Box 23-9 lists guidelines for preventing heart disease.

Non–Drug Treatment. Following a healthy lifestyle is one of the most effective ways to deter the risk of CAD. Smoking, obesity, lack of exercise, and poor dietary habits all increase the risk of CAD. If all efforts fail, then a surgical procedure may be necessary. These include angioplasty or coronary artery bypass graft (CABG). Angioplasty is the insertion and inflation of a small type of balloon into the affected area, which removes and/or stabilizes the plaque. A CABG uses a piece of healthy blood vessel taken from another part of the body

BOX 23-9 AMERICAN HEART ASSOCIATION GUIDELINES TO PREVENT HEART DISEASE

Exercise: A minimum of 30 minutes daily of moderate physical activity is recommended.

Diet: Eat a diet high in fruits, vegetables, grains, fish, nuts, legumes, lean meat, and low-fat dairy products. Avoid saturated and trans–fatty acids.

Stress: Decrease stress through methods such as biofeedback, meditation, and yoga.

Control diabetes: Blood glucose levels should be less than 110 mg/dl and hemoglobin A_{1c} measurements should be less than 7%.

Control blood pressure: BP should be no more than 120/80 mm Hg. BPs for persons who have diabetes should not exceed 130/80 mm Hg.

Control cholesterol: LDL levels less than 100 mg/dl should be sustained.

Quit smoking: Both first-hand and second-hand smoke should be avoided.

Take aspirin: Low-dose aspirin (ASA) should be taken for those persons at high risk of MI (per physician's recommendation).

Tech Note!

Arteriosclerosis is characterized by hardening and loss of elasticity of the arterial vessels. Three forms of this condition are atherosclerosis, sclerosis of the arterioles, and calcific sclerosis of the medial layer of the arteries. Of these three types, atherosclerosis is the most common type, which causes angina, transient ischemic attacks (TIAs), stroke, or even an MI resulting from the formation of a thrombus (clot).

to bypass the affected vessel in the heart. Box 23-9 provides an overview of preventive measures.

Drug Treatment. There are several medications that can control blood pressure, cholesterol, and other symptoms of CAD. These include nitrates, beta-blockers (BBs), calcium channel blockers (CCBs), and bile acid sequestrants.

Thrombosis

The formation of a clot in a vessel that blocks blood flow is known as a thrombosis. Coagulation (blood clotting) is a normal body function aimed at stopping hemorrhage and starting the healing process. Unfortunately, our bodies also can form unwanted blood clots that can appear in other areas. This clotting can occur because of an overactive clotting mechanism (genetic), can result from narrowing of the arteries (such as in persons with atherosclerosis), or may be due to prolonged inactivity. Conditions related to the type of thrombosis are listed in Table 23-5. The body naturally produces chemicals that break up clots. An embolus (plural, emboli) is a blood clot that has broken away from the thrombus (main clot) and has traveled through the body to another area where it can become lodged and create a blockage.

Prognosis. If the embolism is treated within time, the prognosis is good. However, it is important to prevent future clotting that can cause an acute attack. In certain cases warfarin or low-dose heparin may need to be taken for the patient's lifetime.

Non–Drug Treatment. Wearing support stockings and standing and walking on a regular basis to move the blood in the lower extremities are the best way to deter clots from forming.

Drug Treatment. Depending on the severity of the clot, either an anticoagulant (to prevent clotting) or a thrombolytic (breaks up or dissolves clot) should be used. Thrombolytics are given parenterally under the supervision of a physician. These must be used soon after a clot occurs before damage is sustained to the affected organ or tissue. The medications used for a thrombosis are emergency agents that include streptokinase, urokinase, and tissue plasminogen activator (t-PA). The dosage forms of these agents are injectable only and are kept in areas within a hospital such as emergency, surgery, and intensive care units. A patient

TABLE 23-5 **Examples of Types of Embolisms**

Types of Clots: Condition	Affected Area	Symptoms	Causes	Treatment: All Include Lifestyle Changes
DVT	Located in deep veins of legs, arms, or abdominal area	Pain, edema, redness in legs	Sitting or lying for long periods, increased clotting	Warm compresses, leg compression, analgesics and anticoagulants
Pulmonary embolism	Located in a branch of lungs	SOB, blood in sputum, chest pain, elevated heart rate, decreased oxygen saturation	DVT or damage to walls of veins	Oxygen therapy, anticoagulants, and/or thrombolytics
Coronary embolism	Heart (especially dangerous when present in right side of heart, leading to lungs)	Elevated heart rate, heart attack (MI)	Endocarditis, aneurysm, tumor, catheterization, surgery	Oxygen therapy, cardiac arrest agents, anticoagulants, and/or antiplatelet agents or thrombolytics
Brain embolism	Vessels in brain	Confused state, pain in head, altered vision, dizziness; leading to TIA or stroke (CVA)	DVT, cerebral hemorrhage, inflammation of blood vessels	Oxygen therapy, antiplatelet agents, anticoagulants and/or thrombolytics
Fat embolism	Any vessel; may follow trauma to bone or side effect of certain procedures or underlying conditions	Pain, cyanosis, disorientation, tachycardia, tachypnea	Pieces of fat that enter bloodstream and eventually block vein in body	Oxygen therapy, possible anticoagulants and/or thrombolytics

normally does not need more than one dose, and the sooner the drug is administered to the patient, the better the outcome. To prevent blood from coagulating (binding together), anticoagulants may be prescribed.

Anticoagulants. Clots are formed by fibrin, a protein that holds blood cells together to make a blood clot. Heparin inhibits thrombosis by inactivating factor Xa and by preventing the conversion of prothrombin to **thrombin**. This stops the **coagulation** mechanism. Heparin is available in injectable form only. Heparin is prepackaged by manufacturers in 20,000-unit bags of 500 mL or can be made in various units from a wide variety of vial strengths (Box 23-10). Heparin cannot be given orally because stomach acids destroy it. For example, patients who are admitted to the hospital with an MI or stroke may be administered a heparin intravenous drip to prevent blood coagulation. Heparin is effective and is intended for short-term use in a hospital setting. Another use for heparin is to clean the IV line of any coagulating blood; only low concentrations of heparin are used, such as 100 units/mL or less. Because there have been mistakes made in choosing the correct concentrations of heparin, it has caused several deaths, particularly in neonates (see Chapter 14).

Another type of anticoagulant is warfarin. This agent is the only anticoagulant still available in oral dosage form in the United States (the injectable form is used less often). Unlike heparin, orally administered warfarin is indicated for long-term use and is usually taken once daily. Warfarin interferes with the synthesis of vitamin K–dependent coagulation factors (II, VII, IX, and X) in the liver. Prothrombin time and International Normalized Ratio (INR) tests must be done to monitor how long it takes the blood to form clots while the patient is

TABLE 23-6 Examples of Anticoagulants

Generic Anticoagulants	Trade Name	Dosages	Side Effects	Storage
argatroban	argatroban*	IV dose is based on weight, condition, and response to treatment	Minor bleeding, redness, and discomfort	Room temperature; protect from light. Refrigerate for 96 hr after reconstitution
bivalirudin	Angiomax	IV dose is based on weight, condition, and response to treatment	N/V, heartburn, pain, redness, swelling at injection site, H/A, or insomnia	Room temperature. Refrigerate after reconstitution
heparin		Ranges from 5000 to 10,000 units subcutaneously q8h for DVT prevention to weight-based IV infusions given as 18 units/kg/hr IV and adjusted to lab values	Irritation or mild pain at injection site; watch for unusual bleeding or bruising	Room temperature
tinzaparin	Innohep	Subcutaneous dose 175 units/kg/day	Bruising, irritation/bleeding at injection site; pain, swelling, redness	Room temperature
warfarin	Coumadin, Jantoven	Oral dose is based on PT/INR response to drug	Few to none; watch for unusual bleeding or bruising	Room temperature. Protect from light

*No brand name available.

BOX 23-10 HEPARIN CONCENTRATIONS

Generic Name: Heparin Sodium
Vial concentrations
    1000 units/mL
    2000 units/mL
    2500 units/mL
    5000 units/mL
    10,000 units/mL
    20,000 units/mL
    40,000 units/mL

Trade Name: Heplok
10 units/mL
100 units/mL

taking this medication. It is vital that a patient not be overdosed on warfarin or the patient can die from internal bleeding. Warfarin has many interactions with other drugs and with certain foods. Any drug that may increase the potency of warfarin should be avoided unless medically necessary, as well as those agents that counteract the effectiveness of this medication. Patients taking warfarin should wear a medical alert bracelet to notify health care personnel in an emergency. This is due to the severe drug-drug interactions and risks of this drug. Each drug works at a different site within the body and blocks the formation of blood clots. However, once a clot is formed, warfarin (Coumadin or Jantoven) or aspirin cannot be used for active treatment. A **thrombolytic** drug and/or heparin must be administered as soon as possible. Examples of anticoagulants are listed in Table 23-6.

BOX 23-11 ENOXAPARIN (LOVENOX)

Prefilled Injection (PFS)
30 mg per 0.3 mL
40 mg per 0.4 mL
60 mg per 0.6 mL
80 mg per 0.8 mL
100 mg per 1 mL
120 mg per 0.8 mL
150 mg per 1 mL

Low-Molecular-Weight Heparins (LMWHs). Some patients are treated in the hospital and/or discharged home with a low-molecular-weight heparin, such as enoxaparin, which is a subcutaneous injection (Box 23-11). The dosage is dependent on the indication for use and also on the weight of the patient. The patient may be counseled by his or her physician or nurse on how to administer this injectable subcutaneous dose. This low-dose heparin normally is administered for up to 14 days for prophylactic treatment against embolisms. Enoxaparin is just one example of a LMWH; there are many commercially available forms such as Fragmin (dalteparin), Normiflo (ardeparin), and Orgaran (danaparoid).

ANTICOAGULANTS

GENERIC NAME: heparin
TRADE NAME: None
INDICATION: clot treatment and prevention
ROUTE OF ADMINISTRATION: injectable forms only (intravenous, subcutaneous)
SIDE EFFECTS: possible hemorrhage (prothrombin time must be monitored closely)
NOTE: ANTIDOTE: protamine sulfate injection

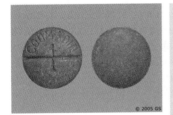

GENERIC NAME: warfarin
TRADE NAME: Coumadin, Jantoven
INDICATION: clot prevention
ROUTE OF ADMINISTRATION: oral, injection (intravenous)
SIDE EFFECTS: possible hemorrhage (prothrombin time or INR must be monitored closely)
AUXILIARY LABELS:
- Avoid alcohol.
- Do not take if you become pregnant.
- Do not take aspirin unless instructed to do so by physician.
- Do not take NSAIDs unless instructed to do so by physician.
NOTE: ANTIDOTE: phytonadione injection (vitamin K)

Antiplatelet Agents. Antiplatelet drugs are used to prevent arterial thrombi, which are made of platelet aggregates (particles). Table 23-7 lists the drugs most commonly used to prevent formation of these types of clots.

Thrombolytics. Streptokinase (Streptase) was an enzyme extracted from bacteria that destroyed clots after they are formed. Urokinase (Abbokinase) is another

TABLE 23-7 **Oral Antiplatelet Agents**

Trade Name	Generic Name	Common Prophylaxis Dosage
Bayer aspirin, others	aspirin	81 to 325 mg/day
Persantine	dipyridamole	75 to 100 mg/day
Ticlid	ticlopidine	250 mg bid with food
Plavix	clopidogrel	75 mg/day
Effient	prasugrel	5 to 10 mg/day

type of lytic agent that is retrieved from a human protein that also reduces thrombosis. Many other thrombolytics are derived through recombinant processes. There are several different thrombolytics, each having their own specific use (Table 23-8). The thrombolytics break down fibrin within a thrombus, dissolving the clot.

Types of Medications Used for Heart Conditions

Because many different agents are used to treat heart conditions (such as coronary artery disease) and their causes (such as hypertension and high cholesterol levels), it is important not only to understand the types of medications but also to comprehend their mechanisms of action and possible side effects. An easy way of remembering the types of medications used to treat the heart conditions discussed in this chapter is to employ the abbreviation "ABCD" (**A**CE inhibitors, **b**eta-blockers, **c**alcium channel blockers, and **d**iuretics). This acronym indicates the common classifications of agents used to treat heart conditions, not the order in which they are prescribed. Although more classifications of agents are available, this is a simplified way to remember them. These classes of drugs are used to treat both CAD and CHF and are discussed next. Diuretics are listed and discussed under CHF because they are one of the main treatments for that condition.

ANGIOTENSIN-CONVERTING ENZYME AGENTS (ACE INHIBITORS)

ACE inhibitors are a group of agents that help reduce blood pressure by causing a decrease of pressure in the arteries. Certain **enzymes** produced by the kidneys ultimately help produce ACE, which increases sodium content. This allows for further increases of fluid retention. ACE inhibitors stop these enzymes from causing vasoconstriction that normally would result in high blood pressure caused by the sodium imbalance. Side effects for ACE inhibitors may include headache, hypotension, and nausea or vomiting (N/V).

ACE INHIBITORS (ACEIs)

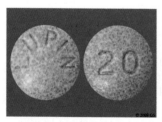

GENERIC NAME: lisinopril
TRADE NAME: Prinivil, Zestril
INDICATION: hypertension, acute MI and post-MI, CHF
ROUTE OF ADMINISTRATION: oral
COMMON ADULT DOSAGE: 10 to 40 mg once daily
SIDE EFFECTS: dizziness, H/A, N/V, diarrhea
AUXILIARY LABEL:

■ May cause dizziness/drowsiness.

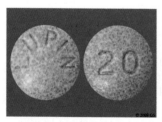

★ **Tech Note!**

To remember the agents used to treat hypertension, use the acronym ABCD (**a**ngiotensin-converting enzyme inhibitors, **b**eta-blockers, **c**alcium channel blockers, and **d**iuretics). Although these agents are not prescribed in this order, it is a way of remembering the classes of drugs.

TABLE 23-8 Examples of Thrombolytics

Generic Thrombolytics	Trade Name	Dose	Side Effects	Storage
streptokinase	Streptase, Kabikinase	Acute MI: 1,500,000 units within 60 min of event	Nausea, dizziness, hypotension, mild fever; potential for bleeding from cuts	Room temperature Use within 8 hr after reconstitution
		(within 7 days) PE:* LD 250,000 units over 30 min, then 100,000 units over 24 hr		
		(within 7 days) Arterial thrombosis: LD 250,000 units over 30 min, then 100,000 units/hr for 24-72 hr		
		(within 7 days) DVT: LD 250,000 units over 30 min, then 100,000 units/hr for 72 hr		
		(within 7 days) Embolism: LD 250,000 units over 30 min, then 100,000 units/hr for 24-72 hr		
urokinase	Kinlytic	Acute MI: LD 4400 units/kg to run at 90 mL/hr × 10 min, then 15 mL × 12 hr	Bleeding from cuts or injection site, fever, hypotension	Refrigerate
		PE: Both LD and continuous infusion are based on weight (kg) of patient; dose ranges between 2,250,000 and 6,250,000 units/kg		
alteplase	Activase (t-PA)	Acute MI: 15 mg IV bolus, then 0.75 mg/kg IV (max: 50 mg) infused over 30 mins, and then 0.5 mg/kg IV (max: 35 mg) over next 60 mins	Bleeding	Refrigerate Protect from light Use within 8 hr after reconstitution
		PE: 100 mg over 2 hr × 1 dose		
		Ischemic stroke: 0.9 mg/kg, max 90 mg over 60 min × 1 dose		
reteplase	Retavase (rPA)	Acute MI: first bolus given over 2 min, second bolus given 30 min after first bolus	Bleeding	Room temperature or refrigerate Protect from light Good for 4 hr refrigerated after reconstitution
tenecteplase	TNKase	Acute MI: dose is based on weight, not to exceed 50 mg	Bleeding	Room temperature or refrigerate
anistreplase	Eminase	Acute MI: 30 units over 2-5 min	Bleeding	Refrigerate Use within 30 min of reconstitution

*LD, Loading dose; PE, pulmonary embolism.

GENERIC NAME: benazepril
TRADE NAME: Lotensin
INDICATION: hypertension
ROUTE OF ADMINISTRATION: oral
COMMON ADULT DOSAGE: 20 to 40 mg once daily or divided twice daily; maximum of 80 mg/day
SIDE EFFECTS: dizziness, H/A, nausea, constipation
AUXILIARY LABEL:
- May cause dizziness/drowsiness.

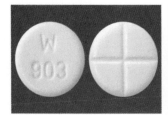

GENERIC NAME: captopril
TRADE NAME: Capoten
INDICATION: hypertension, CHF, post acute MI, diabetic nephropathy
ROUTE OF ADMINISTRATION: oral
COMMON ADULT DOSAGE: 25 to 50 mg two or three times daily; maximum 450 mg/day
SIDE EFFECTS: dizziness, drowsiness, H/A, insomnia, dry mouth, nausea, diarrhea or constipation
AUXILIARY LABELS:
- Take 1 hour before meals.
- May cause dizziness or drowsiness.

GENERIC NAME: fosinopril
TRADE NAME: Monopril
INDICATION: hypertension, CHF
ROUTE OF ADMINISTRATION: oral
COMMON ADULT DOSAGE: 10 to 40 mg once daily
SIDE EFFECTS: dizziness, nausea, cough
AUXILIARY LABELS:
- Take with or without meals.
- Do not take with antacids.
- May cause dizziness.

ANGIOTENSIN II RECEPTOR ANTAGONISTS (ALSO KNOWN AS ANGIOTENSIN RECEPTOR BLOCKERS)

Angiotensin II receptor antagonists work by inhibiting the effects of angiotensin II receptors located in vascular muscles. This in turn lowers blood pressure via antagonistic effects on vasoconstriction. These agents have no major side effects.

ANGIOTENSIN II RECEPTOR ANTAGONISTS

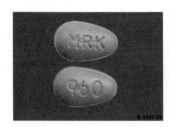

GENERIC NAME: losartan
TRADE NAME: Cozaar
INDICATION: hypertension; diabetic nephropathy
ROUTE OF ADMINISTRATION: oral
COMMON ADULT DOSAGE: 25 to 100 mg once daily or divided twice daily
SIDE EFFECTS: dizziness, muscle cramping
AUXILIARY LABEL:
- Take as directed.

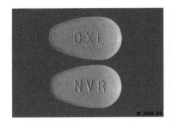

GENERIC NAME: valsartan
TRADE NAME: Diovan
INDICATION: hypertension, heart failure, post-MI
ROUTE OF ADMINISTRATION: oral
COMMON ADULT DOSAGE: 80 to 320 mg once daily
SIDE EFFECTS: dizziness, H/A, fatigue, diarrhea, dry mouth
AUXILIARY LABEL:

■ Take as directed.

BETA-BLOCKING AGENTS

Beta-blockers are a set of agents that are effective because they block both norepinephrine and epinephrine from binding to nerve receptors. Blocking these receptors decreases the heart rate and dilates blood vessels, lowering blood pressure. Beta-blockers act at two sites: the beta$_1$- and beta$_2$-receptor sites. Beta$_1$-receptors are located in the heart, whereas beta$_2$-receptors are located in the lungs and deep arteries. The actions of medications can be specific or nonspecific. Nonspecific agents affect beta$_1$ and beta$_2$ sites.

A nonspecific agent would not be recommended if a person was diagnosed with asthma or another type of respiratory problem. Selective beta-blockers for the heart are preferred in almost all instances of treating heart disease. When beta$_2$ sites are inhibited, respiratory airways can be restricted; therefore the physician must determine the appropriate agent for the patient. Side effects include dizziness, hypotension, and diarrhea.

BETA-BLOCKING AGENTS

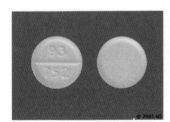

GENERIC NAME: atenolol
TRADE NAME: Tenormin
INDICATIONS: hypertension, angina pectoris, acute and post-MI
ROUTE OF ADMINISTRATION: oral, injection (intravenous)
COMMON ADULT DOSAGE: oral: 25 to 50 mg once daily. Up to 100 mg/day
SIDE EFFECTS: tired feeling, drowsiness or anxiety, nervousness, insomnia
AUXILIARY LABELS:

■ Take as directed.
■ May cause dizziness/drowsiness.
■ Do not discontinue unless advised by physician.

GENERIC NAME: propranolol
TRADE NAME: Inderal, Inderal LA
INDICATIONS: hypertension, angina pectoris, arrhythmias, and migraine prophylaxis
ROUTE OF ADMINISTRATION: oral, injection (IV)
COMMON ADULT DOSAGE: oral (immediate release) for hypertension: 40 to 80 mg three times daily; Inderal LA: 80-160 mg once daily
SIDE EFFECTS: drowsiness, N/V, diarrhea, constipation, insomnia
AUXILIARY LABELS:

■ Take as directed.
■ May cause dizziness/drowsiness.
■ Avoid alcohol.
■ Do not discontinue unless advised by physician.

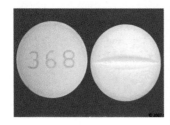

GENERIC NAME: metoprolol
TRADE NAME: Lopressor, Toprol XL
INDICATIONS: hypertension, angina pectoris, acute and post-MI, heart failure
ROUTE OF ADMINISTRATION: oral, injection (intravenous)
COMMON ADULT DOSAGE: oral (immediate release): Initially, 12.5 to 25 mg twice daily. Up to 450 mg/day in divided doses for HTN. 50 to 100 mg twice daily following MI. Toprol XL: 50 to 100 mg per day up to 400 mg/day for HTN
SIDE EFFECTS: drowsiness, insomnia, vomiting or anxiety, nervousness
AUXILIARY LABELS:

- Take as directed.
- Take with food.
- Do not chew or crush tablet.
- Do not discontinue unless advised by physician.

CALCIUM CHANNEL BLOCKERS

Calcium channel blockers act by decreasing calcium intake by the heart and blood vessels. Calcium is used by the heart to stimulate the conduction system (the electrical pump). When the calcium channel is blocked by these agents, the heart rate slows, which decreases stress on the heart muscle. Common side effects include dizziness, drowsiness, constipation, and blurred vision in varying degrees, depending on the specific agent.

CALCIUM CHANNEL BLOCKERS

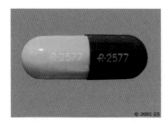

GENERIC NAME: diltiazem
TRADE NAME: Cardizem CD, Cardiazem LA, Cardiazem SR, Dilacor XR, Tiazac
INDICATIONS: angina pectoris, chronic stable angina, essential hypertension
ROUTE OF ADMINISTRATION: oral, injection (intravenous)
COMMON ADULT DOSAGE: for extended-release products: 180 to 240 mg once daily up to 360-420 mg/day for HTN
SIDE EFFECTS: stuffy nose, skin rash or itching, dizziness, headache, tired feeling, nausea
AUXILIARY LABELS:

- May cause dizziness.
- Take with a full glass of water.
- Do not crush or chew (any extended-release dose forms).

NOTE: Tiazac capsules can be either swallowed whole or opened and sprinkled on a spoonful of applesauce.

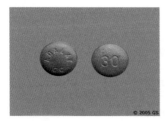

GENERIC NAME: nifedipine
TRADE NAME: Procardia XL, Adalat CC
INDICATIONS: hypertension, chronic stable angina
ROUTE OF ADMINISTRATION: oral
COMMON ADULT DOSAGE: Procardia XL: for hypertension, 30 or 60 mg once daily; Adalat CC: 30 mg once daily. Max: 90 mg/day for HTN
SIDE EFFECTS: dizziness, nausea, constipation, flushing, H/A, fatigue, insomnia
AUXILIARY LABELS:

- Take on an empty stomach.
- Take as directed.
- May cause dizziness/drowsiness.
- Do not crush, chew, or break (for sustained-release tablets).

GENERIC NAME: verapamil
TRADE NAME: Calan, Isoptin, Verelan, Calan SR, Isoptin SR, Verelan PM
INDICATIONS: angina, chronic atrial flutter or fibrillation, essential hypertension
ROUTE OF ADMINISTRATION: oral, injection (intravenous)
COMMON ADULT DOSAGE: oral immediate-release dosage form (Calan, Isoptin, Verelan): 40-120 mg three times daily; Verelan: 240-480 mg once daily; Verelan PM: 200 mg once daily at bedtime; long-acting dosage forms (Calan SR, Isoptin SR): 120 mg once daily to 240 mg every 12 hours
SIDE EFFECTS: dizziness, drowsiness, nausea, constipation, H/A
AUXILIARY LABELS:
- Take with food or milk.
- Take as directed.
- Do not crush or chew (any extended-release dose forms).

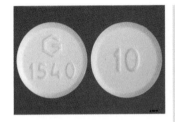

GENERIC NAME: amlodipine
TRADE NAME: Norvasc
INDICATIONS: hypertension, chronic stable angina, variant angina
ROUTE OF ADMINISTRATION: oral
COMMON ADULT DOSAGE: for hypertension, 5 to 10 mg once daily
SIDE EFFECTS: dizziness, drowsiness, H/A, N/V, diarrhea, constipation, insomnia, dry mouth
AUXILIARY LABELS:
- Take as directed.
- May cause dizziness/drowsiness.

Tech Alert!

Remember the following sound-alike/look-alike drugs:

Nicobid versus Nitro-Bid
Cardene versus Cardizem
Cardene SR versus Cardizem SR
nicardipine versus nifedipine versus nimodipine
Lotensin versus Lioresal

GENERIC NAME: felodipine
TRADE NAME: Plendil
INDICATION: hypertension
ROUTE OF ADMINISTRATION: oral
COMMON ADULT DOSAGE: 2.5 to 10 mg once daily
SIDE EFFECTS: dizziness, drowsiness, H/A, nausea, flushing
AUXILIARY LABELS:
- May cause dizziness/drowsiness.
- Take as directed
- Avoid grapefruit juice.
- Do not crush or chew tablet

DO YOU REMEMBER THESE KEY POINTS?

- The location of the heart
- The pathway of blood flow through the heart
- The layers of the heart muscle
- Conditions that affect the heart
- Causes for heart problems such as congestive heart failure, coronary artery disease, and hypertension
- Treatments for conditions affecting the heart
- Common side effects for medications mentioned in this chapter
- Types of diuretics and their mechanism of action
- The effects of over-the-counter medications for persons suffering from hypertension
- The types of angina and the medications used to treat them
- The difference between the use of anticoagulants and thrombolytics
- The difference between atherosclerosis and arteriosclerosis

REVIEW QUESTIONS

Multiple choice questions

1. The average adult heart beats _____ times per minute.
   A. 50
   B. 70
   C. 90
   D. 100

2. The artery responsible for supplying the heart muscle with oxygen is called the:
   A. Pulmonary artery
   B. Aorta
   C. Coronary artery
   D. Myocardial passageway

3. The cardiac conduction system is responsible for:
   A. Providing the electrical charge to the heart muscle
   B. Oxygenating the blood
   C. Receiving blood from the body
   D. None of the above

4. A condition in which fluid builds up within tissues is known as:
   A. Myocardial infarction
   B. Angina pectoris
   C. Congestive heart failure
   D. Hypertension

5. Factor(s) that may affect the condition of atherosclerosis is (are):
   A. Lifestyle
   B. Family history
   C. Smoking
   D. All of the above

6. If Mr. Low has a blood pressure of 165/95 mm Hg, he would have:
   A. Low blood pressure
   B. Normal blood pressure
   C. Slightly high blood pressure
   D. High blood pressure

7. ACE inhibitors is an abbreviation for:
   A. Activating coronary electrical site inhibitors
   B. Altering and converting enzyme inhibitors
   C. Angiotensin-converting enzyme inhibitors
   D. Angina converting enzyme inhibitors

8. Beta-blockers are effective because they work by:
   A. Blocking receptor sites in the heart
   B. Blocking receptor sites in the heart and kidneys
   C. Activating receptor sites in the heart and lungs
   D. Activating receptor sites in the heart and kidneys

9. Calcium channel blockers are effective because they work by:
   A. Blocking channel 1 and 2 receptors
   B. Reducing cardiac conduction
   C. Accelerating the heart rate to pump more blood
   D. None of the above

10. Which instruction is NOT patient information necessary about taking oral nitroglycerin medications?
    A. Take with food.
    B. Keep medication within the original container.
    C. Take as needed for chest pain; maximum 3 times in 15 minutes; if no relief after the first dose, then call 911.
    D. Keep medication out of direct sunlight.

11. Urokinase, Abbokinase, and t-PA are classified as:
    A. Vasoconstrictors
    B. Vasodilators
    C. Prophylaxis thrombolytics
    D. Thrombolytics

12. The common life span of nitroglycerin (once opened) is:
    A. 3 months
    B. 6 months
    C. 12 months
    D. None of the above

13. The four chambers of the heart are:
    A. Right and left: upper and lower atrium
    B. Right and left: atrium and superior and inferior venae cavae
    C. Right and left: atrium and ventricle
    D. None of the above

14. The medication that dissolves blood clots is called:
    A. Heparin
    B. Aspirin
    C. t-PA
    D. Warfarin

15. Heparin cannot be given orally because:
    A. It takes too long to work
    B. It is used only for emergencies
    C. It is degraded by gastric juices
    D. It binds directly to blood products

16. Which of the medications listed below is NOT a calcium channel blocker?
    A. Verapamil
    B. Metolazone
    C. Nifedipine
    D. Diltiazem

17. Which of the medications below is the trade name for amlodipine/valsartan?
    A. Azor
    B. Caudet
    C. Diovan
    D. Exforge

18. Which of the medications listed would be used to treat deep vein thrombosis (DVT)?
    A. Anticoagulants
    B. Thrombolytics
    C. Calcium channel blockers
    D. Both A and B

19. The drug Caduet would be prescribed to:
    A. Lower hypertension
    B. Increase blood pressure
    C. Lower cholesterol
    D. Both A and C

20. Which drug can be taken with grapefruit juice?
    A. Lipitor
    B. Zocor
    C. Mevacor
    D. Pravachol

True/False

If the statement is false, then change it to make it true.

_____ **1.** The heart pumps only oxygenated blood.

_____ **2.** Oxygenated blood returns from the lungs via the pulmonary artery.

_____ **3.** The epicardium is the outer layer of the heart muscle, and it protects the heart.

_____ **4.** The vena cava is the large artery that carries blood to the body system.

_____ **5.** Two major types of lipoproteins that should be monitored are HDL and LDL.

_____ **6.** HDL stands for high-density lipoprotein and is considered bad cholesterol.

_____ **7.** Cholesterol has no benefit to the human body.

_____ **8.** The fibers that control the conduction system are called the pacemaker.

_____ **9.** Congestive heart failure can be cured by surgery.

_____ **10.** Hypertension also is known as the silent killer.

_____ **11.** Nitrates are agents that cause vasoconstriction.

_____ **12.** Aspirin is a thrombolytic agent.

_____ **13.** Calcium channel blockers are often the first line of treatment for angina.

_____ **14.** An embolism is a thrombosis or clot that has moved from its origin.

_____ **15.** Aspirin has more side effects than heparin or warfarin.

_____ **16.** Beta-blockers increase blood pressure, thus helping the heart beat stronger.

_____ **17.** Angiotensin-converting enzyme inhibitors increase blood pressure, thus helping the heart beat faster.

_____ **18.** Nitroglycerin must be kept in a glass container.

_____ **19.** All diuretics cause a loss of potassium through frequent urination.

_____ **20.** Edema is a condition of inflammation of the tissues resulting from hyperlipidemia.

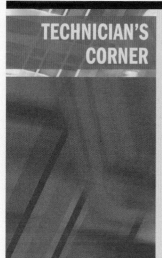

TECHNICIAN'S CORNER

Mrs. Lewis arrives at the pharmacy with several prescriptions. Using a comprehensive drug reference, such as *Drug Facts and Comparisons* or *Mosby's Drug Consult,* look up the medications listed and determine what condition is affecting Mrs. Lewis. In addition, classify each of the medications, and transcribe the prescription into layman terms as though you were preparing a prescription label.

Zocor 5 mg qd, #30
Digoxin 0.125 mg qd, #30
Furosemide 40 mg bid, #60
K-Dur 20 mEq bid, #60
Albuterol INH 1 to 2 puffs prn SOB, #17g
NTG 0.4 mg sl tab prn cp, 1 q 5 min, max 3 tabs over 15 min; call 911 if chest pain unrelieved after first dose, 4/#25s
Atenolol 25 mg qd, #30

BIBLIOGRAPHY

AMA (American Medical Association) *Concise Medical Encyclopedia.* 2006.

Clayton B, Yvonne S, Renae H: *Basic pharmacology for nurses,* ed 14, Philadelphia, 2006, Elsevier Science.

Drug facts and comparisons, ed 63, St Louis, 2008, Lippincott Williams & Wilkins.

Lacy C, et al: *Lexi Comp's drug information handbook,* ed 18, Hudson, 2009, Lexi-Comp.

Heitkemper M, et al: *Medical-surgical nursing: assessment and management of clinical problems*, ed 7, St Louis, 2007, Mosby.

Mosby's 2006 drug consult for nurses, St Louis, 2006, Mosby.

Potter P, Anne P: *Fundamentals of nursing*, ed 6, St Louis, 2004, Mosby.

Professional guide to diseases, ed 9, Ambler, PA, 2009, Lippincott Williams & Wilkins.

Stedman's concise medical dictionary for health professionals, ed 3, Baltimore, 1997, Williams & Wilkins.

WEBSITES

Christian W MD, et al: Arch Neurol 2002;59:1584-1588. Eitology, Duration, and Prognosis of Transient Ischemic Attacks. http://archneur.ama-assn.org/cgi/content/abstract/59/10/1584

Drugs. www.drugs.com

Filtration recommendations summary. www.utmb.edu/rxhome/Operations/Filtrations.htm. Retrieved 10/06

Heart disease: an introduction to coronary artery disease. www.healthcentral.com/heart-disease/what-is-heart-disease-000003_1-145.html?ic=506019

HeartFailure. www.mayoclinic.com/health/heart-failure/DS00061/DSECTION=treatments%2Dand%2Ddrugs

24

Reproductive System

Objectives

UPON COMPLETING THIS CHAPTER, YOU SHOULD BE ABLE TO DO THE FOLLOWING:

- List both trade and generic drug names covered in this chapter.

- Describe the organs of the male and female reproductive tracts and their locations.

- Describe the male and female hormones and their roles in the body.

- List the common conditions affecting the male reproductive system and the medications used to treat these conditions.

- List the common conditions affecting the female reproductive system and the medications used to treat these conditions.

- Describe hormone replacement therapy in the female, and list the medications used for hormone replacement.

- List the different types of oral contraceptives.

- List other types of contraception and the advantages and disadvantages of each.

- Describe the medications that are used as abortifacients.

- List the types of sexually transmitted diseases and their treatments.

TERMS AND DEFINITIONS

Abortifacient *Any treatment that causes abortion of a fetus*

Androgen *Male hormone*

Chloasma *Hyperpigmentation of skin, limited or confined to a certain area*

Depot *An area of the body where a substance can accumulate or be stored for later distribution*

Endometrium *Mucous membrane lining of the uterus*

Fallopian tube *Narrow passage between the ovary and the uterus*

Fertilization *The process by which a sperm unites with an ovum to create a new life*

Gametes *Sex cells, or ova and sperm*

Inert ingredient *An ingredient that has little or no effect on body functions*

Menopause *Cessation of menstruation; a natural phenomenon in which a woman passes from a reproductive state to a nonreproductive state*

Negative feedback *A self-regulating mechanism in which the output of a system has input or control on the process; in this case, the stimulus results in reactions that reduce the effects of the stimulus*

Oocyte or ova *The female reproductive germ cell, more commonly known as an egg*

Palliative *That which brings relief but does not cure*

Sperm or spermatozoa *The male reproductive germ cell*

Teratogen *Any agent causing abnormal embryonic or fetal development*

EXAMPLES OF REPRODUCTIVE SYSTEM DRUGS

Trade Name	Generic Name	Pronunciation	Trade Name	Generic Name	Pronunciation
Androgens			Prempro, Premphase	conjugated estrogens/ medroxyprogesterone	(kon-juh-**gat-ed** **ess**-troe-gens/ me-drox-see-proe -**jess**-teur-owne)
Androderm	testosterone	(tes-**toss**-ter-one)			
Halotestin	fluoxymesterone	(floo-ox-ee-**mes**-ter-one)			
Testred, Android	methyltestosterone	(meth-ill-tes-**toss**-ter-own)			
			Progestins		
Alpha-Adrenergic Blockers			Prometrium	progesterone	(pro-**jess**-teur-owne)
Flomax	tamsulosin	(tam-**sue**-lo-sin)	Micronor	norethindrone	(nor-**eth**-in-drone)
Uroxatral	alfuzosin	(al-**fue**-zoe-sin)	Ovrette	norgestrel	(nor-**jess**-trel)
			Provera	medroxyprogesterone	(me-drox-see-proe- **jess**-teur-owne)
Androgen Hormone Inhibitors					
Avodart	dutasteride	(doo-**tas**-ter-ide)			
Proscar	finasteride	(fin-**ass**-te-ride)	**Oral Contraceptives**		
			Monophasic Combinations		
Estrogens			Alesse, Levlen	ethinyl estradiol/ levonorgestrel	(**eth**-in-ill ess-tra-**dye**-ole/ **lev**-o-nor-**jess**-trel)
Delestrogen	estradiol valerate	(ess-tra-**dye**-ole **val**-er-ate)	Demulen	ethinyl estradiol/ ethynodiol diacetate	(**eth**-in-ill ess-tra-**dye**-ole/ eh-the-no-**dye**-ol di-**as**-ah-tate)
Estrace, Estraderm	estradiol	(ess-tra-**dye**-ole)			
Estratab, Menest	esterified estrogen	(ess-**ter**-i-fide **ess**-troe-gen)	Desogen, Ortho-Cept	ethinyl estradiol/ desogestrel	(**eth**-in-ill ess-tra-**dye**- ole/des-o-**ges**-trol)
Ogen, Ortho-Est	estropipate	(ess-troe-**pye**-pate)	LoOvral, Ovral	ethinyl estradiol/ norgestrel	(**eth**-in-ill ess-tra-**dye**- ole/nor-**jess**-trel)
Premarin	conjugated estrogens	(kon-juh-**gat**-ed **ess**-troe-gens)	Ortho-Cyclen	ethinyl estradiol/ norgestimate	(**eth**-in-ill ess-tra-**dye**-ole/ nor-**jess**-ti-mate)

Continued

EXAMPLES OF REPRODUCTIVE SYSTEM DRUGS—cont'd

Trade Name	Generic Name	Pronunciation	Trade Name	Generic Name	Pronunciation
Ortho Evra Patch	ethinyl estradiol/ norgestimate	(**eth**-in-ill ess-tra-**dye**-ole/ nor-**jess**-ti-mate)	**Infertility Medications**		
Ortho-Novum 1/35	ethinyl estradiol/ norethindrone	(**eth**-in-ill ess-tra-**dye**-ole/ nor-**eth**-in-drone)	Bravelle	urofollitropin (FSH)	(yoor-oh-fol-li-**troe**-pin)
Ortho-Novum 1/50	mestranol/ norethindrone	(**mess**-tra-nol/ nor-**eth**-in- drone)	Clomid	clomiphene	(**kloe**-mi-feen)
Yasmin 28, Yaz	drospirenone/ethinyl estradiol	(dro-**spy**-re-nown/ **eth**-in-ill **ess**-tra-dye-ole)	Crinone, Prochieve, Endometrin	progesterone	(pro-**jess**-teur-owne)
			Follistim AQ	follitropin beta (r-FSH)	(fol-li-**troe**-pin bet-ah)
Biphasic Combination			Luveris	lutropin alfa (r-LH)	(lou-**tro**-peen aal-fa)
Ortho-Novum 10/11	ethinyl estradiol/ norethindrone	(**eth**-in-ill ess-tra-**dye**-ole/ nor-**eth**-in-drone)	Ovidrel	choriogonadotropin alfa (r-HCG)	(kor-ee-**oh**-goe-**nad**- oh-troe-pin aal-fa)
			Parlodel	bromocriptine	(bro-mo-**ckrip**-teen)
Triphasic Combinations			Repronex, Menopur	menotropins	(**men**-o-trop-in)
Ortho Tri-Cyclen/ TriNessa/ Tri-Sprintec	ethinyl estradiol/ norgestimate	(**eth**-in-ill ess-tra-dye-ole/ nor-**jess**-ti-mate)	**Miscellaneous Medications for the Reproductive System**		
			Emergency Contraceptive		
Ortho-Novum 7/7/7	ethinyl estradiol/ norethindrone	(eth-in-ill ess-tra-**dye**-ole/ nor-**eth**-in-drone)	Plan B, NextChoice	levonorgestrel	(**lev**-o-nor-**jess**-trel)
Triphasil	ethinyl estradiol/ levonorgestrel	(**eth**-in-ill ess-tra-dye-ole/ **lev**-o-nor-**jess**-trel)	**Drugs for Endometriosis**		
			Lupron	leuprolide	(loo-**pro**-lide)
Estrophasic Combination			Synarel	nafarelin	(**naf**-a-rell-in)
Estrostep	ethinyl estradiol/ norethindrone	(**eth**-in-ill ess-tra-**dye**-ole/ nor-**eth**-in-drone)	Zoladex	goserelin	(**goe**-ser-a-lin)
			Drugs for Erectile Dysfunction		
Long-Acting Contraceptives			Caverject	alprostadil	(al-**pros**-ta-dil)
Depo-Provera	medroxyprogesterone	(me-drock-see-pro-**jess**-teur-owne)	Cialis	tadalafil	(tah-**dal**-ah-fill)
			Levitra	vardenafil	(var-**den**-ah-fill)
Lunelle	medroxyprogesterone/ estradiol	(me-drock-see-pro-**jess**-teur-owne/ ess-tra-**dye**-ole)	Viagra	sildenafil	(sil-**den**-a-fil)
			Examples of Drugs Used for Reproductive System Infections/Sexually Transmitted Diseases (STDs)		
Mirena IUD	levonorgestrel	(lev-o-nor-jess-trel)	Bicillin LA	penicillin G benzathine	(pen-eye-**cil**-in)
			Flagyl	metrondiazole	(met-row-**nid**-dah-zole)
Spermicidal Contraceptives			Floxin	ofloxacin	(o-**flox**-a-sin)
Delfen, Advantage 24	nonoxynol-9	(non-**ox**-i-nol)	Suprax	cefixime	(sef-**ix**-ime)
			Valtrex	valacyclovir	(val-a-**sye**-kloe-veer)
			Zovirax	acyclovir	(a-**sye**-klo-veer)
			Examples of Drugs for Vaginal Fungal Infections		
			Diflucan	fluconazole	(floo-**koe**-na-zole)
			Vagistat	tioconazole	(**tye**-oh-**kon**-a-zole)

THE MAJOR FUNCTION of the reproductive system is the production of offspring for the survival of the species. This organ system operates interdependently with other systems such as the endocrine system—which provides the necessary hormones responsible for the maturation, development, and regulation of the reproductive system—and the urinary system—which in the male serves as the passageway for both urine and sperm. In men and women, the functions of reproduction are divided between the primary, secondary, and accessory organs. The primary reproductive organs are the gonads (ovaries or testes), which are necessary to produce the gametes or sex cells (ova or sperm, respectively). The gonads are also responsible for the secretion of the hormones that provide gender characteristics of the male or female. The secondary reproductive organs include the structures necessary for transport and sustenance of the **gametes** (ova in females and sperm in males) and those organs necessary for the growth of the developing fetus in the female. Accessory organs include ducts, glands, and external genitalia.

Hormones control the functions of the reproductive system. Estrogen and testosterone are present in both men and women although their effects are somewhat different because of the different concentrations present in each gender. The functions of these hormones and others are outlined in Table 24-1.

The male and female reproductive systems, conditions, and treatments are covered, respectively. A discussion about sexually transmitted diseases (STDs) and their effects on both genders is found at the end of this chapter.

MEDICAL TERMINOLOGY OF THE REPRODUCTIVE SYSTEM

Word Parts (Both Male/Female)	
Cervic	Cervix
Crypt/o	Hidden
Mast/o	Breast
My/o	Muscle
Olig/o	Few, scanty
Urethr/o	Urethra
Zo/o	Animal

Specific to Females	
Hyster/o, metr/o	Uterus
Lact/o	Milk
Men/o	Menstruation
Metri/o, uter/o	Uterus
Oophor/o, ovari/o	Ovaries
Placent/o	Placenta
Salping/o	Fallopian tubes
Vagin/o, colp/o	Vagina
Ves/o	Vessel
Vulv/o	Vulva

Specific to Males	
Orch/o, orchid/o	Testes, testicles
Pen/i, phall/i	Penis
Prostat/o	Prostate gland
Test/i, test/o, testicul/o	Testes, testicles
Vas/o	Vas deferens

Prefixes (Both Male/Female)	
A, an-	Without
Ante-	Forward
Endo-	Within
Peri-	Surrounding
Poly-	Many

Suffixes (Both Male/Female)	
-itis	Inflammation
-ism, -osis	Abnormal condition
-cele	Hernia or protrusion
-ectomy	Surgical removal

Continued

MEDICAL TERMINOLOGY OF THE REPRODUCTIVE SYSTEM—cont'd

-iferous	Carrying
-pause	Stopping
-an	Relating to
-rrhexis	Rupture
-rrhea	Flow or discharge
-dyna, -algia	Pain

Conditions	
Amenorrhea	Absence or suppression of menses
Benign prostatic hypertrophy	Nonmalignant enlargement of prostate gland
Dysmenorrhea	Abdominal pain caused by uterine cramps during menstrual period
Endometriosis	Condition in which tissue resembling endometrium is found outside uterine cavity, usually in pelvic area
Menorrhagia	Abnormally heavy or extended menstrual flow
Metrorrhagia	Bleeding from uterus not associated with menstruation; excessive and irregular bleeding pattern
Nocturia	Excessive urination at night
Oophoritis	Inflammation of ovaries
Polycystic ovary syndrome	Development of cysts due to hormonal imbalance, which causes enlargement of ovaries
Prostatitis	Inflammation of prostate; condition may present with urinary tract infection
Testitis	Inflammation of testes

TABLE 24-1 Hormone Functions

Hormone	Gender	Functions
Androgens	Male	Steroid hormone that stimulates and controls development and maintenance of male characteristics
	Female	Precursor to estrogens in women
Testosterone	Male	Stimulates growth and maturation of male reproductive organs
		Triggers development of secondary sex characteristics: pubic and facial hair, enhanced hair growth on chest and other areas
		Stimulates sperm production
		Responsible for sex drive
		Voice changes
		Skin changes: thicker skin, acne
		Bone and skeletal muscle growth (affects size and mass)
		Affects production of GnRH in hypothalamus
	Female	Responsible for sex drive
Gonadotropin-releasing hormone (GnRH)	Male	Stimulates LH, which then stimulates gonadal secretion of testosterone, estrogen, and progesterone; sex steroids inhibit secretion of GnRH (negative feedback system)
	Female	Same as in male
Luteinizing hormone (LH)	Male	Stimulates secretion of sex steroids from gonads
		Stimulates synthesis and secretion of testosterone; this is converted into estrogen
	Female	Secretion of steroid hormones progesterone and estradiol
Progesterone	Female	Necessary for maintenance of pregnancy and luteinization of ovarian follicles
	Male	Not applicable
Follicle-stimulating hormone (FSH)	Female	Stimulates ovarian follicles, producing many mature gametes (eggs)
	Male	Maturation of sperm production

Male Reproductive System

In the male the reproductive system is closely tied to the urinary system. The urethra passes through the penis, is surrounded by the prostate gland, and is responsible for removal of urine from the body as well as the exit route for sperm. The testicles are responsible for the production of sperm after puberty and for the immediate storage of **sperm** cells (Figure 24-1). Once sperm production begins, it continues throughout the lifetime of the male. After sperm are formed, they mature and are stored in the epididymis (a series of tightly coiled tubes wrapped around the back of the testes) and then travel into the vas deferens (a muscular tube that extends from the epididymis to the ejaculatory duct), where peristaltic movements transport the sperm into the ejaculatory duct.

The prostate is about the size and shape of a walnut. The prostate also encircles part of the urethra, the tube that carries urine out of the bladder and through the penis. The secretions of the prostate gland both enhance the motility and viability of sperm and provide a slightly alkaline environment that will endure the acidic environment of the vagina. Finally, the sperm and fluids pass through the urethra in the penis for ejaculation during sexual intercourse.

Male sex hormones are stimulated by the release of gonadotropin-releasing hormone (GnRH) from the hypothalamus. GnRH then travels to the anterior pituitary and causes it to secrete luteinizing hormone (LH), also called interstitial cell–stimulating hormone in the male, and follicle-stimulating hormone (FSH). Interstitial cell–stimulating hormone then promotes the growth of interstitial cells in the testes and stimulates the cells to secrete testosterone. Testosterone and FSH stimulate spermatogenesis (creation of sperm) in the testicles (Figure 24-2).

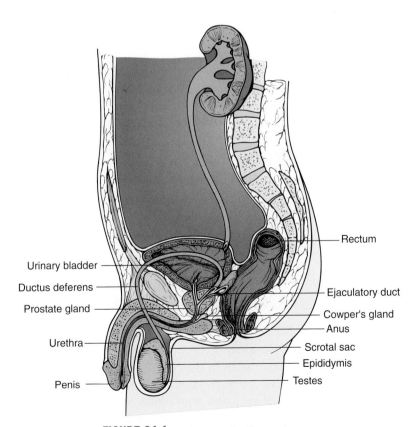

FIGURE 24-1 Male reproductive system.

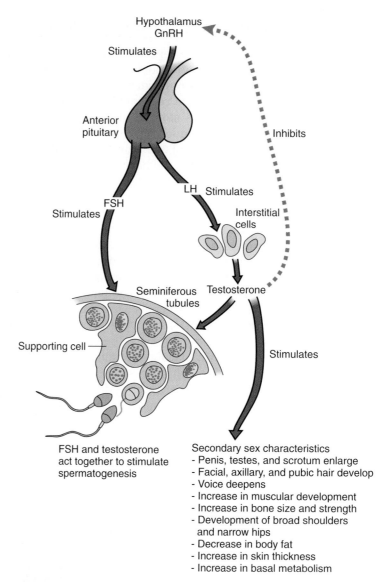

FIGURE 24-2 Function of testes in response to hormone stimulation.

Male sex hormones collectively are called androgens, with testosterone being the most abundant androgen. At puberty, the androgens stimulate the formation of secondary male characteristics, such as increased muscle mass, deepening of the voice, and growth of facial hair. Although females produce testosterone, the androgens play a less significant role in the development of female sexual characteristics and reproduction.

Conditions Affecting the Male Reproductive System

A number of conditions can affect the male reproductive system. With the implementation of diagnostic procedures, many of these conditions can be identified and treated. A wide variety of available medications can cure or mitigate diseases and conditions. A list of various conditions that can affect the male reproductive system is in Table 24-2. In the following section several conditions are outlined that include the prognosis (outlook) as well as drug and non–drug

TABLE 24-2 **Conditions Affecting the Male Reproductive System**

Conditions of the Male	Definition	Treatment
Penis		
Balanitis	Inflammation of tip of penis caused by bacterial or fungal infection or unknown etiology (cause)	Antibiotic or antifungal for infection
Phimosis	Tightness of foreskin of penis that causes nonretractability	Either antibiotics for infection and/or circumcision
Impotence	Inability to achieve or sustain an erection	Change in medication, lifestyle changes, mechanical devices, surgery
Premature ejaculation	Uncontrolled ejaculation either before or immediately after sexual penetration	If diagnosed abnormal, antidepressants (Prozac, Paxil) can be prescribed (an off-label use)
Testicles		
Hypogonadism	Low sperm count attributable to testicular failure or pituitary problem	Hormone replacement (testosterone)
Epididymitis	Infection of epididymal connective tissue, causing inflammation	Antibiotics for infection, analgesics for pain
Testicular cancer	Malignant cancer cells forming in one or both testicles	Chemotherapy, antiemetics for N/V
Orchitis	Inflammation of one or both testicles	Antibiotics (Cipro, Keflex) for infection, NSAIDs* or opiates for pain
Priapism	Uncontrolled erection that lasts for several hours	Vasoconstrictors to reduce blood flow to penis
Prostate Gland		
BPH	Enlargement of prostate gland	Androgen hormone inhibitors and alpha-blockers to decrease size of prostate
Prostate cancer	Malignant cancer cells forming in prostate	Chemotherapy, antiemetics for N/V
Prostatitis	Inflammation of prostate	Antibiotics for infection, analgesics for pain, alpha-blockers for relaxing muscle fibers in bladder neck

*NSAIDs, Nonsteroidal antiinflammatory drugs.

treatments available. In each monograph, information on the medication is given along with common auxiliary labels and side effects. The following abbreviations are used to define side effects:

- H/A, headache
- N/V, nausea and vomiting
- HBP, high blood pressure

COMMON CONDITIONS

Erectile Dysfunction (ED)
Erectile dysfunction is the inability of the male to achieve or maintain an erection, commonly referred to as impotence. This is due to a lack of blood flowing to the penis, rather than a lack of desire. This condition ranges from rare to chronic. As one ages the probability of experiencing ED increases. By the age of 40 years, most men have been affected at one time or another. As men age they have an increased risk of acquiring not only prostate conditions but also other disease states that inadvertently affect the ability to achieve an erection, such as diabetes, atherosclerosis, high blood pressure, and cardiovascular diseases. Additional causes of ED are listed in Table 24-3.

TABLE 24-3 Causes of Erectile Dysfunction

Condition or Cause That Leads to ED	Effects
Prostatism	Enlargement of prostate gland
Prostatitis	Inflammation of prostate gland
Prostatocystitis	Inflammation of prostate gland and bladder
Nerve damage	Injury to NS* caused by trauma, surgery, or disease
Substance abuse	Alcohol leads to atrophy of testes, lowering testosterone levels; other drugs (e.g., heroin, cocaine, marijuana) contribute to ED
Low testosterone levels	Hypogonadism can lower sex drive and cause ED
Medications	Medications can have side effects that may cause sexual dysfunction, including ED, such as certain BBs, CCBs, antidepressants, antihypertensive agents, antihistamines, H_2-antihistamines, antiseizure medications
Depression/anxiety	Depression can cause or worsen ED due to stress, anxiety, low self-esteem, fears, guilty feelings
Cigarette smoking	Smoking can worsen atherosclerosis, which increases possibility of ED

BBs, Beta-blockers; CCBs, calcium channel blockers; ED, erectile dysfunction; NS, nervous system.

Prognosis. In many cases ED only occurs on rare occasions and does not pose a problem. Persistent ED can be a sign of a possible problem with an underlying undiagnosed condition. When a patient complains of ED, it is imperative that the physician identify and treat any underlying conditions. With proper treatment and lifestyle changes the frequency of episodes of ED may be decreased and sexual activity can still occur.

Non–Drug Treatments. There are vacuum devices that can be used to increase blood flow to the penis. Psychotherapy in certain cases can help the male overcome anxieties associated with ED. Most importantly, lifestyle changes should be made, such as decreasing alcohol intake, quitting smoking, losing weight, and participating in an exercise program, to control any underlying condition.

Drug Treatments. Sildenafil (Viagra) was introduced in 1998 for the treatment of erectile dysfunction (ED). This medication initially was researched for use as a cardiovascular agent to lower blood pressure and treat angina pectoris. Today this medication is used for erectile dysfunction; it increases blood flow to the penis and causes penile rigidity. Many other drugs in the same class have been approved for ED as well. The side effects include headaches, flushing of the skin, gastrointestinal symptoms, nasal congestion, and diarrhea. Patients taking nitrates should not take sildenafil or related drugs because of the dangerous decrease in blood pressure that is possible when these agents are combined. Table 24-4 lists medications as well as non–drug treatments used for erectile dysfunction. Any medication used to treat ED has the risk of causing priapism. Priapism is a painful erection that can last for hours. If not treated in a timely fashion priapism can cause scarring and permanent ED or impotency; thus priapism is a medical emergency that requires immediate medical assistance. Suppositories are another option for the treatment of ED although pain is associated with the insertion of the suppository into the urethra. Both injections and suppositories are not used as often as the oral medication.

Benign Prostatic Hypertrophy (Benign Prostatic Hyperplasia or BPH)
Benign prostatic hypertrophy is an overgrowth or enlargement of the prostate gland. The prostate gland is positioned between the bladder and urethra and encircles the urethra. When the prostate becomes enlarged it makes urination difficult.

TABLE 24-4 Medications for Erectile Dysfunction

Generic Name	Trade Name	Indication	Strengths	Dosage Form	Instructions	Side Effects
sildenafil	Viagra	Used for both psychological and physical cause	25, 50, 100 mg	Tab	Taken 1 hr before sexual activity on an empty stomach	H/A, flushing, nausea, diarrhea
vardenafil	Levitra	ED caused by diabetes, post prostate surgery	5, 10, 20 mg	Tab	Taken 1 hr before sexual activity with or without food	H/A, flushing, nasal congestion, dizziness, nausea
tadalafil	Cialis	ED caused by diabetes, post prostate surgery	5, 10, 20 mg	Tab	Taken 1 hr before sexual activity with or without food	H/A, flushing, nasal congestion, indigestion, back pain, muscle aches
alprostadil urethral suppositories	Muse	ED	1 supp	Supp	Inserted before sexual activity; remain standing until erection occurs (15-30 min)	Pain in penis where suppository is inserted, mild urethral bleeding, dizziness
alprostadil	Caverject	ED	Dose determined by physician's order; may be combined off-label with papaverine and phentolamine for injection	Inj	Inject into penis before sexual activity	Pain at injection site, risk of priapism or scarring of penis
yohimbine	Yocon	ED	5.4 mg	Tab	Take three times daily	Dizziness, H/A, irritability, restlessness

This condition occurs in approximately half of men by the age of 50. It is noncancerous and nonlethal although it is disruptive to daily life. The goal of treatment for benign prostatic hypertrophy is to relieve symptoms such as hesitancy on urination, a decrease in the stream of urine, post-voiding dribbling, frequency of urination, and nocturia, and to prevent urinary tract infections.

Prognosis. Although there is no known cause of prostate enlargement there are several treatments that can be effective in lessening the side effects of this condition. Treatments range from lifestyle changes to medication or surgery. There are several procedures as well that may be available to lessen the enlarged prostate gland thus relieving the symptoms of BPH.

Non–Drug Treatment. For mild symptoms of BPH there are steps that can be taken to possibly lessen and/or determine the severity of the condition. This includes avoiding smoking, alcohol, caffeine, OTC antihistamines/decongestants, and to exercise regularly.

Surgery is an option if patients do not respond to medication. The physician physically removes the excess tissue surrounding the prostate gland. Another treatment includes using low-level radiofrequency waves to destroy the excess prostate tissue.

Drug Treatment. There are two classes of drugs used to treat BPH: androgen hormone inhibitors decrease the size of the prostate, although it can take up to 6 months to reach maximum effectiveness. Alpha-blockers act quickly to lessen urinary symptoms of BPH although they do not stop the overall process of prostate enlargement. Most often both types of drugs are used concurrently to give the best results.

Androgen Hormone Inhibitors. These agents block the conversion of testosterone to a more active form that is known to increase the growth of cells (also cancer cells), thus reducing the amount of growth of the prostate tissue.

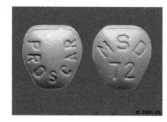

GENERIC NAME: finasteride
TRADE NAME: Proscar
INDICATION: benign prostatic hypertrophy
ROUTE OF ADMINISTRATION: oral
COMMON ADULT DOSAGE: 5 mg once daily
SIDE EFFECTS: mild; change in sex drive or impotence, breast enlargement or tenderness
AUXILIARY LABELS:
- Do not chew or crush.
- Take as directed.
- May cause dizziness.

NOTE: Because this drug causes birth defects, a woman who is pregnant or trying to become pregnant should avoid contact with crushed or broken tablets because the active drug can penetrate through the skin; if contact is made with finasteride, immediately wash hands with soap and water; notify your physician about the exposure.

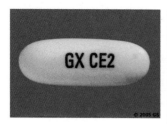

GENERIC NAME: dutasteride
TRADE NAME: Avodart
INDICATION: benign prostatic hypertrophy
ROUTE OF ADMINISTRATION: oral
COMMON ADULT DOSAGE: 0.5 mg once daily
SIDE EFFECTS: mild; change in sex drive or impotence, breast enlargement or tenderness
AUXILIARY LABEL:
- Do not chew or crush.

NOTE: Because this drug causes birth defects a pregnant woman should avoid contact with the capsules because the active ingredient can penetrate through the skin if the capsules are leaking. If contact is made with a leaking capsule, immediately wash hands with soap and water; notify your physician about the exposure.

Alpha-Adrenergic Blockers. These agents work selectively to inhibit alpha$_1$-receptor sites. Some of these agents are less selective for prostate tissue and are also used for the treatment of hypertension. Others (e.g., Flomax) have more targeted activity for the tissues of the prostate. These agents are effective for BPH by relaxing smooth muscle tissue found in the prostate and the bladder neck. This allows urine to flow out of the bladder more easily.

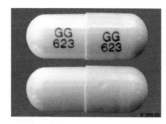

GENERIC NAME: terazosin
TRADE NAME: Hytrin
INDICATION: benign prostatic hypertrophy
ROUTE OF ADMINISTRATION: oral
COMMON ADULT DOSAGE: 1 mg initial dose at bedtime; then increased to 2, 5, and then 10 mg once daily
SIDE EFFECTS: dizziness, drowsiness, blurred vision, puffy hands
AUXILIARY LABELS:
- May cause dizziness/drowsiness.
- Avoid alcohol.
- Do not drive or perform any hazardous tasks until accustomed to side effects.

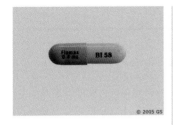

GENERIC NAME: tamsulosin
TRADE NAME: Flomax
INDICATION: benign prostatic hypertrophy
ROUTE OF ADMINISTRATION: oral
COMMON ADULT DOSAGE: 0.4 to 0.8 mg once daily; give ½ hour after the same meal each day
SIDE EFFECTS: dizziness
AUXILIARY LABELS:
- May cause dizziness/drowsiness.
- Avoid alcohol.
- Do not crush or chew capsule.

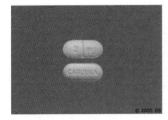

GENERIC NAME: doxazosin
TRADE NAME: Cardura, Cardura XL
INDICATIONS: benign prostatic hypertrophy, mild hypertension
ROUTE OF ADMINISTRATION: oral capsule
COMMON ADULT DOSAGE: immediate release: 1 to 8 mg once daily in the AM or PM; Cardura XL: 4 or 8 mg once daily with breakfast
SIDE EFFECTS: dizziness
AUXILIARY LABELS:
- May cause dizziness/drowsiness.
- Avoid alcohol.
ADDITIONAL LABELS FOR CARDURA XL:
- Do not break, crush, or chew.
- Take with food.

Prostate Cancer

Prostate cancer is a condition in which the cells within the prostate grow (forming tumors) at an uncontrolled rate (Figure 24-3). This blocks the flow of urine through the prostate and if left untreated can metastasize (spread) through the body, causing widespread cancer. Genetics seem to affect the onset of this condition; African American men are more likely to develop prostate cancer as well as those men who have relatives with prostate cancer. Symptoms include nocturia, dysuria, blood in the urine or semen, painful ejaculation, and pain in

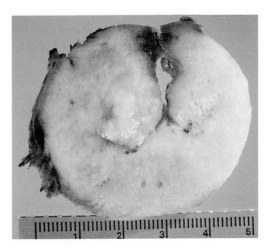

FIGURE 24-3 Prostate cancer. (From Kumar V, Cotran RS, Robbins SL: *Basic pathology,* ed 7, Philadelphia, 2003, Saunders.)

BOX 24-1   STAGES OF PROSTATE CANCER

Stage 1: Cancer is present only in the prostate.
Stage 2: Cancer is more advanced but still located within prostate.
Stage 3: Cancer has spread to local area(s) surrounding the prostate.
Stage 4: Cancer has spread to lymph nodes and possibly to other areas including liver, lungs, bladder, or even the bones.

TABLE 24-5   Prostate Cancer Treatments

Type of Hormone Therapy	Generic Name	Trade Name	Type/Effect in Male
LHRH	leuprolide	Lupron Depot	Blocks hormone production in testes
	goserelin	Zoladex	Blocks hormone production in testes
Antiandrogens	flutamide	Eulexin	Blocks effects of testosterone
	nilutamide	Nilandron	Blocks effects of testosterone

the pelvis or lower back that does not subside. There are four stages of prostate cancer (Box 24-1); staging the cancer is necessary to determine the most effective treatment plan as well as improve the prognosis.

Prognosis. Although prostatic cancer is a serious condition it has become more treatable. Early diagnosis, increased public awareness, and new chemotherapy agents have increased the life span of men diagnosed with prostate cancer (see Chapter 29). If discovered early and treated quickly, there is approximately a 90% chance the condition can be cured. Cure rates are dependent on the person's age, overall health, and preexisting conditions, because all these factors influence treatment success.

Non–Drug Treatment. Changing dietary habits can help to reduce the possibility of prostate cancer. Prostate cancer can be treated by performing surgery that removes the prostate (radical prostatectomy) or the testicles (orchidectomy). A partial removal of prostate tissue (transurethral resection of the prostate, or TURP) may be done to remove some of the cancer. Radiological treatment can be used to treat recurrent or advanced stage prostate cancer. Cryotherapy is less frequently used; in this case a probe is inserted through the rectum and aimed at the prostate; then argon gas or liquid nitrogen is used to literally freeze the tumor.

Drug Treatment. The treatment for prostate cancer is determined by the stage of the cancer. Hormone therapy is the most common medical treatment used for prostate cancer. The activity of hormones can be eradicated or reduced so that the cancerous cells stop reproducing. Antiandrogens and luteinizing hormone–releasing hormone (LHRH) agonists can cause a decrease in hormone activity, and are the most common agents used. All of these treatments are usually started in stage 2 prostate cancer. See Table 24-5 for examples of medications used.

Estrogens were historically used in men for **palliative** treatment of inoperable prostate, breast, and testicular cancers. The increased estrogen in males causes the development of female sexual characteristics, including voice changes, breast enlargement, loss of body hair, testicular and penile atrophy, and impotence. The feminization and impotence of males usually are reversed when the medication is discontinued. Estrogen treatments are not common today.

If the cancer has spread and is no longer responding to hormonal manipulation, then the patient may be treated with various chemotherapy regimens. One of the most common agents used is docetaxel (Taxotere).

Male Hypogonadism

When the body cannot produce enough testosterone, it is referred to as hypogonadism. This condition can occur in the fetus, during puberty, or at any time during adulthood. Hypogonadism can be caused by underdevelopment of the genitals (during fetal development), impaired growth (at puberty), infection (bacterial or viral), or injury (tumors or trauma) to the glands that produce testosterone. Symptoms resulting from the lack of testosterone include fatigue, decreased sex drive, difficulty concentrating, and hot flashes. In adulthood the risk of osteoporosis increases.

Prognosis. If treatment with hormone replacement therapy can be done, this will help to reduce the effects of this condition and the outlook is good.

Non–Drug Treatment. Reducing stress and anxiety can help improve the man's attitude about this condition. There are support groups available that can help men cope with this condition. Osteoporosis can be prevented by taking vitamin D and ensuring proper calcium intake, both of which help to prevent bone loss.

Drug Treatment. Androgens are used to treat hypogonadism or infertility resulting from a low sperm count. The increase in sperm count is achieved through the suppression of **negative feedback**, causing an increased secretion of testosterone, FSH, and interstitial cell–stimulating hormone. Different types of medication delivery systems can be used to promote puberty and development of secondary sex characteristics. Dosage forms include intramuscular (IM), transdermal patch, topical gel, and buccal forms.

Androgens. Testosterones provide a sense of well-being, mental stability, and energy. Testosterone also provides the body with a resistance to fatigue. Natural testosterone that is used for medicinal purposes was originally obtained from the testes of bulls; however, the drug is now chemically synthesized from cholesterol. Androgens that are produced synthetically are called anabolic steroids—medications that can be used to build muscle mass. Because of the misuse and abuse of anabolic steroids, the Drug Enforcement Administration (DEA) has placed all anabolic steroids, including the various testosterone products, on the schedule III list of controlled medications.

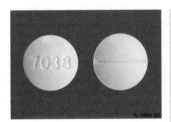

GENERIC NAME: methyltestosterone (C-III)
TRADE NAME: Testred, Android (capsules), and Methitest (tablets)
INDICATIONS: men: androgen replacement therapy, hypogonadism, delayed puberty; women: palliative treatment of metastatic breast cancer (rare)
ROUTE OF ADMINISTRATION: oral
COMMON ADULT DOSAGE: males: 10 to 50 mg daily; some males take 10 mg three times daily
SIDE EFFECTS: acne, breast swelling, baldness, H/A, anxiety, depression, mild nausea, changes in sex drive
AUXILIARY LABEL:
■ Use as directed.

GENERIC NAME: testosterone (C-III)
TRADE NAME: Androderm transdermal system
INDICATIONS: androgen replacement therapy, male hypogonadism
ROUTE OF ADMINISTRATION: 2.5 or 5 mg transdermal patch
COMMON ADULT DOSAGE: apply 5 mg patch once daily
SIDE EFFECTS: itching/burning at patch site, breast swelling/tenderness, acne, hair growth, H/A, depression, changes in sex drive
AUXILIARY LABELS:
■ Topical.
■ Use as directed.

GENERIC NAME: testosterone (C-III)
TRADE NAME: AndroGel
INDICATIONS: men: androgen replacement therapy, male hypogonadism, delayed puberty; women: metastatic breast cancer
ROUTE OF ADMINISTRATION: gel packet or multi-dose pump
COMMON ADULT DOSAGE: apply 5 g once daily (usual max 10 g/day) to the skin on the abdomen, upper arm, or shoulder and rub into skin; cover with cloth
SIDE EFFECTS: temporary stinging at application site, breast enlargement, acne, H/A, HBP, prostate disorder
AUXILIARY LABEL:
■ Use as directed.
NOTE: Flammable; avoid smoking, fire, flames until gel has dried.

GENERIC NAME: testosterone (C-III)
TRADE NAME: Striant
INDICATIONS: male hypogonadism
ROUTE OF ADMINISTRATION: 30 mg buccal striant (curved tablet)
COMMON ADULT DOSAGE: apply striant to the gums every 12 hours; rotate sides of application with each dose
SIDE EFFECTS: bitter taste, gum or mouth irritation, gum tenderness or pain, H/A
AUXILIARY LABEL:
■ Use as directed.

Female Reproductive System

The female reproductive system produces and transports **ova** (or oocytes) from the ovary through the fallopian tube into the uterus, which will house a fertilized ovum. After puberty the female ovary matures an egg each month, although recent studies indicate that more than one egg may mature. At birth the female ovary contains all the eggs available for the woman's lifetime. Thus females do not produce ova throughout life but only mature those that are available. When an egg is mature, it is gathered by the fimbriated end of the infundibulum (funnel-shaped structure or passage) of the **fallopian tube**. The fallopian tubes are in constant motion, but at ovulation their activity increases, and currents in the peritoneal fluid are created to propel the egg into the fallopian tube. During the next 7 days, the ovum is moved down the fallopian tube where it may become fertilized by a sperm. Because an ovum is only viable for 24 to 38 hours, most **fertilization** occurs in the fallopian tube. At the end of the tube is the uterus that either will house the fertilized ovum or slough the ovum and **endometrium** as menses if fertilization has not occurred. This cycle begins at puberty and continues until menopause, or for a period of about 40 years (Figure 24-4).

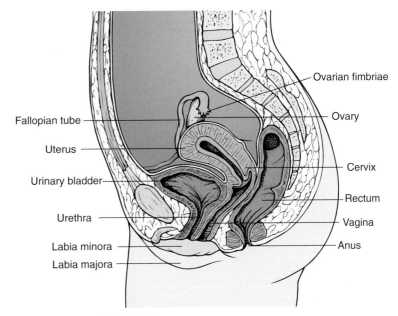

FIGURE 24-4 Female reproductive system.

As in the male, gonadotropin-releasing hormone (GnRH), from the hypothalamus, acts on the anterior pituitary gland to secrete the hormones necessary for ovulation—FSH and LH stimulate the ovaries to secrete estrogen and progesterone. These female hormones are controlled by negative feedback and are secreted in cycles, unlike the continuous secretion of sex hormones in males (Figure 24-5). The levels of female hormones peak when a woman is in her 20s and then gradually decreases throughout life.

The accessory organs of the female reproductive tract are the mammary glands or breasts. Breast tissue also is regulated by hormonal secretions. At puberty the increase in estrogen stimulates the development of glandular tissue, causing an accumulation of adipose tissue, and progesterone stimulates the development of the duct system that is used during milk production.

Conditions Affecting the Female Reproductive System

HORMONAL TREATMENTS

The principal medications that affect the female reproductive system are hormones. Some agents stimulate secretions, whereas others inhibit the action of certain hormones. Medication therapy for conditions of the reproductive tract can be complicated; hormone levels must be considered and must remain constant. Just as female hormones are used to treat certain conditions in males, male hormones are used to treat endometrial or breast cancer, endometriosis, and fibrocystic disease in the female. The inhibition of the natural hormones in either gender is caused by the use of hormones of the other gender, much like negative feedback in which the stimulating hormone is inhibited. Remember that the hypothalamus cannot distinguish between hormones naturally produced by the body and those that are administered as medications; therefore the body will react to synthetic and naturally occurring hormones in the same manner.

Estrogens are the dominant form of medical therapy used to treat conditions such as abnormal uterine bleeding resulting from hormone imbalance, abnormal

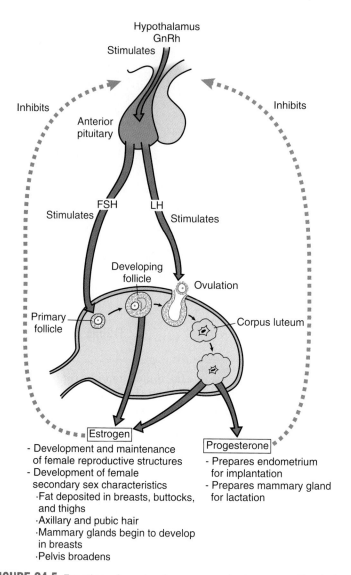

Hypothalamus
GnRh

Stimulates

Inhibits · Inhibits

Anterior
pituitary

FSH   LH
Stimulates   Stimulates

Developing
follicle   Ovulation

Primary
follicle   Corpus luteum

Estrogen   Progesterone

- Development and maintenance
  of female reproductive structures
- Development of female
  secondary sex characteristics
  ·Fat deposited in breasts, buttocks,
   and thighs
  ·Axillary and pubic hair
  ·Mammary glands begin to develop
   in breasts
  ·Pelvis broadens

- Prepares endometrium
  for implantation
- Prepares mammary gland
  for lactation

FIGURE 24-5 Function of ovaries in response to hormone stimulation.

ovulation, and infertility. Estrogens also are used for hormone replacement therapy. One of the main uses of estrogen preparations is for oral contraception. Estrogens also have effects on bone and heart health in females; estrogens support the growth of strong bones and increase levels of high-density lipoproteins (good cholesterol). Estrogens support the development and maintenance of the reproductive organs and the secondary sex characteristics and have profound influences on the menstrual cycle. The naturally occurring estrogens, such as estradiol and estriol, are steroids that are converted to estrone and estrone sulfate by the body.

The primary oral estrogen pharmaceutical products in use are conjugated estrogens (from the urine of pregnant mares or synthetically from yams) or estradiol (produced synthetically). Estrogens are also available in several forms; some forms are unique, such as implants, vaginal inserts, and transdermal systems. The most common forms are oral and injectable (water-based or oil-based) preparations. The oil-based injectable estrogen medications, called depot medications, are prepared to prolong the medication's action by allowing absorption in the fatty tissue for slow distribution. Transdermal preparations are applied to the skin to provide continuous daily release of the medication. Drug-laden vaginal rings are pressed into the vaginal canal for the continuous release of medications into the local tissues. Other locally administered estrogens include vaginal inserts and creams that provide absorption of hormones at the local site. The choice of preparation to be used depends on the reason for use, the benefits versus the risks of treatment, the cost, the reliability of the patient to use it correctly, and the convenience of use. Most estrogens are prescribed at the lowest dose needed to provide the desired effect over the shortest time.

The primary actions of estrogens are to maintain reproductive structures such as ova production and to provide secondary sex characteristics. In women, estrogens are used for a multitude of purposes, and may be used to treat hypogonadism, to increase the possibility of contraception, and to relieve symptoms of menopause (natural or surgical). Adverse effects of estrogens in females may include **chloasma**, photosensitivity, nausea, vomiting, bloating, and risk of gallbladder disease. Dysmenorrhea, breast tenderness and enlargement, and increased susceptibility to thrombotic disease are also common side effects. Although estrogens induce a feeling of well-being, high levels may cause depression that may rarely progress to psychosis. In addition, estrogens may aggravate asthma, epilepsy, migraines, heart disease, diseases of the urinary tract, and diabetes mellitus.

Male hormones can be used for treating certain female breast tumors that grow faster in the presence of estrogen. **Androgens** suppress the effects of estrogen, thus preventing rapid growth of these tumors. Sometimes the medications may even cause the tumor to atrophy (shrink). Other uses of androgens in females are to suppress postpartum breast engorgement and fibrocystic disease by causing atrophy of the breasts; however, these uses are not very common because of the risks to the patient. For the woman with endometriosis, androgens cause suppression of the endometrium and thus prevent the excessive uterine bleeding that is associated with the disease. Women receiving androgen therapy for prolonged periods may have amenorrhea or menstrual irregularities. Hot flashes, headaches, sleep disorders, increased libido, vaginitis, and masculinization also are found. Changes in the voice (lowering of the voice) are often permanent, whereas other symptoms, such as loss of breast mass, increased facial and body hair, and increased muscle mass, may reverse when the testosterone therapy is discontinued. Masculinization does not seem to occur with short-term use of androgens by women with conditions such as postpartum engorgement of the breasts.

COMMON CONDITIONS

Female Hypogonadism

Female hypogonadism is the lack of production of estrogen in the ovaries. In childhood the symptoms include a lack of menstruation and breast development and short height. If this condition occurs during puberty, symptoms include loss of menstruation, hot flashes, loss of body hair, and decreased libido. In adult women, hypogonadism can cause infertility and early menopause. Menopause is a naturally occurring transition between 50 and 60 years of age and is a type of hypogonadism because of the normal decrease in hormone levels. The effects of menopause increase the risk of osteoporosis and heart disease after menopause is complete. Turner's syndrome, one type of female hypogonadism, is caused by a genetic defect in which part of one of the two X chromosomes is partially or entirely missing. Symptoms in infants include swollen hands and feet and a wide, webbed neck. In older females, symptoms may include drooping eyelids, absent or incomplete development at puberty (small breasts, little pubic hair), absence of menstruation, short height, and vaginal dryness.

Prognosis. The outlook is good for many types of female hypogonadism with proper medical treatment.

Non–Drug Treatments. Although the proper functioning of the female reproductive system is not required to sustain the woman's life, most women still desire an effective reproductive tract. The only non–drug treatment would be to prevent or deter possible causes of conditions that result in hypogonadism. In addition, maintaining ideal body weight, eating a healthy diet, refraining from smoking, and adhering to an exercise regimen may improve infertility and reduce cancer risks.

Drug Treatments. There are medications prescribed for hormone replacement therapy and to decrease symptoms of hypogonadism. Estrogen and progestin are used for hormone replacement and may help ovarian stimulation, and low-dose testosterone may increase sex drive. Estrogen is available in tablet form, topical lotions or gels, or as transdermal patches. Testosterone is available in injectable form, gels, or topical patches. In the case of Turner's syndrome, estrogen, progestin, and other hormone therapy are normally started around puberty to trigger breast and pubic hair growth and to ensure proper stature; there is no treatment that will stimulate the production of ova in those with Turner's syndrome. Some of the specific drugs used for the treatment of a variety of causes of hypogonadism are listed under Estrogen Preparations.

Pelvic Inflammatory Disease (PID)

Inflammation of the female reproductive organs is referred to as pelvic inflammatory disease or PID. PID is a severe infection of the uterine lining, fallopian tubes, or ovaries that can cause chronic pain and permanent infertility. Tubal ectopic pregnancy (i.e., the egg attaches and grows in the fallopian tube) occurs 6 to 10 times more often in women who have a history of PID; ectopic pregnancy is normally fatal to the fetus and may be life-threatening to the mother.

Often PID is due to a sexually transmitted disease (STD), although this is not exclusively the case. An untreated infection of the genital tract may result in PID; the use of an intrauterine device (IUD) by a female in a nonmonogamous relationship is also a known risk factor. The length of time for the infection to occur ranges from days to months. Symptoms include abnormal or increased vaginal discharge, bleeding between periods, painful menstruation, painful urination/bowel movements, fever, painful intercourse, and pain in the upper right abdomen. PID can require hospitalization in severe cases, such as for women who do not respond to oral treatment. The following are risk factors for PID:

- History of PID: Prior episodes of PID, especially those caused by gonorrhea and chlamydia, increase the woman's risk for future PID.
- Age: Teenagers are 3 times more likely to develop PID.
- Multiple sex partners: Women who have multiple sex partners or whose partner has multiple sex partners have an increased risk of contracting PID.
- Frequency: Women who have frequent intercourse are at greater risk of contracting infection and PID.
- Use of an IUD (contraceptive): There is an increased risk of developing PID near the time of insertion of an IUD; however, testing for PID or infection before insertion can reduce this risk; use of an IUD when not monogamous also increases PID risks, and IUDs are normally not placed in patients who are not monogamous.
- HIV: Because of a compromised immune system, women with human immunodeficiency virus (HIV) have an increased susceptibility to infection and therefore PID.

Prognosis. Through rapid diagnosis, treatment, and prevention methods, the outlook for PID is good. One third of women who have PID experience an additional episode (womenshealthchannel.com).

TABLE 24-6 PID Treatments

Oral Regimen A*				
Ceftriaxone 250 mg IM × 1 dose	Plus	Doxycycline 100 mg po bid × 14 days	With or without	Metronidazole 500 mg po bid × 14 days
Oral Regimen B*				
Cefoxitin 2 gm IM × 1 & Probenecid 1 gm po × 1	Plus	Doxycyline 100 mg po bid × 14 days	With or without	Metronidazole 500 mg po bid × 14 days
Oral Regimen C*				
Ceftizoxime or Cefotaxime	Plus	Doxycycline 100 mg po bid × 14 days	With or without	Metronidazole 500 mg po bid × 14 days
Parenteral Regimen A*				
Cefotetan 2 gm IV q12h	or	Cefoxitin 2 gm IV qhr	Plus	Doxycycline 100 mg po or IV q 12h
Parenteral Regimen B*				
Clindamycin 900 mg IV q8hr			Plus	Gentamicin LD IV/IM (2 mg/kg), followed by 1.5 mg/kg q8hr
Parenteral A or B to Be Followed with:				
Doxycycline 100 mg po bid × 14 days	or	Clindamycin PO 450 mg qid		
Alternative Parenteral Regimens*				
Ampicillin/Sulbactum (Unasyn) 3 gm IV q6hr			Plus	Doxycycline 100 mg po or IV q12hr

*Regimens are optional for the physician to determine the best course of treatment.
Source: http://www2a.cdc.gov/stdtraining/self-study/pid.asp.

Non–Drug Treatments. The following are some non–drug treatment suggestions to avoid PID: use condoms; have partner(s) tested for STDs; avoid using an IUD if you are prone to STDs, are not in a long-term monogamous relationship, or have a history of PID.

Drug Treatments. Specific antimicrobials are targeted toward the causative microbe (bacteria, protozoa, or fungus). If treated at home, oral medications are typically prescribed. If hospitalization is necessary, therapy is usually initiated with intravenous antibiotics. There are different combinations of medications used to treat PID (Table 24-6).

Menopause

Like testosterone secretion in the male, estrogen and progesterone secretion responds to hormones released from the anterior pituitary gland. Gonadotropin-releasing hormone (from the hypothalamus) stimulates FSH and LH (from the anterior pituitary gland) to cause the ovaries to secrete estrogen and progesterone. Unlike testosterone in the male, these hormones follow cyclical patterns each month beginning at puberty and continuing until menopause, when hormone secretion decreases. During perimenopause, the ovaries gradually decrease estrogen production.

Menopause is a "natural" loss of the production of hormones normally synthesized by the ovaries. Although this is not a "disease," the symptoms associated with menopause can cause unwanted side effects. These can be treated with medications. The bone loss associated with menopause can also be reduced by using medications that lower the risk of osteoporosis.

Prognosis. Uncomfortable but not life-threatening, the symptoms of menopause can last for many years.

Non–Drug Treatments. Some lifestyle changes that can lessen the symptoms associated with menopause include the following: reduce weight if necessary, eat a healthy diet, stop smoking, exercise, use stress reduction techniques, and get enough rest.

Drug Treatments. Estradiol is the major natural estrogen that is produced by the ovaries. Estradiol is used for hormone replacement therapy in the naturally postmenopausal woman or in the woman who is experiencing a surgical menopause. Estradiol usually is combined with a progestin in a woman with an intact uterus because of the increased risk of endometrial overgrowth and the potential risk for endometrial cancer when combination medications are not used. If a patient does not have a uterus, then estrogen alone is prescribed.

The risk and benefits of hormone replacement therapy (HRT) are confusing and complicated. Estrogen replacement therapy is considered the most effective treatment for menopausal symptoms such as hot flashes, mood swings, and night sweats. It has also been shown that HRT can help protect against osteoporosis. However, a 2002 Women's Health Initiative report claimed that HRT poses more risks than benefits to a woman's health. This large study determined that HRT can increase a women's risk of developing breast cancer, stroke, blood clots, and heart disease. Understandably, this report caused confusion among women and health care professionals, with many women discontinuing HRT or deciding not to initiate HRT. The current recommendations for HRT are that HRT is to be used as a short-term therapy to help women with the most severe menopausal symptoms and that the therapy should be discontinued at soon as possible. HRT must be initiated with a thorough understanding of the benefits, risks, family health factors, personal health risks, and preferences of the patient.

Estrogen Preparations. There are many side effects for estrogen therapy; it is advised that the minimal dosage be given for the least amount of time. All estrogens have a Pregnancy Category X rating because of their teratogenicity. **Teratogenic** agents cause birth defects by causing abnormal development of the embryo or fetus during pregnancy.

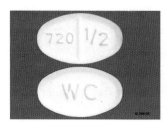

GENERIC NAME: estradiol
TRADE NAME: Estrace, Femtrace, Gynodiol (oral), Estraderm (transdermal), Estring (vaginal ring)
INDICATIONS: menopausal symptoms, female hypogonadism
ROUTE OF ADMINISTRATION: oral, transdermal (patches, lotions, or gels), vaginal
COMMON ADULT DOSAGE: oral, 0.5 to 2 mg once daily or cyclically; transdermal, regimens and application instructions vary with brands of patches (for Estraderm, 0.05 to 1 mg patch replaced twice weekly); vaginal ring, change ring every 3 months; Topical products are also available: Estrogel, Elestrin, Divigel (gels), Evamist (spray), Estrasorb (emulsion lotion), or as an individually tailored strength through a compounding pharmacy; these are applied once daily
SIDE EFFECTS: N/V, swollen breasts/ankles/feet, dizziness, decreased sex drive, breakthrough bleeding
AUXILIARY LABELS:
■ Use as directed.
■ For lotions or gels: external use only.
NOTE: gels and sprays are flammable; avoid smoking, fire, and flames.

GENERIC NAME: esterified estrogen
TRADE NAME: Menest
INDICATIONS: menopausal symptoms, female hypogonadism, palliative treatment for breast cancer
ROUTE OF ADMINISTRATION: oral
COMMON ADULT DOSAGE: 0.3 to 1.25 mg once daily
SIDE EFFECTS: N/V, swollen breasts/ankles/feet, dizziness, decreased sex drive, acne or skin color changes, breakthrough bleeding, depression
AUXILIARY LABELS:
■ Use as directed.
■ Take with food or milk.

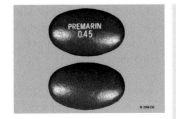

GENERIC NAME: conjugated estrogens
TRADE NAME: Premarin
INDICATIONS: menopausal symptoms, osteoporosis prevention, hypogonadism, atrophic vaginitis, palliative historical treatment for prostate or breast cancer
ROUTE OF ADMINISTRATION: oral, injection, vaginal
COMMON ADULT DOSAGE: oral, 0.3 to 2.5 mg once daily in cycles; vaginal cream, 2 to 4 g vaginally as directed in cycles
SIDE EFFECTS: N/V, swollen breasts/ankles/feet, dizziness, decreased sex drive, breakthrough bleeding
AUXILIARY LABEL:
■ Use as directed.

GENERIC NAME: conjugated estrogens with medroxyprogesterone
TRADE NAME: Prempro, Premphase
INDICATIONS: menopausal symptoms, osteoporosis prevention, hypogonadism, atrophic vaginitis, palliative historic treatment for prostate or breast cancer
ROUTE OF ADMINISTRATION: oral
COMMON ADULT DOSAGE: 0.625 mg/2.5 mg to 0.625 mg/5 mg once daily (for Prempro); Premphase is given cyclically, with part of the cycle estrogen-only and part of the cycle with estrogen/progestin combination tablets
SIDE EFFECTS: H/A, N/V, swollen or tender breasts, changes in weight/appetite, dizziness, decreased sex drive, drowsiness, stomach pain
AUXILIARY LABELS:
■ Take as directed.
■ Take with or without food.

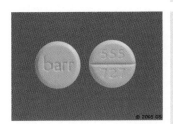

GENERIC NAME: estropipate
TRADE NAME: Ogen, Ortho-Est
ROUTE OF ADMINISTRATION: oral
INDICATIONS: menopausal symptoms, osteoporosis, hypogonadism, palliative historical treatment for prostate or breast cancer
COMMON ADULT DOSAGE: 0.75 to 3 mg once daily in cycles
SIDE EFFECTS: N/V, tenderness in breasts, changes in weight/appetite, dizziness, decreased sex drive, drowsiness, stomach bloating and upset
AUXILIARY LABELS:
■ Take as directed.
■ Avoid alcohol.
■ Avoid prolonged exposure to sunlight.

Infertility

Infertility is defined as the inability to conceive after 1 year of attempting to reproduce. Anovulation is a cause of infertility that can be corrected by pharmaceutical means. Agents are given to promote maturation of the ovarian follicle and to stimulate ovulation. Endometriosis attributable to PID can obstruct the fallopian tubes. Women with irregular menstrual cycles or no menstruation may also have problems with infertility.

Prognosis. The prognosis for infertility is dependent on the ages of the partners, the cause of the condition, the methods of treatment or assisted reproduction techniques employed, and other factors.

Non–Drug Treatment. Surgery may correct fertility problems originating from abnormal conditions in the fallopian tubes, uterus, or ovaries. Another treatment that may help with infertility is assisted reproductive technology (ART), which uses in vitro fertilization, embryo transfer, and both egg and sperm transfer. The likelihood of success depends on several factors including the age of the woman. In the case of ART, hormonal medications are used to control and direct the ovulation and implantation cycles. Male infertility may be treated with medications or by using alternative techniques, such as sperm donation.

Drug Treatment. Hormone treatment is most commonly used to treat infertility; drugs such as Clomid, Pergonal, and other hormones can be used to promote ovulation. Table 24-7 lists examples of drug treatments for infertility.

Ovulation Stimulants

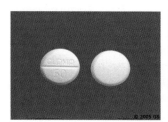

GENERIC NAME: clomiphene
TRADE NAME: Clomid
INDICATION: female infertility
ROUTE OF ADMINISTRATION: oral
COMMON ADULT DOSAGE: one 50-mg tablet once daily for 5 days (initial cycle therapy)
SIDE EFFECTS: blurred vision during or immediately after administration, flushing, bloating, dizziness; increases risk of multiparity (twins)
AUXILIARY LABEL:
- Take as directed.

TABLE 24-7 Infertility Treatments

Generic Name	Trade Name	Uses
bromocriptine	Parlodel	For ovulation problems caused by high levels of prolactin
cetrorelix injection	Cetrotide	Infertility treatment that provides controlled ovarian stimulation; prevents premature ovulation
choriogonadotropin alfa injectable	Ovidrel	Infertility treatment that acts to release mature eggs for fertilization
clomiphene	Clomid	Infertility problems; induces ovulation
danazol	Danocrine	Infertility caused by endometriosis; also used for treatment of cysts or lumps in breast, or for heavy menstrual flow
follitropin alfa injection	Gonal-f	Infertility; used in combination with another hormone to stimulate ovaries
follitropin beta injection	Follistim AQ	Infertility; used in combination with another hormone to stimulate ovaries
gonadotropins, chorionic intramuscular	Pregnyl, Novarel	Infertility; used in combination with other hormones to induce ovulation
menotropins injection	Repronex, Menopur	Infertility; used to stimulate ovaries
metformin	Glucophage	For polycystic ovarian syndrome; lowers insulin resistance, which helps lower high levels of male hormones in women and promotes ovulation
progesterone vaginal gel	Crinone, Prochieve	Infertility caused by progesterone deficiency; used to support early pregnancy

Luteinizing Hormone and Follicle-Stimulating Hormone Stimulants

GENERIC NAME: menotropins
TRADE NAME: Menopur, Repronex
INDICATION: stimulate follicles to produce mature ova
ROUTE OF ADMINISTRATION: injection
COMMON ADULT DOSAGE: 225 units (international units) of FSH/LH activity subcutaneously once daily initially. Adjust to response by no more than 150 units/day. Maximum dose 450 units/day.
SIDE EFFECTS: H/A, mild nausea, cold symptoms
AUXILIARY LABEL:
■ Take as directed.

Ergot Alkaloid

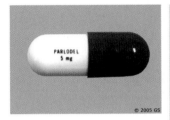

GENERIC NAME: bromocriptine
TRADE NAME: Parlodel
INDICATION: Lowers elevated prolactin levels, reducing a hormonal influence that is prohibiting ovulation
ROUTE OF ADMINISTRATION: oral
COMMON ADULT DOSAGE: 2.5 to 10 mg once daily with food
SIDE EFFECTS: dizziness, drowsiness, H/A, loss of appetite, vomiting
AUXILIARY LABELS:
■ Take as directed.
■ Take with food.
■ May cause dizziness/drowsiness.

PROGESTINS

Progesterone, naturally occurring as progestin, is the female hormone secreted from day 14 through day 28 of the menstrual cycle. This hormone has many functions, including changing the secretions of the cervix, reducing uterine contractility, and maintaining the corpus luteum. Other actions include stimulating the development of ducts and glands of the breasts in preparation of lactation; however, progestin does not cause lactation.

Progestins also may be made synthetically; natural and synthetic forms have similar pharmacological effects on the body. Placentas are one of the natural sources for obtaining progestins. Because the liver rapidly metabolizes progestin preparations, oral administration of natural preparations is not indicated. Injected forms usually are placed in an oil base to delay the absorption and thus prolong effects. Synthetically produced preparations are different from natural progesterone and are called progestins or progestogens. Synthetic forms are used more frequently than natural forms because synthetic forms are more effective. Synthetic forms are either injected or administered orally, and the action of synthetic progestin is prolonged over that of progesterone; oral administration is effective because synthetic progestin is not rapidly metabolized by the liver.

Progestins are used for treating amenorrhea and abnormal uterine bleeding from hormone imbalances, for contraception, in combination with estrogen HRT to prevent endometrial overgrowth if the woman has an intact uterus, and as therapy for renal and endometrial cancer. When combined with oral contraceptive pills with estrogen, the dosage of progestin is measured in milligrams, whereas the estrogen component is measured in micrograms. Used to treat infertility, progesterone and progesterone-like products cause negative feedback and with the gonadotropic hormones stimulate the development of ova and subsequent ovulation.

The side effects of progestins include weight gain, stomach pain and cramping, swelling of the face and legs, headaches, mood swings, anxiety, weakness, rashes, acne, and insomnia. Menstrual changes and breast tenderness may occur, and liver dysfunction and phlebitis are more severe adverse reactions. Glucose intolerance is seen in women who are prone to diabetes mellitus, and fetal teratogenic effects have occurred.

GENERIC NAME: progesterone
TRADE NAME: Crinone
INDICATIONS: secondary amenorrhea (4% or 8% gel); also used in infertility protocols (8% gel)
ROUTE OF ADMINISTRATION: vaginal
COMMON ADULT DOSAGE: initially, 45 mg (4% gel) every other day × 6 doses for secondary amenorrhea
SIDE EFFECTS: dizziness, drowsiness, diarrhea, constipation, bloating, pain during intercourse, mild nausea, vomiting, lost of interest in sex
AUXILIARY LABELS:
- For vaginal use only.
- Use as directed.

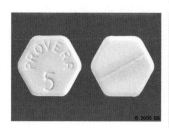

GENERIC NAME: medroxyprogesterone
TRADE NAME: Provera (oral), Depo-Provera (injection), Depo-Subcut Provera 104
INDICATIONS: endometrial hyperplasia, secondary amenorrhea, abnormal uterine bleeding; Depo-Provera, contraception
ROUTE OF ADMINISTRATION: oral, injection
COMMON ADULT DOSAGE: oral: 2 to 10 mg once daily for 5 to 10 days for amenorrhea and abnormal bleeding or cyclically with estrogen HRT; Depo-Provera, 150 mg deep IM q 3 months as a contraceptive or Depo-Subcut Provera 104 mg subcutaneously q 3 months
SIDE EFFECTS: breakthrough bleeding, breast tenderness, increased acne, insomnia, changes in weight or appetite, mild stomach pain, bloating, nausea, osteoporosis with long-term use of contraceptive form
AUXILIARY LABEL:
- Take as directed.

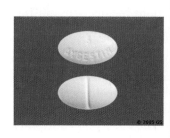

GENERIC NAME: norethindrone
TRADE NAME: Aygestin (hormone replacement), Ortho Micronor (contraceptive)
INDICATIONS: amenorrhea, abnormal uterine bleeding, endometriosis, contraception, prevention of endometrial hyperplasia with estrogen therapy
ROUTE OF ADMINISTRATION: oral
COMMON ADULT DOSAGE: 2.5 to 10 mg in cycles for amenorrhea; 0.35 mg once daily for contraception; 5 mg for prevention of endometrial hyperplasia given cyclically with estrogen HRT
SIDE EFFECTS: unusual menstrual bleeding
AUXILIARY LABEL:
- Take as directed.

MENSTRUAL DISORDERS

There are a wide range of disorders that can affect women's menstrual periods (Box 24-2). The primary agents used to treat these conditions include estrogens, to relieve symptoms of dysmenorrhea, endometriosis, and dysfunctional uterine bleeding.

PROPHYLAXIS MEDICATIONS

Oral Contraceptives (OCs)

Oral contraceptives are used as a means of birth control by preventing fertilization of an ovum and the subsequent pregnancy. Contraception may be

BOX 24-2 MENSTRUAL DISORDERS

Amenorrhea: Absence of menstrual periods
Dysmenorrhea: Abdominal pain attributable to menstrual cramping
Hypomenorrhea: Low menstrual flow over a short menstrual period
Menorrhagia: Heavy menstrual flow over a long menstrual period
Oligomenorrhea: Light and infrequent menstrual periods
Polymenorrhea: Frequent menstruation
Premature menopause: Ovaries lose function before the age of 40
Premenstrual syndrome: A group of symptoms that occur before period (e.g., bloating, edema, H/A, mood swings, and breast discomfort)

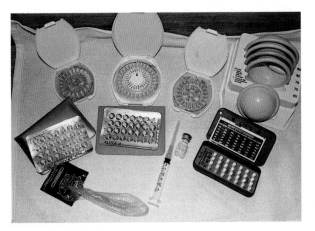

FIGURE 24-6 Common contraceptives, including barrier and medicinal methods: condoms, diaphragm, oral contraceptives, and parenteral contraceptives.

accomplished through pharmacological methods such as oral contraceptives or medication-laden devices such as vaginal rings, patches, or intrauterine devices. Nonpharmacological methods such as surgery, the rhythm method, and mechanical devices also may be used. Of the different methods of birth control, the oral contraceptives have the highest incidence of side effects—from nausea and vomiting to menstrual abnormalities to thrombolytic complications. Barrier methods have the fewest side effects but are not as effective as hormone-based medications (Figure 24-6).

Oral contraceptives are relatively safe when used by nonsmokers who have normal cardiovascular function. Combination oral contraceptives consist of estrogen and progestin to inhibit ovulation. The progestin-only contraceptives are called "mini-pills." The combination contraceptives are the most often prescribed contraceptives and are almost 100% effective. The combination medications are available in monophasic, biphasic, triphasic, and estrophasic formulas. In the monophasic regimen the daily doses of estrogen and progestin remain constant throughout the menstrual cycle. In the biphasic regimen, the estrogen dose remains constant but the progestin dose is increased in the second half of the cycle. The triphasic regimen divides the menstrual cycle into three phases, and the amount of progestin changes in each phase. The estrophasic cycle has a constant amount of progestin, and the estrogen component is increased

Tech Note!

Oral contraceptives should be taken at the same time each day. Oral contraceptives may increase blood glucose levels; thus a person with diabetes mellitus should be monitored closely. Additional methods of contraception should be used during the initial cycle of oral contraceptives. Some oral contraceptives are packaged in 21-tablet packs, whereas others have 21 tablets of the medication and 7 tablets that are an iron preparation or a tablet of an inert ingredient.

gradually throughout the cycle. Phasic oral contraceptives are intended to mimic the female body's natural cycle while lessening the side effects of the birth control pills.

The effectiveness of oral contraceptive use depends on taking the medication as prescribed. Usually, the medication is started on the fifth day of the menstrual cycle and should be taken at the same time of the day for 21 days. If a single dose of a combination oral contraceptive is missed, the chance of ovulation is small. However, the risk of pregnancy increases with each dose missed. If one dose is missed, it should be taken as soon as it is remembered and the next pill should be taken on the regular schedule. This may mean taking two pills in 1 day or in the same dose. If two doses are missed, two tablets should be taken on each of the next 2 days. If three doses are missed, a new cycle of medications should be started 7 days after the last pill was taken, unless the patient is taking the mini-pills, in which case the physician should be consulted. If one active dose is missed take it as soon as possible then continue with daily pills. If two active doses are missed, take both as soon as possible and use additional forms of birth control (such as condoms) for the next 7 days.

Some of the side effects of oral contraceptives include N/V, mood changes, appetite changes, changes in sex drive, and headaches. Women taking combination oral contraceptives may also experience breast tenderness; however, women taking progestin-only pills do not seem to experience as much breast tenderness or nausea. Some of the risks of combination oral contraceptives include thromboembolism, increased susceptibility to myocardial infarction, and stroke; and the risks are often increased in women who smoke. These risks are not as prevalent in women taking the mini-pill; however, the risk for ectopic pregnancy is still present. Both of these types of oral contraceptives can increase blood glucose levels, gallbladder disease, acne, and hirsutism.

Most oral contraceptives are in tablet form, whereas some are available as transdermal patches. Some contraceptives are given by injection, and each injection is effective for 3 months. These injections, used in persons who may be noncompliant with oral dosage forms or who need the convenience of such dosage forms, prevent pregnancy in three ways, depending on the hormones in the injection: by suppressing ovulation, by thickening the cervical mucus, and by altering the endometrium to discourage implantation. Some nontraditional contraceptive dosage forms include the following:

- Seasonale: Similar to traditional OCs except it reduces menstruation cycles to 4 per year
- Today Sponge: Contains spermicide protection up to 24 hours after insertion into the vagina near the cervix
- NuvaRing: Similar to the traditional oral contraceptive, but administered via a ring in the vagina that can be left in place for up to 3 weeks
- Mirena: IUD that contains a progestin; contraceptive action lasts up to 5 years
- ParaGard: Non–hormone-containing IUD; contraceptive action lasts up to 10 years

The contraceptive medications listed are those other than oral cycle packs, which make up most of the contraceptives prescribed. For drugs separated with a slash, the first drug listed is the estrogen component and the second drug is the progestin component. Oral contraceptives provide no protection against STDs; this is an important factor in patient education.

GENERIC NAME: ethinyl estradiol/norelgestromin
TRADE NAME: Ortho Evra
ROUTE OF ADMINISTRATION: topical
COMMON ADULT DOSAGE: transdermal patch applied weekly for 3 weeks; the fourth week is patch-free
SIDE EFFECTS: Mild nausea, unusual or unpleasant taste in mouth, breast pain, increased hair growth, changes in weight, headache, dizziness, decreased sex drive
AUXILIARY LABEL:
■ Apply topically. Take as directed.

Long-Acting Contraceptive

GENERIC NAME: medroxyprogesterone
TRADE NAME: Depo-Provera Contraceptive Injection, Depo-Subcut Provera 104
ROUTE OF ADMINISTRATION: injection
COMMON ADULT DOSAGE: injection every 3 months
SIDE EFFECTS: unpredictable menstrual bleeding
AUXILIARY LABEL:
■ None needed as medication is given by injection by physician

Intrauterine Progesterone Contraception

GENERIC NAME: levonorgestrel intrauterine system
TRADE NAME: Mirena
ROUTE OF ADMINISTRATION: intrauterine
COMMON ADULT DOSAGE: insert one system into the uterus; each system is effective for 5 years, at which time a new system is inserted
SIDE EFFECTS: unusual menstrual bleeding initially; menstruation may cease with continued use or greatly lessen
AUXILIARY LABEL:
■ None needed as device is implanted by physician

Tech Note!

The current recommendation for contraception transdermal patches, such as Ortho Evra, is to apply the patch to the upper arms, back, abdomen, or buttocks. The patch should be applied and worn for 1 week; a new patch should be applied on the same day of the week that the first patch was applied. The fourth week should be patch-free.

Other Contraceptives

Other contraceptives include spermicides that have the active ingredient nonoxynol-9. These contraceptives are available as foam, jelly, gel, cream, suppository, and vaginal film as well as in the Today Sponge. The correct use of a spermicide is essential for contraceptive efficacy. The spermicide must be applied before coitus but no more than 1 hour in advance of sexual intercourse. Spermicides may be purchased without a prescription and must be applied each time intercourse is anticipated. Douching should be postponed for at least 6 hours after intercourse when using spermicides.

Barrier devices are nonpharmacological methods of birth control, although a prescription is written for cervical caps and diaphragms to ensure proper fitting. These devices include male and female condoms, cervical caps, and diaphragms. The most commonly used barrier method is the male condom. Three materials are used in the manufacture of male condoms: latex, polyurethane, and lamb intestine. Lubricants containing mineral oil can decrease the barrier strength of condoms.

Barrier types of contraception for women include the female condom, which is a loose-fitting tubular polyurethane pouch with flexible rings at both ends, and the diaphragm, which is a soft rubber cap with a metal spring that fits over the cervix. Before a diaphragm is inserted, it should be filled with spermicide to block the cervix completely from sperm access. The cervical cap, another contraceptive device, is a small cup-shaped barrier that fits directly over the cervical rim and is held in place by suction.

TABLE 24-8 Contraceptive Methods: Risks, Complications, and Failure

Type	Risks/Potential Complications	Failure Rate (%)
None	Pregnancy	85
Douche	Infection, local irritation	40
Sponge	Allergy, toxic shock (rare), vaginal dryness, vaginal irritation	15-30
Spermicides (alone)	Allergy, local irritation, unpleasant smell/taste	10-25
Diaphragm	Allergy, toxic shock, vaginal irritation, cervical erosion	4-25
Cervical cap	Allergy, toxic shock, vaginal irritation, cervical erosion	4-25
Calendar abstinence	Sexual frustration, unexpected ovulation and pregnancy	9-23
Female condom*	Visibility, loss of spontaneity	21
Male condom*	Allergic reactions, decreased sensitivity, loss of spontaneity	3-15
Periodic abstinence	Sexual frustration, unexpected ovulation and pregnancy	
Withdrawal (coitus interruptus)	Anxiety, frustration, inability to relax, pregnancy	19
Intrauterine devices	Spotting, changes in menstrual bleeding, uterine cramping, pelvic inflammatory disease	1-5
Oral contraceptive (estrogen/progesterone tablets)	Nausea, headaches, dizziness, spotting, weight gain, breast changes, fluid retention, mood changes, cardiovascular problems, thrombosis	1-5
Tubal ligation	Typical abdominal surgical risks	0.4
Injectable progestogen	Menstrual changes, weight gain, headaches, osteoporosis with long-term use	0.3-1
Vasectomy	Bruising, edema, pain, infection	0.15

*Only barrier methods that may reduce risk of transmission of sexually transmitted diseases (STDs).

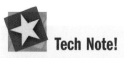

Tech Note!

Birth control vaccines for men and women are currently under development. In testing, the male vaccine has been shown to be 99% effective against sperm production. The vaccine for men requires weekly injections of testosterone.

Table 24-8 provides information on the types of contraception and their efficacy.

A postcoital or emergency form of contraception is commonly known as the "morning-after pill," which prevents conception and pregnancy after intercourse. To be effective, the first dose of morning-after medication must be taken within 72 hours of unprotected sexual intercourse. A second dose then is taken 12 hours after the first dose. These medications should not be used as a routine type of contraception because of the potential side effects, but they are helpful when used for such circumstances as sexual assault or contraception failure.

The morning-after pill regimens are contraceptives formulated of high-dose progestin only or both and estrogen and progestin. The combined form of emergency contraception is about 75% effective, but one almost universal side effect is nausea and vomiting. Thus progestin-only emergency contraception, which is less likely to cause nausea, is more popularly prescribed. The progestin emergency contraception requires two tablets and is packaged under the name of Plan B or NextChoice. The first tablet is to be taken within 72 hours of unprotected intercourse and the second tablet 12 hours later. Only Plan B has been approved for OTC use. Plan B over-the-counter is for women 17 years and older; use in younger women requires a prescription. Progestin-only emergency contraception is more effective than a combined estrogen and progestin regimen, primarily because it is better tolerated. Emergency contraception products do have some risk associated with them and should not be used as a regular means of birth control.

RU-486, or mifepristone (Mifeprex), is more commonly known as the abortion pill. RU-486 acts as an antiprogestin. Because progesterone is necessary for establishment and maintenance of pregnancy, RU-486 acts as an antagonist to progesterone and prevents the maintenance of the pregnancy. For safety, this medication must be used within the first 9 weeks of pregnancy. Because of the **abortifacient** effects of the medication, the administration of RU-486 must be performed by a qualified health care professional and drug distribution is limited to such individuals, and a prescription will not be written for dispensation by a pharmacist.

Sexually Transmitted Diseases (STDs)

STDs have existed for centuries and affect both males and females. Any disease that can be transmitted by sexual intercourse is considered to be an STD. This does not mean that these diseases cannot be transmitted in other ways (nonsexually); it is the difference in terminology. For example, HIV can be spread either by intercourse or by the sharing of needles for injection. Herpes virus can be spread from a mother to a child through childbirth, and pubic lice and scabies can be transmitted from the sharing of towels or bedding as well as by close contact. Because STDs are embarrassing to patients, many do not seek treatment. Additionally, certain STDs (e.g., syphilis, herpes) can remain dormant (latent) for long periods, which results in more transference between partners until the symptoms occur. Even then, many persons are reluctant to provide names of those who may be infected.

STDs are caused by bacterial, viral, fungal, and protozoan organisms (see Chapter 30). If left untreated, some STDs can cause irreversible sterility, blindness, and even death. Several of these diseases, including chlamydia, gonorrhea, hepatitis, autoimmune deficiency syndrome (AIDS), and syphilis, are on the list of Notifiable Infectious Diseases. If a patient is diagnosed as having one of the diseases on this list, the medical practitioner is required by law to notify the local health department. This list of diseases is available from the Centers for Disease Control and Prevention (www.cdc.gov) and is updated once a year. Table 24-9 gives a list of the organisms that cause STDs along with the drug names and dosage forms for the treatment of these diseases.

The symptoms of STDs vary according to disease and severity of infection. Chlamydia caused by the bacterium *Chlamydia trachomatis* can permanently damage a woman's reproductive organs; symptoms may be mild or even absent and is known as the "silent" disease. Gonorrhea caused by the bacterium *Neisseria gonorrhoeae* also may have mild to no symptoms. Both chlamydia and gonorrhea can eventually cause pelvic inflammatory disease (PID) in women and epididymitis in men if left untreated; both painful conditions that can lead to sterility. Early symptoms of HIV typically include fever, headache, fatigue, and rash; as the disease progresses, increased severity of these early symptoms may manifest along with night sweats, chronic diarrhea, and chills. Genital herpes, which can lie dormant for months, years, or decades, causes small red bumps or blisters or a rash on the genitals. Hepatitis, which infects the liver, can cause fatigue, nausea, vomiting, darkening of the urine, or yellowing of the skin.

Many of the symptoms for these diseases are not present in the early stages of the infection, making the transference of the infection more likely. Since infections are typically passed during sexual contact, protection and education are key components to preventing the spread of these diseases. Condoms are available for both men and women and are the most effective method for the prevention of disease. Because the infection is spread either through open sores on the skin, which can be microscopic, or through direct sexual contact, using a condom will create an effective barrier against infection.

Education is also important to prevent the transmission of STDs. Some members of the general public may mistakenly believe that taking oral birth control or using contraceptive gels can protect against STDs, but this is not true. Some vaccines, such as Gardasil, can protect against certain human papillomavirus (HPV) infections but will not protect against all STDs. Research is

TABLE 24-9 **Sexually Transmitted Disease Organisms and Various Drug Therapies**

Organism	Condition	Generic Name	Trade Name
Chlamydia trachomatis	Chlamydia	azithromycin	Zithromax
		erythromycin	E-Mycin
		doxycycline	Vibramycin
		ofloxacin	Floxin
Neisseria gonorrhoeae	Gonorrhea	azithromycin	Zithromax
		cefixime	Suprax
		ceftriaxone	Rocephin
Herpes simplex	Genital herpes	acyclovir	Zovirax
		famciclovir	Famvir
		valacyclovir	Valtrex
Treponema pallidum	Syphilis	erythromycin	E-Mycin
		penicillin G benzathine	Bicillin L-A
		tetracycline	Sumycin
Trichomonas vaginalis	Trichomoniasis vaginalis	metronidazole	Flagyl
Gardnerella vaginalis	Bacterial vaginitis	clindamycin	Cleocin, Cleocin Vaginal
		metronidazole	Flagyl, Metrogel Vaginal
Candida albicans	Vaginal candidiasis	butoconazole	Femstat, Femstat 3
		clotrimazole	Gyne-Lotrimin
		fluconazole	Diflucan
		miconazole	Monistat
		terconazole	Terazol 7, Terazol 3
		tioconazole	Vagistat-1

Tech Alert!

Remember these sound-alike/look-alike drugs:

Cardura versus Coumadin and Cardene
clomiphene versus clomipramine
methyltestosterone versus methylprednisolone
Parlodel versus pindolol
Provera versus Premarin
Yasmin versus Yaz

currently underway to develop a vaccine against HIV; however, at this time there is not a viable vaccine on the market. Because of the large amount of information and misinformation available to the public through a variety of media sources, patients may become confused about how to remain uninfected. The CDC, U.S. Public Health Department as well as each state's public health department prints brochures, produces videos, and maintains a website for up-to-date information.

DO YOU REMEMBER THESE KEY POINTS?

- The hormones mimicked by the medications used in reproductive tract therapy
- The conditions that androgens are used to treat
- The danger of synthetically produced androgens
- The uses of testosterone therapy in the male and estrogen therapy in the female
- The action of medications used to treat benign prostatic hypertrophy
- The forms of oral contraceptive preparations
- The packaging of oral contraceptive for ease of compliance

- The uses of progestin therapy
- The method of wearing transdermal contraceptive patches
- The method of taking oral contraceptives; the method for taking oral contraceptives after missed doses
- The hormones found in combination oral contraceptives
- The forms of contraception other than oral tablets
- The dangers of sildenafil
- Common sexually transmitted diseases and their treatments

REVIEW QUESTIONS

Multiple choice questions

1. The primary reproductive organs in the female are:
   A. Uterus
   B. Ovaries
   C. Testes
   D. Both A and B

2. What are the male sex hormones collectively called?
   A. Estrogens
   B. Androgens
   C. Progestins
   D. Testosterones

3. What is the major natural hormone produced by women?
   A. Estradiol
   B. Androgen
   C. Progestin
   D. All of the above

4. Which one of the following is used to obtain progestin naturally?
   A. Urine of mares
   B. Testes of bulls
   C. Placentas
   D. None of the above

5. Which of the following are classified on the controlled substances list as schedule III drugs?
   A. Estrogens
   B. Androgens
   C. Anabolic steroids
   D. Both B and C

6. Testosterone is used to treat which of the following?
   A. Hypogonadism in females
   B. Hypogonadism in males
   C. Breast and endometrial cancers in females
   D. Both B and C

7. Estrogens are used to treat which of the following?
   A. Menopausal symptoms
   B. Hypogonadism in males
   C. Hypogonadism in females
   D. Both A and C

8. Medications used to treat benign prostatic hypertrophy include:
   A. Antiandrogens
   B. Estrogens
   C. Androgens
   D. Alpha-adrenergic blockers
   E. Both A and D

9. There are four combination forms of oral contraceptives containing estrogen and progestins. In which of the combinations does estrogen level gradually increase throughout the cycle?
   A. Monophasic
   B. Biphasic
   C. Triphasic
   D. Estrophasic
   E. None of the above

10. If two tablets of oral contraceptives are missed and not taken at the correct time, what is the correct procedure?
   A. Do not worry about the missed medication; just discard the medication not taken.
   B. Take the two extra tablets with the next dose of medication.
   C. Take the two tablets with the next two doses at the regular time.
   D. Take the two extra tablets at the end of the cycle.

11. Which medication(s) is (are) prescribed for severe PID?
   A. Metronidazole PO
   B. Ceftriaxone IV
   C. Cefoxitin IV
   D. Clindamycin IV

12. Benign prostatic hypertrophy:
   A. Is enlargement of the prostate gland
   B. Is treated with androgen hormone inhibitors
   C. Is located around the urethra
   D. All of the above are true

13. Pelvic inflammatory disease can be caused by:
   A. Endometriosis
   B. STDs
   C. Bacterial infection
   D. All of the above

14. Gonorrhea may be treated with:
   A. Azithromycin
   B. Valacyclovir
   C. Ciprofloxacin
   D. Both A and B

15. Medications and/or devices used to treat ED include:
   A. Sildenafil, vacuum devices, penile implants
   B. Cialis, Levitra, prostaglandin suppositories
   C. Atenolol, leuprolide, penile implants
   D. Both A and B

True/False

If a statement is false, then change it to make it true.

_____ 1. The female produces ova just as males produce sperm.

_____ 2. Fertilization of the ovum occurs in the uterus.

_____ 3. Patients taking androgens should be told that weight gain may occur because of the accumulation of fluids.

_____ 4. Progestins used with estrogen for contraception are measured in milligrams, and the estrogens are measured in micrograms.

_____ 5. In biphasic oral contraceptives, the progestin level is increased in the first half of the cycle.

_____ 6. Transdermal estrogen patches should be worn on a hairless area of the body such as the upper arms, back, abdomen, or buttocks.

_____ 7. Oral contraceptives are effective against sexually transmitted disease.

_____ **8.** A prescription for RU-486 will be brought to the pharmacy for dispensing.

_____ **9.** Sildenafil is safe for use by all men and may be used as often as necessary.

_____ **10.** All types of contraception have approximately the same effectiveness.

_____ **11.** Both men and women produce testosterone and estrogen.

_____ **12.** Normally, severe cases of PID are treated at home with IV antibiotics.

_____ **13.** Hypogonadism occurs only in males.

_____ **14.** All contraceptives are listed as Pregnancy Category X.

_____ **15.** Morning-after pills can be purchased OTC.

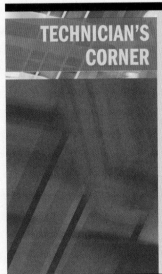

TECHNICIAN'S CORNER

A 55-year-old male patient with diabetes mellitus, hypertension, and coronary artery disease presents a prescription to the pharmacy for sildenafil (Viagra). When you, the pharmacy technician, review his medication history, you find that the following medications are taken regularly:

Glucotrol-XL 5 mg daily
metformin 500 mg tid
Tenormin 50 mg daily
Lipitor 20 mg q AM
Isordil 10 mg bid

Questions: Is the Viagra safe for dispensing with the previously listed medication history? Which of the medications are in a correct dosage? Which medications could be given with sildenafil? Which are contraindicated with sildenafil, if any? What should you as a pharmacy technician do if this prescription is presented for dispensing?

BIBLIOGRAPHY

Applegate E: *The anatomy and physiology learning system*, ed 3, Philadelphia, 2006, Elsevier Health Services.

Clayton B, Yvonne S, Renae H: *Basic pharmacology for nurses*, ed 14, Philadelphia, 2006, Elsevier Science.

Drug facts and comparisons, ed 63, St Louis, 2008, Lippincott Williams & Wilkins.

Fulcher E, Robert F, Cathy S: *Pharmacology: principles and applications*, ed 2, Philadelphia, 2008, Saunders.

Leifer G: *Introduction to maternity and pediatric nursing*, ed 5, Philadelphia, 2006, Saunders.

Mosby's drug consult 2006, ed 16, St Louis, 2005, Mosby.

Mosby's medical nursing & allied health dictionary, ed 6, St Louis, 2002, Mosby.

Stedman's concise medical dictionary for health professionals, ed 3, Baltimore, 1997, Williams & Wilkins.

WEBSITES

www.medicinenet.com/impotence_ed/article.htm

www.prostatecancerfoundation.org/

www.mayoclinic.com/health/male-hypogonadism/DS00300/DSECTION=treatments%2D and%2Ddrugs

www.nlm.nih.gov/medlineplus/ency/article/001195.htm

www.womenshealthchannel.com/pid/treatment.shtml

25

Antiinfectives

Objectives

UPON COMPLETING THIS CHAPTER, YOU SHOULD BE ABLE TO DO
THE FOLLOWING:

- List both trade and generic drug names covered in this chapter.

- Discuss the history of antibiotics and antibacterials.

- Understand the main causes of infections.

- List the various methods of illness transmission.

- Explain the reasons for antibiotic resistance.

- List the various generations of penicillin and cephalosporin antibiotics.

- Describe the differences in the generations of antibiotics.

- Describe the drug action for the various antibiotics discussed.

- List the common side effects of the antibiotics described in this chapter.

- Describe the types of infections caused by bacterial, fungal, and protozoan microbes.

- Describe the types of conditions caused by viruses.

- Distinguish between different antibiotics used for bacterial infections

- Differentiate between helminthic infestations and typical bacterial, fungal, and other parasitic infections.

- List the products used to treat infestations by helminths.

- Distinguish between gram-negative and gram-positive microbes and agents used to treat them.

- Distinguish between bacteriostatic and bactericidal effects of various agents discussed.

TERMS AND DEFINITIONS

Antibiotic *Substance that kills or inhibits the growth of bacteria; a subset of the group of antimicrobials*

Antibiotic spectrum *The variety of microbes that a particular antibiotic can treat. Broad-spectrum agents can treat many different types of organisms, whereas narrow-spectrum agents can treat fewer organisms*

Antimicrobial *Substance that inhibits the growth of or kills microorganisms*

Bacteria *A large group of unicellular, non-nucleated organisms*

ESBLs *Extended-spectrum beta-lactamases*

Inhibit *To stop or hold back; to keep a reaction from taking place*

MRSA *Methicillin-resistant* Staphylococcus aureus

Normal flora *Microorganisms that reside harmlessly in the body and do not cause disease but may aid the host organism*

Nosocomial infection *An infection acquired during a stay in a hospital or other health care service unit or institution*

Parasite *Organism that requires a host for nourishment and reproduction*

Pneumonia *Inflammatory condition of the lungs, most commonly caused by an infection, but may result from a chemical or physical injury as well*

PRSP *Penicillin-resistant* Streptococcus pneumoniae

Symbiotic *A close relationship between two species*

Synthesis *The formation of chemical components within the body system*

VRE *Vancomycin-resistant enterococci*

EXAMPLES OF ANTIINFECTIVES

Trade Name	Generic Name	Pronunciation	Trade Name	Generic Name	Pronunciation
Penicillins			**Cephalosporin Agents**		
First Generation			**First Generation**		
Pfizerpen	penicillin G	(pen-i-**cil**-in)	Ancef	cefazolin	(se-**faz**-oh-lyn)
Pen Vee K	penicillin V	(pen-i-**cil**-in)	Duricef	cefadroxil	(**seff**-ah-**drox**-il)
			Keflex	cephalexin	(sef-ah-**lex**-in)
Penicillinase-Resistant Agents			Velosef	cephradine	(**sef**-rah-deen)
Dicloxacillin	dicloxacillin	(die-klox-ah-**sil**-lin)			
Oxacillin	oxacillin	(ox-ah-**sil**-lin)	**Second Generation**		
Unipen	nafcillin	(naf-**sil**-lin)	Ceclor	cefaclor	(**sef**-ah-klor)
			Cefotan	cefotetan	(**sef**-o-tea-tan)
Second Generation			Ceftin	cefuroxime	(**sef**-ue-**ox**-zeem)
Amoxil	amoxicillin	(a-mox-ah-**sil**-lin)	Cefzil	cefprozil	(sef-**pro**-zil)
Augmentin	amoxicillin/	(a-mox-ah-**sil**-lin/	Lorabid	loracarbef	(lor-a-**kar**-bef)
	clavulanate	**clav**-u-lah-nate)	Mefoxin	cefoxitin	(se-**fox**-eye-tin)
Omnipen	ampicillin	(amp-ah-**sil**-lin)	Monocid	cefonicid	(se-**fon**-eye-sid)
Unasyn	ampicillin/	(amp-ah-**sil**-lin/	Zinacef	cefuroxime	(**sef**-your-**ox**-zeem)
	sulbactam	sul-**back**-tum)			
			Third Generation		
Third Generation Extended-Spectrum Penicillin			Cefizox	ceftizoxime	(**sef**-tah-**zox**-zeem)
Timentin	ticarcillin/	(tie-car-**sil**-lin/	Cefobid	cefoperazone	(sef-o-**pear**-ah-zone)
	clavulanate	**clav**-u-lah- nate)	Fortaz	ceftazidime	(**sef**-taz-eye-deem)
			Omnicef	cefdinir	(sef-**deh**-ner)
Fourth Generation Extended-Spectrum Penicillins			Rocephin	ceftriaxone	(sef-try-**ax**-zone)
Pipracil	piperacillin	(pie-**per**-ah-sil-lin)	Spectracef	cefditoren pivoxil	(sef-deh-**tor**-en)
Zosyn	piperacillin/	(pie-**per**-ah-sil-lin/	Suprax	cefixime	(sef-**ix**-ime)
	tazobactam	taz-oh-**back**-tam)			

Continued

EXAMPLES OF ANTIINFECTIVES—cont'd

Trade Name	Generic Name	Pronunciation
Vantin	cefpodoxime	(sef-poe-**dox**-zeem)
Fourth Generation		
Maxipime	cefepime	(**sef**-eye-peem)
Aminoglycosides		
Amikin	amikacin	(am-ah-**kay**-sin)
Garamycin	gentamicin	(jent-ah-**my**-sin)
Humatin	paromomycin	(par-oh-mow-**my**-sin)
Kantrex	kanamycin	(cane-ah-**my**-sin)
Nebcin, Tobi	tobramycin	(tow-bra-**my**-sin)
Antifungals		
Azole Antifungals		
Diflucan	fluconazole	(flew-**kone**-ah-zole)
Mycelex troche	clotrimazole	(kloe-**trim**-ah-zole)
Monistat	miconazole	(my-**kon**-e-a-zole)
Nizoral	ketoconazole	(kee-toe-**kone**-ah-zole)
Sporanox	itraconazole	(it-trah-**kone**-ah-zole)
VFend	voriconazole	(vor-i-**kone**-an-zole)
Other Antifungals		
Albecet, AmbiSome	amphotericin B, liposomal forms	(am-foe-**ter**-i-sin)
Fulvicin	griseofulvin	(gri-se-oh-**full**-vin)
Fungizone	amphotericin B	(am-foe-**ter**-i-sin)
Lamisil	terbinafine	(**ter**-bin-a-feen)
Mycostatin	nystatin	(ny-**stat**-in)
Mycamine	micafungin	(mic-a-**fun**-jin)
Antiprotozoan Agents		
Aralen	chloroquine	(**klor**-o-kwin)
Biltricide	praziquantel	(pra-ze-**quan**-tell)
Daraprim	pyrimethamine	(pie-rye-**meth**-ah-mean)
Lariam	mefloquine	(**mef**-low-kwin)
Flagyl	metronidazole	(met-row-**nid**-ah-zole)
Primaquine	primaquine	(**prim**-ah-queen)
Vermox	mebendazole	(me-**ben**-dah-zole)
Yodoxin	iodoquinol	(eye-oh-do-**kwin**-ole)
Antituberculin Agents		
Capastat	capreomycin	(**kap**-ree-oh-**mye**-sin)
INH	isoniazid	(**eye**-soe-**nye**-a-zid)
Myambutol	ethambutol	(e-**tham**-byoo-tole)
Paser	aminosalicylic acid	(ah-**mee**-no-**sal**-ih-sill-ik)
Priftin	rifapentine	(**rif**-ah-pen-teen)
Generic only	pyrazinamide	(peer-ah-**zin**-a-mide)
Rifadin	rifampin	(rif-**am**-pin)
Seromycin	cycloserine	(sigh-kloe-**ser**-een)
Generic only	streptomycin	(strep-toe-**my**-sin)
Trecator-Subcut	ethionamide	(e-**thye**-on-am-ide)

Trade Name	Generic Name	Pronunciation
Antivirals		
Abreva	docosanol	(doe-**koe**-san-ole)
Cytovene	ganciclovir	(gan-**sye**-kloe-veer)
Famvir	famciclovir	(fam-**sye**-klo-veer)
Foscavir	foscarnet	(fos-**car**-net)
Relenza	zanamivir	(zan-**am**-i-vir)
Symmetrel	amantidine	(ah-man-**tah**-deen)
Tamiflu	oseltamivir	(os-el-**tam**-eh-veer)
Valcyte	valganciclovir	(val-**gan**-sye-kloe-veer)
Valtrex	valacyclovir	(**val**-ay-**sye**-kloe-veer)
Virazole	ribavirin	(**rye**-ba-**vir**-in)
Zovirax	acyclovir	(a-**sye**-kloe-veer)
Protease Inhibitors		
Aptivus	tipranavir	(tip-**ra**-na-veer)
Crixivan	indinavir	(in-**din**-a-veer)
Invirase	saquinavir	(sa-**kwin**-a-veer)
Lexiva	fosamprenavir	(**fos**-am-pren-a-veer)
Preszista	darunavir	(da-**roon**-a-veer)
Norvir	ritonavir	(rit-**oh**-na-veer)
Reyataz	atazanavir	(a-ta-**zan**-a-veer)
Viracept	nelfinavir	(nel-**fin**-a-veer)
Nucleoside Reverse Transcriptase Inhibitors		
Emtriva	emtricitabine	(em-trye-**sye**-ta-been)
Epivir	lamivudine	(la-**mih**-vyoo-deen)
Hivid	zalcitabine	(zal-**site**-ah-been)
Retrovir	zidovudine	(zye-**doe**-vyoo-deen)
Videx	didanosine	(dye-**dan**-oh-seen)
Zerit	stavudine	(**sta**-vue-deen)
Ziagen	abacavir	(a-**bak**-a-vir)
Non-nucleoside Reverse Transcriptase Inhibitors		
Intelence	etravirine	(**e**-tra-**vir**-een)
Rescriptor	delavirdine	(de-la-**veer**-deen)
Sustiva	efavirenz	(**e**-fa-**vir**-enz)
Viramune	nevirapine	(ne-**vir**-a-peen)
Fusion Inhibitors		
Fuzeon	enfuvirtide	(en-**fyoo**-vir-tide)
Selzentry	maraviroc	(ma-**rav**-i-rock)
Integrase Strand Transfer Inhibitor		
Isentress	raltegravir	(ral-**teg**-ra-vir)
Monolactam		
Azactam	aztreonam	(**az**-tree-oh-nam)
Carbapenems		
Primaxin	imipenem/ cilastatin	(im-eh-**pen**-um/ sye-la-**stat**-in)
Invanz	ertapenem	(er-ta-**pen**-um)
Merrem	meropenem	(mer-o-**pen**-um)
Doribax	doripenem	(dor-i-**pen**-um)

EXAMPLES OF ANTIINFECTIVES—cont'd

Trade Name	Generic Name	Pronunciation	Trade Name	Generic Name	Pronunciation
Quinolones			**Oxazolidinone**		
Avelox	moxifloxacin	(mox-i-**flox**-ah-sin)	Zyvox	linezolid	(lin-eh-**zo**-lid)
Cipro	ciprofloxacin	(ci-pro-**flox**-ah-sin)			
Factive	gemifloxacin	(gem-i-**flox**-ah-sin)	**Tetracyclines**		
Levaquin	levofloxacin	(lee-vo-**flox**-ah-sin)	Achromycin	tetracycline	(tet-ra-**sye**-kleen)
Noroxin	norfloxacin	(nor-**flox**-ah-sin)	Declomycin	demeclocycline	(deme-**klow**-sye-kleen)
			Dynacin	minocycline	(my-noh-**sye**-kleen)
Lincosamides			Vibramycin	doxycycline	(dox-i-**sye**-kleen)
Cleocin	clindamycin	(klin-da-**mye**-sin)			
Lincocin	lincomycin	(lin-koe-**mye**-sin)	**Glycopeptides**		
			Vancocin	vancomycin	(van-koe-**mye**-sin)
Macrolides					
Biaxin	clarithromycin	(cla-**rith**-row-my-sin)	**Glycylcyclines**		
Erythrocin	erythromycin lactobionate	(er-**ith**-row-**my**-sin)	Tygacil	tigecycline	(**tye**-ge-**sye**-kleen)
Zithromax	azithromycin	(a-**zith**-row-**my**-sin)	**Lipopeptides**		
			Cubicin	daptomycin	(**dap**-toe-mye-sin)
Ketolides					
Ketek	telithromycin	(tell-**lith**-row-**mye**-sin)			

THE IMMUNE SYSTEM is the body's built-in defense mechanism that identifies and destroys foreign substances invading the body. However, if a microorganism cannot be destroyed by our immune system, then help from antimicrobials may be necessary. Infections can occur when the invading microorganisms grow rapidly and the body cannot repel the invader. This may be attributable to factors such as a weakened immune system. If the invading organism thrives in spite of our immune response, antibiotics can help resist the organism and return the body to a state of homeostasis. The word **antibiotic** literally means "against life." Antibiotics are made from natural or synthetic substances that can inhibit or destroy microorganisms, specifically bacteria. The term **antimicrobial** refers specifically to substances produced by scientists that are used against the spectrum of microorganisms that result in human infections. However, both terms are commonly used interchangeably in the medical field.

Although it may seem reasonable that bacteria are an unnecessary component for a healthy life, this is actually not true. Within the intestines of a normal human body, billions of microbes reside. We refer to these microbes as the **normal flora,** and their function is a **symbiotic** one; that is, both entities benefit from each other. The human gut provides a warm, nutrient-rich environment for the bacteria to survive, and the bacteria aid in the digestion and absorption of food, from which human beings benefit. Other areas of the human body in which bacteria can be found are in the mouth and throat. However, if the microbial growth becomes unbalanced, then even our own normal flora can cause us to become ill. This can occur if our immune system is weakened and cannot maintain homeostasis.

Antibiotics may have a bacteriostatic or bactericidal effect on microbes. Those agents that arrest the development or stop growth of bacteria are considered bacteriostatic. When antibiotics are "static," they do not kill mature cells. Instead, they inhibit (stop) any new growth, allowing the immune system of the body to destroy the remaining microbes. A bactericidal agent kills the bacteria.

This chapter discusses a brief history of antibiotics, followed by a description of the types of infections most commonly associated with each body system. Finally, the drugs used to treat various conditions are listed along with their drug action, side effects, auxiliary labels, and any special notes with which pharmacy technicians should be acquainted. More information on microorganisms can be found in Chapter 30.

TERMINOLOGY RELATED TO ANTIINFECTIVES

Aerobic	Living or occurring only in presence of oxygen
Anaerobic	Living or occurring in absence of oxygen
Bactericidal	Agent that destroys bacteria
Bacteriostatic	Agent that inhibits bacterial growth
Facultative anaerobic	Ability to survive under certain conditions with oxygen
Fungicidal	Agent that destroys fungus
Fungistatic	Agent that inhibits fungal growth without destroying fungus
Gram negative	Does not hold purple dye when stained by Gram stain because of thinner peptidoglycan layer
Gram positive	Holds purple dye when stained by Gram stain because of thick peptidoglycan layer
Morphology	Describes features of an organism's shape, size, and formation
Mycosis	Infection or disease caused by a fungus
Normal flora	Collection of microorganisms that colonize an animal without causing disease
Species	Classification under genus containing related organisms that can potentially interbreed with one another
Virion	Infective form of virus

Measurements Used for Bacteria, Fungi, Protozoa, and Viruses	
nm	Nanometer (1 billion nanometers = 1 meter)
μm	Micrometer (1 million micrometers = 1 meter)
mm	Millimeter (1 thousand millimeters = 1 meter)

History of Antibiotics

In the 1930s the first antibiotic, sulfa (sulfanilamide), was discovered. This agent was found to cure staphylococcus infections via bacteriostatic action. With the mass production of sulfa drugs, thousands of military personnel were saved from death caused by infections during World War II. Sulfa drugs were the first antibiotics produced and were considered a miracle drug; thus they were used often and without knowledge of the possibility of resistance. Resistance allows a microorganism to decrease the effectiveness of an antibiotic. As patients took their sulfa drugs and began to feel better, they would stop taking their medication. This allowed the remaining microbes to develop a type of immunity to the sulfa drug. The next time the infection appeared, the bacteria were more resistant to the antibiotic. As this trend repeated itself, more bacteria became resistant, eventually making it impossible to kill them with normal antibiotic therapy. Not until decades later did researchers discover that microbes have the ability to alter their genetic composition. Therefore, because of the overuse and misuse of antibiotics, new strains of bacteria made the antibiotic ineffective. By the 1960s sulfa drugs were virtually obsolete; however, they have found a limited yet useful place in antibiotic treatment and are often prescribed for urinary tract infections, certain ophthalmic infections, and certain respiratory tract infections. It is always important to take antibiotics for the full course of treatment, as prescribed.

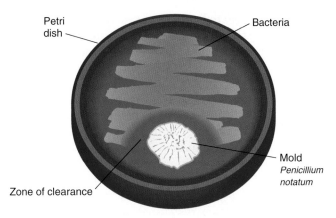

FIGURE 25-1 A Petri dish is prepared with nutrient-rich agar. This nutrient feeds the bacteria that are placed on the plate. The *Penicillium* colony can be seen with an area of clearance where the bacteria cannot grow. This occurs because the *Penicillium* colony inhibits the bacterial growth.

THE DISCOVERY OF PENICILLIN

Most persons associate penicillin with the mold that forms on bread. Alexander Fleming was an English physician who discovered penicillin by accident. As he conducted laboratory experiments, he inadvertently contaminated an agar plate with mold called *Penicillium notatum.* As the mold grew within the agar plate, he observed a ring of clearance being formed around the *Penicillium* species. The ring was produced by chemicals emitted from the mold into the agar plate. The chemicals had destroyed the surrounding microorganisms (Figure 25-1). This is called the zone of clearance. This substance eventually was isolated and became what we now know as penicillin. Penicillin agents have existed since the 1940s and are effective. The earlier generations of these agents had a greater bactericidal effect toward gram-positive bacteria as opposed to gram-negative bacteria; however, later generations of penicillin agents are effective against both types of bacteria.

Advancements in science concerning antiinfectives have increased the current treatments to include more than 12 classifications of antiinfectives and more than 100 individual drugs that are available to combat a range of infections.

GRAM STAIN

A Danish physician named Hans Christian Gram developed the Gram stain procedure in 1883. The procedure is still in use today to determine the morphology of bacteria. The morphology refers to the shape and appearance of microorganisms. Gram-positive bacteria have a thick outer membrane made of peptidoglycan links. Penicillin molecules are incorporated into these links and break them, which kills the microorganism. Gram-negative organisms have a different type of cell wall and are therefore harder to kill. Several antibiotics, especially newer antibiotics, can kill gram-negative microorganisms (see Chapter 30).

MODERN ANTIBIOTICS

The ability of bacteria to resist antibiotics has made the war on infection a life-threatening event to humans and a challenge to drug companies to develop new antiinfectives. During the mid-twentieth century new antibiotic classes were created to combat stronger bacterial infections. During the 1940s and 1950s there were several new classifications added to the arsenal of antiinfectives, which included tetracyclines, aminoglycosides, macrolides, glycopeptides, and chloramphenicol. During the 1960s fewer new drugs were added to the market (quinolones) but many of the antibiotics previously discovered were developed and converted into a useful form, leading to many second-generation antibiotics. The introduction of antibiotics to the general public allowed the human life expectancy to increase by 8 years. This incredible feat allowed for the curing of many childhood and adult illnesses that would have surely killed patients just a few years previously.

The period from 1940 to 1970 is considered to be the "Golden Age of Antibiotics." While there was some evidence as early as 1950 that bacteria could develop resistance to antibiotics, in 1960 the U.S. Surgeon General, William Stewart, announced that "it was time to close the books on infectious diseases." From 1970 through 2000 few novel antibiotics were approved and released into the market; those antibiotics that were developed were later generation or derivative drugs of many older classifications. This means that they were based upon slight chemical changes on existing drugs, usually to expand the drug's spectrum or alter an agent's response to organism resistance. Many of our newer antibiotics in wide use are such agents. One such example is azithromycin. Azithromycin, known by the trade name of Zithromax in the United States, is the most prescribed antibiotic on the market today. This medication is a derivative of erythromycin that was developed and approved for use in the late 1990s.

Up until the 1990s it seemed as though we were winning the war on microbes. It was believed that the amount of resistant strains was so minute that the CDC reported only 0.02% of pneumonia strains were resistant between 1979 and 1987 (http://dwb4.unl.edu/chem/chem869k/chem869klinks/www.fda.gov/fdac/features/795_antibio.html) that there was no urgency to develop new types of antibiotics. Scientists felt that we had time on our side for the development of new antibiotics. Meanwhile, the bacterial organisms were fighting back against antibiotics. It was found that bacterial organisms mutate or adapt much faster than previously believed. They have the ability to share deoxyribonucleic acid (DNA) and thus share resistance through a variety of methods.

This ability to develop bacterial resistance along with the prolific use of antibiotics has now spawned many new "superbugs" that are resistant to most, if not all, antibiotics. By the year 2000 bacteriological resistance to antibiotics was a fact. In 1994 the number of antibiotic-resistant pneumonia cases reported by the Centers for Disease Control and Prevention (CDC) increased to an outstanding 6.6%. Bacteria once manageable with antibiotics, such as *Streptococcus pneumoniae,* were found to be resistant to penicillin. Soon other resistant bacteria, including *Staphylococcus aureus, Salmonella,* and *Escherichia coli,* were discovered. With the emergence of multidrug-resistant strains of bacteria, it became important to discover new and more potent means of controlling bacterial infections.

Today, focus on bacterial control is not only on the development of new and more potent antibiotics but also on the production of agents that will kill the bacteria but leave the host cells intact. Many of the new antibiotics being researched and developed involve either modification of existing antibiotics or semisynthetic agents. Using principles similar to those implemented in fighting cancer, some antimicrobials are being developed as "targeted" therapies. Some viruses that attack bacteria are being investigated as a means to kill infectious bacteria in a manner that would leave healthy cells intact. Methods of "tagging" bacteria with a signal, which would then allow nano-chemicals to destroy the bacteria, are also being investigated. Inhibition of the bacteria's ability to produce essential proteins is also a process being investigated to control infection. The more scientists understand about how bacteria function, the greater will be our ability to fight infection and disease caused by these organisms. Advancements have been made in the treatments for other types of infective agents such as fungal, parasitic, and viral infections.

Certain diagnostic methods are used in the identification of all types of organisms. When identifying bacteria, scientists examine the organism's morphology, Gram stain properties, metabolic behavior (i.e., aerobic, anaerobic, facultative), and DNA sequencing (single or double stranded). Most microbes are only viewed through a microscope at high magnification. An exception is *Thiomargarita namibiensis,* the largest marine bacteria ever discovered, which can reach a size visible by the naked eye. Various parasites are visible to the naked eye.

Microbes that are too small to be seen are measured in micrometers (µm); for example, the size of an average bacterium is 0.5 µm, compared to the size of a dot, which measures 615 µm. Table 25-1 lists examples of infective agents along with their method of identification and conditions or symptoms they cause. Viruses are listed along with microbes, although they are not technically classified as a microbe because of the vast differences in their characteristics. The size of viruses can range from 0.005 µm to 0.3 µm, a virus so small that it requires an electron microscope to visualize. For more information on microbes and viruses, see Chapter 30. Terms and measurements used in microbiology are found in the earlier table entitled Terminology Related to Antiinfectives.

Types of Infections and Their Treatments

Infections can appear anywhere on or within the body. Some infections are more common because of exposure to the environment, food contamination, or direct contact with an infectious individual or substance. The internal body is normally a sterile environment; however, this does not include areas that are open to the outside (air) or those that contain outside substances. Many areas within the body are subject to bacterial, viral, and parasitic infections. Those areas open to the outside are susceptible to infections.

SEXUALLY TRANSMITTED DISEASES

Various bacteria, protozoan organisms, and viruses can cause sexually transmitted diseases (STDs). They can permanently damage internal organs such as the cervix, kidneys, heart, and brain. They can cause sterility and even death if not treated. Men and women differ with respect to the presenting symptoms of various STDs. In certain cases, the patient is asymptomatic (without symptoms). Proper diagnosis and appropriate treatment with the correct antibiotic or antiviral medication are vital. Table 25-2 lists examples of the most common types of sexually transmitted diseases, their symptoms, and treatments.

GASTROINTESTINAL INFECTIONS

The stomach is subjected to food that normally carries many different bacteria. The highly acidic environment within the stomach usually destroys any bacteria; however, if the stomach's lining is injured or the stomach's secretions are not strong enough to destroy microbes, the microbes may accumulate in the gut and result in infections. One of the major infections of the stomach is from the bacterium *Helicobacter pylori,* also known as *H. pylori* (Figure 25-2). Triple drug therapy can eradicate this bacterium. This therapy uses a combination of two different antibiotics to reduce the chance of survival of *H. pylori* as well as an acid-reducing medication to allow the ulceration to heal. The primary antibiotics used include amoxicillin, tetracycline, clarithromycin, or metronidazole. These

TABLE 25-1 Types of Microorganisms and Parasites

Bacterial Infections	Average Size Range	Shapes	Arrangement/ Characteristics	Gram Stain*	Name of Species	Example of Infectious Condition
	0.3-750 µm	Cocci (oval or round)	Diplo (two)	Gram negative	*Neisseria gonorrhoeae*	Gonorrhea
			Strepto (strip)	Gram positive	*Streptococcus pyogenes*	Scarlet fever, rheumatic fever, impetigo
			Staph (clump)	Gram positive	*Staphylococcus aureus*	Toxic shock syndrome, surgical wound infections, food poisoning
		Bacilli (rod-shaped)	Bacillus	Gram negative	*Escherichia coli*	Colitis
		Strepto (strip)	Streptobacillus	Gram negative	*Streptomyces muris*	Endocarditis, pneumonia, metastatic abscesses
		Cocci	Coccobacillus	Gram negative	*Bordetella pertussis*	Whooping cough
		Vibrio (curved)	Vibro	Gram negative	*Vibrio cholerae*	Gram negative: cholera
		Spirochete (spiral)	Spirochete	Gram negative	*Borrelia burgdorferi*	Lyme disease
		Helical	Nonspirochete	Gram negative	*Helicobacter pylori*	Stomach ulcer

Fungal Infections	Average Size Range	Name of Condition	Area Found	Identification	Name of Species	Causes
	1.5-14 µm	Blastomycosis	Soil containing rotting wood, animal droppings, insect remains, and plant material	Dimorphic: does not stain; must be grown in agar and at specific temperatures over several days to weeks for identification	*Blastomyces dermatitidis*	Dermatitis
		Histoplasmosis	Blackbird roosts, chicken houses, and bat guano	Dimorphic: fixation tests: using antigen or antibody	*Histoplasma capsulatum*	Pulmonary disease
		Sporotrichosis	Rose thorns, sphagnum moss, timbers, and soil	Dimorphic: must use special stains to identify	*Sporothrix schenckii*	Chronic infection of skin or subcutaneous tissue

Protozoa	Average Size Range	Name of Condition	Mode of Transmission	Identification	Name of Species	Causes
Flagellates	12-15 µm long, 5-9 µm wide	Traveler's diarrhea	Contaminated water, fecal-oral	Fecal examination	*Giardia lamblia*	Diarrhea, anorexia, nausea, bloating, gas

TABLE 25-1 Types of Microorganisms and Parasites—cont'd

Protozoa	Average Size Range	Name of Condition	Mode of Transmission	Identification	Name of Species	Causes
Amebas	15-20 µm in diameter	Amebiasis	Contaminated water, fecal-oral	Fecal examination or tissue sample from ulcers	*Entamoeba histolytica*	Colitis, dysentery, diarrhea, liver abscess
Ciliates	50-130 µm long by 20-70 µm wide	Swine *B. coli*	Fecal-oral (associated with pigs)	Fecal examination or tissue sample from cyst	*Balantidium coli*	Colitis, diarrhea

Helminths	Size Range	Name of Condition	Mode of Transmission	Identification	Name of Species	Causes
Tapeworm	As long as 12 m	Neurocysticercosis	Contaminated pork	CT, MRI, antibody assay, or stool sample	*Taenia solium*	GI upset; can invade CNS, causing seizures, altered mental status
Roundworm	2 mm	Strongyloidiasis	Soil containing roundworms: penetration via skin	Stool examination	*Strongyloides stercoralis*	Pneumonia
Flukes	7-20 nm	Katayama fever	Contaminated waters such as in pools; enters via skin	Eggs in stool, urine or by biopsy	*Schistosoma japonicum*	Infection of GI or GU system

Viruses	Size	Condition	Transmitted	Diagnostic Methods	Name of Virus	Causes
Poxvirus group	240-320 nm in diameter	Benign viral disease	Cosmetics, shared clothing or towels	Identified by multiple, well-defined papules that measure 2-6 mm in diameter	*Molluscum contagiosum*	Eczema, contagious pustular dermatitis
Reoviridae family: other strains include A and C that infect humans	70 nm	Rotavirus	Fecal-oral, contaminated objects, water or food	Stool examination	Rotavirus B	Enteritis, gastroenteritis
Rhabdovirus family: Specifically RaV (Rabies virus)	100 nm in diameter	Rabies	Direct contact (bite) of wild animals: skunks, raccoons, bats, and foxes	Saliva test	Rabies virus	Early-stage malaise, headache, and fever; acute pain, violent movements, uncontrolled excitement, hydrophobia (fatal it left untreated)
Flaviviridae family	50 nm in diameter	West Nile virus	Mosquitoes	Blood test, MRI scan of head	West Nile virus	Encephalitis, meningitis, poliomyelitis

*Most bacteria can be either gram negative or gram positive while others are hard to identify with traditional Gram staining methods.

TABLE 25-2 Common Sexually Transmitted Diseases and Treatments

Sexually Transmitted Diseases	Species	Symptoms	Drug Treatments
Bacterial			
Chlamydia	*Chlamydia trachomatis*	Men: urethritis and penis discharge Women: vaginal discharge, dysuria	doxycycline, azithromycin
Gonorrhea	*Neisseria gonorrhoeae*	White discharge from penis in men, painful urination, sterility in both genders	ceftriaxone, cefixime, cefpodoxime, doxycycline, gatifloxacin
Syphilis	*Treponema pallidum*	Firm oval sore at site of initial infection Headaches, general aches, and loss of appetite Damages nervous and circulatory systems	penicillin G, procaine penicillin, tetracycline, doxycycline
Trichomoniasis	*Trichomonas vaginalis*	Causes thin, malodorous discharge, often asymptomatic	metronidazole
Viral			
Genital herpes	Most caused by Herpes Simplex Virus (HSV-2)	Fever, headaches, genital blisters (mortality in newborns if active)	acyclovir or famciclovir or valacyclovir
HIV*	Retrovirus (HIV-1)	HIV weakens immune system; when it advances it becomes AIDS	Determined by patient's situation (i.e., pregnancy, treatment exposure, severity of illness, onset, blood tests)
AIDS*	Retrovirus (HIV-1)	AIDS causes severe infections including Kaposi's sarcoma Other illnesses include dementia, shortness of breath, malnutrition, chronic diarrhea	abacavir, atazanavir, delavirdine, didanosine, efavirenz, indinavir, nelfinavir, lamivudine, nevirapine, ritonavir, saquinavir, zalcitabine, zidovudine, others

*HIV/AIDS drug treatments include several agents taken concurrently.

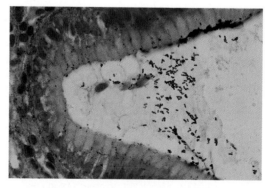

FIGURE 25-2 *Helicobacter pylori,* a bacterium that causes infection of the stomach. (From Kumar V, Abbas AK, Fausto N: *Robbins and Cotran pathologic basis of disease,* ed 7, Philadelphia, 2005, Saunders.)

antibiotics have a bactericidal effect on the bacilli. Other adjacent areas susceptible to infections include the mouth, throat, and trachea.

Microbes also can infiltrate areas of the body that are not exposed to air; these microbes are referred to as anaerobic microbes. Microbes that require oxygen to survive are termed aerobic, those that do not need oxygen to live are called anaerobic, and microbes that can tolerate oxygen to a degree are called facultative anaerobes. The type of antibiotic that is prescribed depends on the type of microbe that is causing the infection.

RESPIRATORY INFECTIONS

Infections of the respiratory system can occur in any part of the respiratory tract. When we breathe, small particles and microorganisms can be inhaled on dust. These microorganisms include bacteria, fungi, and viruses. These can colonize within the airways and cause infection. Common symptoms of a respiratory tract infection include wheezing, coughing, and shortness of breath (see Chapter 18).

One of the most serious respiratory infections is pneumonia, which affects more than 4 million Americans annually. Pneumonia is an infection of the lungs. Bacteria, viruses, fungi, parasites, and chemicals can cause infectious pneumonia. Pneumonia acquired within the hospital or nursing home is referred to as nosocomial pneumonia. Many elderly persons who are bedridden for long periods are at high risk of acquiring pneumonia, as are persons with chronic conditions such as emphysema, bronchitis, asthma, and immunosuppressive disorders.

Unlike pneumonia, tuberculosis is a highly contagious respiratory tract infection that is caused by the bacterium *Mycobacterium tuberculosis*. Tuberculosis causes inflammation, abscesses, necrosis, and fibrosis of the respiratory system and can spread to other parts of the body. Because of the increased prevalence of immunodeficiency attributable to conditions such as human immunodeficiency virus (HIV) and acquired immunodeficiency syndrome (AIDS), the incidence of tuberculosis has been increasing. An estimated 10 million to 15 million Americans have tuberculosis, and more than 1.7 billion persons are infected worldwide. Symptoms include chronic coughing, fever, sweating, and weight loss. Tuberculosis is diagnosed in the United States by a tuberculin skin test, but this must be confirmed by a chest x-ray or sputum test that isolates the bacteria.

Fungal infections of the respiratory tract primarily infect persons with other major illnesses, such as cystic fibrosis, and persons whose immune systems are compromised, such as patients with AIDS, cancer patients receiving chemotherapy, or patients taking multiple antibiotics. Fungal infections normally are acquired while persons are in the hospital or nursing home. The two most common fungal infections of this type are *Candida albicans* and *Aspergillus fumigatus*.

Bacterial infections resulting from chemical exposure include those toxins that are inhaled in fumes. For example, if asbestosis is inhaled, scarring of the lungs can occur, decreasing the capacity of the lungs to assimilate oxygen. This eventually can cause emphysema, pulmonary edema, and even cancer. These conditions in turn can lead to infections within the respiratory system.

NOSOCOMIAL INFECTIONS

Most hospitalizations are a result of illness, trauma, surgery, or diagnostic procedures. Nursing homes are necessary for long-term care of older adults and severely ill persons. Infections that are acquired within hospitals, nursing homes, or other health care facilities or institutions are known as **nosocomial infections**, and they can be deadly. Hand sanitization and hand washing are the major steps for the prevention of nosocomial infections (see Appendix F).

Patients who have conditions weakening the immune system and who are bed-ridden are more susceptible to infection. Whether these nosocomial infections are bacterial, fungal, or viral, they are difficult to combat. With more antibiotics being used to fight infections, more multidrug-resistant organisms are emerging in health care settings.

MULTIDRUG-RESISTANT ORGANISMS (MDROs)

Any bacterium that is resistant to one or more classifications of drug is considered an MDRO. A specific bacterium that is immune to a particular antibiotic is classified by that effect. Multidrug-resistant organisms are increasing as more persons are living longer. More infections may affect older persons who are admitted to hospitals, nursing homes, and long-term care or even those being seen at physicians' offices. Although there are persons who are at high risk for this type of infection, anyone can be susceptible to these deadly microbes. At-risk people include the elderly, dialysis patients, immunocompromised persons, and patients who have undergone urinary catheterization. Hospitals are among the primary areas where resistant microbes can be isolated. Both methicillin-resistant *Staphylococcus aureus* (MRSA) and **vancomycin-resistant enterococci (VRE)** are typically found in nursing homes and long-term care facilities. Penicillin-resistant *Streptococcus pneumoniae* (PRSP) organisms are primarily seen in medical clinics and physicians' offices, primarily in pediatric settings. Because microorganisms have the ability to alter their genetic composition enough to deter the effects of many antibiotics, stronger antiinfectives had to be developed. Antibiotics have been chemically altered to be more effective against resistant microbial infections referred to as "superbugs." Some superbugs are able to resist specific antibiotics such as penicillin while others are resistant to entire classifications of antibiotics. Box 25-1 lists some of the most common MDROs and their acronyms.

These "superbugs" can spread quickly and effectively unless there is strict adherence to guidelines. This includes isolation of the person infected. Careful consideration must be used in prescribing antibiotics. Health care workers need to instruct the patient's family members to pay meticulous attention to hand hygiene, wear gloves whenever contacting the infected person, and wash all of the clothes, towels, or sheets contacted by the infected person separately from those of noninfected family members. The "superbugs" that have been isolated are potentially fatal and are listed in Table 25-3.

BOX 25-1 MDROs

CA-MRSA	Community-associated methicillin-resistant *Staphylococcus aureus*
ESBLs	Extended-spectrum beta-lactamases
GNRB	Gram-negative resistant bacilli
HA-MRSA	Hospital-associated methicillin-resistant *Staphylococcus aureus*
MDR-GNB	Multidrug-resistant gram-negative bacilli
MDROs	Multidrug-resistant organisms
MDRSP	Multidrug-resistant *Streptococcus pneumoniae*
MRSA	Methicillin-resistant *Staphylococcus aureus*
MSSA	Methicillin-susceptible *Staphylococcus aureus*
PRSP	Penicillin-resistant *Streptococcus pneumoniae*
VISA	Vancomycin-intermediate *Staphylococcus aureus*
VRE	Vancomycin-resistant enterococci
VRSA	Vancomycin-resistant *Staphylococcus aureus*

TABLE 25-3 Potentially Fatal "Superbugs"

Species	Common Abbreviation	Gram-Negative/ Gram-Positive
Acinetobacter baumannii	MDR-Acinetobacter	Gram-negative bacilli
Enterococcus species	VRE	Gram-positive bacilli
Klebsiella species	MDR-Klebsiella	Gram-negative bacilli
Pseudomonas aeruginosa	MDRPA	Gram-negative bacilli
Staphylococcus aureus	MRSA	Gram-positive cocci
Streptococcus pneumoniae	MDRSP	Gram-positive cocci

Methicillin-Resistant Staphylococcus aureus (MRSA)

The first case of MRSA was reported in 1968 in the United States; by the 1990s it was responsible for 20% to 25% of *S. aureus* isolates from hospitalized patients. In 1999 MRSA moved into the 50% range for *S. aureus* isolates (Nosocomial Infection Surveillance System [NISS]). The tracking methods of the CDC and other agencies (NISS) have further divided these resistant strains into two types: community-acquired MRSA (CA-MRSA) and hospital-acquired MRSA (HA-MRSA). Each setting has its own obstacles to overcome in the avoidance and/or containment of resistant microbes. Various strains of bacteria may be only partially susceptible to antibiotic treatment, such as vancomycin-intermediate *S. aureus* (VISA) and methicillin-susceptible *S. aureus* (MSSA).

Vancomycin-Resistant Staphylococcus aureus (VRSA)

In 2002 there were eight cases of vancomycin-intermediate *S. aureus* (VISA) identified in the United States. The very first case of VRSA in the United States developed in a 40-year-old patient who suffered from diabetes, peripheral vascular disease, and chronic renal failure. After a toe amputation, the patient developed methicillin-resistant *S. aureus* in an infected skin graft. The infected graft was removed and he was treated with vancomycin and rifampin. Two months later he developed an infection at the dialysis catheter site. A sample taken from the catheter's exit site was found to be infected with an organism resistant to oxacillin and vancomycin. A week later, foot ulcers appeared infected; cultures revealed VRSA, VRE, and *Klebsiella oxytoca*. The patient's infection was treated with aggressive wound care and the antibiotic Septra (sulfa group); the infection responded to treatment (CDC, 2002).

Multidrug-Resistant S. pneumoniae (MDRSP)

According to the *Morbidity and Mortality Weekly Report (MMWR)* the rates of morbidity due to *S. pneumoniae* drug-resistant bacteria in all of 2008 as compared to January to June of 2009 were 1838 and 1593, respectively; 264 deaths (ages < 5 years) occurred in 2008 as compared to 243 in only the first half of 2009. To check the morbidity and mortality weekly report, visit the following website: www.cdc.gov/mmwr/weekcvol.html\. Long-term care facilities are especially concerned about multidrug-resistant *S. pneumoniae* that are resistant to penicillins, macrolides, and fluoroquinolones.

Gram-Negative Resistant Bacilli (GNRB)

Gram-negative bacilli have increased their resistance against broad-spectrum classes of antibiotics such as fluoroquinolones, carbapenems, and aminoglycosides. These agents are among the strongest agents that can be prescribed for severe infections attributable to multidrug-resistant gram-negative bacilli (MDR-GNB). In 1997 it was determined that between 3% and 10% of strains causing pneumonia were resistant to these broad-spectrum antibiotics. Just 6 years later this value increased to 20% of isolates from neonatal intensive care units (ICUs). Specific drug-resistant bacteria include *Pseudomonas aeruginosa* resistant to fluoroquinolones, *Acinetobacter baumannii* strains resistant to carbapenems, and *P. aeruginosa* strains resistant to imipenem. The primary drugs used to treat these strains are becoming obsolete.

Vancomycin-Resistant Enterococcus (VRE)

Similar to the rapid growth of MRSA infections, the number of VRE infections rose from less than 1% in 1990 to 28.5% in 2003. These were found in hospitalized patients in the United States, although cases are found in hospitals worldwide. The infection from VRE can be transferred between humans, animals, and clinical settings to the community (CDC, 2009).

THE CENTERS FOR DISEASE CONTROL AND PREVENTION (CDC)

The mission of the CDC is to monitor dangerous diseases around the world. Because air travel has simplified traveling to and from remote areas of the world, it is necessary to monitor infectious diseases worldwide. Otherwise, a pandemic could occur. Here in the United States, all contagious diseases must be reported to the CDC as soon as they are suspected. This includes all of the resistant strains of microbes. Box 25-2 displays the *Nationally Notifiable Infectious Diseases, United States 2008,* from the CDC's website (www.cdc.gov/ncphi/od/AI/phs/infdis.htm).

INFECTIONS OF THE SKIN

Skin abrasions, cuts, and scrapes are a common occurrence with growing children and should be cleaned and kept free of bacteria that can infect the area and cause disease. Persons with diabetes are at high risk for infections of the skin and tissues if peripheral vascular disease or poor glucose control is present. The decreased blood flow to the extremities in some persons with diabetes causes a lack of sensation due to neuropathy; minor injuries to the feet can go unnoticed resulting in septic infections that can cause cellulitis, which if left untreated, can result in gangrene requiring surgical debridement and/or amputation. For these types of infections, hospitalization and treatment with strong antibiotics may be necessary.

Fungal infections are common on the skin surface because fungi need a high concentration of oxygen to live; fungal infections tend to occur in warm, moist areas, such as the groin and feet. A common fungal infection is tinea pedis, or athlete's foot (Figure 25-3). There are several over-the-counter (OTC) medications available to treat this condition.

INFECTIONS OF THE NOSE AND MOUTH

The nose and mouth are in constant contact with airborne microbes. Colds and the yearly flu (influenza) are common conditions experienced by most persons. For minor colds and flulike symptoms, OTC products can provide some relief of the symptoms. Unfortunately, because viruses cause colds and flu, antibiotics are useless against them; however, antivirals, such as Tamiflu, can limit the duration of the flu. There are no effective antivirals available for treatment of the common cold. It should be noted, however, that viruses are much more likely to mutate and develop resistance to antiviral medications; therefore antiviral medications should be used with discretion. A person who develops a viral infection can become more susceptible to a bacterial infection. If the normal (bacterial) flora within the mouth, nose, or throat multiply unimpeded, antibiotics may be prescribed.

BOX 25-2 NATIONALLY NOTIFIABLE INFECTIOUS DISEASES 2010

Centers for Disease Control

Anthrax
Arboviral neuroinvasive and non-neuroinvasive diseases
    California serogroup virus disease
    Eastern equine encephalitis virus disease
    Powassan virus disease
    St. Louis encephalitis virus disease
    West Nile virus disease
    Western equine encephalitis virus disease
Botulism
    Botulism, foodborne
    Botulism, infant
    Botulism, other (wound and unspecified)
Brucellosis
Chancroid
Chlamydia trachomatis
Cholera
Cryptosporidiosis
Cyclosporiasis
Dengue
    Dengue fever
    Dengue hemorrhagic fever
    Dengue shock syndrome
Diphtheria
Ehrlichiosis/Anaplasmosis
    Ehrlichia chaffeensis
    Ehrlichia ewingii
    Anaplasma phagocytophilum
    Undetermined
Giardiasis
Gonorrhea
Haemophilus influenzae, invasive disease
Hansen's disease (leprosy)
Hantavirus pulmonary syndrome
Hemolytic uremic syndrome, post diarrheal
Hepatitis A, acute
Hepatitis B, acute
Hepatitis B, chronic
Hepatitis B virus, perinatal infection
Hepatitis C, acute
Hepatitis C, chronic
Human immunodeficiency virus (HIV) infection
    Adult/adolescent (age ≥ 13 yr)
    Child (age ≥ 18 months and < 13 years)
    Pediatric (age < 18 months)
Influenza-associated pediatric mortality
Legionellosis
Listeriosis
Lyme disease
Malaria
Measles
Meningococcal disease
Mumps
Novel influenza A virus infections
Pertussis
Plague

Continued

BOX 25-2 NATIONALLY NOTIFIABLE INFECTIOUS DISEASES 2010—cont'd

Poliomyelitis, paralytic
Psittacosis
Q fever
    Acute
    Chronic
Rabies, animal
Rabies, human
Rubella
Rubella, congenital syndrome
Salmonellosis
Severe acute respiratory syndrome–associated coronavirus (SARS-CoV) disease
Shiga toxin–producing *Escherichia coli* (STEC)
Shigellosis
Smallpox
Spotted fever rickettsiosis
Streptococcal toxic shock syndrome
Streptococcus pneumoniae, invasive disease
Syphilis
    Primary
    Secondary
    Latent
    Early latent
    Late latent
    Latent, unknown duration
    Neurosyphilis
    Late, non-neurological
    Stillbirth
    Congenital
Tetanus
Toxic shock syndrome (other than streptococcal)
Trichinellosis (trichinosis)
Tuberculosis
Tularemia
Typhoid fever
Vancomycin-intermediate *Staphylococcus aureus* infection (VISA)
Vancomycin-resistant *Staphylococcus aureus* infection (VRSA)
Varicella infection (morbidity)
Varicella (deaths only)
Vibriosis
Viral hemorrhagic fevers
    Arenavirus
    Crimean-Congo hemorrhagic fever virus
    Ebola virus
    Lassa virus
    Marburg virus
Yellow fever

Source: http://www.cdc.gov/ncphi/disss/nndss/phs/infdis2010.htm

INFECTIONS OF THE EYES AND EARS

The eyes and the ears are susceptible to infections because they are exposed to the environment. The eyes most often are infected by bacteria or viruses. The most common eye infection is conjunctivitis. Conjunctivitis is an inflammation of the lining (i.e., conjunctiva) of the eyelids and cornea. Within the eyelids, styes may appear, as well as a discharge of pus. The eye may swell and close. Seasonal

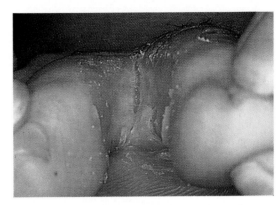

FIGURE 25-3 Tinea pedis, a fungal infection that causes athlete's foot. (From Belchetz PE, Hammond P: *Mosby's color atlas and text of diabetes and endocrinology,* London, 2003, Mosby.)

allergies also can cause conjunctivitis. If an infection of the underlying cornea develops, it is called keratitis.

Otitis media is a common ear infection that many babies and young children experience. Two types of otitis media, or middle ear infection, are acute and chronic. The acute form normally is caused by a bacterial infection that begins as an upper respiratory tract infection and proceeds to infect the ear. The chronic form is caused by repeated infections. Both forms cause inflammation of the tympanic membrane and are painful. Chronic otitis media also may result from rupture of the tympanic membrane. Table 25-4 provides a list of ophthalmic and otic antiinfectives.

ANTIBIOTIC TREATMENTS

Many types of microorganisms can cause infections. Antibiotics are often referred to as either wide-spectrum or narrow-spectrum agents. The spectrum refers to the variety of microorganisms that the antibiotic can inhibit or destroy. A narrow-spectrum antibiotic agent typically is effective against specific families of bacteria, whereas wide-spectrum agents are effective against many gram-positive and gram-negative microorganisms. Another important characteristic is the organism's morphology—the organism's shape (e.g., rod, coccus, spiral, or other). Once the microorganism is identified, a physician can determine the best antibiotic to treat the infection. Several classifications of antibiotics are known. In addition to those agents listed at the beginning of this chapter, there are several more that are effective against specific gram-negative and/or gram-positive microorganisms.

Table 25-5 lists some of the most common types of infections based on their bacterial morphology and their treatments. Details include the Gram stain, the shape of the microbe, and the location of the microbe.

Penicillin

Penicillin antibiotics are taken from two different molds: *Penicillium notatum* and *Penicillium chrysogenum.* These molds are grown in laboratories and are altered synthetically to resist many microorganisms. The drug action of penicillin is bactericidal toward microbes that are currently reproducing. They disrupt the formation of the cell wall so that the bacteria cannot keep a constant osmotic gradient and lyse (break open) the cell wall. Penicillin-type agents are effective against mostly gram-positive organisms. Because oral penicillins are susceptible

Tech Note!

Gram-positive microbes have a different cell wall than gram-negative microbes. Certain antibiotics such as penicillin and its derivatives can destroy bacteria by breaking their cell walls. These antibiotics do not kill human cells because human cells have cell membranes, **not** cell walls.

TABLE 25-4 Otic and Ophthalmic Antiinfectives, Examples

Classification	Generic Name	Trade Name	Indication	Dosage Forms	Auxiliary Label
Otic Agents					
Fluoroquinolone	ciprofloxacin	Cetraxal	External ear infections	Solution	For the ear
Ophthalmic Agents					
Fluoroquinolone	ciprofloxacin	Ciloxan	Broad spectrum of microorganisms	Solution, ointment	For the eye
Fluoroquinolone	ofloxacin	Ocuflox	Conjunctivitis, corneal ulcers caused by susceptible organisms	Solution	For the eye
Macrolide	erythromycin	Ilotycin	Neonatal prophylaxis of *Neisseria gonorrhoeae* or *Chlamydia trachomatis* ocular infections	Ointment	For the eye
Aminoglycoside	gentamicin	Garamycin	Broad spectrum of microorganisms	Solution, ointment	For the eye
Aminoglycoside	tobramycin	Tobrex	Broad spectrum of microorganisms	Solution, ointment	For the eye
Antiviral	idoxuridine	Dendrid	Herpes simplex virus keratitis	Solution, ointment	For the eye
Antifungal	natamycin	Natacyn	Conjunctivitis, keratitis, blepharitis from fungal infection	Solution	For the eye
Triple antibiotic	neomycin, polymyxin B sulfate, bacitracin	Neosporin	Superficial ocular infections	Solution, ointment	For the eye
Sulfonamide	sulfacetamide	Bleph-10, Sulamyd	Susceptible gram-negative organisms	Solution, ointment	For the eye
Antiviral	tifluridine	Viroptic	Herpes simplex virus keratoconjunctivitis	Solution	For the eye
Antiviral	vidarabine	Vira-A	Herpes simplex virus keratoconjunctivitis	Ointment	For the eye

to degradation from stomach acids, it is important that they be taken 1 to 2 hours before or after meals.

For some infections, such as those that can affect the gastrointestinal system, more potent antibiotics are required. In this case, broader-spectrum "cillins" (such as ticarcillin) can kill gram-positive and some gram-negative organisms.

Mild side effects make these agents a good choice. However, if a person has a penicillin allergy, other agents must be used. If penicillin is prescribed to a person suspected of having an allergy, a skin test can be performed to determine whether there is any sensitivity. In some cases, the patient undergoes a desensitization procedure so that the penicillin agent can be administered for a course of treatment. Rash, hives, itching, and swelling of tongue or throat are all indications of an allergic reaction. The following drug monographs list one example of each generation of penicillins along with its individual information. The normal dosage of each drug is the recommended oral adult dosage, unless otherwise indicated.

TABLE 25-5 Examples of Bacterial Morphology, Areas Affected, Treatment, and Conditions

Affected Area	Treatment	Conditions
Gram-Positive Cocci (Spherical-Shaped Microbe): Aerobic and Anaerobic		
Skin, systemic	penicillin G	Throat infections, cuts, septicemia
Systemic, respiratory	penicillin G, penicillin V potassium	Strep throat, pneumonia, septicemia
Blood	penicillin G, ampicillin	Sepsis or endocarditis
Gram-Negative Cocci (Spherical-Shaped Microbe): Aerobic and Anaerobic		
Sexually transmitted disease	ceftriaxone, azithromycin	Gonorrhea
Brain	ceftriaxone, cefotaxime	Meningitis
Respiratory	amoxicillin/sulbactam amoxicillin/clavulanate, levofloxacin	Pneumonia Community-acquired pneumonia
Gram-Positive Bacilli (Rod-Shaped Microbe): Aerobic and Anaerobic		
Respiratory	penicillin G	Pneumonia
Systemic	vancomycin	Sepsis of blood
Peripheral	penicillin G	Necrosis, gangrene
Gram-Negative Bacilli (Rod-Shaped Microbe): Aerobic and Anaerobic		
	cefazolin, cephradine, cefotetan, cefoxitin, cefonicid, gatifloxacin, cinoxacin, doxycycline, sulfa, ampicillin, piperacillin, gentamicin	Urinary tract infections
Sepsis	ampicillin, aminoglycoside carbapenems, cephalosporins	Sepsis, bacteremia, abdominal infections
Respiratory	fourth-generation penicillin, aminoglycosides	Pneumonia

Antibacterial, Penicillins

GENERIC NAME: penicillin V potassium
TRADE NAME: Veetids
GENERATION: first-generation penicillin
ROUTE OF ADMINISTRATION: oral
INDICATION: pneumococcal pneumonia, streptococcal pharyngitis, syphilis
DOSAGE FORMS: tablet, oral solution
COMMON ADULT DOSAGE: 125 to 500 mg PO every 6-8 hours
AUXILIARY LABELS:
■ Take on an empty stomach.
■ Take until gone.
SPECIAL NOTE: Liquid should have a "shake well and refrigerate" auxiliary label and 14-day expiration date after reconstitution if stored in a refrigerator.

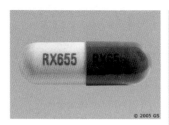

© 2005 GS

GENERIC NAME: amoxicillin
TRADE NAME: Amoxil
GENERATION: second-generation penicillin
ROUTE OF ADMINISTRATION: oral
INDICATION: skin/soft tissue infections, otitis media, sinusitis, respiratory tract infections
DOSAGE FORMS: capsules, suspension
COMMON ADULT DOSAGE: 250 to 500 mg PO every 8 hours
AUXILIARY LABELS:
■ Take on an empty stomach.
■ Take until gone.
SPECIAL NOTE: Suspension should have a "shake well and refrigerate" auxiliary label and 14-day expiration date after reconstitution and is typically recommended to be stored in a refrigerator.

 Tech Note!

Some physicians may prescribe a loading dose of certain antibiotics, such as gentamicin, followed by a lower routine dose. The rationale for a loading dose is to increase the concentration of the antibiotic in the bloodstream to its therapeutic level as quickly as possible.

GENERIC NAME: ticarcillin disodium and clavulanate potassium
TRADE NAME: Timentin
GENERATION: third-generation penicillin
ROUTE OF ADMINISTRATION: injection (intravenous)
INDICATION: drug-resistant or severe skin infections, bone/joint infections, intra-abdominal infections, septicemia, respiratory tract infections, urinary tract infections (UTIs)
DOSAGE FORM: injection only
COMMON ADULT DOSAGE: 3.1 g IV piggyback infusion every 4-6 hours
SPECIAL NOTE: After reconstitution, drug is good for 72 hours if kept in the refrigerator.

Cephalosporins

Oral cephalosporins are less affected by stomach acids; therefore they can be taken with meals. Although cephalosporins are not exactly structured the same as penicillins, there is a 3% to 5% chance of an allergic reaction for those who have penicillin allergies, because the two classes share a beta-lactam–based chemical structure. An example of one cephalosporin from each generation is listed in the following drug monographs. In addition, the common dosage forms and dosages are listed, as well as any special notes of which technicians should be aware.

GENERIC NAME: cephalexin
TRADE NAME: Keflex
GENERATION: first-generation cephalosporin
ROUTE OF ADMINISTRATION: oral
INDICATION: cystitis, skin/soft tissue infections, streptococcal pharyngitis
DOSAGE FORMS: tablet, capsules, suspension
COMMON ADULT DOSAGE: 250 mg to 1 g PO every 12, 8, or 6 hours
AUXILIARY LABEL:
■ Take until gone.
SPECIAL NOTE: Suspension should have a "shake well and refrigerate" auxiliary label and 14-day expiration date after reconstitution if stored in a refrigerator.

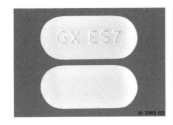

GENERIC NAME: cefuroxime
TRADE NAME: Ceftin (tablet, suspension), Zinacef (injection)
GENERATION: second-generation cephalosporin
ROUTE OF ADMINISTRATION: oral, intramuscular, intravenous
INDICATION: most infections, UTIs, gonorrhea
DOSAGE FORMS: tablet, suspension, injection
COMMON ADULT DOSAGE: 250 to 500 mg PO twice daily
AUXILIARY LABEL:

■ Take until gone.

SPECIAL NOTE: Suspension should have a "shake well and refrigerate" auxiliary label, and a 10-day expiration date after reconstitution if stored in a refrigerator.

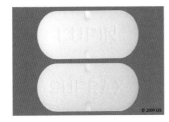

GENERIC NAME: cefixime
TRADE NAME: Suprax
GENERATION: third-generation cephalosporin
ROUTE OF ADMINISTRATION: oral
INDICATION: most infections, gonorrhea
DOSAGE FORMS: tablet, suspension
COMMON ADULT DOSAGE: 400 mg PO once daily or divided every 12 hours
AUXILIARY LABEL:

■ Take as directed

SPECIAL NOTE: Suspension should have a "shake well" auxiliary label. Storage and stability: May be kept at room temperature for up to 14 days.

GENERIC NAME: cefepime
TRADE NAME: Maxipime
GENERATION: fourth-generation cephalosporin
ROUTE OF ADMINISTRATION: intravenous
INDICATION: skin infections, UTIs, moderate to severe pneumonia; wide range of gram-negative bacilli and other microorganisms
DOSAGE FORMS: injection
COMMON ADULT DOSAGE: most infections: 1 to 2 g IV every 12 hours
SPECIAL NOTE: Drug is stable 7 days after reconstitution if refrigerated.

Penicillin and cephalosporins are popular agents used to destroy bacterial infections caused by gram-negative and gram-positive microbes. However, other classes of antibiotics are available, such as those listed in Table 25-6. These medications are prescribed after consideration of the microbe suspected of causing the patient's symptoms or disease presentation, or after isolation of a specific microbe. A culture is taken of the area infected, and by using various laboratory methods, the specific microbe in most cases can be identified (see Chapter 30). In addition, the organism is tested for its sensitivity to various antibiotics; thus the right drug can be used. If the microbe cannot be isolated or the infection is severe, physicians may prescribe a broad-spectrum antibiotic with the hope that it will be effective against the microbe in question. In addition to this alternative type of treatment, a combination of agents can be used to cover many different species of bacterial infections.

Mycobacterium and Mycobacterial Treatment

Two main infections in human beings caused by a mycobacterium are tuberculosis and leprosy. (*Mycobacterium* is related closely to bacteria but is considered a different genus than those that fit into the general Bacteria classification.) Both of these conditions are chronic. Leprosy (Hansen's disease) is a mildly infectious disease that is caused by *Mycobacterium leprae*. In the past, it affected millions of persons across the world, with most cases in Asia and Africa. Recently,

TABLE 25-6 Antibiotics Other Than Penicillins and Cephalosporins

Antibiotic	Trade Name	Generic Name	Effects	Normal Adult Dosage
Aminoglycosides*	Garamycin	gentamicin	Mostly gram-negative microbes: bactericidal	1.5 to 2 mg/kg IV/IM q8h (conventional dosing) OR 5-7 mg/kg q24h (once-daily dosing)
	Amikin	amikacin	Mostly gram-negative microbes: bactericidal	5 to 7.5 mg/kg IV/IM q8h (conventional dosing)
	Nebcin	tobramycin	Mostly gram-negative microbes: bactericidal	1.5 to 2 mg/kg IV/IM q8h (conventional dosing) OR 5-7 mg/kg q24h (once-daily dosing)
Carbapenems	Merrem	meropenem	Broad spectrum: bactericidal	1 g IV q8h
	Primaxin	imipenem/cilastatin	Broad spectrum: bactericidal	500 mg IV q6-8h
Monobactams	Azactam	aztreonam	Broad spectrum: bactericidal	500 mg to 1 g IV q8-12h; 2 g IV q6-8h
Quinolones	Cipro	ciprofloxacin	Broad spectrum: bactericidal	250-750 mg PO q12h; 200-400 mg IV q12h
	Noroxin	norfloxacin	Broad spectrum: bactericidal	200-400 mg PO/q12h
	Levaquin	levofloxacin	Broad spectrum: bactericidal	500-750 mg IV/PO q24h
Lincosamides	Cleocin	clindamycin	Gram-positive microbes; anaerobes: bacteriostatic	150-300 mg PO q6h; 300-600 mg IV q6-12h
	Lincocin	lincomycin	Gram-positive microbes; anaerobes: bacteriostatic	500 mg PO q6-8h; 600 mg IV q12h to daily
Macrolides	Biaxin	clarithromycin	Broad spectrum: bactericidal/ bacteriostatic	250-500 mg PO q12h
	E-Mycin	erythromycin	Broad spectrum: bactericidal/ bacteriostatic	Dosage varies depending on type of erythromycin given: see *Drug Facts and Comparisons*
	Zithromax	azithromycin	Broad spectrum: bactericidal/ bacteriostatic	250-500 mg PO daily
Ketolides	Ketek	telithromycin	Broad spectrum: pneumonia	800 mg PO once daily 7-10 days
Tetracyclines	Achromycin	tetracycline	Broad spectrum: bacteriostatic	250-500 mg PO q6-12h
	Vibramycin	doxycycline	Broad spectrum: bacteriostatic	100 mg PO daily to bid
Vancomycin	Vancocin	vancomycin	Active against gram-positive microbes: bactericidal/ bacteriostatic	125-500 mg PO q6-8h; 1 gram IV q12-24h

*Doses adjusted to peak/trough levels or nomograms; see Drug Facts and Comparisons for more information.

the disease has decreased progressively. The following are some typical symptoms of leprosy: noticeable skin lesions appear; ulceration of the feet and loss of hand function may occur, and corneal abrasions may cause blindness. This condition can be treated with rifampin (bactericidal), along with either dapsone (bacteriostatic) and/or clofazimine (bactericidal). Depending on the severity of the infection treatment can last from 6 months to 24 months.

Tuberculosis is a disease that was known as the wasting disease because it robs a person of breath and strength. Eventually, it results in death. Tuberculosis has been responsible for millions of deaths throughout history, but in the 1960s tuberculosis was disappearing as new drugs were invented to eradicate the disease. Unfortunately, many individuals stopped taking their medication once they felt better; thus the microbe was able to withstand low doses of antibiotics until it became resistant. Today, tuberculosis is once again occurring in

TABLE 25-7 Antituberculin Agents

Generic Name	Trade Name	Dosing Regimen	Common Length of Time
isoniazid	INH	5 mg/kg/day	6-24 months
rifampin	Rifadin	600 mg/day	6-9 months
ethambutol	Myambutol	15 mg/kg/day	6-9 months
pyrazinamide	Generic only	15-35 mg/kg/day	6-9 months
cycloserine	Seromycin	750 mg to 1 g daily	Up to 18-24 months
streptomycin	Generic only	15 mg/kg/day (IM)	Up to 12 months
kanamycin	Kantrex	500 mg to 1 g daily	Up to 12 months

Tech Note!

Visit www.CDC.gov/mmwr *(Morbidity and Mortality Weekly Report)* to see the types of outbreaks that occur in the United States and the world.

staggering numbers. Two thirds of prisoners are estimated to have tuberculosis. Millions of persons are dying each year, and for those persons who acquire the resistant strain, there is no medication available to combat this deadly disease. Tuberculosis is prevalent in the United States and around the world. To view an illustration of a positive TB test, refer to Figure 18-7.

A few antituberculin-type medications are used to treat tuberculosis, but they must be taken for the full course of treatment. The regimens always involve multidrug therapies to combat resistant strains and increase cure rates. Treatment can last from 6 months to years depending on test results and must not be discontinued regardless of how well the person feels. As the number of microbes decreases, the person begins to feel better, but if the medication is stopped, the microbe reappears and is stronger and much harder to destroy (Table 25-7).

Aminoglycosides

Aminoglycosides are bactericidal to many varieties of gram-negative microorganisms. The drug action for parenterally administered aminoglycosides is their ability to bind to the ribosomes of the microorganism, stopping protein **synthesis**, which ultimately causes the death of the organism. Many of these medications are available in parenteral (intravenous) form only and are used mainly in hospitals for severe infections. They are often administered with other antibiotics to further microbial coverage. A serious side effect of high doses of aminoglycosides is possible nephrotoxicity or ototoxicity. Because aminoglycosides have a narrow range between therapeutic and toxic serum levels, careful calculations must be made to determine the appropriate dosage. Monitoring is done by evaluation of the patient's blood levels of antibiotic, drawn at specific times (called peak and trough levels). In this way, the patient's clearance of the aminoglycoside drug can be determined, and changes can be made in the dosage or dosing time if necessary. Patients with renal disease and older adults are more susceptible to toxic levels of these agents because of decreased renal excretion. A sample of the types of agents most commonly encountered by technicians is listed next, along with their specifics.

GENERIC NAME: amikacin
TRADE NAME: Amikin
INDICATION: serious infections such as *Pseudomonas, Proteus, Serratia,* and various gram-positive bacilli that cause bone and respiratory tract infections, endocarditis, and septicemia
DOSAGE FORMS: injection, 50 mg/mL in 2-mL and 4-mL vials; 250 mg/mL in 2-mL and 4-mL vials
COMMON ADULT DOSAGE: based on weight and renal function of patient: normally 5 to 7.5 mg/kg per dose with dosing interval dependent on renal function; once-daily dose regimens also exist
SPECIAL NOTE: Stable for 2 days if refrigerated after mixing into appropriate solution.

GENERIC NAME: gentamicin

TRADE NAME: Garamycin (intravenous), Genoptic (ophthalmic), G-Myticin (topical)

INDICATION: for gram-negative organisms such as *Pseudomonas, Proteus,* and *Serratia* and gram-positive *Staphylococcus;* bone and respiratory tract infections, skin and soft tissue infections, UTIs, abdominal infections, and eye infections caused by susceptible bacteria

DOSAGE FORMS: injection, ophthalmic ointment or solution, topical cream

COMMON ADULT DOSAGE: based on weight and renal function of patient: typically 1.5 to 2 mg/kg per dose IV with interval of dosing dependent on renal function; once-daily dose regimens also exist; ophthalmic: instill ½ inch of ointment 2 to 3 times daily every 3 to 4 hours or 1 or 2 drops in infected eye every 4 hours daily; topical, apply 3 to 4 times per day to affected area(s)

AUXILIARY LABELS:

■ For ophthalmic: For the eye.

■ For topical cream: Topical use only.

SPECIAL NOTE: Intravenous solution does not need to be refrigerated before or after mixing into solution. Stability is 24 hours only after mixing.

GENERIC NAME: tobramycin

TRADE NAME: Nebcin (intravenous), Tobrex (ophthalmic), Tobi (inhalant)

INDICATION: for susceptible gram-negative bacilli including *Pseudomonas aeruginosa;* inhalation used for treatment as well as prophylaxis of *Pseudomonas* colonization in patients with cystic fibrosis; ophthalmic use for superficial infections to the eye from susceptible bacteria

DOSAGE FORMS: injection, ophthalmic ointment or solution, inhalation solution

COMMON ADULT DOSAGE: based on weight and renal function of patient; usually 1.5 to 2 mg/kg per dose IV with dosing interval dependent on renal function; once-daily dose regimens also exist; ophthalmic: instill ointment 2 to 3 times daily every 3 to 4 hours; for inhalation, 60 to 80 mg three times daily

AUXILIARY LABEL:

■ For ophthalmic: For the eye.

SPECIAL NOTE: After reconstitution, intravenous solution is stable for 96 hours if refrigerated.

Drug-Resistant and Miscellaneous Antibiotics

The following agents are commonly used antibiotics for a variety of infections. Their classification, drug action, indications, and generic and trade names are listed in Table 25-8. Only certain antibiotics can be used on the resistant microorganisms.

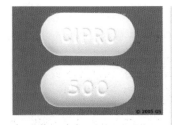

GENERIC NAME: ciprofloxacin

TRADE NAME: Cipro, Cipro XR, Ciloxan

INDICATION: a wide variety of infections and infection sites

DOSAGE FORMS: tablet, suspension, infusion, ophthalmic solution or ointment

COMMON ADULT DOSAGE: oral: 500 mg every 12 hours

SPECIAL NOTE: Ciprofloxacin has bactericidal action against a wide range of gram-positive organisms such as *Staphylococcus epidermidis,* methicillin-resistant strains of *S. aureus,* and gram-negative organisms such as *Escherichia coli*

TABLE 25-8 Antibiotics for Resistant Microorganisms

Class	Generic Name	Trade Name	Indication	Drug Action
Tetracyclines*	doxycycline tetracycline minocycline	Vibramycin Achromycin Minocin	Severe infections such as respiratory, gastrointestinal, and integumentary	Inhibits protein synthesis
Quinolones†	ciprofloxacin levofloxacin ofloxacin norfloxacin	Cipro Levaquin Floxin Noroxin	Respiratory and urinary tract infections	Interferes with bacterial DNA synthesis
Macrolides	azithromycin clarithromycin erythromycin erythromycin ethylsuccinate erythromycin lactobionate	Zithromax Biaxin E-Mycin, Ery-Tab EES Erythrocin	Respiratory, genital, gastrointestinal, and skin infections	Inhibits protein synthesis
Carbapenems	imipenem/cilastatin	Primaxin	Serious infections	Inhibits bacterial cell wall synthesis
Monobactam	aztreonam	Azactam	Wide-spectrum gram-negative aerobic organisms	Inhibits bacterial cell wall synthesis
Vancomycin	vancomycin	Vancocin	Serious/severe infections	Inhibits bacterial cell wall synthesis

*Auxiliary labels: Take on an empty stomach. Take with plenty of water. Avoid dairy products. Avoid antacids. Avoid direct sunlight.
†Auxiliary labels: Do not take antacids. Avoid iron/zinc supplements 4 hours before or 2 hours after taking.

GENERIC NAME: vancomycin
TRADE NAME: Vancocin
INDICATION: staphylococcal and enterococcal infections; also for *Clostridium difficile* in gastrointestinal (GI) tract
DOSAGE FORMS: infusion used for serious staphylococcal infections; orally for GI infections
COMMON ADULT DOSAGE: IV 1 g (15 mg/kg) every 12 hours; regimens adjusted for drug concentrations and renal function
SPECIAL NOTE: Bactericidal for staphylococci and streptococci; also used for resistant staphylococcal infections; orally used for treatment of *Clostridium difficile*.

GENERIC NAME: tigecycline
TRADE NAME: Tygacil
INDICATION: pneumonia, intra-abdominal infections, skin and skin structure infections
DOSAGE FORMS: intravenous infusion
COMMON ADULT DOSAGE: initial dose of 100 mg, then 50 mg every 12 hours
SPECIAL NOTE: Complicated infections caused by MRSA and other resistant organisms; it has no activity against *Pseudomonas*.

ANTIFUNGALS

Fungi are plantlike organisms that can grow on cloth, food, showers, or people, or in any warm, moist environment. They absorb nutrients from the environment or from hosts such as animals and human beings. Most conditions caused by fungi tend to affect the outside of the body and are not life-threatening, but they do cause great annoyance. Antifungal agents, or fungicides, are used to control these infections. The agents used are commonly applied directly to the skin, inserted into the vagina, or used as oral rinses if the infection is relatively superficial and localized. If the infection has not responded or has advanced into the bloodstream or internal tissues, then systemically administered antifungals must be used. Topical agents are available in different dosage forms: lotions, creams, ointments, powders, and sprays. Patients should use the dosage form that they find most convenient as long as they always adhere to the medications' instructions. Many antifungal agents are available OTC to treat mild cases of skin and vaginal mycosis (fungus infections). Some of the agents listed are fungicidal (killing fungi) or fungistatic (inhibiting further growth), depending on the organism for which they are used.

A systemic infection is much more serious. This occurs when the fungus is spread throughout the body by the bloodstream. For these types of infections, more potent agents called fungicides are used intravenously (Table 25-9).

Candida Infections

A common fungal species that resides inside the human body is *Candida albicans*. Although this fungal species is found within a human being's normal flora, if it becomes overpopulated because of a weakened immune system or because of the use of potent antibiotics, it can cause serious effects and discomfort. There are different species of *Candida*. Depending on the specific species, the organism is responsible for infections of the mouth, vagina, skin, blood, or tissues; in addition, it can be found under the fingernails and toenails. The most commonly known *Candida* infection is the vaginal "yeast" infection. Fortunately, there are many products, both prescription and OTC, for the treatment of this infection. *Candida* can also cause certain forms of diaper rash in infants.

TABLE 25-9 Fungal Infections and Their Treatments

Trade Name	Generic Name	Indications	Drug Action
Fungizone	amphotericin B	Systemic mycosis	Lyses fungus cell membrane; both bacteriostatic and bactericidal
Lotrimin, Gyne-Lotrimin	clotrimazole	Vaginal, oral, and topical fungal infections	Alters cell membrane permeability
Diflucan	fluconazole	Esophageal, urinary tract infections, vaginal mycosis	Affects biosynthesis, inhibiting growth; both bacteriostatic and bactericidal
Ancobon	flucytosine	Serious mycosis	Inhibits DNA synthesis and metabolism of pyrimidine; bactericidal
Fulvicin	griseofulvin	Ringworm, toenail/fingernail mycosis	Inhibits cell mitosis; bactericidal
Sporanox	itraconazole	Lung infections	Affects biosynthesis, inhibiting growth; bactericidal
Nizoral	ketoconazole	Systemic mycosis	Affects biosynthesis, inhibiting growth; bactericidal
Monistat, Monistat-Derm	miconazole	Skin, vaginal mycosis	Affects biosynthesis, inhibiting growth; bactericidal
Mycostatin	nystatin	Oral, vaginal, intestinal mycosis	Lyses fungus cell membrane; bactericidal
Lamisil	terbinafine	Skin, toe, and fingernail mycosis	Inhibits cell wall synthesis; bactericidal

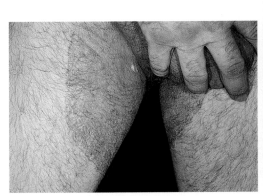

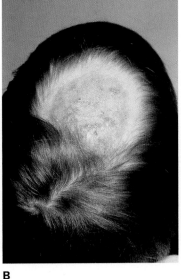

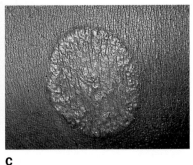

A **B** **C**

FIGURE 25-4 Types of tinea infections. **A,** Tinea cruris. **B,** Tinea capitis. **C,** Tinea corporis. (**A** From Callen JP et al: *Color atlas of dermatology,* ed 2, Philadelphia, 2000, Saunders; **B** from Conlon CP, Snydman DR: *Mosby's color atlas and text of infectious diseases,* London, 2000, Mosby Ltd.; **C** from Zitelli BJ, Davis HW: *Atlas of pediatric physical diagnosis,* ed 5, St Louis, 2007, Mosby.)

BOX 25-3 PARASITIC ORGANISMS AND THEIR DESCRIPTION

> **Cilia:** Hairlike structures that work like oars to move the organism
> **Flagella:** A whiplike tail that propels the organism
> **Pseudopodia:** Footlike protrusions that slowly move the organism
> **Stationary:** A cyst form that waits for an opportunistic environment before regenerating

---

Tinea Infections

One of the most common conditions caused by a fungus is dermatophytosis (fungal infection of the skin of the hands or feet), caused by fungi from the genera *Trichophyton, Microsporum,* or *Epidermophyton.* Tinea pedis (foot) is also known as athlete's foot. If it appears on the scalp, it is known as tinea capitis, and anywhere else on the skin it is commonly called ringworm. If it appears in the groin area, it is called tinea cruris or "jock itch" (Figure 25-4, *A-C*). Onychomycosis is an infection of the nails, usually caused by dermatophytic species; while a few topical treatments are available, systemic treatment with oral medications is often needed to clear fungal nail infections.

PARASITES

Parasites are organisms that benefit at the expense of another. The host is the organism that is being used by the parasite. Under the kingdom Protista, the phylum Sporozoa consists of parasitic organisms. The morphology (characteristics) of an organism depends on whether it is multicellular or unicellular and how it is transmitted. These organisms are distinguished from one another according to several factors, such as morphology and locomotion (movement), as listed in Box 25-3. The life cycles of many of the organisms that affect human beings are explained in Chapter 30. Some major conditions that can occur from protozoa are listed in Table 25-10.

TABLE 25-10 Protozoan Infections and Their Treatments

Species	Disease Name	Transmission	Treatment, Generic	Trade Name
Toxoplasma gondii	Toxoplasmosis	Contaminated food, water, feces of bug or cat; sand flies; tsetse flies also carry this disease	pyrimethamine and sulfadiazine	Daraprim and sulfadiazine(no generic)
			pyrimethamine and sulfamethoxazole/ trimethoprim	Daraprim and Septra or Bactrim
			pentamidine (IV)	Pentam
			azithromycin	Zithromax
			atovaquone	Mepron
Plasmodium vivax	Malaria	Female mosquitoes	chloroquine	Aralen
			artemether/lumefantrine	Coartem
			atovaquone/proguanil	Malarone
			pyrimethamine/sulfadoxine	Fansidar
			hydroxychloroquine	Plaquenil

Protozoa

Many protozoa are human parasites. Amebiasis is an infection caused by the protozoan species *Entamoeba histolytica*. The cyst form is transferred via fecal-oral routes. Symptoms can include abdominal pain, nausea, flatulence, and fatigue. Treatments include iodoquinol, which rids the body of the infestation. Another protozoan disease that is more dangerous to human beings is toxoplasmosis. The species *Toxoplasma gondii* is transferred via uncooked meat or cysts that may be present in cat feces. Although the symptoms may be mild in most adults, they can be deadly to infants and the unborn fetus. Treatment includes pyrimethamine and sulfadiazine. Trichomoniasis is caused by the species *Trichomonas vaginalis*. This disease affects the vaginal area; the cervical area appears red and inflamed. These protozoa also can infect the female and male urethra. Metronidazole is the drug of choice and must be used by both sexual partners.

Helminths (Worms)

Helminths are parasitic worms. They are not microscopic organisms, but the procedures used to diagnose infections from these organisms are performed in a clinical laboratory. These parasites are multicellular. The two major worms that affect Americans are roundworms (Nematoda) and flatworms (Platyhelminthes). Fifty species of roundworms can infect human beings. Many can be transferred in undercooked meat. Some species can lodge in the intestine or lymph nodes, causing harm to the host. Hookworms are another type of roundworm and are transferred through skin contact with feces infected by the worm. For example, if a person walks on soil that has been contaminated with human feces that contains hookworms, the hookworms will enter through the skin of the foot.

Flatworms are divided further into tapeworms and flukes. Many flatworms survive by feeding off dead matter or small organisms and are not harmful to human beings. Tapeworms reside in the intestines of most vertebrates, where they absorb digested food from the host. Eating undercooked meat can transfer them to human beings. Flukes have an interesting life cycle that involves freshwater snails and human beings. Persons who drink water from feces-contaminated water can acquire flukes. Many helminthic diseases are caused by undercooked meat or contaminated water and soil. Most helminthic infections occur in persons

TABLE 25-11 Helminthic Infestations and Their Treatments

	Species or Disease Name	Symptoms	Treatment
Class Nematoda			
Roundworms	*Trichinella spiralis* (trichinosis)	Inflammation	diethylcarbamazine, ivermectin
Hookworms	*Ancylostoma duodenale, Necator americanus*	Anemia, weakness, fatigue	mebendazole, albendazole, pyrantel
Pinworms	*Enterobius vermicularis*	Anal itching; can sometimes see worms with flashlight at night around anal area.	mebendazole, albendazole, pyrantel, praziquantel
Phylum Platyhelminthes			
Tapeworms	*Taenia saginata, Taenia solium*	Diarrhea, weight loss, perforation of intestine	praziquantel, niclosamide, paromomycin
Flukes	Schistosomiasis	Loss of blood in feces	praziquantel

who live in areas where sanitation is nonexistent or in persons who are not aware of the dangers of eating raw meat. Table 25-11 lists the species, symptoms, and treatments for helminthic infestations.

Parasitic Treatments

Parasites can be addressed in only a few ways: destroyed and washed off the body; removed from the body alive or dead; or removed surgically. Whichever mechanism is used, the main goal is to remove them from the body. All medications used to rid the body of parasites are oral dosage forms; therefore hospitalization is rarely necessary. In addition, the dosage regimen is normally short term, and treatment can be done in just a few oral doses.

All parasites can cause damage to the tissues or organs that they invade. Although parasites may weaken the host, most parasites do not kill their host because this would destroy the source of their food and shelter. Table 25-12 lists the main anthelmintic agents and their drug action.

MALARIA

Malaria is a sporozoan infection with symptoms consisting of fever, chills, sweating, headache, and nausea. The cycle of chills, fever, and sweating varies depending on the particular pathogen. The genus *Plasmodium* has four different species that are responsible for malaria. Some cause severe side effects, such as the species *Plasmodium falciparum,* which can cause death. The human body, the site of sporozoan reproduction, is called the reservoir. Transmission is usually via an infected mosquito, but the sporozoa also can be transmitted by infected needles or syringes or by blood transfusion. The incubation period ranges from 1 week to 1 month depending on the species.

Malaria is a major health problem in more than 100 countries. Reported cases of malaria are responsible for more than 1 million deaths annually. Approximately 1200 cases are diagnosed in the United States annually. The prevention and control of malaria consist of controlling mosquitoes by using insect repellents, filling water holes where mosquitoes breed, and using insecticides.

The diagnosis of malaria is made based on blood smears. Chloroquine phosphate is used as treatment when possible. However, if the strain is resistant to chloroquine, other agents such as mefloquine, doxycycline, or primaquine can be used.

TABLE 25-12 Anthelmintic Drug Actions and Common Dosage

Generic Name	Trade Name	Drug Action	Common Dosage
albendazole	Albenza	Prevents glucose intake in worm, causing it to die	400 mg bid or 15 mg/kg/day divided into bid doses
diethylcarbamazine	Hetrazan*	Vermicidal: increases loss of filariae; decreases ability to produce more	2-3 mg/kg PO tid
mebendazole	Generic only	Vermicidal: stops glucose uptake in worm	100 mg PO bid × 3 days
niclosamide	Niclocide	Vermicidal: affects mitochondria; decreases metabolism	8 g × 1 dose or 2 g PO daily × 1 week (depends on type of worm infestation)
ivermectin	Stromectol	Paralysis: causes depolarization and eventual paralysis of worm, which is then flushed out	200 mcg/kg in single dose
praziquantel	Biltricide	Paralysis: causes loss of calcium and eventual paralysis of worm, which is then flushed out	25 mg/kg PO tid × 1 day
pyrantel	Pin-X	Paralysis: causes depolarization and eventual paralysis of worm, which is then flushed out	11 mg/kg PO × 1 dose; may be repeated in 2-3 weeks if necessary
thiabendazole	Mintezol	Vermicidal: inhibits essential enzymes, causing death	25 mg/kg PO bid × 2 days

*Please note: Hetrazan is only available through a CDC protocol.

ANTIVIRALS

Viruses are organisms that cannot live outside their host. They are unlike bacteria or any other organisms because of their structure and design. Viruses are classified by the following criteria:

1. Nucleic acid makeup (single- or double-stranded DNA or ribonucleic acid [RNA])
2. Size
3. Host it infects
4. Enveloped or naked

Debate continues within the scientific community as to whether viruses should be classified as living organisms because they differ in most criteria that are used to classify living organisms. All living organisms replicate or reproduce themselves with their own set of blueprints or DNA; however, viruses cannot reproduce by themselves. They require a host's DNA to replicate. Unlike parasites, viruses use the host cell to replicate and then kill the host by budding. Budding is the process used by a replicated virus to leave the host cell. The virus associates with an area of cell membrane, which forms an envelope around the virus and replaces some of the cell's proteins with virus-coded proteins. Therefore the composition of the virus is closely related to a human being's DNA, and when agents are used to destroy a virus, they inadvertently can destroy human cells along with the virions. Plants and animals can contract many types of viral diseases. For animals, these include chickenpox, colds, influenza, polio, rabies, warts, HIV, AIDS, and some types of cancer.

The following analogy will help explain viral replication. Let us say you have been given the key to an automobile manufacturing plant, but instead of making one of the cars normally made in the plant, you want a truck specialized to fit your needs. You have all the necessary components within the auto shop, but the outcome will be different from what normally is manufactured in the plant. This is the same type of action that a virion (one virus particle) has on your body. The virus invades your cells and uses your components to assemble its own blueprints. The invasion and spread of virions have the following five steps:

1. Attachment: This is a lock-and-key mechanism that allows virions to attach to specific host cells.
2. Injection of nucleic acids: The whole virion enters the cell or it injects its nucleic acids to begin the replication process.
3. Synthesis: The virion assumes control of the cell and begins to use parts of the cell to make its own necessary enzymes and proteins to replicate its RNA or DNA and component parts.
4. Assembly: Once all the parts are made, then the parts are assembled to create a new virion. Millions of new virions are assembled and readied for transport.
5. Spread via lysis or budding: When the assembly is completed, the virions leave the manufacturing plant (host cell) and continue to infect other cells.

Agents can slow down and, in some cases, kill viruses. To interrupt the process outlined in the previous manufacturing plant analogy, an antiviral agent can affect the virus by the processes listed in Box 25-4. In addition, Table 25-13 lists both antiviral and antiretroviral agents and examples of the types of viruses for which they are indicated.

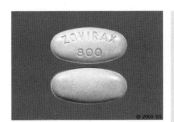

GENERIC NAME: acyclovir
TRADE NAME: Zovirax (Glaxo Wellcome)
INDICATION: herpes zoster (shingles), genital herpes, and chickenpox
DOSAGE FORMS: tablet, capsules, injection, suspension, ointment
COMMON ADULT DOSAGE: 200 to 800 mg PO every 4 hours (5 times daily) for 7 to 10 days, depending upon type and severity of infection.
SIDE EFFECTS: headache, dizziness, rash, nausea
AUXILIARY LABELS:

- Suspension: Shake well.
- Ointment: Topical use only.

SPECIAL NOTE: Suspension is banana flavored.

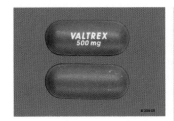

GENERIC NAME: valacyclovir
TRADE NAME: Valtrex
INDICATION: genital herpes, herpes labialis (cold sores), and herpes zoster
DOSAGE FORMS: caplet
COMMON ADULT DOSAGE: 500 mg to 1 g PO every 12 hours, depending upon type and severity of infection
SIDE EFFECTS: headache, nausea, and abdominal pain
AUXILIARY LABELS:

- Medication should be taken with plenty of water
- Finish all medication unless otherwise directed by your physician.

BOX 25-4 ANTIVIRAL MECHANISMS OF ACTION

1. Stop the virus from attaching to the host cell by blocking the receptor sites on the host cell or by blocking the sites on the virion
2. Stop the replication process within the host cell, thus inhibiting the virion from making its necessary components
3. Disrupt the assembly of virion particles as they are being assembled within the host cell, thus rendering an incomplete virion particle

TABLE 25-13 Antiviral and Antiretroviral Agents

Classification	Generic Name	Trade Name	Indications
Antivirals	acyclovir	Zovirax	Herpes simplex, herpes zoster
	amantidine	Symmetrel	Influenza A strains, Parkinson's disease
	famciclovir	Famvir	Herpes zoster, recurrent genital herpes
	foscarnet	Foscavir	Herpes simplex, CMV* retinitis, acyclovir-resistant HSV in immunocompromised patients
	valacyclovir	Valtrex	Herpes zoster, genital herpes, herpes simplex
	docosanol	Abreva	Herpes simplex
	oseltamivir	Tamiflu	Influenza A and B virus
	zanamivir	Relenza	Influenza A and B virus
	influenza virus vaccine	Fluarix, FluMist	Influenza A and B virus (prevention of)
	ribavirin	Virazole	RSV
	valganciclovir	Valcyte	CMV infection
Protease inhibitors	tipranavir	Aptivus	HIV infection
	indinavir	Crixivan	HIV infection
	saquinavir	Invirase	HIV infection
	fosamprenavir	Lexiva	HIV infection
	darunavir	Preszista	HIV infection
	ritonavir	Norvir	HIV infection
	atazanavir	Reyataz	HIV infection
	nelfinavir	Viracept	HIV infection
Nucleoside reverse transcriptase inhibitors	emtricitabine	Emtriva	HIV infection
	lamivudine	Epivir	HIV infection, chronic hepatitis B
	zalcitabine	Hivid	HIV infection
	zidovudine	Retrovir (AZT)	HIV infection, prevention of maternal-fetal transmission
	didanosine	Videx	HIV infection
	stavudine	Zerit	HIV infection
	abacavir	Ziagen	HIV infection
Non-nucleoside reverse transcriptase inhibitors	etravirine	Intelence	HIV infection
	delavirdine	Rescriptor	HIV infection
	efavirenz	Sustiva	HIV infection
	nevirapine	Viramune	HIV infection
Fusion inhibitors	enfuvirtide	Fuzeon	HIV infection
	maraviroc	Selzentry	HIV infection
Integrase strand transfer inhibitors	raltegravir	Isentress	HIV infection

*CMV, Cytomegalovirus; HSV, herpes simplex virus; RSV, respiratory syncytial virus.

GENERIC NAME: oseltamivir
TRADE NAME: Tamiflu
INDICATION: influenza
DOSAGE FORMS: tablet, suspension
COMMON ADULT DOSAGE: 75 mg PO bid
SIDE EFFECTS: headache, nausea, vomiting, and abdominal pain
AUXILIARY LABEL:

■ Take as directed.

NOTE: Suspension should have a "shake well" auxiliary label. The suspension is good for 17 days when refrigerated or 10 days if at room temperature. Write the expiration date on the label.

© 2005 GS

HIV/AIDS

Since the 1980s the incidence of HIV infection (the resulting end-stage disease is called AIDS) has been increasing. HIV is a bloodborne, sexually transmitted virus. Although there are many agents now available to treat HIV infection, there is no cure for this disease. However, effective antiretroviral treatment can delay progression of the infection to AIDS, and prolong life. The virion does not cause death, but instead it eventually renders the host too weak to fight any infection. A person with AIDS will succumb to opportunistic illnesses. The HIV virus attacks the immune system of human beings.

In the beginning stages of HIV, the body weakens because of the virus replication process within the immune system. Specifically, the number of CD4 T lymphocytes decreases; according to the CDC classification system of this disease, the infected person is diagnosed as having AIDS when the CD4 T-cell count is less than 200 per microliter of blood.

The onset of AIDS is estimated to be able to occur up to 20 years after acquisition of HIV. However, the virus is always contagious. All agents that are available to treat HIV and AIDS are aimed at controlling the progression of the disease but cannot cure it. Therefore the only way to avoid this disease is to follow measures that prevent its contraction.

HIV can be transmitted by bodily fluids containing the virus. Simple protective steps, including testing both partners for HIV before sexual activities and wearing condoms, reduce the chances of acquiring HIV via sexual contact. In medical settings, proper use of protective equipment, such as gloves and face shields, helps decrease the risk of contamination. HIV could be transmitted to a nurse or physician via fluids such as blood or even vaginal secretions. New syringes are also now in use to decrease the possibility of needle sticks.

NOTE: Antiretroviral dosages can vary widely, depending on the drug combinations prescribed and the presence of interacting drugs or health conditions. The following are simple examples of adult dosing.

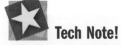

Tech Note!

Remember that HIV is a virus. A positive test result for HIV is considered the precursor to AIDS.

Nucleoside and Nucleotide Reverse Transcriptase Inhibitors (NRTIs)

GENERIC NAME: zidovudine (also known as AZT)
TRADE NAME: Retrovir
INDICATION: treatment of HIV and hepatitis C
DOSAGE FORMS: tablet, capsule, injection, syrup
COMMON ADULT DOSAGE: 200 mg three times daily or 300 mg twice daily
SIDE EFFECTS: headache, weakness, abdominal pain, diarrhea, nausea, anemia
AUXILIARY LABEL:
■ Take as directed.
SPECIAL NOTE: Syrup is strawberry flavored.

Non-Nucleoside Reverse Transcriptase Inhibitors

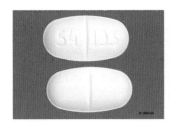

GENERIC NAME: nevirapine
TRADE NAME: Viramune
INDICATION: treatment of HIV
DOSAGE FORMS: tablet, suspension
COMMON ADULT DOSAGE: 200 mg once daily for the first 14 days, then 200 mg twice daily
SIDE EFFECTS: rash, hypersensitivity, and possibility of developing hepatitis
AUXILIARY LABELS:
■ Take as directed.
■ Suspension: Shake well before use.

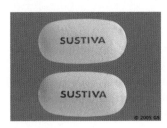

GENERIC NAME: efavirenz

TRADE NAME: Sustiva

INDICATION: treatment of HIV

DOSAGE FORMS: tablet, capsules

COMMON ADULT DOSAGE: 600 mg PO once a day (bedtime dosing on empty stomach recommended)

SIDE EFFECTS: abnormal dreams, changes in body fat, diarrhea, dizziness, drowsiness, headache, trouble concentrating, and trouble sleeping

AUXILIARY LABELS:

- Take as directed.
- Take on an empty stomach.
- May cause drowsiness.
- Do not drink alcohol with this medication.

Protease Inhibitors (PIs)

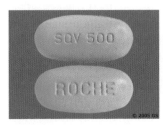

GENERIC NAME: saquinavir

TRADE NAME: Invirase

INDICATION: treatment of HIV

DOSAGE FORMS: capsules, tablet

COMMON ADULT DOSAGE: 1000 mg PO twice daily

SIDE EFFECTS: anxiety, constipation, diarrhea, dizziness, drowsiness, headache, trouble concentrating and trouble sleeping, vomiting, warts, night sweats and dry skin/lips, changes in body fat

AUXILIARY LABELS:

- Take as directed.
- May cause drowsiness.
- Take within 2 hours after a full meal.

NOTE: This medicine is always taken with ritonavir.

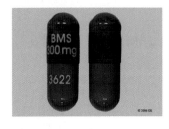

GENERIC NAME: atazanavir

TRADE NAME: Reyataz

INDICATION: treatment of HIV

DOSAGE FORMS: capsules

COMMON ADULT DOSAGE: 300 to 400 mg PO once each day

SIDE EFFECTS: nausea, jaundice, and diarrhea; skin rash can indicate severe allergic reaction and can be fatal; changes in body fat

AUXILIARY LABELS:

- May cause drowsiness.
- Take with food.
- Do not open capsules.

Tech Note!

Did you know that there are even smaller virus-type particles called viroids? They have only a single strand of RNA. Fortunately, they do not affect human beings but have been found in plant species. They are responsible for the destruction of many plants and important food crops.

COLDS/FLU

Colds occur occasionally and without much concern. Because colds are caused by large groups of viruses, there is no cure for the common cold. Viruses mutate very well; therefore they change each year. Some herbal and dietary products claim to decrease the chance or severity of colds; however, these claims have not been evaluated or approved by the FDA and have generally not provided substantial benefit per research trials. The good news is that although a cold is inconvenient, in a healthy person it is not deadly. As discussed in Chapter 18, colds generally affect the upper respiratory system.

Influenza is another type of virus that affects millions of persons each year. Influenza generally affects the lower respiratory system, and this condition, unlike the common cold, causes serious illness or death in many older adults and immunocompromised persons every year. For this reason, vaccines, which contain weakened or dead versions of the virus strains that are most likely to cause influenza that year, are given annually (in late fall or early winter in the United States), especially to persons who are at higher risk or between the ages of 18 and 56 years old. These include older adults, children, pregnant women, health care workers, and immunocompromised persons such as elderly persons and those living in nursing homes, those receiving chemotherapy, and those with HIV or AIDS.

While influenza vaccines do help to reduce the effects and spread of seasonal flu there are times when population vaccination is not enough and influenza outbreaks and pandemics occur. This can happen if the virus does not mutate in a way that follows the strains of the vaccine, if major outbreaks occur before the vaccine becomes available, or if a new strain of influenza virus mutates to become pathogenic in humans. When this happens, resources can be strained and death counts can rise. Fortunately, pharmaceutical companies have researched influenza virus enough to produce antivirals that, if taken in the first 48 hours after flu symptoms appear, can greatly reduce the severity and duration of the illness. It should be noted that influenza virus infection can be severe in susceptible patients, causing pneumonia and occasionally death. Prevention with immunization and good hygiene habits is essential in limiting the impact of the illness.

MISCELLANEOUS VIRAL CONDITIONS

Human Papillomavirus (HPV)

The human papillomaviruses are a group of viruses that cause the common wart and genital warts; different strains are responsible for the different presentations of the disease. Contraction of genital HPV also increases the person's susceptibility to certain cancers, such as cervical cancer. Most common warts disappear without treatment within 6 months. Many agents are available OTC, such as Wart-Off, to treat persistent warts (see Chapter 20 for additional information about OTC drugs in regard to wart treatment).

Herpes Viruses

The three main types of herpes are herpes type 1 (HSV-1 or oral herpes), herpes type 2 (HSV-2 or genital herpes) and herpes zoster (shingles). Their activities within the human body vary, as outlined in Box 25-5.

Herpes type 1 is transmitted through oral secretions causing blisters on the surface of the skin. This virus also can cause blindness if left untreated. Herpes type 2 infections are caused by sexual contact. If a mother has an active case of herpes type 2 when the baby is being born, the neonate can

BOX 25-5 TYPES OF HUMAN HERPES VIRUSES

Herpes Simplex
Type 1: Causes disease of the mouth, face, skin, esophagus, or brain
Type 2: Causes disease of the rectum, genitals, and meninges

Herpes Zoster (Shingles)
Lesions on the skin surface appear on torso, arms, and legs; reactivation of latent varicella infection; vaccine is available for prevention of disease

Varicella Zoster Chickenpox
Childhood disease: the body normally will produce immunity against reinfection; vaccine is available for childhood disease prevention

acquire the virus. Outbreaks can be brought on by the following conditions; note that transference of both types of herpes is possible even when sores are not present.

Fatigue

Physical or emotional stress

Immunosuppression due to AIDS, chemotherapy, or steroids

General illnesses

Trauma to the affected area (includes sexual activity)

Menstruation

The infection chickenpox is caused by the virus herpes zoster. After the infection subsides the virus lies dormant in the nerve roots, often forever. But a weakened immune system can activate the virus which travels along the nerve fiber to the surface of the skin. Persons over the age of 60 years of age are at most risk. Lesions on the skin surface, referred to as shingles, form blisters that eventually ooze the fluid out and heal, usually taking anywhere from 3 to 4 weeks. Shingles is contagious while the sores are open; anyone coming into contact would develop chickenpox; then they will be at risk of a shingles later in life. Because shingles affects the nerve endings, this results in severe pain. Note; when/if the virus becomes active again it can only cause shingles, not chickenpox. For more information and a slide show on shingles go to: http://www.webmd.com/skin-problems-and-treatments/shingles/slideshow-shingles-pictures

Tech Alert!

Remember the following sound-alike/look-alike drugs:

amoxicillin versus
    amoxapine
Diflucan versus Diprivan
cefixime versus cefepime
Rifampin versus rifabutin
Trimox versus Diamox

DO YOU REMEMBER THESE KEY POINTS?

- The generations of penicillins and cephalosporins
- The drug actions of the agents discussed in this chapter
- The types of bacteria that are considered "good" and where they reside
- The procedure used to perform the Gram stain and what it indicates
- The causes of tuberculosis and its treatment
- The names of some of the most common fungal infections
- The way in which viruses proliferate
- The three mechanisms of destroying or stopping viruses

REVIEW QUESTIONS

Multiple choice questions

1. Penicillin agents are most effective against which type of microbes?
   A. Gram positive
   B. Gram negative
   C. Gram positive and fungi
   D. Gram positive and viruses

2. The difference in the "generations" of penicillin and cephalosporin agents is that:
   A. Generations determine the spectrum of gram-negative and gram-positive microbes against which they work
   B. Generations determine the types of microbes against which they work
   C. Generations determine the length and course of treatment
   D. Generations are determined by when they were discovered

3. The following diseases are classified as sexually transmitted diseases EXCEPT:
   A. Chlamydia
   B. Syphilis
   C. Trichomoniasis
   D. Trichinosis

4. The following conditions are *always* caused by viruses except:
A. Colds
B. Warts
C. Acquired immunodeficiency syndrome
D. Pneumonia

5. A person with an allergy to penicillin who has a urinary tract infection most likely would be treated with which of the following agents?
A. Amoxicillin
B. Ampicillin
C. Cephalosporin
D. Aminoglycoside

6. All of the following agents are third-generation cephalosporins EXCEPT:
A. Vantin
B. Cefixime
C. Ceftizoxime
D. Cefprozil

7. Corneal abrasions and progressive skin lesions are symptoms of:
A. Sexually transmitted diseases
B. Tuberculosis
C. Human immunodeficiency virus
D. Hansen's disease

8. The most common treatment for tuberculosis is the combination regimen of:
A. Penicillin G and gentamicin
B. Isoniazid, rifampin, and ethambutol
C. Kanamycin, cycloserine, and isoniazid
D. Amikacin, kanamycin, and rifampin

9. Fungus grows best in or on:
A. Shower floors
B. Very dry environments
C. Clothes
D. Cooked food

10. Antiparasitic agents work by all of the methods listed EXCEPT:
A. Killing the parasite
B. Killing the host
C. Ridding the body of the live parasite
D. Paralyzing the parasite and then flushing it out of the body

11. One way to avoid a parasitic infestation is to:
A. Cook all meat thoroughly
B. Do not drink from rivers or streams
C. Wash your hands before eating
D. All of the above

12. The following anthelmintic agents are vermicidal EXCEPT:
A. Thiabendazole
B. Oxamniquine
C. Praziquantel
D. Mebendazole

13. Malaria is a disease that is caused by:
A. Mosquitoes
B. Blood transfusions
C. Tropical climates
D. Sporozoan species

14. The actions of antiviral agents include all of the following EXCEPT:
A. They can interrupt the attachment of the virion to the host cell
B. They can affect the replication phase of the virion within the host cell
C. They can affect the assembly of the viral parts within the host cell
D. They can lyse the viral particles before they reach the host cell

15. Influenza is most dangerous to all of the following groups of persons EXCEPT:
A. Babies
B. Older adults
C. Immunosuppressed
D. Adults ages 18 to 25 years

16. The type of herpes that is related closely to chickenpox is:
A. Herpes type 1
B. Herpes type 2
C. Herpes simplex
D. Herpes zoster

17. Rabies is most often caused by:
A. Raccoons and skunks
B. Bats and foxes
C. Dogs and cats
D. Both A and B

18. Which of the medications listed below are NOT antiretrovirals?
A. Didanosine
B. Famciclovir
C. Zidovudine
D. Both B and C

19. The CDC has determined that a person has AIDS if:
A. The person has been previously diagnosed with HIV
B. The CD4 T-cell count is less than 200 per microliter of blood.
C. The B-cell count is less than 200 per microliter of blood
D. Both B and C

20. A patient diagnosed with *H. pylori* infection might be treated with:
A. Septra
B. Flagyl
C. Tetracycline
D. All of the above

True/False

If the statement is false, then change it to make it true.

_____ **1.** All microbes cause disease.

_____ **2.** Bacteriostatic agents kill microbes, whereas bactericidal agents only stop the growth.

_____ **3.** Anaerobic organisms need oxygen to survive, whereas aerobic organisms do not.

_____ **4.** A nosocomial infection is an infection within the nose, such as a cold.

_____ **5.** Tinea pedis is a viral infection affecting the feet.

_____ **6.** Terbinafine normally is used to treat fungal infections such as onychomycosis.

_____ **7.** The most common form of fungus found as part of the normal flora is the species *Candida albicans*.

_____ **8.** All parasites cause problems for the host because they benefit at the expense of the host.

_____ **9.** The sexually transmitted disease *Trichomonas vaginalis* is a parasitic infection.

_____ **10.** AIDS causes similar conditions such as HIV.

_____ **11.** Not all herpes viruses are contagious.

_____ **12.** Chickenpox is a childhood disease that will result in passive immunity.

_____ **13.** Passive immunity occurs when a mother passes immunity onto her unborn child.

_____ **14.** Colds can be caused by bacterial infections.

_____ **15.** *Streptococcus pneumoniae, Staphylococcus aureus, Salmonella,* and *Escherichia coli* are all resistant strains of viruses.

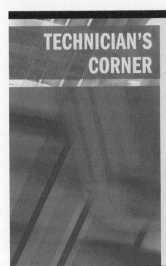

TECHNICIAN'S CORNER

Use a reference book to determine the following information about the listed antiinfective agents:

Use
- Necessary auxiliary label
- Dosage forms
- Routes of administration

Agents
- Zidovudine
- Ethambutol
- Miconazole
- Ticarcillin/clavulanate
- Maxipime

BIBLIOGRAPHY

Center for Disease Control and Prevention: Retrieved January 30, 2002, from www.cdc.gov/travel/., Travelers Health. National Center for Infectious Diseases, Division of Global Migration and Quarantine. 10-24-2006.

CDC/MMWR, July 5, 2002 / 51(26);565-567; www.cdc.gov/mmwr/preview/mmwrhtml/mm5126a1.htm.

CDC Emerging Infectious diseases. EID Journal Home > Volume 15, Number 5–May 2009)www.cdc.gov/eid/content/15/5/838.htm

Drug facts and comparisons, ed 63, St Louis, 2008, Lippincott Williams & Wilkins.

Hardman J, Lee L: *The pharmaceutical basis of therapeutics,* ed 11, New York, 2005, McGraw-Hill.

McKenry L, Evelyn S: *Mosby's pharmacology in nursing,* ed 21, St Louis, 2001, Mosby.

Skidmore-Roth L: *Mosby's drug guide for nurses,* ed 8, St Louis, 2008, Mosby.

Thibodeau G, Kevin P: *Structure and function of the body,* ed 13, St Louis, 2007, Mosby.

Walsh T, Fischbach M: New ways to squash superbugs, Scientific American. July 2009 page 44.

Wilson B, Margaret S, Kelly S: *Prentice Hall nurse's drug guide 2009,* Upper Saddle River, 2008, Prentice Hall.

WEBSITES

www.biomedcentral.com/1471-2334/7/56

http://emedicine.medscape.com/article/999282-overview

http://microbewiki.kenyon.edu/index.php/Microbe

www.medifix.org/safec/index.html

www.nursingceu.com/courses/236/index_nceu.html

www.cdc.gov/ncidod/dhqp/ar_multidrugfaq.html

26

Antiinflammatories and Antihistamines

Objectives

UPON COMPLETING THIS CHAPTER, YOU SHOULD BE ABLE TO DO THE FOLLOWING:

- List both trade and generic names covered in this chapter.
- Describe the symptoms of inflammation.
- Differentiate between steroidal and nonsteroidal antiinflammatories.
- List the major side effects of the agents discussed.
- List the major cells that are activated from the immune system to repair damaged cells.
- List the common inflammatory conditions covered.
- List the drug action of pain receptors.
- List the major medications used in the treatment of arthritis, rheumatoid arthritis, osteoarthritis, and other major conditions.

TERMS AND DEFINITIONS

Analgesic *A drug that relieves pain by reducing the perception of pain*

Anaphylactic shock *A severe allergic reaction that causes a rapid decrease in blood pressure, ventricular tachycardia, and constriction of the airways; a medical emergency that will cause death if not treated immediately*

Antigen *The marker on cell surfaces that identifies the cell as a "self-cell"; it stimulates the production of antibodies*

Antipyretic *Medication that reduces fever*

Bradykinins *Chemicals produced by the body and responsible for inflammation and pain*

Corticosteroid *A steroid produced by the adrenal cortex*

Debride *To remove dead or damaged tissue*

Histamine$_1$ *A substance that interacts with tissues, producing some of the symptoms of an allergic reaction*

NSAIDs *Nonsteroidal antiinflammatory drugs*

Osteoarthritis *Also known as degenerative joint disease*

OTC (over-the-counter) *Medications that can be purchased without a prescription; non–legend medications*

Rheumatoid arthritis *A progressive degenerative and crippling immune disease*

Rhinitis *Inflammation of the lining of the nose; runny nose*

Steroid *Messenger chemical produced by the body that helps fight inflammation and pain*

Systemic *Pertaining to the entire body rather than to individual body parts*

Urticaria *Also known as hives; red welts that arise on the surface of the skin often attributable to an allergic reaction, but may have nonallergic causes*

Vasodilation *Widening of the blood vessels that allows for increased blood flow*

COMMON ANTIINFLAMMATORY AGENTS

Trade Name	Generic Name	Pronunciation	Trade Name	Generic Name	Pronunciation
Salicylates/Nonsteroidal Antiinflammatory Drugs			Orudis, Oruvail	ketoprofen	(**key**-toe-**proe**-fin)
Arthropan	choline salicylate	(**koe**-leen sall-ih-**sa**-late)	Relafen	nabumetone	(nab-**ue**-me-tone)
Bayer	aspirin	(**ass**-pur-in)	Tolectin	tolmetin	(**tole**-met-in)
Trilisate	choline magnesium trisalicylate	(**koe**-leen mag-**knee**-see-um try-sa-**li**-si-late)	Toradol	ketorolac	(**key**-toh-**role**-ak)
			Cyclooxygenase-2 Inhibitors (COX-2 Inhibitors)		
			Celebrex	celecoxib	(**sel**-e-**kox**-ib)
Nonsteroidal Antiinflammatory Drugs			**Analgesic Medications**		
Aleve, Naprosyn, Anaprox	naproxen sodium	(nah-**prox**-sin **sow**-dee-um)	Percocet	oxycodone/ acetaminophen	(**ox**-e-koe-done/ a-**seet**-ah-**min**-oh-fen)
Ansaid	flurbiprofen	(**flur**-bi-**pro**-fin)	Percodan	oxycodone/ aspirin	(**ox**-e-koe-done/ **ass**-pur-in)
Clinoril	sulindac	(suh-lin-**dack**)	Tylenol	acetaminophen	(a-**seet**-ah-**min**-oh-fen)
Daypro	oxaprozin	(**ox**-ah-**pro**-sin)	Tylenol w/ Codeine	acetaminophen/ codeine	(a-**seet**-ah-**min**-oh-phen/ **koe**-deen)
Feldene	piroxicam	(pir-**ox**-i-kam)	Vicodin, Lortab	hydrocodone/ acetaminophen	(hye-droe-**koe**-done/ a-**seet**-ah-**min**-oh-phen)
Indocin	indomethacin	(in-doe-**meth**-ah-sin)			
Lodine	etodolac	(ee-toe-**doe**-lak)			
Meclomen	meclofenamate	(mea-**kloe**-fen-ah-**mate**)			
Mobic	meloxicam	(me-**lox**-i-cam)			
Motrin	ibuprofen	(**eye**-bue-**proe**-fen)			
Nalfon	fenoprofen	(**fen**-oh-**proe**-fen)			

Continued

COMMON ANTIINFLAMMATORY AGENTS—cont'd

Trade Name	Generic Name	Pronunciation	Trade Name	Generic Name	Pronunciation
Antihistamine Drugs (Sedating) OTC			**Antihistamine Drugs Rx**		
Benadryl	diphenhydramine	(dye-fen-**hye**-dra-meen)	Atarax	hydroxyzine HCl	(high-**drox**-eh-zeen)
Chlor-Trimeton	chlorpheniramine	(klor-fen-**ihr**-ah-meen)	Vistaril	hydroxyzine	(high-**drox**-seh-zeen
Dimetane	brompheniramine	(brom-feh-**neer**-a-meen)		pamoate	**pam**-oh-ate)
Tavist	clemastine	(**klem**-aas-teen)			
			Antihistamine Drug (Non-Sedating) Rx		
Antihistamine Drug (Non-Sedating) OTC			Allegra	fexofenadine	(**fex**-oh-**fen**-ah-deen)
Claritin	loratadine	(lor-**a**-tah-dean)			
Antihistamine Drugs (Low-Sedating) OTC					
Zyrtec	cetirizine	(sea-**tir**-a-zeen)			

UNLIKE MANY OTHER CONDITIONS, inflammation can be treated with several over-the-counter medications. With the exception of the common cold, muscle pain resulting from inflammation is one of the leading causes for self-medication. Most pharmacies sell more **over-the-counter (OTC)** nonsteroidal antiinflammatory drugs **(NSAIDs)** and **analgesics** (pain medications) than any other type of agent. This is partially attributable to today's fast-paced lifestyle as well as the accessibility of OTC drugs. Although many OTC drugs are considered safe and effective, they can cause adverse side effects if taken inappropriately, especially when the patient may be taking other medications concurrently or has a preexisting condition. In addition, many legend (prescription) drugs can alleviate pain; however, these too can have serious side effects if not taken correctly.

In this chapter we explore the conditions with which inflammation is associated and the use of steroidal and nonsteroidal medications to treat inflammation. We discuss causes of allergies and asthma, as well as agents used to treat them. An overview is given of the types of associated symptoms of inflammation, such as pain, and the most common agents used to treat them.

The Inflammatory Response

Inflammation can be caused by infection, allergic reactions, or injury. Inflammation is a necessary response if the body is to heal itself.

Along with the obvious swelling effects of inflammation, other effects are felt rather than seen. Thousands of years ago, the Romans described the symptoms of inflammation as redness, swelling, heat, pain, and the eventual loss of function of the affected area. The body tries to repair the damage with the help of blood, cells, and natural chemicals. Some chemicals send messages to the smooth muscles, causing **vasodilation**, allowing more blood to reach the affected area. Because the blood flows rapidly through dilated vessels, the affected area is warmer. Areas surrounding the injury may not be able to adapt to the increase in blood flow, resulting in edema (buildup of fluids) within the surrounding tissues. Specialized cells are sent to the injured area, and the repair process begins. Table 26-1 lists some of the major types of cells that constitute our immune system and describes their effects on the body system.

The cells of the body contain many different chemicals that have a role in inflammation. Each chemical has a specific job to perform. One such chemical found in many cells is an enzyme called cyclooxygenase. This enzyme produces various hormones called prostaglandins, which are responsible for other chemical reactions that cause inflammation, pain, and increased temperature. Aspirin is one agent that inhibits cyclooxygenase pathways and thereby stops the production of prostaglandin.

TABLE 26-1 Immune Cell Responses in Injury

Name of Cell	Type of Cell Involved	Effects
Antibodies	Produced by B lymphocytes in response to an antigen; memory cells previously produced increase in population to fight infection; found in blood	Can neutralize or destroy antigens in different ways, such as by coating or lysing antigen; can stimulate phagocytosis and prevent antigen from adhering to host cells
Fibrinogen	Globulin found in blood plasma	Assist in blood coagulation
Granulocytes	Mature leukocyte cells that contain granules, including neutrophils and other types of immune response cells	Fight infection
Leukocytes	White blood cells formed in bone marrow, including granulocytes and nongranulocytes	Fight infection and tissue damage; destroy foreign organisms and also clean up damaged cells by phagocytosis
Lymphocytes	White blood cells formed in spleen and bone marrow	Adhere to endothelial cells: intensify inflammation by causing direct cell injury and promoting formation of antibodies that increase inflammatory response
Monocytes	Large type of leukocyte	Eventually become macrophages; macrophages are part of first-line defense in inflammatory process
Neutrophils	Mature white blood cells in granulocytic series; make up more than 50% of leukocytes present in body	Adhere to damaged site to protect against infection by destroying infectious microbes; also destroy antigens
Macrophages	Large cells called phagocytes that secrete cytokines	Ingest dead tissue, bacterial cells, or dying cells

Inflammation can occur only in living tissue; therefore if an area undergoes necrosis (death of the tissue), such as necrosis of the hands or feet from frostbite, there will be no apparent swelling of the tissue. Instead, as blood flow diminishes the skin turns black, and because the tissue has no blood supply, the area needs **debriding** to prevent the infection from spreading further.

The two different types of inflammation are acute and chronic. Acute inflammation only lasts a few days, and the body usually can recover without the aid of any medication. Chronic inflammation can arise from an acute case of inflammation or from an injury. Chronic inflammation can occur locally, such as at a cut on the surface of the skin, or **systemically** within areas of the body. When inflammation becomes chronic, the site of injury may swell again, and a low-grade fever can result. Table 26-2 describes types of inflammation.

Chronic inflammation can cause damage to the affected sites or internal organs. As the body heals, it leaves behind scar tissue. This scar tissue can alter the affected area's physiology. For instance, if the heart becomes scarred, its ability to pump or circulate the blood may be adversely affected. If the fallopian tubes are scarred by pelvic inflammatory disease (PID), the woman may become sterile. Inflammation also can damage the kidneys to the extent that the person needs dialysis. Along with inflammation, there can be varying degrees of pain associated with the swelling.

Although the inflammatory conditions listed must be treated with specific medications because of the underlying cause of infection or disease, antiinflammatory agents may be given to reduce the pain and swelling that accompanies the condition. This chapter examines commonly used antiinflammatories, including both over-the-counter (OTC) and prescription drugs. Ancillary drugs used for acute pain associated with inflammation will also be covered. The terminology used for major organs or structures that can become inflamed is presented in the following table.

TABLE 26-2 Types of Inflammatory Conditions

Condition	Common Name	Symptoms	Treatment
Allergic conjunctivitis	Pink eye	Painful, itchy, watery eyes	Mast cell stabilizers, decongestants, antihistamines, NSAIDs
Allergic gastritis	Food allergy to foods like milk, eggs, peanuts, wheat, or seafood. Common problems are celiac disease and cow milk protein allergy	Nausea, cramps, bloating, gas, diarrhea	Antihistamines, proton pump inhibitors, antiemetics
Allergic otitis	Earache	Aching ear, itching	Analgesics, antihistamines, corticosteroids
Allergic rhinitis	Hay fever	Stuffy or runny nose, sneezing, itching, watery eyes	Antihistamines, decongestants, steroidal nasal sprays, cromolyn sodium
Allergic sinusitis	An extension of hay fever into the sinus area	Headache, cough, runny nose, nasal congestion	Decongestants, analgesics, corticosteroids
Dermatitis	Skin hives or rash	Hives, itching, swollen welts, mild or moderate wheezing	Hydrocortisone topical cream or lotion, antihistamines

ANTIINFLAMMATORY AND ANTIHISTAMINE TERMINOLOGY

Medical term	Inflammation of the
Arthritis	Joints
Carditis	Heart
Colitis	Colon
Conjunctivitis	Conjunctiva
Cystitis	Bladder
Dermatitis	Skin
Encephalitis	Brain
Enteritis	Small intestine
Gastritis	Stomach
Hepatitis	Liver
Keratitis	Cornea
Mastitis	Breasts
Meningitis	Meninges
Myringitis	Eardrum
Nephritis	Kidneys
Neuritis	Nerves
Oophoritis	Ovary
Osteitis	Bone
Otitis	Ear
Pancreatitis	Pancreas
Pneumonitis	Lungs
Prostatitis	Prostate
Rhinitis	Nose
Salpingitis	Fallopian tube
Sinusitis	Sinus
Tendonitis	Tendon
Testitis	Testicle
Thymitis	Thymus
Urethritis	Urethra

The Body's Natural Response

GLUCOCORTICOIDS (STEROIDS)

The body produces different types of **steroids**. They are secreted from the endocrine glands and are chemical messengers of the body. The main gland that produces steroids is the adrenal gland. The adrenal cortex synthesizes glucocorticoids and mineralocorticoids; both are referred to as **corticosteroids**. Another steroid, corticotropin, which is secreted by the anterior pituitary gland, is a hormone and is a regulator of the adrenal gland. Steroids have an important role in the maintenance of the body system. The imbalance of normal steroid levels can cause various diseases. Because of the common use of high doses of systemic glucocorticoids, we focus on these agents in this chapter.

Adrenal Effects of Steroid Agents

Glucocorticoids are essential to the wellness of the body. One problem of long-term use of steroids is that the ability of the body to produce glucocorticoids on its own is decreased and eventually may stop altogether. Depending on the length of time that steroids are used, the body can take from days to a year to begin production of glucocorticoids. Steroids must be discontinued slowly (i.e., tapered) to allow the body to initiate production of glucocorticoids; usually steroid dosages are tapered over a month or more. An example of a tapered order is given in Figure 26-1.

Several routes of administration for steroids are oral, parenteral (intravenous, intramuscular, subcutaneous), topical, and inhalation. Prescriptions normally are written for the smallest effective amount of steroids and for the least amount of time necessary to treat the condition. Side effects of oral dosages include gastrointestinal upset; therefore all steroids should have the auxiliary label "take with food." Because dosages are varied based on the severity of the condition and patient's health, they are not included in the drug monographs in this chapter. The following drug monographs are examples of oral, topical, nasal, and injectable agents used to treat inflammation and pain caused by several

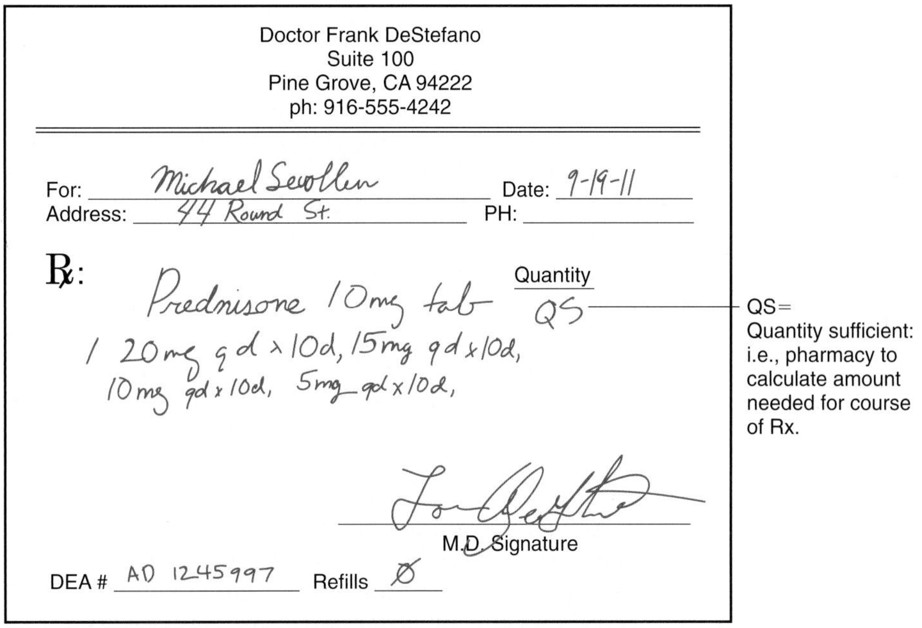

```
            Doctor Frank DeStefano
                  Suite 100
              Pine Grove, CA 94222
                ph: 916-555-4242


  For:  _Michael Sevollen_____   Date: _9-19-11__
  Address: __44 Round St._____   PH: _____

  Rx:                                Quantity
         Prednisone 10mg tab          QS            QS=
      1  20mg qd x 10d, 15mg qd x 10d,              Quantity sufficient:
         10mg qd x 10d, 5mg qd x 10d,               i.e., pharmacy to
                                                    calculate amount
                                                    needed for course
                                                    of Rx.

                          _____
                            M.D. Signature
  DEA # _AD 1245997_  Refills _Ø___
```

FIGURE 26-1 Prednisone-tapered prescription.

BOX 26-1 CORTICOSTEROID DOSAGE FORMS AND USES

Oral dosage forms
    Tablets, capsules, syrups
        Treat arthritis, lupus, inflammatory conditions including asthma and rheumatoid arthritis
Nasal/intranasal forms
    Inhalants, sprays
        Treat allergies and asthma
Topical
    Creams, ointments, roll-ons, pastes
        Treat skin conditions; pastes are used by dentists to relieve mouth and gum diseases
Injection
    Vials
        Treat tendonitis, severe musculoskeletal pain, serious rashes from poison oak/ivy

conditions and injuries. A list of dosage forms and their uses is outlined in Box 26-1.

CORTICOSTEROIDS

The glucocorticoids have two major effects on the body—physiological and pharmacological. When low doses are given, replacement mimics the natural physiological effect (e.g., replacement for treatment of adrenocortical insufficiency). When high doses are given, pharmacological effects are seen that exceed the normal physiological response. This involves the ability of these agents to decrease inflammatory conditions caused by various types of arthritis, such as rheumatoid arthritis and **osteoarthritis**. Other uses include treatment of asthma (Chapter 18) and certain types of cancer and suppression of the immune response in organ transplant recipients.

Because of their strong effects on the immune system, corticosteroids can cause many serious side effects if they are taken over long periods, are taken inappropriately, or are stopped abruptly. To understand why this can happen, we first must review the mechanism of action of high doses of steroids.

Glucocorticoid therapy has the same effects as naturally produced glucocorticoids. Glucocorticoid affects protein, fat, and glucose metabolism within the body by raising the blood glucose levels. One way in which this is accomplished is by decreasing the metabolism of proteins by converting them into glucose. The overall effect reduces muscle mass and bone density and causes thinning of the skin. Glucocorticoid therapy also causes fat redistribution by alteration of fat metabolism. This can lead to the appearance of a "moon face," a symptom of Cushing's disease.

Normally the release of glucocorticoids in the body is regulated by a negative feedback system. For example, when a physiologically stressful event occurs, the brain sends signals to the adrenal glands to release cortisol. Glucocorticoids and other chemicals, such as prostaglandins and leukotrienes, are released into the body system and reduce inflammation.

Although glucocorticoids are effective in reducing inflammation, they can have adverse effects if their secretion is prolonged. Stressful events, such as surgery or high doses or prolonged use of glucocorticoid medications, may cause a suppression of lymphocytes, which may in turn lower resistance to infections. Oral and injectable dosage forms and strengths of corticosteroid agents are listed in Table 26-3.

TABLE 26-3 Examples of Corticosteroidal Agents and Dosage Forms

Generic Name	Trade Name	Dosage Forms	Strengths	Notes
betamethasone	Celestone	Oral solution	0.6 mg/5 mL	
	Celestone Soluspan	Injection	6 mg/mL	
budesonide	Rhinocort Aqua	Intranasal	32 mcg/spray	Crohn's disease
	Entocort EC	Capsule	3 mg	
cortisone	Cortastat, Cortastat LA, Cortastat 10	Tablets		
cortisone acetate	Cortone	Tablets	25 mg	
dexamethasone	Decadron	Tablets	0.75 mg	
	Generic dexamethasone	Tablets	0.25, 0.5, 0.75, 1, 1.5, 2, 4, 6 mg	
	Generic dexamethasone	Oral solution	0.5 mg/5 mL	
	Dexamethasone Intensol	Oral solution concentrate	1 mg/mL	30-mL dropper
dexamethasone sodium phosphate	Generic	Injection	4 mg/mL, 10 mg/mL	Injection
hydrocortisone	Cortef	Tablets	5, 10, 20 mg	
	Generic hydrocortisone	Tablets	10, 20 mg	
hydrocortisone sodium succinate	A-Hydrocort	Injection	100 mg/2 mL	
	Solu-Cortef	Injection	100 mg/2 mL, 250 mg/2 mL, 500 mg/4 mL, 1000 mg/8 mL	
methylprednisolone	Medrol	Tablet	2, 4, 8, 16, 24 mg	
	Generic methylprednisolone	Tablet	4, 8, 16 mg	
methylprednisolone acetate	Depo-Medrol and generic	Injection	20 mg/mL, 40 mg/mL, 80 mg/mL	
methylprednisolone sodium succinate	Solu-Medrol and generic sodium succinate	Injection	40 mg/vial, 125 mg/vial, 500 mg/vial, 1 g/vial	Needs to be reconstituted
prednisolone	Prelone	Tablets	5 mg	
	Prelone	Syrup	15 mg/5 mL	
	Generic prednisolone	Syrup	15 mg/5 mL	
prednisolone sodium phosphate	Pediapred	Oral liquid	5 mg/5 mL	
	Generic prednisolone sodium phosphate	Oral liquid	5 mg/5 mL, 15 mg/5 mL	
prednisolone sodium phosphate	Orapred	Oral liquid	15 mg/5 mL	
prednisolone sodium phosphate	Orapred ODT	Disintegrating tablets	10, 15, 30 mg	
prednisone	Generic prednisone	Tablets	1, 2.5, 5, 10, 20, 50 mg	
triamcinolone acetonide	TAC 3	Injection solution	3 mg/mL	
	Kenalog-10	Injection suspension	10 mg/mL	
	Kenalog-40	Injection suspension	40 mg/mL	

Continued

TABLE 26-3 **Examples of Corticosteroidal Agents and Dosage Forms—cont'd**

Generic Name	Trade Name	Dosage Forms	Strengths	Notes
	Generic triamcinolone acetonide	Injection suspension	10 mg/mL, 40 mg/mL	
	Nasacort AQ	Intranasal	55 mcg/spray	
triamcinolone hexacetonide	Aristospan Intralesional	Injection suspension	5 mg/mL	
	Aristospan Intra-articular	Injection suspension	20 mg/mL	
fludrocortisone acetate	Florinef	Tablets	0.1 mg	
	Generic fludrocortisone	Tablets	0.1 mg	

CORTICOSTEROIDS

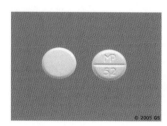

GENERIC NAME: prednisone

TRADE NAME: Deltasone

INDICATIONS: for the treatment of a wide variety of diseases such as adrenocortical insufficiency and respiratory, gastrointestinal, and neoplastic diseases; also used for allergic, inflammatory, and autoimmune conditions, arthritis, colitis, asthma, bronchitis

DOSAGE FORMS: tablets, solution, syrup

COMMON ADULT DOSAGE: oral: 5 to 60 mg once daily

SIDE EFFECTS: H/A, weight gain, stomach pain, increased blood pressure, easy bruising, insomnia, mood swings

AUXILIARY LABELS:

- Take as directed.
- Avoid alcohol.
- Take with food.

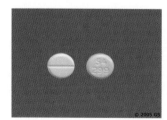

GENERIC NAME: dexamethasone

TRADE NAME: Decadron, Baycadron, DexPak

INDICATIONS: for the treatment of a wide variety of diseases such as arthritis, Crohn's disease, asthma, allergic rhinitis, bronchitis, severe psoriasis

DOSAGE FORMS: tablets, solution, syrup, injection, tablet dose pack (tapered dose)

COMMON ADULT DOSAGE: oral: 0.5 to 9 mg once daily (given in divided doses)

SIDE EFFECTS: dizziness, nausea, indigestion, weight gain, insomnia

AUXILIARY LABELS:

- Take as directed.
- May take with food.

GENERIC NAME: hydrocortisone
TRADE NAME: Cortef
INDICATIONS: types of arthritis (psoriatic, RA, gouty), endocrine disorders, dermatological diseases
DOSAGE FORMS: oral forms: tablet, solution, syrup, suspension, injection
COMMON ADULT DOSAGE: oral: 20 to 240 mg once daily depending on disease being treated
SIDE EFFECTS: depression, insomnia, mood changes, slow wound healing, H/A, dizziness, nausea
AUXILIARY LABELS:
■ Take as directed.
■ Avoid alcohol.
■ May cause dizziness.
■ Take with food.

GENERIC NAME: prednisolone
TRADE NAMES: Prednoral, Prelone, Orapred, Pediapred
INDICATIONS: antiinflammatory conditions: RA, lupus, acute gouty arthritis, ulcerative colitis, Crohn's disease; severe allergic reactions: bronchial asthma, allergic rhinitis, drug-induced dermatitis; also prescribed for severe psoriasis and chronic conditions of the eye
DOSAGE FORMS: solution, syrup, orally dissolving tablets (ODTs), ophthalmic drops
COMMON ADULT DOSAGE: oral: 5 to 60 mg (depending on disease) in divided doses per day
SIDE EFFECTS: H/A, weight gain, increased blood pressure, easy bruising, insomnia, mood swings
AUXILIARY LABELS:
■ Take as directed.
■ Avoid alcohol.
■ Take with food.
■ Do not refrigerate.

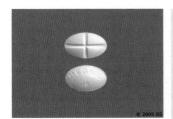

GENERIC NAME: methylprednisolone acetate
TRADE NAMES: Medrol, Medrol Dosepak
INDICATIONS: antiinflammatory or immunosuppressive agents used to treat a variety of diseases; also used after bone marrow transplants, arthritis, lupus, Crohn's disease, ulcerative colitis
DOSAGE FORMS: oral: tablet, tablet dose pack (tapered dose), injection
COMMON ADULT DOSAGE: oral: 4 to 48 mg per day as determined by physician
SIDE EFFECTS: H/A, weight gain, increased blood pressure, easy bruising, insomnia, mood swings
AUXILIARY LABELS:
■ Take as directed.
■ Avoid alcohol.
■ Take with food.
■ Do not refrigerate.

INFLAMMATORY PAIN

Inflammation and pain are closely associated because of the various hormones that the body secretes when damaged. These hormonal chemicals are temporary and as pain receptors continue to be activated, analgesics may be necessary to dull the pain (Figure 26-2).

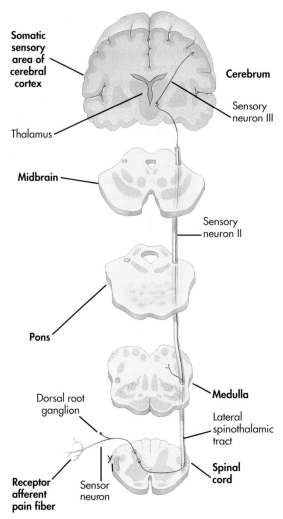

FIGURE 26-2 Pain route. (From Potter PA, Perry AG: *Fundamentals of nursing,* ed 7, St Louis, 2009, Mosby.)

Tech Note!

Acetaminophen (Tylenol) is not an antiinflammatory agent. Although it does affect cyclooxygenase enzymes in an inhibitory way by relieving pain and fever, it does not alleviate inflammation.

Each person has a specific and distinct perception of pain, which cannot be measured by scientific methods. Most pain lasts only a short time. This is referred to as acute pain; however, if the pain is persistent (lasts for 3 months or longer), it is called chronic pain.

When consulting a health care provider, a patient may be asked to rate the severity of pain using a numerical scale from 1 to 10. The number 1 indicates very little pain, and 10 indicates severe pain. From this indicator the physician can make a determination of what, if any, **analgesics** (pain medication) should be prescribed. Most muscle or tendon sprains result in acute pain and last only a few weeks. Several types of medications, mostly combination drugs, can be prescribed to treat pain, inflammation, and even fever that may be associated with injury or chronic pain that affects joints and other areas of the body.

Analgesics can be controlled or non–controlled substances; for controlled agents, various classifications (e.g., C-II, C-III) may be prescribed.

There are two tracks on which pain can be distributed. The fast track, which courses along the spinal cord to the brain, is used by acute pain. Chronic pain moves along the slow track, which results in dull, aching, burning, and cramping pain.

Pain and Inflammation Medications

ASPIRIN

In England in the early 1800s, it was reported that the bark from the willow tree was effective as a pain, fever, and inflammation reducer. Many cultures had known this for centuries, but it was not until the early 1800s that the medical community began to isolate the active ingredients. A French chemist by the name of Henri Leroux determined that a bitter glycoside was responsible for the medicinal properties of the bark. This chemical was referred to as salicin. Salicin can be broken down into two compounds—glucose (sugar) and salicylic alcohol. Salicylic alcohol ultimately can be broken down into acetylsalicylic acid—the active ingredient of aspirin.

Scientists were aware of the effects of salicin and wanted to know exactly how it produced these effects. With regard to salicin's ability to decrease pain, it was determined that salicin inhibits prostaglandins. Prostaglandins, produced naturally by the body, are a group of hormonal chemicals that are responsible for pain, inflammation, and the elevated temperature associated with injury. Although salicin helps decrease inflammation, pain, and the heat associated with injury, it will not lower body temperature caused from normal activities, such as exercising.

As this new information became available, salicin was considered a miracle drug and was used to treat illnesses such as gout, to decrease inflammation from injury, to alleviate pain, and to reduce high fever, which could cause death. The first company to market this miracle agent was the Bayer Company in 1899. They called their new wonder drug aspirin. Since then there have been many new drugs introduced into the marketplace that work similarly; aspirin is still a popular drug because it is effective and inexpensive.

Although aspirin has proven to be an effective agent to treat fever, pain, and inflammation, it should generally not be given to children, especially those with flulike symptoms. This is because taking aspirin is a risk factor for Reye's syndrome. Reye's syndrome, which may occur following chickenpox or an upper respiratory tract viral infection, is a childhood disease that causes vomiting, lethargy, and encephalopathy, which can lead to coma and death. For children suffering from chickenpox or flulike symptoms, acetaminophen (Tylenol) can be given without fear of Reye's syndrome.

Aspirin has a maximum dosing range for adults that should not exceed 4 g per day (Table 26-4). A common side effect is upset stomach. Therefore the

TABLE 26-4 Various Strengths of Aspirin Available

Trade Name	Strength	Dosage Form
Halfprin	165 mg	Enteric-coated* tablet
Arthritis Foundation Pain Reliever	500 mg	Tablet
Aspergum	227.5 mg	Gum tablet
Bayer Adult Low Dose	81 mg	Tablet
Ecotrin Low Strength	81 mg	Tablet
Ecotrin	325 mg	Enteric-coated tablet, caplet
Bayer Extra Strength EC	500 mg	Enteric-coated tablet, caplet
Halfprin	81 mg	Tablet
Heartline	81 mg	Tablet
Bayer Maximum Strength	500 mg	Tablet, caplet
St. Joseph Adult Chewable Aspirin	81 mg	Chewable tablet

*Enteric coated: a film coating protects the stomach from irritation.

auxiliary label "take with food" should be affixed to any aspirin prescription. Aspirin decreases platelet aggregation. Most persons taking anticoagulation agents normally should not take aspirin because it acts synergistically to the anticoagulation effects of the prescribed agent, which may result in internal bleeding; patients should obtain prescriber approval before using aspirin with the anticoagulant. Pharmacists should counsel patients any time an anticoagulant such as warfarin is prescribed. One of the most common uses of aspirin is for the prevention of strokes or heart attacks. If a clot occurs in the brain, it can cause a stroke. If the clot occurs in the blood vessels of the heart, it can cause a heart attack. If it occurs in the lungs, it can cause a pulmonary embolism. All of these conditions are life-threatening.

NONSTEROIDAL ANTIINFLAMMATORY DRUGS (NSAIDS)

Aspirin is a salicylate drug and was the prototype agent for the newer NSAIDs. Although NSAIDs have a different chemical structure than aspirin, a close similarity exists between their structure and the structures of aspirin and aspirin-like drugs. All of these agents have analgesic, **antipyretic**, and antiinflammatory properties that make them popular in the retail marketplace. Other chemicals in the body are able to help with the reduction of inflammation, such as corticosteroids. In contrast, NSAIDs suppress inflammation by inhibiting the enzyme cyclooxygenase, which is responsible for prostaglandin production. By inhibiting prostaglandin synthesis, NSAIDs not only suppress inflammation but also obstruct many of the steps involved in the inflammatory and immune responses.

More than one dozen NSAIDs are available in prescription form, and about four different types of medications are available OTC. In contrast, most aspirin is sold OTC by dozens of different manufacturers in various strengths and dosage forms and in combinations with other drugs. NSAIDs can be used for mild to moderate pain and inflammation. They have several positive effects on the body, such as the following:

- They are not addictive, unlike controlled substances.
- They decrease pain (analgesic).
- They decrease fever (antipyretic).
- They decrease inflammation (antiinflammatory).
- Some may be purchased OTC.

The mechanism of action of NSAIDs includes inhibition of cyclooxygenase, which is the enzyme responsible for the formation of prostaglandins and **bradykinins**. These substances cause pain and inflammation. NSAIDs also have an antipyretic effect by acting on the hypothalamus (the body thermostat). Wide variations have been documented among different NSAIDs, even if they are related and in the same chemical family (e.g., Arylpropionic acids class). Because each type of NSAID tends to work differently, if one brand does not work, another one might.

NSAIDs are used to treat many different types of conditions and chronic illnesses such as the following:

- Muscle pain
- Rheumatoid arthritis (RA)
- Bone pain such as in osteoarthritis
- Dysmenorrhea

Millions of persons use OTC and prescription NSAIDs to treat various inflammatory conditions. However, overuse of these agents can cause major

TABLE 26-5 Nonsteroidal Antiinflammatory Drugs, Cyclooxygenase-2 Inhibitors, and Similar Agents*

Generic Name	Trade Name	Common Adult Dosage	Note
Nonsteroidal Antiinflammatory Drugs			
etodolac	Lodine	200 to 400 mg q6-12h	Max 1.2 g/day
fenoprofen	Nalfon	200 to 600 mg q6h	Max 3.2 g/day
flurbiprofen	Ansaid	50 to 100 mg q6-12h	Max 300 mg/day
ibuprofen	Motrin†	200 to 800 mg q6-8h	Max 1.2 g/day
indomethacin	Indocin	25 to 50 mg q8-12h	Max 200 mg/day
ketoprofen	Orudis†	12.5 to 75 mg q6-8h	Max 300 mg/day
	Orudis SR	100 to 200 mg/day	Max 200 mg/day sustained release
ketorolac	Toradol	15 to 60 mg q6h (IM or IV)	Max 60 mg (IM or IV) not to exceed 5 days total
		10 mg q4-6h	Max 40 mg/day (PO) not to exceed 5 days total
meclofenamate	Meclomen	50 to 100 mg q4-6h	Max 400 mg/day
meloxicam	Mobic	7.5 to 15 mg/day	Max 15 mg/day
nabumetone	Relafen	500 mg to 1 g q12-24h	Max 2 g/day†
naproxen	Naprosyn†	275 to 500 mg q12h	Max 1.25 g/day
piroxicam	Feldene	10 to 20 mg q24h	Max 20 mg/day
sulindac	Clinoril	150 to 200 mg q12h	Max 400 mg/day
tolmetin	Tolectin	200 to 600 mg q6-8h	Max 1.8 g/day
	Tolectin DS	400 mg tid	Max 2 g/day
Cyclooxygenase-2 (COX-2) Inhibitor			
celecoxib*	Celebrex	100 to 200 mg q12-24h	Max 400 mg/day†
Salicylate Agents			
aspirin	Bayer, others†	325 mg to 1 g q4-6h	Max 4 g/day
choline magnesium trisalicylate	Trilisate	500 mg to 1 g bid to tid	Max 3 g/day

*Doses listed are prescription doses. Requires monitoring of plasma salicylate concentrations to avoid toxicity.
†Over-the-counter form available; may have various brand names.
†Higher dose used for prophylaxis of colorectal adenoma.

problems. NSAIDs can worsen stomach problems such as gastroesophageal reflux disease (GERD). They also can cause gastrointestinal ulcers or bleeding. All NSAIDs should be taken with food to prevent stomach irritation. Table 26-5 lists some of the common NSAIDs, COX-2 inhibitors, and aspirin-like agents. Lower dosages of some of these agents are available OTC (see Chapter 8). The following are two prescription NSAIDs used to relieve inflammation and associated pain.

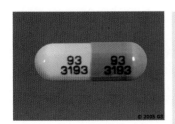

GENERIC NAME: ketoprofen
TRADE NAME: Orudis, Oruvail
ROUTE OF ADMINISTRATION: oral
INDICATIONS: mild to moderate pain, osteoarthritis, RA
DOSAGE FORMS: tablets, capsules, extended-release capsules
COMMON ADULT DOSAGE: immediate release: 50 mg four times daily or 75 mg three times daily; maximum 300 mg/day; extended-release: 100 to 200 mg once daily
AUXILIARY LABELS:
- Take with food.
- May cause dizziness or drowsiness.
- Do not crush or chew extended-release capsules.

GENERIC NAME: nabumetone
TRADE NAME: Relafen
ROUTE OF ADMINISTRATION: oral
INDICATIONS: osteoarthritis, RA, acute or chronic treatment
DOSAGE FORM: tablet
COMMON ADULT DOSAGE: 1000 mg once daily or 500 mg twice daily; maximum 2000 mg/day
AUXILIARY LABELS:

- May cause dizziness or drowsiness.
- Take with plenty of water.
- Avoid prolonged or excessive exposure to sunlight.

CYCLOOXYGENASE-2 INHIBITORS

Cyclooxygenase (COX) is an enzyme involved in the pathway that synthesizes prostaglandins and other compounds. COX is a substance found in all tissues, where it helps regulate many processes. Cyclooxygenase has two forms, COX-1 and COX-2. COX-1 is present in most tissues and assists with many normal body functions, including protecting gastric mucosa and promoting platelet aggregation. COX-2 is found mainly at sites of tissue injury, where it helps sensitize receptors to pain and mediates inflammation. COX-2 also is located within the brain, where it affects fever and pain perception. Therefore COX-1 can be considered as an enzyme involved in maintaining normal metabolic processes whereas COX-2 is associated with processes in which pain and discomfort are present.

First-generation NSAIDs inhibit COX-1 and COX-2 enzymes, which results in a decrease in inflammation, pain, and fever. Unfortunately, inhibiting COX-1 enzymes has serious side effects such as gastric erosion, ulceration, bleeding, and renal damage. However, selectivity for COX-2 has not been shown to be greatly advantageous in reducing NSAID-related side effects. Agents such as rofecoxib (Vioxx) and valdecoxib (Bextra) (both of which are COX-2 inhibitors) were withdrawn from the market because of safety concerns, including the potential for an increased risk of cardiovascular events, such as heart attack and stroke. COX-2 inhibitors are now usually reserved for patients intolerant of traditional NSAID agents. The following is a COX-2 inhibitor that is approved and still marketed for use.

COX-2 INHIBITORS

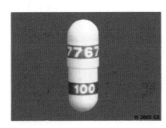

GENERIC NAME: celecoxib
TRADE NAME: Celebrex
ROUTE OF ADMINISTRATION: oral
INDICATIONS: acute or chronic pain, rheumatoid arthritis (RA), or degenerative joint disease (osteoarthritis)
DOSAGE FORMS: capsules
COMMON ADULT DOSAGE: RA: 100 to 200 mg twice daily; degenerative joint disease: 200 mg once daily or 100 mg twice daily. For familial polyposis: 400 mg twice daily
AUXILIARY LABELS:

- May cause dizziness or drowsiness.
- Take with food or milk.
- Do not crush or chew capsules.

CONTROLLED ANALGESICS

These medications, which are mostly from the opioid class, can play an important part in the reduction of pain through their mechanism of action on receptors in the brain. The effects either dull the pain or diminish the perception of pain. The following monographs list schedule II and schedule III agents. They are available in oral and intravenous dosage forms and may be combined with NSAIDs to intensify their effects. Oxycodone combinations are available in immediate and controlled-release dosages. Duragesic (fentanyl) is available in topical form as a patch.

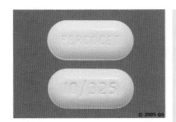

GENERIC NAME: acetaminophen and oxycodone
TRADE NAME: Percocet, Tylox, Roxicet, Endocet, Primalev, Xolox, (C-II)
ROUTE OF ADMINISTRATION: oral
INDICATION: moderate to severe pain
DOSAGE FORMS: tablets, capsules, solution
COMMON ADULT DOSAGE: tablet: 1 tablet or capsule every 6 hours as needed for pain (maximum dose 8 tablets/day)
AUXILIARY LABELS:
- May cause dizziness or drowsiness.
- Do not drink alcohol while taking this medication.
NOTE: Maximum dose of APAP is 4 g/day.

GENERIC NAME: acetaminophen and hydrocodone
TRADE NAME: Vicodin, Lortab, Norco, Maxidone, Xodol, Zydone (C-III)
ROUTE OF ADMINISTRATION: oral
INDICATION: moderate to severe pain
DOSAGE FORMS: tablets, capsules, elixir
COMMON ADULT DOSAGE: tablet: 1 to 2 PO every 4 to 6 hours as needed for pain (maximum dose 8 tablets/day)
AUXILIARY LABELS:
- May cause dizziness or drowsiness.
- Do not drink alcohol while taking this medication.
NOTE: Maximum dose of APAP is 4 g/day.

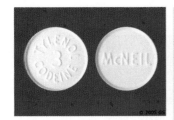

GENERIC NAME: acetaminophen and codeine (C-III)
TRADE NAME: Tylenol w/codeine #2 (300 mg of APAP/15 mg of codeine), #3 (300 mg of APAP/30 mg of codeine), and #4 (300 mg of APAP/60 mg of codeine)
ROUTE OF ADMINISTRATION: oral
INDICATION: moderate to severe pain
DOSAGE FORMS: tablet; solution, suspension, and elixir contain 120 mg of APAP/12 mg of codeine (e.g., Capital with codeine)
COMMON ADULT DOSAGE: tablets: 1 to 2 tabs PO every 4 to 6 hours as needed for pain
SIDE EFFECTS: dizziness, drowsiness, itching, constipation, H/A, N/V
AUXILIARY LABELS:
- May cause dizziness or drowsiness.
- Constipation.
- Avoid alcohol.
NOTE: Maximum dose of APAP is 4 g/day.

GENERIC NAME: hydrocodone/ibuprofen (C-III)
TRADE NAME: Vicoprofen
ROUTE OF ADMINISTRATION: oral
INDICATION: moderate to severe pain
DOSAGE FORMS: tablet
COMMON ADULT DOSAGE: tablets: 1 to 2 tabs PO every 4 to 6 hours as needed for pain.
  Max: 5 tablets/day
SIDE EFFECTS: dizziness, drowsiness, itching, constipation, H/A, N/V
AUXILIARY LABELS:
- May cause dizziness or drowsiness.
- Constipation.
- Avoid alcohol.

Inflammatory Conditions

COMMON CONDITIONS

Osteoarthritis

Osteoarthritis is also known as degenerative joint disease and is a common type of arthritis seen in persons over the age of 45 years. Although osteoarthritis is not as severe as rheumatoid arthritis, it is painful. Because of the degradation of the cartilage between the joints, an overgrowth of bone (such as bone spurs) may occur (Figure 26-3). Extreme pain can result from the wear and tear on the bone itself from constant movement. Eventually, when the bone is smooth from long-term use, the pain may decrease. Treatment of osteoarthritis consists of administration of medication, removal of the synovial membrane (synovectomy), or even replacement of the total joint (arthroplasty).

Prognosis. Although there is no known cure for osteoarthritis, there are many treatments and proactive ways to slow the progression of this disease.

Non–Drug Treatment. Exercise is important because it strengthens the tendons around the joints; an exercise regimen may be performed in conjunction with a physical therapist or the patient can increase his or her overall level of activity. Other actions that have been determined to reduce the adverse effects of osteoarthritis on the body include the following: quitting smoking, eliminating soft drinks, reducing salt intake, limiting alcohol and caffeine intake. Losing weight will reduce the workload on the joints, and applying heat and cold compresses

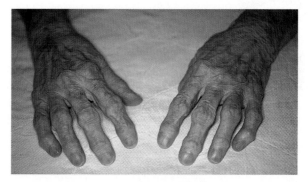

FIGURE 26-3 Severe osteoarthritis. (From Swartz M: *Textbook of physical diagnosis: history and examination*, ed 6, Philadelphia, Saunders.)

to the site can relieve spasms and pain. Classes are offered to help the osteoarthritis patient learn methods to cope with the pain. Surgery is recommended as a last resort, and may include joint replacement, debridement of the joint area, or realigning or fusing of the affected bones to eliminate pain.

Drug Treatment. Treatments include many over-the-counter (OTC) agents and prescription medications if necessary. Acetaminophen (APAP) can be used for pain but it does not reduce inflammation. However, acetaminophen is often the first agent recommended for osteoarthritis. There are NSAIDs available OTC. For severe pain, narcotic analgesics may be prescribed. Another option is steroid injections into the aching joint, although this treatment is for short-term use only because it can damage the joint.

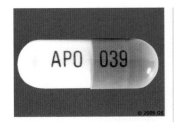

GENERIC NAME: etodolac
TRADE NAME: Lodine, Lodine XL
ROUTE OF ADMINISTRATION: oral
INDICATIONS: inflammation, pain, osteoarthritis
DOSAGE FORMS: tablet, sustained-release tablets, capsules
COMMON ADULT DOSAGE: immediate release: 200-400 mg every 6 to 8 hours; extended-release tablets: 400-1000 mg once daily
AUXILIARY LABELS:
- May cause dizziness or drowsiness.
- Take with food or milk.
- Do not crush or chew extended-release capsules.

GENERIC NAME: ibuprofen
TRADE NAME: Motrin, Advil
ROUTE OF ADMINISTRATION: oral
INDICATIONS: inflammation, pain, osteoarthritis, fever
DOSAGE FORMS: tablet, capsule, liquid-gel, oral suspension, liquid, chewable tablet, drops
COMMON ADULT DOSAGE: 200 to 400 mg every 6 to 8 hours. Max: 3200 mg/day
AUXILIARY LABELS:
- May cause dizziness or drowsiness.
- Take with food or milk.
- Do not crush or chew extended-release capsules.

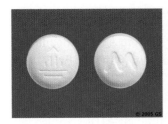

GENERIC NAME: meloxicam
TRADE NAME: Mobic
ROUTE OF ADMINISTRATION: oral
INDICATION: osteoarthritis
DOSAGE FORM: tablet
COMMON ADULT DOSAGE: 7.5 to 15 mg once daily
AUXILIARY LABELS:
- May cause dizziness or drowsiness.
- Do not drink alcohol.
- Take with water.

Rheumatoid Arthritis (RA)

Unlike osteoarthritis, **rheumatoid arthritis** not only is painful but also can be bone-deforming (Figure 26-4). More women than men are afflicted with RA. Although RA can be present in families, it is unknown whether this is a genetic

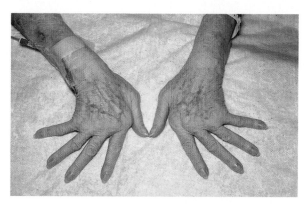

FIGURE 26-4 Severe rheumatoid arthritis. (From Swartz M: *Textbook of physical diagnosis: history and examination*, ed 6, Philadelphia, Saunders.)

condition. RA also affects young adults between the ages of 20 and 30 years and is believed to have a possible viral origin. The cause of rheumatoid arthritis lies within the immune system. As excessive amounts of synovial fluid are produced, the area swells, causing painful inflammation; and the cartilage within the joint area degrades. Bones and cartilage eventually are eroded, making movement extremely painful. If the joint freezes through calcification, it becomes impossible for the person to move the joint. This deformity of the joints is irreversible. Treatment for RA includes physical therapy, medications (antiinflammatories and/or analgesics and disease-modifying antirheumatic drugs [DMARDs]), and diet. The removal of excess synovial fluid may be an option to relieve pain and joint damage.

Prognosis. Because there is no known cure for RA the only recourse is to attempt to slow the progression of this disease and to treat the pain. The speed at which the disease progresses is different for everyone; ultimately, it will deform and cause erosion of the joints.

Non–Drug Treatment. Treatments include increasing mobility and obtaining psychological counseling if necessary. Various assistive devices to assist with daily tasks may help protect joints from erosion and limit pain in task performance. Because RA is a debilitating disease, it is important to keep a positive attitude; therefore psychiatrists or a counselor may be recommended by the physician to deal with the daily problems of RA. Physical therapists can help increase mobility by providing exercise regimens. A treatment called protein A immunoadsorption therapy filters the blood to remove antibodies and agents that cause inflammation, and may be recommended for patients who have failed standard therapies.

Drug Treatment. Medications used to treat RA include NSAIDs, analgesics (non-narcotic and narcotic), steroids, biological response modifiers (BRMs), and disease-modifying antirheumatic drugs (DMARDs). BRMs modify the immune system through inhibition of the proteins (cytokines) that cause inflammation. DMARDs are used in conjunction with other RA medications to slow the destruction of the joint. Examples of both BRMs and DMARDs are provided in the following monographs. DMARDs and BRMs are important because they help slow progression of the disease and preserve joint function. Other agents (NSAIDs and analgesics) are listed under their respective headings.

BIOLOGICAL RESPONSE MODIFIERS

GENERIC NAME: abatacept
TRADE NAME: Orencia
ROUTE OF ADMINISTRATION: intravenous infusion
INDICATIONS: RA
DOSAGE FORMS: injection
COMMON ADULT DOSAGE: IV infusion based on body weight (<60 kg, give 500 mg; 60 to 100 kg, give 750 mg; >100 kg, give 1 g); given every 2 weeks × 2 doses, then every 4 weeks thereafter
SIDE EFFECTS: H/A, nausea, dizziness, runny nose, sore throat
NOTE: IV dose to be given by nurse or physician.

GENERIC NAME: adalimumab
TRADE NAME: Humira, Humira Pen
ROUTE OF ADMINISTRATION: subcutaneous
INDICATIONS: RA, juvenile idiopathic arthritis, psoriatic arthritis
DOSAGE FORMS: injection
COMMON ADULT DOSAGE: RA: 40 mg subcutaneously every other week
SIDE EFFECTS: H/A, stuffy nose, sinus pain, nausea, stomach pain
AUXILIARY LABEL:
■ Dispose of properly.
NOTE: Dosage may be given in stomach or thigh; dose to be given by nurse or physician or patient may use Pen form at home.

GENERIC NAME: etanercept
TRADE NAME: Enbrel, Enbrel PFS (pre-filled syringe)
ROUTE OF ADMINISTRATION: subcutaneous
INDICATIONS: RA, psoriatic arthritis
DOSAGE FORMS: injection
COMMON ADULT DOSAGE: RA, 25 mg subcutaneously twice per week (3 to 4 days apart)
SIDE EFFECTS: N/V, H/A, diarrhea, stomach pain, cold symptoms
AUXILIARY LABEL:
■ Dispose of properly.
NOTE: Dose to be given by nurse or physician. PFS may be given at home.

GENERIC NAME: infliximab
TRADE NAME: Remicade
ROUTE OF ADMINISTRATION: intravenous infusion
INDICATIONS: RA, psoriatic arthritis, ulcerative colitis, Crohn's disease
DOSAGE FORMS: injectable
SIDE EFFECTS: stuffy nose, sinus pain, mild stomach pain, skin rash, H/A
COMMON ADULT DOSAGE: RA: 3 mg/kg IV infusion, followed by 3 mg/kg given at 2 and 6 weeks after first dose, and repeated every 8 weeks; dose may be increased slowly up to 10 mg/kg every 4 to 8 weeks if needed
NOTE: IV dose to be given by nurse or physician.

DISEASE-MODIFYING ANTIRHEUMATIC DRUGS

GENERIC NAME: methotrexate
TRADE NAME: Rheumatrex
ROUTE OF ADMINISTRATION: oral
INDICATIONS: lower doses: RA, psoriasis; higher doses: cancer
DOSAGE FORMS: tablet
COMMON ADULT DOSAGE: RA: 7.5 mg PO once weekly or 2.5 mg PO every 12 hours for 3 doses once weekly
SIDE EFFECTS: dizziness, fatigue, nausea, mouth ulcers, chills/fever, abdominal pain and upset
AUXILIARY LABELS:
- Do not take if pregnant.
- Avoid alcohol.

NOTE: Check prescription label carefully before giving to patient; make sure label has weekly directions, not daily, if patient has RA or psoriasis. Otherwise, patient will get an overdose.

GENERIC NAME: azathioprine
TRADE NAME: Imuran, Azasan
ROUTE OF ADMINISTRATION: oral, intravenous
INDICATIONS: RA
DOSAGE FORMS: tablet, injection
COMMON ADULT DOSAGE: RA: initial dose 1 mg/kg (50 to 100 mg) orally in 1 to 2 divided doses; maximum after titration 2.5 mg/kg/day
SIDE EFFECTS: nausea, diarrhea, loss of appetite, hair loss, skin rash, mild upset stomach
AUXILIARY LABELS:
- Take with food.
- Take with water.
- Take as directed.

Allergies

The first time the body is exposed to an antigen, it produces immunoglobulin E antibodies that attach to mast cells. These sensitized mast cells are found in tissues of the gastrointestinal tract, skin, and the respiratory tract. They attach to the mast cells throughout the body, waiting for the next exposure to the antigen. **Histamine$_1$-receptors** are located in the lower respiratory tract and skin, whereas histamine$_2$-receptors are located in the gastrointestinal tract. With the second exposure to the **antigen**, the antigen binds to the immunoglobulin E antibodies on the mast cells (Figure 26-5). This binding causes a release of the contents of the mast cells. Histamine is released and binds to histamine receptor sites in tissues, causing an allergic response that commonly includes coughing, sneezing, wheezing, and **urticaria** (i.e., hives). More severe reactions can include decreased blood pressure, migraine headache, bronchiolar constriction, increased heart rhythm, and **anaphylactic shock** (Figure 26-6). Box 26-2 lists the most common allergenic substances.

Histamine can produce a drop in blood pressure because it can dilate small blood vessels and capillaries. This dilation then can stimulate pain receptors in the head, causing severe headaches or migraines. Histamine also causes bronchoconstriction, making it difficult to breathe. In extremely severe reactions, the airways can become swollen and close; this is called anaphylactic shock. This systemic effect can result in death if not treated immediately.

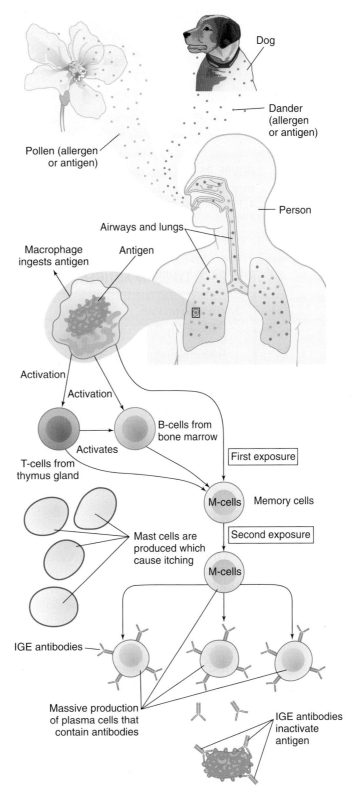

FIGURE 26-5 Asthma: airways become obstructed by mucus and edema, causing dyspnea.

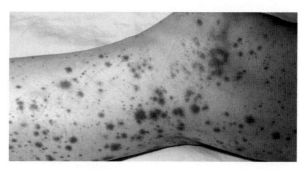

FIGURE 26-6 Events that take place in an allergic reaction, from the first exposure to an antigen to the allergic response. (From Lookingbill D, Marks J: *Prinicples of dermatology*, ed 4, Philadelphia, 2006, Saunders.)

BOX 26-2 TYPES OF ANTIGENS

Synthetic Chemicals
  Detergents, cleaners
  Drugs
  Topical agents such as soaps, lotions, and creams
Naturally Occurring Chemicals
  Heavy-molecular-weight compounds such as blood or dextran
  Pollen
  Venom from snakebites or bee stings
Miscellaneous
  Animal dander
  Dust
  Large lacerations

When an allergic reaction takes place, antihistamines decrease the release of histamines by binding the antigen to the mast cells. Allergic reactions can be blocked in two ways:

1. Mast cells are prevented from releasing histamine.
2. Histamine$_1$-receptors are blocked from interacting with histamine.

Antihistamine drugs specifically block histamine$_1$-receptors. These agents commonly are found in cold and cough medications because of their ability to dry secretions (some antihistamines work against cholinergic responses of the nervous system). These agents are classified as anticholinergics (see Chapter 16).

Histamine$_2$-receptors are located in the gastrointestinal tract—the stomach and intestines. Foods that cause an allergic reaction can result in vomiting, diarrhea, and cramps. A different class of drugs is used to treat this type of allergic reaction. The histamine$_2$-blockers, called H$_2$-antagonists, block the receptor sites within the gastrointestinal tract (see Chapter 21).

Allergic Conditions and Their Treatments

Millions of people, both young and old, suffer from seasonal allergies, as well as allergies from other common substances. Although there is no cure for allergies, there are many OTC medications available to relieve allergic symptoms. These agents can be used as a short-term remedy to treat seasonal allergies attributable to pollen, molds, and other airborne allergens. Box 26-3 lists allergic conditions.

The first-generation drugs are considered nonspecific antihistamines. They were found to bind to histamine$_1$- and histamine$_2$-receptors. Many can cause sedation because of their effect on the central nervous system if used in higher concentrations. Some of the first-generation agents also decrease nausea, vomiting, and motion sickness by their actions on the central nervous system. Second-generation antihistamines became available more recently. These agents can affect histamine$_1$-receptors specifically; thus they do not cause the same amount of sedation.

BOX 26-3 ALLERGIC CONDITIONS

Allergic Rhinitis
Inflammation of the nasal mucosa caused by molds, dust, animal dander, hay fever

Mold spores: indoor/outdoor
  Indoor: fabrics, rugs, stuffed animals, books, wallpaper, damp locations
    (e.g., bathroom, basement)
  Outdoor: soil, compost, damp vegetation
Animal dander: skin scales, cat saliva
Hay fever: trees, grasses, ragweed
Dust mites: bedding and mattresses

Symptoms of Allergic Rhinitis:
  Coughing, difficulty breathing, sneezing, wheezing
  Hives, rash
  Redness of the eyes, tearing
  Pruritus (itching)
  Excessive mucus production
  Sinus pressure

Contact Dermatitis
Inflammation of the skin caused by direct contact with an irritant/allergen

Poison ivy, poison oak
Miscellaneous plants
Cosmetics, fragrances, and perfumes
Detergents, solvents, and other chemicals
Fabric and clothing
Adhesives

Symptoms of Contact Dermatitis:
  Pruritus (itching)
  Skin redness and inflammation
  Tenderness of area exposed
  Warmth of area exposed
  Skin lesion or rash at the site of exposure

Atopic Dermatitis
Irritation of the skin leading to long-term inflammation; tends to occur in families

Exposure to environmental irritants
Exposure to water
Stress
Dry skin
Temperature

Continued

BOX 26-3 ALLERGIC CONDITIONS—cont'd

Symptoms of Atopic Dermatitis:
   Weeping blisters/lesions and crusting
   Dry, leathery skin areas
   Intense itching
   Skin redness or inflammation
   Ear discharge or bleeding

Drug Allergies
Sulfa drugs
Penicillins
Anticonvulsants
Insulin (animal sources)
Anesthetics
Iodine (x-ray contrast agents)

Symptoms of Drug Allergies:
   Hives
   Skin rash
   Itching of skin or eyes
   Wheezing
   Inflammation of the face, tongue, lips
   Anaphylaxis (severe allergic reaction; life-threatening)

Food Allergies
Eggs
Milk
Peanuts and tree nuts
Shellfish
Soy
Wheat and corn products

Symptoms of Food Allergies:
   Abdominal or stomach pain
   Inflammation of the face, lips, tongue, throat, mouth
   Itching of the mouth, throat, skin, eyes
   Difficulty swallowing
   Diarrhea
   Nausea/vomiting
   Runny nose

ANTIHISTAMINES AND COMBINATION DRUGS

Antihistamine agents are used to decrease inflammation and irritation from allergens. Allergens are also known as antigens. They are substances that are capable of stimulating an immune response. Medications that can be taken to prevent an allergic response by stabilization of the mast cell membranes include cetirizine (Zyrtec) and fexofenadine (Allegra) (Table 26-6). Many formulations combine both antihistamines with decongestants for oral, nasal, and ophthalmic use.

Antihistamines are most effective when taken before an allergic reaction because they can block histamine from interacting with histamine receptors. Depending on the type of allergies experienced there are several choices of antihistamines available OTC; stronger agents can be prescribed if necessary (Table 26-7). In addition to antihistamines, decongestants can be part of a com-

TABLE 26-6 Ophthalmics for Allergic Inflammation (Mast Cell Stabilizers)

Generic Name	Trade Name	Dosage Form	Strength
pemirolast	Alamast	Solution	0.1%
nedocromil	Alocril	Solution	2%
lodoxamide tromethamine	Alomide	Solution	0.1%
cromolyn sodium	Crolom	Solution	4%
	Generic cromolyn sodium	Solution	4%

TABLE 26-7 Examples of Oral Antihistamines

Generic Name	Trade Name	Dosage Forms	Strengths	OTC/Rx
First Generation (Nonselective)				
brompheniramine maleate	LoHist 12	Tablet: extended release	6 mg	Rx
	Lodrane 24	Tablet: extended release	12 mg	Rx
	VaZol	Liquid	2 mg/5 mL	Rx
brompheniramine tannate	BroveX	Suspension	12 mg/5 mL	Rx
chlorpheniramine	Chlor-Trimeton Allergy Relief	Tablet	4 mg	OTC
	Chlor-Trimeton Allergy 8 Hour	Tablet: extended release	8 mg	OTC
	Chlor-Trimeton Allergy 12 Hour	Tablet: extended release	12 mg	OTC
	Efidac 24	Tablet: extended release	16 mg	OTC
	Generic chlorpheniramine	Capsule: sustained release	8, 12 mg	Rx
	Aller-Chlor	Syrup	2 mg/5 mL	OTC
clemastine	Tavist Allergy	Tablet	1.34 mg	OTC
	Generic clemastine	Tablet	1.34, 2.68 mg	OTC; 2.68 mg is Rx
		Syrup	0.5 mg/5 mL	Rx
cyproheptadine	Periactin	Tablet	4 mg	Rx
		Syrup	2 mg/5 mL	Rx
dexchlorpheniramine	Generic only	ER tablet	4 mg	Rx
		Syrup	2 mg/5 mL	Rx
diphenhydramine	Children's Benadryl Allergy FastMelt	Tablet: orally disintegrating	12.5 mg	OTC
	Triaminic	Strips: orally disintegrating	12.5, 25 mg	OTC
	Banophen Allergy	Elixir	12.5 mg/5 mL	OTC
	Benadryl Children's Allergy	Liquid	12.5 mg/5 mL	OTC
	Hydramine Cough	Syrup	12.5 mg/5 mL	OTC
	Diphenhist	Capsule	25 mg	OTC
	Dytan	Suspension	25 mg/5 mL	OTC
	Benadryl Dye-Free Allergy Liqui-Gels	Capsule	25 mg	OTC
	Benadryl	Tablet: chewable	12.5 mg	OTC
Second Generation (Peripherally Selective, Low-Sedating, and Non-Sedating Agents)				
cetirizine	Zyrtec	Tablet	5, 10 mg	OTC
	Zyrtec	Tablet: chewable	5, 10 mg	OTC
	Zyrtec	Syrup	5 mg/5 mL	OTC

Continued

TABLE 26-7 **Examples of Oral Antihistamines—cont'd**

Generic Name	Trade Name	Dosage Forms	Strengths	OTC/Rx
desloratadine	Clarinex	Tablet	5 mg	Rx
	Clarinex Reditabs	Tablet: rapidly disintegrating	2.5, 5 mg	Rx
		Syrup	2.5 mg/5 mL	Rx
fexofenadine	Allegra	Tablet	30, 60, 180 mg	Rx
	Allegra	Capsule	60 mg	Rx
loratadine	Claritin	Tablet	10 mg	OTC
	Claritin Reditabs	Tablet: rapidly disintegrating	5 mg, 10 mg	OTC
	Claritin	Syrup	5 mg/5 mL	OTC

TABLE 26-8 **Oral Combination Antihistamine/Decongestant OTC Agents**

Generic Combinations	Trade Name	Dosage Forms
brompheniramine/phenylephrine	Dimetapp	Syrup, chewable tablets
chlorpheniramine/phenylephrine	Rynatan	Tablets, chewable tablets
chlorpheniramine/phenylephrine	Allerest PE	Tablets
diphenhydramine	Benadryl-D	Tablets SR, capsules SR, liquid, chewable tablets, strips
diphenhydramine/phenylephrine	Dytan-D	Suspension
fexofenadine/pseudoephedrine	Allegra-D 12hr and 24hr	Tablets ER (Rx only)
loratadine/pseudoephedrine	Alavert-D, Claritin-D	Tablets
triprolidine/phenylephrine	Actifed	Tablets

bination drug for the relief of a runny nose (Table 26-8). Other agents include OTC nasal sprays and drops (Table 26-9), and those stronger agents (steroids) that must be prescribed are listed in Table 26-10 to treat rhinitis. Ophthalmic agents to treat inflammation and itchiness (i.e., pruritus) of the eyes are listed in Table 26-11. For moderate to severe dermatitis, most topical antiinflammatory drugs are steroidal and must be prescribed because of their side effects (Table 26-12).

Nasal agents are used for seasonal allergies or chronic inflammation of the nasal mucosa (i.e., rhinitis). The oral dosage forms are not listed because those are used for asthma or prophylaxis treatment.

DRUG INTERACTIONS

The effects of drugs that suppress the central nervous system will increase if used with first-generation antihistamines. Alcohol should not be consumed if one is taking antihistamines because it can intensify drowsiness. All first-generation antihistamines should be given an auxiliary label that states, "May cause drowsiness." All OTC antihistamines have labeling that cautions consumers of the medication's ability to cause drowsiness. The only OTC nondrowsy antihistamine is Claritin, and this can cause drowsiness if not taken according to the recommended dosage. Some antibiotics such as macrolides, ketoconazole, and itraconazole can intensify the effects of second-generation antihistamines.

Antihistamines

Side effects may include dizziness, drowsiness, headache, stomach pain, dry mouth, vision changes, or loss of appetite. Drowsiness and other side effects are lessened if a non-sedating or low-sedating agent is selected.

TABLE 26-9 Nasal OTC Decongestant Agents

Generic Name	Trade Name	Dosage Form	Strength	Recommended Adult Dosage
Levmetamfetamine (L-desoxyephedrine)	Vicks Vapor Inhaler	Nasal spray	0.25%	2 inhalations into each nostril q2h (max 6 doses/24 hr)
naphazoline	Privine	Nasal spray or drops	0.05%	1-2 sprays into each nostril (max 4 doses/24 hr)
oxymetazoline	Afrin	Nasal spray	0.05%	2-3 sprays into each nostril q12h (max 2 doses/24 hr)
phenylephrine	Neo-Synephrine 4-hour (mild, regular, extra strength)	Nasal spray or drops	0.25%, 0.5%, 1%	2-3 sprays into each nostril (max 6 doses/24 hr)
sodium chloride	Salinex	Nasal drops or mist	0.4%	1-2 sprays into each nostril (max for 3 days)
sodium chloride	Simply Saline	Nasal spray	0.9% (normal saline)	1-2 sprays into each nostril prn (max for 3 days)
tetrahydrozoline	Tyzine	Nasal spray or drops	0.05%, 1%	3-4 sprays into each nostril (max 8 doses/24 hr)
xylometazoline	Natru-Vent	Nasal spray or drops	0.1%	1-3 sprays into each nostril (max 3 doses/24 hr)

TABLE 26-10 Intranasal Prescription Steroids

Generic Name	Trade Name	Strength	Recommended Adult Dose	Rhinitis from Seasonal Allergies; used for
beclomethasone	Beconase AQ	42 mcg	1-2 sprays into each nostril bid	Relief of symptoms
budesonide	Rhinocort Aqua	32 mcg	1 spray into each nostril daily	Relief of symptoms
flunisolide	Nasarel	25 mcg	2 sprays into each nostril bid	Relief of symptoms
fluticasone	Flonase	50 mcg	1-2 sprays into each nostril daily	Relief of symptoms
mometasone furoate	Nasonex	50 mcg	2 sprays into each nostril daily	Prophylaxis and relief of symptoms
triamcinolone	Nasacort AQ	55 mcg	2 sprays into each nostril daily	Relief of symptoms
ciclesonide	Omnaris	50 mcg	2 sprays into each nostril daily	Relief of symptoms
azelastine	Astelin	137 mcg	2 sprays into each nostril bid	Relief of symptoms
olopatadine	Patanase	665 mcg	2 sprays into each nostril bid	Relief of symptoms

TABLE 26-11 Ophthalmic Steroidal Prescription Agents

Generic Name	Trade Name	Dosage Form	Strength
fluorometholone	FML	Suspension	0.1%
	Generic fluorometholone	Suspension	0.1%
	FML Forte	Suspension	0.25%
	FML S.O.P.	Ointment	0.1%
prednisolone	Pred Mild	Suspension	0.12%
	Econopred Plus	Suspension	1%
	Pred Forte	Suspension	1%
dexamethasone	Generic dexamethasone	Solution	0.1%
	Maxidex	Suspension	0.1%

TABLE 26-12 Topical Steroidal Treatment

Generic Name	Trade Name	Dosage Form	Strength
betamethasone dipropionate augmented	Diprolene (all Rx)	Gel	0.05%
		Lotion	0.05%
betamethasone dipropionate	Del-beta (all Rx)	Ointment	0.05%
		Cream	0.05%
		Aerosol	0.10%
clobetasol propionate	Temovate (all Rx)	Ointment	0.05%
		Cream	0.05%
		Gel	0.05%
dexamethasone	Decaspray (Rx)	Aerosol	0.04%
fluocinolone acetonide	Synalar (all Rx)	Ointment	0.025%
		Cream	0.01%, 0.025%
		Solution	0.01%
fluocinonide	Lidex (all Rx)	Cream	0.05%
		Ointment	0.05%
		Solution	0.05%
		Gel	0.05%
fluticasone propionate	Cutivate (all Rx)	Cream	0.05%
		Ointment	0.005%
		Lotion	0.05%
hydrocortisone	Cortizone-5 (OTC)	Ointment	0.5%
	Cortizone-10 (OTC)	Ointment	1%
	Hydrocortisone (Rx)	Ointment	2.5%
	Cortizone for Kids (OTC)	Cream	0.5%
	Cortizone-10 (OTC)	Cream	1%
	Hydrocortisone (Rx)	Cream	2.5%
	Hydrocortisone (OTC)	Lotion	1%
	Hytone (Rx)	Lotion	2.5%
	Alcortin (Rx)	Gel	2%
	Texacort (Rx)	Solution	1%
	Texacort (Rx)	Solution	2.5%
	Maximum Strength Cortaid (OTC)	Pump spray	1%
	Maximum Strength Cortaid Fastick (OTC)	Stick, roll-on	1%
triamcinolone (all Rx)	Kenalog (All Rx)	Ointment	0.025%, 0.1%, 0.5%
	Kenalog	Cream	0.025%, 0.1%, 0.5%
	Kenalog	Lotion	0.025%, 0.1%
	Delta-tritex (Rx)	Ointment	0.1%
	Kenalog	Aerosol	2-sec spray

Commonly Used Antihistamines

GENERIC NAME: loratadine
TRADE NAME: Claritin, Claritin Reditab
ROUTE OF ADMINISTRATION: oral
INDICATION: seasonal rhinitis
DOSAGE FORMS: oral tablet, orally disintegrating tablet, syrup, chewable tablets (for young kids)
COMMON ADULT DOSAGE: 10 mg once daily
NOTE: No auxiliary labels needed, OTC form.

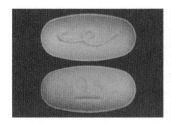

GENERIC NAME: fexofenadine
TRADE NAME: Allegra (Rx)
ROUTE OF ADMINISTRATION: oral
INDICATIONS: rhinitis and allergies
DOSAGE FORMS: oral tablet, orally disintegrating tablet, suspension
COMMON ADULT DOSAGE: 60 mg twice daily or 180 mg once daily
AUXILIARY LABELS:
- Do not take with food.
- Do not use if breast-feeding.
- Take as prescribed.
- Suspension: Shake well before each use.

GENERIC NAME: cetirizine
TRADE NAME: Zyrtec
ROUTE OF ADMINISTRATION: oral
INDICATIONS: rhinitis and allergies
DOSAGE FORMS: oral tablet, chewable tablet, syrup
COMMON ADULT DOSAGE: 10 mg once daily
NOTE: No auxiliary labels needed, OTC form.

Common Nasal Corticosteroids

GENERIC NAME: budesonide
TRADE NAME: Rhinocort Aqua
ROUTE OF ADMINISTRATION: nasal
INDICATION: seasonal and perennial allergic rhinitis
DOSAGE FORMS: nasal spray, 32 mcg per spray
COMMON ADULT DOSAGE: 1 spray into each nostril each day; up to 4 sprays/nostril per day
AUXILIARY LABELS:
- For the nose.
- Shake well before using.

GENERIC NAME: flunisolide
TRADE NAME: Nasalide
ROUTE OF ADMINISTRATION: nasal
INDICATION: rhinitis
DOSAGE FORMS: nasal spray, 25 mcg per actuation
COMMON ADULT DOSAGE: 2 sprays into each nostril twice daily in the morning and evening
AUXILIARY LABELS:
- For the nose.
- Shake well before using.

Tech Alert!

Many generic drug names are similar. Do not confuse flunisolide with fluticasone or dexamethasone with beclomethasone. Also, make sure you double-check the route of administration because these agents have several different dosage forms!

GENERIC NAME: fluticasone
TRADE NAME: Flonase
ROUTE OF ADMINISTRATION: nasal
INDICATION: seasonal and perennial allergic rhinitis in patients 12 years or older
DOSAGE FORMS: nasal spray, 50 mcg per spray
COMMON ADULT DOSAGE: 1-2 sprays into each nostril once daily; use lowest effective dose
AUXILIARY LABELS:
- For the nose.
- Shake well before using.

ANAPHYLAXIS

Anaphylaxis is the most severe case of an allergic reaction; it can be deadly if not treated immediately. For most people allergies are inconvenient but not life-threatening; for others, a reaction can cause swelling of the airways within minutes. Most people have an allergic reaction from one agent or another within their lifetime and it may occur more than once. Anaphylaxis can occur even upon first contact with an antigen. For the most severe reactions that cause swelling of the airways, epinephrine is given either by inhalation or, if necessary, by injection. Persons who know they can suffer anaphylactic shock from a bee sting or other allergic reaction should always carry an epinephrine autoinjector (e.g., EpiPen and EpiPen Jr.) in case they are stung or have an allergic exposure. There are packs of two injectors per kit in 1.5 mg (for children) and 3 mg strengths (for adults). For a video demonstration of the use of EpiPen, visit the website www.epipen.co.uk/video-demo-uk.htm.

DO YOU REMEMBER THESE KEY POINTS?

- The commonly used agents for each of the conditions discussed in this chapter
- The chemicals produced by the body that cause inflammation
- The chemicals that can be used to reduce inflammation
- The risks of taking steroids and why dosages must be tapered
- The difference between osteoarthritis and rheumatoid arthritis
- When histamine 1 versus histamine 2 agents are prescribed
- The manner in which steroid use should be discontinued
- The process responsible for the symptoms of seasonal allergies
- The names of some OTC remedies available to treat allergies
- The side effects of most agents used to treat allergies
- Why children should not take aspirin

REVIEW QUESTIONS

Multiple choice questions

1. Inflammation is caused by all of the following EXCEPT:
   A. Infection
   B. Temperature
   C. Allergic reactions
   D. Injury

2. All of the following symptoms accompany inflammation EXCEPT:
   A. Swelling
   B. Pain
   C. Redness
   D. Dizziness

3. Nonspecific antihistamines are used for all of the following symptoms EXCEPT:
   A. Sleepiness
   B. Motion sickness
   C. Allergies
   D. All of the above

4. The enzyme that is responsible for pain, inflammation, and fever is:
   A. Prostaglandin
   B. Acetylsalicylic acid
   C. Cyclooxygenase
   D. Inflammatory disease

5. Histamine$_1$-receptors are located in the:
   A. Gastrointestinal system
   B. Skin
   C. Bronchioles
   D. Both B and C

6. Aspirin should not be given to children because:
   A. It can cause Reye's syndrome in children with flulike symptoms
   B. It can cause vomiting
   C. It can cause lethargy
   D. All of the above

7. Aspirin often is given to patients who have had a TIA because:
   A. It stops inflammation and infection
   B. It lowers body temperature
   C. It decreases chances of blood clotting
   D. It speeds up the flow of blood

8. Common side effects of steroidal use include:
   A. Increased ability to bruise
   B. Increased susceptibility to infections
   C. Increased heart rate
   D. All of the above

9. Those cells that contain histamine are called:
   A. Immunoglobulin E antibodies
   B. Antihistamines
   C. Mast cells
   D. Immune cells

10. Corticosteroids are available in all dosage forms EXCEPT:
   A. Injection
   B. Inhalant
   C. Liquid
   D. Tablet
   E. All of the above

11. Dermatitis can be treated with:
   A. Corticosteroids
   B. Salicylic agents
   C. Leukotrienes
   D. Xanthenes

12. Antihistamine common side effects may include:
   A. Headache, stomach pain, and decreased blood pressure
   B. Increased blood pressure, headache, and drowsiness
   C. Drowsiness, nausea, and vomiting
   D. All of the above

13. Osteoarthritis is considered:
   A. An immune system disease
   B. A degenerative joint disease
   C. An acute allergic reaction
   D. All of the above

14. The classification of drugs used to treat gastritis would include:
   A. Proton pump inhibitors
   B. NSAIDs
   C. Antihistamines
   D. All of the above

15. Which of the drug(s) below are NOT first-generation antihistamines?
   A. Chlor-Trimeton, Tavist, Triaminic
   B. Benadryl, Optimine
   C. All of the above are first-generation antihistamines
   D. None of the above are first-generation antihistamines

True/False

If the statement is false, then change it to make it true.

_____ **1.** All antiinflammatory agents are legend drugs.

_____ **2.** Edema is a result of blood rushing to the damaged tissue or organ.

_____ **3.** Promethazine suppositories are used commonly for allergies.

_____ **4.** Acetylsalicylic acid increases inflammation.

_____ **5.** All aspirin strengths are available over-the-counter.

_____ **6.** All nonsteroidal antiinflammatory drugs work the same; therefore if one does not work, none of them will.

_____ **7.** Corticosteroids are used solely for asthma patients.

_____ **8.** Alpha-Adrenergic agents affect the bronchioles by causing dilation.

_____ **9.** Asthma is a genetically acquired condition, or only affects persons who smoke.

_____ **10.** Antihistamine agents bind to mast cells and stop all allergic reactions.

_____ **11.** Prophylactic antihistamines are used for asthmatic attacks.

_____ **12.** NSAIDs are used topically for severe dermatitis.

_____ **13.** Osteoarthritis and rheumatoid arthritis are both treated with steroids to reduce inflammation.

_____ **14.** Alcohol should not be consumed if one is taking antihistamines because it can intensify drowsiness

_____ **15.** All antihistamines can cause drowsiness.

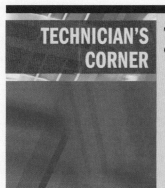

TECHNICIAN'S CORNER

Transcribe the following order into layperson terms and answer the following questions. Prednisone order as follows:

Give orally 30 mg bid × 2 days, 25 mg bid × 2 days, 20 mg bid × 2 days, 15 mg bid × 2 days, 10 mg qd × 2 days, 5 mg bid × 2 days, 5 mg qd × 2 days, stop.

How many tablets and which strength will you use to fill this order?

What auxiliary label(s) will you need to apply, if any?

The patient should be consulted by the pharmacist about which side effects?

BIBLIOGRAPHY

Clayton B, Stock Y, Harroun R: *Basic pharmacology for nurses*, ed 14, Philadelphia, 2006, Elsevier Science.

Drug facts and comparisons, ed 63, St Louis, 2008, Lippincott Williams & Wilkins.

Hardman J, Limbird L: *The pharmaceutical basis of therapeutics*, ed 11, New York, 2005, McGraw-Hill.

Koda-Kimble M, Guglielmo J: *Applied therapeutics: the clinical use of drugs*, ed 9, Philadelphia, 2008, Lippincott Williams & Wilkins.

Potter P, Perry A: *Fundamentals of nursing*, ed 6, St Louis, 2004, Mosby.

Rang H, et al: *Rang and Dale's pharmacology*, ed 6, Philadelphia, 2007, Churchill Livingstone.

Rosdahl C, Kowalski M: *Textbook of basic nursing*, ed 9, Philadelphia, 2008, Lippincott Williams & Wilkins.

Leon S, et al: *Comprehensive pharmacy review*, ed 7, Baltimore, 2009, Lippincott Williams & Wilkins.

Stedman's concise medical dictionary for health professionals, ed 3, Baltimore, 1997, Williams & Wilkins.

WEBSITES

www.mayoclinic.com/health/osteoarthritis/DS00019
http://health.discovery.com/centers/allergyasthma/allergy/guide/allergy-medicine.html
www.ra.com/
www.macalester.edu/psychology/whathap/ubnrp/audition/site/pain%20pathway.htm
www.healthprofessor.com/landers/allergies.php?
www.healthprofessor.com/landers/allergies.php
keywords=allergic+rhinitis&referrer=Yahoo&camp=HealthProfessor

27

Vitamins and Minerals

Objectives

UPON COMPLETING THIS CHAPTER, YOU SHOULD BE ABLE TO DO THE FOLLOWING:

- List the conditions that can occur from a deficiency of the vitamins covered in this chapter.

- Explain the functions of vitamins and minerals.

- Describe the differences between water-soluble and fat-soluble vitamins.

- List the recommended daily allowance of each vitamin.

- List the trace elements and explain the importance of each element.

- List the most common minerals.

- Write the chemical symbols for the most commonly used minerals.

- Describe the adverse effects of overuse of vitamins and minerals.

- List the foods that contain the common elements listed in this chapter.

Anemia *A condition marked by the presence of an abnormally low number of red blood cells*

Avitaminosis *Any disease caused by vitamin deficiency or deficiency in metabolic conversion of a vitamin*

Coenzyme *A compound that activates an enzyme*

Cofactor *A non-protein chemical compound that is bound to a protein and is required for the protein's biological activity*

Fat-soluble vitamin *A vitamin that is soluble in fat and therefore is stored in body fat; vitamins A, D, E, and K are fat-soluble vitamins*

Hemoglobin *The iron-containing pigment on red blood cells that carries oxygen to the tissues*

Hypervitaminosis *A disorder caused by the intake of too many vitamins; more common with fat-soluble vitamins*

Intrinsic factor *A naturally produced protein that is necessary for the absorption of vitamin B_{12}*

Supplement *An additive intended to compensate for a dietary deficiency, such as specific vitamins and minerals*

Trace elements *Minerals that are required by the body in very small quantities*

VITAMINS

A	Retinol, β-carotene	B_9	Folic acid
B_1	Thiamine	B_{12}	Cyanocobalamin
B_2	Riboflavin	C	Ascorbic acid
B_3	Nicotinic acid, niacin	D_2	Ergocalciferol
B_5	Pantothenic acid	D_3	Cholecalciferol
B_6	Pyridoxine	E	α-Tocopherol
B_7	Biotin	K	Phytonadione

MINERALS

Name	Chemical symbol (example of form found in drug preparations)
Major Minerals	
Calcium	Ca (calcium carbonate, calcium acetate, many others)
Chlorine	Cl (available as a mineral chloride)
Magnesium	Mg (magnesium sulfate, magnesium chloride)
Phosphorus	P (sodium phosphate, potassium phosphate)
Potassium	K (potassium chloride, salt substitute, others)
Sodium	Na (NaCl, table salt)
Sulfur	S (available as a mineral sulfate)
Trace Mineral Elements (10 Currently Known to Be Essential in Human Beings)	
Chromium	Cr
Cobalt	Co
Copper	Cu (cupric sulfate)
Fluorine	F
Iodine	I (iodized table salt)
Iron	Fe (ferrous sulfate, ferrous fumarate, ferrous gluconate, iron dextran, iron sucrose, carbonyl iron, and others)

Continued

MINERALS—cont'd

Name	Chemical symbol (example of form found in drug preparations)
Manganese	Mn
Molybdenum	Mo (not currently available as separate supplement because of its toxicity)
Selenium	Se
Zinc	Zn (zinc sulfate, zinc acetate)

LIKE HERBAL SUPPLEMENTS, MOST VITAMINS and minerals in small quantities are considered **supplements** and do not require a prescription. They are sold over-the-counter in pharmacies, in grocery markets, and in herbal stores. Because there can be adverse interactions between these agents and medications, it is recommended that persons consult with their physicians before taking any vitamin or mineral supplements. In addition, taking too many vitamins and minerals can cause toxicity in some cases.

Vitamins and minerals are termed "essential" if disorders occur when they are not present in sufficient amounts. Many vitamins are essential, such as vitamins A, B, C, D, and E. Examples of important essential minerals found in the body are calcium, chlorine, magnesium, potassium, phosphorus, and sodium. **Trace elements** are elements required for the completion of various enzymatic reactions; however, they are needed only in extremely small amounts. Examples of trace elements are cobalt, copper, iodine, selenium, manganese, and zinc.

Vitamins and minerals are necessary for proper growth and development. A healthy, well-balanced diet typically contains most vitamins and minerals. If a person consumes a well-balanced diet, then all the daily nutritional requirements normally are met.

Many fat- and water-soluble vitamins function as **coenzymes**; that is, they assist enzymes in the completion of important chemical reactions. Fat-soluble vitamins act in several ways. Vitamin D acts on the nucleus of the cell to cause a normal physiological change in the cell. Vitamin K acts as a coenzyme to produce four factors that enable the blood to clot. Vitamin A becomes incorporated in the rod cells of the eyes, enabling us to see at night. Vitamin E and other vitamins bind to free radicals that would otherwise damage cells.

The mineral elements usually are called "minerals" in the body, and are found in very large to extremely small quantities. Most minerals found in the body in large quantities form structures, such as the calcium and phosphate in bone, or compose a large portion of essential ions in body fluids, such as sodium, chloride, potassium, and calcium. When a trace mineral element combines with another molecule to enable that molecule to function in a particular manner, the element is called a **cofactor**. For example, calcium also combines with several separate clotting factors that, when activated, enable the blood to clot. Many of the trace elements are cofactors for different enzymes.

This chapter discusses the functions, interactions, conditions caused by overuse or underuse, and recommended amounts in the daily diet of vitamins, mineral elements, and trace mineral elements.

History of Regulation of Vitamin and Mineral Supplements

Before World War II, deficiencies in vitamins were common. In 1941 the Food and Drug Administration (FDA) established regulations governing the labeling of vitamins in foods; however, there were no restrictions both on the amounts that could be added and on the advertising claims that could be made by manufacturers of both vitamins and dietary supplements. It was not until 1962 that the FDA was able to revise the earlier regulation to include a recommended daily allowance (RDA). The establishment of dietary intake recommendations was important because overconsumption of both vitamins and minerals could have severe consequences on a person's health. The FDA unfortunately had no control over false claims made from manufacturing companies. In 1973 the FDA request to impose further regulations on these additives was revoked because of congressional support both of manufacturing companies and of Section 411 of the Federal Food, Drug, and Cosmetic Act. This act prohibited the FDA from establishing standards that would limit the potency of vitamins in food supplements or regulate them based on potency alone. As a result of limited regulation, the FDA did not have control over the manufacturing practices of supplements, which led to the "Tryptophan Incident" in 1989. The FDA had warned consumers not to use L-tryptophan for insomnia or premenstrual problems, but not before it was too late.

Between 1980 and 1985, a specific supplement was often being used to treat premenstrual problems, insomnia, and depression. It was sold over-the-counter (OTC) and was stocked primarily in health food stores. In late 1989 physicians started to observe certain patients with a previously unseen combination of symptoms, termed eosinophilia-myalgia syndrome (EMS). EMS caused sharp muscle pain, fever, rashes, and fatigue. With the assistance of the Centers for Disease Control and Prevention (CDC) it was determined that the symptoms were due to L-tryptophan (an amino acid). The specific L-tryptophan formulation responsible for EMS was primarily produced by a company based in Japan that supplied their product worldwide. More than 1500 cases of EMS were reported; 38 people died before the product could be recalled. After all L-tryptophan formulations were removed from the market, no new or delayed cases were reported. The FDA was able to ban L-tryptophan as an OTC agent. A different form, 5-hydroxy-L-tryptophan, is still available OTC and is now monitored by the FDA. This consumer safety incident demonstrated that the dangers of dietary supplements are very real.

Further regulation changes continue to occur with respect to dietary supplements. Under the Dietary Supplement Health and Education Act (DSHEA), Congress ruled that manufacturers of dietary supplements are limited to the types of claims they can make pertaining to their supplement. Manufacturers may not claim their product treats, cures, or prevents any disease. However, under DSHEA, it is the FDA's responsibility to prove a supplement is unsafe before the agency can take action against a manufacturer. The act limits the scope of the FDA with regard to ensuring the safety of supplements. Even so, manufacturers do need to label their product with some restrictions (Box 27-1).

The responsibility of supervising food products containing supplements now is generally divided between the U.S. Department of Agriculture (USDA) and the FDA. The USDA oversees the labeling and inspection of products such as meat, eggs, and poultry. The Department of Commerce is another government agency involved and is responsible for supervising the labeling and inspection of some seafood. The USDA and Department of Commerce grade products according to taste, texture, and appearance, not the nutritional value of the food item. The FDA developed recommended daily allowance (RDA) standards for vitamins and minerals from recommendations by the Institute of Medicine (IOM) Food and Nutrition Board of the National Academy of Sciences National Research Council. The regulatory guidelines are updated every 10 years and are used to inform consumers of the necessary nutritional requirements of average healthy persons of all ages. As of 2009 the FDA changed RDA to daily recommended intake (DRI), which provides a comprehensive listing for 26 vitamins

BOX 27-1   FOOD AND DRUG ADMINISTRATION REGULATORY REQUIREMENTS FOR DIETARY SUPPLEMENTS AND NONREGULATED ITEMS

Regulatory Requirements:

Manufacturers must notify the Food and Drug Administration (FDA) of any "new" dietary ingredient that is not already present in a food substance.

Label information must state the following:

- The agent that is a food supplement
- The name and address of the manufacturer (packer or distributor)
- A complete list of all ingredients
- The net contents of the package
- A "supplement facts" panel listing each ingredient within the package, or ingredients may be listed in the "other ingredient" area below the panel
- All products must print the following statement pertaining to the effectiveness of the agent(s):
  - "This statement has not been evaluated by the FDA. This product is not intended to diagnose, treat, cure, or prevent any disease." This is to ensure that consumers do not believe it is a medication approved by the FDA.

The Manufacturers Must Also State on All Containers:
- "Not Regulated by the FDA"
- The safety of the ingredients within the container (FDA only regulates the safety of prescription medications)
- Specific quantity of supplement in a tablet or capsule
- Disclosure of proprietary information pertaining to the supplement (such as the formulation used to make a vitamin tablet). Proprietary information would include, for example, the filler used in making a tablet or capsule and the chemical coating on a tablet, or a proprietary blend of herbs, with the ingredients, but not the specific recipe of the blend, disclosed.

and minerals according to gender and five age groups. Using the DRI and daily reference values (DRVs), manufacturers are required to list on food labels a single value, known as the Daily Value (DV). The DRVs pertain to several nutrients and food components. The following are included in these product labels:

- Fats
- Saturated fats
- Unsaturated fats
- Cholesterol
- Carbohydrates
- Fiber
- Sodium
- Potassium

The FDA considers all vitamins, minerals, herbs, amino acids, and extracts as dietary supplements. Dietary supplements, however, are regulated under DSHEA. Unfortunately, in contrast to the procedures for the approval of prescription and new over-the-counter drugs, products containing dietary supplements do not need to be reviewed by the FDA before they are marketed. It is the FDA's responsibility to prove a supplement is unsafe before the product is restricted or removed from the shelves. If an illness or accident concerning a supplement occurs, it can be reported to the FDA. An inspection of the manufacturing plant, formulation, or processing method can be assessed by the FDA if warranted. This is the only time that a dietary supplement manufacturer may be inspected and a product scrutinized, at which time the FDA can alert the consumer via the website and news programs. The information obtained by the FDA is also available online for consumers. For reporting problems, the FDA has MedWatch. This program can be accessed by a telephone hotline (1-800-FDA-1088); written complaints can be mailed or can be accessed and filed online at FDA.gov. All health care providers and consumers can report problems concerning supplements, medical foods, devices, and drugs; all information is kept confidential.

Tech Alert!

Fat-soluble vitamins (e.g., vitamins A and E) and minerals (e.g., iron) can accumulate in the body system and cause great illness and even death. This must be taken into consideration, especially when the technician prepares intravenous preparations that contain these types of additives.

Vitamins

When supplementing a diet with vitamins, one must make an important distinction between the fat-soluble and water-soluble types. Vitamin B (including all of the B complex) and vitamin C are water-soluble. Any excess B or C vitamins are usually excreted in the urine. In contrast, **fat-soluble vitamins**—vitamins A, D, E, and K—may be stored by the body in the liver and lipids of cells. These vitamins accumulate instead of being excreted. As these vitamins accumulate in a cell, they may reach such a high level that they interfere with the function of the cell. This makes fat-soluble vitamins a greater source of potential toxic effects when they are taken in excess.

FAT-SOLUBLE VITAMINS (A, D, E, AND K)

Fat-soluble vitamins are stored in the liver and body fat, which is why they do not need to be replaced on a daily basis. There is no loss of these vitamins in cooked foods. Most people do not need supplements for these vitamins if they eat a well-balanced diet. If supplementation is required, then only a small amount is necessary, because the liver will store any excess until it is needed. Sources of fat-soluble vitamins and their functions are discussed, including conditions caused by deficiencies of specific vitamins. There are interactions that can occur when taken with other agents. Table 27-1 lists fat-soluble vitamins and conditions caused by an overdose as well as their interactions. The DRI values for fat-soluble vitamins are listed in Table 27-2.

TABLE 27-1 Drug Interactions of Fat-Soluble Vitamins

Vitamin	Chemical Name	Overdose	Drug Interactions
A	Retinol, β-carotene	Nausea, vomiting, diarrhea	Mineral oil, Alli, Xenical (decreases oral absorption of vitamin)
D	Ergocalciferol (vitamin D_2), cholecalciferol (vitamin D_3)	Weakness, nausea, vomiting, headache, dry mouth, hypercalcemia	Thiazides may cause an increased risk of hypercalcemia; mineral oil, Alli, Xenical (decreases oral absorption of vitamin)
E	α-Tocopherol	Anemia	Mineral oil, Alli, Xenical (decreases oral absorption of vitamin); higher doses of vitamin E may increase bleeding risk if patient is taking anticoagulants
K	Phytonadione	Excessive bleeding	Mineral oil, Alli, Xenical (decreases oral absorption of vitamin); decreases warfarin's effectiveness

TABLE 27-2 DRI Values for Fat-Soluble Vitamins

Age Category	A (mcg)	D (mcg)	E (mg)	K (mcg)
Children				
1-3 yr	300	5	6	30
4-8 yr	400	5	7	35
Males				
9-13 yr	600	5	11	60
14-18 yr	900	5	15	75
19-30 yr	900	5	15	120
31-50 yr	900	5	15	120
51-70 yr	900	10	15	120
>70 yr	900	15	15	120
Females				
9-13 yr	600	5	11	60
14-18 yr	700	5	15	75
19-30 yr	700	5	15	90
31-50 yr	700	5	15	90
51-70 yr	700	10	15	90
>70 yr	700	15	15	90
Pregnancy				
14-18 yr	750	5	15	75
19-30 yr	770	5	15	90
31-50 yr	770	5	15	90
Lactation				
14-18 yr	1200	5	19	75
19-30 yr	1300	5	19	90
31-50 yr	1300	5	19	90

Vitamin A

Vitamin A is also called β-carotene or retinol. Vitamin A has four primary functions. First, vitamin A is an important part of the visual pigment for rods in the retina of the eye. Rods enable us to see in dim light. Because rods have no color pigment, there is no color perception in dim light. Without an adequate intake of vitamin A, individuals with a severe deficiency may suffer from keratomalacia (night blindness) and have little or no vision in dim light, which can over time result in total blindness. The second function of vitamin A is to protect against cancer in the skin and other epithelial (surface) cell types in the respiratory and digestive tracts, urinary bladder, and breast. People who are deficient in vitamin A may be more susceptible to these types of cancer. A third major function is to stimulate the immune system so that bacterial, viral, and parasitic infections are addressed efficiently and the organisms eventually are destroyed. The final, most important, function is that vitamin A acts as an antioxidant, absorbing free radicals that could be dangerous to cells. Free radicals are atoms with an odd or unpaired number of electrons. The full extent of damage that free radicals can cause is unknown, but they have been implicated in cancer, Alzheimer's disease, and aging. Vitamin A is necessary for proper bone growth, renal function, and digestive activity, and it is associated with normal reproductive function in both genders.

Sources of Vitamin A. Vitamin A sources include dairy products (e.g., whole milk, butter, cheese, and egg yolks), liver, and fish. Vitamin A is also present in yellow and green fruits and vegetables. Many dairy products, such as butter substitutes and all forms of milk, are fortified with vitamin A.

Hypervitaminosis A. Excessive ingestion of vitamin A may result in a condition known as **hypervitaminosis A.** Symptoms include headaches, vomiting, peeling of the skin, loss of appetite (i.e., anorexia), irritability, atrophy of bone mass, and, in fatal cases, destruction of the liver. Birth defects also can occur in children whose mothers ingested large amounts of vitamin A during the first 3 months of pregnancy. Simply stopping the use of too much vitamin A will elevate the symptoms.

Vitamin D

The two precursors of vitamin D are cholecalciferol and ergocalciferol. Cholecalciferol (vitamin D_3) is produced by the skin in the presence of ultraviolet light. The ultraviolet light changes modified cholesterol present in the skin (vitamin D_3). Vitamin D_2 can be synthetically manufactured by exposing ultraviolet radiation to a yeast product found in bread and milk, called ergosterol. This form of vitamin D is added to dairy products and bread. Ingested ergocalciferol or cholecalciferol absorbed through the skin is transported to the liver where the hormone calciferol is formed. Calciferol then is transported to the kidney where the final product, a hormone called calcitriol (also called vitamin D hormone), is produced.

Calcitriol increases phosphorus absorption and calcium intake. Calcitriol is also necessary for providing adequate calcium and phosphate to mother and child during pregnancy and lactation.

Sources of Vitamin D. Dairy foods such as milk, cheese, and eggs contain vitamin D in the form of ergocalciferol. Natural and artificial sunlight provide ultraviolet radiation that synthesizes vitamin D in the skin.

Deficiency of Vitamin D. A deficiency of vitamin D in children can result in bone weakness and deformities, a condition known as rickets (Figure 27-1). Vitamin

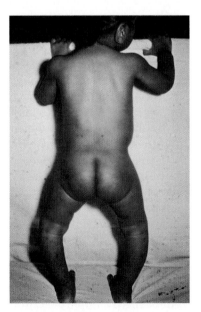

FIGURE 27-1 Rickets. (From Kumar V, Abbas AK, Fausto N: *Robbins and Cotran pathologic basis of disease,* ed 7, Philadelphia, 2005, Saunders.)

D deficiency in adults can cause a similar weakened bone structure called osteomalacia. In osteomalacia there is also a reduction in bone mass called osteoporosis. Osteoporosis also can occur in postmenopausal women and in older men if vitamin D and calcium intake is not sufficiently high.

Hypervitaminosis D. Vitamin D excess may cause hypercalcemia (higher than normal calcium blood levels). Toxic effects of vitamin D can result in calcium deposits in various areas, such as in soft tissue and joints, causing muscle weakness or pain. In severe cases, convulsions or even death can occur.

Drug Interactions. Thiazide diuretics and vitamin D can cause hypercalcemia. Mineral oil may antagonize the oral absorption of vitamin D.

Vitamin E
Vitamin E has been promoted extensively over the past decade as a potent antioxidant. Vitamin E is essential for normal metabolism and protection of the skin, eyes, tissues, and muscles. Vitamin E also seems to protect red blood cells from oxidative damage.

Sources of Vitamin E. Vitamin E can be found in whole grains such as wheat and rice germ, nuts, corn, vegetables, and dairy products (eggs and butter).

Deficiency of Vitamin E. A vitamin E deficiency may cause **anemia** and cardiovascular disease.

Hypervitaminosis E. Fully documented cases of hypervitaminosis E have not been reported in the literature.

Drug Interactions. The use of mineral oil may decrease the oral absorption of vitamin E.

Vitamin K (Phytonadione)
Vitamin K is responsible for the formation of blood coagulation factors.

Sources of Vitamin K. Vitamin K can be found in wheat, legumes, egg yolks, milk, and vegetables such as broccoli and spinach. Certain bacteria in the intestine also produce vitamin K as a by-product of their metabolism.

Deficiency of Vitamin K. Deficiency of vitamin K can cause an increased tendency to bleed. The bleeding may be manifested as repeated nosebleeds, blood in the sputum without coughing, spontaneous bruising (i.e., bruising not caused by injury) in several parts of the body, or blood in the urine. Patients with severe liver disease may be deficient in vitamin K, contributing to coagulopathy (a failure of blood to clot). In addition, excess bleeding may be a sign that the patient has taken an overdose of anticoagulation medication. For example, if a patient misses a dose or doses of warfarin (an oral anticoagulant) and takes double or triple the normal dose to compensate, excessive bleeding may occur. Alternatively, if a patient takes several doses of aspirin for a headache and is also taking warfarin, additive effects may be experienced.

WATER-SOLUBLE VITAMINS (B AND C)

The B vitamins are referred to as B complex because there are several types. All of the B complex vitamins are water-soluble. This includes B_1 (thiamine), B_2 (riboflavin), B_3 (nicotinic acid [niacin]), B_5 (pantothenic acid), B_6 (pyridoxine), B_7 (biotin), B_9 (folic acid), and B_{12} (cyanocobalamin) as well as vitamin C. These are

TABLE 27-3 DRI Values for Water-Soluble Vitamins

Age Category	C (mg)	B_1 (mg)	B_2 (mg)	B_3 (mg)	B_5 (mg)	B_6 (mg)	B_{12} (mcg)	Biotin (mcg)	Choline (mg)	Folic Acid (mcg)
Children										
1-3 yr	15	0.5	0.5	6	2	0.5	0.9	8	200	150
4-8 yr	25	0.6	0.6	8	3	0.6	12	12	250	200
Males										
9-13 yr	45	0.9	0.9	12	4	1	1.8	20	375	300
14-18 yr	75	1.2	1.3	16	5	1.3	2.4	25	550	400
19-30 yr	90	1.2	1.3	16	5	1.4	2.4	30	550	400
31-50 yr	90	1.2	1.3	16	5	1.3	2.4	30	550	400
51-70 yr	90	1.2	1.3	16	5	1.7	2.4	30	550	400
>70 yr	90	1.2	1.3	16	5	1.7	2.4	30	550	400
Females										
9-13 yr	45	0.9	0.9	12	4	1	1.8	20	375	300
14-18 yr	65	1	1	14	5	1.2	2.4	25	400	400
19-30 yr	75	1.1	1.1	14	5	1.3	2.4	30	425	400
31-50 yr	75	1.1	1.1	14	5	1.3	2.4	30	425	400
51-70 yr	75	1.1	1.1	14	5	1.5	2.4	30	425	400
>70 yr	75	1.1	1.1	14	5	1.5	2.4	30	425	400
Pregnancy	85	1.4	1.4	18	6	1.9	2.6	30	450	600
Lactation	120	1.4	1.4	17	7	2	2.8	35	550	500

TABLE 27-4 Water-Soluble Vitamins: Overdose and Drug Interactions

Vitamin	Generic/Chemical Name	Overdose	Drug Interactions
B vitamins	Thiamine	B_1: none	B_1: none
	Riboflavin	B_2: none	B_2: none
	Nicotinic acid	B_3: liver damage, heartburn, nausea, vomiting, diarrhea	B_3: inhibits effects of sulfinpyrazone; may increase risk of myopathy with statins
	Pantothenic acid		
	Pyridoxine	B_6: ataxia, neuropathy	B_5: none
	Cyanocobalamin		B_6: decreases effect of levodopa; interferes with altretamine
			B_{12}: proton pump inhibitors (PPIs) decrease B_{12} absorption over time
C	Ascorbic acid	Damage to heart and kidneys, fatigue, nausea	Warfarin (decreases effects ONLY if vitamin C taken in large doses, >5 g/day); iron (increases absorption)

not stored in the liver and body fat; rather, they are excreted through the urine, which is why they need to be replaced daily. Their levels are also reduced to some extent by the cooking process, unlike the fat-soluble vitamins. Table 27-3 lists the DRI values of water-soluble vitamins. Table 27-4 covers both interactions and overdose information.

B Vitamins

Sources of B Vitamins. B vitamins can be found in foods such as peas, beans, red meats, flour, and yeasts. Table 27-5 lists seven common B vitamins and their sources. Depending on which B vitamins are deficient, different side effects can occur. These effects are discussed in the following section.

TABLE 27-5 B Vitamins: Sources, Function, and Deficiency States

Vitamin	Chemical Name	Food Sources	Function	Deficiency
B_1	Thiamine	Grains, cereals, beans, pork, liver	Metabolism	Beriberi (wet and/or dry forms)
B_2	Riboflavin	Cereals, eggs, dark green vegetables, milk, liver	Maintains mucous membranes, metabolic energy pathways	Discolored tongue and dry scaling and fissuring of lips
B_3	Nicotinic acid	Nuts, beans, peas, wheat, rice, grains	Fat synthesis, protein metabolism, electron transport	Pellagra, diarrhea, dementia, depression, characteristic skin dermatitis
B_5	Pantothenic acid	Vegetables, cereals, yeast, liver	Coenzyme	Fatigue, headaches, nausea, skin disorders
B_6	Pyridoxine	Meat, liver, chicken, salmon, trout, beans, rice, whole grains	Amino acid and fatty acid metabolism	Dizziness, weakness, depression, nausea, impaired vision and nerve function
B_9	Folic acid	Green vegetables, liver	Production of red blood cells	Glossitis, megaloblastic anemia, pancytopenia
B_{12}	Cyanocobalamin	Meats, liver, chicken, dairy products	Formation of red blood cells	Pernicious anemia

Deficiencies of B Vitamins. Persons at high risk of vitamin B deficiencies include older adults who have poor diets and pregnant or lactating (breast-feeding) women, because of the additional requirements of the fetus. Anyone who suffers from a poor diet is prone to be deficient in many other vitamins and minerals.

Persons who may be more susceptible to vitamin B deficiencies, as well as a wide variety of other vitamin deficiencies, include alcoholics, smokers, and those persons with any disease that may affect intake or processing of necessary vitamins and/or minerals. Deficiencies may remain unnoticed for several years until illness occurs. Fortunately, many medications can be taken to replace the necessary amounts of the B vitamins.

B vitamins enable proper cellular functioning of the body system. They accomplish this by acting as coenzymes that combine with the protein portions of enzymes to form the complete enzymes. The enzymes enable important reactions to occur within the cell. If the body becomes vitamin B deficient, the enzymes will not work and the cells will not function properly. Some of the important enzymatic reactions that fail to occur include those involved in the immune system, carbohydrate metabolism, protein synthesis, neurotransmission, and blood formation.

Vitamin B_1 (Coenzyme). Thiamine has three major functions that help maintain the body system. First, thiamine is important for proper carbohydrate metabolism so that energy can be produced from ingested carbohydrates. In this process the carbohydrates are broken down and energy in the form of adenosine triphosphate is produced; this energy is transferred by carrier molecules to the mitochondria of the cell. Water is a by-product of this process, and some of this water is excreted as urine or perspiration. The other two roles of thiamine involve its importance in the well-being of the nervous system and the cardiovascular system.

Deficiency of Vitamin B_1. A deficiency in vitamin B_1 can cause a condition known as beriberi. The symptoms include wasting of the muscles and malfunctioning of the nervous system. Other signs of a deficiency include anorexia, constipation, nausea, mental confusion, and depression. A common cause of thiamine deficiency, along with deficiency of other B vitamins, is chronic alcoholism.

Drug Interactions with Vitamin B₁. Medications such as digoxin, and certain diuretics (furosemide) can result in the heart cells inability to both absorb and use thiamine. Some patients who take phenytoin (Dilantin) can experience in lower levels of thiamine in the blood.

Vitamin B₂ (Coenzyme). Riboflavin is another important component for proper enzymatic activity in the metabolism of carbohydrates and the resultant production of energy for the body system. Riboflavin is necessary for proper growth and maintenance of the body.

Deficiency of Vitamin B₂. A deficiency of vitamin B₂ can lead to anemia, affect the nervous system, and cause depression. In addition, because part of vitamin B₂ is involved in the maintenance of healthy mucous membranes, a deficiency of B₂ can cause drying and soreness of the tongue, mouth, eyes, and skin. Headaches, burning sensations of the skin (especially the feet), cracking of the corners of the mouth, and seborrheic dermatitis are other symptoms of vitamin B₂ deficiency.

Vitamin B₃ (Coenzyme). Nicotinic acid is also known as niacin. This vitamin is used in tissue respiration and metabolism. Although there are two related compounds, nicotinic acid and nicotinamide, they are used in much the same way in the body because nicotinic acid eventually is converted to nicotinamide. However, when nicotinic acid and nicotinamide are taken orally, they do behave differently shortly after ingestion. Nicotinic acid has been found to reduce levels of low-density lipoprotein ("bad" cholesterol). Nicotinic acid also releases histamine and causes peripheral vasodilation, resulting in flushing of the skin. Its counterpart, nicotinamide, does not have these effects. Nicotinic acid and nicotinamide are also necessary for lipid metabolism, proper nerve functioning, and overall maintenance of cells.

Deficiency of Vitamin B₃. A deficiency of niacin can cause a condition known as pellagra. The symptoms include a characteristic dermatitis, diarrhea, weakness, lethargy, dementia, mouth sores, and gastrointestinal disturbance.

Vitamin B₅ (Coenzyme). Pantothenic acid is another compound that is a coenzyme and thus affects body metabolism. Pantothenic acid is incorporated into a coenzyme or into the enzyme itself, where it is used to synthesize important compounds in the body such as fatty acids, steroid hormones, and other molecules necessary for protein and carbohydrate metabolic processes. Pantothenic acid is produced by bacteria within the gastrointestinal tract of many animals and can be found in plant cells.

Deficiency of Vitamin B₅. It is rare for this deficiency to be seen and diagnosed clinically. Symptoms may include headache, sleep disturbances, muscle cramps, and fatigue. The medication used to replace pantothenic acid is calcium pantothenate.

Vitamin B₆ (Coenzyme). Pyridoxine functions in the metabolism of carbohydrates, proteins, and fats in the diet. The increased metabolic rate that is a side effect of vitamin B₆ is the main reason this vitamin is added to diet preparations. Increased metabolism reduces the breakdown of carbohydrates so that they are not absorbed by the body. Pyridoxine also helps in the absorption of vitamin B₁₂ and is a component needed for the production of many different amino acids,

Tech Note!

Riboflavin generally is taken orally each day. It may turn the urine yellow to orange.

Tech Note!

One of the most common side effects of taking immediate-release forms of niacin is flushing of the face (i.e., the face turns red). In addition, a slight drop in blood pressure may cause mild dizziness.

including a major amino acid neurotransmitter found in the brain and spinal cord.

Deficiency of Vitamin B$_6$. A vitamin B$_6$ deficiency causes skin problems such as seborrheic-type lesions, stomatitis, and even seizures, depending on the severity. A deficiency can cause dwarfism, blindness, dementia, depression, and osteoporosis.

Drug Interactions with Vitamin B$_6$. Agents that may cause pyridoxine deficiency include penicillamine and isoniazid (INH); supplements of pyridoxine should be taken with these medications. Because pyridoxine may also antagonize the effect of levodopa (when used without carbidopa), which is used to treat Parkinson's disease. However, levodopa is usually combined with carbidopa.

Vitamin B$_7$ (Biotin). Biotin is important for proper functioning of the body's enzymes. Enzymes are essential for the metabolism of fatty acids and carbohydrates into energy. This conversion allows the production of fats and the excretion of protein by-products. Vitamin B$_7$ is found in a wide variety of foods such as beans, egg yolks, and cauliflower, with even higher concentrations present in both liver and nuts.

Deficiency of Vitamin B$_7$. Symptoms of biotin deficiency include lethargy, weakness, fatigue, and hair loss. In severe cases eczema or swelling of the tongue may occur.

Vitamin B$_9$ (Coenzyme). Folic acid is an essential vitamin for deoxyribonucleic acid (DNA) synthesis and the creation of cells in areas that have high growth turnover. These areas include the bone marrow, where red and white blood cells are formed, and the gastrointestinal tract. Folic acid can be found in green vegetables such as broccoli, avocado, and beets. Other sources include orange juice and meats such as liver. Folic acid is metabolized in the liver and then is used in the bone marrow cells.

Deficiency of Vitamin B$_9$. Vitamin B$_9$ deficiencies cause anemia, diarrhea, weight loss, weakness, sore mouth, irritability, and behavior disorders.

Interactions with Vitamin B$_9$. Drug interactions can occur when vitamin B$_9$ is taken with phenytoin, estrogen, or nitrofurantoin.

Vitamin B$_{12}$ (Coenzyme). Cyanocobalamin is obtained mainly from dietary intake. Cyanocobalamin is required by the body for red blood cell production, myelin sheath production (myelin accelerates the conduction of nerve impulses in the nervous system), and nucleic acid synthesis. Smokers have an increased need for vitamin B$_{12}$.

Deficiency of Vitamin B$_{12}$. Persons deficient in vitamin B$_{12}$ may experience anemia, dementia, depression, hair loss, poor growth rate (in children), and loss of appetite. One type of megaloblastic anemia is specific to vitamin B$_{12}$ deficiency and is called pernicious anemia. The term *pernicious* means "serious" or "severe" and does not relate to a particular cell type. *Megaloblastic* means that the red blood cells (RBCs) are not formed in sufficient quantity and the RBCs that are produced are immature in function and increased in size (macrocytic). Pernicious anemia results from the loss of intrinsic factor, a protein produced by the same stomach cells that produce hydrochloric acid. Normally, vitamin B$_{12}$ is bound to intrinsic factor, enabling vitamin B$_{12}$ to be absorbed into the blood. If there is no intrinsic factor produced, vitamin B$_{12}$ is not absorbed. Persons suffering from disorders of the stomach or those who have undergone gastric surgery procedures such as gastrectomy (removal of the stomach) may develop vitamin B_{12} deficiency attributable to the lack of intrinsic factor. Most cases of pernicious anemia are autoimmune, in which the body develops antibodies against the cells that produce intrinsic factor. As a result, the cells are destroyed and not replaced. Eventually, there are insufficient cells remaining to produce intrinsic factor, and pernicious anemia develops. Persons who cannot absorb vitamin B_{12} require lifetime administration of agents that bypass oral administration, such as intranasal vitamin B_{12} or vitamin B_{12} injections. If there are some stomach cells left that produce intrinsic factor, there may be limited oral absorption; in those cases, injectable or intranasal routes are usually preferred. Vitamin B_{12} is available over-the-counter in an oral form and by prescription for the intranasal and injectable forms.

Vitamin C

Vitamin C also is known as ascorbic acid and is a well-known antioxidant. The main function of vitamin C is the formation of the connective tissue that is found in skin, bones, teeth, and gums. It also aids in wound healing.

Deficiency of Vitamin C. Vitamin C cannot be synthesized by the body; therefore this vitamin must be consumed daily. Vitamin C deficiency results in the disease known as scurvy. This condition causes excessive bleeding in the skin and gums as well as loosening of the teeth. Vitamin C is important for the proper nutrition of cells and their permeability (i.e., the ease with which molecules can penetrate the cell membrane). A deficiency can decrease the ability of the immune system to produce T cells. These cells aid in fighting infection. Vitamin C is found in citrus fruits and a wide variety of vegetables.

ANTIOXIDANTS

Many of the vitamins that are popular are advertised as being antioxidants. Antioxidants are composed of certain enzymes and vitamins that bind to free radicals, which are responsible for damage to the cells and tissues inside the body. The main antioxidant vitamins are vitamins A, C, and E. Although significant research about antioxidants has been conducted, whether antioxidants actually can increase the life span is still a subject of much debate. Antioxidants are added to foods to counteract the detrimental effects of oxygen, which decays food products.

Minerals

Minerals are inorganic elements (i.e., they do not contain carbon) and are the ingredients of the earth's crust. Only small amounts are necessary for proper functioning of many metabolic steps within the body. Each type of trace element has specific functions and consumption of too much of any element can be harmful (Table 27-6). Table 27-7 lists the DRI values of many minerals and trace elements. Table 27-8 lists the sources of trace elements.

ZINC

Zinc is important for promoting normal growth, ensuring the sense of smell and taste, and maintaining the skin's integrity. Zinc also helps heal wounds. A deficiency of zinc will be noted by impairment of taste, a poor immune response, and poor wound healing. If zinc is taken in excess, side effects can range from nausea, vomiting, and diarrhea to pulmonary edema, hypotension, and tachycardia.

TABLE 27-6 Common Minerals and Trace Elements, Their Actions, and Deficiencies

Mineral/Trace Element	Functions	Deficiency	Overdosage
Calcium	Bone formation, cell transport, nerve and muscle functions	Osteoporosis, rickets	Frequent urination and kidney stones/damage, heart rate changes, muscle weakness, impaired muscle function
Copper	Iron utilization, skin pigmentation, nervous system functions	Poor bone growth, nausea, liver failure, kidney failure, nervous system disorders, poor response of immune system	Jaundice
Magnesium	Normal muscle and heart function; necessary for vitamin C and calcium metabolism	High blood pressure, kidney and heart problems, mental confusion	Muscle and generalized weakness, hypotension, cardiac arrhythmias, drowsiness, CNS depression, decreased alertness/concentration
Phosphorus	Necessary for healthy bones and teeth; component of phospholipids*	Muscle weakness, defective bone function, arthritis	May be associated with hypoparathyroidism, diabetic ketoacidosis, kidney failure
Potassium	Cellular transport; normal muscle, heart, kidney, and nervous system functions	Muscle weakness, lethargy, poor growth, cardiac disturbance	Cardiac arrhythmias, cardiac arrest
Iron	Hemoglobin/oxygen transport	Anemia, poor growth, confusion, loss of appetite	Gastrointestinal disturbance, pulmonary edema, black stools, circulatory shock, coma
Selenium	Proper immune functioning and growth	Heart and bone disease	Gastrointestinal disturbance, liver damage
Manganese	Necessary for bone formation and for metabolism of amino acids, lipids, and cholesterol	Poor growth of hair and nails, osteoporosis	None known
Zinc	Proper growth and reproduction; helps heal wounds	Decreased vitamin D absorption, nausea, hair loss, birth defects, decreased immune response, decreased sperm count	Blurred vision, decreased consciousness, tachycardia

*Phospholipids are required for the formation of cell membranes.

Drug Interactions

Penicillamine is a chelator, a drug that binds to metals and treats heavy metal toxicity. Zinc taken with penicillamine may decrease the amount of drug that is absorbed, thus lessening its effectiveness. Zinc and penicillamine should be taken at least 2 hours apart.

IRON

Iron (ferrous sulfate, ferrous fumarate, and ferrous gluconate) is also an important mineral that plays a role in the transport of oxygen within the blood. Within the red blood cell, iron in **hemoglobin** binds tightly to the oxygen molecule,

TABLE 27-7 DRI Values for Minerals and Trace Elements

Minerals	Calcium (mg)	Chloride (mg)	Chromium (mcg)	Copper (mcg)	Iodine (mcg)	Magnesium (mg)	Manganese (mg)	Molybdenum (mcg)	Phosphorus (mg)	Potassium (mg)	Selenium (mcg)	Sodium (mg)	Zinc (mg)
Children													
1-3 yr	500	1500	11	340	90	80	1.2	17	460	3000	20	1000	3
4-8 yr	800	1900	15	440	90	130	1.5	22	500	3800	30	1200	5
Males													
9-13 yr	1300	2300	25	700	120	240	1.9	34	1250	4500	40	1500	8
14-18 yr	1300	2300	35	890	150	410	2.2	43	1250	4700	55	1500	11
19-30 yr	1000	2300	35	900	150	400	2.3	45	700	4700	22	1500	11
31-50 yr	1000	2300	35	900	150	420	2.3	45	700	4700	55	1500	11
51-70 yr	1200	2000	30	900	150	420	2.3	45	700	4700	55	1300	11
>70 yr	1200	1800	30	900	150	420	2.3	45	700	4700	55	1200	11
Females													
9-13 yr	1300	2300	21	700	120	240	1.6	24	1250	4500	40	1500	8
14-18 yr	1300	2300	24	890	150	360	1.6	43	1250	4700	55	1500	9
19-30 yr	1000	2300	25	900	150	310	1.8	45	700	4700	55	1500	8
31-50 yr	1000	2300	20	900	150	320	1.8	45	700	4700	55	1500	8
51-70 yr	1200	2000	20	900	150	320	1.8	45	700	4700	55	1200	8
>70 yr	1200	1800	20	900	150	320	1.8	45	700	4700	55	1200	8
Pregnancy	1000	2300	30	1000	220	360	2	50	700	4700	60	1500	11
Lactation	1000	2300	45	1300	290	320	2.6	50	700	5100	70	1500	12

TABLE 27-8 Mineral Sources

Mineral	Sources
Calcium	Dairy products, broccoli, dark leafy greens such as spinach and rhubarb, and fortified products such as orange juice, soy milk, and tofu
Chromium	Some cereals, beef, turkey, fish, beer, broccoli, and grape juice
Copper	Organ meats, oysters, clams, crabs, cashews, sunflower seeds, wheat bran cereals, whole-grain products, and cocoa products
Fluoride	Fluorinated water, teas, marine fish, and some dental products
Iodine	Processed foods and iodized salt
Magnesium	Whole-grain products, leafy green vegetables, almonds, peanuts, hazelnuts, lima beans, black-eyed peas, avocados, bananas, kiwifruit, shrimp, and chocolate
Manganese	Pecans, almonds, legumes, green and black tea, whole grains, and pineapple juice
Molybdenum	Legumes, grain products, and nuts
Phosphorus	Dairy products, beef, chicken, halibut, salmon, and whole-wheat breads
Potassium	Broccoli, potatoes (with skins), prune juice, orange juice, leafy green vegetables, bananas, raisins, and tomatoes
Selenium	Organ meats, shrimp, crabs, salmon, halibut, and Brazil nuts
Zinc	Red meat, fortified cereals, oysters, almonds, peanuts, chickpeas, soy foods, and dairy products

TABLE 27-9 Iron Sources

Heme iron sources	Beef, chicken, cod, flounder, pork, salmon, shrimp, tuna, turkey
Non-heme iron sources	Almonds (raw), apricots (dried), bagels, breads, broccoli, dates, molasses (blackstrap), peas (frozen), prune juice, raisins (not packed), rice, spinach, pastas (macaroni, spaghetti), beans (kidney, lima), supplements

thus allowing oxygen to be transported throughout the body. Iron gives blood its red color. Much of the iron within the body is found in hemoglobin. Iron is used in other metabolic body functions, and iron is found in all muscles (it gives muscles their red color). Iron also is stored in the liver, giving that organ its color.

Although iron is found in many different food sources (Table 27-9), its availability differs within the body system. Iron's availability is dependent on whether the iron is present in heme or non-heme form. Sources of heme iron are found only in fish, meat, and poultry. This type of iron is more easily absorbed than non-heme iron, found in foods such as fruits, vegetables, nuts, grains, and dried beans. Ways to increase iron absorption include adding a vitamin C supplement to the diet, eating both heme and non-heme foods together, or cooking non-heme foods in a cast iron skillet. Likewise, there are foods that will inhibit the effectiveness of iron, including calcium supplements and large amounts of tea or high-fiber foods, all of which bind to iron and lessen its absorption.

TABLE 27-10 DRI for Elemental Iron

Age Limit	Iron
Infants 0-6 mo	0.27 mg
Infants 7-12 mo	11 mg
Children 1-3 yr	7 mg
Children 4-8 yr	10 mg
Males 9-13 yr	8 mg
Males 14-18 yr	11 mg
Males 19-30 yr	8 mg
Males 31-50 yr	8 mg
Males 51-70 yr	8 mg
Males 70+ yr	8 mg
Females 9-13 yr	8 mg
Females 14-18 yr	15 mg
Females 19-30 yr	18 mg
Females 31-50 yr	8 mg
Females 51-70 yr	8 mg
Females 70+ yr	8 mg
Pregnancy	27 mg
Females during lactation	9 mg
Vegetarians, men	14 mg
Vegetarians, women	33 mg

From www.bloodindex.org/iron_rich_food.php.

Iron Deficiency

Iron deficiency anemia is one of the most common types of anemia, and it affects more than 30% of the world's population. Iron deficiency can occur for many reasons:

- Lack of iron in the diet. For example, vegetarians consuming high-fiber diets often need more iron in the diet to reduce the risk of iron deficiency. Recommended amounts are as follows: women, 33 mg/day; men, 14 mg/day.
- Pregnancy: As a result of increased metabolic demands, pregnant women typically require 12 mg more iron per day than nonpregnant women.
- Inadequate intestinal absorption
- Excessive blood loss
- Certain forms of kidney failure in which the kidneys fail to produce erythropoietin*
- Alcoholism
- Females are typically affected more than males, primarily because of blood loss during menstruation

Symptoms of iron deficiency include hair loss, shortness of breath, anemia, lethargy, and even heart palpitations. The toxic effects of an overdose are severe and include acidosis, liver and kidney impairment, and coma. Iron poisoning is one of the leading causes of poisoning death in children; all vitamin and mineral products containing iron must be packaged in special child-resistant packaging. Table 27-10 gives the daily recommended allowance values for iron among different age groups.

---

*Erythropoietin is a hormone necessary to synthesize red blood cells. Epoetin is available in injectable form and normally is given to dialysis patients but also can be administered to patients with severe anemia.

DO YOU REMEMBER THESE KEY POINTS?

- The main vitamins required by the body and their functions
- The names of water-soluble vitamins
- The names of fat-soluble vitamins
- The main minerals required by the body and their functions
- The cause of pernicious anemia
- The DRI for vitamins
- The manner in which iron is used in the body
- The causes of iron deficiencies
- The supposed effects of free radicals and how antioxidants are used to counteract damage from them

REVIEW QUESTIONS

Multiple choice questions

1. All of the following vitamins are water-soluble EXCEPT:
   A. Vitamin C
   B. Vitamin E
   C. Vitamin B
   D. Ascorbic acid

2. Cyanocobalamin is the chemical term for _____ and is important for avoiding _____.
   A. Vitamin B_{12}, pernicious anemia
   B. Vitamin K, anemia
   C. Vitamin C, free radicals
   D. Vitamin E, immunity problems

3. Two important minerals that human beings require are:
   A. Ascorbic acid and pyridoxine
   B. Zinc and phytonadione
   C. Folic acid and calcitriol
   D. Iron and zinc

4. All of the following vitamins have antioxidant properties EXCEPT:
   A. Vitamin A
   B. Vitamin C
   C. Vitamin E
   D. Vitamin D

5. The FDA considers all of the following substances as food ingredients EXCEPT:
   A. Amino acids
   B. Vitamins
   C. Minerals
   D. Aspirin

6. All of the following statements are true concerning retinol EXCEPT:
   A. It also is called vitamin A
   B. It is an antioxidant
   C. It aids in the absorption of vitamin D
   D. It can be found in several dairy products, fruits, and vegetables

7. The vitamin most associated with proper blood clotting is:
   A. Phytonadione
   B. Niacin
   C. Thiamine
   D. Vitamin A

8. Of the statements listed, which is NOT true concerning the condition pernicious anemia?

A. It can be caused by a lack of vitamin B.

B. It commonly is experienced by individuals with a deficiency of intrinsic factor.

C. Intrinsic factor is caused by hydrochloric acid.

D. It is a fatal disease.

9. Iron deficiency can be caused by the following reasons EXCEPT:

A. Alcoholism

B. Pregnancy

C. Coffee

D. Kidney failure

10. Calcium deficiency can cause the following condition(s)?

A. Rickets

B. Osteoporosis

C. Osteomalacia

D. All of the above

True/False

If the statement is false, then change it to make it true.

_____ **1.** All minerals are natural and do not have to be taken through supplements if a proper diet is eaten.

_____ **2.** All vitamins are water-soluble; therefore all can be taken as often as needed or wanted.

_____ **3.** The initials "FDA" stand for the "Federal Department of Agriculture."

_____ **4.** The FDA considers all over-the-counter vitamins and minerals as food supplements.

_____ **5.** Iron is a main component of hemoglobin and is responsible for oxygen content.

_____ **6.** A deficiency of vitamin D can cause rickets.

_____ **7.** Goiter can be caused by too much iodine.

_____ **8.** Antioxidants are agents that combine with and reduce free radicals.

_____ **9.** Vitamin A is responsible for normal metabolism.

_____ **10.** Nicotinic acid is believed to be active in lowering cholesterol.

TECHNICIAN'S CORNER

An elderly female patient arrives at the pharmacy window with the following questions: She is currently taking vitamins A, B, C, D, and E. She would like to know if that is okay.

1. What do you know about these vitamins?
2. What would you tell her?

BIBLIOGRAPHY

Bryant B, Knights K, Salerno E: *Pharmacology for health professionals*, St Louis, 2003, Mosby.

Hillman R, Ault K: Hematopoietic agents: growth factors, minerals, and vitamins. In Hardman JG, Gilman AG, Limbird LE: *Goodman and Gilman's the pharmacological basis of therapeutics*, ed 10, New York, 2001, McGraw-Hill.

Marcus R: Agents affecting calcification and bone turnover: calcium, phosphate, parathyroid hormone, vitamin D, calcitonin, and other compounds. In Hardman JG, Gilman AG, Limbird LE: *Goodman and Gilman's the pharmacological basis of therapeutics*, ed 10, New York, 2001, McGraw-Hill.

Marcus R, Coulston A: The fat-soluble vitamins: vitamins A, K, and E. In Hardman JG, Gilman AG, Limbird LE: *Goodman and Gilman's the pharmacological basis of therapeutics*, ed 10, New York, 2001, McGraw-Hill.

Marcus R, Coulston A: The vitamins: introduction. In Hardman JG, Gilman AG, Limbird LE: *Goodman and Gilman's the pharmacological basis of therapeutics*, ed 10, New York, 2001, McGraw-Hill.

Marcus R, Coulston A: The water-soluble vitamins: the vitamin B complex and ascorbic acid. In Hardman JG, Gilman AG, Limbird LE: *Goodman and Gilman's the pharmacological basis of therapeutics*, ed 10, New York, 2001, McGraw-Hill.

Mason J: Consequences of altered micronutrient status. In Goldman L, Bennett J: *Cecil textbook of medicine*, ed 21, Philadelphia, 2000, Saunders.

McKenry L, Salerno E: *Mosby's pharmacology in nursing*, ed 22, St Louis, 2005, Mosby.

Schlenker E, Long S: Williams' essentials of nutrition and diet therapy, ed 9, St Louis, 2006, Mosby.

WEBSITES

Mineral RDA: www.cellinteractive.com/ucla/vitamins_minerals/vits_mins1.html
www.mckinley.illinois.edu/Handouts/dietary_sources_iron.html
Food and Drug Administration: www.fda.gov

Objectives

UPON COMPLETING THIS CHAPTER, YOU SHOULD BE ABLE TO DO THE FOLLOWING:

- Describe the importance of vaccines.

- Explain how vaccines are produced.

- List the most common vaccines.

- Explain how the body develops immunity against diseases.

- Describe where immune cells are produced and discuss the functions of immune cells.

- Differentiate between active and passive immunity.

- List the schedule for administering vaccines.

- Explain why some vaccines need boosters.

- Explain under which circumstances adults should receive vaccines.

Acquired immunity *Immunity acquired by active infection, by vaccination (active immunity), or by the transfer of products (usually antibodies) from a donor (passive immunity). Acquired immunity is in contrast to innate immunity (natural immunity system), which provides natural barriers and defenses to infection but does not confer long-lasting immunity*

Active immunity *A form of acquired immunity in which the body produces its own antibodies against disease-causing antigens*

Antibodies *Complex molecules (immunoglobulins) that are made in response to the presence of an antigen (such as a protein of bacteria or other infecting organism) and that neutralize the effect of the foreign substance*

Antigen *A substance that prompts the generation of antibodies and that can produce an immune response*

Attenuated *An altered or weakened live vaccine made from the disease organism against which the vaccine protects*

Contagion *The transfer of a disease from one individual to another; a contagious disease*

Globulin *Protein that is insoluble in water; immune globulins protect against disease*

Immunity *A type of resistance to infection caused by an immune response from the body following exposure to antigens or administration of vaccines*

Immunosuppressive agents *Agents that prevent or lessen the activity of the immune system; immunosuppressive drugs are used frequently to prevent organ rejection or to treat certain autoimmune or inflammatory diseases*

Lymph node *A structure that consists of many small, oval nodules that filter lymphatic fluid and fight infection; lymphocytes, monocytes, and plasma cells are formed in lymph nodes*

Passive immunity *Resistance to a disease that has been acquired through a transfer of antibodies from another person or animal or from mother to child*

Toxoid *A type of vaccine where a toxin has been rendered harmless but still invokes an antigenic response, improving immunity against the active toxin at some future date*

Vaccine *A biological preparation that improves immunity to a particular disease by invoking an immune response and a "memory" of the response for future use*

Virion *A virus particle*

Virus *A microscopic organism that replicates exclusively inside the host's cell, using parts of the host cell including DNA, ribosomes, and proteins*

TYPES OF VACCINES

	Pronunciation		Pronunciation
Immune Globulins		Hepatitis B immune globulin (HBIG)	(hep-ah-**ty**-tiss **B** im-**myoon glob**-yoo-lin)
Botulism immune globulin (BIG)	(**bot**-ue-lizm im-**myoon glob**-yoo-lin)	Rabies immune globulin (RIG)	(**ray**-beez im-**myoon glob**-yoo-lin)
Cytomegalovirus immune globulin (CMV-IG)	(sye-toe-**meg**-a-lo-vye-rus im-**myoon glob**-yoo-lin)	Respiratory syncytial virus immune globulin (RSV-IG)	(res-pi-rah-tory sink-**tee**-ahl vye-rus im-**myoon glob**-yoo-lin)
Immune globulin G (IgG)	(im-**myoon glob**-yoo-lin)		

TYPES OF VACCINES—cont'd

	Pronunciation		Pronunciation
Tetanus immune globulin (TIG)	(**tet**-n-us im-**myoon** **glob**-yoo-lin)	Rotavirus oral	(**roe**-ta-vye-ris)
Vaccinia immune globulin (VIG)	(vax-**in**-ee-a im-**myoon** **glob**-yoo-lin)	Smallpox (vaccinia)	(**small** pox)
		Varicella (chickenpox)	(var-ih-**sel**-a)
Varicella-zoster immune globulin (VZIG)	(var-ih-**sel**-ah-**zos**-ter im-**myoon glob**-yoo-lin)	Herpes zoster (varicella-zoster)	(her-**pees zos**-ter)

Antitoxins | | **Inactivated Viral Vaccines** |
Botulinum antitoxin	(**bot**-ue-li-um an-ti-**tok**-sin)	Avian influenza	(**a**-vee-an in-floo-**enz**-a)
Diphtheria antitoxin	(**dip**-theer-ee-a an-ti-**tok**-sin)	Hepatitis A	(hep-ah-**ty**-tiss **A**)
Tetanus antitoxin	(**tet**-n-us an-ti-**tok**-sin)	Hepatitis B	(hep-ah-**ty**-tiss **B**)
		Human papillomavirus (HPV)	(hyoo-man **pap**-i-**lo**-ma-**vye**-rus)
Antivenins		Inactivated influenza virus injectable	(in-**ak**-ti-vay-ted in-flu-**en**-za **vye**-rus)
Black widow spider antivenin	(an-tee-**ven**-in)	Japanese encephalitis virus	(**jap**-a-**neez** en-**cef**-a-**lye**-tis **vye**-rus)
Coral snake antivenin	(an-tee-**ven**-in)	Inactivated poliovirus (IPV)	(in-**ak**-ti-vay-ted **poe**-lee-oh-**vye**-rus)
Rattlesnake antivenin	(an-tee-**ven**-in)	Swine flu	(**swy**-neen **flew**)
		Yellow fever	(yel-**oh** fee-**ver**)
Toxoids		
Botulinum	(**bot**-ue-**lye**-num)	**Vaccines against Bacterial Illness**	
Diphtheria	(**dip**-theer-ee-a)	Anthrax vaccine	(**anth**-rax vax-**een**)
Tetanus	(**tet**-n-us)	*Haemophilus influenzae*	(hee-**maw**-fil-liss in-flew-**en**-za)
		Lyme disease	(**lime** dis-**ese**)
Live (Attenuated) Viral Vaccines		Meningococcal	(me-**nin**-je-**kok**-al)
Influenza intranasal	(in-**floo**-enz-a in-**tra**-naz-al)	Plague	(**pla**-gwe)
Measles, mumps, rubella (MMR)	(**mee**-zels, **mumps**, roo-**bel**-a)	Pneumococcal	(**noo**-moe-**kok**-al)
Poliovirus oral (OPV)	(**poe**-lee-oh)	Typhoid	(**tye**-foid)

SYSTEMIC IMMUNOSUPPRESSIVE AGENTS (EXCLUDES CORTICOSTEROIDS)

Trade Name*	Generic Name	Pronunciation	Trade Name*	Generic Name	Pronunciation
Azasan, Imuran	azathioprine	(ay-za-**thye**-oh-preen)	**Biological Response Modifiers used for Immunosuppression**		
CellCept, Myfortic	mycophenolate	(**mye**-koe-**fen**-oh-late)	Orthoclone OKT3	muromonab-CD3	(**mue**-roe-**moe**-nab)
Cytoxan	cyclophosphamide	(**sye**-kloe-**fos**-fa-mide)	Simulect	basiliximab	(bass-ih-**lix**-ih-mab)
Gengraf, Neoral, Sandimmune	cyclosporine	(**sye**-kloe-**spor**-en)	Zenapax	daclizumab	(dah-**klye**-zue-mab)
Prograf	tacrolimus	(ta-**kroe**-li-mus)			
Rapamune	sirolimus	(sir-**oh**-li-mus)			
Trexall	methotrexate	(meth-oh-**trex**-ate)			

*Listing of trade names on the same row does not indicate that products are interchangeable in patient treatment regimens.

HUMAN BEINGS HAVE ALWAYS BEEN plagued by bacterial and viral microbes that have caused disease and even death. In addition to outside invaders, the body may need to address internal assailants, such as cancer cells or a misdirected attack from the immune system (i.e., autoimmune disease). Fortunately, highly organized defense mechanisms work specifically on eliminating unwanted entities.

Several factors contribute to the overall wellness of a person. The development of vaccines to prevent infections has contributed directly to the current longevity of human beings. However, specific regions of the earth, such as Third

World countries, still face a higher risk of contracting bacterial and viral infections.

This chapter describes the major functions of the immune system and then focuses on the various types of bacteria and viruses that can affect the body. This chapter also explains the schedule for immunizations. In addition, the immunological malfunctions of the body and the agents prescribed to treat them are discussed.

Lymphatic System

The body has an innate defense mechanism that helps protect it from invading organisms. From birth, one of the most important functions of the body is to defend against invasion. The lymphatic system is a primary source of immune cell production and commonly is referred to as the immune system. The lymph nodes produce our natural arsenal of weapons. The many lymph nodes serve the body by destroying bacteria and cancer cells, using various methods to stop them from entering the bloodstream. Although many lymphoid tissues and small vessels are located throughout the body, a few main production centers are responsible for much of the immune arsenal. The thymus, tonsils, and spleen are larger organs of the lymphatic system, each having specific functions (Figure 28-1).

THYMUS

The thymus is an important organ located in the upper chest and in the middle of the neck region. The primary function of the thymus is to produce lymphocytes, which ultimately circulate through **lymph nodes** and lymphatic tissues and help provide **immunity**. The thymus begins producing these lymphocytes before birth, and the organ is much larger in childhood than in adulthood.

TONSILS

Other important lymphoid tissues are the tonsils and the adenoids, located in the throat and nose, respectively. The tonsils help fight infection by filtering bacteria and other infective material. The adenoids, located at the back of the nose above the tonsils, function as part of the lymphatic system by stopping disease-causing microorganisms from entering the body through the nose and mouth.

SPLEEN

The spleen is located in the left side of the upper abdomen. The spleen is also the largest lymphatic organ in the body. The function of the spleen is to filter large amounts of blood cells as they reach the end of their life cycle. Macrophages within the spleen help in the removal of cellular debris. The result is the destruction of old blood cells, bacteria, and any foreign bodies.

TYPES OF IMMUNE CELLS

The many nodes and tissues located throughout the body produce some of the cells responsible for the immune system's defense mechanisms. When first contact is made with a foreign body (antigens), **antibodies** are formed. Certain immune system cells remember that specific **antigen** until the next time contact is made, enabling faster production of more antibodies. The body, having equipped its arsenal, then has the necessary forces to defend against an antigen invader.

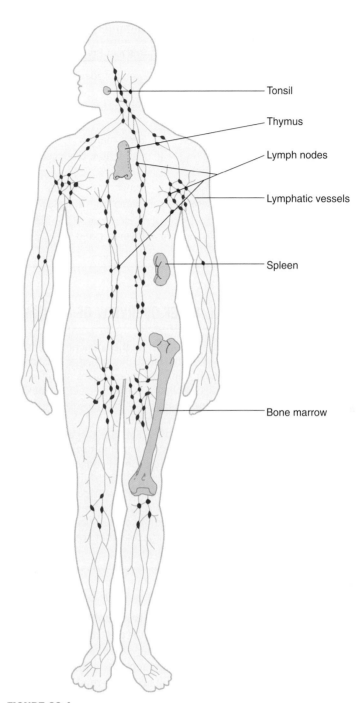

Tonsil

Thymus

Lymph nodes

Lymphatic vessels

Spleen

Bone marrow

FIGURE 28-1 Overview of the major lymphatic organs within the body.

A major portion of the immune system's attack cells are lymphocytes. They patrol the body by circulating through the bloodstream. Many lymphocytes reside in lymph nodes and tissues, waiting to attack foreign bodies. The two types of lymphocytes are B cells and T lymphocytes. B cells and their products—immunoglobulins—contribute to humoral immunity, also known as antibody-mediated immunity. B cells typically reside in the lymph nodes and can multiply into many thousands of the same type of cells. When activated, they become plasma cells that initiate immunoglobulins or an antibody-mediated response to invading antigens (some of the B cells also become memory cells that "remember" the invasion for a future date); this response is mediated by T lymphocytes

TABLE 28-1 Major Immune Response Cells

Major Cell Types	Origin of Production	Location in Body	Function
T lymphocytes	Lymph nodes	Lymph nodes	Produces more T lymphocytes that are sensitized to specific antigens
B lymphocytes	Bone marrow (prenatal, produced in liver)	Lymph nodes	Produce specific antibodies
Plasma cells	Lymph from B cells	Bloodstream	Produce antibodies
Memory cells	Lymph from B cells	Lymph nodes	Create memory antibody
T cells	Thymus gland	Bloodstream, lymph nodes	Binds to specific antigen

BOX 28-1 BRIEF OVERVIEW OF ALL IMMUNE CELLS

T Cells: Contribute to the immune defense in two ways—by regulating the immune system or by directly attacking and destroying infected cells.

Cytokines: Chemical messengers secreted by cells of the immune system. Binding to specific receptors on target cells, cytokines recruit many other cells to the area. Cytokines encourage cell growth, promote cell activation, and destroy target cells, including cancer cells.

Phagocytes: Large white cells that engulf and digest foreign invaders; include monocytes and macrophages found in tissues throughout the body.

Neutrophils: Are considered phagocytic and granulocytic; circulate through the blood but move into tissues when they are needed to destroy foreign invaders; granulocytes contain granules filled with potent chemicals that work to destroy microorganisms and play a role in acute inflammatory reactions. Other types of granulocytes include eosinophils and basophils. Mast cells are also granule-containing cells in tissues.

Macrophages: Large cells that scavenge waste materials inside the cell; also play a role in T cell activation.

and their products—lymphokines. Lymphokines, which include interleukins and interferons, are important in determining the class of immunoglobulins made by B cells. T lymphocytes also are located in the lymph nodes and remain there until an antigen attaches to their surface protein at specific receptor sites. These T cells then perform a cell-mediated immune response. This response can be a direct destruction of the attached cell and antigen, or the T cells can release a chemical signal that enlists the help of macrophages to destroy the invading cells. Table 28-1 lists major immune cells along with their location and primary function. Box 28-1 gives a brief overview of all immune cells.

Immunizations

For diseases such as whooping cough, tetanus, and polio, a weakened form of the agent (which acts as an antigen in the body) is given as an immunization to stimulate the production of antibodies, which protect the body from the disease. It is important that children receive the course of vaccinations recommended by the Centers for Disease Control and Prevention Advisory Committee on Immunization Practices (ACIP) because they are at risk for contracting diseases such as measles, mumps, rubella, chickenpox, whooping cough, and polio. Without the benefit of immunizations, many children may contract these childhood diseases. Historically, thousands of children have died from diseases such as measles and mumps or have been physically scarred by the effects of polio. Although children still can contract these diseases today, they are seen less commonly, and death is rare because of the widespread use of immunizations.

By immunizing children and adults, society is better protected against diseases such as chickenpox, measles, and influenza. Those persons with weakened immune systems, such as older adults, chemotherapy patients, transplant recipients, and persons with acquired immunodeficiency syndrome, are also at higher risk to develop and even die from these diseases. Another high-risk group is persons from countries where immunizations are not available. In addition, many diseases can be transmitted through blood or other body fluids. Therefore anyone sharing needles or having unprotected sex with an infected person is at risk. Unfortunately, not all communicable conditions may be detected. Many newly infected persons do not know that they are infected or how they contracted the disease.

TYPES OF IMMUNITY

Active Immunity

Active natural immunity occurs when the body is exposed to a disease, actively produces antibodies to respond to the disease, and then recovers. Upon subsequent exposure to the same antigen, the memory cells produced from the first encounter are able to rapidly destroy the antigen and prevent the disease process.

Active acquired immunity occurs when a vaccine is administered. Vaccines can be either live or inactive. Live vaccines must be **attenuated** (weakened). When live vaccines are used, there is a small risk of developing the infection. However, once the body manufactures antibodies against the injected antigen, it has long-lasting immunity. For vaccines that are made from killed or inactive antigens, the risk of infection is lower. The disadvantage is that booster shots are needed to maintain a sufficiently high level of antibodies.

Passive Immunity

Passive immunity does not require any action by the body. The body receives protection from outside sources, such as by administration of immune **globulin** in passive acquired immunity or by transfer of immunity from mother to child as in passive natural immunity.

HOW VACCINES ARE PREPARED

Viral Vaccines

A **virus** or any foreign substance that causes a disease or allergy can be referred to as an antigen. When a vaccine is injected or absorbed systemically into the body, the immune system responds by manufacturing antibodies. Antibodies are complex molecules produced by the lymph tissue in response to the presence of an antigen. Millions of antibodies overcome the small number of antigens injected in the vaccine. Table 28-2 gives examples of major types of viral vaccines.

Some available vaccines (e.g., measles, mumps, rubella [MMR]; oral polio; oral rotavirus; intranasal influenza; smallpox [vaccinia]; and varicella [chickenpox]) contain live viruses that have been attenuated before they are given to patients. The **virions** taken are weakened or defused so that they do not cause the full extent of the disease. The attenuated virus may replicate, but at a very slow rate. A person with an active immune system quickly begins to make a full complement of antibodies and antigen-induced reactions that produce immunity. The advantage of live vaccine administration is the durable and complete

Tech Note!

It is important to follow the manufacturer's instructions on storing vaccines. **Vaccines** are always kept either in the refrigerator or freezer at the pharmacy to prevent loss of potency. There must be a thermometer in the refrigerator and/or freezer and the temperature must be documented daily to ensure stability.

TABLE 28-2 Common Viral Vaccines, Diseases Treated, and Route of Administration

Vaccine Agents	Disease Treated	Route of Administration
Attenuvax	Measles	Subcutaneous (Subcut)
Engerix-B, Recombivax-HB	Hepatitis B	Intramuscular (IM)
Fluzone	Influenza	IM
Havrix	Hepatitis A	IM
IPOL	Polio	Subcut or IM
Meruvax II	Rubella	Subcut
MMR II	Measles, mumps, and rubella	Subcut
Mumpsvax	Mumps	Subcut
Varivax	Chickenpox	Subcut
YF-VAX	Yellow fever	Subcut

TABLE 28-3 Common Toxoids and Route of Administration

Toxoid Agents	Disease Treated	Route of Administration
Tetanus toxoid	Tetanus	Subcutaneous Intramuscular
Diphtheria and tetanus	Diphtheria, tetanus	Intramuscular
DPT	Diphtheria, pertussis, tetanus	Intramuscular

immunity produced. However, if a person is immunocompromised, live vaccines could carry a risk of disease and other problems, so they are to be avoided. See the list at the beginning of the chapter for examples of medications that cause immunosuppression; administration of vaccines to immunosuppressed patients should be avoided.

An inactivated viral vaccine is one in which the virus products are grown in culture and then the virus is destroyed so it cannot replicate and cause disease. While much of the virus is destroyed, the viral capsid proteins (outer shells) remain intact and are easily recognized by the immune system. Because the capsule or outer shell of the antigen does not continually reinforce the response needed for the body to resist further attacks, boosters must be given to remind the body to develop antibodies within the immune system.

Bacterial Vaccines
Live, attenuated bacterial vaccines include typhoid vaccine. Some vaccines are referred to as **toxoids;** these are inactivated bacterial toxins. Although the bacterial cell has been altered so that it cannot cause disease, it still can induce an antibody response within the body. Table 28-3 lists major toxoids.

Many persons believe that after 18 years of age immunizations are not necessary. However, there are vaccines, such as the tetanus toxoid, that also should be given to adults. Although tetanus immunizations are given to children combined with diphtheria and pertussis, tetanus booster immunizations should be given every 10 years throughout a person's lifetime. Tetanus is a disease caused by a toxin-secreting bacterium that can be contracted through scrapes and cuts from dirty objects.

Miscellaneous Vaccines
Although the two most common vaccines are inactivated (killed) or live-attenuated (weakened), there are other less common types of vaccines available,

BOX 28-2 THREE TYPES OF LESS COMMON VACCINES AND THEIR SPECIFIC CHARACTERISTICS

Antiidiotypic Vaccines

This newer type of vaccine is based on using an antibody that is shaped like the antigen. When the antibody is administered, the body will react as though it were the antigen. The immune system will create antibodies to fight the disease. In effect, the body is making an antibody against the injected antibody. This second antibody then can be injected to act as the vaccine and will create a third antibody. In the future, this method may make it possible to kill deadly viruses such as human immunodeficiency virus.

Subunit Vaccines

Subunit vaccines are small pieces of the genetic code that originate from the disease microbe. These pieces are injected into a bacterium or yeast and then grown. They are then harvested and used as a vaccine to stimulate the body to produce an immune response. Because there are only pieces of the original virion or antigen, they do not carry the full extent of immunity provided by a complete antigen. Hepatitis B is a subunit vaccine that is grown in yeast cells and then is given as a vaccine.

Acellular and Conjugated Vaccines

When a vaccine is disassembled or fragmented to isolate specific antigens from entire cells, it is referred to as an acellular vaccine. Pertussis is one type of vaccine made in this manner. Bacterial cells that have been altered and mixed with toxoids to increase their overall effectiveness are called conjugated vaccines. Such is the case with tetanus or diphtheria.

as shown in Box 28-2. These vaccines are slightly different in their composition from the usual types.

Unfortunately, the only two types of vaccines that are available are those that protect against viruses and bacterial microbes. Immunizations for diseases caused by a parasite, such as malaria, and for fungal infections have not been developed.

DEVELOPMENT OF VACCINES

To develop a vaccine, researchers must collect a large number of contagious cells. Most vaccine development has involved the use of laboratory animals. For instance, the rabies vaccine was first grown in the nervous systems of rabbits. Most vaccines, however, were created to protect against bacterial microbes or those viruses that could be grown in or on animal tissue. In the beginning of vaccine research, this was difficult to accomplish if the diseases only occurred in human beings. Since then, scientists have discovered how to retrieve culture cells from human beings. This led to the development of vaccines against polio, mumps, and measles.

Currently, research continues on a vaccine for the human immunodeficiency virus (HIV), the virus that causes acquired immunodeficiency syndrome (AIDS). Although the viral particles can be grown in monkey tissue, and monkeys become infected with HIV and similar viruses, monkeys do not develop AIDS. Even if researchers succeed in developing a vaccine, administration of the vaccine can be dangerous. This is because the presence of any live virus particles in the vaccine could cause infection in the recipient. Table 28-4 lists some vaccine-preventable diseases.

TABLE 28-4 Vaccines That Prevent Diseases

Vaccine	Series of Doses	Persons Who Should Have Vaccine Coverage	Comments
Anthrax	Series of 6 injections	Anyone who has a high risk of infection	
Varicella (chickenpox)	Series of 2 injections	Given at 12 months with second dose between ages 4 and 6 yr	
Hepatitis A	Series of 2 injections	Children 12 months old with second dose 6 months after first dose	Adults who travel to countries where HepA is prevalent should be vaccinated
Hepatitis B	Series of 3 injections	Dose 1, at birth; dose 2, 4 weeks after birth; dose 3, 8 weeks after birth	All adults at high risk: multiple sex partners, chronic liver/kidney disease, dialysis patients, infected sex partner, HIV
Haemophilus influenza type B	Series of 4 injections	Dose 1, 6 weeks of age; dose 2, 4 weeks after dose 1; dose 3, 8 weeks after dose 2; dose 4, 8 weeks after dose 3	Some older children or adults with special health conditions; conditions include sickle cell disease, HIV/AIDS, removal of spleen, bone marrow transplant, or cancer treatment with drugs
Human papillomavirus	Series of 3 injections	Dose 1, girls 11-12 yr; dose 2, 2 months after dose 1; dose 3, 6 months after dose 2	Prevents 4 types of HPV infection
Influenza	Doses given annually	Approved for ages 2-49 yr (live intranasal) for those in good health; age 6 months and older (including >50 yr) for trivalent inactivated injection	Two dosage forms of vaccines: intranasal spray and injection
Japanese encephalitis	Series of 3 injections	People who live or travel in certain rural parts of Asia should be vaccinated; laboratory workers at risk of exposure to JE virus should also be vaccinated	Children 1-3 yr receive smaller dose than older children and adults
Diphtheria, tetanus, pertussis	Series of 4 or 5 injections	Dose 1, 6 weeks old; dose 2, 4 weeks after dose 1; dose 3, 4 weeks after dose 2; dose 4, 6 months after dose 3; dose 5, 6 months after dose 4	Dose 5 not necessary if dose 4 was administered at age of 4 yr or older
Meningococcal	1 injection	Given between 11 and 18 yr of age; should be given to people 2-55 yr of age in high-risk groups only	Prevents 4 types of meningococcal disease
Measles, mumps, rubella (MMR)	Series of 2 injections	Dose 1, at 12 months old; dose 2, 4 weeks after dose 1	If not previously vaccinated those persons between ages 7-18 yr can be vaccinated; two injections should be 28 days apart
Pneumococcal (PVC7)	Series of 4 doses	Children between 2 and 15 months old	Prevents 7 types of pneumococcal viruses prevalent in children

TABLE 28-4 Vaccines That Prevent Diseases—cont'd

Vaccine	Series of Doses	Persons Who Should Have Vaccine Coverage	Comments
Pneumococcal (PPSV)	1 injection	Ages 65 yr and older or ages 2-64 yr if high risk	Prevents 23 types of pneumococcal viruses prevalent in adults and children at high risk
Poliomyelitis	IPV: series of 4 doses	Children 2 months to 4 yr	3 doses for adults never vaccinated
Rabies	Series of 4 doses	Given to persons at high risk or who have been bitten by animal with rabies	
Rotavirus	Series of 3 oral doses	2-6 months of age	
Rubella		See MMR	
Shingles	1 injection	In adults 60 yr and older	
Smallpox	1 vaccination	For all exposed to smallpox: eradicated in U.S. since 1977	CDC has enough vaccine stockpiled for every U.S. citizen in case it is needed
Tetanus		See Diphtheria	Tetanus booster recommended every 10 yr
Typhoid fever	Injection or oral	1 vaccination and 1 every 2 yr afterwards for high-risk persons	Oral should not be given to children <6 yr
Yellow fever	1 injection	9 months and older: initial shot given for high-risk persons (traveling to countries that have yellow fever)	Boosters to be given (if necessary) every 10 yr thereafter

TABLE 28-5 Childhood Immunization Schedule

Vaccine	1 Month	2 Months	4 Months	6 Months	12 Months	15 Months	1½ Years	2 Years	4-6 Years	11-12 Years	13-18 Years
Hepatitis B	X	X	X	X	X	X	X				
DPT*		X	X	X		X	X		X		
HiB		X	X	X	X	X					
Polio		X	X	X	X	X	X		X		
MMR					X	X			X	X	X
Varicella					X	X	X	X	X	X	X

*DPT, Diphtheria, pertussis, tetanus; HiB, Haemophilus influenzae type B; MMR, measles, mumps, rubella.

CHILDHOOD IMMUNIZATION

Because children are at a high risk for catching and spreading many communicable diseases, a series of immunizations has been recommended to protect children and to promote community health and protection against the spread of disease. In the United States, children cannot register for school unless they have proof of their immunizations, or have obtained and filed appropriate medical or religious exemptions. Table 28-5 gives a recommended schedule for immunizations for children through 18 years of age.

National Childhood Vaccine Injury Act of 1986

In rare cases, any vaccine may cause an allergic reaction. Therefore it is important to observe for any severe reactions after vaccination. With most vaccinations, a vaccine information statement (VIS), published by the Centers for Disease Control and Prevention (CDC), is issued to the patient or legal caregiver of the patient receiving the vaccine. The VIS contains important information regarding the vaccine and its potential side effects. The law requires that the VIS be made available for certain vaccinations.

In 1986 the U.S. Congress passed the National Childhood Vaccine Injury Act. This act provided a National Vaccine Injury Compensation Program for those persons who may have been injured after receiving a routine vaccine. These vaccines include measles, mumps, or rubella (or any combination thereof) and tetanus toxoid, pertussis, polio, influenza, varicella, rotavirus vaccine, and/or pneumococcal vaccines. Studies have shown that a small number of vaccinated persons had severe side effects. More information can be found on the website www.vaccineinjury.org.

Autism and Vaccines

Autism is a spectrum of disorders characterized by various degrees of communication difficulties, social impairments, and repetitive types of behavior. There is no known cure for these conditions. Many parents have concerns regarding vaccine safety and autism; the concerns have been magnified by the media and the positing of personal experiences rather than scientific evidence on websites. Many studies have examined whether there is a direct relationship between childhood autism and vaccines, specifically those vaccines containing the preservative thimerosal (thimerosal has been removed from routine childhood vaccines). To date, all scientifically sound studies have failed to find an association between vaccines and the occurrence of autism. After review of the available evidence, the Centers for Disease Control and Prevention (CDC) concluded that there is no relationship between the two, and the CDC continues to support the advancement of research into the possible causes of autism and effective treatments (www.cdc.gov/vaccinesafety/Concerns/Autism/Index.html).

Diphtheria, Pertussis, and Tetanus Infections and Vaccines

Diphtheria is a disease that is transmitted by contact with infected respiratory droplets (e.g., coughing and sneezing by the infected person). Symptoms of the disease normally appear from 2 to 5 days after infection. Symptoms include breathing problems resulting from thick mucus covering the back of the throat.

Pertussis is also known as whooping cough because of the traumatic coughing spasms it can cause; a distinctive "whooping" sound is often made by the infected person as air is inspired. Pertussis is a disease of the respiratory tract caused by the bacterium *Bordetella pertussis*. Coughing can be so severe that it is hard to eat, drink, or even breathe. Pertussis may lead to pneumonia and possibly death, especially in infants. Pertussis is an illness that has been increasing in both adults and children, prompting new vaccine development for booster doses in adolescents and adults.

Tetanus is known commonly as lockjaw because the infected person's jaw locks in place as skeletal muscle contraction progresses. Tetanus is acquired through exposure to the bacterium *Clostridium tetani,* which is normally present in soil. Infection can occur through an open wound or deep puncture wound caused by a cut, insect bite, or dirty nails. The symptoms of the disease are due to a neurotoxin produced by the bacteria. Tetanus is not transmitted from person to person. Symptoms include difficulty eating and swallowing because of muscle spasms initially in the jaw; however, if the disease progresses, it can cause generalized seizure-like activity. If left untreated it can cause death.

Vaccines for Diphtheria, Pertussis, and Tetanus Infections. Vaccines for diphtheria, pertussis, and tetanus can be given together in five separate doses. These doses are extended over several years. Children receive doses at 2, 4, 6, and 15 to 18 months, and again at 4 to 6 years. Children older than the age of 7 years should not receive the combination diphtheria, pertussis, and tetanus vaccine; they should receive the diphtheria and tetanus vaccine. Because pertussis spreads easily by coughing and sneezing, older children and adults are advised to obtain a booster shot (e.g., tetanus-pertussis) even though the condition is less severe in these age categories than in young children and infants. The pertussis booster dose in adolescents and adults helps limit the exposure of older persons and young children to the illness. Tetanus boosters must be given every 10 years throughout life to maintain protection against tetanus.

Side effects include fever and soreness at the injection site.

Polio

Polio was once a common disease affecting many persons in America. The main symptom of polio is paralysis of the muscles of the legs and respiratory system. Many children and adults who contracted this disease died. Some who survived had to wear leg braces to help them walk. The oral polio vaccine was developed in the mid-1950s and soon was given to all persons free of charge by placing the liquid vaccine on a sugar tablet. Persons went to nearby schools, where the vaccine was provided for all adults and children. Because of this effective vaccine, polio was eradicated totally from the United States. Unfortunately, we still must immunize against this disease because some countries have not had the same success in eradicating the disease.

Vaccine for Polio. Until recently, oral polio vaccines were routine, but an oral dose has been made with live vaccine and can cause polio in 1 in 2.4 million persons. Today only the injectable form (IPV) is used in U.S. immunization schedules because polio has been essentially eradicated within the United States and the IPV does not carry any risk of active infection. Children should receive the series of four immunizations at 2 months, at 4 months, between 6 and 18 months, and finally a booster between 4 and 6 years of age. Because all children have been administered the polio vaccine since the mid-1950s, most adults do not need to receive it because they already are immunized.

Some soreness at the injection site is common.

Measles, Mumps, and Rubella

Measles is a serious disease that begins with flulike symptoms and fever (Figure 28-2, *A*). If the symptoms are ignored, the disease can progress to a major infection, causing pneumonia, brain damage, or even death. Throughout history, this disease has been responsible for thousands of deaths among both children and adults.

Mumps is a disease that affects the parotid glands (Figure 28-2, *B*). These glands become visibly enlarged, and the disease is accompanied by a fever. Mumps also may cause meningitis and deafness.

Rubella also is known as German measles (Figure 28-2, *C*). This is an acute, mildly contagious viral disease. Symptoms include a 3-day rash and inflammation of the lymph nodes. Normally rubella occurs in children ages 5 to 9,

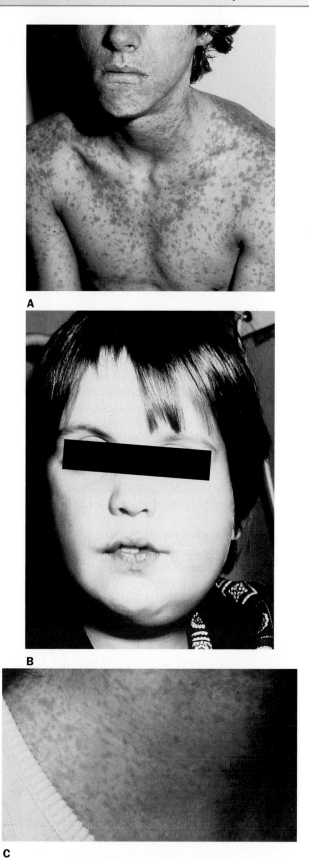

FIGURE 28-2 A, Measles. Symptoms include rash, consisting of both papules and macules, that spreads over the body and lasts 3 to 5 days. **B,** Mumps. Glands become swollen, causing pain when chewing or drinking liquids. Symptoms last approximately 24 hours. **C,** Rubella. Lymph nodes enlarge, and a fine red rash occurs. Symptoms last approximately 2 to 3 days. (From Zitelli BJ, Davis HW: *Atlas of pediatric physical diagnosis,* ed 5, St Louis, 2007, Mosby. **A** and **C,** Courtesy Dr. Michael Sherlock; **B,** Courtesy Dr. G.D.W. McKendrick.)

adolescents, and young adults. The incubation period is 14 to 21 days. It typically presents as a rash on the face (although not always) that may spread to the trunk; other symptoms include headache, malaise, low-grade fever, coryza (upper respiratory tract condition), swelling of the lymph nodes, and in some cases conjunctivitis. In pregnant women, this contagious disease can cause birth defects in the unborn child or even a miscarriage. For this reason, women should be given this vaccine 3 months before becoming pregnant if they have never had rubella. Complications in children are rare and can be treated with an analgesic/antipyretic such as acetaminophen for joint pain and fever.

Vaccine for Measles, Mumps, and Rubella. Immunization against measles, mumps, and rubella is given together as one vaccination (MMR). Normally two vaccinations are administered: the first between 12 and 15 months of age and the second between 4 and 6 years of age.

The most common side effects include fever and rash. In some cases, allergic reactions can cause problems that are more serious; however, these are rare.

Chickenpox

Varicella vaccine is known more commonly as the chickenpox vaccine (Figure 28-3). Adults who never received the chickenpox vaccination (first marketed in 1995) may have contracted chickenpox when they were a child from other children via airborne droplets or by touching the fluid from the skin blisters of infected children. This is a contagious disease, and may cause serious complications in young children. Typical non-serious symptoms include skin blisters, fever, and an itchy rash. Some persons can experience more severe effects, such as brain damage, pneumonia, infection, or (rarely) even death. If chickenpox is contracted by a pregnant female, the disease can be severe and require hospitalization. Also, the same virus that causes chickenpox (varicella-zoster) can remain latent and reappear later as shingles, another significant cause of illness.

Vaccine for Chickenpox. The first dose of the varicella vaccine is recommended between 12 and 18 months of age, and a booster dose is given at 4 to 6 years of age. However, anyone can be given this vaccine, even adults. Persons who should not be vaccinated include pregnant mothers or those who are immunocompromised.

If the disease is contracted through immunization, only a mild form of disease results. After the injection, there can be soreness at the injection site and mild fever.

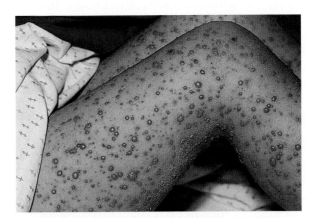

FIGURE 28-3 Chickenpox. Rash begins with macules, which turn into severe papules. Symptoms can last from a few days to 2 weeks. (From Callen JP, et al: *Color atlas of dermatology,* ed 2, Philadelphia, 2000, Saunders.)

This vaccine must be continuously frozen until time of use at −15° C (5° F) or colder.

Herpes Zoster. Another disorder caused by the same virus that causes chickenpox (herpes zoster) is shingles, which may appear in adulthood in a person who had childhood chickenpox. After lying dormant for several years, the virus may become activated and cause acute inflammation of the dorsal root ganglia. Symptoms include painful lesions along the nerves. Treatment for shingles includes medications such as valacyclovir (Valtrex), which can be given orally or intravenously. Acyclovir (Zovirax) also may be used over a 7-day period to reduce pain and promote healing. In 2006 a single-dose vaccine was introduced for adults older than age 60. The vaccine prevented shingles in about half the subjects tested and can reduce the pain associated with this condition. It is given as a single dosage.

HEPATITIS INFECTIONS AND VACCINES

Viral hepatitis is a common systemic disease marked by hepatic (liver) cell destruction. In most patients, hepatic cells eventually regenerate; however, old age and other underlying disorders can make complications more likely to occur. The prognosis is not good if edema and hepatic encephalopathy develop. There are several types of hepatitis forms: types A, B, C, D, E, F, and G. These forms are the result of an infection attributable to a virus. Box 28-3 lists the forms that currently have no vaccine.

Hepatitis A Virus (HAV)

Hepatitis A is caused by contaminated fecal matter that is ingested in food or water. HAV is contagious. The incubation period is short (15 to 45 days) with a rapid, acute onset that often affects children and young adults. Complete recovery is possible for this type of hepatitis.

Vaccine. Although this type of hepatitis is rare, there is a vaccine available. If the infection arises in a non-vaccinated person, immune globulin injection is given to the infected person as well as all persons who have contacted the infected person.

Hepatitis B Virus (HBV)

Hepatitis B has a long incubation period (30 to 180 days) and can affect all age groups. HBV can cause many serious side effects, including diarrhea, vomiting, jaundice, and lack of energy. Infection can lead to liver damage or even death if left untreated. This virus is contagious via blood and body fluids. Hepatitis B can be contracted by having unprotected sex, sharing syringes, or being stuck with an infected needle. The virus also can be transferred from the mother to the newborn at birth. The incubation period for HBV is between 45 and 180 days; after this time it becomes infectious.

BOX 28-3 HEPATITIS INFECTIONS WITH NO AVAILABLE VACCINES

Hepatitis E: Caused by food or water infected with fecal matter; a vaccine has been in development because of its worldwide prevalence as a source of hepatitis infection
Hepatitis F: A rare form of hepatitis that has a rapid and severe onset of pain
Hepatitis G: Transmitted via blood from transfusions, hemodialysis, or IV drug users; causes mild symptoms

Vaccine. The vaccine for hepatitis B is given in a series of three to four doses depending on the age at which the initial dose is given. Newborns receive their first immunization soon after birth. The second dose is given about 1 month after the first. The third is given at 4 months, followed by the last dose when the child is approximately 6 months old.

Usual side effects of the hepatitis B vaccine include soreness at the injection site and sometimes a slight fever.

Active Treatment. Chronic disease is treated with antiretroviral medications, such as adefovir, entecavir, lamivudine, and tenofovir.

Hepatitis C Virus (HCV)

Hepatitis C accounts for about 20% of all viral hepatitis and for most post-transfusion cases. Many people infected with hepatitis C show no symptoms for years. In fact, symptoms may not occur until there is already cirrhosis of the liver. HCV is typically transmitted by contacting infected blood, receiving an infected blood transfusion (before 1992, blood was not screened for HCV), or sharing needles or straws (for snorting drugs) between drug users. A less common way of transmission is by sexual intercourse or via sharing of personal items (toothbrush, razor) with an infected person; it is also possible to acquire HCV by being born to an infected mother. Those patients on long-term kidney dialysis also seem to have an increased risk.

Vaccine. No vaccine is currently available for HCV.

Active Treatment. Two drugs are used to treat hepatitis C: an injectable agent called peginterferon alfa-2a (Pegasys) and an oral agent called ribavirin, which is taken twice daily. The goal of these medications is to inhibit the hepatitis virus, reducing liver inflammation and preventing scarring and fibrosis. Patients must avoid alcohol when taking these medications.

Hepatitis D Virus (HDV)

Hepatitis D has a rapid onset (4 to 12 weeks on average). People infected with hepatitis D are contagious early in the incubation period. HDV occurs only concurrently with hepatitis B infection and is transmitted in the same manner as HBV.

Vaccine. The only way to avoid HDV is through vaccination with the HBV series.

OTHER VIRUSES AND VACCINES

Human Papillomavirus

Human papillomavirus (HPV) is common around the world and affects both genders. There are 100 types of HPV. It is estimated that approximately 50% of sexually active persons will contract HPV at some time. The CDC reports that nearly 2.6 million persons are diagnosed yearly with HPV. The most vulnerable age category is females in their teens up to the early twenties. Certain strains of this virus can cause cervical cancer and genital warts.

Vaccine. The vaccines (i.e., Gardasil and Cervarix) are used in females between the ages of 9 and 26 years. The best time to receive the vaccine is before any sexual activity is initiated. Gardasil is given in three injections over a 6-month period—the second injection is given 2 months after the first and the final injection is given 6 months after the first. This provides protection against four types of HPV that are responsible for 70% of the cases of cervical cancer and 90% of the cases of genital warts. The only side effect is brief soreness at the injection site. The vaccine is not safe in pregnant women. Research on a vaccine for older women (>26 years) is being explored at this time. In 2010, the Gardisil regimen was approved for use in boys and men 9 years of age and older to reduce the incidence of genital warts.

Pneumonia

Pneumococcal conjugate vaccine is given for *Streptococcus pneumoniae,* which causes pneumonia and meningitis. This serious disease still affects children, causing pneumonia, brain damage, and death. Children younger than the age of 5 years are at the highest risk for this bacterial infection, as are the elderly.

Vaccine. The vaccine results in immunity for 3 years, and it is given in three doses spaced at 2, 4, and 6 months and a fourth dose between 12 and 15 months of age. Older children who might be at high risk of infection also can be given the vaccine. The total number of doses may vary. Older children and adults can receive another type of vaccine to protect them from meningitis and pneumonia—pneumococcal polysaccharide vaccine.

Side effects include redness or tenderness at the injection site, and some children have a slight fever.

Haemophilus influenzae Type B

The *Haemophilus influenzae* type B vaccine is given to prevent the bacterial infection *Haemophilus influenzae* type B. Children younger than 5 years can contract this bacterial infection from other children or adults. The symptoms can be mild if the infection remains in the nose or throat. However, the infection may spread into the lungs. Pneumonia, meningitis, brain damage, and infection of the entire body (known as systemic infection) can occur, and death can result. Children and infants less than 5 years old are most at risk for serious disease; serious disease from this organism is rare after these ages.

Vaccine. A series of four shots is given to children at 2, 4, and 6 months and between 12 and 15 months of age.

Common side effects include redness and swelling at the injection site and sometimes a fever.

Influenza

Flu vaccines are popular because they effectively protect various groups of persons who are at higher risk of becoming ill with influenza. The common months of transmittance of influenza (in the United States and other areas of the northern hemisphere) are between October and April each year. For best coverage persons should be immunized as soon as the vaccine becomes available in the fall (as early as September). The vaccines are approximately 90% effective at reducing serious influenza disease.

Vaccines. In 2003 the Food and Drug Administration approved a new intranasal spray vaccine containing cold-adapted live virus (FluMist). This vaccine allows the virus to grow in the cooler temperature of the nasal mucosa but not the warmer temperature of the body, so it cannot produce influenza pneumonia. Mild side effects such as runny nose, nasal congestion, headache, sore throat, chills, and cough may occur for a few days. The intranasal live influenza vaccine can be used only on healthy children over 5 years and adults up to age 49 years. Others who should not receive the live vaccine are those who are immunosuppressed, pregnant women, and those with a chronic condition such as asthma, diabetes, or cardiovascular disorders. In addition to these individuals, the nasal spray vaccine should be avoided in health care workers and other persons who may come into contact with immunocompromised individuals. According to the Centers for Disease Control and Prevention, the only influenza vaccine that can be given to persons 50 years and older is the killed trivalent influenza vaccine (the flu "shot").

The inactivated (killed) trivalent vaccine (Fluvin and Fluzone, the flu "shot") can be injected intramuscularly. Side effects found with this vaccine are soreness at the injection site, fever, myalgia, and malaise. The Fluzone vaccine is available in a pediatric version that can be given to children 6 to 23 months of age. The vaccine is also safe for ages from 2 years to those older than 50 years of age. Other persons who can receive this injectable vaccine safely include health care workers, caregivers, nursing mothers, and pregnant women after the first trimester. Neither type of influenza vaccine can be given to infants less than 6 months old or to persons with a history of egg allergy or a history of Guillain-Barré syndrome.

Swine Flu (H1N1)

In 2009 a new influenza virus appeared that was very different from previous human seasonal influenza viruses. By late summer of 2009 the World Health Organization (WHO) recognized the virus as a pandemic because it had spread to many countries. The virus is transmitted by inhaling infected airborne droplets that have been expelled by coughing or sneezing. Symptoms are similar to those experienced with seasonal influenza, including fever, cough, headache, muscle and joint pain, sore throat, runny nose, and sometimes diarrhea. The virus has also caused severe illness and deaths, especially in high-risk groups such as those with preexisting conditions such as cardiovascular and respiratory disease, diabetes, and cancer. Pregnant women also seem to have an increased risk for a more severe type of infection, especially those in the second and third trimesters. To prevent the transfer of this virus, the following actions are recommended: cover mouth and nose when coughing and/or sneezing, stay at home when or if symptoms appear, wash hands regularly, and avoid crowded areas if possible.

Vaccine. The following groups are recommended to receive the H1N1 vaccination:

- Pregnant women
- Household contacts and caregivers for children younger than 6 months of age
- Health care and emergency medical service personnel
- All people from 6 months to 24 years of age
- Persons 25 years through 64 years who have health conditions associated with higher risk of medical complications from influenza

Although these persons should be vaccinated first (because of the higher risk of infection), the vaccine should be made available to all persons over the age of 65 and others who are at lower risk.

When the H1N1 strain is likely to be circulated, future yearly influenza vaccines will incorporate protection against the strain into the annual flu regimen.

PASSIVE IMMUNITY

Immune globulins are different from vaccines because they are not prepared in a laboratory, but must be obtained from a human or animal donor. γ-Globulins contain antibodies that can be passed to the recipient, giving the recipient

TABLE 28-6 Types of Vaccines

Vaccine	Organism	Recommendation
Cholera	*Vibrio cholerae*	Persons living or traveling to endemic areas where disease occurs; military
Plague	*Yersinia pestis*	Persons protecting against wild rodents in endemic areas; military
Yellow fever	*Flavivirus*	Persons living in or traveling to endemic areas; military
Anthrax	*Bacillus anthracis*	Military only at this time

passive immunity. Immune globulins are administered for immediate protection against a specific virus. Compared to **active immunity**, passive immunity has a shorter duration of protection. Examples of common globulins are the following:

- Cytomegalovirus immune globulin
- γ-Globulin
- Hepatitis B immune globulin
- Tetanus immune globulin
- Varicella-zoster immune globulin

TRAVEL MEDICINE AND IMMUNIZATIONS

Many adults receive immunizations when they are planning to travel outside of the United States. The U.S. military immunizes all troops against the 12 top **contagions** that exist across the world. On a smaller scale, persons who are traveling to foreign countries often get specific vaccines to guard against contagions common to the area of interest. Other persons who may need a specific vaccine are scientists, researchers, those who work in close contact with a disease (such as those caring for laboratory animals), or those who live in regions that are likely to have an epidemic outbreak. Table 28-6 lists the types of vaccines available and explains when they should be administered.

ANTITOXINS AND ANTIVENINS

Antitoxins and antivenins are yet another form of passive immunity that can provide short-term, immediate protection from serious symptoms. These agents contain antibodies that can neutralize dangerous toxins. For example, stepping on a rusty nail may allow the pathogen *Clostridium tetani* to enter through the wound and pass into the bloodstream, where it may develop into the dangerous condition called tetanus. By administration of the tetanus antitoxin, the victim can be protected against this life-threatening condition. Antivenins are also given to counteract poison from creatures such as snakes and spiders. Common antitoxins include those for diphtheria, rabies, and botulism. Common antivenins include antivenin for the black widow spider (*Latrodectus mactans*) and Crotalidae polyvalent antivenin for rattlesnake venom.

STORAGE OF VACCINES

The Centers for Disease Control and Prevention have guidelines on the storage of vaccines in order to preserve their effectiveness. Most vaccines should be kept at temperatures between 2° and 8° C (i.e., between 36° and 46° F), but some require freezing until the time of use. For example, the cold-adaptive FluMist (an intranasal live influenza vaccine) can be frozen if packed in a specially made

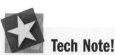

Tech Note!

Adults also need immunizations to confer immunity to communicable diseases. Many vaccinations routinely given in childhood may also be used in adults needing immunity to specific diseases. Information regarding vaccine schedules for adults can be found at the CDC website www.immunize.org/catg.d/p2011.pdf.

TABLE 28-7 Examples of Biological/Immune Therapies

Generic Name	Trade Name	Indication
Immunostimulants		
etanercept	Enbrel	Crohn's disease, psoriasis, rheumatoid arthritis
interferon alfa-2b	Intron A	Hairy cell leukemia, hepatitis, Kaposi's sarcoma
anakinra	Kineret	Rheumatoid arthritis
infliximab	Remicade	Crohn's disease, rheumatoid arthritis, psoriasis ankylosing spondylitis, ulcerative colitis
erlotinib	Tarceva	Pancreatic cancer, metastatic non–small cell lung cancer
gefitinib	Iressa	Head and neck cancers, non–small cell lung cancer
Immunosuppressives		
cyclosporine	Sandimmune	Transplant rejections, rheumatoid arthritis, severe psoriasis
tacrolimus	Prograf, Protopic	Organ rejections, severe psoriasis, atopic dermatitis (ointment)
auranofin	Ridaura	Rheumatoid arthritis, psoriatic arthritis

Tech Note!

Tuberculosis vaccine is routinely administered in many countries, such as the Philippines. Pharmacy technicians should be tested annually for exposure to tuberculosis. Although there is a vaccine for tuberculosis, it is not used in the United States because a tuberculosis vaccine does not guarantee immunity. If a vaccine is given, antibodies are developed against the antigen; therefore all tuberculosis tests would show positive results and a chest x-ray film would be necessary to rule out active tuberculosis. Chapter 18 discusses the microbe that causes tuberculosis.

Tech Alert!

Remember these sound-alike/look-alike drugs:

cyclosporine versus cycloserine or cyclophosphamide
interleukin-2 versus interferon-2
erlotinib versus gefitinib
Ridaura versus Cardura
Protopic versus Protonix, Protopam, or Protropin

freeze box (32° F) issued by the manufacturer. Varicella vaccine must be kept frozen until time of use.

IMMUNE THERAPIES

Immune therapy, also known as biological therapy or biotherapy, is an effective form of treatment for persons with specific conditions. Depending on the type of condition affecting the patient, certain biological response modifiers (BRMs) may be able to suppress or stimulate the immune system.

The body normally produces small amounts of BRMs that respond to infections and/or a disease. Scientists have been able to synthesize large amounts of BRMs in the laboratory. These then can be used in the treatment, for example, of cancer, rheumatoid arthritis, and Crohn's disease, and in the prevention of organ rejection following transplant surgery.

This type of therapy is not without side effects such as loss of appetite, nausea, vomiting, and diarrhea. Other effects include fever, chills, and muscle aches. If side effects are severe, the patient may be admitted into the hospital for the course of the treatment. The good news is that these side effects usually are present only for the duration of treatment.

Table 28-7 gives a brief list of examples of biologic/immunologic medications used, along with their indications.

SPECIAL SITUATIONS FOR VACCINATION—PREGNANCY

Pregnancy can pose unique challenges to vaccination, given the risks of contraction of the illness by both mother and baby. If a pregnant mother should contract hepatitis, there is a high risk of transmitting the disease to the fetus. Therefore physicians weigh the potential risk of the mother contracting the disease from the vaccine and causing damage to the fetus against the possibility of catching the disease if the vaccine is not given. Vaccines such as diphtheria and tetanus, hepatitis B, and influenza may be given to high-risk women. If a mother has not been given the rubella vaccine previously, she must wait until the child is born before receiving the vaccine because of the risk of contracting a mild case of rubella, which could be harmful to the fetus.

DO YOU REMEMBER THESE KEY POINTS?

- The various types of immunity
- The way in which vaccines are produced
- The names of vaccines that require several series
- The side effects of vaccines
- The common childhood diseases
- The diseases each immunization covers
- The major types of adult immunizations that are given and why they are available
- The location in the pharmacy where most vaccines are kept
- The diseases that can be prevented from vaccinations

REVIEW QUESTIONS

Multiple choice questions

1. The most common side effects from vaccinations are:
- A. Fever
- B. Soreness at the injection site
- C. Vomiting
- D. Both A and B

2. The vaccine given to protect against *Streptococcus pneumoniae* is:
- A. *Haemophilus influenzae* type B vaccine
- B. Varicella-zoster vaccine
- C. Pneumococcal conjugate vaccine
- D. None of the above

3. Shingles is related to the childhood disease:
- A. Measles
- B. Mumps
- C. Rubella
- D. Chickenpox

4. Vaccines can protect human beings against all of the following organisms EXCEPT:
- A. Viruses
- B. Fungi
- C. Bacteria
- D. All of the above

5. The two basic types of immunity are:
- A. Bacterial and viral
- B. Live and inactive
- C. Active and inactive
- D. Active and passive

6. Vaccines can be altered by which of the following ways?
- A. Attenuated or weakened
- B. Inactivated or killed
- C. Attenuated or activated
- D. A and B

7. When the body comes into contact with a contagious disease, it causes:
- A. Antibodies to be produced
- B. Antigens to be produced
- C. A body rash
- D. No reaction

8. Which of these statements is true concerning toxoids?
- A. Toxoids are bacterial toxins that have been inactivated.
- B. All bacterial vaccines are toxoids.
- C. Both A and B are true.
- D. None of the above is true.

9. Vaccines that are composed of small pieces of genetic code harvested from bacteria or yeast are:
   A. Acellular vaccines
   B. Conjugated vaccines
   C. Subunit vaccines
   D. Toxoid vaccines

10. Most adults need vaccines for all of these reasons, EXCEPT:
    A. They never got them as children
    B. They are in the military
    C. They are health care workers
    D. Adults need vaccines for any of the above reasons

True/False

If the statement is false, then change it to make it true.

_____ **1.** The thymus helps provide immunity.

_____ **2.** Most vaccinations have no side effects.

_____ **3.** Hospital technicians must have an annual tuberculosis test.

_____ **4.** Polio vaccine is given routinely in an oral form rather than by injection.

_____ **5.** Hepatitis B is a serious condition affecting the kidneys.

_____ **6.** Pertussis vaccine normally is combined with diphtheria and tetanus vaccines.

_____ **7.** Attenuated vaccines often can give protection for a lifetime.

_____ **8.** Tetanus vaccine should be given every 5 years.

_____ **9.** When vaccines are injected, antibodies are produced by the body to fight the injected antigens.

_____ **10.** Many Third World countries do not immunize children.

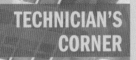

TECHNICIAN'S CORNER Visit the website of the Centers for Disease Control and Prevention at www.cdc.gov and print the most recent list of suggested immunizations for children and adults.

BIBLIOGRAPHY

Gardner P, Pabbatireddy S: Vaccines for women age 50 and older. Emerging Infectious Diseases 10(11). Retrieved 11/05, from www.cdc.ogv/nicdod/EID/wol10no11/04-0469.htm.

McKenry L, Salerno E: *Mosby's pharmacology in nursing*, ed 22, St Louis, 2005, Mosby.

Nathan JP, Rosenberg JM: Who should get the flu vaccine and who shouldn't? *Drug Topics* 147:28, 2003.

National Immunization Program: HPV vaccine. 8/02/06. Retrieved 11/06 from www.cdc.gov/nip/vaccine/hpv/hpv-facts.htm.

Tortora G, Funke B, Case C: *Microbiology: an introduction*, ed 8, Redwood City, 2003, Benjamin Cummings.

WEBSITES

MMR information: www.who.int/en/
H1N1 vaccine. www.cdc.gov/h1n1flu/vaccination/acip.htm
www.cdc.gov
www.ncbi.nlm.nih.gov
www.vaccineinjury.org
www.webmd.com
www.cdc.gov/vaccines/pubs/vis/default.htm#mening

Oncology Agents

Objectives

UPON COMPLETING THIS CHAPTER, YOU SHOULD BE ABLE TO DO
THE FOLLOWING:

- List both trade and generic drug names covered in this chapter.

- List common types of cancer.

- Describe how cancer spreads.

- Describe the methods used to diagnose cancer.

- Explain the method of action for each classification of drugs listed
  in this chapter.

- Define oncology terms.

- Describe the stages of normal cell reproduction.

- List the types of agents that are vesicants and the precautions
  technicians need to take when preparing them.

- Describe the most common side effects of chemotherapy.

- List the treatments used in fighting cancer.

- Differentiate between acute lymphocytic leukemia and
  myelogenous leukemia.

- Describe how nuclear medicine is used in oncology.

TERMS AND DEFINITIONS

Antineoplastic *An agent used to prevent the development, proliferation, or growth of neoplastic cells; a medication used in treatment of abnormal cells*

Benign *A tumor or growth that is not life-threatening*

Biopsy *A procedure in which a piece of tissue is removed from a patient for examination and diagnosis; the tissue is a sample of the whole*

Bolus *A single dose of drug*

Cancer *A general term used to describe malignant neoplasms or tumors*

Carcinogen *A substance or chemical that can increase the risk of developing cancer*

Chemotherapy *The treatment of a disease with toxic chemical substances to slow the disease process or to kill cells*

Deoxyribonucleic acid (DNA) *The complex nucleic acids that are bases for genetic continuance*

Invasive *The tendency for a tumor or mass to move into tissues and/or organs in proximity; when referred to as invasive surgery, cutting through skin is performed*

Lymphoma *A term used to describe a malignant disorder of lymphoid tissue*

Malignant *An invasive and destructive pattern of rapid, abnormal cell growth; often fatal*

Melanoma *A malignant neoplasm of the pigmented cells of skin; it may metastasize to other organs*

Metastasis *The movement or spread of cancerous cells through the body to organs in distant areas*

Mitosis *Cellular reproduction that creates two identical daughter cells from the DNA of the parent cell*

Mortality *Death; being susceptible to death*

Mortality rate *The number of deaths that occur in a specific time period*

Mutation *An unexpected change in the molecular structure within the DNA, causing a permanent change in cells*

Neoplasm *An abnormal tissue growth*

Oncogene *A gene that when mutated or expressed at high levels can help transform a normal cell into a cancerous one*

Oncologist *A specialist in the area of cancer and cancer treatment*

PCA *Patient-controlled analgesia*

Remission *The span of time during which a disease, such as cancer, is not spreading and may even be diminished or cured; this may be permanent or temporary*

Stage *Describes the extent of cancer within the body and its distribution to other areas*

Survival rate (absolute) *The number of patients still alive after diagnosis within a certain period; normally based on 5 years after diagnosis (when cancer statistics are reported)*

CHEMOTHERAPEUTIC AGENTS

Trade Name	Generic Name	Pronunciation
Abraxane	albumin-bound paclitaxel	(al-**bue**-men-bound-pack-lee-**tax**-el)
Adriamycin	doxorubicin	(dox-oh-**ru**-bi-sin)
Adrucil	fluorouracil, 5-FU	(flure-oh-**your**-a-sil)
Afinitor	everolimus	(**e**-ver-**oh**-li-mus)
Alkeran	melphalan	(**mel**-fa-lan)
Alimta	pemetrexed	(pem-e-**trex**-ed)
Arranon	nelarabine	(nel-**ar**-a-been)
BiCNU	carmustine, BCNU	(kar-**mus**-teen)
Blenoxane	bleomycin	(blee-oh-**my**-sin)
Busulfex	busulfan	(byoo-**sul**-fan)
Camptosar	irinotecan	(eye-rih-no-**tee**-can)
Carac, Efudex	fluorouracil topical	(**floor**-oh-**ure**-a-sil)
CeeNU	lomustine, CCNU	(low-**mus**-ten)
Cerubidine	daunorubicin	(daw-**now**-roo-bi-sin)
Clolar	clofarabine	(kloe-**far**-a-been)
Cosmegen	dactinomycin	(**dak**-tin-oh-**mye**-sin)
Cytosar-U	cytarabine	(sye-**tare**-ah-bean)
Cytoxan	cyclophosphamide	(sye-kloe-**fos**-fah-mide)
DaunoXome	liposomal daunorubicin	(daw-**noe**-roo-bi-sin)
DepoCyt	liposomal cytarabine	(sye-**tare**-ah-bean)
Doxil	liposomal doxorubicin	(dox-oh-**roo**-bi-sin)
Droxia	hydroxyurea	(hy-drox-ee-yoo-**ree**-uh)
DTIC-Dome	dacarbazine	(da-**carb**-ah-zine)
Ellence	epirubicin	(**ep**-i-**roo**-bi-sin)
Eloxatin	oxaliplatin	(ox-**al**-ih-**pla**-tin)
Emcyt	estramustine	(**es**-tra-**mus**-teen)
Fludara	fludarabine	(flew-**dare**-ah-been)
FUDR	floxuridine	(flox-**yoor**-eye-deen)
Gemzar	gemcitabine	(gem-**sit**-ah-been)
Gleevec	imatinib	(im-**ma**-ta-nib)
Gliadel Wafer	carmustine, BiCNU	(car-**muh**-steen)
Hexalen	altretamine	(all-**treh**-tah-mean)
Hycamtin	topotecan	(toe-po-**tee**-can)
Hydrea	hydroxyurea	(high-drox-ee-yoo-**ree**-uh)
Idamycin	idarubicin	(eye-da-**roo**-bi-sin)
Ifex	ifosfamide	(i-**fos**-fa-myde)
Iressa	gefitinib	(gee-**fi**-ti-nib)
Ixempra	ixabepilone	(**ix**-ab-**ep**-i-lone)
Leukeran	chlorambucil	(klor-**am**-byoo-sil)
Leustatin	cladribine	(**klad**-ri-been)
Lysodren	mitotane	(**mye**-toe-tane)
Matulane	procarbazine	(pro-**kar**-ba-zeen)
Methotrex	methotrexate	(meth-oh-**trex**-ate)
Mustargen	mechlorethamine	(me-klor-**eh**-tha-meen)
Mutamycin	mitomycin	(mye-toe-**my**-sin)
Myleran	busulfan	(byoo-**sul**-fan)
Mylocel	hydroxyurea	(hy-drox-ee-yoo-**ree**-uh)
Navelbine	vinorelbine	(vin-**nor**-ell-been)
Nipent	pentostatin	(pen-toe-**sta**-tin)
Novantrone	mitoxantrone	(mi-to-**zan**-trone)
Oncovin	vincristine	(vin-**kris**-teen)
Onxol	paclitaxel	(pak-li-**tak**-sel)
Paraplatin	carboplatin	(**car**-bow-pla-tin)

Trade Name	Generic Name	Pronunciation
Platinol	cisplatin	(**sis**-pla-tin)
Purinethol	mercaptopurine	(mer-kap-toe-**pur**-een)
Targretin	bexarotene	(beks-**air**-oh-teen)
Taxol	paclitaxel	(**pak**-li-**tax**-el)
Taxotere	docetaxel	(doc-e-**tax**-el)
Tabloid	thioguanine	(thye-oh-**gwah**-neen)
Temodar	temozolomide	(**tem**-oh-**zoe**-loe-mide)
Thioplex	thiotepa	(**thye**-oh-**tep**-a)
Toposar	etoposide	(**eh**-toe-**poh**-side)
Treanda	bendamustine	(**ben**-da-**mus**-teen)
Trexall	methotrexate	(meth-oh-**trex**-ate)
Valstar	valrubicin	(val-**roo**-bi-sin)
Velban	vinblastine	(vin-**blas**-teen)
VePesid	etoposide	(e-teh-**poh**-side)
Vesanoid	tretinoin	(**tret**-i-noin)
Vidaza	azacitidine	(ay-za-**sye**-ti-deen)
Vincasar	vincristine	(vin-**kris**-teen)
Vumon	teniposide	(ten-nye-**poe**-side)
Xeloda	capecitabine	(**kap**-e-**sye**-ta-been)
Zanosar	streptozocin	(strep-toe-**zoe**-sin)
Zolinza	vorinostat	(vor-**in**-o-stat)

Monoclonal Antibodies
Avastin	bevacizumab	(bev-a-**ciz**-oo-mab)
Bexxar	tositumomab/ iodine-131	(tos-**it**-too-moe-mab)
Campath	alemtuzumab	(al-em-**tooz**-oo-mab)
Erbitux	cetuximab	(se-**tux**-i-mab)
Herceptin	trastuzumab	(tras-**too**-zoo-mab)
Rituxan	rituximab	(ri-**tuk**-si-mab)
Vectibix	panitumumab	(pan-i-**tue**-moo-mab)
Zevalin	ibritumomab/tiuexetan	(eye-bri-**toom**-oh-mab)

Immune Response Modifier
Aldara	imiquimod	(i-**mi**-kwi-mod)

Antiangiogenesis Agent
Thalomid	thalidomide	(tha-**lid**-o-mide)

Fusion Protein
Ontak	denileukin diftitox	(de-ni-**loo**-kin **dif**-ti-toks)

Signal Transduction Inhibitors
Gleevec	imatinib	(im-**ma**-ta-nib)
Nexavar	sorafenib	(sor-a-**fen**-ib)
Sprycel	dasatinib	(da-**sat**-in-ib)
Sutent	sunitinib	(soo-**nit**-in-ib)
Tarceva	erlotinib	(er-**loe**-ti-nib)
Tasigna	nilotinib	(nye-**loe**-ti-nib)
Tykerb	lapatinib	(la-**pa**-tin-ib)
Velcade	bortezomib	(bor-**tez**-oh-mib)

Alpha-Interferon
Intron-A	interferon alfa-2b	(**in**-ter-**fear**-on **al**-fa)

Interleukin
Proleukin	aldesleukin, IL-2	(**al**-des-**loo**-kin)

CONTROLLED OPIOID ANALGESICS COMMONLY USED FOR CANCER PAIN

Trade Name	Generic Name	Pronunciation	Trade Name	Generic Name	Pronunciation
Codeine	codeine	(**koe**-deen)	OxyContin	oxycodone	(ox-e-**koe**-done)
Demerol	meperidine	(me-**pear**-eye-deen)	Percocet	oxycodone/	(ox-e-**koe**-done/a-sea-tah-
Dilaudid	hydromorphone	(hye-droe-**mor**-fone)		acetaminophen	**men**-oh-phen)
Duragesic	fentanyl	(**phen**-tah-nill)	Percodan	oxycodone/aspirin	(ox-e-**koe**-done/**ass**-peh-rin)
Duramorph	morphine sulfate	(**mor**-feen **sul**-fate)	Vicodin	hydrocodone/	(hye-droe-**koe**-done/a-sea-
Hycodan	hydrocodone	(hye-droe-**koe**-done)		acetaminophen	tah-**men**-oh-phen)
Lorcet	hydrocodone/	(hye-droe-**koe**-done/a-sea-	Vicoprofen	hydrocodone/	(hye-droe-**koe**-done/eye-bu-
	acetaminophen	tah-**men**-oh-phen)		ibuprofen	**pro**-fen)

NOT LONG AGO the diagnosis of **cancer** meant certain death. A sense of hopelessness was associated with a cancer diagnosis, partially because of the lack of understanding of the cancer process, but also because of the sparse number of treatments available. Over the past decade, much progress has been made, including better understanding of the human genome, stem cells, and proteins as well as the development of many innovations in cancer treatment. As a result of this progress, new agents have been developed that can be used to treat specific types of cancers.

This chapter discusses the process by which cancer develops, the manner and location(s) of cancer **metastasis** (i.e., spreading or growing), and the medications used to treat some of the most common cancers. Common side effects from chemotherapeutic agents and other cancer therapies also are described. Much of the information pertaining to the preparation of chemotherapeutic agents is found in Chapter 12.

Cancer can strike any area of the body. The incidence of certain common cancers, such as skin cancer and leukemia, may be decreased. However, even with all the advancements that have occurred, the prevention of cancer is not an exact science.

One of the frustrating aspects of headline news stories regarding cancer is the continuous inference that every conceivable food product or eating habit may lead to cancer. In reality, moderation appears to be a key component in protection from cancer, both in the food we ingest and in the substances to which we are exposed. However, two factors that can increase the likelihood of cancer are environment and genetics. At this point in time the genetic factor cannot be altered. Although much research and testing are being done by geneticists to modify genes, gene therapy is currently not a treatment for cancer. In the meantime, the most effective way to fight cancer is to lessen the risk by treating the body in a responsible manner and by following preventive measures, such as self-examination and routine visits to the physician.

What Is Cancer?

Under normal circumstances, cells within the body proliferate, especially in the intestinal epithelium and within the bone marrow. Our body constantly replicates cells to replace old or damaged cells or to increase the cell population. The normal life cycle of cells is required if the body is to remain in homeostasis (equilibrium). Cells normally follow a set of steps. An important step, in addition to replication of new cells, is their eventual death. If control of cellular

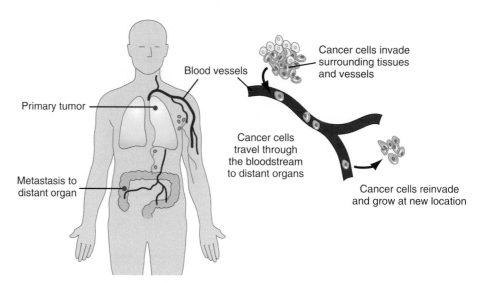

FIGURE 29-1 Metastasis of cancer. Diagram shows how lung cancer may metastasize to other areas of the body.

proliferation malfunctions, the cells grow much faster than normal and do not stop reproducing. This may cause tumors to form and eventually spread to other areas of the body (Figure 29-1).

Benign tumors are noncancerous and do not disperse throughout the body system. Tumors that grow and spread are referred to as **malignant** tumors, or simply referred to as cancer. A cancer tumor has three main characteristics: (1) it grows aggressively and the growth is not limited, (2) it invades surrounding tissues, and (3) it may metastasize (spread to other body areas). For example, if a patient is diagnosed with a **melanoma** (type of skin cancer) and it continues to grow, it may metastasize (spread) and colonize at new sites within the body.

It is important for the patient to participate in his or her cancer treatment; understanding the options, getting a second opinion, and continually reading educational materials can help the patient cope with the disease. The outcome of cancer treatments is determined by the **stage** at which it is diagnosed, the type of treatment prescribed, and the genetics and, notably, the attitude of the patient. There are many terms used specifically when discussing cancer; some of these terms are listed below.

MEDICAL TERMINOLOGY

Prefixes	
Neo-	New
Cyto-	Cell
Malign-	Bad/harmful
Onco-	Mass or tumor
Chemo-	Chemicals

Suffixes	
-ologist	Specialist
-ectomy	Surgical removal
-oma	Tumor
-emia	Blood

MEDICAL TERMINOLOGY—cont'd

Combining forms and terms	
Aden/o	Gland
Blast/o	Immature stage of development
Carcin/o	Cancer
Immun/o	Immune system
Leuk/o	White
Lymph/o	Lymph glands
Melan/o	Black
Sarc/o	Connective tissue, flesh, or muscle

Conditions	
Adenoma	Benign tumor of a gland
Carcinoma	Malignant tumor in epithelial tissue that tends to infiltrate other tissues and metastasize
Hodgkin's lymphoma	One of the types of lymphoma—cancer of lymphatic system
Kaposi's sarcoma	Rare cancerous tumors of/on skin, mucous membranes, lymph nodes, and internal organs; most commonly occurs in patients with AIDS
Leukemia	Cancer that starts in blood-forming tissue such as bone marrow and causes large numbers of blood cells to be produced and enter bloodstream; there are several variants
Myeloma	Cancerous tumor composed of blood-forming tissues of bone marrow
Myoma	Cancerous tumor of muscle
Neuroma	Benign tumor consisting of nerve tissues

What Causes Cancer?

The three different risk factors that may influence the rate of cancer (in addition to genetics) are environmental contaminants, radiation, and viruses. Many different environmental contaminants, known as **carcinogens**, can cause cancer. For example, cigarette smoking may cause cancer because of the many additives contained in tobacco that have been isolated, tested, and proved to cause cancer in laboratory animals. Another causative agent of cancer is radiation. Any type of radiation that breaks the bonds of **deoxyribonucleic acid** (DNA) can lead to **mutations**. For example, radiation in the form of sunlight or x-rays may lead to mutations that cause the cell to alter its DNA, potentially forming versions that promote cancerous cell growth if the body is sufficiently exposed. Other types of carcinogens (i.e., cancer-causing agents) include radioactive materials, asbestos, coal, soot, and certain dyes. Viruses are also responsible for certain forms of cancer. Viruses replicate by using the components of their host. The host is the person who has contracted the virus. The virus inserts itself into human DNA and creates proteins from the host's DNA to build new virions. The normal genes are affected by the virus, and the newly mutated genes are referred to as **oncogenes**. Oncogenes are small pieces of genes that are normally present in cells and that are not dangerous unless they are not inactivated through normal reactions. The following list provides some of the possible factors that may increase the risk of cancer:

- Aging
- Tobacco use
- Sunlight
- Ionizing radiation

- Certain chemicals and other substances
- Some viruses and bacteria
- Certain hormones
- Family history of cancer (genetics)
- Alcohol use
- Poor diet, lack of physical activity, or being overweight

Types of Cancer

More than 100 known cancers affect the human body. The stage of a cancer's growth is used to determine the treatment prescribed. **Invasiveness** refers to the cancer's tendency to spread; some cancers grow very slowly while others grow rapidly. Many cancers are named after the area of origination; the cancers listed in Box 29-1 describe the five main areas where they occur. Table 29-1 presents an in-depth look at common forms of cancer.

Text continued on page 976.

BOX 29-1 TYPES OF CANCER AND WHERE THEY OCCUR

Carcinoma: Originates in the skin or in tissues lining organs
Sarcoma: Found in bone, fat, muscle, cartilage, blood vessels, and associated tissues
Leukemia: Starts in the bone marrow, where blood cells are made, and then travels into the bloodstream
Lymphoma: May occur anywhere in the lymph system or in other organs that create immune cells
CNS cancer: Starts in the brain and/or spinal cord

TABLE 29-1 Types of Cancer

Types of Cancer	Location of Organ or Parts of Organ Where Cancer May Occur	Symptoms*	Traditional Treatments Include	Additional Treatments and/or Comments
Adrenal cortical carcinoma	Adrenal glands, located above kidneys	Weight loss, edema, excess facial or body hair in women, pain	Surgery, radiation therapy, chemotherapy	Mitotane blocks glands from making hormones and destroys cancer; 80% of patients benefit from this drug
Anal cancer	Anus is about 1.5 inches long; starts at end of large intestine and runs to outside of body	Bleeding or itching around anus, pain in anal area, change in width of stool (may be more narrow), abnormal discharge	Surgery, radiation therapy, chemotherapy	Most common treatment is CRT,[†] when surgery is omitted
Bile duct cancer	Bile duct is thin tube (4-5 inches long) that extends from liver to small intestine	Jaundice, itching, abdominal pain, weight loss, light-colored stools or dark urine, N/V	Surgery, radiation therapy, chemotherapy	If cancer cannot be removed, liver transplant may be option, although it is rare

TABLE 29-1 Types of Cancer—cont'd

Types of Cancer	Location of Organ or Parts of Organ Where Cancer May Occur	Symptoms*	Traditional Treatments Include	Additional Treatments and/or Comments
Bladder cancer	Bladder is located below kidneys and ureters; cancer affects outside layers of bladder	Blood in urine, changes in bladder habits, such as urge to urinate but cannot urinate or frequent urination (both symptoms are indicative of many noncancerous conditions)	Surgery, immunotherapy, radiation therapy, chemotherapy	Intravesical therapy: BCG (bacteria) is an example of immunotherapy; agent is placed into bladder through catheter; body's immune system is attracted to BCG and attacks cancer
Bone cancer	Any part of bones, including bone marrow, cartilage, outside layers Osteoblasts are cells that form bone; osteoclasts are cells that dissolve bone	Bone pain, swelling in painful area, common fractures of bone, weight loss, fatigue (bone pain and swelling are common symptoms of injury or arthritis)	Surgery: includes those that require amputation as well as limb-sparing surgery, curettage (removes tumor, leaving a hole in bone)	Radiation and chemotherapy are more commonly used when bone cancer has spread to other areas of body
Breast cancer in women	Areas affected include ducts, lobules (milk glands); not all breast cancers have lumps	Breast swelling, skin irritation or dimpling, pain, redness, thickening of nipple or skin, discharge or lump in underarm area	Surgery (lumpectomy or mastectomy), radiation, chemotherapy, hormone therapy, targeted therapy (immunotherapy)	Hormone therapy is used to lower estrogen levels, which decreases cancer cell growth Targeted therapy includes trastuzumab (Herceptin) and lapatinib (Tykerb) protein suppressors, which stop cancer cell growth
Breast cancer in men	Composed mostly of tissue ducts and a few lobules	Lump or swelling (may be painless), skin dimpling or puckering, nipple retraction, redness/scaling of skin and discharge	Surgery (lumpectomy or mastectomy), radiation, chemotherapy, hormone therapy, targeted therapy (immunotherapy)	Antibody bevacizumab (Avastin) stops cancer cells from growing new blood vessels
CNS cancer in adults	Brain or spinal cord tumors cause harm whether benign or malignant because they apply pressure to areas within brain; rarely metastasize to other areas of body	Dependent on location of tumor: seizures, numbness, weakness, abnormal movements of parts of body, language problems, personality changes, vision or balance changes	Surgery, radiation therapy, chemotherapy, targeted therapy	Targeted therapy with the antibody bevacizumab (Avastin) prevents tumors from developing new blood vessels, which they need to grow

Continued

TABLE 29-1 Types of Cancer—cont'd

Types of Cancer	Location of Organ or Parts of Organ Where Cancer May Occur	Symptoms*	Traditional Treatments Include	Additional Treatments and/or Comments
CNS cancer in children	Areas affected are normally different than those in adults; some tumors have mixture of cell types	Dependent on area of tumor; symptoms may include seizures, pain, poor school performance, fatigue, personality changes, irritability, vomiting, loss of appetite, developmental delay, decreased motor abilities	Surgery, radiation, chemotherapy	Children tend to respond better to chemotherapy than adults and side effects are less than those seen in adults. Specialized centers that have teams of health care professionals are often used for support services: psychologists, social workers, child life specialists, nutritionists, rehabilitation/physical therapy, and educators for entire family
Cervical cancer	Lower part of uterus; cervix connects body of uterus to vagina	Unusual discharge from vagina, blood spots or light bleeding (not from period), bleeding or pain after sex, douching, or pelvic exam	Radiation, chemotherapy, or surgery; types of surgery include cryosurgery (freezing cancer cells), laser, conization (cone-shaped piece of tissue removed), hysterectomy (simple or radical)	Newer surgery called trachelectomy: removes cervix and upper part of vagina and replaces it with artificial opening of cervix inside uterus; allows women to become pregnant
Childhood Non-Hodgkin's lymphoma	Lymphatic tissue located in lymph nodes and vessels; spleen, thymus, adenoids, and tonsils all contain lymph tissue	Symptoms vary depending on where it is located: swelling of affected area, fever, chills, night sweats	Chemotherapy or monoclonal antibody treatment	Monoclonal antibody treatments are similar to normal antibodies made by body but they attack cancer cells; rituximab (Rituxan) is an example
Colon cancer	Any part of large intestine, which is about 5 feet long	Diarrhea, constipation, narrow stools produced for several days, rectal bleeding, dark stools, blood in stools, cramping or stomach pain, weakness or fatigue	Surgery, radiation therapy, chemotherapy, targeted therapies	Monoclonal antibody treatments are similar to normal antibodies made by body but they attack cancer cells

TABLE 29-1 Types of Cancer—cont'd

Types of Cancer	Location of Organ or Parts of Organ Where Cancer May Occur	Symptoms*	Traditional Treatments Include	Additional Treatments and/or Comments
Endometrial cancer	Inner lining of uterus	Unusual bleeding, spotting, or discharge; pelvic pain; weight loss	Surgery, radiation, chemotherapy or hormonal therapy	Hormonal therapy includes progestins (slow growth), tamoxifen, GnRH, aromatase inhibitors (lower estrogen levels)
Esophageal cancer	Muscular tube that extends from mouth to stomach, about 12 inches long	Dysphagia (trouble swallowing), pain or pressure, weight loss, hoarseness, hiccups, pneumonia, high calcium levels	Surgery, radiation, chemotherapy, other treatments	Other treatments include PDT (harmless chemical collects in tumor; then laser light is used to change chemical into a cancer cell killer)
Eye cancer	Range from intraocular cancers to orbital cancers	Decreased vision, loss of field of vision, changes in eye movement, floaters in field of vision, flashes of light, bulging of eye	Surgery, radiation, laser therapy, chemotherapy, monoclonal therapy	Laser therapy uses high-energy light beam to burn tissue near optic nerve, which causes less nerve damage than radiation
Gallbladder cancer	Pear-shaped organ located under right lobe of liver, 3 to 4 inches long and approximately 1 inch wide	Jaundice, abdominal pain, N/V	Surgery, radiation, chemotherapy	Surgery is most accepted way of treating gallbladder cancer
GI carcinoid tumors	Located within inner lining of digestive system	May not have symptoms; if symptoms present, may include facial flushing, severe diarrhea, wheezing, rapid heart rate	Surgery, radiation, chemotherapy, other treatments	Other treatments include use of octreotide (related to natural hormone and may slow cancer growth) and interferons (activate immune system and slow tumor cell growth)
GI stromal tumors	Located in wall of digestive system (rare type of cancer)	Abdominal pain or discomfort, bleeding into intestinal tract, weakness, fatigue, vomiting blood, nausea, weight loss	Surgery, radiation, chemotherapy, targeted therapy	Targeted therapy includes use of imatinib (Gleevec) to block cell growth or sunitinib (Sutent) if imatinib ineffective or side effects too severe
Hodgkin's disease	Areas include lymph nodes and tissue; nodes are small bean-shaped organs found throughout body	Lumps under skin, night sweats, weight loss, fever, itching, fatigue, coughing or trouble breathing	Chemotherapy or radiation therapy	In general, Hodgkin's disease in children is different than that in adults; children respond better to chemotherapy treatment

Continued

TABLE 29-1 Types of Cancer—cont'd

Types of Cancer	Location of Organ or Parts of Organ Where Cancer May Occur	Symptoms*	Traditional Treatments Include	Additional Treatments and/or Comments
Kaposi's sarcoma	Cells that line lymph or blood vessels	Skin, mouth, or throat lesions; depending on where lesions occur; soreness, bleeding, and pain may be present	Chemotherapy, radiation, local therapy	Local therapy involves application of medicine to site of lesion or using cryosurgery Biological therapy involves immune system cells made in lab that attack cancer cells and prevent them from replicating; example is interferon alfa
Kidney cancer	Two kidney bean–shaped organs located in abdomen behind rib cage, to right and left of spine	Blood in urine, low back pain on one side, mass on side or lower back, fatigue, weight loss, fever, swelling of ankles and legs	Surgery, radiation, chemotherapy, biological therapy, targeted therapy, other types of therapy	Other types of therapy include cryotherapy (use of extreme cold to destroy tumor), radiofrequency (uses high-energy radio waves to heat tumor), arterial embolization (blocks artery that feeds kidney affected by cancer (used before surgery to kill cancer cells and reduce bleeding)
Laryngeal and hypopharyngeal cancer	Larynx (voice box or Adam's apple) found in neck as well as surrounding tissue (hypopharynx), which is part of esophagus (swallowing tube)	Persistent sore throat and coughing, pain or trouble swallowing or breathing, weight loss, hoarseness or voice changes, mass in neck	Surgery, radiation, chemotherapy, targeted therapy	Cetuximab (Erbitus) is only example of targeted therapy currently approved for this type of cancer
Leukemia (all types)	Location of this type of cancer originates in bone marrow that spreads into bloodstream	Because there are several types of leukemia, general symptoms include weight loss, fever, loss of appetite, increased infections, dizziness, SOB, easy bruising, bleeding (nose, gums)	Chemotherapy, radiation therapy, surgery	Surgery is used only to deliver treatment via a venous access device that is left in place to allow for administration of drugs and/or removal of blood samples

TABLE 29-1 Types of Cancer—cont'd

Types of Cancer	Location of Organ or Parts of Organ Where Cancer May Occur	Symptoms*	Traditional Treatments Include	Additional Treatments and/or Comments
Liver cancer	Shaped like a pyramid; two lobes are located under right rib cage below right lung	Weight loss, lack of appetite, N/V, fever, mass on right side, ongoing stomach pain, stomach swelling, jaundice, swollen veins on stomach	Surgery, liver transplant, tumor ablation and embolization, radiation, targeted therapy, chemotherapy	Tumor ablation involves local treatment; embolization places material in artery that blocks blood flow to tumor Radioembolization is injection of small radioactive beads into artery that feeds liver; beads attach to cancer cells and destroy them
Lung cancer, non–small cell	Sponge-like organs found in chest behind rib cage on either side of spinal cord; lining of bronchi or other parts of lung	Persistent cough; chest pain; painful breathing, coughing, or laughing; weight loss; blood in saliva or phlegm; SOB; wheezing	Surgery, radiation, chemotherapy, targeted therapies, other local treatments	Local treatment: PDT uses a light-activated drug injected into vein; within 2 days enough drug has attached to cancer cells; a light tube is placed into lung to activate drug, which kills cancer cells
Lung cancer, small cell	Starts in bronchi near center of chest; cells are small but multiply quickly	Same as in non–small cell lung cancer	Surgery, radiation, chemotherapy	VATS is a new surgical procedure that uses a tiny camera placed into chest to see tumor; surgeon makes two small holes in skin and tumor is removed
Lung carcinoid tumor	Typical carcinoids: tumors form in walls of large airways (bronchi) Atypical carcinoids: tumors form in narrower airways along edges of lungs	Coughing up bloody sputum, wheezing, SOB, chest pain; large carcinoids cause partial or complete blockage of airways, pneumonia	Surgery, radiation therapy	Radiation therapy includes external beam radiation or radioactive drugs Drugs used include octreotide, which attaches to cancer cells, delivering higher doses of radiation
Non-Hodgkin's lymphomas (NHLs)	Bean-sized organs located throughout body; cells look different from Hodgkin's type lymphoma cells There are approximately 30 different types of NHL	*If cancer site is:* Abdomen: swollen stomach, pain, N/V, reduced appetite Chest: SOB, coughing, swelling of head and arms Brain: H/A, trouble thinking, moving, seizures, personality changes Skin: itchy, red/purple lumps under skin	Surgery, radiation, chemotherapy, biological therapy	Biological therapy includes monoclonal antibodies such as rituximab (Rituxan); they may have radioactive agent attached to them Interferon is a protein that may cause cancer cells to shrink

Continued

TABLE 29-1 Types of Cancer—cont'd

Types of Cancer	Location of Organ or Parts of Organ Where Cancer May Occur	Symptoms*	Traditional Treatments Include	Additional Treatments and/or Comments
NHL: malignant mesothelioma	Cells that line areas such as chest, abdomen, and heart or testicles	If cancer site is in chest: pain in lower back or side of chest, SOB, trouble swallowing, hoarseness, cough, fever, sweating, weight loss, swelling of face and arms If cancer is in abdominal cavity: abdominal pain, weight loss, N/V, fluid or lump in abdomen	Surgery, radiation, chemotherapy	Radiation therapy includes external x-rays or implanted radiation, where radioactive agents are placed inside tumor
NHL: multiple myeloma	Plasma cells in bone marrow	Bone pain, weakness, SOB, dizziness, frequent infections, thirsty, frequent urination, loss of appetite, constipation, drowsy, confusion, nerve pain, muscle weakness and/or numbness	Surgery, radiation, chemotherapy, biological therapy, bisphosphonates	Bisphosphonates slow progression of bones dissolving because of cancer cells
Nasal cavity and paranasal cancer	Nasal cavity extends along roof of mouth to throat; paranasals are sinus cavities	Pain above or below eyes, persistent nasal congestion, nosebleeds, decreased sense of smell, numbness or pain of teeth, pain or pressure in ear(s), loss of vision, trouble opening mouth, swelling of lymph nodes in neck	Surgery	Surgery is difficult because of massive blood vessels and nerves in proximity to centers for eyesight, chewing, swallowing; therefore it is used sparingly
Neuroblastoma	Primitive developing nerve cells found in embryo or fetus	Lump, weight loss, pain, bladder and/or bowel problems, difficulty breathing, droopy eyelids, inability to move or feel arms/legs; all symptoms dependent on location of tumor	Surgery, chemotherapy, radiation therapy, combination therapy	Combination therapy involves high-dose chemotherapy and radiation therapy prior to replacing bone marrow cells Most often used on children who have not responded to previous treatments

TABLE 29-1 Types of Cancer—cont'd

Types of Cancer	Location of Organ or Parts of Organ Where Cancer May Occur	Symptoms*	Traditional Treatments Include	Additional Treatments and/or Comments
Oropharyngeal cancer	Cancer develops in part of throat behind mouth, including back of tongue, roof of mouth, and side and back walls of throat (i.e., throat cancer)	Pain, sore throat, trouble chewing/ swallowing/moving tongue, swelling of jaw, loosening of teeth, mass in neck or cheek, voice changes, weight loss	Surgery, radiation, chemotherapy, targeted therapy	Targeted therapy involves cetuximab (Erbitux), which blocks growth factor receptors in oral area; when these are blocked cancer cell growth is controlled
Osteosarcoma	Cancer cells in bone, specifically long bones of legs around knee or thigh; arm bones near shoulder are most common starting points	Bone pain that may be worse at night or with activity, swelling, lump(s)	Surgery, radiation, chemotherapy	Surgery may involve amputation or replacement of bone with metal rod In children rod may be able to lengthen as child grows
Ovarian cancer	Ovaries are located on each side of uterus in pelvis; cancer may occur inside or outside	Swelling or bloating of abdomen, pelvic pressure or pain, trouble eating, frequent urination	Surgery, radiation, chemotherapy	Surgery may involve removing ovaries, both fallopian tubes, and omentum (fatty tissue covering stomach area)
Penile cancer	Skin, nerves, smooth muscle, blood vessels of penis	Skin changes including color, thickness, ulcer-type sores or lump on penis that may include bleeding	Surgery, radiation, chemotherapy, immune therapy	Immune therapy uses imiquimod, which boosts immune system and is applied topically to treat genital warts and cancer of penis
Pituitary tumor	Pituitary gland is located in skull above nasal passages and is linked to hypothalamus Cancer cells can invade pituitary gland or tissue	Gland: paralysis of eye movement, loss of peripheral vision, sudden blindness, H/A, dizziness, fainting Tissue: nausea, weakness, weight loss or gain, amenorrhea, erectile dysfunction	Surgery, radiation, medicines	Medicines: both bromocriptine (Parlodel) and cabergoline (Dostinex) prevent cancer cell growth; octreotide inhibits growth hormone secretion that affects cancer cells
Prostate cancer	Prostate is walnut-sized gland that surrounds urethra	Trouble having or keeping erection; blood in urine; pain in spine, hips, ribs, or other bones; weakness/numbness in legs or feet; loss of bladder or bowel control	Surgery, radiation, chemotherapy, cryosurgery, hormone therapy	Hormone therapy includes leuprolide (Lupron Depot), which lowers testosterone levels; antiandrogens used to block androgens

Continued

TABLE 29-1 Types of Cancer—cont'd

Types of Cancer	Location of Organ or Parts of Organ Where Cancer May Occur	Symptoms*	Traditional Treatments Include	Additional Treatments and/or Comments
Retinoblastoma	Retina is inner layer of back of eye; made of nerve cells sensitive to light	Because of eye changes, eye emits white glare after photo is taken rather than normal "red-eye" Eye pain, redness of eye, and pupil that does not change size	Surgery, radiation, chemotherapy, laser therapy, cryotherapy, thermotherapy	Cryotherapy uses ultrasound, microwaves, or infrared rays to apply heat to eye
Rhabdomyosarcoma	Cancer cells that develop in skeletal muscles of body	Depending on area of cancer: Tumor in trunk, extremities, groin: mass Tumor around eye: cross-eyed Tumor in ear/nasal sinuses: earache or sinus infection Tumor in bladder: difficult or painful urination and/or bowel movements	Surgery, radiation, chemotherapy	Chemotherapy agents include vincristine, dactinomycin, cyclophosphamide
Salivary gland cancer	Three salivary glands are located inside and near mouth	Mass and/or pain in face, neck, or mouth; numbness or muscle weakness in face; trouble swallowing	Surgery, radiation, chemotherapy	Surgery is performed to remove affected gland and may involve taking surrounding tissue, which may affect facial nerves
Sarcoma	Soft tissue type cancer develops in fat, muscle, nerves, fibrous tissues, blood vessels, or deep skin tissues that are found in all areas of body	Lump or growing lump anywhere on body, abdominal pain, blood in stool or vomit, black tarry stools	Surgery, radiation, chemotherapy	Radiation may be delivered either externally or internally—small pellets of radioactive material are placed into cancerous tumor Both treatments may be used together
Skin cancer, basal and squamous cell	This cancer is located either in upper epidermis (squamous cell) or in lowest layer of epidermis (basal cell)	New skin growth, spot or bump that is growing, sore that does not heal within 3 months	Surgery, radiation, chemotherapy, other forms of treatment	Other treatments include cryosurgery, PDT, topical chemotherapy
Skin cancer, melanoma	This cancer affects epidermis layer of skin where melanocytes are located	Mole that is asymmetrical, irregular border, uneven color, large diameter	Surgery, radiation, immunotherapy	Surgery is most common treatment and may include simple excision, wide-excision, amputation, lymph node removal in area of cancer cells

TABLE 29-1 Types of Cancer—cont'd

Types of Cancer	Location of Organ or Parts of Organ Where Cancer May Occur	Symptoms*	Traditional Treatments Include	Additional Treatments and/or Comments
Small intestine cancer	Located in one of three areas of small intestine: duodenum (25 cm long), jejunum and ileum (together >6 m long)	Pain in abdomen, weight loss, weakness and fatigue, N/V, black stools	Surgery, radiation, chemotherapy	Surgery may involve placing a stent (hollow tube) through blocked area of intestine to allow food to pass
Stomach cancer	This type of cancer normally starts in mucosa (outer lining) or cells that form inner lining of stomach	Lack of appetite, weight loss, N/V, swelling of abdomen, pain in abdomen, heartburn	Surgery, radiation, chemotherapy	Surgery may involve removal of tumor, part of stomach, or entire stomach and adjacent lymph nodes, spleen, and other organs (i.e., gastrectomy)
Testicular cancer	Tumors may grow in all areas of testes	Lump or swollen testes, loss of sex drive, breast growth or tenderness; in children, growth of hair on face/body at young age	Surgery, radiation, chemotherapy	Surgery may involve removal of one or both testes and lymph nodes behind abdomen; in young adults sperm may be frozen for future use and testicular prosthesis implanted
Thymus cancer	Located behind breast bone and between lungs	SOB, cough (may be bloody), chest pain, trouble swallowing, weight loss, fever	Surgery, radiation, chemotherapy	Chemotherapeutic agents used include doxorubicin, cisplatin, carboplatin, cyclophosphamide, ifosfamide, vincristine, etoposide, paclitaxel, pemetrexed, 5-fluorouracil, gemcitabine
Thyroid cancer	Located in front part of neck	Lump or swollen neck, pain in front of neck, hoarseness or voice changes, trouble swallowing, difficulty breathing, continuous coughing	Surgery, hormone therapy, radiation, chemotherapy	Hormone therapy involves administering high levels of TH to decrease levels of TSH, which causes cancer cell growth
Uterine sarcoma	Sites within uterus include connective tissue of endometrium or muscles in wall of uterus (myometrium)	Abnormal bleeding, vaginal discharge, pelvic pain or mass	Surgery, radiation therapy, chemotherapy, hormone therapy	Hormone therapy is used primarily for endometrial cancer cells and includes progestins (megestrol, medroxyprogesterone), GnRH (goserelin, leuprolide), aromatase inhibitors (letrozole, anastrozole, exemestane, and tamoxifen)

Continued

TABLE 29-1 Types of Cancer—cont'd

Types of Cancer	Location of Organ or Parts of Organ Where Cancer May Occur	Symptoms*	Traditional Treatments Include	Additional Treatments and/or Comments
Vaginal cancer	Located from lower part of uterus to vulva; 3 to 4 inches in length	Abnormal bleeding, vaginal discharge, mass, pain during intercourse	Surgery, radiation, chemotherapy, laser therapy, topical therapy	Laser therapy uses high-energy light to vaporize abnormal tissue Topical therapy may include applying fluorouracil to lining of vagina to kill cancer cells or imiquimod cream applied to boost immune response
Vulvar cancer	Located on outer part of female genitalia	Persistent itching, skin color change in area affected	Surgery, radiation, chemotherapy	Chemotherapeutic agents most often used include fluorouracil, mitomycin, and cisplatin; fluorouracil may be applied directly to area affected
Waldenström's macroglobulinemia	Cancer of B cells of immune system	Weakness, loss of appetite, fever, neuropathy (nerve pain), swollen lymph nodes or abdomen	Surgery, radiation, chemotherapy, biological therapy, immunotherapy	Immune therapy helps body fight cancer cells; drugs used include rituximab and alemtuzumab; immunomodulating agent (thalidomide) is used to treat multiple myelomas
Wilms' tumor	Location is in kidneys; more common in children	Stomach pain, fever, loss of appetite, constipation, blood in urine, high blood pressure	Surgery, radiation, chemotherapy	Surgery may involve removing part or both kidneys, which requires dialysis and eventual transplant

*Many of the symptoms listed are common to noncancerous conditions and indicate early signs and symptoms of cancer.
†*BCG*, Bacille Calmette-Guérin; *CNS*, central nervous system; *CRT*, chemoradiotherapy; *GI*, gastrointestinal; *GnRH*, gonadotropin-releasing hormone; *H/A*, headache; *N/V*, nausea/vomiting; *PDT*, photodynamic therapy; *SOB*, shortness of breath; *TH*, thyroid hormone; *TSH*, thyroid-stimulating hormone; *VATS*, video-assisted thoracic surgery.

Hodgkin's **lymphoma**, or Hodgkin's disease, is a cancer of the lymphatic cells that are located in the lymph nodes. This disease was named after Thomas Hodgkin, the physician who first described its features (Figure 29-2).

Non-Hodgkin's lymphoma is not Hodgkin's disease but is named after Hodgkin's lymphoma because it also affects the lymphatic system. This cancer may have a nodular or diffuse pattern that spreads; non-Hodgkin's lymphoma may have a low, moderate, or high rate of malignancy. Its morphology is different from that of Hodgkin's disease.

Prostate cancer is a slow but progressive adenocarcinoma of the prostate gland. The incidence of this type of cancer increases with age. As the cancer grows, it obstructs the urethra and affects urination. If left untreated it can metastasize into other areas of the body.

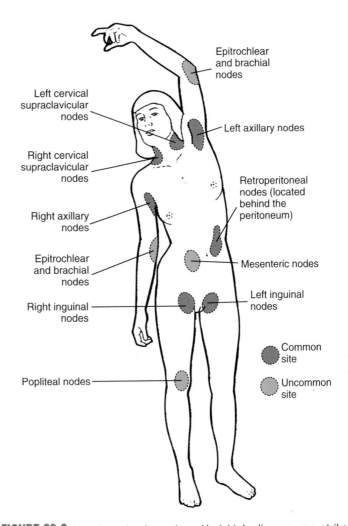

FIGURE 29-2 Lymph node sites where Hodgkin's disease can strike.

Kaposi's sarcoma is a rare type of cancer that affects the skin and is marked by brownish-purplish skin lesions that can spread to internal organs. Persons who are most likely to acquire this type of cancer are those who suffer from acquired immunodeficiency syndrome (AIDS). Because the immune system is compromised, the body is more susceptible to a variety of diseases (Figure 29-3).

Leukemia arises in the bone marrow and lymphatic system. Malfunctioning bone marrow produces abnormal leukocytes (white blood cells [WBCs]). These leukocytes can suppress normal blood cell production; the disease is often fatal. Two major groups of leukemias are lymphocytic leukemia and myelogenous leukemia. Each group is subdivided into many different types of cancer, two of the subtypes being the following:

- Acute lymphocytic leukemia: The cure rate for this type of leukemia is more than 90%. This form of leukemia usually affects children, although it has also been diagnosed in adults. Approximately 75% of those with the disease will enter a period of **remission**. Remission is when the disease disappears for months to years but may reoccur at a later time.
- Acute myelogenous leukemia: This type of leukemia is the most common among adults, with 10% to 20% of those affected being children. The increase in the number of WBCs, in addition to a decreased production of red blood cells, makes the body more susceptible to infection. In fact, the cause of death

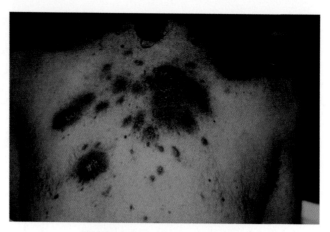

FIGURE 29-3 Kaposi's sarcoma.

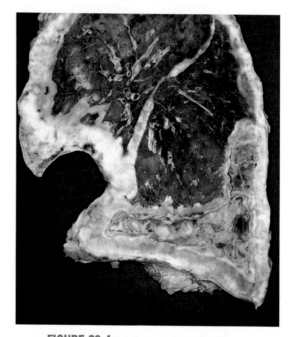

FIGURE 29-4 Malignant mesothelioma.

is usually an invading microorganism rather than the disease itself. The disease progresses rapidly, and a person can succumb to it in less than 6 months.

The primary risk factor for lung cancer is cigarette smoking. Other risk factors include exposure to asbestos and other environmental factors, as well as family history of the disease (genetics). There are several different types of lung cancer, which determine prognosis and response to treatment. Small cell lung cancer tends to be diagnosed long after it has metastasized, making it more difficult to treat.

Meningioma is a cancerous tumor of the meninges—the membranes that surround the brain and spinal cord. This type of cancer grows slowly and occurs mostly in the brain. The lesions invade the brain, causing bone erosion and pressure on parts of the brain tissue. Meningiomas occur mainly in adults.

Mesothelioma is a rare tumor that occurs in the pleura or peritoneum and is associated with exposure to asbestos. Persons affected by this disease have a poor prognosis because most treatments are ineffective (Figure 29-4).

BOX 29-2 CHARACTERISTICS OF CANCER GROWTH AND TREATMENT

Morphology: The morphology of a cell or organism is its shape characteristics. Most cancerous cells have rigid edges or edges that are not smooth, unlike noncancerous cells that tend to be smooth and round. Cancer cells also can form large masses or may remain as small cells. Normal cells tend to have an appearance of flattened cells, whereas cancer cells tend to be more stacked.

Growth pattern: Cell types have different characteristics. Some of the patterns that identify types of cancer include the speed of growth of cancer cells and the time it takes for them to travel to different parts of the body. When cancer cells are grown in a culture dish, they tend to form multiple layers because they do not follow the same growth pattern as normal cells. Normal cells form a single layer.

Karyotype: The actual mutation of a cancer cell is contained in the karyotype. Within the DNA of the cell is the mutation or cancer gene that initiates uncontrollable growth. Included in the DNA are also various components that can help accelerate growth. Normal cells have the capability to divide between 20 and 60 times before they are too old to continue; however, cancer cells have been observed to divide thousands of times, furthering their unruly nature. This rate of reproduction may decrease the effectiveness of the medication or treatment given to kill the cancer cells.

Response to therapy: Because different cancers have different morphologies, growth patterns, and karyotypes, they may or may not be responsive to treatment. Many times, multiple agents are used to treat the growth of cancer cells.

Diagnosis of Cancer

Although cancer can strike any area of the body, this chapter discusses the most common types of cancer and their progression. Many cancers can be identified and treated with the use of the following methods: x-rays, regular physical exams by a physician, self-examination, laboratory testing for tumor markers, magnetic resonance imaging (MRI), sonograms, biopsies, and radiopharmaceuticals. A pathologist determines the level or grade of the tumor based on its appearance when observed under a microscope or in a culture plate. The stage or severity of the cancer is diagnosed by the **oncologist** (a physician who specialize in the treatment of cancer). Detection of precancerous cells allows early initiation of treatment, which helps avoid more invasive and lengthy future treatment. These types of precancerous cells are referred to as carcinoma in situ. As the diagnosis is being determined, several aspects of the cancer must be considered, such as the morphology, growth pattern, karyotype, and response to chemotherapy agents. Box 29-2 explains each consideration.

Ordinarily, if a cancer is diagnosed in the early stages, when its growth is limited to a specific locale, it may be removed surgically. If there is no recurrence within 5 years, the cancer normally is considered cured. With new advancements in the treatment of cancers, some cancers can be cured even if they are discovered in later stages. For example, many leukemias are curable, especially in children. Other cancers such as skin melanomas are being detected in the early stages through routine skin cancer screening. This can be attributed to public education. For example, breast cancer and prostate cancer are cured more frequently than other forms of cancer because individuals are performing self-examinations and having checkups to detect cancerous masses before they metastasize.

Treatments for Cancer

There are more treatments available to treat cancer today than ever before; they include surgery, radiation therapy, implanted radioactive isotopes,

TABLE 29-2 Combination Therapies for Cancer

Disease	Drug Set	Agents
Ovarian cancer	CC	carboplatin, cyclophosphamide
Breast cancer	CFM	cyclophosphamide, fluorouracil, mitoxantrone
Lung cancer	CDV	cyclophosphamide, doxorubicin, vincristine
Testicular cancer	BEP	bleomycin, etoposide, cisplatin
Hodgkin's lymphoma (pediatric)	CVMP	cyclophosphamide, vincristine, methotrexate, prednisone
Sarcoma	DI	doxorubicin, ifosfamide, mesna
Non-Hodgkin's lymphoma	MIV	mitoxantrone, ifosfamide, etoposide

chemotherapy, biological therapy, targeted therapy, topical therapy, and photodynamic therapy. New advancements in each type of treatment have lessened the risk of recurrence and have altered expected side effects.

Treatment guidelines are based on how, where, and when a cancer cell is attacked. For example, certain chemotherapeutic drugs can destroy cancer cells either within specific phases of the cell cycle or throughout the entire cell cycle. The cell has four basic cycles in the replication process. Depending on the type of cancer present, oncologists refer to a protocol (a set of guidelines) that recommends multiple agents used simultaneously to treat cancer. The protocol combines agents that are effective during a specific part of the cell cycle with other agents that are effective throughout the entire cell cycle; in this way, the best coverage is given to eliminate the cancer. Table 29-2 lists examples of combination therapy.

Age is an important factor that must be considered in patients who will undergo cancer treatments. The possibility of cancer increases in individuals older than age 65. Age can increase the risks of cancer treatment because older adults tend to have preexisting disease conditions. In children, cancer can reproduce quickly because children are growing rapidly. However, children tend to respond to chemotherapy and recuperate more quickly than older patients.

SURGERY

Surgery is frequently used in the diagnosis and treatment of cancer. The diagnostic phase begins with excision of a piece of the cancerous tumor or cells (i.e., a **biopsy**). Microscopy is then used to determine the type of cancer. In this way, physicians can measure the degree to which the cancer has spread—a process called staging. Markers are one diagnostic indicator that can be used to determine the type of cancer. Markers are substances that may be found in tumor tissue or released from a tumor into the bloodstream or other body fluids. A high level of a tumor marker may indicate that a certain type of cancer is present. The following three important markers used in staging help determine the treatment plan:

1. The original tumor size and its extent of distribution
2. The presence of dissemination of the cancer to adjacent lymph nodes
3. The presence of metastasis of the cancer to distant areas of the body

These criteria are used in addition to other diagnostic techniques (such as laboratory testing) and imaging studies (such as MRI, computerized tomography [CT] scans, and x-rays) to gather the maximum amount of information on the type of cancer. Not all cancers can be staged. An example is leukemia; this is

BOX 29-3 FORMS OF TREATMENT

Preventive
Removal of precancerous tissue such as rectal polyps; removal of an organ (e.g., a breast) that has a high risk of cancer because of genetics

Staging
The physical exam to determine the stage or severity of the cancer

Curative
Removal of a tumor that has not spread

Debulking
Removal of a part of a tumor that cannot be totally removed, because of location, for example

Palliative
Does not remove cancer but helps relieve side effects caused by the cancer

Supportive
Procedure where catheter ports are surgically placed into a large vein for drug delivery

Restorative
Reconstructive surgery performed to correct appearance after cancer surgery

Laser
High-powered light energy used to cut cancerous tissue or to vaporize

Cryosurgery
Use of liquid nitrogen to kill cancer cells

Electrosurgery
High-frequency electrical current used to kill cancer cells

Laparoscope
A flexible tube that is inserted into a small incision for observation, biopsy, or organ removal

Thoracoscope
A rigid tube with a camera inserted into a small incision in the thorax for observation, biopsy, or removal of small tumors

Stereotactic
Not true surgery; uses a precise high-intensity radiation dose applied to a small tumor area

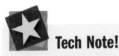

Tech Note!

A bone marrow transplant typically has a much greater chance of curing adults and children with leukemia who do not respond to traditional treatments. The bone marrow is transplanted by intravenous infusion, using marrow that is free from cancer cells. The new bone marrow naturally attaches to the patient's bones and alters the defective bone marrow by making healthy red blood cells (RBC) and white blood cells (WBC).

because the cancer is present throughout the body, including highly sensitive brain tissue.

Several types of procedures and treatments are available to cancer patients, ranging from tumor removal to reconstructive surgery. Various treatments are listed in Box 29-3.

RADIATION

Radiation can be used to diagnose or treat certain diseases. For example, x-ray imaging, computed tomography scans, and radioisotope scans use electromagnetic waves to project images as the waves pass through the body. Although radiation also is known to be a carcinogen, if used correctly it can kill cancer cells. In cancer treatment, radiation is categorized by the intensity of the rays. These are α-(alpha), β-(beta), and γ(gamma)-rays. Both α- and β-rays normally are used to treat superficial lesions, whereas γ-rays are stronger and can treat deeper lesions.

Side Effects of Radiation Therapy

The side effects of radiation therapy differ widely from person to person, and may be dependent on the area of the body treated, the dose and type of radiation

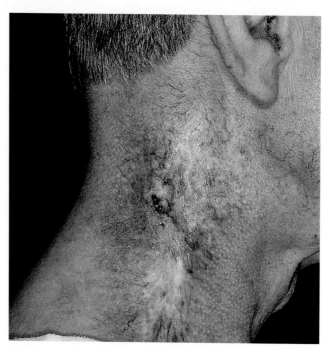

FIGURE 29-5 Radiation dermatitis from exposure to radiation treatment for cancer.

used, and the size of the radiation field. Certain effects can occur soon after treatment while other side effects may take a few weeks to appear. One of the early side effects is fatigue, either physically, mentally, and/or emotionally, possibly worsening as treatment continues. Skin changes include a red, swollen, blistered, sunburned, or suntanned appearance that tends to disappear just a few weeks after treatment ends. Dermatitis caused by exposure to radiation may not appear until several weeks after cessation of treatment and may include sloughing of the skin, blistering, and changes in skin pigmentation (Figure 29-5). There are many supportive treatments for these side effects. Other side effects include hair loss, low white blood cell count, low levels of platelets, and eating problems (usually attributable to difficulty swallowing from esophageal or mouth irritation). Reactions are variable and are dependent on the location exposed to radiation.

RADIOACTIVE ISOTOPES

Certain cancers may require alternative types of treatment because of their location or nature. Brachytherapy is a type of radiation treatment that uses an internal device, such as a seed or wire, to deliver radiation. In this case, implants can be placed directly into the cancer site. This may be effective in cancers of the tongue or the cervix. The implants may remain in the body from hours to a few days.

CHEMOTHERAPY

Many different types of medications are used to treat cancers. Table 29-3 lists some of these agents. Often, these agents are effective at eradicating cancer cells. The disruption caused by interfering with the normal metabolism of cancer cells causes cell death. Other agents commonly prescribed during the treatment of cancer are palliative; that is, they relieve symptoms of cancer or the side effects of chemotherapeutic agents, such as hair loss, emesis (vomiting), fatigue, weight loss, and pain.

TABLE 29-3 Common Types of Chemotherapeutic Agents

Generic Name	Trade Name	Classification	Indication	Route of Administration
bleomycin	Blenoxane	Antibiotic	Lymphomas, squamous cell carcinomas	IV*
busulfan	Myleran	Alkylating agent	Leukemia	PO, IV
carboplatin	Paraplatin	Alkylating agent	Ovarian cancer and tumors	IV
carmustine	BiCNU	Alkylating agent	Brain tumors, Hodgkin's and non-Hodgkin's lymphomas	IV, wafer
chlorambucil	Leukeran	Alkylating agent	Leukemia, lymphomas	PO
cisplatin	Platinol	Alkylating agent	Ovarian/testicular tumor	IV
cyclophosphamide	Cytoxan	Alkylating agent	Leukemias, Hodgkin's disease, lymphomas	PO, IV
cytarabine	Cytosar-U	Antimetabolite	Myelocytic leukemias	IV
dacarbazine	DTIC-Dome	Alkylating agent	Melanoma, Hodgkin's disease	IV
dactinomycin	Cosmegen	Antibiotic	Wilms' tumor	IV
doxorubicin	Adriamycin	Antibiotic	Leukemias, tumors	IV
etoposide	VePesid	Plant extract	Lung and testicular cancer	PO, IV
fludarabine phosphate	Fludara	Antimetabolite	Leukemia	IV
fluorouracil	Adrucil	Antimetabolite	Cancer of colon, rectum, pancreas, breast, stomach	IV
fluorouracil	Efudex	Antimetabolite	Skin cancers, stomach cancer	Topical
gefitinib	Iressa	Antineoplastic	Non–small cell lung cancer	PO
gemcitabine	Gemzar	Miscellaneous antineoplastic antimetabolite	Adenocarcinoma of pancreas	IV
hydroxyurea	Hydrea	Miscellaneous antineoplastic	Leukemia, recurrent cancer of ovary	PO
idarubicin	Idamycin	Antibiotic	Adult leukemias	IV
ifosfamide	Ifex	Alkylating agent	Sarcoma, cancer of testes	IV
mechlorethamine	Mustargen	Alkylating agent	Hodgkin's disease, lymphomas	IV
melphalan	Alkeran	Alkylating agent	Multiple myelomas	PO, IV
methotrexate	Methotrex	Antimetabolite	Leukemia, psoriasis, rheumatoid arthritis	PO, IV
paclitaxel	Taxol	Antimitotic	Ovarian/breast cancer	IV, intraperitoneal
streptozocin	Zanosar	Alkylating agent	Cancer of pancreas	IV
teniposide	Vumon	Plant extract	Childhood leukemia	IV
topotecan	Hycamtin	Topoisomerase I inhibitor	Ovarian cancer	IV
trastuzumab	Herceptin	Targets HER2/neu protein	Breast cancer	IV
vinblastine	Velban	Antimitotic	Hodgkin's disease, tumors	IV
vincristine	Oncovin	Antimitotic	Leukemia, tumors	IV
vinorelbine	Navelbine	Antimitotic	Lung cancer	IV

*IV, Intravenous; PO, oral.

TABLE 29-4 Routes of Administration of Chemotherapeutic Agents

Abbreviation	Definition	Location
Traditional		
PO	By mouth	Orally
TOP	Topical	Onto skin
IM	Intramuscular	Into muscle
IT	Intrathecal	Into intrathecal space
IV	Intravenous	Into vein
Newer Routes		
Infusion pumps	Syringe pump	Portable pump worn by patient that administers preset amount of drug through catheter inserted into tumor
Implants	Wafers/tablets/capsules	Implanted into cancerous area where medication can be dispersed over set time

Chemotherapy is normally given in cycles that can range from 1 day to weekly for several weeks to months. Routes of administration vary depending on the agent used. Not all chemotherapy drugs are given intravenously. Table 29-4 lists the different routes of administration of chemotherapeutic agents. Certain agents are administered over a short period or over several hours depending on the drug. Some chemotherapy agents are administered through a central line that is surgically placed for the delivery of the chemotherapy, referred to as supportive surgery.

TARGETED THERAPY

Targeted therapy is a newer form of chemotherapy that specifically targets cancer cells. Just as the name implies, the therapy given targets a site or type of cancer, infiltrates the cell, and kills the cancer. Unlike chemotherapy, which destroys both healthy and cancerous cells, this type of treatment decreases the severe side effects that can result from traditional chemotherapy. Each type of targeted therapy differs in the way it attacks a cancer cell. The drugs recognize the difference between a cancer cell and a normal healthy cell. Targeted therapy can be used to treat conditions/diseases other than cancer. Targeted agents can also be used in conjunction with chemotherapeutic agents because of their different mechanism of action.

Antiangiogenesis is a type of targeted therapy that works in a unique way. Cancer cells are thought to possibly create their own blood vessels, thereby providing the cancer cells with nourishment and an avenue to proliferate and spread. Antiangiogenesis inhibits the formation of new blood vessels, specifically in cancer cells. When the cells' source of nourishment is terminated, the cells die.

AGENTS USED IN THE TREATMENT OF NEOPLASTIC DISEASES

Antimetabolite Agents

Nucleic acids, often referred to as bases, are a part of the structure of each DNA molecule. These bases form the fundamental configuration of DNA. The structure of antimetabolites is similar to that of the bases that form DNA strands, but because they are not identical, antimetabolites prevent the completion of cell division, or **mitosis**. Therefore the cells into which antimetabolites are introduced are not able to replicate. Antimetabolites often are used to treat leukemia. The most common side effects include nausea, vomiting, fever, anorexia, bone marrow depression, and jaundice. Antimetabolites include the following:

- Cytarabine
- Floxuridine
- Fludarabine
- Fluorouracil
- Mercaptopurine
- Methotrexate
- Thioguanine

Antibiotics

The antibiotics used to treat cancers are not in the same category as those used to treat infections. They are specific to tumors that cause cancer. These antibiotics bind directly to the DNA of the cancer cells and prevent the synthesis of any new cells. These agents are not used to treat infections because of their toxic side effects. Instead, they are used to destroy newly formed cancer cells. Because they also destroy normal cells along with the cancer cells, they produce side effects that include severe emesis (vomiting), nausea, diarrhea, red urine, and hair loss. Agents of this type include the following:

- Bleomycin
- Dactinomycin
- Daunorubicin
- Doxorubicin
- Idarubicin
- Mitomycin
- Mitoxantrone
- Pentostatin
- Plicamycin

Mitotic Inhibitors

Mitotic inhibitors prevent mitosis at the metaphase stage. Mitosis is the process of cell division that all cells must perform (Figure 29-6). The agents used to

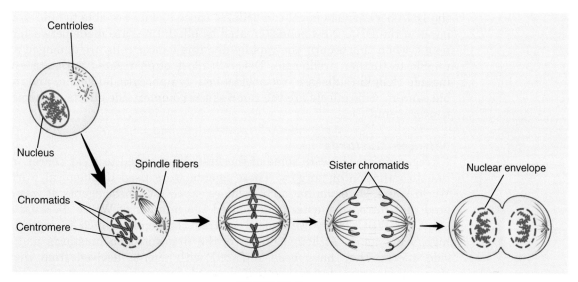

FIGURE 29-6 Mitosis.

prevent this cellular reproduction are a group of alkaloids derived from plants. Diseases such as Hodgkin's disease and various cancers that may not respond to other medications often are treated with mitotic inhibitors. Side effects may include appetite loss, back pain, diarrhea, hair loss, increased sweating, nausea, vomiting, voice changes, and blue or purple discoloration of the skin. These agents include the following:

- Etoposide
- Teniposide
- Vinblastine
- Vincristine
- Vinorelbine

Each cell that produces the next generation of cells leaves a part of its genetic makeup behind. Genes are contained within the chromosomes of DNA, located in the nucleus of the cell. The process of producing new cells is referred to as replication. When a cell replicates, it copies all the chromosomes (all of the genes of the cell are replicated). As the chromosomes are duplicated, they are divided evenly into two daughter cells (or new cells) and are contained within the new nuclei. Mitosis is the process by which the nucleus of the cell is divided. The entire process of mitosis starts with prophase, followed by metaphase, anaphase, and then telophase. This process of mitosis is sometimes referred to as the "M" phase. Each part of the process is specific and lasts a certain time. The last stage, called cytokinesis, is the separation of the daughter cells. The mitotic phase and cytokinesis are the end processes of the life span of the cell. After cytokinesis takes place, the new cell enters a much longer phase referred to as interphase. The interphase process has three parts, the first of which is called G1. The replication process begins in this stage as the centrioles pull apart chromosomes, preparing for mitosis once again. Centrioles anchor to the chromosomes at opposite ends of the cell and separate them. The second part of interphase is the S phase, in which DNA replication starts. Lastly, the G2 phase of interphase prepares the cells for the mitotic phase, and the entire process is repeated.

Alkylating Agents
The two major types of alkylating agents are the nitrogen mustards and nitrosoureas. Although their structures are similar, their methods of action and side effects are different. Because alkylation is a normal reaction that takes place in the DNA between chemical compounds, these agents are able to bind to certain bases of the DNA. New bonds (created by alkylation) are made between components; when this occurs, the rapidly dividing cancer cells are damaged and are unable to further proliferate. Diseases most often treated with these agents include Hodgkin's disease, retinoblastoma, lymphocytic leukemia, and inoperable cancers. Side effects are the same as the common side effects of chemotherapeutic agents.

Nitrogen Mustards
Nitrogen mustards were some of the first agents used to treat cancer in addition to radiation or surgery. These agents were used in chemical warfare in World War I. On examination of soldiers exposed to these agents, it was discovered that nitrogen mustards decreased the number of WBCs. Because of this effect on WBCs, they were used to treat leukemia, which is marked by a high WBC count. Although effective, the first nitrogen mustards had severe side effects; they have been replaced with agents derived from the same chemical structure but are better tolerated. Side effects may include low blood counts, nausea, vomiting, mouth sores, hair loss, darkening of veins used for

infusion, and loss of fertility. Examples of nitrogen mustard agents include the following:

- Chlorambucil
- Cyclophosphamide
- Ifosfamide
- Mechlorethamine
- Melphalan

Nitrosoureas

These agents cross the blood-brain barrier that surrounds the central nervous system. Because of this ability, they can be used to treat cancers within the brain. Side effects of these agents may include nausea, vomiting, intense flushing of the skin, reddening of the eyes, headache, or rash. The following drugs are nitrosoureas:

- Carmustine
- Lomustine
- Streptozocin

Other Antineoplastic Agents

Various other **antineoplastic** agents commonly are used to treat cancer. One group, the hormones and hormone modifiers, includes corticosteroids, androgens, and antiandrogens. Most hormone agents are indicated for cancers that are influenced by hormonal control. Corticosteroids can be useful in treating leukemia and lymphomas. They also work to decrease inflammation and edema in vital areas. Antiandrogens are used to treat prostate cancer.

Other agents do not fall neatly into the categories previously discussed. One such agent is interferon, a natural protein found in the body. When used in treatment, it boosts immune cells, which are then better able to attack cancer cells. Interferon also changes the structure of the cells, making them less "cancer like" and more "normal" in their behavior. Interferon is used for a special form of leukemia known as hairy cell leukemia. Table 29-5 lists the specific actions of other miscellaneous agents used to treat cancer, along with the types of cancers for which they are used.

SIDE EFFECTS OF CHEMOTHERAPY AND BIOLOGICAL TREATMENTS

Because cancer is caused by a malfunction of our own cells, it is difficult for medication aimed at destroying cancer cells to distinguish between normal and

Tech Note!

When preparing chemotherapeutic agents, special chemotherapy gloves must be worn or the technician must double-glove to protect the skin; gowns and masks are also advised if the technician is preparing agents that must be compounded, reconstituted, or admixed. Such agents are prepared in a special laminar flow hood to prevent unwanted exposure. If a chemotherapeutic agent spills on the gloves, the top gloves can be removed and discarded into an appropriate container for hazardous waste, and a new pair of gloves can be worn. Always follow the appropriate procedures for the type of agent handled.

Often the policies and procedures of an institution require that one pharmacist checks the orders, dosage, and preparation of all chemotherapy agents and that a second pharmacist, who was not involved in the preparation and first check of the dosage, independently rechecks the computer entries, orders, medication preparations, and labels. These "pharmacist double check" procedures help reduce medication errors, which could be devastating to a patient receiving cancer treatments. For more on chemotherapy preparation, see Chapter 12.

TABLE 29-5 Other Cancer Treatment Agents

Agent	Mechanism of Action	Types of Cancer
Asparaginase	Depletes asparagine (necessary for cell survival)	Lymphocytic leukemia
Dacarbazine	Inhibits synthesis in G2 phase	Hodgkin's disease
Docetaxel	Inhibits activity of microtubules in G1 phase	Breast cancer
Gemcitabine	Inhibits specific DNA synthesis	Adenocarcinoma of pancreas
Hydroxyurea	Inhibits specific DNA synthesis	Head, neck, and ovarian cancers; melanoma
Paclitaxel	Antimicrotubule agent in G2 phase	Metastatic ovarian cancer
Procarbazine	Inhibitor in S phase	Hodgkin's disease

defective cells. The components are the same in both. On the other hand, antibiotics used to treat microbial infections can differentiate between diseased and healthy cells.

When fighting cancer cells, the only way to ensure full remission is to destroy all the cancer cells. Unfortunately, healthy cells are also destroyed with the cancer cells, especially fast-growing cells such as those responsible for hair growth and those found in mucosal areas. Fortunately, hair will regrow over time.

The following are some common side effects of chemotherapy:

- Anemia
- Diarrhea
- Dry skin or skin tone discoloration
- Fatigue
- Hair loss and change in the appearance of the nails
- Increased chance of bruising and/or bleeding
- Infertility
- Mouth sores
- Nausea and vomiting (N/V)
- Risk of infection
- Taste and smell changes

Each person is affected differently; some people experience few, if any, side effects. In addition, the duration of the side effects differs for each patient, and may range from short-term to long-term. Each type of chemotherapy has specific common side effects; some have many, and others have very few. Several techniques can be used to treat many of the side effects as shown in Table 29-6.

ADJUNCTIVE AGENTS

Chemotherapeutic agents may destroy not only cancer cells but also the cells of the immune system. Patients treated with chemotherapeutic agents often become anemic or, because of a reduction of WBCs, they develop leukopenia and anemia. Because WBCs are essential in protecting the body from various infections, and red blood cells (RBC) are important for tissue oxygenation, special medications may be prescribed to boost the WBC count and/or the RBC count. Two main agents used to treat chemotherapy side effects are erythropoietin and filgrastim. Both agents are used to stimulate specific bone marrow production of blood cells; erythropoietin stimulates red blood cell production, and filgrastim stimulates WBC production. Levels of RBCs and/or WBCs in the patient's blood serum must be monitored to dose these medications properly. The manufacturer's storage instructions require these agents to be refrigerated between 2° and 8° C. They must not be shaken or frozen.

Erythropoietin

Erythropoietin is used primarily to treat anemia in patients with malignant **neoplasms** who acquire anemia during chemotherapy. Erythropoietin also may be used to treat persons with human immunodeficiency virus infection or end-stage renal disease. Normal doses of erythropoietin range from 2000 to 10,000 units/mL; the dosage is adjusted on the basis of the patient's hemoglobin levels and response to treatment. A normal dosing regimen is 150 units/kg three times a week.

Filgrastim

Filgrastim binds to bone marrow cells and stimulates growth of neutrophils. Neutrophils are key components of the immune system. They are part of the

TABLE 29-6 Treatment of Chemotherapy Side Effects

Symptom	Treatment
Nausea/vomiting	Eat frequent small meals.
	Eat and drink slowly.
	Avoid foods high in sugar and fats; avoid fried foods.
	Try dry toast or crackers for early morning nausea.
	Avoid bad odors.
	Suck on ice cubes, mints, or tart candies.
	Breathe deeply when feeling nauseated.
	Distract yourself with music, TV, conversation.
Hair loss	Cut hair length; hair will look thicker.
	Use mild shampoos.
	Use soft brushes.
	Avoid rollers, blow dryers, hair dye, or permanents.
	Use a sunscreen, hat, or wig to protect scalp from sun.
Fatigue	Get plenty of rest; allow for rest periods throughout day.
	Exercise regularly.
	Limit activities; get help from friends and/or family.
	Rise slowly from sitting or lying position to avoid dizziness.
Low blood cell count	Do not take any medication without consulting physician.
	Do not drink alcohol.
	Use an extra-soft toothbrush.
	Avoid dental floss and blowing nose with force.
	Avoid cutting or burning oneself.
	Avoid contact sports.
	Use an electric shaver instead of a razor.
Sore mouth and gum problems	See dentist before chemotherapy treatment.
	Use a fluoride rinse/gel to prevent cavities.
	Brush after every meal with an extra soft toothbrush.
	Rinse toothbrush and store in a dry place.
	Avoid commercial mouthwashes.
Mouth and throat problems	For dry mouth use artificial saliva.
	Drink plenty of liquids.
	Chew sugarless gum.
	Moisten dry foods with butter, margarine, gravy, or sauces.
	Eat soft and pureed foods.
	Use lip balm if lips become dry.
	Suck on ice chips, popsicles, or sugarless hard candies.
Skin and nail problems	Apply cornstarch to affected area.
	Take short warm showers, not long hot baths.
	Apply creams/ointments while skin is still moist from shower.
	Avoid perfumes, cologne, or aftershave agents.
	Keep face, hands, and feet clean and dry.

WBC defense mechanisms and often are destroyed by chemotherapy treatment. When this happens, a condition known as leukopenia may occur, increasing the risk of infection to the patient. The normal dosage of filgrastim is 5 mcg/kg per day. The dosage is given when the number of WBCs decreases below a certain level and may be given daily until the WBC levels increase to a normal level. The concentration of the injection is 300 mcg/mL, which either is given subcutaneously or is diluted before intravenous administration.

Cytoprotective Agents

Mesna is a cytoprotective agent used to treat the side effect of hemorrhagic cystitis caused by the chemotherapeutic agent ifosfamide. Mesna is given intravenously at a concentration of no more than 20% of the ifosfamide dose. Another agent used to alleviate side effects is amifostine. This agent is administered along with the chemotherapy agent cisplatin to prevent its toxic effects.

OTHER TYPES OF TREATMENT

Chemoradiotherapy (CRT)

The use of both chemotherapy and radiation is another option that can be effective in various cancers. It can be used both preoperatively and postoperatively or in cases where tumors cannot be easily removed. Although there are many studies being done to prove the effectiveness of this type of treatment, many initial studies show that both chemotherapy and radiation done concurrently is more effective than radiation therapy followed by chemotherapy (Mayo Clinic, 2009).

RADIOPHARMACEUTICALS

The agents used in nuclear pharmacy are referred to as radiopharmaceuticals. These agents are used as diagnostic tools and for treatments and may be administered to the patient in oral, intravenous, or inhaled forms. Just as chemotherapy agents must be handled carefully when being prepared in the pharmacy, so must nuclear medications. Radiopharmaceuticals are isotopes that can be seen on radiographs as small specks as they participate in the cell activity within the body system. Box 29-4 lists the types of nuclear medicine scans.

A nuclear pharmacy technician is expected to help prepare and label the medications as well as perform quality control testing under the direction of a licensed pharmacist. For safety purposes, each person in the nuclear pharmacy must wear a dose meter, which provides a measurement of radioactive levels to which the person is exposed. In addition, each medication package is labeled with a monitor that gives a reading of radioactive level. If the contents are damaged, the meter will reflect the level of exposure. Compliance with the proper handling of the radioisotopes during preparation and disposal is imperative for all personnel. All medications are prepared in a vertical

BOX 29-4 EXAMPLES OF RADIOPHARMACEUTICALS AND THEIR USE

Chromium-51 sodium chromate
  For labeling red blood cells for examination
Indium-111 capromab
  For prostate cancer imaging
Iodine-131 sodium iodide
  For thyroid imaging
Strontium-89
  For treatment of pain from bone cancer
Technetium-99m
  For determination of coronary artery disease
Gallium scan
  To evaluate infections of the kidney and certain tumors; used in brain, gastrointestinal bleeding, bone, liver, gallbladder, thyroid gland, lung, and heart scans

flow hood (see Chapter 12) and are disposed in a special lead container. The half-life of the radioisotope determines the time required for the isotope to decay.

BIOLOGICAL THERAPY

Also known as immunotherapy, biological therapy is a type of cancer treatment that uses natural substances or substances produced in the laboratory. These substances stimulate the body's own immune system to resist cancer. They can stop or slow the growth of cancer cells and keep cancer from spreading as well. Certain cancers are affected by this type of therapy. They are often used in conjunction with chemotherapy and radiation therapy. Biological therapy can be used to treat diseases other than cancer.

HYPERTHERMIA

The term hyperthermia refers to a body temperature that is higher than normal. This occurs naturally when we develop a fever from an infection. Although heat treatment is not a new concept, newer devices and methods are used to precisely control the heat source so that cancer cells can be destroyed. Hyperthermia can be administered either locally or regionally. Local hyperthermia heats a very small area to a very high temperature. This can be done either by externally heating the skin or by directly inserting a needle into a tumor and heating the needle's tip until the cancer cells are destroyed. Regional hyperthermia involves heating a larger area, such as a limb or body cavity. The blood in the area to be treated is isolated by pumping that blood to a heating device and then back to the limb or cavity. In this way the whole body is not affected. This form of treatment is used with chemotherapy drugs; they are circulated in the isolated heated blood only within the area designated. Radiation is another treatment that may be used along with hyperthermia.

PHOTODYNAMIC THERAPY

Photodynamic therapy uses specialized photosensitized agents to destroy cancer cells. These agents are activated upon exposure to certain kinds of light. The agents can be injected into the bloodstream or applied topically. After the agent is absorbed by the cancer cells, a light source is aimed over the diseased area, which activates the agent. The activated agent reacts with oxygen and destroys the cancer cells. There are different agents used for different cancers. This type of therapy can only be used for cancers that can be exposed to the light source.

COMPLEMENTARY AND ALTERNATIVE MEDICINE

CAM is also referred to as alternative medicine (Chapter 9) and is another option for many cancer patients who believe in a more natural approach to cancer treatment or who have exhausted traditional medications and treatments. Most herbal remedies are not prescribed by physicians because they have not proven their effectiveness through clinical trials or have not been endorsed by the FDA. Certain CAM methods have proven effective in treating symptoms of cancer; for example, ginger or peppermint may relieve nausea, and relaxation therapies can lessen stress and anxiety. It is important to ask the physician about taking various CAM agents because they can cause more harm than good as a result of interactions with chemotherapeutic and other cancer agents.

PAIN CONTROL

Many medications can be used to control acute and chronic cancer pain. These medications include schedule II and schedule III controlled substances that can be given in a variety of dosage strengths and forms. This enables patients to manage their pain at home or outside the hospital. Dosage forms may be oral liquids, tablets, capsules, patches, or suppositories. In the hospital, injectable analgesics may be given intramuscularly or intravenously. A patient-controlled analgesic (or **PCA**) pump also may be ordered; it dispenses a predetermined amount of drug at set times from a preloaded syringe. The patient also has the ability to push a button for an additional amount of medication for maximum pain relief. The patient-controlled analgesia is preset for **bolus** doses so that regardless of how many times the patient may push the button, the pump will release only the preset dose. In this way the patient cannot overdose. The amount of medication must be monitored closely by the physician based on the severity of the patient's pain.

Tech Alert!

Remember the following sound-alike/look-alike drugs:

cyclophosphamide versus cyclosporine
Cytoxan versus Cytosar
cisplatin versus carboplatin
VePesid versus Versed
Leukeran versus leucovorin

Cancer Survival Rates

Cancer is the second most common cause of death in the United States; only heart disease is responsible for more deaths. More than ½ million Americans die annually from cancer, which is more than 1500 people per day. The **mortality rate** is relatively evenly distributed between genders. The most common type of cancer, according to the American Cancer Society, is skin cancer. More than 1 million unreported cases in 2009 alone were expected. The rate of survival is directly related to the type and stage of the cancer; however, overall the 5-year **survival rate** for all cancers has increased from 50% (from 1975 to 1977) to 66% (from 1996 to 2004), a 16% increase. For a list of cancer types and death rates, refer to Table 29-7.

TABLE 29-7 Estimated Deaths Attributable to Cancer for 2009

Cancer	Estimated New Cases (2009)	Estimated Deaths (2009)	Estimated Death Rates in 2009 (%) (Rounded to Nearest Whole Number)
Bones and joints	2,570	1,470	57
Brain and CNS	22,070	12,920	56
Breast	194,280	40,610	21
Digestive system	275,720	135,830	49
Endocrine system	39,330	2,470	6
Eye and orbit	2,350	230	10
Genital system	282,690	56,160	20
Leukemia	44,790	21,870	49
Lymphoma	74,490	20,790	28
Myeloma	20,580	10,580	51
Oral cavity and pharynx	35,720	7,600	21
Respiratory system	236,990	163,790	69
Soft tissue (includes heart)	10,660	3,820	36
Urinary system	131,010	28,100	21

DO YOU REMEMBER THESE KEY POINTS?

- The types of factors that may cause cancer
- Ways to decrease the possibility of acquiring certain cancers
- The diagnostic tools used to determine the type and stage of cancer
- The definition of leukemia, as well as the various types of leukemia
- The process used by cancer to replicate
- The types of treatments available to cancer patients
- The main types of chemotherapy treatments
- The reasons side effects of chemotherapy are similar
- The way nuclear pharmacy is used in the diagnosis and treatment of cancer
- The method of action for each of the chemotherapeutic agents discussed in this chapter
- Terminology used to describe cancer and its treatments

REVIEW QUESTIONS

Multiple choice questions

1. Which of the following cell processes is not normally seen in cells?
   A. Replication
   B. Mitosis
   C. Death
   D. Metastasis

2. The term used to define the spread of cancer cells into other areas of the body is:
   A. Melanoma
   B. Cancerous
   C. Malignant
   D. Metastasis

3. Factors that are taken into account when diagnosing cancer include:
   A. Etiology
   B. Karyotype
   C. Morphology
   D. All of the above

4. The small sections of a gene that usually perform normally within a cell but when altered by a retrovirus can produce cancerous cells are referred to as:
   A. Oncogenes
   B. Tumors
   C. Neoplasms
   D. None of the above

5. A type of cancer that affects the lymphatic system and may or may not have a high grade of malignancy is referred to as:
   A. Leukemia
   B. Hodgkin's disease
   C. Non-Hodgkin's disease
   D. Kaposi's sarcoma

6. Which of the following chemotherapeutic agents are NOT used to treat cancer?
   A. Antimetabolites
   B. Mitotic inhibitors
   C. Nitrogen mustards
   D. Analgesics

7. The process of mitosis is a set of stages that begins with:
   A. G2 phase
   B. Cytokinesis
   C. S phase
   D. G1 phase

8. When preparing radiopharmaceuticals, guidelines require:
   A. The use of a radioactive meter
   B. Specialized containers for disposal
   C. Preparation within a vertical flow hood
   D. All of the above

9. Which of the following persons may be at higher risk for acquiring cancer?
   A. Persons who have family members who have been diagnosed with cancer
   B. Persons exposed to excessive radiation such as those caused by sunburns
   C. Persons who smoke
   D. All of the above

10. Which of the following side effects are seen most commonly after chemotherapy treatment?
    A. Nausea and vomiting
    B. Diarrhea
    C. Immunosuppression or anemia
    D. All of the above

True/False

If the statement is false, then change it to make it true.

_____ 1. Cancer can be caused by a virus.

_____ 2. Preventive measures can eliminate any chance of acquiring cancer.

_____ 3. Only pharmacists can prepare radiopharmaceuticals.

_____ 4. Surgery does not necessarily eliminate cancers; it is normally followed with radiological therapy and/or chemotherapy.

_____ 5. Radioactive isotopes often are implanted directly into the cancer site for treatment.

_____ 6. Anticancer agents that alter normal hormone levels include corticosteroids.

_____ 7. Vesicant agents must be prepared by a pharmacist.

_____ 8. Chemotherapy drugs are administered intravenously or intramuscularly only.

_____ 9. Erythropoietin is used to promote growth of neutrophils.

_____ 10. Traditional antibiotics can be used to treat cancer.

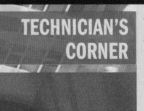

TECHNICIAN'S CORNER

Using a comprehensive drug textbook, such as *Drug Facts and Comparisons* or *Mosby's Drug Consult,* research the following chemotherapy agents and list their trade names, routes of administration, and preparation guidelines:

idarubicin
doxorubicin
mitomycin

BIBLIOGRAPHY

Drug facts and comparisons, ed 63, St Louis, 2008, Lippincott Williams & Wilkins.

Fremgen B, Frucht S: *Medical terminology*, ed 2, Upper Saddle River, NJ, 2002, Prentice Hall.

Hardman J, Limbird L: *The pharmaceutical basis of therapeutics*, ed 11, New York, 2005, McGraw-Hill.

Malarkey L, McMorrow M: *Nurse's manual of laboratory tests and diagnostic procedures*, ed 2. Philadelphia, 2000, Saunders.

Mosby's medical, nursing, & allied health dictionary, ed 6.

Stedman's concise medical dictionary for health professionals, ed 3. Baltimore, 1997, Williams & Wilkins.

WEBSITES

www.cancer.org/docroot/home/index.asp?level=0

Cancer Statistics: Source: Estimated new cases are based on 1995-2005 incidence rates from 41 states and the District of Columbia as reported by the North American Association of Central Cancer Registries (NAACCR), representing about 85% of the US population. Estimated deaths are based on data from US Mortality Data, 1969-2006.

Head and Neck Trials. CliniCal Trials. Mayo Clinic, 2009. Available at www.mayoclinic.org/head-neck-tumors/clintrials.html.

National Center for Health Statistics, Centers for Disease Control and Prevention, 2009.

www.mayoclinic.org/head-neck-tumors/clintrials.html

www.cancer.org/docroot/MBC/MBC_2x_RadiationEffects.asp?sitearea=MBC

www.cancer.gov/cancertopics/biologicaltherapy#1

www.cancer.org/docroot/MBC/content/MBC_2_2X_Will_My_Skin_Be_Affected.asp?sitearea=MBC

Basic Sciences for the Pharmacy Technician

30

Microbiology

Objectives

UPON COMPLETING THIS CHAPTER, YOU SHOULD BE ABLE TO DO
THE FOLLOWING:

- Describe the golden age of microbiology and its importance in the medical field.

- List the five kingdoms.

- List at least two different types of organisms within each kingdom.

- Differentiate between prokaryotic and eukaryotic cells.

- List the major components of the eukaryotic cell.

- Describe the functions of the major components of eukaryotic cells.

- List the steps required to perform a Gram stain.

- Describe the characteristics of bacterial cell walls of gram-positive and gram-negative microbes.

- Differentiate between gram-positive and gram-negative results.

- Describe the differences between microbes and viruses.

- List some of the most common conditions caused by species within each kingdom.

- Explain how and why bacteriophages are used to protect against viruses.

TERMS AND DEFINITIONS

Aerobic *A term that describes organisms that need oxygen to survive*

Anaerobic *A term that describes organisms that live in the absence of oxygen*

Binary fission *The method of non–sexual reproduction by which a single cell divides into two separate cells, each with the potential to grow to the size of the original cell; method of bacterial reproduction*

Biology *The study of life*

Enzyme *A protein that accelerates a reaction by reducing the amount of energy required to initiate a reaction; also called a biological catalyst*

Facultative anaerobe *A microorganism that can live with or without oxygen*

Heterotrophic *The ability to reproduce asexually.*

Microbial *Refers to microorganisms (very small organisms) not visible without a microscope*

Microbiology *The study of microscopic organisms*

Morphology *Appearance of organisms, including shape, size, structure, and Gram stain characteristics; studying the structure of organisms without studying the function of organisms*

Peptidoglycan *The polymer substance that comprises bacterial cell walls, specifically of gram-negative and gram-positive microbes*

Species *Of Latin origin meaning "kind"; in biology the term describes the basic rank in taxonomic classification*

Taxonomy *The science of classification; with respect to biology, taxonomy is a hierarchical structure for the nomenclature (naming) and classification of organisms*

Vector *An entity by which infections are transferred, but the entity of transference does not have the disease and does not need to be living. For example, a mosquito bite transfers malaria. In this case, the mosquito is the vector*

Virology *The study of viruses*

Virus *A microscopic organism that replicates exclusively inside a host's cell, using parts of the host cell including DNA, ribosomes, and proteins*

EXAMPLES OF ORGANISMS AND DISEASES THEY CAUSE

Organism	Genus and Species	Condition(s)
Protozoa	*Plasmodium falciparum*	Malaria
Fungi	*Candida albicans*	Candidiasis
	Epidermophyton	Skin and nail infections
	Microsporum	Hair and skin infections
	Trichophyton	Hair, skin, and nail infections
Bacteria	*Borrelia burgdorferi*	Lyme disease
	Clostridium botulinum	Botulism
	Clostridium tetani	Tetanus
	Helicobacter pylori	Stomach ulcers
	Haemophilus influenzae	Meningitis
	Mycobacterium leprae	Leprosy
	Mycobacterium tuberculosis	Tuberculosis
	Neisseria gonorrhoeae	Gonorrhea
	Staphylococcus aureus	Skin infections, pneumonia, bacteremia, osteomyelitis
	Streptococcus pneumoniae	Meningitis, pneumonia, otitis media
	Streptococcus pyogenes	Scarlet fever

Continued

EXAMPLES OF ORGANISMS AND DISEASES THEY CAUSE—cont'd

Organism	Genus and Species	Condition(s)
Helminths	Hookworm	Severe anemia
	Roundworms	Fever, cough, diarrhea, muscle weakness
	Flatworms (Flukes)	Rash, fever, chills, diarrhea, abdominal pain
	Pinworms	Itching around the anus
	Tapeworms	Abdominal discomfort, diarrhea, and loss of appetite
Viruses	Human immunodeficiency virus	Acquired immunodeficiency syndrome (AIDS)
	Herpesvirus	Herpes
	Influenza A and B viruses	Influenza
	Poliovirus	Polio
	Varicella-zoster virus	Chickenpox
	Rabies virus	Rabies
	Rhinoviruses or coronaviruses	Common cold

BIOLOGY IS THE STUDY OF LIFE. Some forms of life cannot be seen without the aid of a microscope. **Microbiology** is the study of very small organisms, or microorganisms. This includes bacteria, some forms of fungus, and protists. **Viruses** are even smaller than bacteria. **Virology** is the study of viruses. Special microscopes and techniques are needed to view viruses because of their small size. An understanding of how microbes work is important in order to appreciate how antibiotics and other agents fight infections and other conditions that affect the human species. To understand the world of microbes, we first must have some background on how life has been explained scientifically. From the dawn of humankind, human beings have tried to define life. We must understand life forms because these forms interact with each other.

As scientific techniques advance, so does our insight into the mysterious world of **microbial** life forms. Because of the strange and bizarre life forms that have been discovered on this planet, scientists believe now, more than ever, that life may exist on other planets. Microbes have been found in fossils dating back more than 3 billion years before the beginning of humankind. They have adapted to the drastic and harsh changes in the environment since the beginning of their existence. Microbes can live regardless of adverse conditions. Bacteria and other life forms have been a part of human evolution. Human beings benefit from bacteria in many ways. This chapter explores the positive and negative effects of bacteria on humans.

Charles Darwin (Evolution)

In 1831 Charles Darwin traveled to the Galapagos Islands and studied the various **species** on each island. He discovered that evolution plays a key role in the survival of the fittest by allowing adaptations of species in response to their environments. Darwin's observations of the animals on the Galapagos Islands made him question the theories of how species inhabited islands far from the mainland.

Darwin found that the species on the islands were not very different and yet they were not the same as the species on the mainland. His research directed him in another direction. From all his recorded notes and from previous research by animal researchers, Darwin found that tortoises, birds, insects, and even plants living on the many islands were similar to one another. However, even though they lived in proximity to one another, the species were different between islands. Darwin believed that the reason for this major difference was that each species followed a different evolutionary path. The various animals and organisms living on each island developed into different species altogether. Only those species that survived the changes on each island would reproduce. Therefore, only the fittest survived. Darwin formed taxonomic categories based on the phylogenetic (evolutionary relationships) relationship between offspring from previous generations, contributing to our understanding of biology. He is considered the Father of Evolution.

The Golden Age of Microbiology

Until the invention of the microscope in the 1600s, scientists did not know that organisms were made of cells nor did they know about microscopic organisms (see Chapter 1). An English eyeglass maker by the name of Robert Hooke is considered the father of microscopy; he devised the first compound microscope. Around 1665 he used a crude type of microscope to observe the cells of a simple cork. He described them as tiny boxes or "cells." This was the beginning of the study of microscopic organisms. In 1674 Anton van Leeuwenhoek invented a more sophisticated microscope and documented the observation of tiny microbes in a drop of water and teeth scrapings; Hooke later confirmed these scientific findings. van Leeuwenhoek referred to these small organisms as "animalcules" or "little animals"; he was the first to see bacteria. Although many microbes were now being discovered, debate continued in the scientific world regarding the origins of these microbes.

In the beginning of microbiology, most scientists believed in spontaneous generation. The idea was that some organisms were generated from other organisms or their by-products. For example, it was believed that flies were generated from manure, maggots were produced from decaying corpses, and mice and snakes developed from common soil. In the 200 years after the invention of the microscope, these inaccurate beliefs were disproved by scientific methods. They were replaced by the understanding that new life arises from preexisting living organisms (biogenesis). Scientific methods were established, and these methods are still used today to prove or disprove hypotheses. Figure 30-1 illustrates a time line of major advances in the field of microbiology.

LOUIS PASTEUR

The French scientist Louis Pasteur (1822-1895) is probably most well known for his development of the pasteurization process—used today to slow the spoilage of milk and other dairy products. Pasteur devised experiments in 1861 that would set the standards for scientific research in the future. He proved that unseen microorganisms exist in the air rather than in nonliving material, such as broth. Using broth-filled, long-neck glass flasks that were made to trap airborne microbes, he proved that the broth could be kept free from contamination. Therefore spontaneous generation of organisms could not exist within the broth. His experiments proved the presence of biogenesis. He also was able to show through his experiments that bacteria were responsible for spoilage of certain beverages, and thus paved the way for our understanding of germs.

Many advances in scientific knowledge occurred after Pasteur's experiments— from discovering new bacteria to understanding the theory of evolution. It is no wonder that this period (approximately 1857 to 1914) was called the golden age of microbiology. Most of the discoveries made during this time included the development of vaccines, such as anthrax and rabies. With the acceptance of the existence of bacteria and other microbes, scientists and physicians were able to

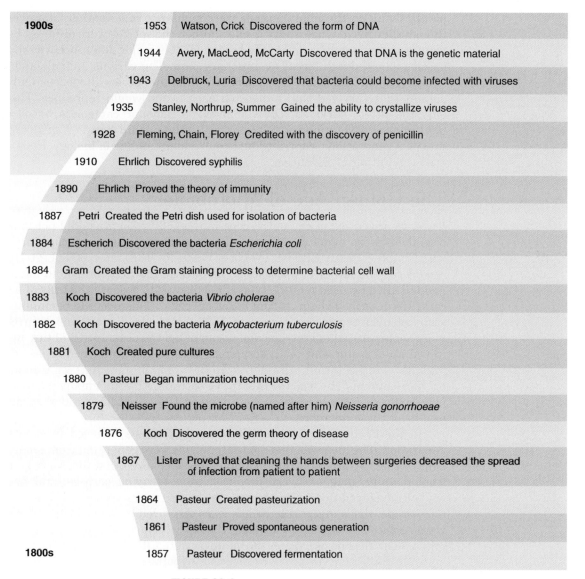

1900s	1953	Watson, Crick Discovered the form of DNA
	1944	Avery, MacLeod, McCarty Discovered that DNA is the genetic material
	1943	Delbruck, Luria Discovered that bacteria could become infected with viruses
	1935	Stanley, Northrup, Summer Gained the ability to crystallize viruses
	1928	Fleming, Chain, Florey Credited with the discovery of penicillin
	1910	Ehrlich Discovered syphilis
	1890	Ehrlich Proved the theory of immunity
	1887	Petri Created the Petri dish used for isolation of bacteria
	1884	Escherich Discovered the bacteria *Escherichia coli*
	1884	Gram Created the Gram staining process to determine bacterial cell wall
	1883	Koch Discovered the bacteria *Vibrio cholerae*
	1882	Koch Discovered the bacteria *Mycobacterium tuberculosis*
	1881	Koch Created pure cultures
	1880	Pasteur Began immunization techniques
	1879	Neisser Found the microbe (named after him) *Neisseria gonorrhoeae*
	1876	Koch Discovered the germ theory of disease
	1867	Lister Proved that cleaning the hands between surgeries decreased the spread of infection from patient to patient
	1864	Pasteur Created pasteurization
	1861	Pasteur Proved spontaneous generation
1800s	1857	Pasteur Discovered fermentation

FIGURE 30-1 The golden age of microbiology.

devise means to fight infection, most notably aseptic techniques. The average life span of an adult in the 1600s was 40 years; in contrast, midlife today is 40 years and many persons live into their 80s and 90s.

In 1887 Louis Pasteur founded the Pasteur Institute in Paris, France. The Pasteur Foundation funds the Pasteur Institute, whose mission is to improve public health by contributing to the prevention and treatment of infectious diseases. The institute accomplishes this through research, teaching, and treatment of infectious diseases. Notable diseases such as the autoimmune deficiency syndrome (AIDS) virus were first discovered by the researchers at the Pasteur Institute, and they developed a test to detect the H1N1 virus as recently as 2009.

Classifications of Organisms (Taxonomy)

Scientists have classified organisms into seven different groups. These groups are based on structural similarities, and the groups clarify how different organisms survive and interact with each other. This knowledge serves to aid scien-

TABLE 30-1 Kingdoms, Cell Characteristics, and Examples

Kingdom	Eukaryote/ Prokaryote	Method of Nutrition	Types of Organisms
Plantae	Eukaryote	Photosynthesis	Mosses, ferns, woody and nonwoody flowering plants
Animalia	Eukaryote	Ingest food	Sponges, worms, fish, mammals, reptiles, insects, amphibians, birds
Protista	Eukaryote	Absorb, ingest, and photosynthesize food	Algae, water molds, amebae
Fungi	Eukaryote	Absorb food	Molds, yeasts, fungi, mushrooms, mildews
Monera	Prokaryote	Absorb food	Bacteria, blue-green algae, spirochetes

tists in understanding evolutionary changes. In biology, the study of naming and classifying organisms is called **taxonomy**. Taxonomy is a difficult area of study because it can be hard to classify new organisms in a specific group when they may have similarities to more than one group.

ROBERT WHITTAKER (THE FIVE KINGDOMS)

The five kingdoms—Plantae, Animalia, Fungi, Protista, and Monera—were conceived by the scientist Robert Whittaker and are still in use today (Table 30-1). Four of the five kingdoms (Plantae, Animalia, Fungi, and Protista) consist of eukaryotic organisms, whereas Monera consists of prokaryotic organisms, including bacteria. Within each kingdom, the organisms are next divided into different phyla, followed by classes, orders, families, genera, and then finally species. The use of these specific classifications aids in identifying organisms, because as one proceeds from kingdom to species the organisms become more similar. The following list presents a brief overview of each of the seven classifications (using humans as an example) and provides examples of similarities within each group:

- Kingdom: This is the largest group; it is composed of five different categories for living things, Animalia being one of them.
- Phylum: There are about 20 phyla for animals. All animals with a backbone belong to the phylum Chordata. Humans are in the subphylum Vertebrata (because we have vertebrae).
- Class: Animals belong to the class Mammalia. All mammals share at least three characteristics: three middle ear bones, hair, and use of mammary glands to produce milk.
- Order: Animals that primarily eat meat are in the order Carnivora. Primates, bats, dolphins, and whales are in the same order.
- Family: Animals are grouped into families. Humans are in the Canidae family.
- Genus: Humans are in the genus *Homo*. Most organisms in this genus have a prominent face and jaw; nostrils are close together and facing forward and downward. Chimps, gorillas, orangutans, and humans are in this genus.
- Species: A species is a group of organisms with similar physical characteristics, including the ability to interbreed with viable offspring. The species of humans is *sapiens*.

Caroleus Linnaeus introduced the use of binomial nomenclature to identify organisms; in the case of humans we are referred to as *Homo sapiens* (the combination of genus and species).

These seven different classifications are used to organize all the known living organisms on planet Earth. Each kingdom, of course, contains many different types of organisms.

Viruses are not included in the five kingdoms. Scientists differ on the classification of viruses because they do not completely fit into the characteristics of a "life form." Viruses are discussed at the end of this chapter.

Eukaryotic and prokaryotic organisms have different characteristics. The most obvious difference is that in contrast to prokaryotes, eukaryotes have a nucleus that binds deoxyribonucleic acid (DNA). Also, eukaryotes do not have a cell wall structure as seen in prokaryotes. One way antibiotics can kill bacteria is by their ability to attach to the bacterial cell wall, where they break down the organism and destroy it. Because eukaryotes do not have this cell wall, antibiotics cannot attach themselves. This difference makes it possible for antibiotics to kill microbes without harming the cells of the human body. Each eukaryotic kingdom is differentiated from the others by the following four main criteria:

1. Pattern of development
2. Nutritional requirements
3. Tissue differentiation
4. Possession of flagella (form of locomotion)

We briefly review each of the five kingdoms, specifically discussing organisms that may have an adverse effect on human beings. In addition, a brief discussion of viruses covers their unique characteristics and abilities to inflict harm—knowledge that can help us in the ever-growing battle against infection.

Plantae

The kingdom Plantae includes land (terrestrial) and water plants (aquatic). They are mainly multicellular and are classified further based on their photosynthetic pigmentation. Plants are eukaryotic organisms that obtain their food and energy supply from the sun through photosynthesis. They include mosses, ferns, flowers, conifers, and an array of other organisms. Human beings have a special relationship with plants; we need them for nutrition and protection from inclement weather; they also generate oxygen from carbon dioxide, continuously renewing air that we breathe. We use parts of plants to build homes and make clothing and to treat various medical conditions. For example, digoxin is taken from the plant foxglove and is used to treat heart conditions. A drug used to treat ovarian cancer, Taxol, is derived from the bark of the Pacific yew *(Taxus brevifolia)*. More recently, *Ginkgo biloba*, part of the ginkgo tree, has been used to support memory (see Chapter 9).

Plant Cell Structure. Plant cells contain many of the same structures as animal cells. However, plant cells are different from animal cells in the manner that they acquire energy. Figures 30-2 and 30-3 illustrate the differences between animal and plant cells. Plants have chloroplasts that are used to convert sunlight into energy, which then is stored. In addition, plants have a cell wall that is composed of cellulose, which maintains cell shape. Vacuoles (fluid-filled cavities found in the cytoplasm of a cell) of plant cells are also much larger than those found in animal cells.

Communicable diseases are not transmitted easily by plants to humans; however, plants may cause contact irritations in humans or toxicity upon ingestion. Because plants are linked in many ways to animal survival, we have

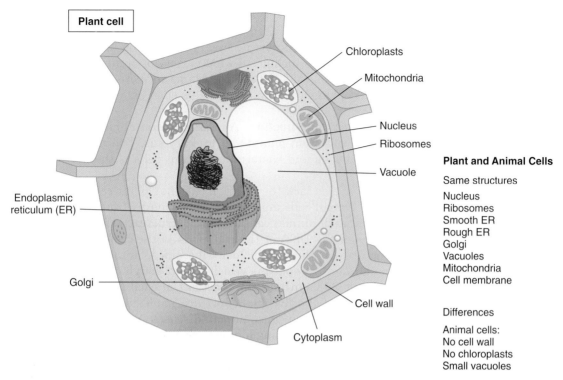

Plant cell

Chloroplasts
Mitochondria
Nucleus
Ribosomes
Vacuole

Endoplasmic
reticulum (ER)

Golgi

Cell wall

Cytoplasm

Plant and Animal Cells

Same structures

Nucleus
Ribosomes
Smooth ER
Rough ER
Golgi
Vacuoles
Mitochondria
Cell membrane

Differences

Animal cells:
No cell wall
No chloroplasts
Small vacuoles

FIGURE 30-2 Major components of a plant cell.

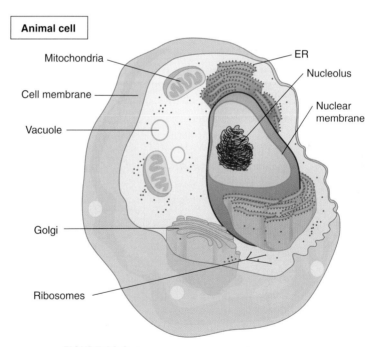

Animal cell

Mitochondria
Cell membrane
Vacuole

ER
Nucleolus
Nuclear
membrane

Golgi

Ribosomes

FIGURE 30-3 Cell composition of an animal cell.

benefited from many plants, using them for food, flavorings, and colorings (dyes) and to treat various conditions.

Animalia
The kingdom Animalia contains more species than any other kingdom. Species in this kingdom are more complex physiologically than other species and rely

on many motor skills and sensory organs. Ingested food must be broken down through a series of complicated steps before it can be used. Nervous systems that are more complex may be necessary, depending on the species of animal. The Animalia kingdom includes a wide variety of organisms, ranging from the more simplistic sponges, jellyfish, and clams to more complex organisms such as spiders, frogs, kangaroos, and mammals such as humans.

Animal: Eukaryotic Cell Structure. Animal cells contain different structures than those found in cells from plants and prokaryotes. The most obvious difference between animal cells and bacterial and plant cells is the lack of a cell wall in animal cells.

Animal cells also lack the chloroplasts that plant cells use to store energy from the sun. Animal cells must derive their energy from food rather than from the sun. Inside each animal cell are many structures that work in unison. The nucleus contains the DNA of the cell. This is the genetic code of the animal. Other structures in the cell include ribosomes, mitochondria, golgi complex, plasma membrane, cytoplasm, vesicles, and rough and smooth endoplasmic reticulum. Table 30-2 outlines the functions of each structure.

Because four of the five kingdoms are made up of eukaryotic organisms, many types of species can cause human diseases. Various organisms in the Animalia, Fungi, or Protista kingdom can be transmitted to human beings from various vectors. Plants can transfer toxins if ingested or contacted (e.g., poison oak/ivy). Vectors are the carriers of disease organisms. The way the organism moves through various environments during its life cycle ultimately reveals actions to avoid contact, as explained under Human Diseases and Conditions later in this chapter.

TABLE 30-2 Characteristics and Structure of an Animal (Eukaryotic) Cell

Cell Component	Structure	Description
Centrosomes	Rod-like structures	Contain centrioles, which are symmetrical in design; they are needed at beginning of reproduction
DNA	Double helix	Genetic code responsible for many characteristics
Endoplasmic reticulum (ER)	Membranous network	Contained throughout cytoplasm; provides surface area for production, transportation, and storage of molecules within cell; attached ribosomes involved in lipid and protein synthesis
Golgi complex	Flat membranous stacks of sacs	Serves as a transport system for enzymes and proteins; some proteins have carbohydrates added to structure before they are moved out of cell
Lysosomes	A single sac filled with digestive juices	Digestive sacs that dispose of unwanted particles within cell; they then are emptied outside of cell
Mitochondria	Cell-like structure with membranous material	Responsible for making adenosine triphosphate, that then is carried to places within cell where energy is needed to produce enzymes and so forth; cells contain many mitochondria that are located near production areas such as ER
Nucleus	Envelope containing DNA	Contains DNA and nucleolus; nucleolus manufactures substances (such as ribosomes) used in cytoplasm
Ribosomes	Small, dot-like structures	ER that contains ribosomes is referred to as rough ER; it produces proteins such as enzymes
RNA	Chain	A messenger for coding proteins
Smooth ER	Membranous network	Produces various lipid substances; has no ribosomes

Protista

Most of the organisms in the kingdom Protista are unicellular; all are eukaryotic and although diverse in their makeup they have common characteristics with one another. Most are found in aquatic or semi-aquatic environments, most need air to survive, most have either flagella or cilia to propel themselves, and most are able to produce cysts at some point in their life cycle that is resistant to harsh conditions such as drought or freezing. They are composed of many different plant-like and animal-like organisms. The plant-like organisms such as algae, molds, diatoms, and dinoflagellates make their own food much like plants do, whereas many protozoans are animal-like organisms that catch and swallow food from outside sources. All are **heterotrophic**, which means they reproduce asexually. Some cause diseases in other organisms.

Algae and water molds can be found in and around coastal waters. Certain forms of algae are macroscopic, reaching lengths from a few meters up to 50 meters. Whether living in large brown kelp beds off the coast to growing in trees, algae prefer moist to wet areas and need light to survive. They produce chlorophyll, which they use as a food source. Some protists, such as brown algae or lichens, anchor themselves to a surface. Other organisms, such as euglenoids and green algae, propel themselves by means of a flagellum, a whip-like structure that moves them through water.

Protozoans can live in water or soil, and they live off bacteria and other organic particles. Protozoans can be a part of the "normal flora" of an animal, and most do not cause disease. There are four classes of protozoans: sarcodines, ciliates, flagellates, and sporozoans. Sarcodines are gelatin-like in appearance, and they move using the fluids inside their cell to flow in the direction they are moving, ciliates have cilia (small hair-like structures) surrounding them that push the organism from one place to another, and flagellates use a whiplike tail to propel themselves. Sporozoans cannot move themselves but rather depend on their host for transportation. Figure 30-4 shows the three modes of locomotion used by protozoa.

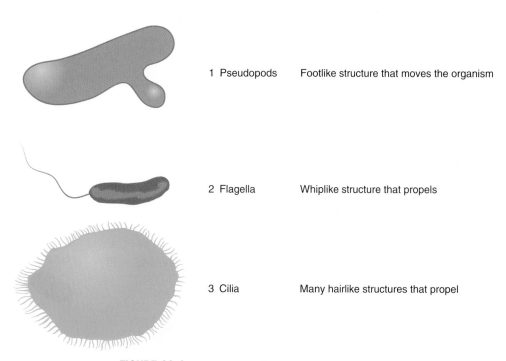

1 Pseudopods Footlike structure that moves the organism

2 Flagella Whiplike structure that propels

3 Cilia Many hairlike structures that propel

FIGURE 30-4 Three forms of locomotion in protozoa.

How Parasites Are Transmitted. The ameba *Entamoeba histolytica* is a parasitic organism that feeds on red blood cells. It is transmitted among humans via ingestion of cysts that are excreted in the feces. The **vector** or carrier of these disease-causing microorganisms includes human beings and mosquitoes.

Trichomonas vaginalis is another protozoan that causes infections in the male urinary tract and in the vagina of females. The organism is transferred mostly by sexual intercourse.

Dysentery is caused by another protozoan ciliate, *Balantidium coli,* and is transferred by ingestion of contaminated cysts present in feces. When the cysts are ingested, they travel to the colon and replicate.

Sporozoa, such as *Plasmodium vivax,* are responsible for the disease malaria. Their life cycle involves an infected female mosquito. The sporozoa in the salivary glands of the mosquito easily move into the human bloodstream once the mosquito bites the human being. From the bloodstream, the sporozoa pass to the liver, where they replicate and move into the bloodstream. As the parasites are released into the bloodstream, their toxic by-products cause illness in the host. When an uninfected mosquito bites an infected human being, the cycle is repeated (Figure 30-5).

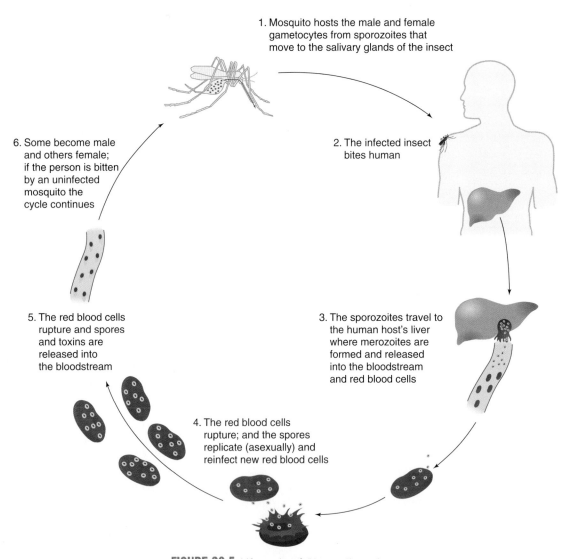

1. Mosquito hosts the male and female gametocytes from sporozoites that move to the salivary glands of the insect

2. The infected insect bites human

3. The sporozoites travel to the human host's liver where merozoites are formed and released into the bloodstream and red blood cells

4. The red blood cells rupture; and the spores replicate (asexually) and reinfect new red blood cells

5. The red blood cells rupture and spores and toxins are released into the bloodstream

6. Some become male and others female; if the person is bitten by an uninfected mosquito the cycle continues

FIGURE 30-5 Life cycle of *Plasmodium vivax.*

Helminths (worms) are also protists but are categorized under different phyla (headings) than protozoa (single-celled organisms). Two types of helminths are Platyhelminthes (flatworms) and Aschelminthes (roundworms). These worms are multicellular eukaryotic organisms that have many of the same organ systems found in humans; they have digestive, circulatory, nervous, excretory, and reproductive systems. Flatworms and roundworms live in soil and feed on organic material. Those that lack a digestive system remain parasitic. They must absorb digested nutrients from a host. Other differences between free-living and parasitic helminths are that parasitic helminths may lack means of locomotion and they have a simple nervous system because they do not need to be sensitive to their environment. The parasitic helminth life cycle is complex, which requires a more sophisticated reproductive system. Table 30-3 lists some parasitic diseases that can be contracted by humans. All forms of these parasites can be avoided by using the following precautions:

- Always cook meat thoroughly.
- Wear shoes when walking outside on soil.
- Never drink from a stream or other freshwater because it may be contaminated with feces from animals upstream.
- Wash your hands after touching animals or after cleaning cat litter boxes.

TABLE 30-3 Parasitic Diseases Contracted by Human Beings

Organism	Species	Life Cycle
Phylum: Platyhelminthes		
Trematodes (flukes)	*Paragonimus westermani*	Miracidium swims and imbeds in snail; then develops into next form, cercaria, that invades lobster. Person eats lobster and contracts adult fluke. Defecation into water continues cycle.
Cestodes (tapeworms)	*Taenia saginata*	Proglottids containing eggs are found in feces defecated onto grass. Cattle ingest proglottids containing eggs. They hatch and bore into muscle and form cyst. Cysts are ingested by humans in uncooked meat, and cycle continues
	Echinococcus granulosus	Humans ingest eggs excreted in feces. Eggs hatch within small intestines, and larvae migrate to liver or lungs. Cyst is formed. In the wild, host may be eaten by another animal, and cycle continues.
Phylum: Aschelminthes		
Nematodes (roundworms)	*Enterobius vermicularis*	This species spends its entire life in human host. Adult pinworms deposit eggs around perianal region, where they can be transferred via exposure to contaminated clothing.
	Ascaris lumbricoides	Adult form lives in small intestines of human host. Eggs are excreted and can survive in soil until ingested by another host. Eggs hatch in intestines, travel to lungs to mature stage, and then migrate to intestine to continue cycle.
	Necator americanus	Adult lives in small intestines of human beings; eggs are excreted and live in soil. Worm infects host by penetrating through skin of feet, from where it is carried to lungs via blood. It is coughed up and then ingested into stomach, where it enters intestine.
	Trichinella spiralis	Undercooked pork or beef containing cyst form enters human digestive tract, where cysts reproduce live nematodes. They migrate to various muscles and tissues and remain to be parasites of host.

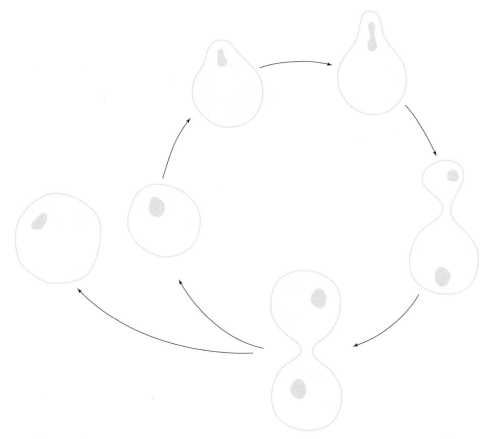

FIGURE 30-6 The budding process of replication of yeast cells. Yeast multiplies asexually by budding or sprouting a new cell that then breaks away from the mother cell.

Tech Note!

Yeast (facultative anaerobe) usually is associated with baking bread and making beer. As the species *Saccharomyces cerevisiae* (bakers' yeast) buds, it expands and the bread dough rises. The yeast in beer disperses carbon dioxide as a by-product and also gives beer its unique taste.

Fungi

The Fungi kingdom is divided into true fungi and slime molds. Many have a complex reproductive cycle. Lichens are a specialized type of fungi that can grow in the most inhospitable environments.

Fungi are different from bacteria. The DNA of a fungus is contained within a nuclear membrane. Some of the organisms that belong in the kingdom Fungi include fleshy-type fungi (such as mushrooms), yeasts, and certain types of molds. Fungi are aerobes (need oxygen to survive) or facultative anaerobes (require some oxygen to survive). Yeasts are the only fungi that are not multicellular, but they too absorb nutrients from plants. They are round or oval and may be found on leaves of plants. Each single cell replicates by the process of budding (splitting into two pieces) (Figure 30-6).

Molds may have long filaments called hyphae and may form a mass large enough to be seen by the naked eye. Molds can infect and ultimately destroy (spoil) plants and food. Fungi play an important role in the environment because they are responsible for decomposing plant organisms. They use dead plants as a food source while cleaning the environment. Compared to humans, plants are more susceptible to fungal infections. Many fungi do not cause illness; however, human beings can become infected from specific species.

The following sections describe the characteristics of prokaryotic cells, the conditions caused by these organisms, and the ways in which antibiotics are used to treat them. Please refer to Chapter 25 for specific antimicrobial actions of antibiotics and their side effects.

Prokaryotic cell size	Description of basic form			Description of basic cocci or bacilli shapes	
Coccus	oval or round	1. 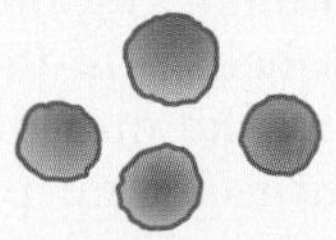		diplococcus diplobacilli	5. 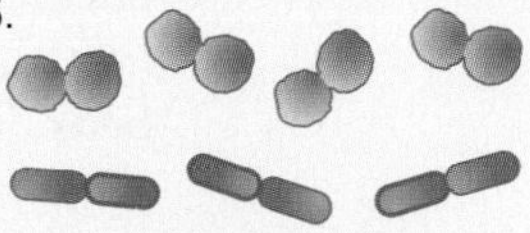
Bacillus	rectangular, rod shaped	2. 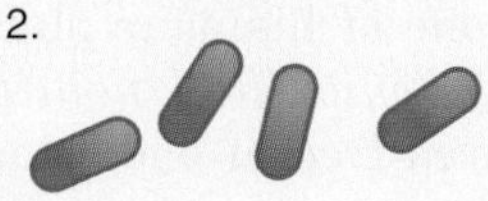		streptococcus streptobacilli	6. 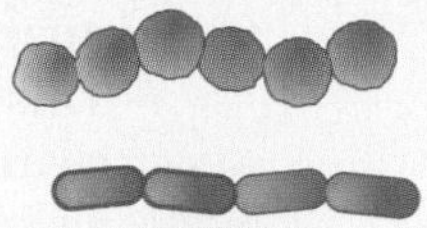
Spirilla	twisted, helical, corkscrew, spiral	3. 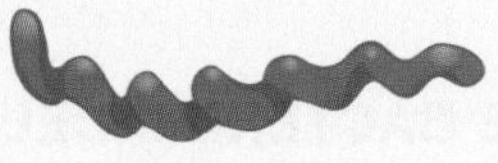		staphylococci staphylobacilli	7. 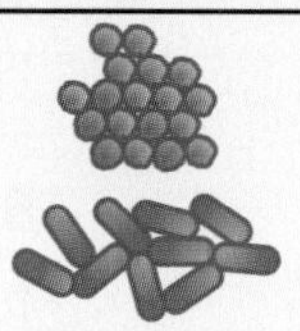
Vibrios	resemble commas	4. 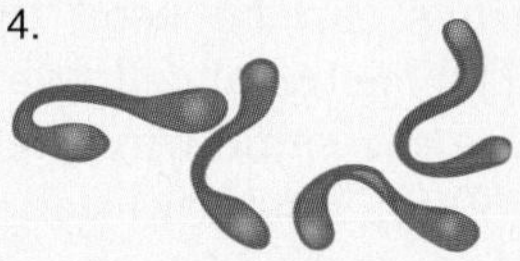			

FIGURE 30-7 Morphology of prokaryotic organisms. Pictures *1* to *6* show the various morphologies or shapes of microbes. The most common shapes include the following: *1*, coccus; *2*, bacilli; *3*, spirilla; *4*, vibrios. Picture *5* shows cocci microbes that are found in sets of two, called diplococci or diplobacilli. Those microbes found in strips are shown in picture *6*: streptococci or streptobacilli. Picture *7* shows staphylococci and staphylobacilli, which are found in clusters.

Monera

Monera, the smallest organisms (in size) of the five kingdoms, may be the simplest in physiology but are the most abundant worldwide. Fossils of bacteria have been dated back 3.5 billion years; in contrast, eukaryotic cells date back only 1.5 billion years. The cell structure of prokaryotes is less complicated than that of eukaryotes. Bacteria are classified further depending on how they derive their energy, as well as other characteristics.

Characteristics and Structure of Prokaryotes. Until now, we have explored a few of the many different types of eukaryotic cell organisms. Many basic differences exist between prokaryotic and eukaryotic cell structures. The visual characteristics of bacteria and other microbial organisms are used to describe the **morphology** or appearance of the organism (Figure 30-7).

Other characteristics specific to prokaryotes are that they can reproduce by **binary fission** (divide in two), they do not have a nuclear envelope, and, amazingly, they have the ability to live in the most inhospitable environments, adding to their prevalence. Prokaryotes may be anaerobic or aerobic. Before the discovery of these minute life forms, the effects of bacteria were attributed to other causes, such as evil spirits.

Brief History of Antibiotics

Bacteria reside just about everywhere in the world. Environments that contain bacteria range from hot springs, to the bottom of the ocean, to deep in the earth's crust, to the mouths and intestinal systems of humans. Bacteria that require oxygen to survive are called **aerobic**, whereas those that grow only in the absence of oxygen are called **anaerobic**. Some bacteria, called **facultative**

anaerobes, can survive without oxygen or with only small amounts of oxygen. The relationship that some bacteria have with animals is mutually beneficial. This means that both organisms benefit from one another. For instance, various bacteria reside within the human gut, including *Escherichia coli* and *Lactobacillus;* they assist in the metabolism of food so that it can be absorbed into the body. The bacteria benefit by the nutrient-rich environment. In the laboratory, they easily grow on nutrient-rich agar plates.

In 1928 Alexander Fleming, a scientist who was studying crops plagued by infections, noticed that one of his agar plates was contaminated with a mold. This mold, later named *Penicillium notatum,* was surrounded by a zone of clearance—that is, an area free of bacteria. It took many years to isolate the active component within the mold—penicillin. Penicillin destroys bacteria by interacting with **enzymes** that are present within the bacterial cell wall.

STRUCTURE OF THE BACTERIAL CELL WALL

Because bacteria have many characteristics that are different from cells present in the body, certain drugs can be used to attack and kill bacteria without harming human cells. The bacterial cell has a wall or barrier made of **peptidoglycan** that protects it in the same way that our skin protects us from damage and intrusion (Figure 30-8). Bacterial cell walls are made of a finely woven network of two forms of protective barriers. Penicillin disrupts the barrier and causes the bacteria to lyse or break open. Because human cells are surrounded by a cell membrane, not a cell wall, they are not harmed.

Bacteria are categorized as either gram-positive or gram-negative. This basis is determined by a Gram stain, which differentiates cell walls on the basis of their composition. There are several differences between gram-positive and gram-negative bacteria. Cell walls of gram-positive bacteria consist of thick peptidoglycan layers linked by teichoic acids to the inner membrane. In contrast, a gram-negative cell wall has few peptidoglycan layers. Gram-negative cells also differ in other aspects of their components; for example, gram-negative cells have an outer membrane that enables them to withstand certain antibiotics, such as penicillin, as well as detergents, digestive enzymes, and certain dyes. In addition, gram-negative cell walls contain a lipid that becomes toxic (endotoxins) when in the bloodstream of the host. Openings on the surface of the outer cell membrane of the gram-negative cell allow some chemicals to penetrate the cell. These openings are responsible for the difference shown between gram-negative and gram-positive bacteria on the Gram stain; thus laboratory technicians can differentiate between the two types of organisms (Table 30-4).

Exterior of Bacterial Cell Walls

Glycocalyx is a sticky substance that surrounds many different types of bacteria. This thick layer is composed of different materials, depending on the species. The purpose of glycocalyx is to protect the bacteria from being destroyed by the immune system cells of the host. This sticky substance enhances the ability of bacteria to adhere to surfaces. This increases the chance of bacterial survival.

ANTIBIOTIC SPECTRUM AND RESISTANCE

Certain antibiotics destroy bacteria by breaking down the cell walls of bacteria. To choose the right drug to destroy specific bacteria, the type of microbe must be determined. The first step in this process is to determine whether the bacteria are gram-positive or gram-negative.

Most penicillins are effective at destroying the cell walls of gram-positive microbes. However, many forms of bacteria are not destroyed by penicillin because they secrete enzymes that break bonds within the penicillin structure,

Bacterial cell

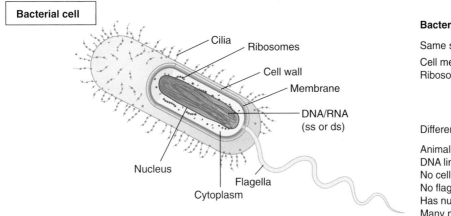

Cilia
Ribosomes
Cell wall
Membrane
DNA/RNA (ss or ds)
Nucleus
Flagella
Cytoplasm

Bacterial and Animal Cells

Same structures

Cell membrane
Ribosomes

Differences

Animal cell:
DNA linear only DS
No cell wall
No flagella, cilia
Has nuclear envelope
Many more structures

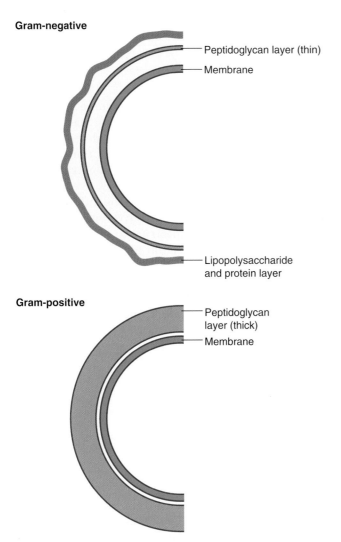

Gram-negative

Peptidoglycan layer (thin)
Membrane
Lipopolysaccharide and protein layer

Gram-positive

Peptidoglycan layer (thick)
Membrane

FIGURE 30-8 Bacterial cell walls.

TABLE 30-4 Classes of Microorganisms within the Kingdom Monera

Common Name	Examples	Characteristics
Wall-less prokaryotes	Mycoplasmata	Smallest known bacteria that can live outside host cells; lipid-type barrier helps protect them
Typical gram-positive cell wall	Rods, cocci Actinomycetes	Thick walls made of peptidoglycan
Typical gram-negative cell wall	Anaerobic photosynthetic bacteria Cyanobacteria Nonphotosynthetic bacteria	Thin walls made of peptidoglycan
Altered cell wall type	Archaebacteria	Walls not composed of peptidoglycan but polysaccharides or proteins

thus rendering it useless against the bacteria. The name for this bacterial enzyme is penicillinase (just one of many beta-lactamases). Special additives can be included with penicillin-type agents to prohibit their destruction. Additives such as sulbactam added to ampicillin (Unasyn) inhibit the beta-lactamases, allowing the antibiotic to break bacterial bonds and penetrate the bacterial cell wall.

As the antibiotic spectrum broadens, so does the effectiveness against microbes; thus broad-spectrum antibiotics are effective against more microbes than narrow-spectrum antibiotics. Narrow-spectrum antibiotics normally affect gram-positive microbes, whereas broad-spectrum antibiotics may affect gram-negative microbes additionally. Broad-spectrum agents such as aminoglycosides are much more effective against gram-negative bacteria. Another important aspect of bacterial organisms is their ability to live in the presence or absence of oxygen; some antibiotics are effective against anaerobic bacteria and some are not.

Some agents are very specific, killing one type of bacteria preferentially. This is why it is important to choose the correct antibiotic. Table 30-5 provides examples of common types of conditions caused by bacteria.

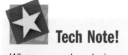 **Tech Note!**

When a word ends in *-ase,* it means that it is an enzyme.

Human Diseases and Conditions

DISEASES CAUSED BY ORGANISMS WITHIN THE PLANTAE KINGDOM

While many plant species are harmless, several have inherent mechanisms for self-protection. For this reason it is important to know which plants are potentially dangerous if contact is made or if they are ingested. Several types of common garden and household plants can be extremely dangerous if eaten by children and animals. In certain instances emergency treatment is necessary; physicians may use an oral agent such as activated charcoal to absorb the toxins in the stomach. An example of poisonous plants is given in Box 30-1.

• Poison ivy/oak: Both types of plants can cause an allergic reaction in some people when the sap of the plant is touched. Symptoms include rash, itching

TABLE 30-5 Commonly Caused Bacterial Conditions

Organism	Disease	Morphology
Borrelia burgdorferi	Lyme disease	Difficult to Gram stain*
Clostridium botulinum	Botulism	Anaerobic, gram-positive rods
Clostridium tetani	Tetanus	Anaerobic, gram-positive rods
Escherichia coli	Cystitis (an opportunistic bacteria of GI tract)	Gram-negative rods
Haemophilus influenzae	Meningitis, respiratory tract infections, septicemia	Aerobic, gram-negative rods
Helicobacter pylori	Stomach ulcers	Aerobic, gram-negative rods
Mycobacterium leprae	Leprosy	Difficult to Gram stain*
Mycobacterium tuberculosis	Tuberculosis	Difficult to Gram stain*
Neisseria gonorrhoeae	Gonorrhea	Aerobic, gram-negative cocci
Staphylococcus aureus	Boils, carbuncles, abscesses	Aerobic, gram-positive cocci
Streptococcus pneumoniae	Pneumonia	Aerobic, gram-positive cocci
Streptococcus pyogenes	Scarlet fever	Aerobic, gram-positive cocci group A beta-hemolytic

*For those microbial organisms that cannot be grown on artificial media agar plates, other means are used, such as acid-fast staining or an immunological test to determine whether the disease is present.

BOX 30-1 EXAMPLES OF COMMON PLANTS THAT CAN CAUSE HARM TO HUMANS AND ANIMALS

Azaleas (all parts)
Fatal; produces nausea/vomiting, depression, difficulty breathing, prostration, and coma

Foxglove (leaves)
Large amounts can cause dangerously irregular heartbeat/pulse, digestive upset, and mental confusion; may be fatal

Bleeding heart (foliage, roots)
May be poisonous in large amounts; has proven fatal to cattle

Irises (underground stems)
Severe digestive upset

Mistletoe (berries)
Fatal; both children and adults have died from eating the berries

Oleander (leaves, branches)
Extremely poisonous; affects the heart, produces severe digestive upset, and has caused death

Larkspur (young plant, seeds)
Digestive upset, nervous excitement, depression; may be fatal

Rhubarb leaves (leaf blade)
Fatal; large amounts of raw or cooked leaves can cause convulsions, coma, followed rapidly by death

Wisteria (seeds, pods)
Mild to severe digestive upset; many children are poisoned by this plant

(i.e., pruritus), blisters, burning and redness of the skin, and swelling. A more severe (life-threatening) form of allergic reaction can occur if smoke from a burning poison ivy/oak plant is inhaled. Preventive agents, such as IvyBlock, may act as skin barriers when applied before gardening and may decrease the risk of contact. Topical contact usually can be treated at home although care should be taken because the sap (if left on clothing, for

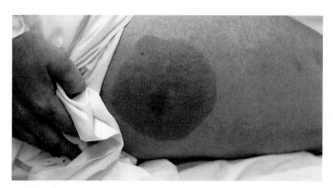

FIGURE 30-9 Poison oak infection.

example) can be transferred to others. The most common treatment after contact with these plants is the use of antihistamines, such as oral diphenhydramine (i.e., Benadryl), or topical treatments, such as Caladryl Pink (which contains Calamine Lotion). It is also imperative that the skin be kept clean and dry (Figure 30-9). Topical antihistamines, such as Caladryl Clear (contains diphenhydramine), are not recommended because of the risk of skin sensitization.

- Digitalis and cardiac glycosides: Common garden plants known as foxglove or oleander can be very dangerous if the flowers, leaves, or seeds are eaten by children or animals. Symptoms of ingestion include blurred vision, confusion, depression, hallucinations, fainting, irregular heartbeat, lethargy, low blood pressure, rash or hives, stomach pain, nausea/vomiting, and weakness. Death can occur if large amounts are consumed. Treatment may include activated charcoal and/or the antidote Digibind.

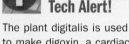

Tech Alert!

The plant digitalis is used to make digoxin, a cardiac medication.

DISEASES CAUSED BY ORGANISMS WITHIN THE ANIMALIA KINGDOM

Most diseases carried by animals are bacterial or viral in nature. Only those that produce their own toxins are truly animal diseases. Contact with the venom of animals can cause illness (rather than disease) ranging from minor to severe. Certain venoms result in death. Examples with figures are listed below.

Lice (i.e., the head louse) are parasites that cause disease. They are wingless insects that live on birds and mammals for their lifetime; different lice species infest different animals. Both adult lice and their eggs can transfer among humans by direct contact. Treatment must be given to all persons living in the same home environment. The primary drug used in the treatment of lice is a pediculicide; many are available either over-the-counter (OTC) (e.g., Rid, Triple X, Nix) or by prescription (e.g., Ovide, Lindane). A second treatment is normally necessary, as most pediculicides are not ovicidal.

The brown recluse spider is a venomous spider that causes a necrotic lesion on the skin at the bite site. Symptoms include pain, nausea, fever, and chills. The bite mark may swell with a pimple-like lesion that expands over the next 24 hours; after filling with blood it bursts and leaves a black scar (Figure 30-10). Treatment consists of topical antibiotic such as Neosporin to prevent infection, diphenhydramine for pruritus, analgesics (e.g., Tylenol) for pain, and a tetanus immunization.

Jellyfish such as the box jellyfish are among some of the most venomous animals that can cause damage to humans by the mere touch of their venom-containing tentacles. Symptoms include red welts on the skin where the tentacles touched, pain, nausea, weakness, nasal discharge, muscle spasms,

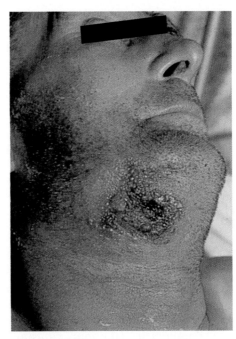

FIGURE 30-10 Brown recluse spider bite.

perspiration, and difficulty breathing. Treatment involves antihistamines (e.g., diphenhydramine) or topical cream (e.g., hydrocortisone 1%) for pruritus, analgesics (e.g., ibuprofen, acetaminophen) for pain, and antiseptics (e.g., Neosporin) to prevent infection. If severe reactions occur, a physician should be consulted immediately.

DISEASES CAUSED BY ORGANISMS WITHIN THE PROTISTA KINGDOM

Leishmania tropica is a protozoan that can be transmitted to humans either by the bite of sand flies (that carry the protozoan) or through the sharing of needles. Symptoms include sores on the skin and then ulceration of the mouth. This condition is prevalent mostly in the Middle East and Latin America. Pentavalent antimony (available from the Centers for Disease Control and Prevention [CDC]) is the treatment of choice. Other treatment includes amphotericin B, pentamidine, and other agents.

Malaria is caused by many species of protozoa. *Plasmodium falciparum* is the most severe type of malaria that humans can contract. Female mosquitoes transfer this disease when they bite the skin. It is contained in their saliva. Symptoms include chills, fever, anemia, enlarged spleen, arthralgia, weakness, and vomiting. Malaria occurs mostly in Central America, Africa, and Asia. Depending on the severity of the disease the patient may be treated at home. Various drugs used include chloroquine, quinine, doxycycline, mefloquine, and atovaquone/proguanil (Malarone). For more information on antibiotics used in the treatment of malaria refer to Chapter 25.

Toxoplasma gondii are parasitic cysts that are transferred to humans through uncooked meats infected with the cysts. If the cysts are transferred to humans, they produce toxoplasmosis. Cats are another carrier for the cysts; persons who change cat litter may come into contact with the cysts. If these are ingested by contact with cat feces or close cat contact, the infection can be quite severe for the fetus in pregnant women. The organism can cross the placenta, causing hydrocephaly, deafness, seizure, cerebral palsy, damage to the retina, and mental retardation. Stillbirths can also occur in some pregnancies. Treatment for nonpregnant patients includes a 6-week regimen consisting of pyrimethamine and sulfadiazine; sulfadiazine may be substituted with azithromycin, clindamycin, or atovaquone. Pregnant patients will receive spiramycin, and 3 weeks of pyrimethamine and sulfadiazine or leucovorin. Patients with AIDS are treated with pyrimethamine, folinic acid, and sulfadiazine followed by life long suppressive therapy.

DISEASES CAUSED BY ORGANISMS WITHIN THE MONERA KINGDOM

Anthrax is caused by the organism *Bacillus anthracis.* It resides in the soil as a spore where it can be inhaled by animals; the spores are viable for decades. Anthrax is an acute infectious disease caused by bacteria that reside in cattle, goats, and sheep. If the animal is eaten before it dies of disease, the bacteria are transferred via inhalation or through contact (e.g., open wound). Symptoms include internal bleeding, muscle pain, headache, fever, nausea, and vomiting. More than 95% of anthrax cases are transmitted cutaneously and are rarely lethal; however, inhalation of anthrax usually results in death within 1 to 3 days. Treatment examples include penicillin, doxycycline, meropenem, imipenem, daptomycin, rifampin, vancomycin, erythromycin, aminoglycosides, and first-generation cephalosporins.

Toxocariasis results from infection with larvae of the bacterium *Toxocara canis,* often found in roundworms carried by dogs. A similar form of this bacterium is carried by cats *(Toxocara cati).* When the eggs of infected roundworms are ingested by humans (from soil), the larvae spread throughout the body. Symptoms include respiratory problems, enlarged liver, skin rashes, and delayed ocular lesions.

Rocky Mountain spotted fever is a tick-borne infectious disease caused by Rickettsia rickettsii. Symptoms include chills, fever, severe headache, mental confusion, and rash. This rash spreads quickly over the whole body (Figure 30-11).

Lyme disease is a multisystem disorder caused by *Borrelia burgdorferi* (spirochete), which is carried by ticks in the Ixodidae family. Lyme disease occurs when a tick injects saliva into the bloodstream of a person. After incubating for 3 to 32 days, the spirochetes migrate to the skin, causing lesions. They also move to other areas and organs through the bloodstream or lymphatic system. The spirochetes may survive for years in the joints or they may trigger an inflammatory response in the host and then die. Lyme disease has three stages; the

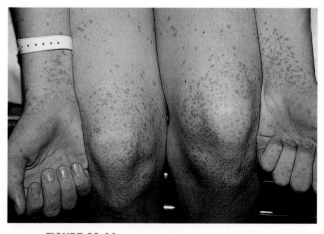

FIGURE 30-11 Rocky Mountain spotted fever.

first stage is marked by the development of skin lesions that can spread. The second stage (typically weeks to months after infection) is manifested by neurological abnormalities (such as facial palsy) and cardiomegaly (enlargement of the heart). The third stage (persistent infection) may begin weeks to years after initial infection and is characterized by arthritis in approximately 80% of patients. Migrating musculoskeletal pain leads to arthritis and severe swelling of the joints and may cause both cartilage and bone erosion. Treatment consists of antibiotics such as doxycycline (for adults) or amoxicillin (for children) for a 28-day course. Other antibiotics that can be used include cefuroxime and ceftriaxone. IV therapy is normally used in the third stage of this condition.

Pneumocystosis is caused by *Pneumocystis carinii,* a bacterial microbe that causes infection of the lungs. This condition is usually seen in people with weakened immune systems, such those suffering from AIDS or transplant recipients. Symptoms include fever, cough, shortness of breath, and rapid breathing. Treatment is with antibiotics such as trimethoprim/sulfamethoxazole (Septra, Bactrim), pentamidine, clindamycin, primaquine, and atovaquone. In addition, corticosteroids are used to reduce inflammation and pain. There is a high degree of mortality in untreated patients or in moderate to severe infections in immunocompromised patients.

DISEASES CAUSED BY FUNGUS

The species *Candida albicans* is a yeast-like organism that is part of the normal flora in the mouth and genitourinary tract of human beings. The organism is kept in check by the bacterial flora also present in the mouth and genitourinary areas. When antibiotics are taken that destroy the normal bacterial flora of these areas, the fungus *C. albicans* can proliferate and cause an infection. Other conditions caused by fungi are athlete's foot, lung and vaginal infections, and even sepsis. Fungus prefers warm, moist environments; however, some species of fungi can grow under low-moisture conditions. A disease caused by a fungus is called mycosis. The types of agents used to kill fungi are called antifungal agents (see Chapter 25). Many conditions are caused by fungi, as shown in Box 30-2.

Amanita phalloides is a species of poisonous mushroom that causes hallucinations, gastrointestinal (GI) upset, and pain that can be followed by liver, kidney, and central nervous system damage. It is commonly found in the woods of hilly to middle mountain regions across all continents except Antarctica. Ingesting less than 1 cap of this mushroom can cause death. Treatment must begin within 36 hours and requires administering several doses of activated charcoal and/or gastric lavage (pumping the stomach) as well as keeping the patient well hydrated. After 36 hours the liver may fail, leading to death unless a liver transplant can be performed.

Athlete's foot is the common term for *tinea pedis,* a fungal infection of the foot that occurs between the toes and on the soles. It is common worldwide and can develop when areas of the foot are not kept dry. Symptoms include itching, scaling, and red skin. Wearing constrictive shoes and having sweaty feet can

---

BOX 30-2 CONDITIONS CAUSED BY FUNGI

Candida albicans: Multiple conditions
Tinea pedis: Athlete's foot
Pneumocystis carinii: Pneumonia
Tinea cruris: Jock itch
Tinea unguium: Cutaneous infection
Tinea capitis: Ringworm

worsen the condition. Treatment using fungal foot powders along with keeping the feet dry helps to destroy the fungus. OTC products such as tolnaftate or miconazole can be used and are available in both topical powders and creams.

Candidiasis is due to a bacterial infection that affects various areas of the body; each infected area has a specific name for the condition (for example, skin [diaper rash], vagina [yeast infection], and mouth [thrush]). In rare instances it may pass into the bloodstream, affecting internal organs Symptoms include pruritus, bleeding, peeling skin, and a white exudate. Treatment for yeast infections can be provided by using over-the-counter antifungal medications such as clotrimazole or miconazole or, in severe cases, prescription strength forms of amphotericin B or fluconazole may be required. Diaper rash can be treated using barrier creams and ointments along with frequent diaper changing and keeping the area dry; however, if the rash does not respond, antifungal treatment may be necessary.

Viruses

One of the major disagreements in the scientific community is how to classify viruses. They do not fit nicely into any of the kingdoms outlined previously. In fact, viruses have their own field of study called virology (the study of viruses). Viruses not only infect animals but also infect plants and even bacteria. Plant viruses are responsible for destroying many food crops, impacting both people and livestock.

CLASSIFICATION OF VIRUSES

Viruses can be categorized into the following three types:

1. Animal viruses
2. Plant viruses
3. Bacterial viruses

Morphology and Characteristics of Viruses

Viruses may have a double or single strand of DNA. They are different from other organisms because they also can have a double or single strand of ribonucleic acid (RNA).

The classification of viruses is basically determined by their outer covering and any additional coating they may contain, as shown in Figure 30-12. Unenveloped viruses are covered by capsids; capsids are protective coverings made of proteins called capsomeres. Enveloped viruses have a capsid plus a covering of proteins, fats, and carbohydrates. Different viruses have different appearances; sometimes they resemble small space capsules.

Other ways to classify viruses or virions include according to their method of replication. This is probably one of the characteristics that is most different from the characteristics of organisms in any of the five kingdoms. As shown in Figure 30-13, viruses do not seem to replicate in any of the previously described methods; instead, they assemble themselves, just as cars are assembled in a processing plant. In all living organisms except viruses, DNA is double stranded. RNA is replicated from the DNA information. Viruses invade a host cell and assume control of this replication process to make more viral DNA or RNA.

Other differences between viruses and organisms of the other kingdoms include the way that viruses survive. Most organisms obtain nutrition from organic means or from the sun by photosynthesis; in addition, most organisms replicate by fission (splitting into two), sexual reproduction, or asexual reproduction. Viruses do not fit any of these categories. They are closer to parasites,

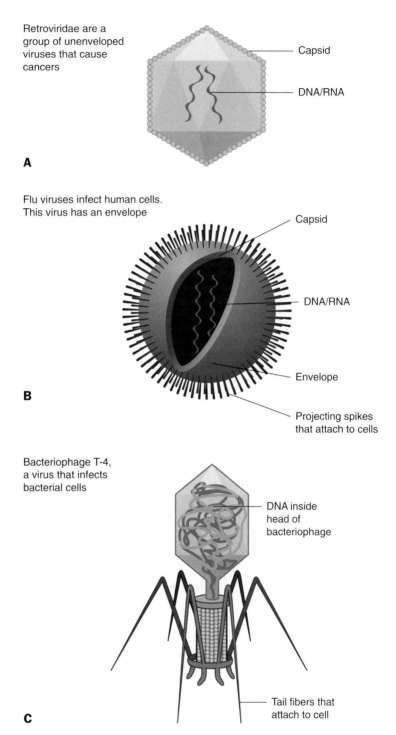

Retroviridae are a group of unenveloped viruses that cause cancers

Capsid

DNA/RNA

A

Flu viruses infect human cells. This virus has an envelope

Capsid

DNA/RNA

Envelope

Projecting spikes that attach to cells

B

Bacteriophage T-4, a virus that infects bacterial cells

DNA inside head of bacteriophage

Tail fibers that attach to cell

C

FIGURE 30-12 Viral composition. **A,** Unenveloped (capsomeres). **B,** Enveloped virus. **C,** Bacteriophage.

although, unlike viruses, most parasites do not kill their hosts. Viruses assemble new virions by using the cell parts from their hosts. Some viruses can travel from host to host by way of blood, body fluids, or even the air. Thus, although they do have some similarities with other organisms, they do not behave as entities that can replicate without the components of the cells that they invade. All viruses are so small that they cannot be seen with a light microscope. To isolate and identify viruses, different methods must be used.

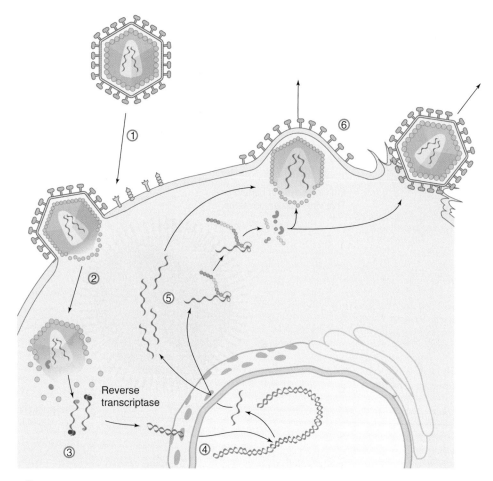

① HIV virus attaches to host cell

② The capsid releases viral RNA into cytoplasm

③ The host's enzyme is used to replicate viral RNA into DNA

④ During latency period the viral DNA stays in the host cell's DNA

⑤ The virus's DNA is activated where it codes for proteins and RNA strands to be assembled

⑥ The newly formed viral cells either bud off or lyse out of the host cell releasing free HIV

FIGURE 30-13 Human immunodeficiency virus replication. Diagram of the replication process of viruses. Each component is made independently inside the host cell. All materials are made from the host cell. Once the parts are made, they are assembled.

ANALYSIS OF VIRIONS

Viruses that infect bacteria (such as bacteriophages) can be grown on agar plates. However, those that cannot be grown on agar plates must be grown in animals or on animal tissues, such as mice, rabbits, or other laboratory animals, to observe their characteristics. Once the animal is infected, the tissue can be analyzed. To view the morphology of a virus an electron microscope (a very high-powered microscope) is used. The most common way to identify viruses is by their reaction with antibodies. When the human body comes into contact with a foreign substance, it makes antibodies in response to the antigen (foreign body), as shown in an experiment aimed at determining antibody formation (Figure 30-14).

Some human viruses, such as human immunodeficiency virus (HIV), cannot be grown in laboratory animals. Although chimpanzees can be infected

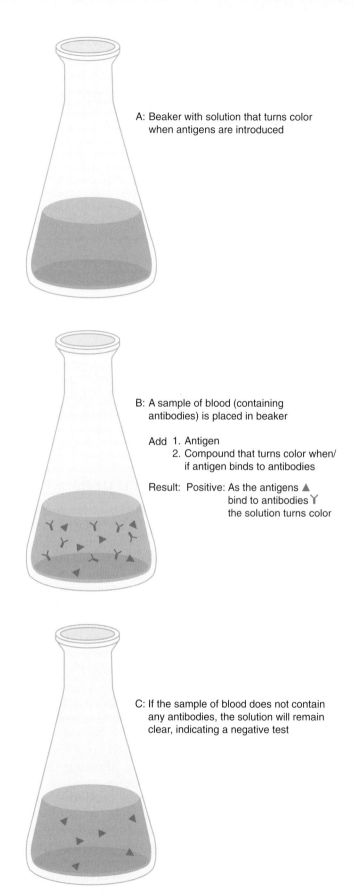

A: Beaker with solution that turns color when antigens are introduced

B: A sample of blood (containing antibodies) is placed in beaker

Add 1. Antigen
2. Compound that turns color when/ if antigen binds to antibodies

Result: Positive: As the antigens ▲ bind to antibodies Y the solution turns color

C: If the sample of blood does not contain any antibodies, the solution will remain clear, indicating a negative test

FIGURE 30-14 Determination of antibody formation: antibody test using bacteriophages. This proves whether a person has formed antibodies against a certain antigen. **A,** A sample of blood (containing an antibody, O) is placed in a beaker. Two components are added to this beaker: a complement (color when bound to antigen and antibody) and the antigen (A) to the antibody. **B,** The result would be that O and A bind, resulting in a color that makes this test positive. **C,** A sample of blood (with no antibody) is placed in a beaker. The two components are then added to the beaker. The result in this case is negative because there is no antibody present to complete the color change. Thus the blood has no previous contact with that specific antigen.

TABLE 30-6 Well-Known Viral Diseases

Virus	Human Disease
Herpesvirus	Herpes
HIV retrovirus	Acquired immunodeficiency syndrome
HPV	Human papillomavirus
Poliovirus	Polio
Varicella-zoster virus	Chickenpox
Rabies virus	Rabies
Rhinovirus	Common cold

with one strain of HIV, they do not display any symptoms of the disease. Thus it is more difficult to study or perform tests on the HIV virus in a laboratory setting.

Another problem with the study of viruses is that viruses are made of the same components as their hosts. This means that they are more difficult to kill because the antiviral agent will harm the healthy cells too, although researchers have discovered that viruses can be manipulated to work for them rather than against them. Examples of well-known viral diseases are shown in Table 30-6.

Diseases Caused by Viruses

Influenza virus is a contagious infection of the respiratory system. It is transmitted in air droplets and can occur as an isolated case or as a pandemic condition affecting thousands worldwide. Symptoms include sore throat, cough, fever, weakness, and pain in the muscles. The incubation period is only 1 to 3 days; then the onset is rapid as the body reacts with fever, chills, headache, respiratory symptoms, and extreme fatigue. Young children, the elderly, and immunocompromised persons may experience a higher risk of complications and a longer recovery time than the normal 3 to 10 days. There are three main strains of influenza: A, B, and C. When new strains develop they are named after the geographical region where they first appeared, such as the Asian flu. Treatment is based on the severity of the symptoms. Patients are advised to get plenty of rest, drink fluids, and use acetaminophen for fever.

Polio is caused by one of three polioviruses—asymptomatic (without symptoms), mild (infection of the meninges), and paralytic forms. The virus is highly contagious and is spread from person to person through oral contact, fecal contact, and contaminated food and water. Once infection occurs the virus spreads throughout the body, affecting the nervous system by destroying afferent neurons and sometimes causing paralysis (i.e., the paralytic form). Symptoms begin with fever, headache, neck and back stiffness, and constipation. Loss of the use of limbs on one or both sides of the body can occur suddenly. There is no cure for polio, only a preventive vaccine. Treatment is limited to analgesics for pain and portable ventilators for breathing in conjunction with moderate exercise and a well-balanced diet. Although polio has been eradicated in many countries through the polio vaccine, certain countries such as India still have outbreaks of polio. There is great concern that polio may once again infect people around the world because of the ease of travel.

Rabies is a virus found worldwide that is transmitted from animals to humans through the saliva of an infected animal. The most common animal carriers are dogs (originating in feral dogs) although other animals carry the virus, including cats, raccoons, bats, skunks, and wolves. Most cases of rabies that result in death occur in Asia and Africa. Many of the deaths include children that are scratched or bitten by a domestic animal that has become infected. Once symptoms appear, rabies is fatal to both humans and animals. Symptoms include respiratory and gastrointestinal and/or nervous system problems followed by paralysis that leads to coma and then death. A vaccine is available but is only recommended for high-risk groups, such as veterinarians and those who frequently handle animals. Treatment after exposure requires thorough cleansing of the wound area followed by the first dose of the rabies vaccine series (100% effective), along with rabies immunoglobulin (RIG) to provide immediate protection against the virus.

H1N1, also known as the swine flu, is a common virus found in most countries around the world. The virus is transmitted by inhaling infected airborne droplets that have been expelled by coughing or sneezing. Symptoms are similar to those experienced in seasonal influenza, including fever, cough, headache, muscle and joint pain, sore throat, runny nose, and sometimes diarrhea. The virus has also caused severe illness and deaths, especially in high-risk groups such as those with preexisting conditions such as cardiovascular and respiratory diseases, diabetes, and cancer. Pregnant women also seem to have an increased risk for a more severe type of infection, especially those in the second and third trimesters. The H1N1 vaccine can be given to all age categories. For more information on H1N1 see Chapter 25.

HOW VIRAL INFECTIONS ARE STOPPED

Many viral infections can be avoided because of the vaccines that have been created; this includes polio, measles, mumps, rubella, and others. Certain viral infections that do not have a vaccine available can be halted or delayed by the use of a variety of antiviral medications (Chapter 25). Although research has expanded our knowledge about viruses, only a handful of agents currently are being used to treat various conditions caused by viruses. Each drug must be specific in its mechanism of action to lessen the adverse effects on normal human cells. There are four main mechanisms of action that antivirals can use to overcome viral synthesis and eventual dissemination. These mechanisms are shown in Figure 30-15 and are listed in Box 30-3. Most agents are aimed at disruption of the DNA of the virus or a closely related component of the newly synthesized DNA viral strand. Drugs such as zidovudine cause inhibition of the viral replication of HIV; this drug becomes part of the viral DNA to halt the continued synthesis of new viral DNA. Other agents, such as acyclovir, inhibit viral DNA polymerase, ultimately halting the synthesis of new viral DNA; acyclovir is used against herpes simplex and varicella-zoster viruses. Non-nucleoside reverse transcriptase inhibitors cause the premature termination of the growing viral DNA strand by interfering with specific enzymes of the virus.

USING VIRUSES TO FIGHT DISEASE

One of the most studied types of viruses is the bacteriophage. These viruses can be loaded with a vaccine and then used to immunize human beings. For example, by removing the DNA inside the capsid (head) of the bacteriophage, a non–disease-causing strain of poxvirus can be inserted. The virus then is injected into the human bloodstream, where the virus vaccine can attach easily to human cells and stimulate immunity to the poxvirus.

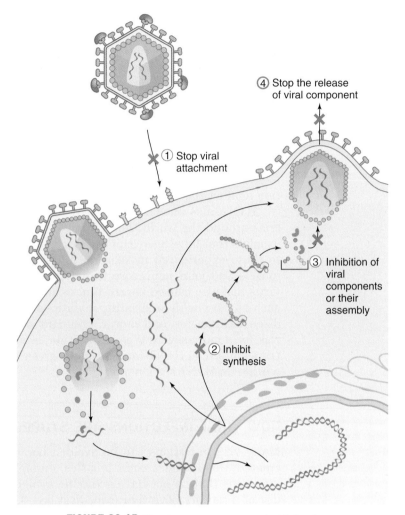

FIGURE 30-15 The four ways to stop viral infections.

BOX 30-3 METHODS OF VIRAL INHIBITION

1. Inhibit the ability of the virus to attach to the host cell. If an antibody can be made to fit the viral coating, then it may be possible to inhibit the attachment of the virion to a host cell.
2. Inhibit replication by suppressing synthesis of viral DNA/RNA. By interjecting an antiviral agent that attaches itself to the DNA of the host cell, it may disrupt the replication process that codes the important proteins and enzymes used by the virion. Other components include disruption of specific nucleic acids, DNA polymerase, and other critical enzymes necessary for formation of viral DNA/RNA strands.
3. Inhibit the ability of the virus to assemble itself properly. If protein synthesis is disrupted, the virion may not be able to build a necessary component that is needed to continue infecting new hosts.
4. Inhibit the ability of the virus to break out of the host cell. If the assembly process is disrupted or altered, it may be possible to inhibit the virion from assembling its components in the proper order or manner. This faulty virion cannot attach itself to the cell wall of the host to move out of the cell and reinfect new host cells.

DO YOU REMEMBER THESE KEY POINTS?

- The names of the five kingdoms
- The categories into which kingdoms are divided
- The person who was responsible for the theory of evolution
- The contributions of Louis Pasteur to microbiology
- The way the golden age of microbiology changed history
- The characteristics of and differences between animal, plant, and bacterial cells
- The components of an animal cell and their functions
- The types of diseases/conditions spread by the organisms discussed in this chapter
- The morphological characteristics used to distinguish between organisms
- The importance of the Gram stain in determining morphology of bacteria
- The composition of bacterial cell walls and the way in which antibiotics affect them
- The types of environments in which bacteria can be found
- The differences between microorganisms and viruses
- The way viruses replicate
- The ways to prevent the replication and dissemination of viruses
- The components of viruses

REVIEW QUESTIONS

Multiple choice questions

1. Charles Darwin is best known for:
   A. Evolution
   B. Genetics
   C. Taxonomy
   D. Classification

2. Of the groups of organisms listed, which one is not eukaryotic?
   A. Fungi
   B. Bacteria
   C. Animalia
   D. Plants

3. Of the five-kingdom classification system, which of those listed include bacteria?
   A. Plantae
   B. Animalia
   C. Protista
   D. Monera

4. Viruses can contain which of the following types of nucleic acids?
   A. Double-stranded DNA
   B. Single-stranded DNA
   C. Double- or single-stranded RNA
   D. All of the above

5. Which of the microbes listed is (are) part of a person's "normal flora"?
   A. *Candida albicans*
   B. *Borrelia burgdorferi*
   C. *Streptococcus pyogenes*
   D. Both A and C

6. Alexander Fleming is best known for the:
   A. Discovery of viruses
   B. Discovery of penicillin
   C. Classification of drugs
   D. Development of the scientific method

7. The disease malaria is caused by the microbe:
   A. *Entamoeba histolytica*
   B. *Plasmodium vivax*
   C. *Trichomonas vaginalis*
   D. *Balantidium coli*

8. The function of the Golgi complex is to:
   A. Transport proteins through the cell membrane
   B. Tag proteins to help them reach their final destination
   C. Produce adenosine triphosphate, the power source for the cell
   D. Produce proteins

9. The main types of locomotion of protozoa are:
   A. Pseudopods
   B. Flagella
   C. Cilia
   D. All of the above

10. Some microbes can resist antibiotics because of specific enzymes that are called:
    A. Antimicrobials
    B. Penicillinase
    C. Antienzymes
    D. Antibiotics

True/False

If the statement is false, then change it to make it true.

_____ 1. Only animals can catch viruses.

_____ 2. All cells have the same components.

_____ 3. The mitochondria within each cell are analogous to a powerhouse.

_____ 4. Gram-negative bacteria have a thicker layer of polypeptide bonds.

_____ 5. The primary difference between smooth endoplasmic reticulum (ER) and rough ER is the absence of ribosomes on smooth ER.

_____ 6. Protists include algae, water molds, and amebae.

_____ 7. Plants use chloroplasts for the same purpose that animals use mitochondria.

_____ 8. Spontaneous generation was believed to explain how life begins.

_____ 9. Cocci, bacilli, and spirilla are the three main morphologies of bacteria.

_____ 10. Animal and plant cells multiply by binary fission.

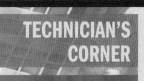

TECHNICIAN'S CORNER Following the steps outlined in the workbook, perform a Gram stain of the cheek cells from inside your mouth. Locate and describe the morphology of the cells. Compare your cells to those bacterial cells listed in a lab book.
To learn more about microbiology visit the website www.cellsalive.com.

BIBLIOGRAPHY

Campbell N, Reese J: *Biology*, ed 8. Redwood City, 2007, Benjamin/Cummings.
Greulach V, Chiappetta V: *Biology: the science of life*. Morristown, 1977, Silver Burdett.
Malarkey L, McMorrow M: *Nurse's manual of laboratory tests and diagnostic procedures*, ed 2. Philadelphia, 2000, Saunders.
Tortora G, Funke B, Case C: *Microbiology: an introduction*, ed 8. Redwood City, 2003, Benjamin Cummings.
Voet D: *Biochemistry*, ed 3. New York, 2004, Wiley.

WEBSITES

http://pedsinreview.aappublications.org/cgi/content/extract/18/5/162 (toxic plants)

www.ansci.cornell.edu/plants/php/plants.php?action=indiv&byname=common&
keynum=22

www.ncbi.nlm.nih.gov/books/bv.fcgi?rid=mmed.chapter.4093 (protozoa)

http://emedicine.medscape.com/article/829613-overview (Anthrax)

www.healthcentral.com/encyclopedia/408/312.html (Candidiasis)

www.polio.com/?fa=learn/polio/disease

www.who.int/rabies/human/en/

https://www.msu.edu/course/lbs/158h/manual/Protistans.pdf

http://www.medical-look.com/Parasitic_diseases/Roundworms.html

http://www.merck.com/mmhe/sec17/ch196/ch196o.html

31

Chemistry

Objectives

UPON COMPLETING THIS CHAPTER, YOU SHOULD BE ABLE TO DO THE FOLLOWING:

- Name the 10 basic ions necessary for proper electrolyte balance and describe the role of each ion in maintaining homeostasis.

- Define the terms *atom, molecule, proton, neutron,* and *electron.*

- Distinguish between ionic and covalent bonds.

- List the types of molecules that are formed from various nucleic acids.

- List the 20 amino acids necessary in a balanced diet.

- Distinguish between acids and bases.

- Distinguish between anions and cations.

- Describe how sodium bicarbonate balances pH.

- Explain how chemistry plays an important part in the action and reactions of drugs.

- Describe how enzymes and proteins are used in the body.

- Define the terms *inorganic* and *organic* as related to chemistry, giving an example of each.

- Define metabolism in terms of anabolism and catabolism.

T FIRST, it may not seem as though chemistry is relevant to the health care field. However, this is not true. Chemistry is at the heart of the discovery of new medicines and treatments and the understanding of chemical interactions in the body. It is important for pharmacy technicians to become acquainted with the body's basic chemical reactions and interactions. The goal of this chapter is to present the basics of chemistry, discuss reasons that drugs interact, and explain the importance of these reactions within the body system.

Parts of an Atom

Atoms are made up of smaller particles called **protons** (positively charged), **electrons** (negatively charged), and **neutrons** (no charge). The center of the atom, the nucleus, contains the protons and neutrons. In 1968 scientists discovered new particles inside the proton called quarks. The quarks are held together by particles called gluons. The electrons of a specific atom **orbit** around the nucleus in much the same way that the planets in our solar system orbit around the sun (Figure 31-1).

The nucleus of an atom is very small. Most of the atom is empty space. Most atoms have an equal number of positively charged protons and negatively charged electrons, giving them a net charge of zero. If an atom has more or fewer electrons than protons, it becomes charged and is called an **ion**. The structure of each atom is determined by the number of electrons that it has in the outer orbit.

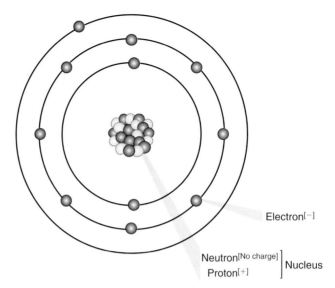

FIGURE 31-1 Electron orbit.

1	2	3	4	5	6	7	8	9	10	11	12	13	14	15	16	17	18
$_1$H																	$_2$He
$_3$Li	$_4$Be											$_5$B	$_6$C	$_7$N	$_8$O	$_9$F	$_{10}$Ne
$_{11}$**Na**	$_{12}$**Mg**											$_{13}$Al	$_{14}$Si	$_{15}$P	$_{16}$S	$_{17}$**Cl**	$_{18}$Ar
$_{19}$**K**	$_{20}$Ca	$_{21}$Sc	$_{22}$Ti	$_{23}$V	$_{24}$Cr	$_{25}$Mn	$_{26}$Fe	$_{27}$Co	$_{28}$Ni	$_{29}$**Cu**	$_{30}$Zn	$_{31}$Ga	$_{32}$Ge	$_{33}$As	$_{34}$**Se**	$_{35}$Br	$_{36}$Kr

FIGURE 31-2 Periodic table of elements. The elements K, Na, Cl, Mg, Se, and Cu are highlighted.

Tech Note!

The periodic table of elements is a chemical chart that lists all known natural and manmade elements. In the periodic table of elements, a period refers to the row across the table, whereas a group indicates the vertical column. Each element is assigned a symbol; below the symbol is the atomic number.

Two common types of bonding between atoms are **ionic bonds** and **covalent bonds**. When two atoms are in close contact with each other, the nucleus (positively charged) of the first atom is attracted to the **electrons** (negatively charged) of the other atom, and vice versa. These two atoms can exchange or transfer electrons, forming ionic bonds, or they can share the electrons, forming covalent bonds. Covalent bonds are stronger than ionic bonds because the electrons are held in a tighter arrangement. The joining of two or more different types of atoms can create different **molecules,** such as salts, carbohydrates (sugars), lipids (fats), proteins (e.g., meat), and nucleic acids (e.g., DNA). Sometimes, when two oppositely charged ions combine, such as sodium (Na$^+$) and chloride (Cl$^-$), some of their charges are excluded because they form an ionic bond (NaCl). Not all charges are dropped when ions combine; in many cases there are charges remaining, which usually are indicated at the right of the chemical name with a plus or minus sign.

The periodic table of elements has all of the known elements strategically placed according to their properties (Figure 31-2). The table has seven horizontal rows of elements. All of the elements are placed in a specific box next to elements to which they are closely related; for example, across the top of the table are numbers 1 to 18. Looking down the first column of the chart, there are three important alkali metals: lithium, sodium, and potassium. They are in the same

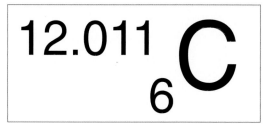

FIGURE 31-3 Carbon, represented by the letter C. Below the element is the atomic number. Above is the atomic weight.

column because of their similarities. They have one electron in their outer shell, and they are white, soft, and very reactive metals.

Elements also are listed in order based on their chemical properties and size. As you can see, there are numbers assigned to each element. In Figure 31-3, carbon is the sixth element on the table, indicated with the number 6. Above the number 6 in the table is the value 12.011, indicating the atomic weight of the atom. The entire periodic table of elements categorizes elements by their elemental properties, such as weight and types of bonds that they form. This makes it easier to learn their properties. Although the table lists each element by itself, in nature they are not necessarily isolated. For instance, the metal sodium by itself is highly reactive and would explode if it were exposed to oxygen. The same can be said of chloride. Even as a solid, chloride emits deadly vapors when isolated. However, if you combine these two elements, you have NaCl, or sodium chloride (i.e., table salt). NaCl is also used in hospital intravenous solutions and irrigation solutions into which antibiotics and other medications are added for administration to patients. Highlighted within the periodic table in Figure 31-2 are the elements most often used in the pharmacy. Many of these are also elements contained in the body that are measured in laboratory blood tests.

Charges are grouped in pairs: any excess of electrons appears as a negative sign (−), whereas any deficiency of electrons appears as a positive sign (+). For example, in a molecule of water, each hydrogen atom has one electron that can be shared or bonded. Oxygen has eight electrons. This number indicates the total number of electrons in oxygen. Oxygen has two electrons in its inner shell and six in its outer shell. Oxygen is able to accept another two electrons in its outer shell. When joined with two hydrogen molecules, there is no overall charge (neutral), as shown in Figure 31-4.

Some common atoms form tight bonds with other atoms to make substances such as water (oxygen and hydrogen) and common table salt (sodium chloride). Table 31-1 lists some of these compounds.

MOLECULES

Two distinct areas of study in chemistry are inorganic chemistry and organic chemistry. Inorganic chemistry is the study of all types of molecules that do not contain carbon atoms. Examples include some metals and gases such as iron (Fe) and oxygen (O). Together, the molecule FeO_2 makes ferric oxide, also known as rust. Organic chemistry is the study of substances that contain carbon as one of the components of a molecule. What contains the most important carbon-based substances? The human body.

Enzyme Activators and Inhibitors

Enzymes are proteins that can regulate the speed of reactions. They can accelerate an action or inhibit (stop) reactions from taking place. They can be inactive

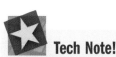

Tech Note!

If you attempt to determine the method of action of a specific drug and you read "unknown," it is because science still cannot explain how that drug functions in the human body.

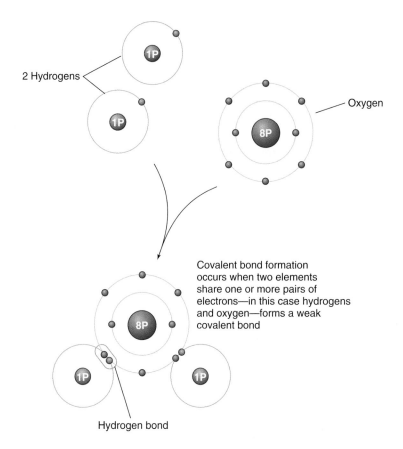

2 Hydrogens

Oxygen

Covalent bond formation
occurs when two elements
share one or more pairs of
electrons—in this case hydrogens
and oxygen—forms a weak
covalent bond

Hydrogen bond

FIGURE 31-4 Water molecule formation. Water is one of the most important compounds on earth. Water composes approximately 65% to 75% of all living cells.

TABLE 31-1 Chemical Charges of Compounds

Substance	Positive Charge	Negative Charge	Chemical Symbol
Acetate	$2\ C^{4+}$, $3\ H^+$	O_2^{2-}	$C_2H_3O_2^-$
Ammonia	$3\ H^+$	N^{3-}	NH_3
Bicarbonate	H^+, C^{4+}	O_3^{2-}	HCO_3^-
Ferrous sulfate	Fe^{2+}, S^{4+}	O_4^{2-}	$FeSO_4^-$
Hydrochloric acid	H^+	Cl^-	HCl
Magnesium hydroxide	Mg^{2+}, H^+	O^{2-}	$MgOH$
Potassium chloride	K^+	Cl^-	KCl
Potassium phosphate	K^+, P^{4+}	O_4^{2-}	KPO_4^{3-}
Sodium bicarbonate	Na^+, H^+, C^{4+}	O_3^{2-}	$NaHCO_3$
Sodium chloride	Na^+	Cl^-	$NaCl$
Water	$2\ H^+$	O^{2-}	H_2O

until they encounter certain elements (called ions). For example, elements or ions such as chloride, zinc, iron, and magnesium can serve as activators of the digestive enzyme pepsin. Once pepsin is activated, it helps break down food to be absorbed by the intestines. Another enzymatic reaction is the bubbling reaction of hydrogen peroxide when placed on a cut or scrape. Pharmacology includes the study of these types of reactions. An example of an inhibitory reaction occurs when a drug such as famotidine (Pepcid), which is taken for gastric secretion, inhibits specific histamine receptors. The result is that the levels of stomach acids are decreased.

Metabolism: Anabolism and Catabolism

The foods we eat must be broken down into usable molecules (**catabolism**) and built up into other new useful molecules (**anabolism**). **Metabolism** is all the chemical reactions that take place in the body; the reactions can be divided into a series of steps or cycles. This cycle is the systematic process of the transformation of molecules, such as fatty acids, **amino acids**, and carbohydrates, into other molecules necessary to the body. A series of reactions are possible because of the interactions between ions and enzymatic reactions. This allows the body to break down and/or build up substances as needed. Metabolism is necessary for such processes as hormonal control, protein synthesis, pH (acid/base) balance, and regulation of lipid (fat) and glucose (sugar) levels. This area of study is called biochemistry; biochemistry plays an important role in the study of pharmacology.

The human body needs certain nutrients daily. These are essential for proper growth and overall maintenance of the body. Diagnostic blood tests can reveal to a physician and a pharmacist (when tests are performed in a hospital) any deficiencies of essential nutrients that may affect the health of a patient. Laboratory tests may help ensure that the proper dosage of medication and/or replacement therapy is given.

A pharmacist will look for specific values depending on the type of medication that the patient is taking. For instance, when a patient is receiving an aminoglycoside, such as gentamicin (antiinfective), the pharmacist will have drug concentrations drawn (taken by blood samples) at certain times after the gentamicin has been administered intravenously. The results will inform the pharmacist how fast the patient's body is clearing the drug (excretion). The condition of the patient's kidneys affects the amount of drug that should be administered. If a patient is older, he or she naturally will have a decrease in the rate of drug clearance. If an aminoglycoside is dosed at too high a level, it can build up in the blood and tissues. This adds an additional strain on the body system. Patients who may be at high risk are those with kidney failure, older adults, children, and those with an existing medical problem.

ELECTROLYTE AND MINERAL REPLACEMENT

Electrolyte levels are another type of laboratory test result encountered frequently by pharmacists. Certain patients may receive intravenous infusions or oral medications that contain needed electrolytes or they may require complete intravenous nutritional supplementation, such as hyperalimentation (or hyperal).

Two types of ions are cations (those with a positive charge) and anions (those with a negative charge). Many cations and anions form bonds between one another, producing various molecules such as proteins, amino acids, and many different types of enzymes. Remember, enzymes are proteins that regulate reactions. The following list describes the role of some of these important ions (electrolytes and minerals) in the human body:

- K: Potassium is found mostly inside the cell (i.e., intracellular fluid), as opposed to outside the cell (i.e., extracellular fluid) where many other ions are found. Potassium is the principal cation of intracellular fluid and is necessary for homeostasis. Potassium plays a major role in the maintenance of muscle function, such as the heart, and the conduction of nerve impulses. A deficiency can cause a wide range of side effects, including cardiac irregularities (arrhythmias). An excess of potassium can cause impaired conduction of the heart, and may lead to cardiac arrest.

- Na: Sodium is a key component in the transfer of water between areas of the body and is found mostly in the extracellular fluid of the body. Sodium is the most abundant cation in extracellular fluid. There are many processes in the body that require sodium for proper functioning; this includes the nervous system and musculoskeletal system, which both require electrical signals for communication. Excess or insufficient levels of sodium can cause cells to malfunction and in extreme cases can be fatal.

- Cl: Chloride is found inside and outside the cells of the body. Chloride has a negative charge, which makes it an anion. Chloride is the most abundant anion in extracellular fluid. It also contributes to osmotic pressure. The combination of sodium (cation) and chloride (anion) makes up more than 65% of the acidic ions of the blood. Hydrogen and chloride (HCl) is another important combination in the body, especially in the digestion of food in the stomach. Chloride is also important for the health of the heart muscle and helps the body in maintaining a normal balance of fluids. Too much chloride can cause kidney and parathyroid gland malfunctions.

- Mg: Magnesium is found in bones and the soft tissues of the body. Magnesium is used in the synthesis of adenosine triphosphate (ATP) and the release of energy from ATP. Magnesium plays a part in the overall maintenance of muscles of both the heart and the skeletal system as well as tissues of the nervous system. Magnesium is also a component in combination with other ions that helps promote proper bone growth. Too much magnesium can lead to symptoms such as diarrhea, nausea, abdominal cramps, low blood pressure, difficulty breathing, and irregular heartbeat. Too little magnesium can cause muscle cramps, seizures, and abnormal heart rhythms. Low blood levels of calcium and potassium may also occur as magnesium regulates these at a cellular level.

- Cu: Copper is a metal that the body uses in minute amounts. This ion helps maintain healthy blood vessels, hair, and skin. Copper also is believed to play a role, along with iron, as a component of hemoglobin. Copper deficiency can affect the number of white blood cells. Too much copper can cause diarrhea, liver destruction, and even death.

- P: Phosphorus is found mainly in the bones. Phosphorus participates in the synthesis of certain enzymes, including ATP. This important enzyme is responsible for supplying the energy that human cells require. Excessive levels of phosphorus may be seen mostly in persons who have end-stage renal failure or hypervitaminosis D; the adverse effects include reduced calcium absorption and calcification of tissues, especially in the kidneys. Insufficient levels of phosphorus (rarely seen in most people) can cause anorexia, anemia, muscle weakness, bone pain, confusion, and increased susceptibility to infection; this condition may be seen in persons near starvation, chronic users of aluminum-containing antacids, and alcoholics.

- Fe: When you think of iron, you may think of cast iron or you may think of good, healthy blood. The iron in the body is the same type of iron used in construction, but in very small amounts. Iron is necessary to help hemoglobin bind to the oxygen molecules that we breathe. If iron is deficient, anemia (iron deficiency anemia) may result. As the amount of hemoglobin decreases, the amount of oxygen carried by the blood decreases as well. Because iron is fat-soluble, excessive iron intake can cause a toxic buildup, leading to severe side effects including brain damage, coma, or even death. This is especially true in children.

- Ca: We have been told that calcium is important because it helps children grow big and strong, which is why it is important for children to drink enough milk. However, calcium not only helps growing children but also is important as we grow older. Calcium must be activated by vitamin D to be absorbed. Calcium is necessary to maintain appropriate acid-base balance and also is a factor in blood coagulation. A decrease in calcium levels can cause cramping or twitching of the muscles. As we age, the body decreases its production of many necessary vitamins and minerals. Some drugs increase the absorption of calcium, whereas other drugs may decrease the absorption. This is one of the details that a pharmacist notes when giving a patient consultation. For example, tetracycline should not be taken with calcium supplements because they decrease the effectiveness of the antibiotic. Not enough calcium in the body contributes to weak bones and muscles. This is especially true in older adults. Many older citizens have osteoporosis, which is directly related to many years of calcium deficiency. Too much calcium can contribute to heart and kidney disease. In addition to proper bone growth, calcium helps the muscles by increasing electrical impulses.

- Zn: Zinc is only needed in minute amounts. Zinc is a vital component of the enzyme carbonic anhydrase found in hemoglobin. This enzyme helps in the stabilization of the pH of the blood. Zinc must always be given in combination with other chemicals. Too much zinc can cause stomach cramps, nausea, and vomiting. Over several months, it can cause anemia and damage to the pancreas. If too little zinc is ingested by the body, symptoms may include a loss of appetite, decreased sense of taste and smell, decreased immune function, slow wound healing and skin sores. If a pregnant woman does not obtain enough zinc, the baby may have birth defects.

- Mn: Manganese is an essential nutrient involved in many chemical processes in the body, including the formation of connective tissue, bones, blood clotting factors, and sex hormones. Manganese also plays a role in fat and carbohydrate metabolism, calcium absorption, and blood sugar regulation. It is also necessary for normal brain and nerve functions. Although the occurrence of low levels of manganese is rare, it can contribute to infertility, bone malformation, weakness, and seizures. Too much manganese can cause neurological disorders that mimic Parkinson's disease with symptoms such as tremors or facial spasms.

- I: Iodine is necessary for the proper functioning of the thyroid gland and metabolism of cells (converting food into energy). A shortage of iodine can lead to goiter (enlargement of the thyroid gland). Because salt sold in the United States is iodized, goiters are rare. A deficiency of iodine has been linked to cretinism (rare in the United States). Too much iodine in the diet (also rare in the United States) can reduce the function of the thyroid gland.

HYPERALIMENTATION EXAMPLE: ELECTROLYTES IN CLINICAL PRACTICE

Hyperalimentation may be given as total parenteral nutrition (TPN, administered through a large central vein) or peripheral parenteral nutrition (PPN, given through a smaller peripheral vein; see Chapter 10). An intravenous bag is hung daily as a nutritional supplement if the patient cannot eat food, is healing from a stomach or intestinal operation, or is about to undergo surgery to the stomach or intestines. Ingredients of a hyperalimentation bag include electrolyte, vitamin, and mineral replacement. This preparation is calculated by the pharmacist or the physician after laboratory values for the patient and other nutritional assessments have been obtained.

In either case, the technician may be responsible for pulling the necessary electrolyte and/or parenteral medications to be placed in the hyperalimentation bag and for preparation of the bag. The size of the bags can range from 1 L up to 3 L for an adult. Regardless of the size of the hyperalimentation bag or the dosing, a new bag must be hung daily to ensure sterility of the solution. Electrolyte replacement commonly consists of the ions potassium, sodium, chloride, phosphate, calcium, and magnesium. In addition, most hyperalimentation bags include an assortment of vitamins and trace elements added daily. A standard formulated hyperalimentation bag usually is given to patients until their laboratory results are received by the pharmacy. Except for the bag provided on the first day, each daily bag of hyperalimentation usually is tailor-made to the patient's specific needs.

CHEMISTRY IN CLINICAL PRACTICE: DRUG AND FOOD CHEMICAL REACTIONS

Virtually every medication has side effects, some of which are due to chemical interactions specifically with metal ions such as copper, zinc, potassium, and iron. After extensive laboratory testing, consumers are notified of these interactions by their health care providers, pharmacists, nurses, or manufacturing companies. When specific interactions are recognized, a prescription bottle will have an auxiliary label placed on the outside to alert the patient. Pharmacies also use prepared information sheets to inform patients of potential risks from taking a medication as well as supplements that should be avoided while taking the medication. Examples of common interactions that occur between ion metals and medications are listed in Table 31-2.

ACID-BASE REACTIONS

Many of the reactions that occur naturally in the body or after administration of medications are acid-base reactions. This is evident with antacids such as Maalox. These agents reduce heartburn by neutralizing stomach acid with a base—in the case of Maalox, magnesium/aluminum hydroxide. Acid-base reactions within the bloodstream are some of the most important reactions because they can make the difference between life and death. The pH scale is a repre-

TABLE 31-2 Interactions between Ions and Medications

Ion Supplements	Medication/Drug Classifications
Calcium	Alendronate absorption is decreased.
	Antacids that contain aluminum can have increased concentrations in the blood.
	Corticosteroids taken over long periods may deplete calcium levels and a supplement may be recommended.
	Estrogens may increase calcium levels.
	Diuretics: Thiazides can raise calcium levels while loop diuretics decrease calcium levels.
	Reduces absorption of tetracycline.
Iron	Levothyroxine absorption is decreased.
	Oral contraceptives may increase iron levels.
	Tetracyclines and quinolones may decrease absorption of iron.
	ACE* inhibitors may decrease absorption of iron.
Potassium	Potassium levels can be increased by NSAIDs, ACE inhibitors, heparin, cyclosporine, trimethoprim, beta-blockers.
	Potassium levels can be decreased by diuretics, corticosteroids, antacids, insulin, theophylline, laxatives, amphotericin B.
Aluminum hydroxide	Phosphorus levels may be decreased.
	Interferes with absorption of bisphosphonates.
Sodium	Diuretics can lower sodium levels.

*ACE, Angiotensin-converting enzyme; NSAID, nonsteroidal antiinflammatory drug.

Tech Note!

Sodium bicarbonate has historically been kept on a crash cart for emergency situations, such as cardiac arrest. It is no longer a first-line agent to be administered in cardiac arrest, because its administration has not been proven to improve patient outcome and in some cases may complicate treatment. Sodium bicarbonate is injected into the bloodstream to stabilize the blood pH in any of the following emergency situations:

· Treat preexisting metabolic acidosis
· Treat hyperkalemia (high blood potassium levels)
· Treat tricyclic antidepressant or barbiturate overdosage
· After prolonged cardiac arrest, when first-line methods of the life support protocols have failed to produce a response

sentation of the amount of hydrogen in water. pH is a logarithmic function. This means that one unit represents a tenfold increase in hydrogen concentration. The pH ranges from 1 (the most acidic) to 14 (the most basic). The normal pH of human blood is 7.4. If the pH of the blood changes by 0.4, such as to 7.8 or 7.0, the person could suffer life-threatening consequences. The body works hard to maintain the pH at a steady 7.4 by making buffers such as sodium bicarbonate. Remember, the ions that form **molecules** (as described previously) drive reactions that can change pH balance.

Amino Acids

Molecules form amino acids that perform different functions (Figure 31-5). These amino acids include neurotransmitters (see Chapter 16) and metabolic intermediates. Each one of these amino acids can form long chains by binding the amino group of one amino acid to the carboxyl group of another amino acid.

When this bond is formed, a reaction called dehydration takes place (the loss of a water molecule). When many amino acids joined, proteins are made. The overall molecule will not be a straight chain. Amino acid chains can range from a few interconnected amino acids (**micro**molecules) to more than 1 thousand (**macro**molecules) combined amino acids. Their behavior is based on their shape, size, and chemical structure.

A hemoglobin molecule has 547 individual amino acids in its 4 amino acid chains. Amino acids play an important role in everyday life because they are the components of proteins, many of which are enzymes. Enzymes are necessary for reactions to occur. A total of 20 amino acids compose almost every protein known in the animal kingdom as well as many nutrients required by the human body. The rings (called benzene rings) within amino acids are a shortcut representation of a specific chemical arrangement, as shown in Figure 31-6. Each corner of the ring represents a carbon atom and its adjoining hydrogen atom. The catabolism of various amino acids allows the body to produce energy (i.e., ATP) to power bodily functions, such as moving, working, and playing.

Mitochondria are the powerhouses of the human body; they produce energy much the same way that a hydroelectric plant produces energy with the use of turbines and generators. The mitochondria (see Chapter 30) are contained within human cells and produce much of the power we use. For instance, alanine, cysteine, glycine, serine, and threonine (all amino acids) are converted

FIGURE 31-5 Amino acid structure.

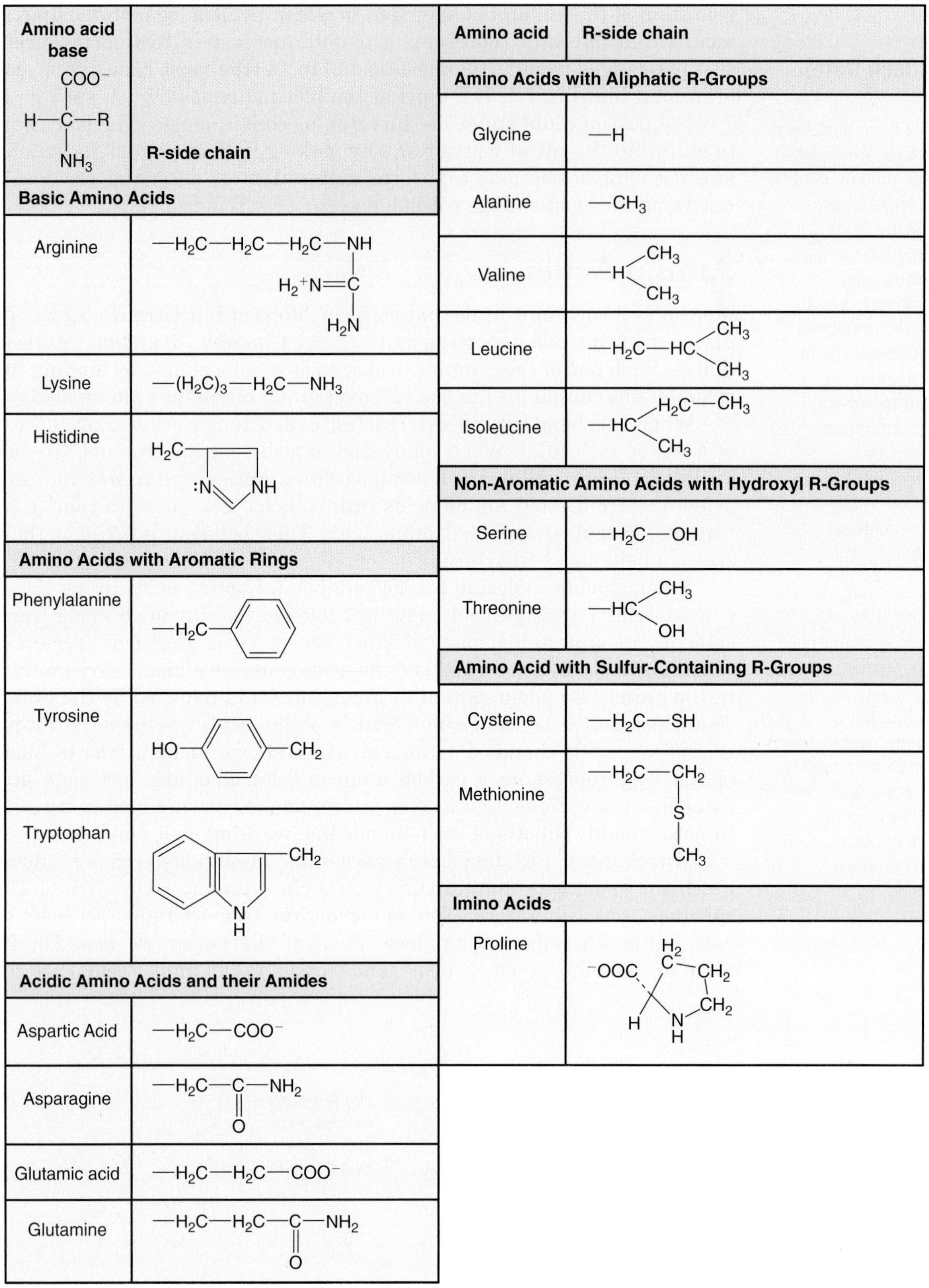

Amino acid base $$\begin{array}{c} COO^- \\ | \\ H-C-R \\ | \\ NH_3 \end{array}$$	R-side chain
Basic Amino Acids	
Arginine	$-H_2C-H_2C-H_2C-NH$, $H_2{}^+N=C$, H_2N
Lysine	$-(H_2C)_3-H_2C-NH_3$
Histidine	H_2C ... $:N$ NH
Amino Acids with Aromatic Rings	
Phenylalanine	$-H_2C-$ (benzene ring)
Tyrosine	$HO-$ (benzene ring) $-CH_2$
Tryptophan	(indole ring) $-CH_2$, N , H
Acidic Amino Acids and their Amides	
Aspartic Acid	$-H_2C-COO^-$
Asparagine	$-H_2C-\underset{\underset{O}{\|}}{C}-NH_2$
Glutamic acid	$-H_2C-H_2C-COO^-$
Glutamine	$-H_2C-H_2C-\underset{\underset{O}{\|}}{C}-NH_2$

Amino acid	R-side chain
Amino Acids with Aliphatic R-Groups	
Glycine	$-H$
Alanine	$-CH_3$
Valine	$-H\underset{CH_3}{\overset{CH_3}{<}}$
Leucine	$-H_2C-HC\underset{CH_3}{\overset{CH_3}{<}}$
Isoleucine	$-HC\underset{CH_3}{\overset{H_2C-CH_3}{<}}$
Non-Aromatic Amino Acids with Hydroxyl R-Groups	
Serine	$-H_2C-OH$
Threonine	$-HC\underset{OH}{\overset{CH_3}{<}}$
Amino Acid with Sulfur-Containing R-Groups	
Cysteine	$-H_2C-SH$
Methionine	$-H_2C-CH_2$, S , CH_3
Imino Acids	
Proline	^-OOC ... $\underset{H_2}{C}-CH_2$, CH_2 , H N H

FIGURE 31-6 Essential amino acids for human life. They are the basis for proteins that are responsible for normal body functions.

Tech Note!

When you work with certain chemicals, you will see the term *millimoles*. A **mole** is a standard unit used when describing the concentration of a specific substance; 1 millimole is equal to 1/1000 mole. The abbreviation for millimole is mmol.

into pyruvate. Pyruvate then enters the mitochondria (the cellular powerhouse) and undergoes many more changes, eventually producing three molecules of ATP, which powers the metabolism of the body with further reactions. ATP is essential for life, as are many other complex molecules.

Conclusion

The human body is composed of millions of molecules that participate in a complex series of actions and reactions within the body. External factors—including diet, drugs, ambient temperature, stress, and even the air we breathe—also affect the body's chemistry. The complexity of the human body is so great that researchers have only begun to understand how it functions. Chemical reactions make life happen; thus the types of bonds, charges, reactions, and molecules formed are important in understanding life, disease, and other biological effects.

DO YOU REMEMBER THESE KEY POINTS?

- The major chemical elements that are essential to human beings
- The difference between ionic and covalent bonds
- The difference between an anion and a cation
- The composition of an element
- The composition of a molecule
- The definition of an enzyme and the importance of enzymatic reactions
- The measurements used in chemistry and in pharmacy
- The pH of the blood that is necessary for human life
- The properties that determine whether a substance is an acid or base

REVIEW QUESTIONS

Multiple choice questions

1. Organic chemistry is the study of:
   A. Metals
   B. Carbon-based matter
   C. Water
   D. All of the above

2. Which of the following statements is true concerning the parts of an atom?
   A. Protons are negatively charged, electrons are positively charged, and neutrons are neutral in charge.
   B. Neutrons are negatively charged, electrons are positively charged, and protons are neutral in charge.
   C. Protons are positively charged, neutrons are negatively charged, and electrons are neutral in charge.
   D. Protons are positively charged, electrons are negatively charged, and neutrons are neutral in charge.

3. Which of the following molecules is not essential to life?
   A. Carbohydrates
   B. Lipids
   C. Proteins
   D. All are important

4. The elements in the periodic table of elements are listed in order of all of the following criteria EXCEPT:
   A. According to properties and number of protons
   B. According to size
   C. According to their shapes
   D. According to weight of the atoms

5. Which of the chemicals listed has no charge when combined into a compound?
   A. Sodium chloride
   B. Sodium bicarbonate
   C. Ferrous sulfate
   D. Both A and B

6. Symptoms including stomach cramps, nausea, and vomiting and eventual anemia and/or damage to the pancreas would be associated with too little:
   A. Calcium
   B. Zinc
   C. Potassium
   D. Manganese

7. Of the elements listed, which element is not monitored by the pharmacy when preparing hyperalimentation bags for patients?
   A. Potassium
   B. Sodium
   C. Magnesium
   D. Hydrogen

8. Which chemicals listed is (are) a component of the enzyme adenosine triphosphate?
   A. Fe
   B. K
   C. P
   D. Both B and C

9. A blood pH of 7.9 is considered:
   A. Acidic
   B. Basic
   C. Normal
   D. Buffered

10. Pyruvate is a key component in the making of:
    A. Amino acids
    B. Sugars
    C. The citric acid cycle
    D. ATP

True/False

If the statement is false, then change it to make it true.

_____ 1. Proteins are made up of amino acids.
_____ 2. Dehydration is the loss of a water molecule when amino acids combine.
_____ 3. Sodium chloride is a buffer.
_____ 4. Iron and zinc play key roles in the hemoglobin count of blood.
_____ 5. Peripheral parenteral nutrition may be ordered for a person who is unable to eat.
_____ 6. Most intravenous solutions are placed into isotonic solutions such as NaCl.
_____ 7. Anions are positive, whereas cations are negative.
_____ 8. Enzymes always make reactions move forward.
_____ 9. Metabolism is the making of molecules.
_____ 10. Ionic and covalent refer to the two types of bonds that atoms form.

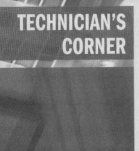

TECHNICIAN'S CORNER

A customer comes into the pharmacy to have a prescription for ferrous sulfate tablets filled. She is taking the following drugs:

Tetracycline
Milk of Magnesia
Cimetidine

The pharmacist will give a consultation to the patient, letting her know whether there is any problem, but you want to know for yourself whether there is any contraindication. What, if any, interactions are there between ferrous sulfate and the patient's current medications?

Look up the answer in *Drug Facts and Comparisons*.

BIBLIOGRAPHY

www.umm.edu/altmed/articles/iron-000964.htm (iron supplements)

Appendices

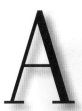

A

Review for the PTCB Examination

THE FOLLOWING PRACTICE EXAM IS formatted in the same fashion as the Pharmacy Technician Certification Board (PTCB) exam. The PTCB exam has 100 multiple-choice questions divided into 3 areas of pharmacy competencies. The first portion of the exam, Assisting the Pharmacist in Serving Patients, accounts for 66% of the questions. Question topics include processing new prescriptions, assisting the pharmacist, record keeping, and preparing controlled substances for delivery. Other competencies tested include understanding a formulary, preparing and/or repackaging medications, calibrating equipment, and performing calculations. The first 80 questions in the following practice exam will cover these types of questions that may be asked on the PTCB exam.

The next 22% of the exam is Maintaining Medication and Inventory Control Systems. This portion of the exam tests your knowledge on inventory concerns, such as proper storage of medications, compounding, repackaging, medication recalls, and hazardous wastes. Also tested are record keeping, understanding policies and procedures, and performing quality assurance tests on compounded medications.

The last 12% of the exam involves Participating in the Administration and Management of Pharmacy Practice. This section contains information on refills, insurance claims, prescription tracking, and audits. Other areas include understanding both federal and state laws, adhering to The Joint Commission standards, and knowing procedures for proper use of laminar flow hoods, equipment maintenance, automated systems, and computer software information.

The PTCB test is now computerized and is offered on a daily basis at testing centers around the country. Applicants can find more information about the test, testing procedures, and test scheduling at www.ptcb.org.

The following practice examination consists of 125 questions that represent the same topics and proportions as found on the PTCB exam.

1. When a prescription inhaler is dispensed, how often should a patient package insert be given to the patient?
   A. Only if the patient asks for one
   B. The first time the prescription is filled
   C. Every time the prescription is filled
   D. Every 6 months

2. Which of the following DEA numbers is correct for Dr. Paul J. Hanson?
   A. BH 1234575
   B. BH 1234567
   C. APH 8494783
   D. BH 1234631

3. A patient requests valid refills of AcipHex tablets and Ventolin HFA inhaler. Which two medications would be filled?
   A. Rabeprazole and albuterol
   B. Tapazole and metaproterenol
   C. Atenolol and ipratropium
   D. Rabeprazole and beclomethasone

4. Trace elements are used in the following solutions:
   A. Antibiotics
   B. Insulin drips
   C. Sterile water
   D. Total parenteral nutrition (TPN)

5. Which of the following OTC agents has limitations on quantities purchased?
   A. Sudafed
   B. Claritin
   C. Robitussin DM
   D. Hydrocortisone 1% cream

6. A prescription with directions to instill iii qtt OS qod would require the label to read:
   A. Inject 3 mL into left side every day
   B. Instill 3 drops into the eyes twice daily
   C. Instill 3 drops into the left eye every other day
   D. Instill 3 drops into both eyes every other day

7. A prescription for Tylenol with Codeine #4 contains how much codeine?
   A. 7.5 mg
   B. 15 mg
   C. 30 mg
   D. 60 mg

8. Which of the drugs listed below is not a cephalosporin?
   A. Ceftriaxone
   B. Zinacef
   C. Clarithromycin
   D. Cefazolin

9. Refills of Schedule III agents have the following limitations:
   A. The prescription must be written on a specialized DEA prescription form.
   B. They can be refilled up to 5 times within 6 months from the date the prescription was written.
   C. They have no limitations on refills although the patient has only 1 year to fill all medication refills.
   D. There are no limitations on C-III agents, only C-II agents.

10. How many doses of Zinacef 500 mg can be prepared from a 10-g bulk vial?
    A. 20 doses
    B. 50 doses
    C. 100 doses
    D. 200 doses

11. Estraderm is available in which type of dosage form?
   A. Oral tablets
   B. Implant
   C. Vaginal ring
   D. Topical patch

12. A prescription is written for Pen Vee K susp 500 mg PO qid for 10 days. What volume of a 250 mg/5 mL suspension will need to be dispensed to fill the order for 10 days?
   A. 100 mL
   B. 400 mL
   C. 500 mL
   D. 1000 mL

13. What volume of a 2% erythromycin solution can be made from 15 g of erythromycin powder?
   A. 250 mL
   B. 500 mL
   C. 750 mL
   D. 900 mL

14. You receive an order for 10 mEq of magnesium sulfate to be added to a TPN. You have a 50-mL vial of 4 mEq/mL magnesium sulfate in stock. How much do you need to inject into the TPN?
   A. 1 mL
   B. 2.5 mL
   C. 5 mL
   D. 50 mL

15. If you have a 70% dextrose solution, how many grams are in 50 mL of solution?
   A. 5 mg
   B. 5 g
   C. 35 mg
   D. 35 g

16. Which of the following IV drugs needs to be prepared in a horizontal laminar flow hood?
   A. Tobramycin
   B. Cefazolin
   C. Ampicillin
   D. All of the above

17. Of the drugs listed below, which one is not indicated to lower cholesterol?
   A. Pravachol
   B. Zaroxolyn
   C. Lipitor
   D. Zocor

18. Which auxiliary label(s) would need to be attached to the drug Orap?
   A. Do not take if you are breast-feeding.
   B. Do not take with grapefruit juice.
   C. Avoid sunlight while taking this medication.
   D. Both labels A and B should be attached.

19. The drug Prilosec is classified as a(n):
   A. H_2-blocker
   B. NSAID
   C. Beta-blocker
   D. Proton pump inhibitor

20. The four middle numbers of the NDC represent:
   A. The package size
   B. The manufacturer
   C. The product name, strength, and dosage form
   D. The package size, manufacturer, and dosage form

21. A prescription is given to you for a medication that has the following sig: Take 1 tab SL prn cp. This translates into:
   A. Take one tablet sublingually daily for pain.
   B. Take one tablet sublingually as indicated for complications.
   C. Take one tablet sublingually as needed for chest pain.
   D. Take one tablet sublingually as directed by physician.

22. The type of measuring device used to dispense 2.5 mL of oral solution (most accurately) would be:
   A. A 1-mL oral dropper
   B. A 5-mL teaspoon
   C. A 20-mL oral dose syringe
   D. A 10-mL oral dose syringe

23. When insulin is added to a TPN, which type is used?
   A. Lente insulin
   B. Ultralente insulin
   C. Regular insulin
   D. Insulin cannot be added to TPN

24. A patient complaining of headaches asks you to recommend a good brand of aspirin. She is also picking up her prescriptions of the following medications:
   Lasix 40 mg tabs
   KCl 20 mEq tabs
   Coumadin 2.5 mg tabs
   Plavix 10 mg tabs
   What should you do and why?
   A. Tell her to call her physician because only he/she can recommend an OTC medication when the patient is taking a prescription drug.
   B. Notify the pharmacist because there is a possible interaction between Coumadin, Plavix, and aspirin.
   C. Notify the pharmacist because there is a possible interaction between Coumadin and aspirin.
   D. Tell the patient the names of several agents because you stock the pharmacy and know the names of many aspirin agents.

25. A prescription is ordered for clindamycin suspension. You have 75 mg/5 mL in stock. How many milliliters are needed for a 300-mg dose for 7 days?
   A. 70 mL
   B. 140 mL
   C. 150 mL
   D. 450 mL

26. You have a vial of heparin 20,000 units/mL. How many milliliters are needed for a 12,500-unit dose?
   A. 0.025 mL
   B. 0.265 mL
   C. 0.625 mL
   D. 0.1 mL

27. The Roman numeral CL is equivalent to:
   A. 1050
   B. 150
   C. 50
   D. None of the above

28. How many ounces are contained in 1 pt?
   A. 8 oz
   B. 12 oz
   C. 16 oz
   D. 24 oz

29. The following drug would not be used for constipation:
  A. Metamucil
  B. Colace
  C. Bisacodyl
  D. Imodium

30. Which of the following drugs requires an auxiliary label stating that "This drug may cause discoloration of the urine"?
  A. Septra
  D. Sinemet
  C. Doxycycline
  D. Pyridium

31. How many grams of 0.45% normal saline and 5% dextrose are in a 1-L bag of IV solution?
  A. 4.5 g of 0.45% NS; 5 g of 5% dextrose
  B. 4.5 g of 0.45% NS; 50 g of 5% dextrose
  C. 0.45 g of 0.45% NS; 0.5 g of 5% dextrose
  D. None of the above

32. A prescription order for neomycin 0.75 g PO bid × 30 days is submitted. In stock you have 500-mg tablets. How many tablets will the patient use per day?
  A. ½ tablet daily
  B. 1½ tablets daily
  C. 3 tablets daily
  D. 3½ tablets daily

33. You need to prepare a dose of lidocaine 500 mg with your supply, which is a 10-mL vial of 2% lidocaine. How much should you draw up into a syringe?
  A. 2.5 mL
  B. 12.5 mL
  C. 25 mL
  D. 250 mL

34. You receive an order for doxycycline 100 mg IV. After preparation and check-off by the pharmacist but before delivery of the IV bag, what should you do?
  A. Place a DO NOT REFRIGERATE label on the doxycycline bag.
  B. Place the doxycycline bag in a light-protected bag.
  C. Place the doxycycline bag in a chemo bag and mark VESICANT.
  D. Nothing needs to be done for doxycycline.

35. A physician prescribes his patient Vasotec 7.5 mg PO bid × 30 days. You have 5-mg tablets in stock. How many tablets will it take to fill this script?
  A. 15 tablets
  B. 45 tablets
  C. 84 tablets
  D. 90 tablets

36. Which of the following devices must be checked daily and documented to ensure storage requirements are met for medications?
  A. The temperature of the pharmacy room
  B. The temperatures of the refrigerator and freezer
  C. The temperature of the laminar flow hood
  D. Both A and B

37. Using your penicillin injectable stock of 125,000 units/mL, how many milliliters will it take to prepare 1 million units?
  A. 500 mL
  B. 125 mL
  C. 80 mL
  D. 8 mL

38. A physician orders ampicillin 3 mg/kg/day for a 75-lb child. How many milligrams will the child receive per day? You have in stock ampicillin 80 mg/mL.
   A. 10.22 mg/day
   B. 22.5 mg/day
   C. 102.3 mg/day
   D. 225 mg/day

39. An oral suspension is available as 100 mg/5 mL. The physician orders 0.25 g PO tid. How many milliliters will this patient receive per dose?
   A. 4.2 mL
   B. 12.5 mL
   C. 25 mL
   D. 37.5 mL

40. You receive an order for 1500 mL of 5% dextrose to run at 125 mL per hour. How long will this bag last?
   A. 4.5 hours
   B. 10 hours
   C. 12 hours
   D. 24 hours

41. To prepare 500 mL of a 5% dextrose solution, you must use your available stock of 2% and 10% dextrose. How much of each available solution will you need to prepare the order?
   A. 187 mL of 2%; 312.5 mL of 10%
   B. 312.5 mL of 2%; 187.5 mL of 10%
   C. 340.9 mL of 2%; 159.1 mL of 10%; then qs with water to equal 1000 mL
   D. 250 mL of 2%; 250 mL of 10%

42. How many milliliters of 35% acetic acid must be mixed with 5% acetic acid to give 1000 mL of 10% acetic acid?
   A. 125 mL of 35%; 875 mL of 5%
   B. 875 mL of 35%; 125 mL of 5%
   C. 222.2 mL of 35%; 777.8 mL of 5%
   D. 777.8 mL of 35%; 222.2 mL of 5%

43. How many grams of drug are in 500 mL of solution if it is labeled 40% solution?
   A. 20 g
   B. 0.125 g
   C. 0.200 g
   D. 200 g

44. To which programs can medication errors be reported?
   A. MERP
   B. MedWatch
   C. Better Business Bureau
   D. Both A and B

45. An order calls for 500 mg/250 mL to be infused at 50 mL per hour. How much drug will be infused per hour and how many hours will the bag last?
   A. 25 mg for 5 hours
   B. 100 mg for 5 hours
   C. 500 mg for 1 hour
   D. 500 mg for 5 hours

46. Which medication is packaged in an amber-colored glass container to protect drug degradation?
   A. Nitroglycerin
   B. Amoxicillin suspension
   C. Phenytoin
   D. Cardura

47. The amount of hydrocortisone powder needed to prepare 8 oz of 2% hydrocortisone cream is:

A. 0.24 g

B. 0.48 g

C. 2.4 g

D. 4.8 g

48. You receive a prescription for a 5-year-old patient for Cipro 500-mg tablets with a Sig: Take 1 tab bid × 10 days. Would you bring this to the attention of the pharmacist? Why?

A. Yes; because this medication does not come in this dosage form

B. Yes; because the dosage form of the drug may not be appropriate for a child

C. Yes; because the strength of this drug is not written for a long enough time

D. No; nothing is wrong with this prescription

49. KCl is an abbreviation for:

A. Sodium chloride

B. Iodine chloride

C. Phosphate chloride

D. Potassium chloride

50. If a patient is allergic to penicillin and gives you a prescription for Keflex, what would you do?

A. Notify the registered pharmacist. The patient will have a severe allergy to this medication as well.

B. Notify the registered pharmacist. The patient might have an allergic reaction to this medication as well.

C. Do not notify the registered pharmacist. The patient most likely will not have an allergic reaction.

D. Do not notify the registered pharmacist. The patient will not have an allergy to this medication.

51. Which of the books listed below is available in a removable hard-bound form to allow pages to be updated?

A. *PDR*

B. *Drug Facts and Comparisons*

C. *Red Book*

D. *Ident-A-Drug*

52. The acronym of the accrediting body of hospitals and other patient institutions is:

A. TJC

B. FDA

C. MEDICARE

D. All of the above

53. Which act requires that all patient information within the pharmacy be on a need-to-know basis and must be protected from public knowledge?

A. The Joint Commission's Patient Rights Act

B. The Board of Pharmacies Patient Amendments Rights Act

C. Individual to each pharmacy's standard policies

D. Health Insurance Portability and Accountability Act

54. The drug metronidazole is available in which dosage forms?

A. Tablets and capsules

B. Injectable

C. Lotion, cream, and gel

D. All of the above

55. The drug Auralgan would be used in the:

A. Ears and eyes

B. Ears; not in the eyes

C. Eyes; not in the ears

D. Ears and mouth

56. Which of the following statements include three examples of where and/or when medication errors may occur?

A. A different dosage form for a prescribed medication is typed into the computer system, misinterpretation of a drug order causes a patient to be dosed only 2 times a day instead of 3, nurse administers a patient's medication 5 minutes later than prescribed.

B. A patient takes the wrong amount of a drug at home, a patient shares prescription medications with others, a patient does not discontinue an old prescription after being prescribed new medication.

C. A person misses a dose at the time prescribed, a technician doses a medication as a prn dose rather than a tid dose (as intended), the wrong quantity of medication is filled at the pharmacy.

D. All of the above are examples of potential medication errors.

57. The abbreviation *Rx* means:

A. Prescription

B. Drug

C. Narcotic

D. Pill

58. Which drug is a potassium-sparing diuretic?

A. Lasix

B. Hydrochlorothiazide

C. Aldactone

D. Bumex

59. The main indication for the drug phenytoin is:

A. Anticonvulsant

B. Antidepressant

C. Antianxiety

D. Diabetes

60. Tall man lettering is being used on various medications because:

A. The lettering is easier to read for the elderly

B. The lettering can reduce drug errors from occurring in look-alike drugs

C. The lettering is enlarged to fit the size of its container

D. Both A and B

61. Which of the drugs below would require a DO NOT DRINK GRAPEFRUIT JUICE auxiliary label?

A. Sertraline

B. Nimodipine

C. Quinidine

D. All of the above

62. Which drug listed below is an antiviral?

A. Cisplatin

B. Biaxin

C. Zovirax

D. Neurontin

63. Which drug listed below is not an SSRI?

A. Elavil

B. Prozac

C. Zoloft

D. Paxil

64. Extemporaneous compounding is when:

A. Water is added to an antibiotic for reconstitution

B. A tablet is crushed with a mortar and pestle and added to a sweetening and suspending agent to make a liquid medication

C. A laminar flow hood is used to remove 2.5 mL of medication from a stock bottle and placed in a 50-mL bag of sterile saline

D. TPN medications are made

65. If a nitroglycerin SL tablet 1/200 grains was ordered, what strength would you take from the shelf to fill this order?
A. 0.2 mg
B. 0.3 mg
C. 0.4 mg
D. 0.6 mg

66. Of the following drug combinations, which would result in a drug-drug interaction?
A. Aspirin and codeine
B. Digoxin and penicillin
C. Coumadin and aspirin
D. Estrogen and Mobic

67. Of the diagnostic devices listed below, which one is used for urinalysis?
A. One Touch
B. First Choice
C. Glucostix
D. Diastix

68. The term *prophylaxis* means:
A. A weak immune system
B. To treat with medications at home
C. Preventive treatment
D. To treat after a condition has been determined

69. The term *half-life* refers to:
A. The life of a medication on the shelf
B. The amount of time it takes a chemical concentration in the body to be decreased by half
C. The amount of time it takes a chemical to begin to become effective
D. Certain medications only last half as long in the body system

70. If a dose of medication is to be given at 0600, 1400, and 2200, the doses are given at what times?
A. 6 AM, 4 PM, and 2 AM
B. 6 AM, 2 PM, and 2 AM
C. 6 AM, 4 PM, and 2:20 PM
D. 6 AM, 2 PM, and 10 PM

71. Which of the drugs listed below is a Schedule IV drug?
A. Codeine
B. Oxycodone/ASA
C. Ativan
D. Percocet

72. Nosocomial infections are found to originate in:
A. The nose
B. Third World countries
C. Hospitals
D. Laboratories

73. How many milliliters are contained in 1½ tbsp of liquid?
A. 15 mL
B. 22.5 mL
C. 37.5 mL
D. 45 mL

74. Which drugs listed are examples of lipid-lowering agents?
A. Crestor, Pravachol
B. BuSpar, Zoloft
C. Plendil, Procardia
D. Viagra, Cialis

75. An order of insulin is added to a TPN bag. The directions are to add 100 units of regular insulin. You draw up 10 mL of insulin to push into the bag. Is there anything wrong with this scenario?
    A. Only a pharmacist can add insulin.
    B. You cannot add insulin after a TPN is made.
    C. You have added 10 times more insulin than ordered.
    D. You have not added enough insulin to the bag.

76. A prescription for a buccal tablet would be labeled:
    A. Place in the rectum.
    B. Chew the tablet.
    C. Place under the tongue.
    D. Place against the inside of the cheek.

77. A person weighing 67 kg is how many pounds?
    A. 30.5 lb
    B. 147.4 lb
    C. 134 lb
    D. 200 lb

78. Cyanocobalamin is the chemical name for which vitamin?
    A. Vitamin A
    B. Vitamin B_6
    C. Vitamin K
    D. Vitamin B_{12}

79. Of the needles listed below, which is in order from smallest to largest and used in pharmacy?
    A. 14 gauge; 16 gauge; 18 gauge; 20 gauge
    B. 27 gauge; 19 gauge; 18 gauge; 16 gauge
    C. 1 gauge; 2 gauge; 3 gauge; 4 gauge
    D. None of the above gauges are used in pharmacy.

80. Of the following intravenous medications, which cannot be mixed with NS?
    A. Cefazolin
    B. Ampicillin
    C. Primaxin
    D. All of these can be mixed with NS.

81. The recommended storage temperature for unopened Xalantin is:
    A. 20° to 25°C (68° to 77°F)
    B. 2° to 8°C (36° to 46°F)
    C. 15° to 30°C (59° to 86°F)
    D. −20° to −10°C (−4° to 14°F)

82. When an investigational drug expires, you should:
    A. Do nothing; only a pharmacist can handle investigational drugs
    B. Remove the drug from the shelf and place it in the hazardous waste bin
    C. Record the quantity and lot number, and return it to the manufacturer
    D. Record the quantity and lot number, and return to the FDA

83. Which of the following forms is needed for pharmacy to dispense controlled substances?
    A. Form 222
    B. Form 224
    C. Form 225
    D. Form 363

84. When unit dosing a tablet, what is the necessary labeling for each unit dose label?
    A. Trade name of drug, strength, color, expiration date
    B. Trade and generic names of drug, strength, manufacturer lot number, and expiration date
    C. Generic and trade names of drug, dosage form, strength, pharmacy lot number, and expiration date
    D. Name of drug, dosage form, color, strength, lot number, and expiration date

85. A glass compounding slab is used for:
    A. A hard, clean surface to mix all compounding products
    B. A smooth surface to mix ointments
    C. A smooth surface to mix ointments and creams
    D. A smooth surface to mix all topical medications

86. Empty capsules used in compounding range in the following sizes (from large to small):
    A. 5 to 000
    B. 5 to 0
    C. 0 to 5
    D. 000 to 5

87. When adding weights to a Class A balance, you should use tweezers because:
    A. The weights are irregularly shaped and hard to pick up
    B. The tweezers have a better grip than your fingers
    C. The oils from your skin will dirty and alter the actual weights
    D. You do not need to use tweezers

88. A prescription says to prepare a medication and qs solution to 100 mL. This means:
    A. Quickly make enough solution to equal 100 mL
    B. Add the appropriate solution to the medication to equal 100 mL
    C. To pour off any medication over 100 mL
    D. None of the above

89. Which of the following drugs should not be stocked on an adult crash cart?
    A. Nitroglycerin patches
    B. Sodium bicarbonate PFS
    C. Epinephrine PFS
    D. Atropine PFS

90. PCA is used to:
    A. Administer antibiotics to children
    B. Administer D_5W only
    C. Administer controlled analgesics
    D. Administer anticonvulsants

91. Lipids should be stored:
    A. At room temperature
    B. In the refrigerator
    C. In the freezer
    D. In a fireproof cabinet

92. When stocking shelves with new stock, you should:
    A. Remove all outdated stock first
    B. Rotate stock, placing the longer expiration dates to the back
    C. Place new stock in a different container next to the older stock
    D. Both A and B

93. Which of the following explanations best defines formulary?
    A. A set of rules and guidelines for pharmacy personnel
    B. A list of drugs that are approved by the pharmacy management
    C. A list of drugs that are approved by the pharmacy and therapeutics committee
    D. A set of guidelines for nurses on how to use medications

94. Which drug below is not available in the dosage form described?
    A. Heparin injectable
    B. Warfarin 2.5-mg tablets
    C. Prednisone 1 mg/mL suspension
    D. Morphine sulfate 15 mg CR tablets

95. A prescription calls for amoxicillin suspension to be reconstituted. What auxiliary label(s) will you place on the container?
A. Keep refrigerated after opening.
B. Keep refrigerated; take until gone.
C. Keep refrigerated; take until gone; shake well before using; see expiration date.
D. Keep refrigerated; shake well before using; see expiration date.

96. Of the medications listed below, which one is a C-II drug?
A. Clonazepam
B. Valium
C. Meperidine
D. Lortab

97. A C-II drug can be refilled:
A. As many times as the refill indicates
B. A maximum of 5 times or within 6 months from the original order, whichever comes first
C. Only twice
D. A new prescription is needed for each prescription fill

98. When a drug is recalled and is considered a Class 1 recall, this means:
A. This is the lowest level used for products that may have a minor defect
B. This is when the drug may cause serious but reversible harm
C. This is the highest level of recall for products that could cause serious and/or irreversible illness or may even be fatal
D. None of the above

99. When repackaging medications into unit dose containers, which of the listed required information does not need to be recorded in a logbook?
A. The dosage form
B. The person who repackaged the medication
C. The date the medication was prepared
D. The patient's name and medical record number

100. Within the policies and procedures manual, the requirement for pharmacists to counsel patients on medications they have not taken before is listed under which law?
A. Durham-Humphrey Amendment
B. Kefauver-Harris Amendment
C. Prescription Drug Marketing Act
D. OBRA '90

101. The program under the FDA that allows health care professionals to report any adverse reactions is:
A. DEA Form 222
B. MedWatch
C. Pharmacist in Charge
D. AARP

102. As new stock arrives at the pharmacy, the technician should check the following information on the stock against the invoice:
A. Name, strength, and quantity
B. Name, strength, dosage form, and quantity
C. Name, strength, dosage form, quantity, and expiration date
D. Name, strength, dosage form, quantity, expiration date, and delivery person's name

103. Which of the following automated systems is used specifically in hospitals to stock PAR levels of medications on nursing floors?
A. Baker Cell systems
B. Pyxis
C. Robot systems
D. All of the above

104. A drug manufacturer is required by law to recall any product that has been found to violate any of the following guidelines except:
A. Labeling is wrong
B. Drug batch was contaminated
C. Any change that causes the drug to fall outside the FDA's or manufacturer's guidelines
D. The drugs sent to the pharmacy were damaged in transit

105. Where should phenol be stored?
A. In the refrigerator
B. On a shelf at room temperature
C. On the bottom shelf behind cabinet doors
D. Locked in the narcotics room

106. Grinding tablets into a fine powder in a porcelain mortar is an example of:
A. Flocculation
B. Emulsification
C. Levigation
D. Trituration

107. Which drug agency is responsible for regulating medical devices?
A. FDA
B. DEA
C. EPA
D. OSHA

108. Which of the following medications is available as an inhaler for asthma?
A. Propranolol
B. Albuterol
C. Nasonex
D. Both B and C

109. Transdermal nitroglycerin would be kept in which section of the pharmacy?
A. The topicals
B. The oral medications
C. The liquids
D. In the refrigerator

110. A pregnant patient arrives with a prescription for temazepam 15 mg q hs. What do you do?
A. Fill the prescription.
B. Label the medication with "take at bedtime" and "may cause drowsiness."
C. Alert the pharmacist because this is a Pregnancy Category X medication.
D. Alert the pharmacist because this is a Pregnancy Category A medication.

111. A STAT order is called into the pharmacy by a nurse in the hospital unit. What do you do?
A. You can take the order orally, and then let the pharmacist know about it.
B. You should tell the nurse that she must send the order in writing.
C. You should give the phone to the pharmacist, alerting him or her to a stat order.
D. You should fill the order immediately because it is a stat order.

112. What is the proper procedure for cleaning a laminar flow hood?
A. Spray the inside of the entire hood and clean all areas.
B. Clean the hood starting from the front and working toward the back.
C. Clean the hood starting from the back, using side-to-side motions and moving top to bottom toward the front.
D. Wash the whole hood using a circular motion.

113. Which of the agencies listed below is responsible for accreditation of an institutional facility?
    A. APhA
    B. DEA
    C. TJC
    D. ASHP

114. The main purpose of OSHA is to:
    A. Write laws pertaining to the workplace for employees
    B. Ensure the safety of drugs for patients
    C. Ensure the safety of air quality for patients
    D. Ensure the safety of the workplace for employees

115. The MSDS contains what type of information?
    A. Drug ingredients
    B. How to work safely
    C. How to file a complaint about an incident
    D. The ingredients and specifics of all types of chemical products

116. A computer program used for dispensing medication in the pharmacy setting is referred to as:
    A. Hardware
    B. Software
    C. Medware
    D. Disks

117. Materials management refers to:
    A. Inventory control
    B. Drug storage
    C. The drug procurement process
    D. All of the above

118. If a pharmacy pricing formulary is the AWP plus $4.50 and the AWP is $90 for 100 tablets, what is the charge to the customer for a prescription of 30 tablets?
    A. $27.50
    B. $30.50
    C. $31.50
    D. $94.50

119. The cost of 100 tablets of a bottle of aspirin is $1.50. What would the dispensing charge be to yield a 50% gross profit?
    A. $2.00
    B. $2.10
    C. $2.25
    D. $2.50

120. Which of the programs listed below is administered by individual states?
    A. Medicare
    B. Medicaid
    C. Medicare Part A
    D. Medicare Part D

121. AWP can be found in which book?
    A. *Red Book*
    B. *PDR*
    C. *American Drug Index*
    D. *United States Pharmacopoeia*

122. If a manufacturer's invoice totals $520.00 with the terms 2% net, what amount should be remitted if it is paid within 30 days?
    A. $490.00
    B. $509.60
    C. $520.00
    D. $530.40

123. When choosing between state and federal requirements, which take precedence?
   A. The state's requirements
   B. The federal government's requirements
   C. The requirements of the institution that is your employer
   D. The most stringent requirements

124. A person who is older than 65 years of age, who is disabled, or who has kidney failure would be covered by _____ insurance.
   A. Medicaid
   B. HMO
   C. Medicare
   D. PPO

125. Online processing of a third-party claim to determine payment is called:
   A. Reconciliation
   B. Processing degree
   C. Adjudication
   D. Authorization

Answer Key

   1. B. The first time the prescription is filled (Chapter 7)
   2. A. BH 1234575 (Chapter 2)
   3. A. AcipHex (Chapter 21) and Ventolin (Chapter 18)
   4. D. TPNs (Chapter 10)
   5. A. Sudafed (Chapter 2)
   6. C. Instill three drops into the left eye every other day (Chapter 5)
   7. D. 60 mg (Chapter 4)
   8. C. Clarithromycin (Chapter 25)
   9. B. Can be refilled up to 5 times within 6 months from the date it was written (Chapter 2)
   10. A 20 doses (Chapter 4)
   11. D. Topical patch (Chapter 24)
   12. B. 400 mL (Chapter 4)
   13. C. 750 mL (Chapter 4)
   14. B. 2.5 mL (Chapter 4)
   15. D. 35 g (Chapter 4)
   16. D. All of the above (Chapter 10)
   17. B. Zaroxolyn (Chapter 22)
   18. D. Both A and B (Chapter 15)
   19. D. Proton pump inhibitor (Chapter 20)
   20. C. The product name, strength, and dosage form (Chapters 2 and 14)
   21. C. Take one tablet sublingually as needed for chest pain (Chapter 5)
   22. D. A 10-mL oral dose syringe (Chapter 2)
   23. C. Regular (Chapter 13)
   24. B. Notify the pharmacist because there is a possible interaction between Coumadin, Plavix, and aspirin (Chapter 23)
   25. B. 140 mL (Chapter 4)
   26. C. 0.625 mL (Chapter 4)
   27. B. 150 (Chapter 4)
   28. C. 16 oz (Chapter 4)
   29. D. Imodium (Chapter 21)

30. D. Pyridium (Chapter 21)

31. B. 4.5 g of 0.45% NS; 50 g of 5% dextrose (Chapter 4)

32. C. 3 tablets daily (Chapter 4)

33. C. 25 mL (Chapter 4)

34. B. Place the doxycycline in a light-protected bag (Chapter 4)

35. D. 90 tablets (Chapter 4)

36. B. The temperatures of the refrigerator and the freezer (Chapter 13)

37. D. 8 mL (Chapter 4)

38. C. 102.3 mg/day (Chapter 4)

39. B. 12.5 mL (Chapter 4)

40. C. 12 hours (Chapter 4)

41. B. 312.5 mL of 2%; 187.5 mL of 10% (Chapter 4)

42. A. 166.7 mL of 35%; 833.3 mL of 5% (Chapter 4)

43. D. 200 g (Chapter 4)

44. D. Both A and B (Chapter 14)

45. B. 100 mg for 5 hours (Chapter 4)

46. A. Nitroglycerin (Chapter 23)

47. D. 4.8 g (Chapter 4)

48. B. Yes; because the dosage form of the drug may not be appropriate for a child (Chapters 4 and 14)

49. D. Potassium (Chapter 31)

50. B. The patient MIGHT have an allergic reaction to this medication as well. Notify the registered pharmacist (Chapter 25)

51. B. *Drug Facts and Comparisons* (Chapter 6)

52. A. TJC (Chapter 2)

53. D. HIPAA patient confidentiality act (Chapter 2)

54. D. All of the above (Chapter 25)

55. B. Ears; not in the eyes (Chapter 19)

56. C. A person who missed a dose at the time prescribed, a technician who doses a medication as a prn dose rather than a tid dose (as intended), the wrong quantity of medication was filled at the pharmacy (Chapter 14)

57. A. Prescription (Chapter 5)

58. C. Aldactone (Chapter 5)

59. A. Anticonvulsant (Chapter 17)

60. B. The lettering can reduce the occurrence of drug errors (Chapter 14)

61. D. All of the above (Chapters 17 [sertraline] and 23 [nimodipine, quinidine])

62. C. Zovirax (Chapter 29)

63. A. Elavil (Chapter 17)

64. B. When a tablet is crushed with a mortar and pestle and added to a sweetening and suspending agent to make a liquid medication (Chapter 14)

65. B. 0.3 mg (Chapter 4)

66. C. Coumadin and aspirin (Chapter 8)

67. D. Diastix (Chapter 22)

68. C. Preventive treatment (Chapter 5)

69. B. The amount of time it takes a chemical to be decreased by half of its strength (Chapter 5)

70. D. 6 AM, 2 PM, and 10 PM (Chapter 4)

71. C. Ativan (Chapter 2)

72. C. In hospitals (Chapter 10)

73. B. 22.5 mL (Chapter 4)

74. A. Crestor, Pravachol (Chapter 23)

75. C. You have added 10 times too much insulin (Chapters 4, 7, and 14)

76. D. Place against the inside of the cheek (Chapter 5)

77. B. 147.4 lb (Chapter 4)

78. D. Vitamin B_{12} (Chapter 27)

79. B. 27 gauge; 19 gauge; 18 gauge; 16 gauge (Chapter 12)

80. D. All of these can be mixed with NS (Chapter 25)

81. B. 2° to 8°C (36° to 46°F) (Chapters 13 and 19)

82. C. Record the quantity and lot number, and return it to the manufacturer (Chapter 4)

83. B. Form 224 (Chapter 2)

84. C. Generic and trade names of drug, dosage form, strength, lot number, and expiration date (Chapter 10)

85. C. A smooth surface to mix ointments and creams (Chapter 11)

86. D. 000 to 5 (Chapter 5)

87. C. The oils from your skin will dirty and alter the actual weights (Chapter 11)

88. B. Add the appropriate solution to the medication to equal 100 mL (Chapter 4)

89. A. Nitroglycerin patches (Chapter 10)

90. C. Administer controlled analgesics (Chapter 2)

91. A. At room temperature (Chapter 11)

92. D. Both A and B (Chapter 14)

93. C. A list of drugs that are approved by the pharmacy and therapeutics' committee (Chapter 10)

94. C. Prednisone 1 mg/mL solution (Chapter 25)

95. C. Keep refrigerated; take until gone; shake well before using; see expiration date (Chapter 8)

96. C. Meperidine (Chapter 2)

97. D. A new prescription is needed for each prescription fill (Chapter 2)

98. C. This is the highest level of recall for products that could cause serious illness or may even be fatal (Chapter 2)

99. D. The patient's name and medical record number (Chapter 13)

100. D. OBRA '90 (Chapter 2)

101. B. MedWatch (Chapter 2)

102. C. Name, strength, dosage form, quantity, and expiration date (Chapter 13)

103. B. Pyxis (Chapters 10 and 14)

104. D. The drugs sent to the pharmacy were damaged in transit (Chapter 13)

105. C. On the bottom shelf behind cabinet doors (Chapter 13)

106. D. Trituration (Chapter 12)

107. A. FDA (Chapter 2)

108. B. Albuterol (Chapter 18)

109. A. The topicals (Chapter 22)

110. C. Alert the pharmacist because this is a Pregnancy Category X (Chapter 7)

111. C. You should give the phone to the pharmacist (Chapter 7)

112. C. Clean the hood starting from the back, using side-to-side motions and moving top to bottom toward the front (Chapter 12)

113. C. TJC (Chapter 11)

114. D. Ensure the safety of the workplace (Chapter 2)

115. D. The ingredients and specifics of all types of chemical products (Chapter 6)

116. B. Software (Chapter 6)

117. D. All of the above (Chapter 14)
118. C. $31.50 (Chapter 4)
119. C. $2.25 (Chapter 4)
120. B. Medicaid (Chapter 2)
121. A. *Red Book* (Chapter 6)
122. B. $509.60 (Chapter 4)
123. D. The most stringent (Chapter 2)
124. C. Medicare (Chapter 2)
125. C. Adjudication (Chapter 13)

B

200 Top Selling Trade Name Drugs for 2009

Trade Name	Generic Name	Indication/Use	Trade Name	Generic Name	Indication/Use
1. Lipitor	atorvastatin	Hyperlipidemia	31. Lantus	insulin glargine	Insulin-dependent diabetes
2. Singulair	montelukast	Asthma	32. Viagra	sildenafil	Erectile dysfunction
3. Lexapro	escitalopram	Depression	33. Altace	ramipril	High blood pressure
4. Nexium	esomeprazole	GERD	34. Yasmin 28	drospirenone/ethinyl estradiol	Oral contraceptive
5. Synthroid	levothyroxine	Hypothyroidism			
6. Plavix	clopidogrel	CAD	35. Levoxyl	levothyroxine	Hypothyroidism
7. Toprol XL	metoprolol	High blood pressure	36. Adderall XR	amphetamine/ dextroamphetamine	Attention deficit/ hyperactivity disorder
8. Prevacid	lansoprazole	GERD			
9. Vytorin	ezetimibe/simvastatin	Hyperlipidemia			
10. Advair Diskus	fluticasone/salmeterol	Asthma	37. Lotrel	amlodipine/benazepril	High blood pressure
11. Zyrtec	cetirizine	Allergies	38. Actonel	risedronate	Osteoporosis
12. Effexor XR	venlafaxine	Depression	39. Ambien CR	zolpidem	Insomnia
13. Protonix	pantoprazole	GERD	40. Cozaar	losartan	High blood pressure
14. Diovan	valsartan	High blood pressure	41. Coreg	carvedilol	CAD; heart failure
15. Fosamax	aldendronate	Osteoporosis	42. Valtrex	valacyclovir	Viral infection
16. Zetia	ezetimibe	Hyperlipidemia	43. Lyrica	pregabalin	Fibromyalgia; neuropathy
17. Crestor	rosuvastatin	Hyperlipidemia			
18. Levaquin	levofloxacin	Bacterial infection	44. Concerta	methylphenidate	Attention deficit/ hyperactivity disorder
19. Diovan HCT	valsartan/ hydrochlorothiazide	CAD			
			45. Ambien	zolpidem	Insomnia
20. Klor-Con	potassium chloride	Potassium replacement	46. Risperdal	risperidone	Bipolar disorder; schizophrenia
21. Cymbalta	duloxetine	Depression	47. Digitek	digoxin	Heart failure; cardiac arrhythmia
22. Actos	pioglitazone	Non–insulin- dependent diabetes mellitus			
			48. Topamax	topiramate	Epilepsy
23. Premarin Tabs	conjugated estrogens	Menopause	49. Chantix	varenicline	Smoking cessation
24. ProAir HFA	albuterol	Asthma	50. Avandia	rosiglitazone	Non–insulin- dependent diabetes mellitus
25. Celebrex	celecoxib	NSAID, COX-2 inhibitor subtype			
26. Flomax	tamsulosin	Benign prostatic hyperplasia	51. Lamictal	lamotrigine	Epilepsy
			52. Ortho Tri-Cyclen Lo	norgestimate/ethinyl estradiol	Oral contraceptive
27. Seroquel	quetiapine	Bipolar disorder; schizophrenia	53. Xalatan	latanoprost	Glaucoma
28. Norvasc	amlodipine	High blood pressure	54. AcipHex	rabeprazole	GERD
29. Nasonex	mometasone	Nasal allergies			
30. Tricor	fenofibrate	Hyperlipidemia			

Continued

Trade Name	Generic Name	Indication/Use	Trade Name	Generic Name	Indication/Use
55. Hyzaar	losartan/ hydrochlorothiazide	High blood pressure	95. Lidoderm	lidocaine	Fibromyalgia
56. Spiriva	tiotropium	COPD	96. Strattera	atomoxetine	Attention deficit/ hyperactivity disorder
57. Wellbutrin XL	bupropion	Depression			
58. Lunesta	eszopiclone	Insomnia	97. Aviane 28	levonorgestrel/ethinyl estradiol	Oral contraceptive
59. Benicar	olmesartan	High blood pressure			
60. Benicar HCT	olmesartan/ hydrochlorothiazide	High blood pressure	98. Patanol	olopatadine	Allergic conjunctivitis
61. Aricept	donepezil	Alzheimer's disease	99. Proventil HFA	albuterol	Asthma
62. Avapro	irbesartan	High blood pressure	100. Clarinex	desloratadine	Allergies
63. Detrol LA	tolterodine	Urinary incontinence	101. Thyroid, Armour	thyroid	Hypothyroidism
64. TriNessa	norgestimate/ethinyl estradiol	Oral contraceptive	102. Astelin	azelastine	Allergies
			103. Zyrtec-D	cetirizine/ pseudoephedrine	Allergies
65. Cialis	tadalafil	Erectile dysfunction			
66. Combivent	ipratropium/albuterol	COPD	104. Tussionex	hydrocodone/ chlorpheniramine	Cough-antitussive agent
67. Budeprion XL	bupropion	Depression			
68. Yaz	drospirenone/ethinyl estradiol	Oral contraceptive	105. Caduet	amlodipine/ atorvastatin	High blood pressure with hyperlipidemia
69. GlycoLax	polyethylene glycol	Constipation			
70. Imitrex Oral	sumatriptan	Migraine	106. Avodart	dutasteride	Benign prostatic hyperplasia
71. Evista	raloxifene	Osteoporosis			
72. NuvaRing	etonogestrel/ethinyl estradiol	Oral contraceptive,	107. Keppra	levetiracetam	Epilepsy
			108. Januvia	sitagliptin	Non–insulin-dependent diabetes mellitus
73. Omnicef	cefdinir	Bacterial infection			
74. Niaspan	niacin	Hyperlipidemia			
75. Tri-Sprintec	norgestimate/ethinyl estradiol	Oral contraceptive	109. Kariva	desogestrel/ethinyl estradiol	Oral contraceptive
76. Boniva	ibandronate	Osteoporosis	110. Prempro	conjugated estrogens/ medroxyprogesterone	Menopause
77. Flovent HFA	fluticasone	Asthma			
78. Avelox	moxifloxacin	Bacterial infection	111. Rhinocort Aqua	budesonide	Nasal allergies
79. Abilify	aripiprazole	Schizophrenia			
80. Avalide	irbesartan/ hydrochlorothiazide	High blood pressure	112. Levitra	vardenafil	Erectile dysfunction
			113. Ortho Evra	norelgestromin/ethinyl estradiol	Oral contraceptive
81. Requip	ropinirole	Parkinson's disease; restless legs syndrome	114. Low-Ogestrel	norgestrel/ethinyl estradiol	Oral contraceptive
82. Zyrtec Syrup	cetirizine	Allergies	115. Vivelle-DOT	estradiol	Menopause
83. Coumadin	warfarin	Anticoagulant	116. Apri	desogestrel/ethinyl estradiol	Oral contraceptive
84. Zyprexa	olanzapine	Bipolar disorder; schizophrenia	117. Loestrin 24 Fe	norethindrone/ethinyl estradiol/ferrous fumerate	Oral contraceptive
85. Depakote ER	divalproex	Migraine			
86. Nasacort AQ	triamcinolone	Nasal allergies	118. Levothroid	levothyroxine	Hypothyroidism
87. Skelaxin	metaxalone	Musculoskeletal relaxant	119. Necon 1/35	norethindrone/ethinyl estradiol	Oral contraceptive
88. Allegra-D	fexofenadine/ pseudoephedrine	Allergies	120. Fosamax Plus D	alendronate/ cholecalciferol	Osteoporosis
89. Humalog	insulin lispro	Insulin-dependent diabetes mellitus	121. Byetta	exenatide injection	Non–insulin-dependent diabetes mellitus
90. Vigamox	moxifloxacin	Bacterial conjunctivitis			
91. Endocet	oxycodone/ acetaminophen	Pain	122. Pulmicort Respules	budesonide	Asthma
92. Budeprion SR	bupropion	Depression	123. Paxil CR	paroxetine	Depression
93. Depakote	divalproex delayed release	Bipolar disorder; epilepsy	124. GlipiZIDE XL	glipizide	Non–insulin-dependent diabetes mellitus
94. Namenda	memantine	Alzheimer's disease			

Trade Name	Generic Name	Indication/Use	Trade Name	Generic Name	Indication/Use
125. Provigil	modafinil	Narcolepsy; sleep apnea; attention deficit/ hyperactivity disorder	156. Avandamet	rosiglitazone/ metformin	Non–insulin-dependent diabetes mellitus
126. Trileptal	oxcarbazepine	Epilepsy	157. Lanoxin	digoxin	Congestive heart failure; atrial fibrillation
127. Humulin N	isophane insulin (NPH)	Insulin-dependent diabetes mellitus	158. Travatan	travoprost	Glaucoma
128. Lumigan	bimatoprost	Glaucoma	159. Zoloft	sertraline	Depression
129. Alphagan P	brimonidine	Glaucoma	160. Bactroban	mupirocin	Bacterial skin infections
130. Xopenex HFA	levalbuterol	Asthma	161. Tamiflu	oseltamivir	Influenza
131. Tobradex	tobramycin/ dexamethasone	Bacterial eye infection	162. Guaifenex PSE	guaifenesin/ pseudoephedrine	Cold/flu symptoms
132. Trivora-28	levonorgestrel/ethinyl estradiol	Oral contraceptive	163. Differin	adapalene	Acne vulgaris
133. Atacand	candesartan cilexetil	Hypertension	164. Premarin Vaginal	conjugated estrogens	Hormone replacement
134. Xopenex	levalbuterol	Asthma	165. Pseudovent 400	pseudoephedrine/ guaifenesin	Cold/flu symptoms
135. Cosopt	dorzolamide/timolol	Glaucoma	166. Vagifem	estradiol	Menopause
136. Geodon Oral	ziprasidone	Bipolar disorder; schizophrenia	167. Levora	levonorgestrel/ethinyl estradiol	Oral contraceptive
137. Micardis	telmisartan	Hypertension	168. Relpax	eletriptan	Migraine
138. Lovaza	omega-3-acid ethyl esters	Hypertriglyceridemia	169. Allegra-D 24 Hour	fexofenadine/ pseudoephedrine	Allergies
139. Micardis HCT	telmisartan/ hydrochlorothiazide	Hypertension	170. Methylin	methylphenidate	Attention deficit disorder
140. Focalin XR	dexmethylphenidate	Attention deficit/ hyperactivity disorder	171. AndroGel	testosterone	Male hypogonadism
			172. Aggrenox	aspirin/dipyridamole	Stroke prophylaxis
141. OxyContin	oxycodone controlled release	Moderate to severe pain	173. Propecia	finasteride	Alopecia
			174. Asmanex	mometasone	Asthma
142. Mirapex	pramipexole	Parkinson's disease; restless legs syndrome	175. NovoLog Mix 70/30	70% insulin aspart protamine/30% insulin aspart (rDNA)	Insulin-dependent diabetes mellitus
143. Prometrium	progesterone	Menopause; infertility; PMS	176. Uroxatral	alfuzosin	Benign prostatic hyperplasia
144. Humulin 70/30	70% insulin isophane (NPH)/30% insulin regular	Insulin-dependent diabetes mellitus	177. Estrostep Fe	norethindrone acetate/ethinyl estradiol	Oral contraceptive
145. Ciprodex Otic	ciprofloxacin/ dexamethasone	Infections of external ear	178. Sular	nisoldipine	High blood pressure
146. Restasis	cyclosporine	Ocular inflammation	179. Lescol XL	fluvastatin	Hyperlipidemia
147. Suboxone	buprenorphine/ naloxone	Opioid dependence	180. Novolin 70/30	insulin isophane (NPH)/insulin regular	Insulin-dependent diabetes mellitus
148. Zymar	gatifloxacin	Bacterial conjunctivitis	181. EpiPen	epinephrine auto injector	Anaphylactic reaction
149. Arimidex	anastrozole	Breast cancer	182. Actoplus Met	pioglitazone/ metformin	Non–insulin-dependent diabetes mellitus
150. Sprintec (28)	norgestimate/ethinyl estradiol	Oral contraceptive			
151. Dilantin Kapseals	phenytoin	Epilepsy	183. M-Oxy	oxycodone	Moderate to severe pain
			184. Rozerem	ramelteon	Insomnia
152. Fluzone	influenza virus vaccine	Seasonal influenza prevention	185. Enablex	darifenacin	Urinary incontinence
153. BenzaClin	clindamycin/benzoyl peroxide	Acne vulgaris	186. Jantoven	warfarin	Anticoagulant
			187. Catapres-TTS	clonidine	High blood pressure
154. VESIcare	solifenacin succinate	Urinary incontinence	188. Junel Fe	norethindrone acetate/ethinyl estradiol/ferrous fumarate	Oral contraceptive
155. Asacol	mesalamine	Ulcerative colitis			

Continued

Trade Name	Generic Name	Indication/Use	Trade Name	Generic Name	Indication/Use
189. Coreg CR	carvedilol	CAD, heart failure	194. Aldara	imiquimod	Superficial basal cell carcinoma; genital warts
190. Ortho Tri-Cyclen	norgestimate/ethinyl estradiol	Oral contraceptive			
191. PrimaCare One	vitamin supplement	Prenatal supplement	195. Necon 0.5/35E	norethindrone/ethinyl estradiol	Oral contraceptive
192. Zovirax Topical	acyclovir	Cold sores, genital herpes	196. Arthrotec	diclofenac/misoprostol	Osteoarthritis
			197. Ultram ER	tramadol	Moderate chronic pain
193. TriLyte	polyethylene glycol/ sodium chloride/ sodium bicarbonate/ potassium chloride	Bowel cleansing	198. Ceron-DM	chlorpheniramine/ dextromethorphan/ phenylephrine	Cold symptoms
			199. EtheDent	sodium fluoride	Cavity prevention
			200. Elidel	pimecrolimus	Atopic dermatitis

C

Top 30 Herbal Remedies

Common Name	Scientific Name	Common Reported Uses	Common Name	Scientific Name	Common Reported Uses
Aloe vera (leaf)	*Aloe* spp.	Wound and burn healing	Ginkgo (root)	*Ginkgo biloba*	Support of memory, increased blood flow to brain, prevention of dementia
American ginseng (root)	*Panax quinquefolius*	Energy, stress, immune system support			
Bilberry (berry)	*Vaccinium myrtillus*	Eye and vascular support	Ginseng	*Panax quinquefolius, Panax ginseng*	Increase physical endurance and concentration, lessen fatigue
Black cohosh (root)	*Cimicifuga racemosa*	Menopause, PMS*			
Cascara sagrada (aged bark)	*Rhamnus purshiana*	Laxative	Glucosamine	Nutriceutical	Osteoarthritis
Cat's claw (root, bark)	*Uncaria tomentosa*	Antiinflammatory, immune system support	Goldenseal (root)	*Hydrastis canadensis*	Chest congestion, cystitis
			Grapeseed (seed, skin)	*Vitis vinifera*	Support circulation
Chondroitin	Nutriceutical	Osteoarthritis			
Cranberry (berry)	*Vaccinium macrocarpon*	Urinary tract infection prevention	Green tea (leaf)	*Camellia sinensis*	Cancer prevention, antioxidant, lower cholesterol, weight maintenance
Dong quai (root)	*Angelica sinensis*	Energy (females), menopause, dysmenorrhea, PMS			
Echinacea (flower, root)	*Echinacea purpurea* *Echinacea angustifolia*	Support of common cold, immunostimulant	Isoflavones (soy)	Nutriceutical	Cancer prevention, decreased bone loss, hot flashes
			Kava (root)	*Piper methysticum*	Anxiety, sedation
Evening primrose (seed oil)	*Oenothera biennis*	PMS, menopause	Melatonin	Nutriceutical	Insomnia
Feverfew (leaf)	*Tanacetum parthenium*	Antiinflammatory, migraine prevention	Milk thistle (seed)	*Silybum marianum*	Antioxidant, liver support
			Saw palmetto (berry)	*Serenoa repens*	Benign prostatic hyperplasia
Fish oils	Nutriceutical	Lower triglycerides, heart health	Siberian ginseng (root)	*Eleutherococcus senticosus*	Athletic performance, stress, immune builder
Garlic (bulb)	*Allium sativum*	Antimicrobial, lower cholesterol	St. John's wort (flowering buds)	*Hypericum perforatum*	Depression, anxiety
Ginger (root)	*Zingiber officinale*	Antiemetic, gastrointestinal distress, dyspepsia	Valerian (root)	*Valeriana officinalis*	Sedative, muscle spasms
			Wild yam (tuber)	*Dioscorea villosa*	Female vitality

*PMS, Premenstrual syndrome.

Glossary

Abortifacient Any treatment that causes abortion of a fetus

Absorption The taking in of nutrients and drugs from food and liquids

Absorption (gastrointestinal) The processes describing the movement of nutrients, fluids, and medications from the gastrointestinal tract into the bloodstream

Accommodation The change that occurs in the ocular lens when it focuses at various distances

Acidification The conversion to an acidic environment

Acidosis The increase in acid content of the blood resulting from the accumulation of acid or loss of bicarbonate; the pH of blood is lowered

Acne vulgaris Commonly known as pimples, acne occurs when the pores of the skin are clogged with oil or bacteria

Acoustic nerve The cranial nerve that controls the senses of hearing and equilibrium and eventually leads to the cerebellum and medulla

Acquired immunity Immunity acquired by active infection, by vaccination (active immunity), or by the transfer of products (usually antibodies) from a donor (passive immunity). Acquired immunity is in contrast to innate immunity (natural immunity system), which provides natural barriers and defenses to infection but does not confer long-lasting immunity

Act A statutory plan passed by Congress or any legislature that is a "bill" until it is enacted and becomes law

Active immunity A form of acquired immunity in which the body produces its own antibodies against disease-causing antigens

Addison's disease Condition resulting in a decrease in adrenocortical hormones, such as mineralocorticoids and glucocorticoids, which cause symptoms including muscle weakness and weight loss

Adjudication Electronic insurance billing for medication payment

Adulteration The mishandling of medication that can lead to contamination/impurity, falsification of contents, or loss of drug quality or potency. Adulteration may cause injury or illness to the consumer

Aerobic A term that describes organisms that need oxygen to survive

Afferent The direction of neuronal impulse from the body toward the central nervous system

Alexander Fleming Discovered penicillin, the first antibiotic

Aliquots Part or portion of a medicine and/or ingredient that has the same volume or weight

Alkalosis The increase of alkalinity of the blood resulting from the accumulation of alkali or reduction of acid content; the pH of blood is raised

Alligation A mathematic method of solving problems that involve the mixing of solutions or mixtures of solids possessing different percentage weights

Amendment A change in the original act or law

American Association of Pharmacy Technicians (AAPT) First pharmacy technician association; founded in 1979

American Pharmacists Association (APhA) Oldest pharmacy association; founded in 1852

American Society of Health-System Pharmacists (ASHP) Pharmacy association founded in 1942

Amino acids Molecules that make up proteins

Anabolism To build up; the construction phase of metabolism

Anaerobic A term that describes organisms that live in the absence of oxygen

Analgesic A drug that relieves pain by reducing the perception of pain

Anaphylactic shock A severe allergic reaction that causes a rapid decrease in blood pressure, ventricular tachycardia, and constriction of the airways; a medical emergency that will cause death if not treated immediately

Androgen Male hormone

Anemia A condition marked by the presence of an abnormally low number of red blood cells

Antibiotic spectrum The variety of microbes that a particular antibiotic can treat. Broad-spectrum agents can treat many different types of organisms, whereas narrow-spectrum agents can treat fewer organisms

Antibiotic Substance that kills or inhibits the growth of bacteria; a subset of the group of antimicrobials

Antibodies Complex molecules (immunoglobulins) that are made in response to the presence of an antigen (such as a protein of bacteria or other infecting organism) and that neutralize the effect of the foreign substance

Antiemetic Agent that stops nausea and vomiting

Antigen A substance that prompts the generation of antibodies and that can produce an immune response

Antihypertensive Agent that decreases blood pressure

Antiinflammatory A drug that reduces swelling, redness, and pain and promotes healing

Antimicrobial Substance that inhibits the growth of or kills microorganisms

Antineoplastic An agent used to prevent the development, proliferation, or growth of neoplastic cells; a medication used in treatment of abnormal cells

Antipyretic Medication that reduces fever

Antiseptic A substance that slows or stops growth of microorganisms on surfaces such as skin

Antitussive A drug that can decrease the coughing reflex of the central nervous system

Apothecary system A system of measurement once used in the practice of pharmacy to measure both volume and weight; has been replaced by the metric system

Apothecary Latin term for pharmacist. Also, a place where drugs are sold

Aqueous humor The fluid found in the anterior chamber of the eye, in front of the lens

Aristotle Greek scientist, philosopher

Artery A vessel that carries oxygenated blood from the heart to the tissues of the body

ASA Acetylsalicylic acid (aspirin)

Asclepius Early physician and hero in Greece who was eventually considered the God of healing and medicine

Aseptic technique The procedures used to eliminate the possibility of a drug becoming contaminated with microbes or particles

Atom The smallest unit of an element, composed of a nucleus surrounded by electrons

Atomic orbit The rotational path of electrons around the nucleus

Attention deficit/hyperactivity disorder (ADHD) A physiological brain disorder that affects the ability to engage in quiet, passive activities or to focus one's attention because of an imbalance of neurotransmitters in the brain

Attenuated An altered or weakened live vaccine made from the disease organism against which the vaccine protects

Auditory canal A 1-inch segment of tube that runs from the external ear to the middle ear

Auditory ossicles The set of three small bony structures in the middle ear: malleus, incus, and stapes

Autocrine Denoting a mode of hormone action in which a hormone binds to receptors on the cell and affects the function of the cell type that produced it

Autoimmune disease Condition in which a person's tissues are attacked by his or her immune system; abnormal antigen-antibody reaction

Automated dispensing system (ADS) Computerized, automated machines that hold a supply of various medications that can be accessed by authorized individuals to provide prescription fills in community or institutional pharmacy and also used to dispense patient medications near to the point of care in an institutional setting

Autonomic nervous system Division of the nervous system that controls the involuntary body functions; consists of sympathetic and parasympathetic divisions

Autonomic Self-controlling or involuntary

Auxiliary label An adhesive label that is attached to a container with specific instructions or information pertaining to the medication inside

Average wholesale price (AWP) The average price at which a drug is sold; the data are compiled from information provided from manufacturers, distributors, pharmacies. The AWP is often used in calculations related to medication reimbursement

Avitaminosis Any disease caused by vitamin deficiency or deficiency in metabolic conversion of a vitamin

Avoirdupois system A system of measurement previously used in pharmacy for determination of weight, in which ounces and pounds were used; has been replaced by the metric system

Axon The part of a nerve cell that conducts impulses away from a cell body

Ayurveda A holistic traditional medical system originating in India; in the system the prevention of disease is emphasized

Bacteria A large group of unicellular, non-nucleated organisms

Barbiturate A drug derived from barbituric acid; a barbiturate acts as a central nervous system depressant. Barbiturates are often employed in the treatment of seizures and as sedative and hypnotic agents

Behind-the-counter Nonprescription drugs that are kept behind the pharmacy counter and may have limited amounts sold or require the permission of a pharmacist to purchase

Benign A tumor or growth that is not life-threatening

Binary fission The method of non–sexual reproduction by which a single cell divides into two separate cells, each with the potential to grow to the size of the original cell; method of bacterial reproduction

Bioavailability The degree to which a drug or other substance becomes available to the target tissue after administration

Bioequivalence The relationship between two drugs that have the same dosage and dosage form and that have similar bioavailability. Generic versions of a medication must show bioequivalence to the innovator product as a requirement of drug approval

Biology The study of life

Biopsy A procedure in which a piece of tissue is removed from a patient for examination and diagnosis; the tissue is a sample of the whole

Blister pack Container usually made of plastic that holds a single-dose tablet or capsule

Blood-brain barrier (BBB) A barrier formed by special characteristics of capillaries that supply the brain cells to prevent certain solutes or chemicals from moving to the brain from the blood

Blood urea nitrogen (BUN) A test that measures the amount of nitrogen in the blood in the form of urea

Bloodletting The practice of draining blood; believed to release illness

Board of pharmacy (BOP) State-governed agency that licenses pharmacists and may either register or license pharmacy technicians to work in pharmacy. The board of pharmacy also regulates the practice of pharmacy within the state

Bolus A single dose of drug

Boxed warning Drug warning that is placed in the prescribing information or package insert of the product and that indicates a significant risk of potentially dangerous side effects. It is the strongest warning the FDA can give. It is common in the pharmacy profession to call these warnings "Black Box Warnings" because of their appearance on a drug label; the warning is often enclosed in a black outlined box to draw attention to the content

Bradykinins Chemicals produced by the body and responsible for inflammation and pain

Brand/trade name Trademark of a drug or device held by the originating manufacturing company

Bubble pack A preformed card with depressions that can hold medications, they are sealed with a foil card backboard

Bulk forming Fiber used to treat constipation or to cause a feeling of fullness to decrease appetite

Caduceus Often confused as the symbol of the medical field; it is a staff with two entwined snakes and two wings at the top

Calibration The markings on a measuring device

Cancer A general term used to describe malignant neoplasms or tumors

Capillary Extremely small vessel that connects the ends of the smallest arteries (arterioles) to the smallest veins (venules), where exchange of nutrients and wastes, O_2 and CO_2, occurs; blood vessels at cellular level

Carbohydrates Organic compounds consisting of carbon, hydrogen, and oxygen; examples include sugars, glycogen, starches, and cellulose

Carcinogen A substance or chemical that can increase the risk of developing cancer

Catabolism To break down; the destruction phase of metabolism

Cataract Loss of transparency of the lens of the eye

Catecholamines The hormones made in the brainstem, nervous system, and adrenal glands. They help the body respond to stress and prepare the body for the "fight or flight" response. They are important to heart rate, blood pressure, and nervous system functions

Cell body The main part of a neuron from which axons and dendrites extend

Central nervous system Consists of the brain and spinal cord; acts to coordinate sensory and motor control of body functions

Cerebrospinal fluid A fluid that fills the ventricles of the brain and also lies in the spaces of the brain or spinal cord and the arachnoid layer of the meninges

Certified pharmacy technician A technician who has passed the national certification examination; the technician can use the abbreviation CPhT after his or her name

Cervical Pertaining to the neck region of the spinal cord; the region begins at the base of the skull and consists of the first seven vertebrae

Chemical structure The shape of molecules and their location to one another in a given compound

Chemotherapy The treatment of a disease with toxic chemical substances to slow the disease process or to kill cells

Chiropractic Manual manipulation of the joints and muscles

Chloasma Hyperpigmentation of skin, limited or confined to a certain area

Chyme The soupy consistency (semifluid consistency) of food after mixing with stomach acids and digestive enzymes as it passes into the duodenum (first part of small intestine)

Clean room As it pertains to pharmacy, a contained and controlled environment within the pharmacy that has a low level of environmental pollutants such as dust, airborne microbes, aerosol particles, and chemical vapors; the clean room is used for preparing sterile medication products

Closed door pharmacy A pharmacy that fills and delivers medications prescribed by institutions such as long-term care facilities; these pharmacies may also provide mail-order prescriptions; closed pharmacies are not open to the public

Closed formulary In a closed formulary, medication use is tightly restricted to those medications provided within the formulary list. Medications that are NOT listed as pre-approved drugs per the health plan provider or pharmacy benefits manager are not reimbursed except under extenuating circumstances and with proper documentation

Coagulation To solidify or change from a fluid state to a solid state, as in forming a blood clot

Coenzyme A compound that activates an enzyme

Cofactor A nonprotein chemical compound that is bound to a protein and is required for the protein's biological activity

Cognition Activities associated with thinking, learning, and memory

Colloid An agent that contains small particles (1 to 1000 nm in diameter) that do not precipitate under the influence of gravity but remain distributed throughout either in a suspension or in an emulsion

Comedone A blackhead; a plug of keratin and sebum within a hair follicle that is blackened at the surface

Communication The ability to express oneself in such a way that one is readily and clearly understood

Community pharmacy Also known as an outpatient or retail pharmacy; pharmacies that serve patients in their communities; consumers can walk-in and purchase a prescription or OTC drug

Competency The capability or proficiency to perform a function

Compounded Sterile Products (CSPs) Preparations prepared in a sterile environment using nonsterile ingredients or devices that must be sterilized before administration

Compounding The act of mixing, reconstituting, and packaging a drug

Computerized physician order entry (CPOE) Computer order entry

Cones Photoreceptors in the retina of the eye responsible for color perception (daylight vision)

Confidentiality To keep privileged customer information from being disclosed without the customer's consent

Conjunctiva Transparent protective mucous membrane that lines the underside of the eyelid

Contagion The transfer of a disease from one individual to another. A contagious disease

Continuing education (CE) Education beyond the basic technical education, usually required for license or certification renewal

Controlled substance Any drug or other substance that is scheduled I through V and regulated by the Drug Enforcement Administration

Co-pay The portion of the prescription bill that the patient is responsible for paying

Cornea The transparent tissue covering the anterior portion of the eye

Corticosteroid A steroid produced by the adrenal cortex

Cough reflex Response of the body to clear air passages of foreign substances and mucus by a forceful expiration

Covalent bond The sharing of electrons between two atoms

Crash carts Also known as code carts. A moveable cart containing trays of medications, administration sets, oxygen, and other materials that are used in life-threatening situations such as cardiac arrest

Cream A hydrophilic base

Cretinism Condition in which the development of the brain and body is inhibited by congenital lack of thyroid hormone secretion

Cushing's disease Condition causing an increase in secretion of adrenocortical hormones; includes symptoms such as a moon face (moon facies) and deposits of fat (buffalo hump)

Cushing's syndrome May have multiple causes (e.g., corticosteroid therapy), whereas Cushing's disease is specifically an adenoma of the pituitary gland causing an increase in ACTH secretion and elevations in cortisol levels

Debride To remove dead or damaged tissue

Decongestant An adrenergic drug that reduces swelling of the mucous membranes by constricting dilated blood vessels; reduces blood flow to nasal tissues, thus reducing nasal congestion

Dendrite The part of a neuron that branches out to bring impulses to the cell body

Deoxyribonucleic acid (DNA) The complex nucleic acids that are bases for genetic continuance

Depot An area of the body where a substance can accumulate or be stored for later distribution

Depression A mental state characterized by sadness, feelings of loss and grief, and loss of appetite and that may include suicidal thoughts

Dermis A thick layer of connective tissue that contains collagen

Desquamation A process of shedding the top layer of the skin, also known as exfoliation; this process may be a normal process or may be associated with a disease

Diabetes mellitus A complex disorder of carbohydrate, fat, and protein metabolism that is primarily a result of a deficiency or complete lack of insulin secretion from cells within the pancreas. Three primary types include: type 1 diabetes mellitus, an autoimmune process, dependent on insulin to prevent ketosis; type 2 diabetes mellitus, adult-onset diabetes and/or ketosis-resistant diabetes that are non–insulin-dependent; gestational diabetes mellitus, occurs in women that become glucose intolerant during pregnancy

Diagnosis A physician's recognition of a condition or disease based on its outward signs and symptoms and/or confirming tests or procedures

Dialysis The passage of a solute through a semipermeable membrane to remove toxic materials and to maintain fluid, electrolyte, and pH levels of the body system when the kidneys are not working properly

Digestion The mechanical, chemical, and enzymatic action of breaking food into molecules that can be used in metabolism

Diluent An inert product, either liquid or solid, that is added to a preparation and that reduces the strength of the original product

Dilution The process of adding a diluent or solvent to a compound, resulting in a product of increased volume or weight and lower concentration

Distribution (medication) The location of a medication throughout the bloodstream, organs, and tissues after administration

Distribution (urinary system) Within the kidneys, the mechanism by which substances are sent throughout the body system

Diuretic An agent that increases urine output and excretion of water from the body

Dogma Code of beliefs based on ideology, religion, or authoritative tradition rather than factual evidence

Drug classification Categorization based on various characteristics, including the chemical structure of a drug, the action of a drug, and/or the therapeutic or anatomical use of a drug

Drug diversion The intentional misuse of a drug intended for medical purposes; the Drug Enforcement Administration usually defines diversion as the recreational use of a prescription or scheduled drug. Diversion can also refer to the channeling of the prescription drug supply away from legal distribution and to the illegal street market

Drug Enforcement Administration (DEA) Federal agency within the U.S. Department of Justice that enforces U.S. laws and regulations related to controlled substances

Drug Facts and Comparisons Reference book found in pharmacies that contains detailed information on medications

Drug Topics Red Book Reference book listing NDC numbers, manufacturers, and average wholesale pricing of drug products. Note that pharmacies often include this type of product and pricing information in their online database systems, which are provided by companies such as First DataBank and Gold Standard

Drug utilization evaluation (DUE) or review (DUR) The process by which pharmacists ensure proper medication utilization

Dystonia Symptoms that include twisting, repeated jerking movements, and/or abnormal posture

Efferent The direction of a neuronal impulse from the central nervous system toward the body

Electroconvulsive therapy Also known as shock therapy; a carefully calibrated electrical current is administered to the patient after induction of anesthesia, causing a brief seizure that can relieve certain symptoms, such as depression

Electrolyte Charged elements called cations (which have positive charges) and anions (which have negative charges); in the human body, some key electrolytes are sodium, chloride, potassium, calcium, and magnesium

Electron The smallest subset of an atom that contains a negative charge

Electronic medication administration record (E-MAR) Medication orders that are transcribed listing drug name, strength, dose, dosage form, and dosing time. Nurses record time and initials of when the dose was given

Elixir A base solution that is a mixture of alcohol and water

Embolism The formation of a clot from any foreign substance that obstructs a vessel

Emulsification To make into an emulsion, or bind together

Endocardium The thin inner lining of each chamber of the heart

Endometrium Mucous membrane lining of the uterus

Enzyme A protein that accelerates a reaction by reducing the amount of energy required to initiate a reaction; also called a biological catalyst

Epicardium The outer layer of the heart wall; the inner layer of the pericardium

Epidermis The outermost layer of the skin composed of the stratum corneum (or horny layer), the keratinocytes (squamous cells), and the basal layer; also contains melanin, which gives skin its color

E-Prescribing Electronically sent prescription from prescriber's computer or mobile device transmitted directly to the pharmacy

ESBLs Extended-spectrum beta-lactamases

Ethics The values and morals that are used within a profession

Eustachian tube A tubular structure within the middle ear that extends to the nasopharynx (throat); it functions to equalize pressure and to drain mucus

Excipient Inert substance added to a drug to form a suitable consistency for dosing

Excretion (drug) The final elimination of a drug or other substance from the body via normal body processes, such as kidney elimination (urine), biliary excretion (bile to stool), sweat, respirations, or saliva

Excretion (urinary system) Elimination of waste products and other remnants of metabolism, primarily through stools and urine

Exophthalmos Prominence (protrusion) of the eyeball out of the orbit; bilateral presentation commonly caused by increased levels of thyroid hormone

Expectorant A drug that aids in the removal of mucous secretions from the respiratory system; it loosens and thins sputum and bronchial secretions for ease of expectoration

Extrapyramidal symptoms Often result from taking antipsychotic medications and include parkinsonism, dystonia, and tremors

Facultative anaerobe A microorganism that can live with or without oxygen

Fallopian tube Narrow passageway between the ovary and the uterus

Fat-soluble vitamin Vitamin that is soluble in fat and therefore is stored in body fat; vitamins A, D, E, and K are fat-soluble

FDA Food and Drug Administration

Fertilization The process by which a sperm unites with an ovum to create a new life

Flocculation The process by which a solute comes out of a solution in the form of flakes or precipitation; the solute then can be filtered out of the solution

Food and Drug Administration (FDA) The agency within the U.S. Department of Health and Human Services responsible for ensuring the safety, efficacy, and security of human and veterinary drugs, biological products, medical devices, the national food supply, cosmetics, and radioactive products

Formulary A list of preferred drugs to be stocked by the pharmacy; also a list of drugs covered by an insurance company

Galen Greek physician

Gametes Sex cells, or ova and sperm

Gauge The size of the needle opening

Generic name Name assigned to a medication or nonproprietary name of a drug

Gerhard Domagk Discovered sulfonamide, the first synthetic antibiotic

Globulin Protein that is insoluble in water; immune globulins protect against disease

Glucose Also known as simple sugar, a very important carbohydrate in biology; it is the primary source of energy fuel for cells and is measurable in the blood

Goiter Condition in which the thyroid gland is enlarged because of a lack of iodine, known as simple goiter; if develops because of a tumor, known as toxic goiter

Good manufacturing practice (GMP) Federal guidelines that must be followed by all entities that prepare and package medications or medical devices

Granules A small particle or grain of either individual ingredients or the entire composition of the agent

Graves' disease Condition caused by hypersecretion of thyroid hormones; symptoms include diffuse goiter, exophthalmos, and skin changes

Gregor Mendel Scientist and monk known as the father of genetics

Half-life (1) The amount of time it takes for the concentration of a chemical to be decreased by half. (2) The time required for half the amount of a substance, such as a drug in a living system, to be eliminated or disintegrated by natural processes. (3) The time required for the concentration of a substance in a body fluid (blood plasma) to decrease by half

Health Insurance Portability and Accountability Act (HIPAA) Federal act for protecting patients' rights, establishing national standards for electronic health care communication, and the security and privacy of health data

Hemoglobin The iron-containing pigment on red blood cells that carries oxygen to the tissues

Herb Any nonwoody (herbaceous) plant that is valued for its aromatic, medicinal, flavorful, or other properties

Heterotrophic Requiring complex carbon and nitrogen for metabolic synthesis

Hippocrates Greek physician and philosopher; considered to be the father of medicine

Hippocratic Oath An oath taken by physicians concerning the ethics and practice of medicine

Histamine$_1$ A substance that interacts with tissues, producing some of the symptoms of an allergic reaction

Homeopathy A system of therapy based on the belief that dilutions of medicinal substances that cause a specific symptom can be used to treat an illness that yields the same symptoms; homeopathic remedies are regulated by the FDA under the Food, Drug, and Cosmetic Act

Homeostasis The equilibrium pertaining to the balance of the body with respect to fluid levels, pH level, osmotic pressures, and concentrations of various substances

Homogeneous A uniform composition throughout the medication mixture

Horizontal laminar flow hood Environment for the preparation of sterile products that uses air originating from the back of the hood moving forward across the hood out into the room

Hormones Chemical substances produced and secreted by an endocrine duct into the bloodstream that result in a physiological response at a specific target tissue

Household system A system of measurement commonly used in the United States; measures volumes using household utensils

Hydrophilic Water loving; any substance that easily mixes with water

Hydrophobic Water hating; any substance that does not mix in water

Hyperalimentation Parenteral (intravenous) nutrition for patients who are unable to eat solids or liquids

Hypercalcemia Elevated concentration of calcium in the blood

Hyperglycemia Elevated concentration of glucose in the blood

Hypervitaminosis A disorder caused by the intake of too many vitamins; more common with fat-soluble vitamins

Hypocalcemia Low concentration of calcium in the blood

Hypoglycemia Low concentration of glucose in the blood

Immunity A type of resistance to infection resulting from an immune response from the body in response to an antigen exposure or from agents such as vaccinations

Immunosuppressive agent Agents that prevent or lessen the activity of the immune system. The immunosuppressive drugs used frequently to prevent organ rejection or to treat certain autoimmune or inflammatory diseases

Inert ingredient An ingredient that has little or no effect on body functions

Influenza A respiratory tract infection caused by an influenza virus

Ingestion The act of taking in food, liquid, or other substances (e.g., medications)

Inhibit To stop or hold back; to keep a reaction from taking place

Inpatient pharmacy A pharmacy in a hospital or institutional setting

Insomnia Difficulty falling or staying asleep

Instill To place into; instillation instructions are commonly used for ophthalmic or otic drugs, as examples

Institute for Healthcare Improvement (IHI) A nonprofit organization working toward the improvement of health care by promoting promising concepts through safety, efficiency, and other patient-centered goals

Institute for Safe Medication Practices (ISMP) A nonprofit organization devoted entirely to safe medication use and the prevention of medication errors. Gathers information on drug errors and suggests new safer standards to avoid such errors

Institute for the Certification of Pharmacy Technicians (ICPT) National board for the certification of pharmacy technicians

Institute of Medicine (IOM) Established under the National Academies and a component of the National Academy of Science, this nonprofit organization provides scientifically informed analysis and guidance regarding health and health policy. Projects include studies of drug safety systems within the U.S. and recommendations for patient safety

Institutional pharmacy A pharmacy in a hospital or institutional setting; this type of pharmacy may or may not provide retail services

International System of Units (SI) The prefixes for the modern metric system are taken from the French Le Système International d'Unités and were adopted to provide a single worldwide system of weights and measures. This system of measurement is based upon multiples of 10

International time A 24-hour method of keeping time in which hours are not distinguished between AM and PM but are counted continuously throughout the entire day

Intrinsic factor A naturally produced protein that is necessary for the absorption of vitamin B_{12}

Invasive The tendency for a tumor or mass to move into tissues and/or organs in proximity; when referred to as invasive surgery, cutting through the skin is performed

Investigational drug A drug that has not been approved yet by the FDA for marketing but is in clinical trials; can also pertain to an FDA-approved drug that is seeking a new indication for use

Ion An atom or a group of atoms with a leftover unbalanced charge

Ionic bond The transfer of electrons between two atoms

Iris Colored part of eye seen through cornea; consists of smooth muscles that regulate pupil size

Keratolytic A drug that causes shedding of the outer layer of the skin

Kidney stones Solid mineral deposits that form in the urinary tract

Labyrinth A bony maze composed of the vestibule, cochlea, and semicircular canals of the inner ear

Laminar flow hood Environment for the preparation of sterile products

Laudanum A mixture of opium and alcohol used to treat dozens of illnesses during the 1800s

Leeches A type of segmented worm with suckers that attaches to the skin of a host and engorges itself on the host's blood

Legend drug Drug that requires a prescription for dispensing

Lens Flexible, clear covering of the retina that focuses on images

Levigate To make into a smooth paste or into a fine powder, depending on the agent used

Licensed pharmacy technician A pharmacy technician who is licensed by the state board; licensing ensures that the individual has at least the minimum degree of competency required by the profession, unlike a registered pharmacy technician

Lumbar The region of the spine that includes five vertebrae in the area between the ribs (thoracic spine) and the pelvis (sacral spine); also used to describe the area of the back around the waist

Lymph node Composed of many small oval structures that filter the lymph and fight infection. In addition, where lymphocytes, monocytes, and plasma cells are formed

Lymphoma A term used to describe a malignant disorder of lymphoid tissue

Macro Large

Macula Yellow spot in the center of the retina responsible for central and high-acuity vision. The macula contains a pit in its center known as the fovea centralis, which contains ganglion cells and a high concentration of cones. Any damage to the macula results in loss of central visual capacity

Maggots Fly larvae that feed on dead tissue; used in medicine to clean wounds not responding to routine antibiotics

Malignant An invasive and destructive pattern of rapid, abnormal cell growth; often fatal

Mania A mood state characterized by excessive excitement, elevated mood, and exalted feelings; most often associated with bipolar disorder, where episodes of mania alternate (or cycle) with episodes of depression

Material safety data sheets (MSDSs) A document providing chemical product information. A MSDS includes the product name, composition (chemicals in the product), hazards, toxicology, and other information regarding the proper steps to take with spills, accidental exposure, handling, and storage of the product. The filing of MSDSs within the pharmacy or workplace is usually a requirement to meet Occupational Safety and Health Administration (OSHA) standards

Medicaid Federal- and state-managed insurance program that covers health care costs and prescription drugs for low-income children, adults, elderly, and those with disabilities

Medicare Federal- and state-managed insurance program that covers health care costs and prescription drugs for individuals older than age 65, those younger than age 65 with long-term disabilities, or those persons with end-stage renal disease

Medicare Modernization Act (MMA) The enactment of prescription drug coverage to be paid out for persons covered under Medicare; sets limitations on payments

Medication error prevention Methods used by pharmacy, medicine, nursing, and other allied health professionals to prevent medication errors

Medicine The science and art dealing with the maintenance of health and the prevention, alleviation, or cure of disease

MEDMARX A national Internet-accessible database that hospitals and health care systems use to track adverse drug reactions and medication errors

MedWatch FDA's program for drug and medical product safety alerts and label changes; the program also provides a voluntary adverse event reporting system for medications, medical products, and devices

Melanoma A malignant neoplasm of the pigmented cells of skin; it may metastasize to other organs

Menopause Cessation of menstruation; a natural phenomenon in which a woman passes from a reproductive state to a nonreproductive state

Metabolism The physical and chemical changes that take place within an organism

Metabolism (drug) The processes by which the body breaks down or converts medications to active or inactive substances. The primary site of drug metabolism in humans is the liver; however, select drugs are metabolized through other processes

Metastasis The movement or spread of cancerous cells through the body to organs in distant areas

Metered dose inhaler A device for supplying a predetermined dosage of medication(s) to the lungs through inhalation

Metric system The approved system of measurement for pharmacy in the United States based on multiples of 10. The basic units of measurement are the gram (g) for weight, the liter (L) for volume, and the meter (m) for length

Micro Small

Microbial Refers to microorganisms (very small organisms) not visible without a microscope

Microbiology The study of microscopic organisms

Micturition Urination

Miosis Contraction of the pupil

Misbranding Labeling of a product that is false or misleading; label information must include directions for use; safe and/or unsafe dosages; manufacturer, packer, or distributor; quantity; and weight

Mitosis Cellular reproduction that creates two identical daughter cells from the DNA of the parent cell

Mole Used to measure carbon; Avogadro's number = 6.02×10^{23} atoms, molecules, or ions

Molecule The smallest particle of a compound

Monoamine oxidases (MAOs) Enzymes (includes MAO-A and MAO-B) found in the nerve terminals, the neurons, and liver cells; they inactivate chemicals such as tyramine, catecholamines, serotonin, and certain medications

Monograph Comprehensive information on a medication's actions within that class of drugs. Also lists generic and trade names, ingredients, dosages, side effects, adverse effects, how the patient should take the medication, and foods or other drugs (e.g., OTC medications, herbals) to avoid while taking the medication

Morals Ethics; honorable beliefs

Morphology Appearance, including shape, size, structure, and Gram stain characteristics of organisms; studying the structure, not function, of organisms

Mortality Death; being susceptible to death

Mortality rate The number of deaths that occur in a specific time period

Mortar and pestle A bowl and rounded knob used to grind substances into fine powder or to mix liquids

MRSA Methicillin-resistant *Staphylococcus aureus*

Mucilage A sticky substance that binds ingredients together

Mutation An unexpected change in the molecular structure within DNA, causing a permanent change in cells

Mydriasis Dilation of the pupil

Myocardium The muscle tissue layer of the heart

Myxedema Condition associated with a decrease in overall thyroid function in adults; also known as hypothyroidism

Narcotic A nonspecific term to describe a drug (such as opium) that in moderate doses dulls the senses, relieves pain, and induces profound sleep, but in excessive doses causes stupor, coma, or convulsions, and may lead to addiction. From the standpoint of U.S. law, opium, opiates (derivatives of opium), and opioids, as well as cocaine and coca leaves, are "narcotics"

National Association of Boards of Pharmacy (NABP) National organization for members of state boards of pharmacy

National Coordinating Council for Medication Error Reporting and Prevention (NCC MERP) Founded by the *USP*, this is an independent council of more than 25 organizations gathered to address interdisciplinary causes of medication errors and strategies for prevention

National Drug Code (NDC) A 10-digit number given to all drugs for identification purposes. In health and drug databases, the NDC is represented as an 11-digit number, where placeholder zeros are inserted in the proper order within the code for the purpose of standardizing data transmissions

National Healthcareer Association (NHA) Organization of health care professionals that works with educational institutions in developing curriculum, competency testing, and preparation for certification exams. Offers certifications in 14 different fields of health care

National Pharmacy Technician Association (NPTA) Pharmacy association primarily for technicians; founded in 1999

National Provider Identifier (NPI) Number assigned to any health care provider; used for the purpose of standardizing health data transmissions

Negative feedback A self-regulating mechanism in which the output of a system has input or control on the process; a factor within a system that causes a corrective action to return the system to normal range

Negligence A legal concept that describes an action taken without the forethought that should have been taken by a reasonable person of similar competency

Neoplasm An abnormal tissue growth

Nephrons The filtering unit of the kidneys

Nerve terminal The end portion of the neuron where nerve impulses cause chemicals to be released; these chemicals (called neurotransmitters) cross a small space (called the synaptic cleft) to carry the impulse to another neuron

Neuroblastomas Tumors of the neural crest; neuroblastomas often originate in the adrenal glands

Neuron The functional unit of the nervous system, which includes the cell body, dendrites, axon, and terminals

Neurosis Mental disorder arising from stress or anxiety in the patient's environment without loss of contact with reality; phobias can be listed in this category; behavior usually does not deviate from social norms

Neurotransmitter Chemicals that are transmitted from one neuron to another as electrical nerve impulses

Neutron A subset of an atom that does not contain a charge

NKA No known allergies

NKDA No known drug allergies

Non-formulary A list of drugs that are not normally stocked by the pharmacy; these drugs may not be covered by an insurance company unless specific conditions are met

Non-formulary medications Drugs that are not approved for use within the institution unless specific exceptions are filed and approved by the institutional protocols

Nonproductive cough A cough that does not produce mucous secretions from the respiratory tract

Normal flora Microorganisms that reside harmlessly in the body and do not cause disease but may aid the host organism

Nosocomial infection An infection acquired during a stay in a hospital or other health care service unit or institution

NSAIDs Nonsteroidal antiinflammatory drugs

Nucleic acid The bases contained within DNA

Occupational Safety and Health Administration (OSHA) U.S. government-managed agency that oversees safety in the workplace; created MSDS requirements

Ointment A hydrophobic product such as petroleum jelly

Oleaginous base Ingredient used in compounding that does not dissolve in water

Omnibus Budget Reconciliation Act (OBRA '90) Congressional act that changed reimbursement limits and mandated drug utilization evaluation, pharmacy patient consultation, and educational outreach programs

Oncogene A gene that when mutated or expressed at high levels can help transform a normal cell into a cancerous one

Oncologist A specialist in the area of cancer and cancer treatment

Oocyte or ova The female reproductive germ cell; more commonly known as an egg

Open formulary A formulary list that is essentially unrestricted in the types of drug choices offered or that can be prescribed and be reimbursed under the health provider plan or pharmacy benefit plan

Ophthalmic Pertaining to the eye

Opioid Any agent that binds to opioid receptors

Opium An analgesic that is made from the poppy plant

Orbit Eye socket

Osmosis The diffusion of water from low solute concentrations to higher solute concentrations, across a semipermeable membrane

Osteoarthritis Also known as degenerative joint disease

Osteoporosis Condition associated with the decrease of bone mass and softening of bones, resulting in the increased possibility of bone fractures

OTC Over-the-counter; medications that do not require a prescription and may be purchased by customers at any retail outlet

Otic Pertaining to the ear

Outpatient pharmacy Pharmacies that serve patients in their communities; pharmacies that are not in inpatient facilities

Over-the-counter (OTC) medication Medication that can be purchased without a prescription; non–legend medications

Package insert The official prescribing information for a prescription drug; medication information sheet provided by the manufacturer that includes side effects, dosage forms, indications, and other important information

Paget's disease A focal disorder of bone remodeling resulting in weakened, deformed bones of increased mass and associated fractures

Palliative That which brings relief but does not cure

PAR Periodic automatic replenishment; replacement of stock levels to a certain number of allowed units

Paracelsus Swiss physician, philosopher, and scientist

Paracrine Denoting a type of hormone function in which hormone synthesized in and released from one cell signals and binds to its receptor on other types of adjacent cells

Parasite Organism that requires a host for nourishment and reproduction

Parasympathetic nervous system Division of the autonomic nervous system that functions during restful situations; "breed or feed" part of the autonomic nervous system

Parenteral medication Medication that bypasses the digestive system but intended for systemic action; the term parenteral most commonly describes medications given by injection, such as intravenously or intramuscularly

Passive immunity Resistance to a disease that has been acquired through a transfer of antibodies from another person or animal or from mother to child

Patient profile A document listing necessary patient personal and health information, including comprehensive information on the medications the patient is taking

PCA Patient-controlled analgesia

Peptidoglycan The polymer substance that comprises bacterial cell walls, specifically of gram-negative and gram-positive microbes

Pericardium The fluid-filled membrane that surrounds the heart

Periodic automatic replenishment (PAR) A minimum set amount of stock that needs to be kept on hand

Peripheral nervous system The division of the nervous system outside the brain and spinal cord

Peripheral parenteral Injection of a medication into the veins located on the periphery of the body system instead of a central vein or artery

Peristalsis The contraction and relaxation of the tubular muscles of the esophagus, stomach, and intestines that moves substances from the mouth to the anus

Pharmacist Person who dispenses drugs and counsels patients on medication use and any interactions it may have with food or other drugs

Pharmacists Pharmacy students and technicians practicing in hospitals and health care systems, including home health care; ASHP has a long history of advocating patient safety and establishing best practices to improve medication use

Pharmacokinetics The study of the absorption, metabolism, distribution, and excretion of drugs

Pharmacy Drug or remedy (Greek word *pharmakon*); place where drugs are sold

Pharmacy and Therapeutics Committee (P&T Committee) Medical staff composed of physicians and pharmacists who provide necessary information and advice to the institution or insurer on whether a drug should be added to a formulary

Pharmacy clerk Person who assists the pharmacist at the front counter of the pharmacy; the person who accepts payment for medications

Pharmacy technician Person who assists the pharmacist by filling prescriptions and performing other nondiscretionary tasks

Pharmacy Technician Certification Board (PTCB) Offers national certification for pharmacy technicians in the United States

Pharmacy Technician Educators Council (PTEC) U.S. organization that promotes teachers' strategies in instructing pharmacy technician students

Pheochromocytoma Tumors of the adrenal gland that produce excess adrenaline (epinephrine) and norepinephrine

Phobias A continuous irrational fear of a thing, place, or situation that causes significant distress

Physicians' Desk Reference (PDR) One of the many reference books of medications, this reference compiles and publishes select manufacturer-provided package inserts and prescribing information useful for health professionals

Placebo Inert compound believed by the patient to be an active agent

Placebo effect When a person suffering symptoms from illness experiences relief through faith in a treatment that provides no tangible medicinal or treatment value

Pneumonia Inflammatory condition of the lungs; most commonly caused by an infection, but may result from a chemical or physical injury as well

POS Point of sale or service; where the sale or service takes place

Precipitate To separate from solution or suspension

Pregnancy Category A system in use by the FDA to describe five levels of assessment of the fetal effects caused by a drug, a required section of current prescription drug labeling. First introduced in 1979, the system is currently under reevaluation for usefulness and inclusion in the prescription label

Prior authorization Insurance-required approval for a restricted, non-formulary or non-covered medication before the time of prescription or refill

PRN Latin term (pro re nata) meaning "as needed"

Productive cough Cough that expectorates mucous secretions from respiratory tract

Professionalism Conforming to right principles of conduct (work ethics) as accepted by others in the profession

Prophylaxis Treatment given before an event or exposure to prevent the occurrence of a condition or symptom

Protected health information (PHI) A term used to describe a patient's personal health data. Under HIPAA this information is protected from being shared or distributed without permission

Protocol A set of standards and guidelines within which a facility operates

Proton A subatomic particle of an atom that holds a positive charge

PRSP Penicillin-resistant *Streptococcus pneumoniae*

Pruritus Itching

Psychosis A mental illness characterized by loss of contact with reality; psychosis may be a true mental illness, be attributable to an underlying medical condition (e.g., dementia, drug withdrawal syndromes), or be induced by substances such as medications, recreational drugs, or poisons

Psychotherapy Professional therapy that includes helping the patient work through personal problems that affect emotions and behaviors

Punch method Filling of capsules by hand with powdered medication that has been premeasured

Pupil Circular opening in the iris that allows light to enter

PYXIS An automated dispensing system often used in hospitals

Reconstitute To add a diluent such as saline or sterile water to a powder

Reconstitution To mix a liquid and a powder to form a suspension or solution

Red Book (Drug Topics) Also called *Drug Topics Red Book;* reference book listing NDC numbers, manufacturers, and average wholesale pricing of drug products. Note that pharmacies often include this type of product and pricing information in their online database systems, which are provided by companies such as First DataBank and Gold Standard

Registered pharmacy technician A pharmacy technician who is registered through the state board of pharmacy; the registration process helps maintain a list of those working in pharmacy and usually requires a background check through the legal system; the registration process does not guarantee degree of registrant's knowledge or skills

Remission The span of time during which a disease, such as cancer, is not spreading and may even be diminished or cured; this may be permanent or temporary

Renal absorption Within the kidneys: the intake of liquids, solids, and gases

Renal artery One of the pair of arteries that branch from the abdominal aorta. Each kidney has one renal artery

Renal failure The inability of the kidneys to function properly

Renal fascia The membranous tissue that surrounds and supports the kidneys

Renal metabolism Within the kidneys: the mechanism by which chemical transformation takes place

Renal vein The blood vessel by which filtered blood from the kidneys is sent back into the body's circulatory system. Each kidney has one renal vein

Repackaging The act of reducing the amount of medication taken from a bulk bottle; unit dosing is a form of repackaging

Retina Innermost layer of the eye; a complex structure that is considered part of the central nervous system (CNS); the retina contains photoreceptor cells (rods and cones) that transmit impulses to the optic nerve, as well as the macula lutea (a yellow spot in the center of the retina)

Rheumatoid arthritis A progressive degenerative and crippling immune disease

Rhinitis Inflammation of the lining of the nose; runny nose

ROA Route of administration

Rods Photoreceptors in the retina of the eye that respond to dim light and are responsible for black and white color perception (night vision)

Roger Bacon English scientist responsible for scientific methods

Rx Latin abbreviation for "recipe," meaning "to take"; it is commonly used to mean "prescription" and is often found as a symbol on the header of a prescription

Sacrum The large triangular bone at the base of the spine; it connects superiorly with the last vertebra of the lumbar spine and inferiorly with the coccyx (tailbone). It is wedged between the two hip bones and helps form the pelvis

Satellite pharmacy A smaller pharmacy located in a hospital away from the central pharmacy

Schizophrenia A group of mental disorders characterized by inappropriate emotions and unrealistic thinking

Sclera White of the eyes

Script A common slang term describing a medical prescription

Sebaceous glands Skin glands responsible for secretion of oil called sebum

Sebum An oily/waxy substance that lubricates the skin and retains water to provide moisture

Shaman A person who holds a high place of honor in a tribe as a healer and spiritual mediator

Sig From the Latin "signa," which means to write; medication directions written on a prescription

that describe how a medication should be taken or used

Simmonds' disease A pituitary disorder that is a form of panhypopituitarism in which all pituitary secretions are deficient; usually caused by postpartum necrosis of the anterior pituitary

Skin protectant A substance that acts as a barrier between the skin and an irritant

Solute The ingredient that is dissolved into a solution

Solution A water base in which the ingredient or ingredients dissolve completely

Solvent The greater part of a solution that dissolves a solute

Somatic The motor neurons of the peripheral nervous system that control voluntary actions of the skeletal muscles and provide sensory input (touch, hearing, sight)

Spatulation The act of manipulating a material into a homogeneous mass using a spatula

Species Of Latin origin meaning "kind"; in biology the term describes the basic rank in taxonomic classification

Sperm or spermatozoa The male reproductive germ cell

Spermatogenesis The process by which immature germ cells (spermatogonia) mature into spermatozoa (mature sperm); the process normally begins in puberty

Sputum Fluid (mucus) that is coughed up from the lungs and bronchial tissues

Staff of Asclepius The symbol of the medical profession; it is a wingless staff with one snake wrapped around it

Stage Describes the extent of cancer within the body and its dissemination to other areas

Standard operating procedures (SOPs) Written guidelines and criteria that list specific steps for various competencies

Standard Precautions (i.e., Universal Precautions) A set of standards that lowers the possibility of contamination and lowers the risk of transmission of infectious disease; used throughout a health care facility, including to prepare medications

Stat order A medication order that must be filled as soon as possible, usually within 5 to 15 minutes

Steroid Messenger chemical produced by the body that helps fight inflammation and pain

Strip pack A strip of heat-sealed packets each holding one tablet or capsule; used in the repackaging process

Subcutaneous layer The deepest layer of the skin that consists of fat cells and collagen and serves to protect the body and conserve heat

Sunscreen A substance that protects the skin from ultraviolet light, which causes sunburn; skin protection factor (SPF) rates a sunscreen's effectiveness; the FDA regulates sunscreens as nonprescription drug products that adhere to specialized regulations to ensure safety and efficacy

Supplement An additive taken to compensate for a deficiency such as in vitamins and minerals

SureMed An automated dispensing system often used in hospitals

Survival rate (absolute) The number of patients still alive after diagnosis within a certain period; normally based on 5 years after diagnosis when cancer statistics are reported

Suspension A solution in which the powder does not dissolve into the base and which must be shaken before use

Sweat glands Found in the dermis; activated in response to increased body temperature to cool the body

Symbiotic A close relationship between two species

Sympathetic nervous system Division of the autonomic nervous system that functions during stressful situations; "fight or flight" part of the autonomic nervous system

Syndrome A set of conditions

Synthesis The formation of chemical components within the body system

Synthetic medicine Medication made in a laboratory from chemical processes

Syrup A sugar-based liquid

Systemic Pertaining to the entire body rather than to individual body parts

Tardive dyskinesia A type of dyskinesia (unwanted, involuntary rhythmic movements) attributed to potential side effects of taking dopamine antagonists such as phenothiazines or other medications (e.g., metoclopramide); the symptoms may continue even after discontinuation of the offending drug

Taxonomy The science of classification; with respect to biology, taxonomy is a hierarchical structure for the nomenclature (naming) and classification of organisms

Teratogen Any agent causing abnormal embryonic or fetal development

The Joint Commission (TJC) An independent nonprofit organization that accredits hospitals and other health care organizations in the United States. Accreditation is required to accept Medicare and Medicaid payment

Thoracic Pertaining to the thorax area or the chest; essentially the region between the neck and abdomen; also describes the region of the spine that includes 12 vertebrae in the area between the neck (cervical spine) and lumbar (lumbar spine) regions

Thrombin An enzyme that is formed in coagulating blood from prothrombin; this enzyme reacts with fibrinogen, converting it into fibrin, which is essential in the formation of blood clots; thrombin level tested by performing a prothrombin time or partial thromboplastin time blood test

Thrombolytic Medication used to break up a thrombus or blood clot

Thyroxine (T_4) A thyroid hormone derived from tyrosine (amino acid); it influences metabolic rate

Tincture An alcoholic extract of plant materials or nonvolatile substances

Tort To cause harm or injury to a person intentionally or because of negligence

Total parenteral nutrition Large-volume intravenous nutrition administered through the central vein (subclavian vein), which allows for a higher concentration of solutions

Toxoid A type of vaccine in which a toxin has been rendered harmless but still invokes an antigenic response to improve immunity against the active toxin at some future date

Trace elements Minerals that are required by the body in very small quantities

Trade, brand, or proprietary drug name The name a company assigns to a commercial drug product for marketing and identification purposes; most brand names are trademarked and belong to originator products; the named products are often protected, for a time, by patents

Treatment authorization request (TAR) Similar to preauthorization form but is the process used for Medicare and Medicaid

Trephining A practice of making an opening in the head to allow disease to leave the body

Triiodothyronine (T_3) A thyroid hormone that helps regulate growth and development and helps control metabolism and body temperature. Mainly produced through the metabolism of thyroxine (T_4)

Triturate To grind or crush a powder such as a tablet into fine particles

Troche A flat disklike tablet that dissolves between the gum and cheek

Tubular reabsorption The conservation of protein, glucose, bicarbonate, and water from the glomerular filtrate by the tubules

Tubular secretion A function of the nephron where ions, toxins, and water are secreted into the collecting duct to be excreted

Tympanic membrane A thin membranous piece of skin that separates the external ear from the middle ear; also known as the eardrum

Unit dose A single dose of a drug

United States Pharmacopeia (USP) An independent nonprofit organization that establishes documentation on product quality standards, drug quality and information, and health care information on medications, over-the-counter products, dietary supplements, and food ingredients to ensure the appropriate purity, quality, and strength are met

United States Pharmacopeia-National Formulary (USP-NF) A publication of the *USP* that contains standards for medications, dosage forms, drug substances, excipients, medical devices, and dietary supplements

Urea The main nitrogenous constituent of urine and final product of protein metabolism; formed in the liver

Ureter The tube that carries urine from the kidneys to the bladder; each kidney has one ureter

Urethra The tube that carries urine from the bladder to the urethral sphincter for elimination from the body

Urticaria Also known as hives; red welts that arise on the surface of the skin; often attributable to an allergic reaction but may have nonallergic causes

Vaccine A biological preparation that improves immunity to a particular disease by invoking an immune response and a "memory" of the response for future use

Vasodilation Widening of the blood vessels, which allows for increased blood flow

Vector An entity by which infections are transferred, but the entity of transference does not have the disease and does not need to be a living organism. For example, a mosquito bite transfers malaria. In this case, the mosquito is the vector

Vein A blood vessel that carries deoxygenated blood to or toward the heart

Vena cava The large veins that carry deoxygenated blood from the upper (superior vena cava) and lower (inferior vena cava) parts of the body to the right atrium of the heart

Vertical laminar flow hood Environment for the preparation of chemotherapeutic and hazardous agents where air originating from the roof of the hood moves downward (over the agent) and is captured in a vent located on the floor of the hood

Virion A virus particle

Virology The study of viruses

Virus A microscopic organism that replicates exclusively inside a the host's cell by using parts of the host cell, including DNA, ribosomes, and proteins

Viscosity The thickness of a solution or fluid

Vitreous humor Gel-like substance that fills the posterior cavity of the eye, between the lens and retina; helps to maintain shape of the eye

Volume The amount of liquid enclosed within a container

VRE Vancomycin-resistant enterococci

Index